Surgery of the Skull Base

Surgery of the Skull Base

Editor

Paul J. Donald, MD

*Professor, Department of Otolaryngology—
Head and Neck Surgery
Director, UCDMC Center for Skull Base Surgery
University of California, Davis
Sacramento, California*

Illustrations by Nelva B. Richardson

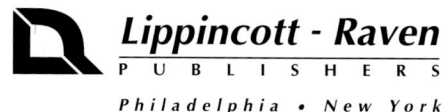

Philadelphia • New York

Acquisitions Editor: Danette Knopp
Developmental Editor: Anne M. Sydor
Manufacturing Manager: Tim Reynolds
Production Manager: Cassie Moore
Production Editor: Rita Madrigal
Cover Designer: Karen Quigley
Indexer: Deana Fowler
Compositor: Maryland Composition

©1998, by Lippincott–Raven Publishers. All rights reserved. This book is protected by copyright. No part of it may be reproduced, stored in a retrieval system, or transmitted, in any form or by any means—electronic, mechanical, photocopy, recording, or otherwise—without the prior written consent of the publisher, except for brief quotations embodied in critical articles and reviews. For information write **Lippincott-Raven Publishers, 227 East Washington Square, Philadelphia, PA 19106-3780.**

Materials appearing in this book prepared by individuals as part of their official duties as U.S. Government employees are not covered by the above-mentioned copyright.

Printed and bound in China

9 8 7 6 5 4 3 2 1

Library of Congress Cataloging-in-Publication Data
Skull base surgery/editor, Paul J. Donald; illustrations by Nelva
  B. Richardson.
      p.   cm.
    Includes bibliographical references and index.
    ISBN 0-397-51289-9
    1. Skull base–Surgery. 2. Face–Surgery. I. Donald, Paul J.
    [DNLM: 1. Skull Base Neoplasms–surgery. 2. Skull Base–surgery.
  3. Surgical Procedures, Operative–methods. WE 707 S6289 1998]
  RD529.S746   1998
  617.5'14–dc21
  DNLM/DLC   98-9868
  for Library of Congress   CIP

Care has been taken to confirm the accuracy of the information presented and to describe generally accepted practices. However, the authors, editors, and publisher are not responsible for errors or omissions or for any consequences from application of the information in this book and make no warranty, expressed or implied, with respect to the contents of the publication.

The authors, editors, and publisher have exerted every effort to ensure that drug selection and dosage set forth in this text are in accordance with current recommendations and practice at the time of publication. However, in view of ongoing research, changes in government regulations, and the constant flow of information relating to drug therapy and drug reactions, the reader is urged to check the package insert for each drug for any change in indications and dosage and for added warnings and precautions. This is particularly important when the recommended agent is a new or infrequently employed drug.

Some drugs and medical devices presented in this publication have Food and Drug Administration (FDA) clearance for limited use in restricted research settings. It is the responsibility of the health care provider to ascertain the FDA status of each drug or device planned for use in their clinical practice.

To my loving and perpetually supportive family.
To my dear wife, Roz, who encouraged me to pursue skull base surgery,
and to my children, their spouses and my grandchildren:
Alison and Dan Corfee and their children Ben and Lizzie;
Scott and Leslie Donald and their children Jack and Anna;
Heather and Scott Fuller;
and finally, my youngest son, Andy.

Contents

Contributing Authors ... xi
Preface ... xv
Acknowledgments ... xvii

I. INTRODUCTION

1. History of Skull Base Surgery ... 3
   Paul J. Donald

2. Surgical Anatomy of the Skull Base ... 15
   Bernard M. Lyons

3. Pathology of Skull Base Tumors ... 31
   Regina Gandour-Edwards, Silloo B. Kapadia, and Leon Barnes

4. Pathophysiology of Skull Base Malignancies ... 51
   Keith Jackson, Paul J. Donald, and Regina Gandour-Edwards

5. Presentation and Preparation of Patients with Skull Base Lesions ... 73
   Paul J. Donald

6. Imaging of the Skull Base ... 87
   Alfred L. Weber and Hugh D. Curtin

7. Carotid Artery Assessment and Interventional Radiologic Procedures Before Skull Base Surgery ... 105
   William R. Nemzek

8. Nursing Care of Skull Base Surgery Patients ... 119
   Ann E. F. Sievers and Denise Borcyckowski

9. Intraoperative Neurophysiologic Monitoring ... 137
   Robert J. Sclabassi, Jeffrey R. Balzer, and Donald N. Krieger

II. ANTERIOR FOSSA APPROACHES

10. Transfacial Approach ... 165
    Paul J. Donald

11. Facial Degloving Approach ... 195
    João J. Maniglia and Ricardo Ramina

12. Extended Unilateral Maxillotomy Approach ... 207
    Edwin W. Cocke, Jr. and Jon H. Robertson

13. Subcranial Extended Anterior Approach for Skull Base Tumors: Surgical Procedure and Reconstruction ... 239
    Joram Raveh, Kurt Laedrach, Tateyuki Iizuka, and Franz Leibinger

14. Cranioorbital Approach 263
    Alfred P. Bowles, Jr. and Vinod K. Anand

15. Extended Transfacial Subcranial Approach 287
    Paul J. Donald

16. Infratemporal Fossa–Middle Cranial Fossa Approach 309
    Paul J. Donald

17. Transmandibular Approach 341
    Jack L. Gluckman, Lyon L. Gleich, and Keith M. Wilson

18. Anterior Subcranial (Transbasal–Derome) Approach 347
    Ricardo Ramina, João J. Maniglia, Ari A. Pedrozo, and Murilo S. Meneses

19. Work-up and Management of the Internal Carotid Artery in Neoplastic and Vascular Lesions 359
    Laligam N. Sekhar and Sorin D. Bucur

III. POSTERIOR FOSSA APPROACHES

20. Temporal Bone Resection 377
    Aongus J. Curran, Patrick J. Gullane, Manohar L. Bance, and Paul J. Donald

21. Transcervicomastoid Approach 409
    Gale L. Gardner, Edwin W. Cocke, Jr., and Jon H. Robertson

22. Petroclival Approach 423
    Madjid Samii and Marcos Tatagiba

23. Evaluation and Management of Vestibular Schwannomas 443
    Hilary A. Brodie and Pamela Bohrer

24. Approaches to Jugulotympanic Paragangliomas 473
    Rick A. Friedman and Derald E. Brackmann

IV. MIDLINE APPROACHES

25. Extreme Lateral Transcondylar Approach to the Craniocervical Junction 491
    Chandranath Sen and Peter J. Catalano

26. Transoral Approach to the Clivus and Upper Surgical Spine 507
    Paul J. Donald

27. Management of the Vertebral Artery 533
    Bernard George

28. Lesions of the Sella Turcica 555
    Andrew E. Sloan, Keith L. Black, and Donald P. Becker

V. ADJUNCTIVE CONSIDERATIONS

29. Complications 585
    Paul J. Donald

30. Postoperative Management 599
    Bernard M. Lyons

31. Free Flaps in Skull Base Surgery 607
Jonathan E. Aviv and Mark R. Sultan

32. Reconstruction of the Skull Base with Regional Flaps and Grafts 623
James L. Netterville and C. Gary Jackson

Subject Index 641

Contributing Authors

Vinod K. Anand, MD
*Professor and Chief, Division of Otolaryngology
Department of Surgery
University of Mississippi Medical Center
2500 North State Street
Jackson, MS 39216-4505*

Jonathan E. Aviv, MD, FACS
*Associate Professor and Director,
Division of Head and Neck Surgery
Department of Otolaryngology—Head and Neck
  Surgery
College of Physicians and Surgeons, Columbia
  University
Columbia–Presbyterian Medical Center
630 West 168th Street
New York, NY 10032*

Jeffrey R. Balzer, PhD
*Assistant Professor
Department of Neurology
University of Pittsburgh Medical Center
200 Lothrop Street
Pittsburgh, PA 15213*

Manohar L. Bance, Bsc, MB, ChB, Msc, FRCS(C)
*Assistant Professor
Department of Otolaryngology
The Toronto Hospital and The University of
  Toronto
EN7-221
200 Elizabeth Street
Toronto, Ontario
M5G 2C4 Canada*

Leon Barnes, MD
*Professor of Pathology and Otolaryngology
Department of Pathology
University of Pittsburgh School of Medicine
200 Lathrop Street
Pittsburgh, PA 15213*

Donald P. Becker, MD
*Professor and Chief
Division of Neurosurgery
University of California, Los Angeles Medical
  Center
10833 Le Conte Avenue
Los Angeles, CA 90095-7039*

Daniel R. Benson, MD
*Department of Orthopedic Surgery
University of California, Davis Medical Center
2230 Stockton Boulevard
Sacramento CA 95817*

Keith L. Black, MD
*Director, Neurosurgical Institute
Department of Surgery
Cedars-Sinai Medical Center
8635 West Third Street, Suite 490
Los Angeles, CA 90048*

Pamela Bohrer, MD
*Department of Otolaryngology
Kaiser Permanente Medical Group
401 Bicentennial Way
Santa Rosa, California 95403*

Denise Borcyckowksi, RN
*Clinical Nurse III, Team Leader, CORLN
Departments of Patient Care Services and
  Otolaryngology—Head and Neck Surgery
University of California, Davis
2315 Stockton Boulevard
Sacramento, CA 95817*

Alfred P. Bowles, Jr., MD
*Assistant Professor
Department of Neurosurgery
University of Mississippi Medical Center
2500 North State Street
Jackson, Mississippi 39216-4505*

Contributing Authors

Derald E. Brackmann, MD
Clinical Professor of Otolaryngology—Head and Neck Surgery
University of Southern California, Los Angeles
House Ear Clinic, Inc.
2100 West Third Street, 1st Floor
Los Angeles, CA 90057

Hilary A. Brodie, MD, PhD
Associate Professor/Acting Chairman
Department of Otolaryngology
University of California, Davis Medical Center
2521 Stockton Boulevard, Room 7200
Sacramento, CA 95817

Sorin D. Bucur, MD
Fellow
Department of Neurosurgery
George Washington University Medical Center
2150 Pennsylvania Avenue, NW
Washington, D.C. 20037

Peter J. Catalano, MD, FACS
Associate Professor of Otolaryngology, Neurosurgery, and Oral Surgery
Department of Otolaryngology
The Mount Sinai Medical Center
1 Gustave L. Levy Place
New York, NY 10029

Edwin W. Cocke, Jr., MD
Clinical Professor
Department of Otolaryngology, Head and Neck Surgery
The University of Tennesee, Memphis
The Health Science Center
951 Court Avenue
Baptist Memorial Hospital
899 Madison Avenue
Memphis, TN 38103

Aongus J. Curran, MB, FRCSI
Head and Neck Surgical Oncology Fellow
Department of Otolaryngology—Head and Neck Surgery
University of Toronto
The Toronto Hospital
200 Elizabeth Street
Toronto, Ontario
M5G 2C4 Canada

Hugh D. Curtin, MD
Associate Professor
Harvard Medical School
Department of Radiology
Massachusetts Eye and Ear Infirmary
243 Charles Street
Boston, MA 02114

Paul J. Donald, MD, FRCS(C)
Professor, Department of Otolaryngology—Head and Neck Surgery
Director, Center for Skull Base Surgery
University of California, Davis
2521 Stockton Boulevard, #7200
Sacramento, California 95817

Rick A. Friedman, MD
House Ear Clinic, Inc.
2100 West Third Street, 1st Floor
Los Angeles, CA 90057

Regina Gandour-Edwards, MD
Assistant Professor
Department of Pathology
University of California, Davis
2315 Stockton Boulevard
Sacramento, CA 95817

Gale L. Gardner, MD
899 Madison Avenue
Memphis, TN 38103

Bernard George, MD
Professor of Neurosurgery
Department of Neurosurgery
Hôpital Lariboisiere
2, rue Ambroise Paré
75010 Paris
France

Lyon L. Gleich, MD
Assistant Professor
Department of Otolaryngology—Head and Neck Surgery
University of Cincinnati
6308 Medical Sciences Building, Room #528
Cincinnati, OH 45267

Jack L. Gluckman, MD
Professor and Chairman
Department of Otolaryngology—Head and Neck Surgery
University of Cincinnati
University Hospital, Inc.
231 Bethesda Avenue, ML0528
Cincinnati, OH 45267-0528

Patrick J. Gullane, MB, FRSC(C)
The Toronto Hospital
Eaton WN 7-242
200 Elizabeth Street
Toronto, Ontario
M5G 2C4 Canada

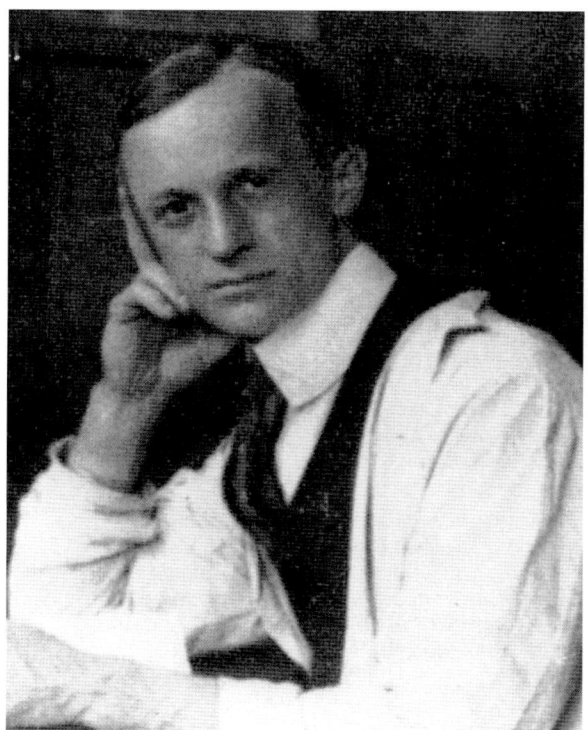
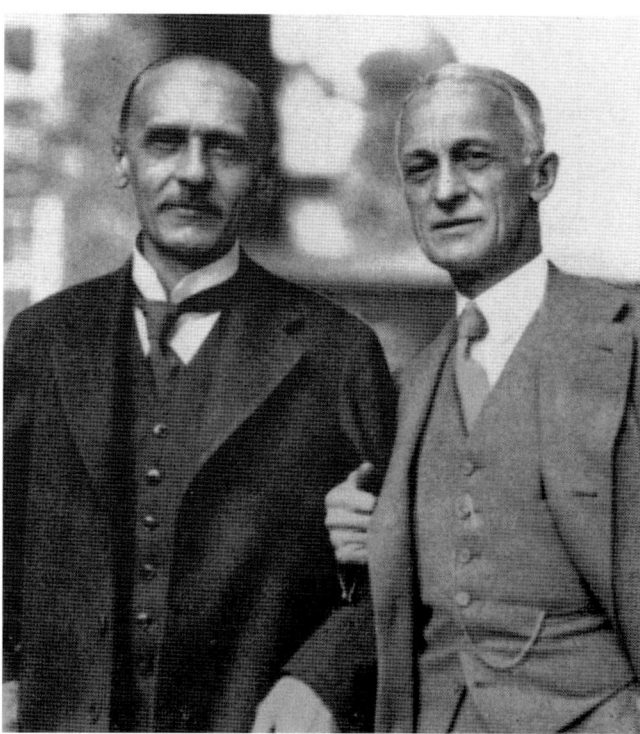

FIG. 4. Harvey Cushing. **A:** In the Hunterian Laboratory, Baltimore, Maryland, in 1912. **B:** With Otfrid Foerster, 1930 (Cushing to the left of Foerster). (From Horrax GT. Neurosurgery: an historical sketch. Publication no. 117 of the American Lecture Series. In: DeBakey ME, Spurling RG, eds. *American lectures in surgery*. Springfield, IL: Charles C Thomas Publishers, 1952:73 **[A]**, 105 **[B]**.)

At the same time that Cushing described the transnasal route to the pituitary, a similar approach was being used by the Viennese otolaryngologist, Oskar Hirsch (13,14). Initially, the procedure was done entirely transnasally in three stages (see Fig. 3). Eventually, in 1911, he combined the stages through a midline sublabial approach. Hirsch emigrated to the United States in the 1930s and, in 1952, published his results (15) of 425 such procedures, with a 65% success rate and a 5.4% mortality rate.

Subsequent developments in skull base surgery occurred on a number of different fronts. The first recorded anterior craniofacial resection for a tumor was by Dandy (Fig. 5) in 1941 (16). While removing an orbital tumor through an anterior cranial fossa approach, he entered the ethmoid bloc in an attempt to improve exposure and achieve complete resection. In 1943, Rae and McLean (17) reported a transorbital/transcranial removal of a retinoblastoma. However, the landmark article in anterior cranial base surgery that involved a coordinated transfacial and transcranial approach to tumor removal was published done in 1954. Klopp, a head and neck oncologic surgeon from Washington, DC, teamed up with Smith and Williams (18) to do a planned procedure to remove what was described as a cancer of the frontal sinus. The author found that his resection was not well accepted by his peers—not an uncommon finding in the early days of skull base surgery, as well as in many other innovative procedures that have been attempted through the history of medicine. Even the pioneering Semmelweis was committed by his colleagues to an insane asylum for proselytizing the principles of antisepsis.

The definitive report that truly launched skull base surgery for malignant disease was a paper by Ketcham et al. on their

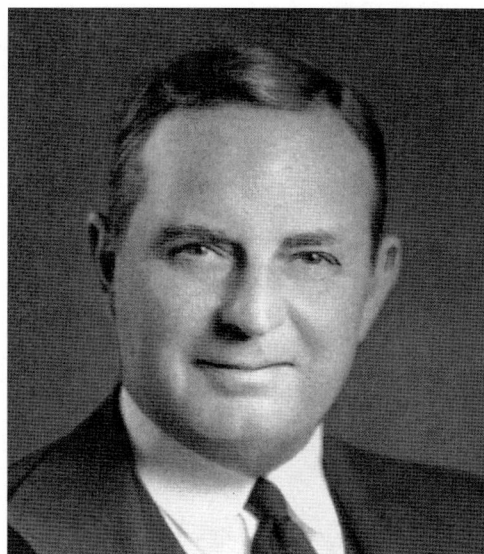

FIG. 5. Walter E. Dandy. (From Horrax GT. Neurosurgery: an historical sketch. Publication no. 117 of the American Lecture Series. In: DeBakey ME, Spurling RG, eds. *American lectures in surgery*. Springfield, IL: Charles C Thomas Publishers, 1952:93.)

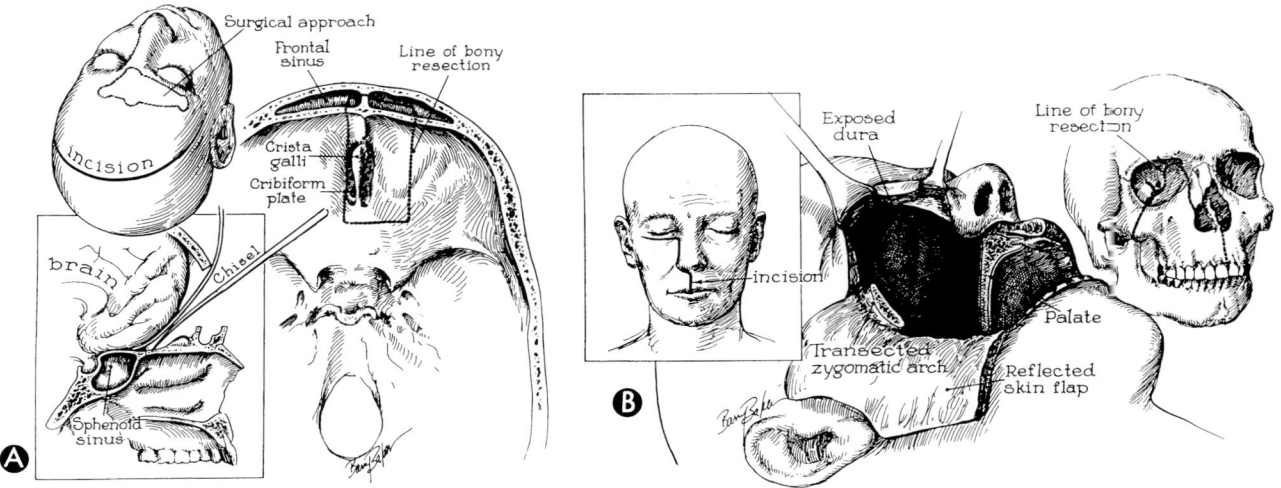

FIG. 6. The anterior skull base approach as described by Ketcham et al. **A:** Transfacial approach. **B:** Transcranial approach. (From Ketcham AS, Chretien PB, Schour L, Herdt JR, Ommaya AK, Van Buren JM. Surgical treatment of patients with advanced cancer of the paranasal sinuses. In: *Neoplasia of the head and neck: a collection of papers presented at the seventeenth annual Clinical Conference on Cancer, 1972*. Sponsored by and held at the University of Texas System Cancer Center, M. D. Anderson Hospital and Tumor Institute, Houston, Texas. Chicago: Year Book Medical Publishers, 1974:192.)

experience with 19 patients who had an anterior craniofacial resection for cancer of the nasal cavity and paranasal sinuses (19). They evaluated 30 patients with advanced paranasal sinus cancer, 22 of whom were failures of past surgery or irradiation. Six of the patients were rejected for surgery because of radiographic evidence of erosion of the sphenoid ridge or pterygoid plates. Two refused surgery, and three were considered incurable at the time of craniotomy because of brain invasion or cranial floor involvement in the region of the optic chiasm. The anterior craniotomy and Weber Fergusson exposure they used are the basis for many anterior fossa approaches today (Fig. 6). Of the 19 patients operated on, 7 were not cured of their disease, 9 were disease free at 2 to 75 months' follow-up, and 3 died of other causes. By 1966, the same group reported on the complications experienced in a group of 31 patients operated on over a 10-year period (20).

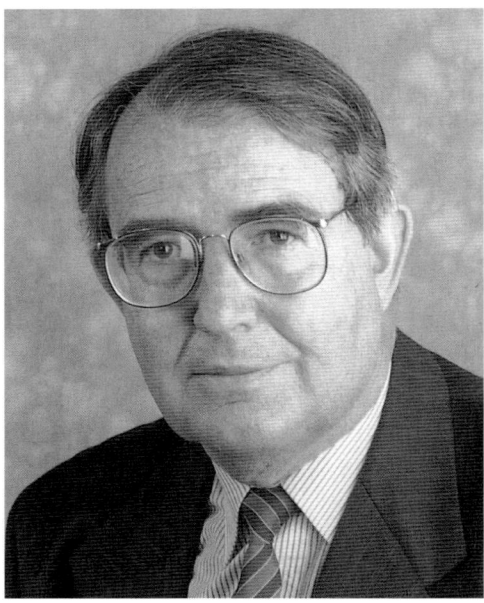

FIG. 7. A. D. Cheesman, a head and neck surgeon and pioneer in skull base surgery who described the "key hole" craniotomy for tumor exposure.

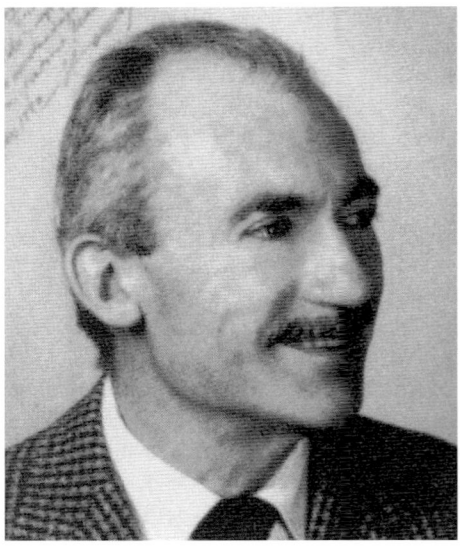

FIG. 8. Paul Tessier, a plastic surgeon, the father of modern craniomaxillary surgery for congenital anomalies.

The 3-year and longer survival rate in this group was 61%. Approximately 80% of patients sustained some form of complication. In 1976, Sisson et al. (21) reported on their 15-year experience with craniofacial resection for sinus malignancies. They had used craniofacial resection for only 8 cases in a series of over 100 malignancies of the sinuses. Three of these patients died of recurrent disease, three were long-term survivors (2–8 years), and two were being followed and were disease-free for less than 1 year. In 1973, Millar et al. (22) reported on three cases of ethmoid cancer done in Australia. In 1980, Bridger (23), also from Australia, reported on 15 cases of craniofacial resection for tumors at this same site. In Bridger's series, seven patients were alive and disease free at 2 years or more. In 1986, Cheesman et al. (Fig. 7) from Great Britain reported their 10-year experience with craniofacial resection for ethmoid carcinomas with intracranial spread using a small "window craniotomy" (24). They had a 60% 5-year cure rate.

Attempts were made to improve the exposure of the anterior fossa, especially in its most posterior extent. This often was difficult to achieve without severe retraction of the frontal lobes using the standard craniotomy. Based on the removal of a frontoorbital bandeau used in craniofacial surgery for congenital craniomaxillary anomalies developed by Tessier et al. (25) (Fig. 8) and the low frontoorbital technique for sphenoethmoid tumors described by Derome et al. (26), various skull base surgical teams devised more direct approaches. The extended anterior subcranial approach was developed by Raveh (Fig. 9) in 1978 to manage intracranial trauma (27) and then adapted it to tumor resection (28), and is excellent for midline lesions. A wider exposure was afforded

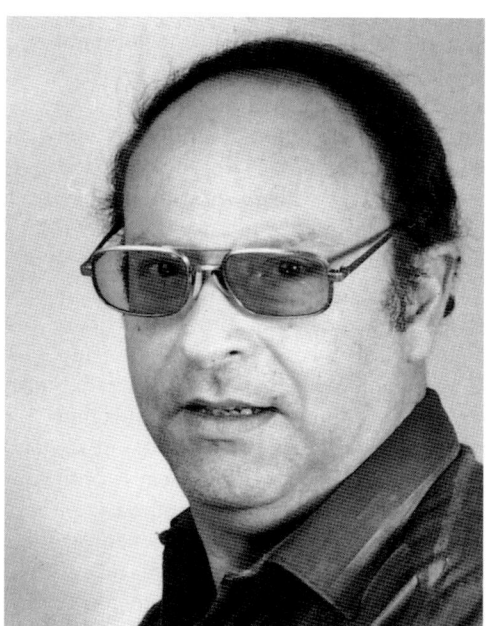

FIG. 9. Joram Raveh, a head and neck and maxillocranial surgeon who described the unique transcranial subcranial approach to the anterior midline skull base.

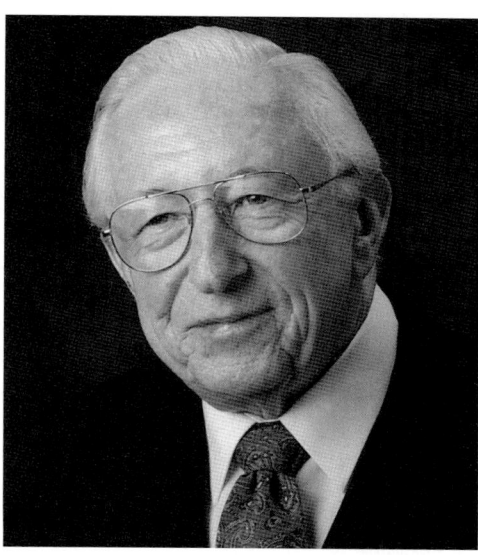

FIG. 10. Edwin W. Cocke, Jr., one of the founders of the Society for Head and Neck Surgeons, who in his mid-70s described a novel approach to the skull base through a Le Fort I osteotomy.

by the technique developed by Maniglia and Ramina (29), in which the entire frontal bandeau was removed.

Many others, including Janecka, Cocke (Fig. 10), Robinson, Panje, and Catilano, have produced variations on these midline approaches, many of which are described in detail in this book.

POSTERIOR FOSSA–ACOUSTIC TUMORS

Another major area in skull base surgery development concerns lesions of the posterior cranial fossa. In the early 20th century, the removal of acoustic neuromas was first done in a systematic manner by Harvey Cushing, the previously mentioned skull base pioneer in pituitary surgery. According to House (30), the early reports of removal of this tumor were "meager and sketchy," and the surgery itself was usually incomplete and attended by a high mortality and morbidity rate. Horsley, Krause, and Von Eiselsberg (30) were names frequently associated with these early attempts. In London in 1894, Ballance (31) and Beevor reported the removal of an acoustic tumor with a favorable result. In America the year before, Starr and McBurney (32) teamed up for a posterior fossa exploration for such a tumor, but were unsuccessful. In the years before Cushing's resections of these lesions, a common practice was to insert a dissecting finger between the tumor and the pons in an attempt to enucleate it. In his own report, Cushing (33) found that with increasing experience, his mortality rate diminished from the death of his first patient to 20% after he had done 30 cases. This was in vivid contrast to the almost 100% mortality in other patients operated on by the surgeons of the time. However, Cushing's greatest contribution probably was the lucid and comprehensive description of the signs, symptoms, and natural history of acoustic tumors. Cushing's student, Walter Dandy (see Fig. 5), is reputed to be one of if not the greatest technological neurosurgeon of this century (30). Disappointed by the incomplete removals and frequent complications of Cushing's finger dissection technique, Dandy developed a more refined, painstaking removal of the tumor and its surrounding capsule. He resected 23 patients in this fashion in his first 9 years of practice and had 5 complete cures, an unheard-of track record at that time (34). Dandy's 1942 description (35) of acoustic tumor removal remained the standard approach until the development of the operating microscope in 1961. Unfortunately, however, this technique resulted in a total facial nerve paralysis in every case. For a more detailed and fascinating account of the development of acoustic tumor surgery, House's excellent section in his two-volume monograph on acoustic tumors should be consulted (31).

The operating microscope was first used in clinical surgery by Nylén (Fig. 11) in 1921 (36) to drain an acute suppurative otitis media by myringotomy. This was a unilocular microscope that lacked the three-dimensional visualization surgeons enjoy today. Holmgren (37), who had been doing labyrinthine procedures for otosclerosis, quickly developed the binocular microscope for middle ear surgery in 1922. In 1953, the Zeiss Company produced the prototype of the operating microscope that is universally used today. From its original use in otology, the microscope rapidly became incorporated into ophthalmologic surgery, neurosurgery, and finally plastic surgery—all specialties that were to become important elements of the skull base surgery team. The microscope revolutionized otology and was one of the single greatest catalysts to modern otologic and neurootologic surgery.

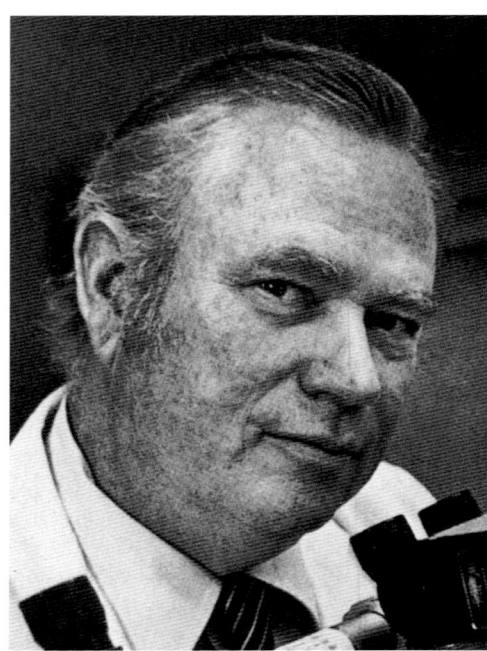

FIG. 12. W. F. House, the first modern otoneurosurgeon.

However, it was not technology that spawned modern neurootology. Credit must undoubtedly be given to the courageous, pioneering genius of William House (Fig. 12). Disturbed by the disappointing results of the standard approach to acoustic tumors developed by Dandy, he strove to design an operation that would extirpate the tumor while saving the function of the facial nerve. After practicing on cadaveric specimens in a makeshift temporal bone laboratory that he and his brother, Howard, constructed in their garage, he set out to do the first otomicroscopic approach to an acoustic neuroma. Attempts using the transtemporal approach had been made in the past. In 1904, Panse (38) developed an approach through the temporal bone, beginning with a radical mastoidectomy, followed by removal of the labyrinth, cochlea, and facial nerve, done with a mallet and gouge. Heavy bleeding and cerebrospinal fluid leakage predictably accompanied these procedures. Buix, Zange, and Schmiegelow (30) were among the few surgeons over the next 13 years who performed a small number of these dangerous procedures through the ear. At this time, a few heroic surgeons (34) did a combined postoccipital and translabyrinthine procedure, but, because of the high mortality rate, this approach was discontinued.

In 1961, House and B. B. Doyle, a neurosurgeon, did the first resection of an acoustic neuroma using the operating microscope. Because it was unprecedented for an otolaryngologist to do this type of surgery, the neurosurgery community presented no little resistance to House's desire to remove this tumor. After considerable debate, the first otoneurosurgical skull base team did the operation through

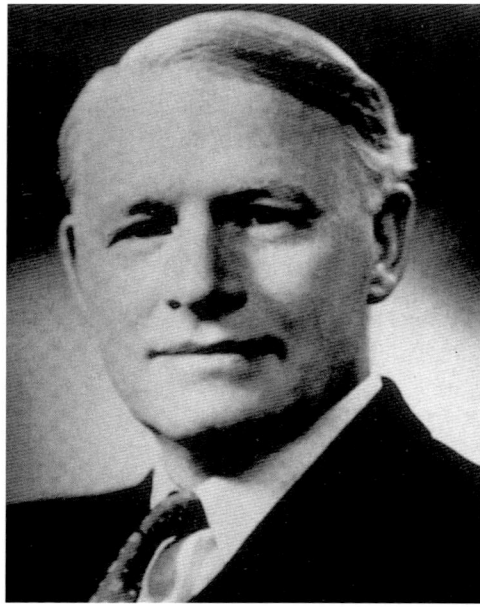

FIG. 11. C. O. Nylén, an otologic surgeon who was the first to describe the operating microscope.

the middle fossa approach. The tumor was incompletely removed and a combined suboccipital and middle fossa transotic approach was unsuccessful on two successive occasions, and the patient died 6 years later. The middle fossa appeared at the time to be a good route for facial nerve exposure, but inadequate for tumor removal. After eight attempts at the middle fossa route, sometimes accompanied by the suboccipital approach, House decided to redesign the operation and modified the original approach of Panse using the microscope, drill, and suction irrigation. He was able to preserve the facial nerve, the posterior canal wall, and the tympanic membrane. House and Doyle came to a serious disagreement over approaches, and their association dissolved in 1963. William Hitselberger (Fig. 13) then joined with House to form a solid, long-lasting relationship that was the nucleus of the first true skull base team.

The history of the evolution of acoustic tumor surgery would be incomplete without the story of the return to the modified Dandy approach by modern neurosurgeons and neurootologists. The transotic approach, by its very nature, destroys hearing; the removal of the bony and membranous labyrinth eliminates all vestiges of hearing on that side. In days gone by, when by the time the diagnosis was made most patients had little or no useful hearing in the affected ear, the loss of remaining hearing acuity was of little consequence (a position voiced by numerous otologists even today). As clinicians became more aware of this diagnosis, and computed tomography and magnetic resonance imaging improved, their ability to detect small tumors in patients whose hearing was intact markedly improved. Hearing preservation now became more important.

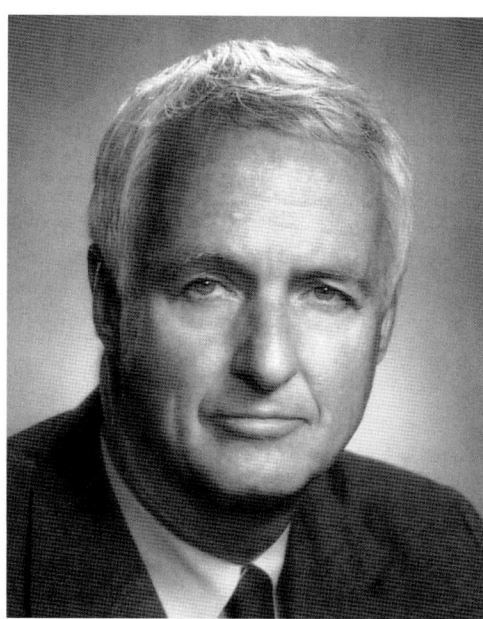

FIG. 14. Mansfield F. W. Smith, an otologist who was among the first to adapt the posterior fossa approach to acoustic tumor removal and preserve hearing.

The reactivation of interest in the suboccipital retrosigmoid approach was stimulated by a desire to salvage hearing. The translabyrinthine approach developed by House preserved facial nerve function in most cases. Dandy, in his report in 1941 on 46 cases operated on with his modification of Cushing's suboccipital approach, reported that 34 of these patients had "good hearing" (36). However, most patients had no postoperative facial nerve function. Rand and Kurze (39, 40) modified Dandy's operation, preserving the facial nerve in 100% of cases when tumors were less than 2 cm in diameter, and reported these results in 1965. They called their operation the "suboccipital transmeatal approach." They also described preserving the vestibular and cochlear nerves in small intercanalicular tumors (41), but questioned the advisability of the operation in such small neoplasms. Sterkers (42) began hearing preservation surgery in 1969 and reported only a 10% favorable hearing result when he and his team used either the middle fossa or retrosigmoid approach. Smith (Fig. 14) et al. (43) modified the Rand procedure and began to popularize it in the early 1970s. Since then, considerable controversy has continued to surround the question of the optimal approach for acoustic neuroma removal, and the quality and utility of hearing when preservation is done.

MIDDLE FOSSA

A history of modern skull base surgery would be very much amiss without mention of one of the premier skull base surgeons of our time, Ugo Fisch (Fig. 15). With his background in head and neck oncologic surgery, he extended the limits of otologic surgery into the area of the infratemporal

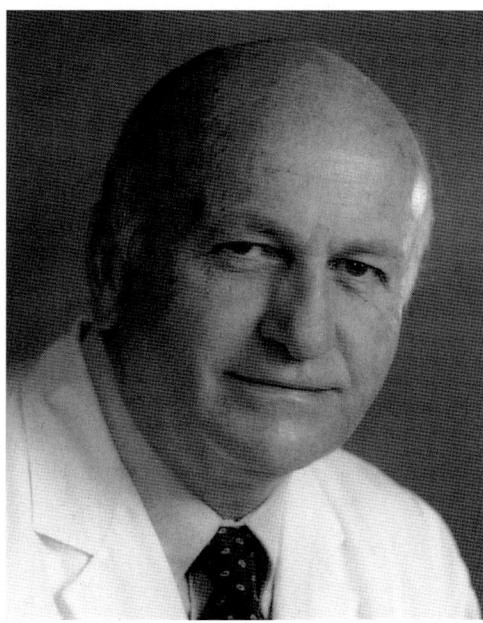

FIG. 13. William Hitselberger, the neurosurgeon who with House created the first skull base surgery team in North America.

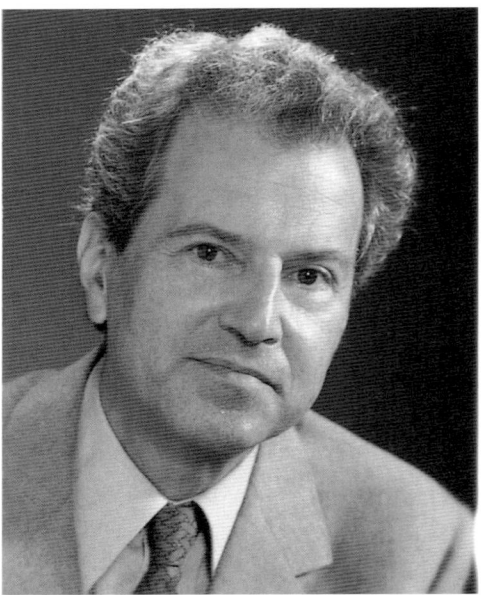

FIG. 15. Ugo Fisch, a head and neck surgeon/otologist who developed the infratemporal fossa approach.

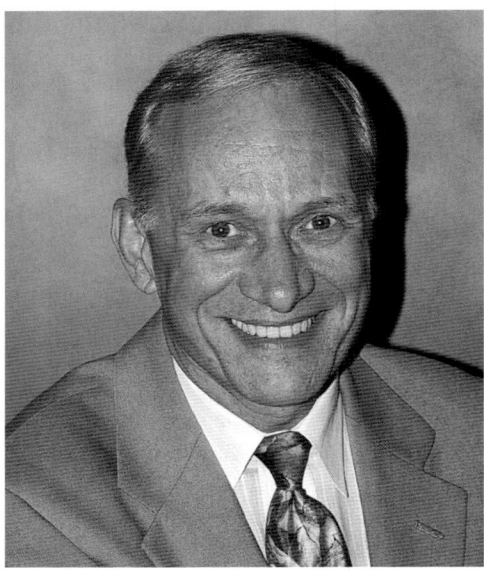

FIG. 17. Victor L. Schramm, a head and neck surgeon who pioneered the middle fossa/infratemporal fossa approach to skull base tumors.

fossa. He and his neurosurgical colleague, Gazi Yasargil (Fig. 16), combined their skills to develop an approach through the infratemporal fossa to lesions that approached or invaded middle fossa dura. The uniqueness of this approach lay in that the lesion could be adequately exposed and resected with minimal temporal lobe retraction. Fisch is particularly noted for his pioneering work in the resection of juvenile nasopharyngeal angiofibroma with massive infratemporal fossa and middle fossa extension. He then turned his attention to resection of jugular foramen tumors, producing a workable classification of glomus jugulare tumors and a systematic solution to their extirpation.

A number of modifications of Fisch's approach have been made, the most notable by Victor Schramm (Fig. 17) and

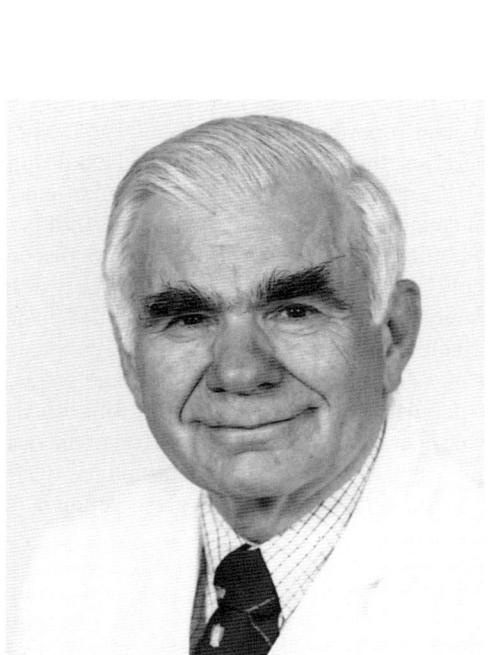

FIG. 16. Gazi Yasargil, a neurosurgeon who along with Fisch developed the middle fossa/infratemporal fossa approach.

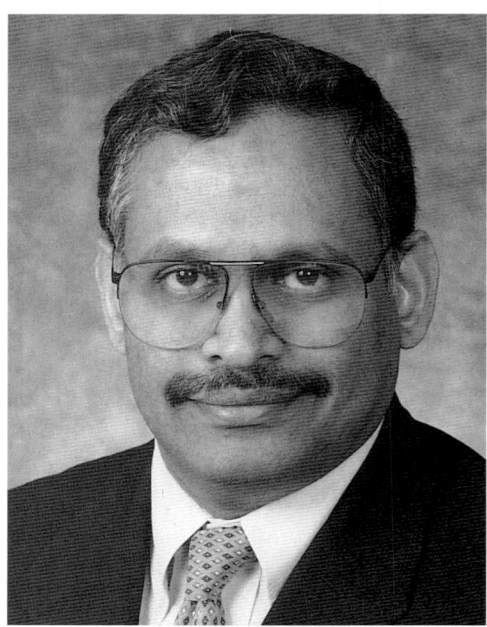

FIG. 18. Laligam N. Sekhar, a neurosurgeon who together with Schramm created the first comprehensive skull base surgery program in North America.

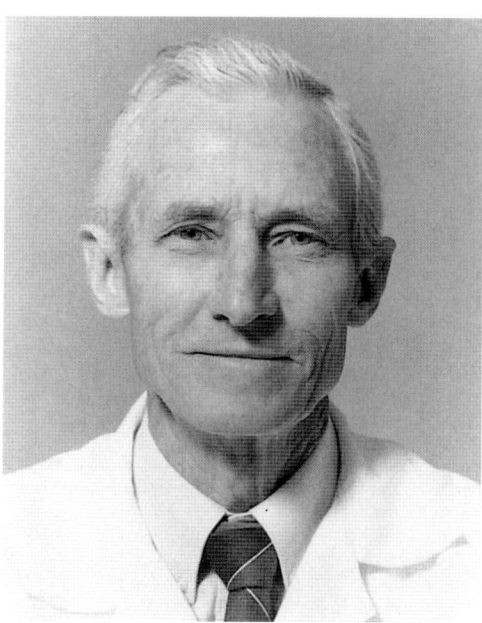

FIG. 19. Dwight Parkinson, neurosurgeon and pioneer in cavernous sinus surgery.

Laligam Sekhar (Fig. 18) when they were together at the University of Pittsburgh. They were the prime movers of the first, organized, academically based skull base surgery center in the United States. Their refinements of Fisch's technique enabled wider exposure and more definitive resection of invasive meningiomas of the anterior and middle cranial fossae with extracranial extension and carcinomas arising in the upper aerodigestive tract invading the intracranial cavity.

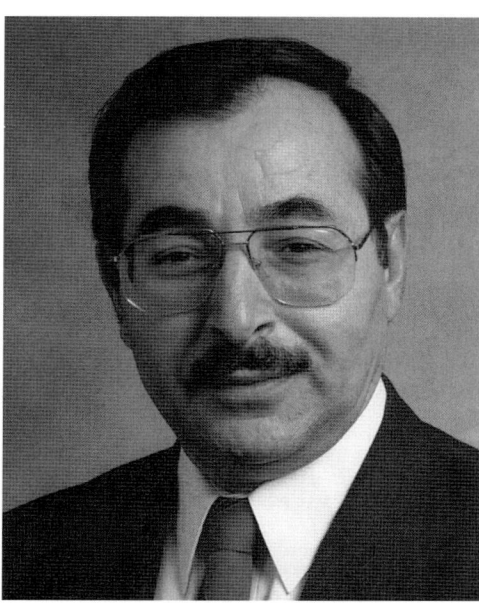

FIG. 20. Ossama Al-Mefty, the neurosurgeon who developed the zygomaticofrontal approach to skull base lesions.

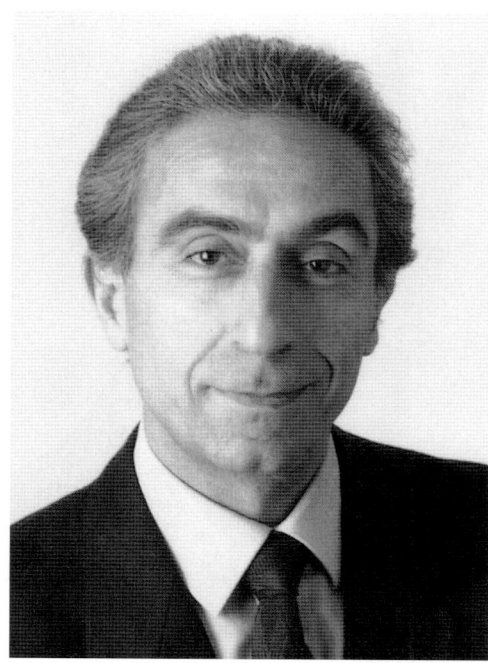

FIG. 21. Madjid Samii, the neurosurgeon responsible in large part for the worldwide development of skull base surgery.

Forays into the middle fossa to resect invasive neoplasms inevitably led adventurous surgeons to chase such tumors into the cavernous sinus. Such resections were unheard-of until the courageous and innovative work of Dwight Parkinson (Fig. 19). In 1860, Holmes (44) was the first to describe a lesion at this site, a giant aneurysm; Bartholow (45) was the first to present an account of signs and symptoms of such lesions involving the sinus. Peet (46) gives Krogius credit for the first operation on a mass, presumably a neuroma, at this site, operated on in 1896. Parkinson's pioneering paper in 1965 (47) led the way for the further elaboration of anatomy and development of approaches by current experts such as Dolenc, Kawasee, Rhoton, Sekhar (see Fig. 18), Al-Mefty (Fig. 20), Samii (Fig. 21), and others.

CENTRAL SKULL BASE

Surgeons have striven to elucidate more direct attacks on intracranial and skull base pathologic processes. The central skull base and adjacent intracranial structures are very difficult to approach through the three cranial fossae. The transoral approach to the upper cervical spine and clivus was first suggested by Scoville and Sherman (48) in 1951. A transoropharyngeal route was used in 1957 by Southwick and Robinson (49) to remove a tumor in the body of the second cervical vertebra (C-2). This was based on the experience of otolaryngologic colleagues who successfully and routinely used this route to drain the retropharyngeal space of abscesses at this site. However, the first description of the transoral approach applied to the cervicocranial junction did not

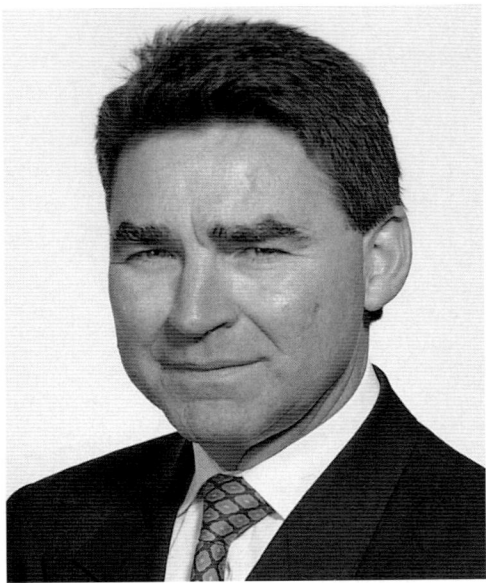

FIG. 22. Alan Crockard, a neurosurgeon who refined and perfected the transoral approach to the lower clivus and upper cervical spine.

appear until the presentation by Fang and Ong (50) at the PanPacific Surgical Society in 1962. In 1966, Stevenson et al. (51) used this approach to remove a clivus chordoma and expose the brainstem. In 1978, Haselden and Bryce (52) used this route to manage a basilar aneurysm. It remained for Crockard (53) (Fig. 22) to refine and perfect this approach for the optimal midline approach to the lower one third of the clivus and the upper two cervical vertebrae. Contributions to the transoral approach have been made by a number of head and neck surgeons. The median labiomandibular glossoptomy developed by Conley (54) provides excellent exposure, but is rarely necessary. The refinements described by Donald (55), Crumley and Gutin (56), and Woods et al. (57) have made the transoropharyngeal approaches easier and safer.

CONCLUSIONS

All of us who practice the challenging discipline of skull base surgery owe much to the early, pioneering efforts of our surgical predecessors. They have enabled us to apply techniques that previously were thought of as outrageously foolhardy, refine them, and use them to the betterment of our patients. Although it is an area of endeavor accepted by our medical peers, only time will reveal the verdict of society—beset by the restrictions of health maintenance organizations, the insurance industry, and governmental control—on the implementation and development of cranial base surgery. Skull base surgery offers a reasonable and significant chance for cure to patients previously abandoned as hopelessly incurable. Let us hope that we can continue to pursue this challenging and rewarding surgical enterprise.

REFERENCES

1. Johnson HC. Surgery of the hypophysis. In: Walker AE, ed. *A history of neurological surgery*. Baltimore: Williams & Wilkins, 1951:152.
2. McDonald TJ, Laws ER. Historical aspects of the management of pituitary disorders with emphasis on transphenoidal surgery. In: Laws ER, Randall RV, Kern EB, Aboud CF, eds. *Management of pituitary adenomas and related lesions with emphasis on transsphenoidal microsurgery*. New York: Appleton Century Crofts, 1982:1–2.
3. Caton R, Paul FT. Notes of a case of acromegaly treated by operation. *Br Med J* 1893;2:1421.
4. Horsley V: On the technique of operations on the nervous system. *Br Med J* 1906;2:411.
5. Landolt AM, Wilson CB. Tumors of the sella and parasellar area in adults. In: Youmans JR, ed. *Neurological surgery*. Vol. 5. 2nd ed. Philadelphia: WB Saunders, 1982:3138.
6. Killiani OGT. Some remarks on tumors of the optic chiasm with a proposal how to reach the same by operation. *Ann Surg* 1904;40:35.
7. Frazier CH. An approach to the hypophysis through the anterior cranial fossa. *Ann Surg* 1913;57:145.
8. Giordano. *Compendio di chirurgia operatorio Italiana*. 2:100, 1897.
9. Schloffer H. Zur frage der operation en an der hypophyse. *Beitrage zur Klinische Chirurgie* 1906;50:767.
10. Von Eiselsberg AF. My experience about operation upon the hypophysis. *Transactions of the American Surgical Association* 1910;28:55.
11. Cushing H. Partial hypophysectomy for acromegaly: with remarks on the function of the hypophysis. *Ann Surg* 1909;50:1002.
12. Killian G. Die submucöse fensterresektion des nasenscheidewand. *Arch Laryngol Rhinol* 1904;16:362.
13. Hirsch O: Demonstration eines nach eines neuen method operiten hypophysentumors. *Verhandlungen der Deutschen Gesellschaft fur Chirurgie* 1910;39:51.
14. Hirsch O. Eine neuen methode der endonasalen operation von hypophesen-tumoren. *Wien Med Wochenschr* 1952;59:636.
15. Hirsch O. Symptoms and treatment of pituitary tumors. *Archives of Otolaryngology* 1952;55:268.
16. Dandy WE. *Orbital tumor: results following the transcranial operative attack*. New York: Oskar Piest, 1941:168.
17. Rae BS, McLean JM. Combined intracranial and orbital operation for retinoblastoma. *Arch Ophthalmol* 1943;30:437.
18. Smith RR, Klopp CT, Williams JM. Surgical treatment of cancer of the frontal sinus and adjacent areas. *Cancer* 1954;7:991–994.
19. Ketcham AS, Wilkins RH, Van Buren JM, Smith RR. A combined intracranial facial approach to the paranasal sinuses. *Am J Surg* 1963;106:698–703.
20. Ketcham AS, Hoyle RC, Van Buren JM, Johnson RH, Smith RR. Complications of intracranial facial resection for tumors of the paranasal sinuses. *Am J Surg* 1966;112:591–596.
21. Sisson GA, Bytell DE, Becker SP, Ruge D. Carcinoma of the paranasal sinuses and craniofacial resection. *J Laryngol Otol* 1976;1:59–68.
22. Millar HS, Petty PG, Wilson WF, Hueston JT. A combined intracranial and facial approach for excision and repair of cancer of the ethmoid sinuses. *Aust N Z J Surg* 1973;43:179–183.
23. Bridger PG. Radical surgery for ethmoid cancer. *Archives of Otolaryngology* 1980;106:630–634.
24. Cheesman AD, Lund VJ, Howard DL. Craniofacial resection for tumors of the nasal cavity and paranasal sinuses. *Head and Neck Surgery* 1986;8:429–435.
25. Tessier P, Guiot G, Rougerie J. Ostéotomies cranio-naso-orbito-faciales hypertélorisme. *Annales de Chirurgie Plastique* 1967;12:103–118.
26. Derome PJ, Akerman M, Anguez L, et al. Les tumeurs sphéno-ethmoidales: possibilités d'exérese et de reparation chirurgicales. *Deurochirurgie* 1972;18[Suppl 1]:1–164.
27. Raveh J. Das einzeitge vorgehan bei der widerherstellung von frontobasal-mittelgesichtsfrakturen modifikatinen und behandlungsmodalitäten. *Chirurgie* 1983;54:677–686.
28. Raveh J, Laehach K, Speiser M, et al. The subcranial approach for fronto-orbital and anterior-posterior skull base tumors. *Arch Otolaryngol Head Neck Surg* 1993;119:385–393.
29. Donald PJ. Cranial facial surgery for head and neck cancer. In: Johnson JT, ed. *American Academy of Otolaryngology—Head and Neck Surgery: Instruction course*, Vol. 2. St. Louis: Mosby, 1989: 225–253.
30. House WF. A history of acoustic tumor surgery. In: House WF, Luetje

CM, eds. *Acoustic tumors*. Vol. I. *Diagnosis*. Baltimore: University Park Press, 1979:3–41.
31. Ballance C. *Some points in the surgery of the brain and its membranes*. London: MacMillan and Company, 1907:276.
32. McBurney C, Starr M. A contribution to cerebral surgery: diagnosis, localization, and operation for removal of three tumors of the brain; with some comments upon the surgical treatment of brain tumors. *American Journal of Medical Science C.V.* 1893;xx:361–387.
33. Cushing H. *Tumors of the nervus acusticus and the syndrome of cerebellopontine angle*. 2nd ed. New York: Hafner Publishing Company, 1917.
34. Dandy WE. An operation for the total removal of cerebellopontine angle (acoustic) tumors. *Surg Gynecol Obstet* 1925;41:129–148.
35. Dandy WE. Results of removal of acoustic tumors by the unilateral approach. *AMA Archives of Surgery* 1942;42:1026–1033.
36. Nylén CO. The microscope in aural surgery, its first use and later development. *Acta Otolaryngol Suppl (Stockh)* 1954;116:226–240.
37. Holmgren G. Some experiences in surgery for otosclerosis. *Acta Otolaryngol (Stockh)* 1924;5:460.
38. Panse R. Ein gliom des akustikus. *Arch Ohrenh* 1904;61:251–255.
39. Rand RW. *Microsurgery for acoustic tumors in Neurosurgery*. St. Louis: CV Mosby, 1969:126–155.
40. Rand RW, Kurze T. Facial nerve preservation by posterior fossa transmeatal microdissection in total removal of acoustic tumors. *J Neurol Neurosurg Psychiatry* 1965;28:311–316.
41. Rand RW, Dirks DD, Morgan DE, Bentson JR. Acoustic neuromas. In: Youmans JR, ed. *Youman's neurological surgery*. Vol. 5. 2nd ed. Philadelphia: WB Saunders, 1982:2967–3003.
42. Sterkers JM. Acoustic neurilemma otologic approaches. In: Sekhar L, Janecka I, eds. *Surgery of the cranial base*. New York: Raven Press, 1993:715–724.
43. Smith MFW, Miller RN, Cox DJ. Suboccipital microsurgical removal of acoustic neuromas of all sizes. *Ann Otol Rhinol Laryngol* 1973;82:407.
44. Holmes T. Aneurysms of the internal carotid artery in the cavernous sinus. *Transactions of the Pathology Society, London* 1860–61;12:61.
45. Bartholow R. Aneurysms of the arteries at the base of the brain: their symptomatology, diagnosis and treatment. *Am J Med Sci* 1872;64:374–386.
46. Peet MM. Tumors of the gasserian ganglion: with the report of two cases of extracranial carcinoma infiltrating the ganglion by direct extension through the maxillary division. *Surg Gynecol Obstet* 1927;44:202–207.
47. Parkinson D. A surgical approach to the cavernous portion of the carotid artery: anatomical studies and case reports. *J Neurosurg* 1965;23:474–483.
48. Scoville WB, Sherman IJ. Ptalybasia: report of 10 cases with comments on familial tendency, a special diagnostic sign and the end result of operation. *Ann Surg* 1951;133:496–502.
49. Southwick WO, Robinson RA. Surgical approaches to the vertebral bodies in the cervical and lumbar regions. *J Bone Joint Surg Am* 1957;39:631.
50. Fang HSY, Ong GB. Direct approach to the upper cervical spine. *J Bone Joint Surg Am* 1962;44:1588–1604.
51. Stevenson GC, Storey RJ, Perkins RK, Adams JE. A transcervical transclival approach to the ventral surface of the brain stem for the removal of a clival chordoma. *J Neurosurg* 1966;24:544–551.
52. Haselden FG, Bryce JG. Transoral clivectomy. *Journal of Maxillofacial Surgery* 1978;6:32.
53. Crockard HA. Transoral approach to intra/extradural tumors. In: Sekhar LN, Janecka IP, eds. *Surgery of cranial base tumors*. New York: Raven Press, 1993:225–234.
54. Conley J. *Concepts in head and neck surgery*. New York: Grune & Stratton, 1970:117.
55. Donald PJ. Infratemporal fossa and skull base. In: Donald PJ, ed. *Head and neck cancer: management of the difficult case*. Philadelphia: WB Saunders, 1984:306–311.
56. Crumley R, Gutin P. Surgical access for clivus chordoma. *Archives of Otolaryngology* 1989;115:295–300.
57. Woods BG, Sadar ES, Levine HL, Dohn DF, Tucker HM. Surgical problems of the base of the skull: An interdisciplinary approach. *Archives of Otolaryngology* 1980;106:1–5.

CHAPTER 2

Surgical Anatomy of the Skull Base

Bernard M. Lyons

There is no more complex display of human anatomy than that which exists at the skull base. The surgery of tumors in this area can be difficult because of restricted access, distortion of normal anatomy, and the proximity of vital structures. The good results and low morbidity of most major series of skull base resections can be achieved only with a thorough understanding and respect for the anatomy in this region. It is essential to have a detailed, three-dimensional appreciation of skull base anatomy, and this can be gained only by spending many hours in the cadaver dissection laboratory. Tumors can distort and destroy already complex anatomy. Anatomic knowledge not only allows adequate tumor resection and preservation of vital structures, but enables the surgeon to maintain function and cosmesis better. Patterns of tumor spread can also be predicted if the clinician is familiar with the myriad basal foramina and preexisting pathways for tumor spread.

Discussion of anatomy in this chapter focuses on practical surgical anatomy, but detailed descriptions of vital structures are presented where appropriate. The three subdivisions of the skull base—anterior, middle, and posterior—are dealt with separately. Each subdivision is discussed in terms of the osteology of the skull base region and its foramina, the intracranial contents, and the subbasal regional anatomy. The latter is important when considering the type of surgical approach to the region.

ANTERIOR SKULL BASE

Osteology

The anterior cranial fossa is enclosed anterolaterally by the frontal bone. The frontal crest is a midline ridge anteriorly to which is attached the falx cerebri. This ridge can be quite prominent and can make separation of the dura and sagittal sinus tedious during anterior approaches (Fig. 1).

B. M. Lyons: Department of Otolaryngology—Head and Neck Surgery, St. Vincent's Hospital, and Royal Victorian Eye and Ear Hospital, East Melbourne 3002, Australia.

Most of the floor of the anterior cranial fossa is made up of the orbital process of the frontal bone, which is grooved by the frontal lobe gyri. It is mainly convex. The central portion of the anterior fossa is much deeper and is formed by the ethmoid bone, with the central area being the cribriform plate and the lateral being the fovea ethmoidalis—the roof of the ethmoid sinus. The anterior central cribriform landmark is the crista galli. Between this and the frontal crest lies the foramen cecum. Fibrous dural attachments usually plug this foramen, although rarely an anterior nasal emissary vein may persist into adult life. The cribriform plate has multiple perforations that transmit the olfactory nerve filaments and their dural and subarachnoid extensions. Tumor spread can occur through these perforations and nerve sheaths. Anterolaterally lies the cribroethmoid foramen, which transmits the anterior ethmoid artery and nerve. The posterior ethmoid artery passes the posterior portion of the plate.

The posterior anterior fossa floor is formed by the sphenoid bone. Centrally, behind the cribriform plate lies the planum or jugum sphenoidale, a flat plate of bone that is an important landmark for the sphenoid sinus and optic nerve in anterior fossa surgery (Fig. 2). This is bordered posteriorly by the chiasmatic sulcus, a groove for the optic chiasm (Fig. 3). Posterolateral is the lesser wing of the sphenoid, which roofs the optic canal and forms a sharp posterior bony border related to the lateral cerebral sulcus and sphenoparietal sinus. Medially, the lesser wing of sphenoid forms the anterior clinoid process, an important landmark for the optic nerve and supracavernous internal carotid artery (ICA). The sphenoid bone is surgically best considered with the anterior fossa, but anatomically it is part of the middle fossa.

Intracranial Contents of the Anterior Skull Base

The dura mater of the anterior fossa is firmly attached in the regions of the crista galli, cribriform plate, and lesser wing of sphenoid. Anteriorly, it forms the falx cerebri, which contains the superior and inferior sagittal sinuses. The supe-

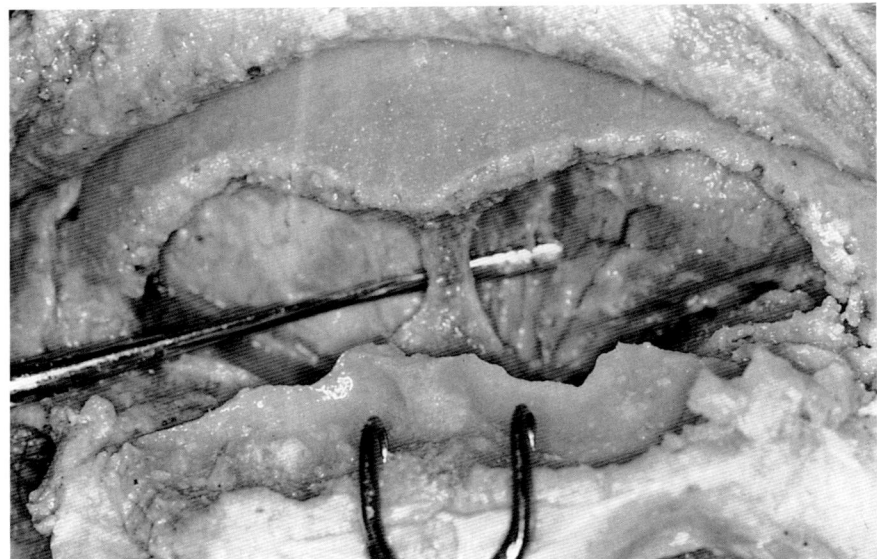

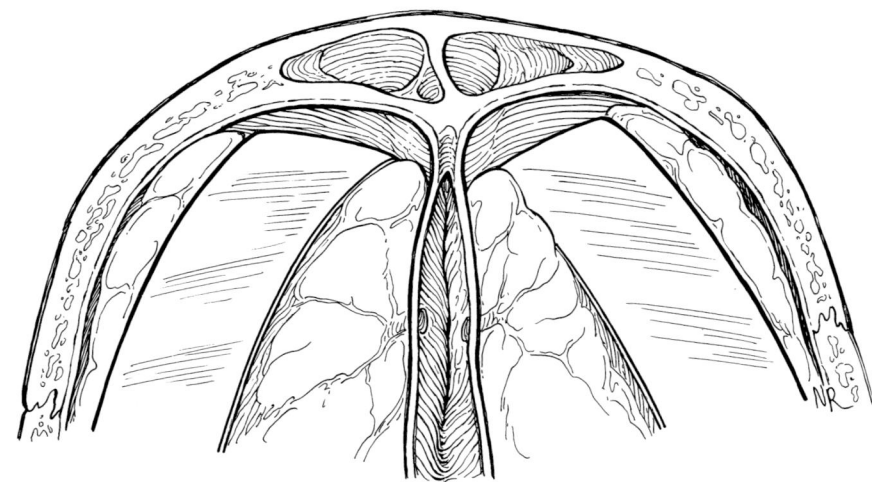

FIG. 1. A: Osteoplastic flap approach to the anterior cranial fossa. Elevator is separating sagittal sinus from frontal crest. **B:** Diagram showing the anterior crest and superior sagittal sinus.

rior sagittal sinus drains the superior cerebral veins and the frontal diploic veins of Breschet and grooves the frontal crest. It is an important posterior relation to the frontal sinus (Fig. 4). The sagittal sinus usually can be safely ligated anterior to the coronal suture. In the region of the crista galli, the sagittal sinus is very tenuous or usually nonexistent.

The frontal lobes occupy the anterior fossa. The inferior surface of the frontal lobe is related to the roof of the orbit and sinonasal tract. As such, it may be involved by tumors in this area. It is marked by the olfactory sulcus, which is occupied by the olfactory bulb and tract (Fig. 5). The olfactory tract lies above the cribriform plate and planum sphenoidale (Fig. 6). The most medial frontal lobe gyrus is the gyrus rectus, a relatively "silent area" of the brain that can be resected if involved with tumor.

Subcranial Relationships of the Anterior Skull Base

The most important subcranial or extracranial relationships of the anterior fossa are the paranasal sinuses and the orbit. The detailed anatomy of the paranasal sinuses is beyond the scope of this chapter, but is dealt with adequately elsewhere (1).

The ethmoid sinuses are directly related to the orbit laterally, the anterior fossa superiorly, and the cribriform plate medially (Fig. 7). The sphenoid sinus is related superiorly to the anterior cranial fossa and is described in detail in the section on the middle fossa. The frontal sinus lies between the two plates of the frontal bone and is often used as a portal of entry in anterior craniofacial resection because of its direct proximity to the anterior fossa. Its thin posterior wall is related to the frontal lobe dura and superior sagittal sinus.

The orbit is important anatomically because it is often involved by tumors in the region and is a portal for the intracranial or extracranial spread of tumors. The bony orbit is related on three sides to the paranasal sinuses and superiorly to the anterior cranial fossa. It is roughly pyramidal in shape, although the orbital apex is closer to the medial wall than the lateral. The medial wall is made up of the orbital process of the frontal bone, and the lacrimal, ethmoid, and sphenoid

SURGICAL ANATOMY OF THE SKULL BASE / 17

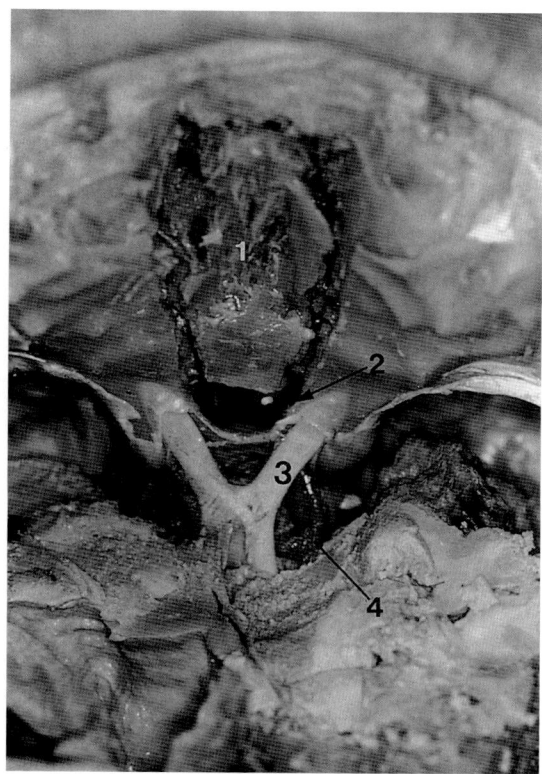

FIG. 2. Cadaver dissection demonstrating bone cuts for anterior craniofacial resection extending into sphenoid sinus and protecting optic nerves. *1*, Cribriform plate; *2*, sphenoid sinus; *3*, optic nerve; *4*, internal carotid artery.

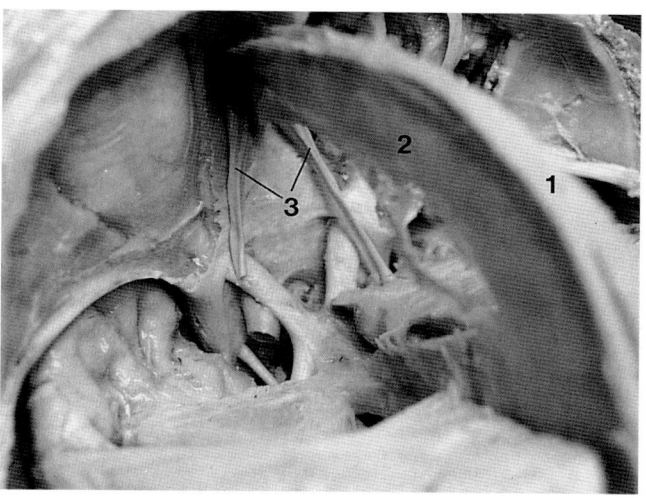

FIG. 4. Cadaver dissection demonstrating relationship of falx cerebri and sagittal sinus to the frontal bones. (Falx and sinus artistically enhanced). *1*, Sagittal sinus; *2*, falx cerebri; *3*, olfactory tracts.

bones. The foramina in this medial wall can be quite variable. The foramina for the anterior and the posterior ethmoid arteries lie 24 and 12 mm behind the anterior lacrimal crest, respectively. The optic foramen lies 6 mm behind that of the posterior ethmoid artery (2). The orbital floor is formed by the maxilla and anterolaterally by the zygoma. It contains the infraorbital groove. The lateral wall consists of the frontal

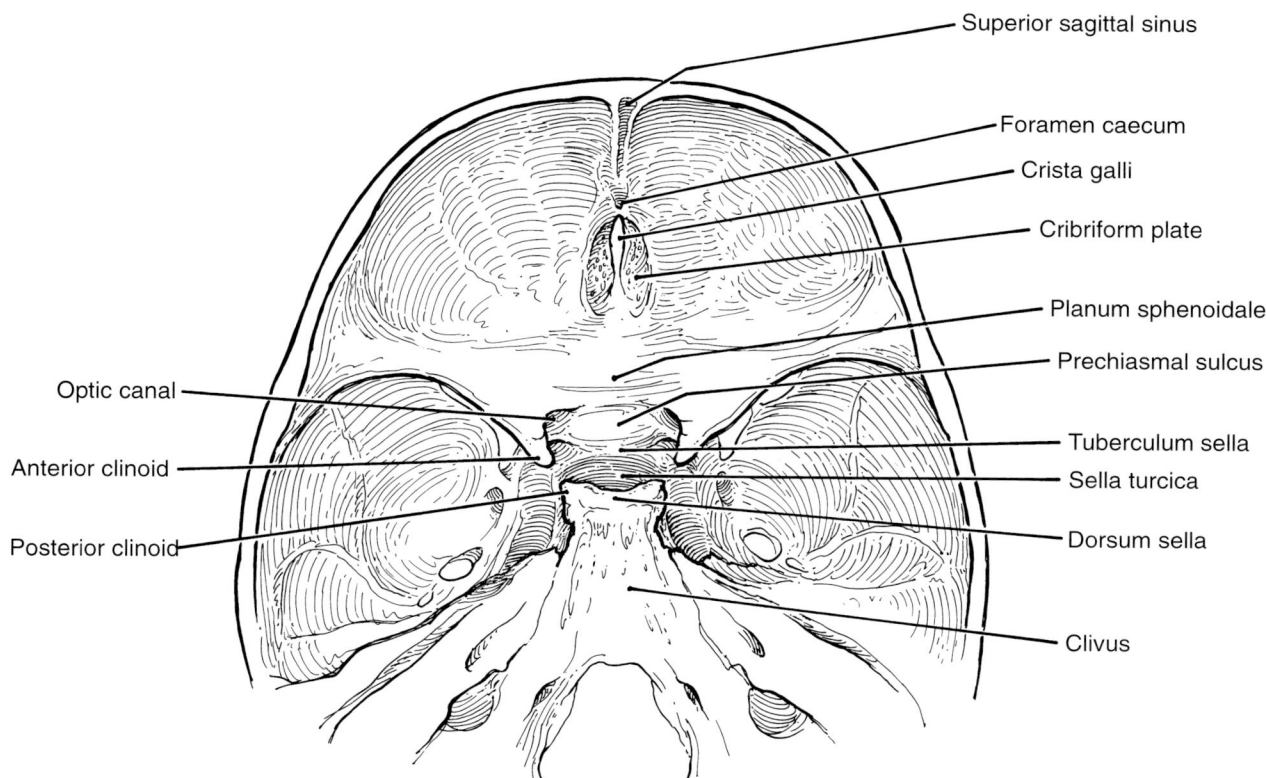

FIG. 3. Anterior cranial fossa and body of sphenoid.

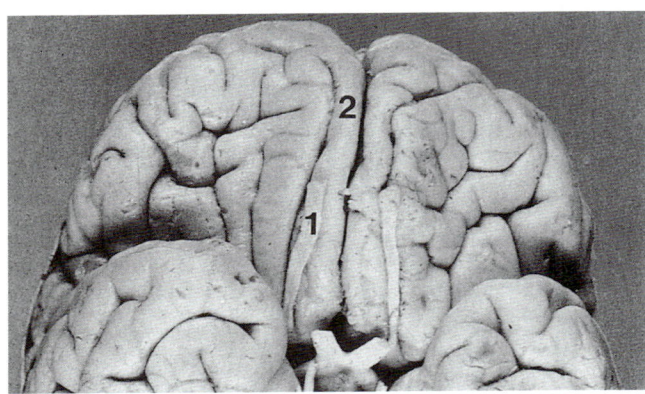

FIG. 5. View of orbital surface of frontal lobes. *1*, Optic tract; *2*, gyrus rectus.

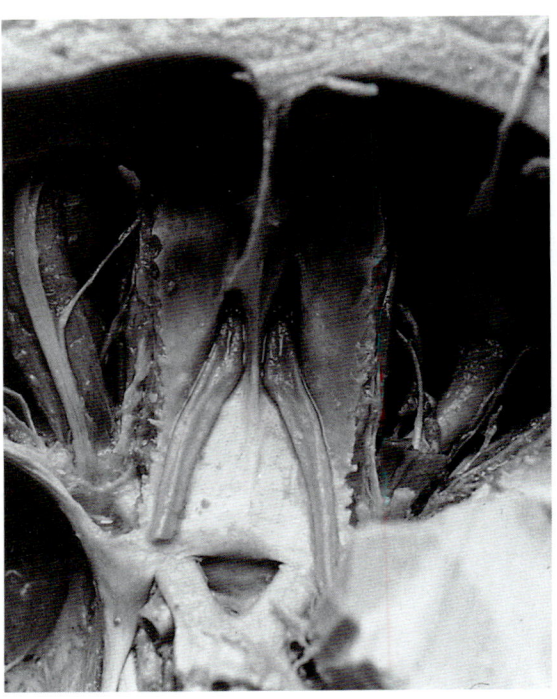

FIG. 6. The olfactory bulbs and tracts are seen here overlying the cribriform plate and planum sphenoidale. The orbit is dissected on both sides.

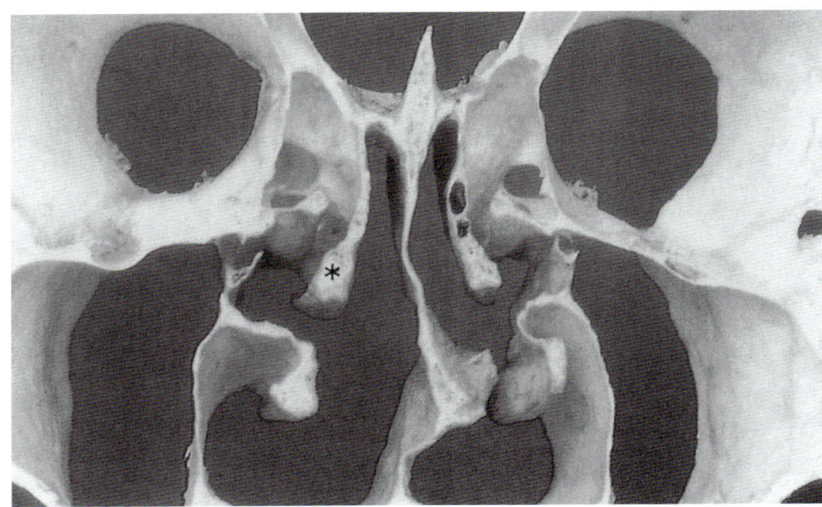

FIG. 7. Coronal section through orbit and ethmoid (*asterisk* on middle concha).

process of the maxilla and greater and lesser wings of sphenoid separated by the superior orbital fissure (Fig. 8). Anteriorly lies Whitnall's tubercle, to which the suspensory ligaments of the orbit attach.

It is important to realize that anteriorly the lateral wall is related to the temporalis muscle, but more posteriorly it forms the anterior wall of the middle cranial fossa and is thus related to the anterior horn of the temporal lobe. The roof is mainly formed by the orbital process of the frontal bone, with a small posterior contribution by the lesser wing of sphenoid. Detailed knowledge of the intraorbital anatomy is necessary only when removing intraorbital tumors. The lateral and superior anatomy is most important in these cases.

The motor nerves most at risk are the lacrimal nerve and the levator palpebrae superioris nerve, which arises from the superior division of the oculomotor nerve and runs medial to or through the superior rectus muscle.

Orbital apex anatomy is complex and important. It consists of three important portals: the optic canal and the superior and inferior orbital fissures. These portals are compartmentalized by the annulus of Zinn, a condensation of the tendons of the rectus muscles and levator palpebrae superioris.

The lateral part of the superior orbital fissure transmits the lacrimal, frontal, and trochlear nerves with the superior ophthalmic vein. Within the annulus, in the medial superior fissure, run the superior and inferior divisions of the oculomotor nerve and the nasociliary and abducens nerves. In the superomedial compartment of the annulus is the optic canal, which transmits the optic nerve and the ophthalmic artery. The optic canal in 40% to 80% of cases indents the lateral wall of the sphenoid, and in 7% to 13% can be encompassed completely in the posterior ethmoid cells (3).

The ophthalmic artery arises from the ICA medial to the anterior clinoid process. It runs medial to the optic nerve, within its dural sheath, and then crosses under the nerve and in the orbit lies lateral and then crosses superior to the optic nerve. In a small percentage of cases it may enter the orbit through a separate foramen (4).

The superior and inferior ophthalmic veins drain the orbit and communicate with facial veins and the pterygoid plexus. The inferior vein usually joins the superior ophthalmic vein at the orbital apex and passes through the superior orbital fissure, lateral to the annulus, and enters the cavernous sinus.

MIDDLE SKULL BASE

Osteology

The central portion of this region is formed by the body of the sphenoid. The tuberculum sellae is a transverse ridge that separates the chiasmal sulcus anteriorly from the sella turcica posteriorly. The sella turcica is a rounded hollow that cradles the pituitary gland (Fig. 9). The sides of the body of the sphenoid slope downward and laterally to meet the floor of the middle fossa. They are grooved by the sigmoid curve of the ICA as it courses from the petrous apex through the cavernous sinus. The anterior and posterior clinoid processes are important landmarks and areas of dural attachment. Occasionally a middle clinoid process exists that can be bridged to the anterior clinoid, so forming a caroticoclinoid foramen, through which passes the ICA (5).

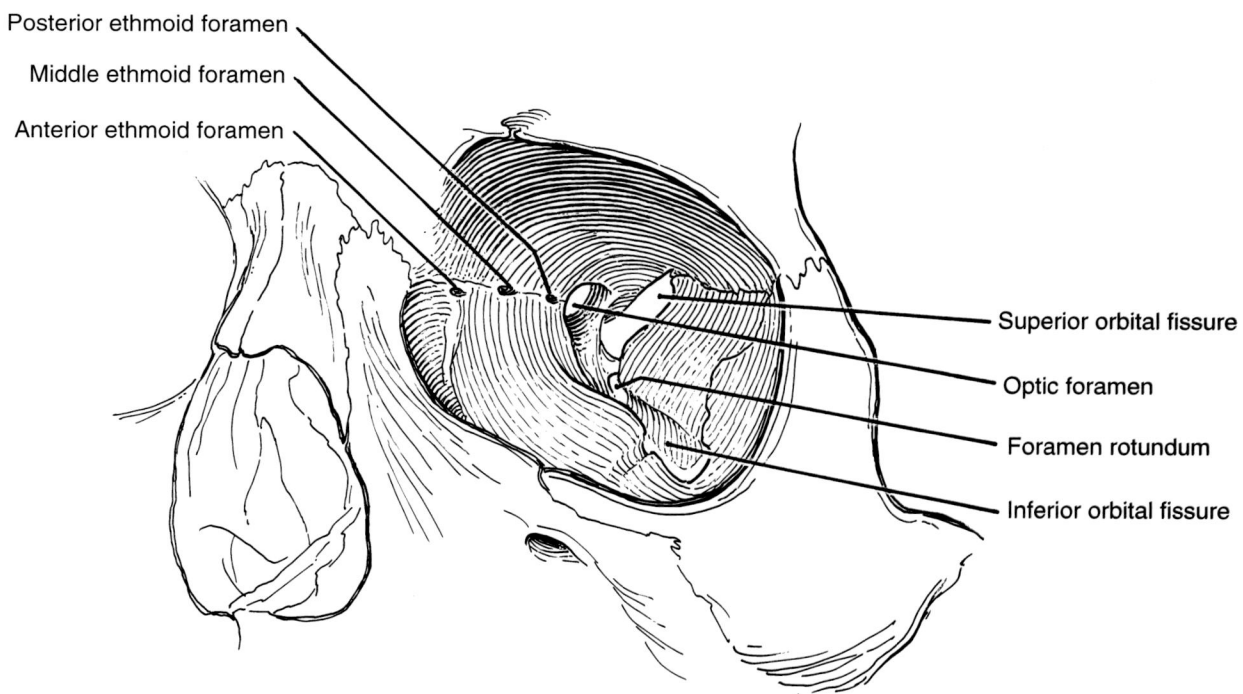

FIG. 8. Orbital apex.

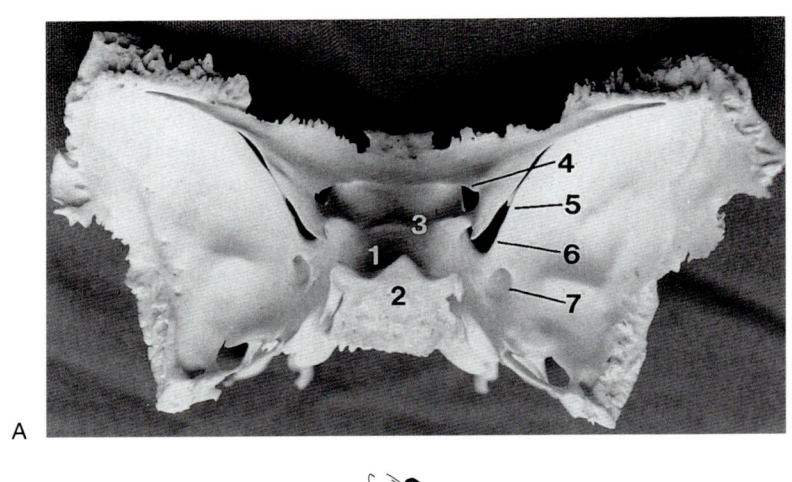

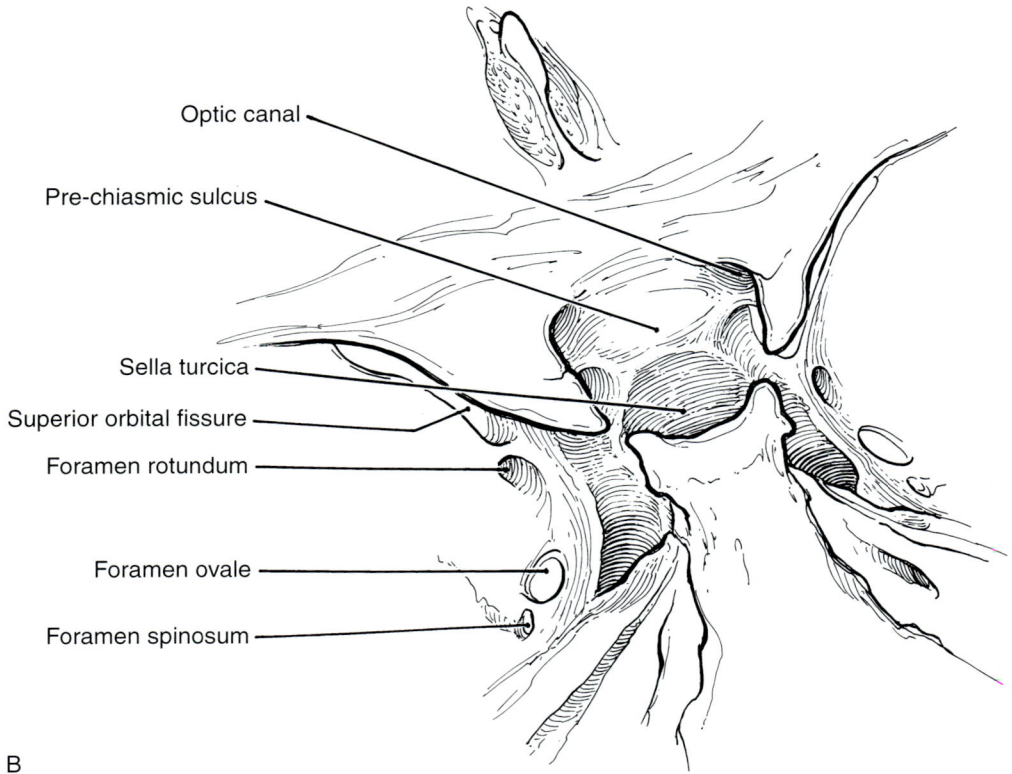

FIG. 9. A: Sphenoid bone from posterior view. *1*, Sella turcica; *2*, dorsum sellae; *3*, tuberculum sellae; *4*, optic canal; *5*, superior orbital fissure; *6*, inferior orbital fissure; *7*, foramen rotundum. **B:** From oblique view B.

The lateral recesses of the middle skull base are the middle cranial fossae proper. They are roughly triangular in shape. They are limited by the sphenoid ridge anteriorly and petrous ridge posteriorly. The anterior wall is formed by the greater wing of the sphenoid. The floor is made up of the greater wing of the sphenoid anteriorly and the petrous ridge of the temporal bone posteriorly. Laterally and between these two, the squamous temporal bone forms part of the floor. The lateral wall is made up of the greater wing of the sphenoid anteriorly and the squamous temporal bone posteriorly. The floor and lateral bony walls are grooved by the middle meningeal artery, curving anteriorly from the foramen spinosum to the region of the pterion, where it courses backward. The pterion is an H-shaped suture marking the confluence of the frontal bone, greater wing of the sphenoid, and the squamous temporal and parietal bones.

The superior surface of the petrous ridge has several important markings. Medially, near the apex, is an impression for the trigeminal ganglion, as it lies in Meckel's cave (Fig. 10). The ICA runs directly under this area and frequently its bony canal may be dehiscent. Dural elevation in this region should be undertaken with caution.

Laterally lies the flattened thin portion of the tegmen tympani, roofing the middle ear and mastoid. Anteromedially

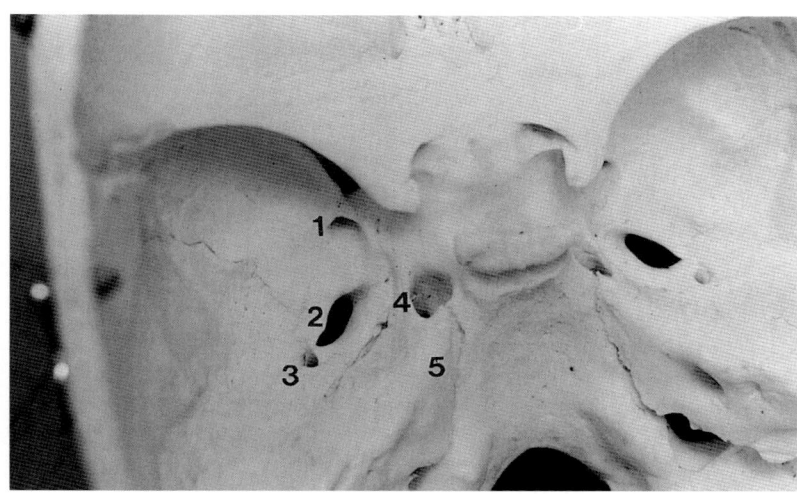

FIG. 10. Middle fossa osteology. *1*, Foramen rotundum; *2*, foramen ovale; *3*, foramen spinosum; *4*, carotid canal; *5*, trigeminal impression.

lies the arcuate eminence, which overlies the superior semicircular canal. Further anteromedially lie the canals for the greater and lesser superficial petrosal nerves.

The arcuate eminence and the hiatus for the greater superficial petrosal nerve (GSPN) are important landmarks in middle fossa approaches to the internal auditory canal (IAC). The superior semicircular canal lies within an arc of 60 degrees to the IAC (6) or the GSPN can be traced to the geniculate ganglion and facial nerve in the IAC (7). The bone of the middle fossa floor may be dehiscent over the geniculate ganglion. The petrous ridge is longitudinally grooved by the superior petrosal sinus, where the tentorium cerebelli attaches.

Foramina of the Middle Fossa

Anteriorly lies the superior orbital fissure, which leads to the orbital apex. The foramen rotundum lies behind and inferior to the superior orbital fissure and transmits the maxillary division (VII) of the trigeminal nerve. The canal is approximately 4 mm long.

Posterolateral to the foramen rotundum is the foramen ovale, which transmits the mandibular division (VIII) of the trigeminal nerve, the accessory meningeal artery, the lesser superficial petrosal nerve (LSPN), and emissary veins to the pterygoid plexus.

The foramen spinosum lies posterolateral to the foramen ovale and transmits the middle meningeal artery and the meningeal branch of cranial nerve VII. There are two inconstant foramina in this region. The innominate foramen lies medial to foramen spinosum and may transmit the LSPN. The foramen of Vesalius lies medial to the foramen ovale in 40% of skulls and transmits an emissary vein from the cavernous sinus (8).

The petrous apex articulates with the sphenoid and occipital bone medially and so forms a rounded opening to the carotid canal. This opening is the cranial counterpart of the foramen lacerum on the undersurface of the skull base.

Intracranial Contents of the Middle Fossa

The dural arrangement in the middle skull base is complex. It is densely adherent in the regions of the clinoid processes, the petrous and sphenoid ridges, and around the basal foramina. In the midline it forms a transverse dural plate, the diaphragma sellae, which bridges between the tuberculum sellae and dorsum sellae. It roofs the pituitary fossa and is perforated by the pituitary stalk. Laterally the dural plate forms the roof of a basin beside the body of the sphenoid, the cavernous sinus (Fig. 11).

Cavernous Sinus

The cavernous sinus is complex but critical to understand when performing skull base surgery. It is a plexus of veins that lies within the layers of the dura beside the sphenoid sinus. The lateral border of the roof is the anterior petroclinoid fold and the posterior border is the posterior petroclinoid fold.

The ICA is the main structure of importance within the cavernous sinus. It runs in an S-shaped curve forward in close relation to the lateral wall of the sphenoid sinus. It gives off two to six caroticocavernous branches. These supply the hypophysis and anastomose with middle meningeal branches.

The abducens nerve (VI) is the only cranial nerve within the cavernous sinus. This pierces the dura over the clivus and enters Dorello's canal. This leads to the cavernous sinus, where the nerve runs in close apposition to the lateral wall of the ICA.

The other cranial nerves are contained in the lateral wall of the cavernous sinus enclosed by two layers of dura. The oculomotor nerve (III) pierces the transverse plate of the dura, with accompanying sheaths of arachnoid and dura, and passes forward in the lateral wall. Anteriorly it divides into superior and inferior divisions. The trochlear nerve (IV) enters in the angle between the anterior and posterior petrocli-

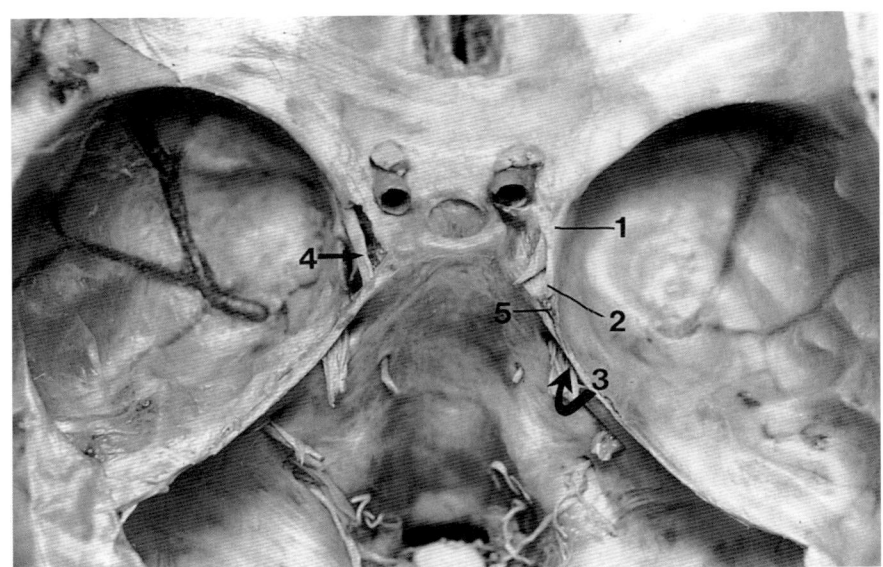

FIG. 11. Cadaver dissection of the dura mater of middle cranial fossa and cavernous sinus. *1*, Anterior petroclinoid fold; *2*, posterior petroclinoid fold; *3*, Meckel's cave; *4*, abducens nerve and Dorello's canal; *5*, trochlear nerve.

noid folds and runs in the lateral wall. The ophthalmic (VI), maxillary (V2), and mandibular (V3) divisions of the trigeminal nerve also run in the lateral wall of the cavernous sinus. Cranial nerves III, IV, and VI are variably related to each other in the lateral wall of the cavernous sinus. Parkinson has described these variations in detail and outlined triangles that can be used to gain access safely to the cavernous sinus between these cranial nerves (9).

Anterior venous connections are the superior ophthalmic vein and the sphenoparietal sinus. Superiorly the cavernous sinus drains the superficial middle cerebral and inferior cerebral veins. Medially it connects with anterior and posterior intercavernous plexuses to form the circular sinus. Inferiorly, emissary veins pass to the pterygoid plexus. Posteriorly it drains into the superior and inferior petrosal sinuses and into the basilar plexus, between the dural layers over the clivus.

The motor and sensory roots of the trigeminal nerve pass underneath the free edge of the tentorium cerebelli and into Meckel's cave. This contains the motor root and the trigeminal (Gasserian) ganglion on the sensory root, which overlies the petrous apex and ICA. The ganglion is variably enclosed by subarachnoid space and cerebrospinal fluid. Cranial nerves VI, V2, and V3 pass from the ganglion into the lateral wall of the cavernous sinus. The motor route passes with V3 through the foramen ovale.

The temporal lobe fills most of the rest of the middle fossa and extends to a variable degree under the anterior cranial fossa.

Consideration of the venous drainage is important in middle fossa surgery. The inferior anastomotic vein (of Labbé) connects the superficial middle cerebral vein to the transverse sinus just before it becomes the sigmoid sinus. Interruption of this vein may result in cerebral infarction. The superior anastomotic vein (of Trolard) connects the middle cerebral vein to the superior cerebral veins.

The GSPN and the LSPN run along the floor of the middle fossa beneath the dura. The LSPN lies parallel but rostral to the GSPN. The GSPN parallels the course of the anterior edge of the petrous bone as it runs to the foramen lacerum to form the nerve of the pterygoid canal with the deep petrosal nerve. In the floor of the middle fossa it may be stretched during dural elevation, resulting in facial nerve paralysis. It is also a landmark for the ICA, which lies just deep and parallel to it in the temporal bone.

The temporal bone itself contains several important structures that should be considered at this point. The sigmoid sinus ends in the jugular bulb, which is considered in more detail with the posterior fossa. The facial (VII) and vestibulocochlear (VIII) nerves enter the porus acusticus and IAC. Cranial nerve VIII ends at the inner ear, whereas the facial nerve traverses the middle ear and mastoid. The eustachian tube arises at the protympanum and runs anteromedially and inferiorly. The tube is one third bony and two thirds cartilaginous. Directly medial to the origin of the bony eustachian tube lies the ICA, and the bone may be dehiscent here. The eustachian tube needs to be traversed before reaching the ICA.

Internal Carotid Artery

Many vital structures are at risk in skull base surgery, but the most important is the ICA. Landmarks in the neck and temporal bone need to be recognized. The course of the ICA can be divided into four parts: cervical, intratemporal, cavernous, and supracavernous (Fig. 12).

The cervical portion of the ICA arises at the level of the third and fourth cervical vertebrae. The artery runs superiorly, posteromedial to the external carotid and deep to the digastric muscle and styloid apparatus. The styloid process and scroll of the temporal bone lead directly deeply to the carotid canal, which lies anteromedial to the jugular foramen. The glenoid fossa is a bony landmark for the higher parts of the

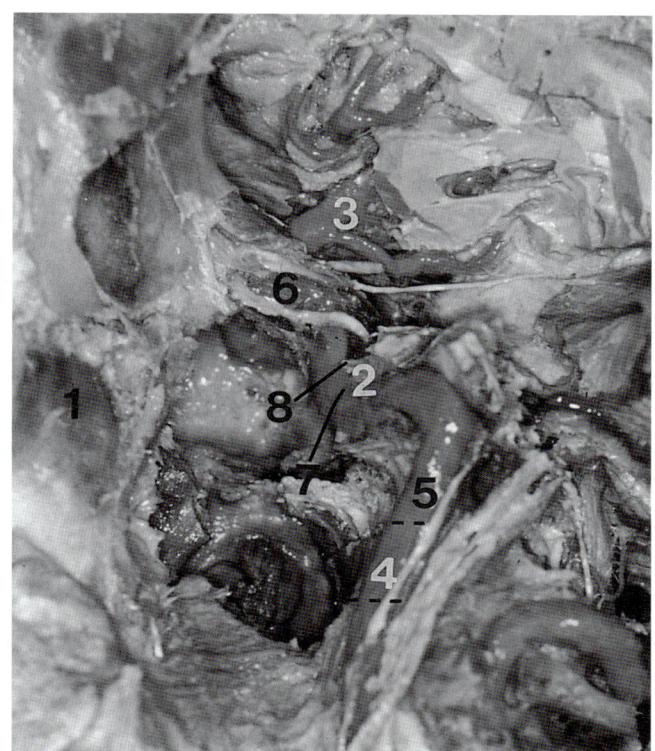

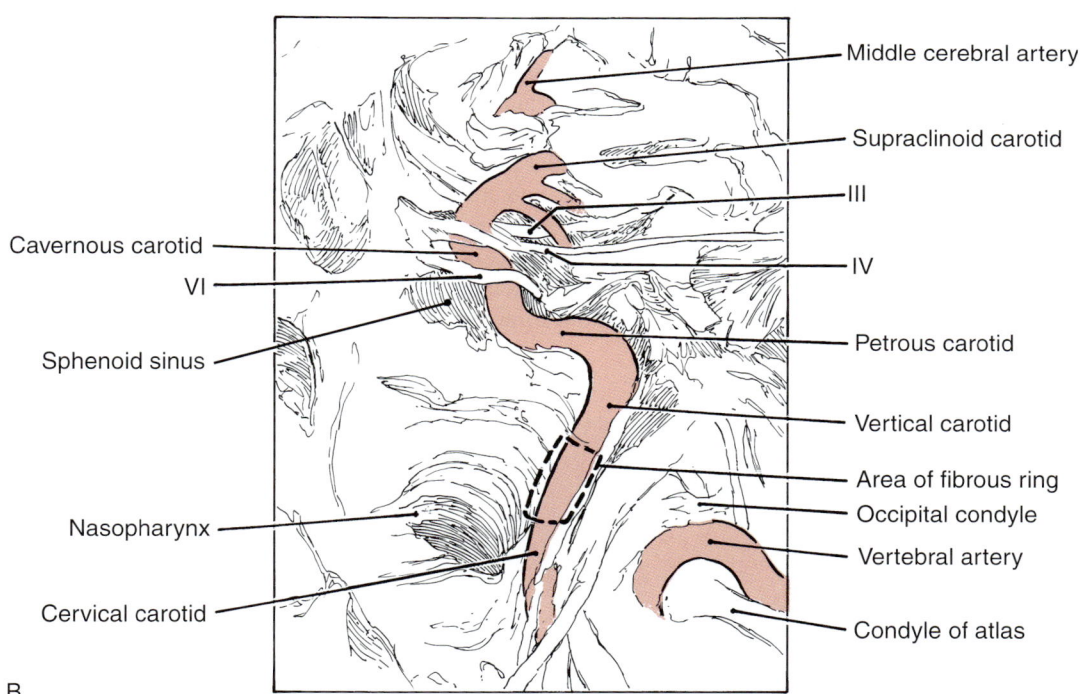

FIG. 12. A: Cadaver dissection demonstrating course of internal carotid artery. *1*, Sphenoid sinus; *2*, horizontal petrosal part; *3*, supracavernous; *4*, area of fibrous ring; *5*, vertical petrosal part; *6*, abducens nerve; *7*, foramen lacerum part; *8*, cavernous part. **B:** Diagram of course internal carotid artery.

ICA at eustachian tube level. The cervical portion has no branches.

The intratemporal ICA has a vertical and a horizontal segment. The vertical segment begins at the carotid canal, where it is anchored very firmly by a fibrous ring and is difficult to mobilize (Fig. 13). It ascends for 5 mm and then turns anteromedially into the horizontal portion. Here it lies medial to the eustachian tube and anterolateral and slightly inferior to the cochlea. It then runs forward in the petrous bone at an angle of 45 degrees to the mid-sagittal plane. It is directly related anterolaterally to the eustachian tube in this portion. The middle fossa relationships of this portion have already been considered. This segment gives off caroticotympanic and pterygoid branches. The artery here is thin walled but

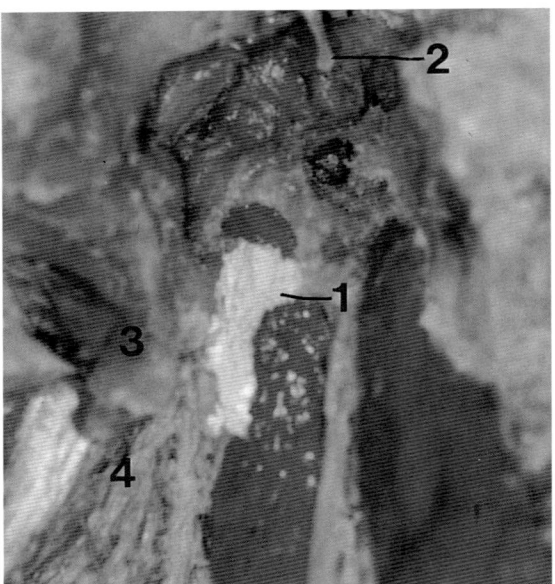

FIG. 13. Cadaver dissection of ascending internal carotid artery and fibrous ring. *1*, Fibrous ring; *2*, malleus; *3*, spine of sphenoid; *4*, mandibular division of the trigeminal nerve.

coated by a thick protective layer of periosteum and vessels.

The cavernous portion of the ICA has already been considered with the cavernous sinus. The artery in this segment is very thin walled.

The supracavernous portion of the ICA begins as the artery pierces the dura in the roof of the cavernous sinus medial to the anterior clinoid process. It passes backward below the optic nerve to the anterior perforated substance, where it ends in the circle of Willis. Branches are the ophthalmic, anterior and middle cerebral, posterior communicating, and anterior choroid arteries.

Subcranial Relationships of the Middle Skull Base

Lateral Subcranial Structures

The undersurface of the middle cranial fossa is the infratemporal fossa, and this provides access to medial skull base areas such as the nasopharynx. Many important structures lie in this area, but they lie deeply, protected by several bony and soft tissue barriers.

The first of these structures are the parotid gland and facial nerve (Fig. 14). The branch of the nerve most at risk in surgery of this area is the frontalis branch, and this can be protected by dissecting in a plane deep to the superficial layer of the temporalis fascia and so reflecting the nerve forward and downward. The nerve lies superficial to the fascia (10,11).

Two bony barriers then present themselves, the zygomatic arch and the condyle of the mandible (Fig. 15). The fan-shaped temporalis muscle arises from the temporal fossa and inserts onto the coronoid process of the mandible. When this is reflected downward, access is obtained to the infratemporal fossa proper. Care is needed on the deep surface because its blood supply, the deep temporal arteries from the maxillary artery, lie here and can be damaged. This may preclude the use of this muscle in reconstruction (Fig. 16).

A three-dimensional understanding of the infratemporal fossa is important, and this can be aided by the concept of the "subtemporal trapezoid" as described by Donald (12). All of the important structures emerging from the basal foramina are encompassed by imaginary lines joining (a) the base of the medial pterygoid plate anteromedially, (b) the articular eminence anterolaterally, (c) the occipital condyle and foramen magnum posteromedially, and (d) the mastoid tip posterolaterally (Fig. 17).

Immediately posterior to the styloid process lies the stylomastoid foramen, where the facial nerve exits the mastoid.

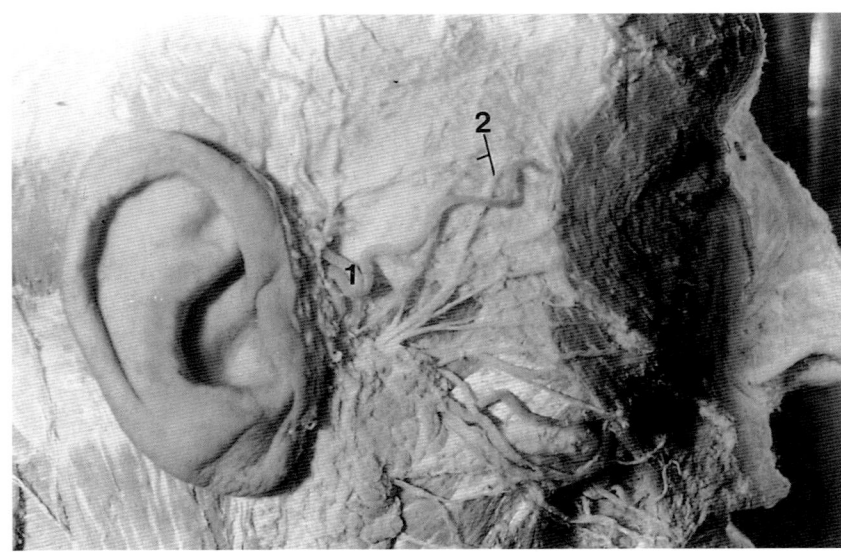

FIG. 14. Facial nerve dissection. 1, Superficial temporal artery; 2, frontalis branches of the facial nerve.

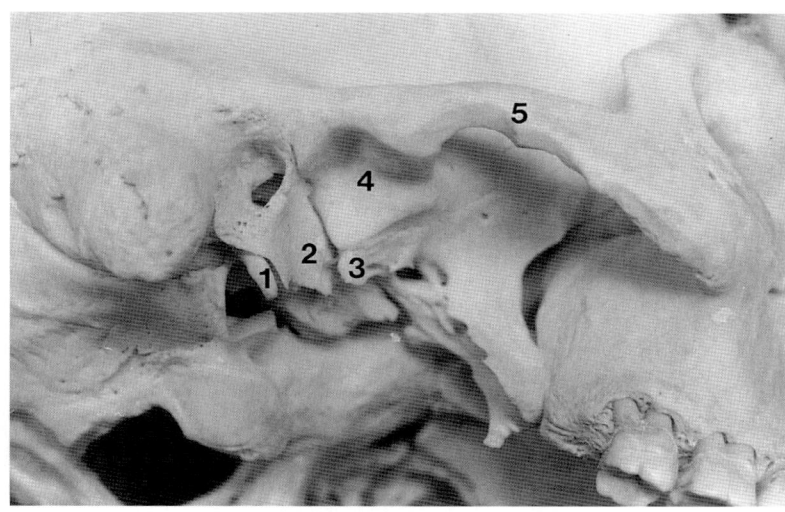

FIG. 15. Osteology of bony barriers to infratemporal fossa. *1*, Styloid process; *2*, vaginal process of temporal bone; *3*, spine of sphenoid; *4*, glenoid fossa; *5*, zygomatic arch.

From here the tympanic portion (vaginal process) of the temporal bone leads anteromedially, and just medial to its tip lies the carotid canal. Directly posterolateral lies the jugular foramen, where cranial nerves IX, X, and XI become intimately related to the great vessels in the neck. Posteromedial to the carotid canal lies the occipital condyle and under its lip, the hypoglossal canal, where cranial nerve XII exits into the neck.

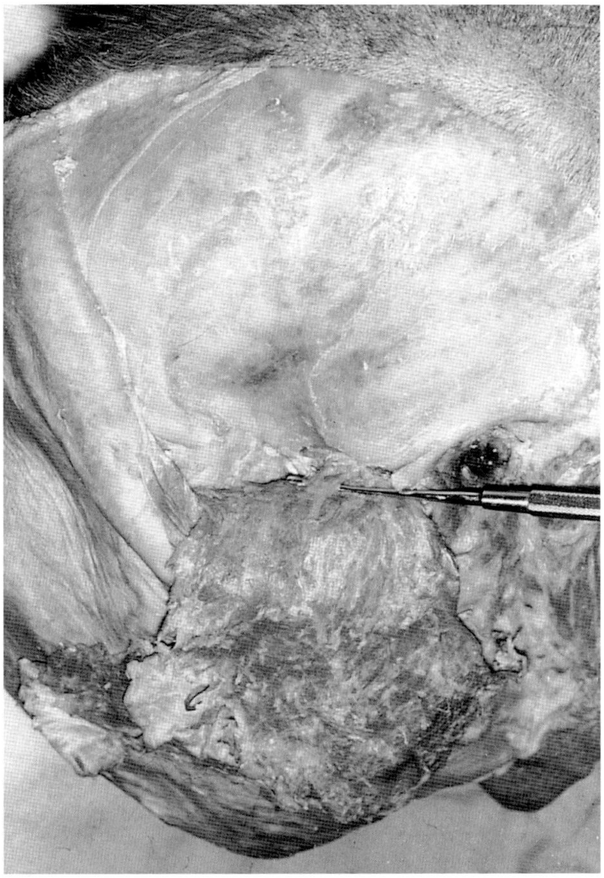

More anteriorly in the trapezoid lies the glenoid fossa. Directly medial to this lies (a) the petrotympanic fissure, where the chorda tympani exits, and (b) the spine of the sphenoid, which is an important landmark for the anteriorly situated foramen spinosum and middle meningeal arteries.

Drilling medially through the glenoid fossa leads straight into the bony eustachian tube and superiorly into the middle cranial fossa, because the bone here is very thin. Anteromedial to the foramen spinosum is the foramen ovale, where the mandibular division of the trigeminal nerve exists. Further medially lies the cartilaginous eustachian tube and more medially the carotid artery and foramen lacerum.

The orientation of these structures can be readily appreciated as three parallel lines running at 45 degrees to the midsagittal plane (along the axis of a line joining the mastoid tip to the medial pterygoid plate). The most superficial line incorporates the foramen spinosum, foramen ovale, and the lateral pterygoid plate. The middle line incorporates the eustachian tube and the deepest line the ICA and foramen lacerum (Fig. 18).

The bulk of the infratemporal fossa is occupied by the lateral and medial pterygoid muscles, which arise from the pterygoid plates and infratemporal surface of the skull. Intimately related to these are the branches of the mandibular division of cranial nerve V, the pterygoid plexus of veins, and the branches of the maxillary arteries. Deeper, arising from the skull base and cartilaginous eustachian tube, are the tensor and levator veli palatini muscles (Fig. 19). At the deepest, most anterior part of the infratemporal fossa lies the pterygoid process and, more anteriorly, the pterygomaxillary fissure. This leads into the pterygomaxillary fossa. The vidian nerve enters this through the vidian canal and the maxillary nerve through the foramen rotundum (Fig. 20). Branches of these two nerves interdigitate through the sphenopalatine ganglion. The maxillary artery enters the fossa between the two heads of the lateral pterygoid muscle.

FIG. 16. Reflected temporalis muscle demonstrating entry point of blood supply on its deep surface.

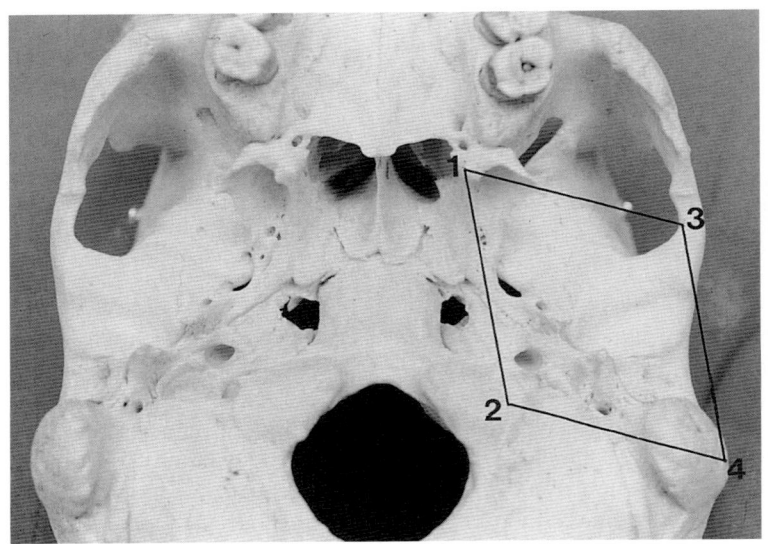
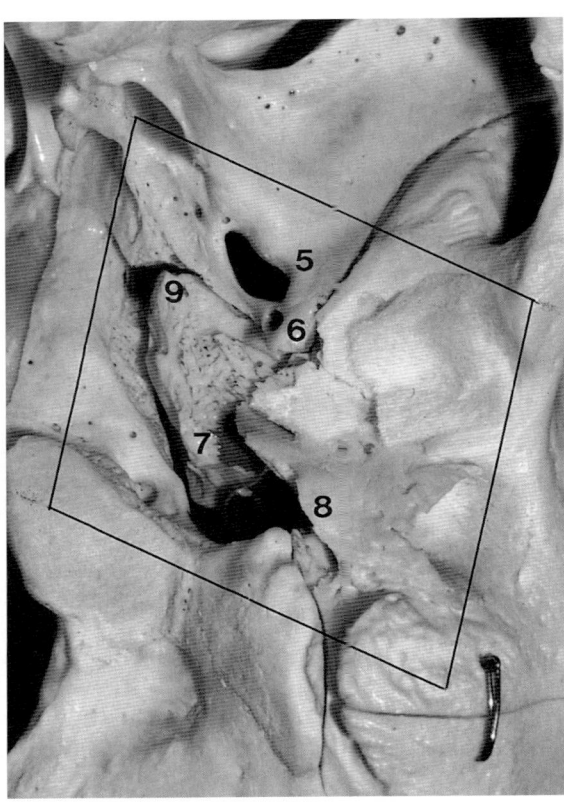

FIG. 17. A: "Subcranial trapezoid." *1,* Medial pterygoid plate; *2,* occipital condyle; *3,* articular eminence; *4,* mastoid tip. **B:** Close-up view. *5,* Foramen ovale; *6,* foramen spinosum; *7,* carotid canal; *8,* jugular foramen; *9,* foramen lacerum.

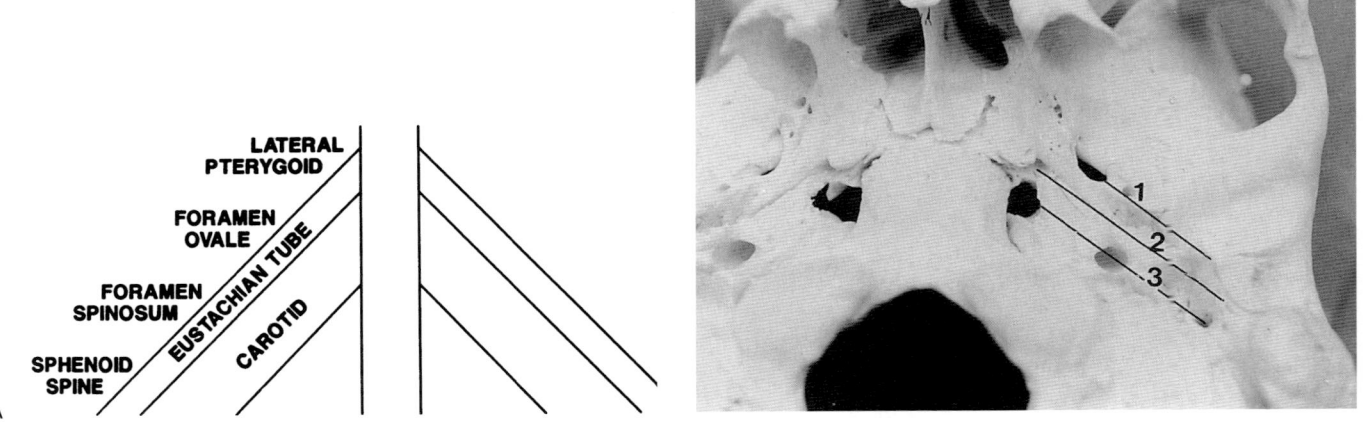

FIG. 18. A: Orientation lines at skull base. **B:** Orientation lines superimposed on skull. *Line 1,* Foramen ovale, foramen spinosum, styloid process; *line 2,* eustachian tube line; *line 3,* carotid canal, internal carotid artery, foramen cecum.

The pterygomaxillary fossa is a pathway for turnouts to spread into the infratemporal fossa. The inferior orbital fissure lies at the most anterior limit. This is formed by the greater wing of the sphenoid and the maxillary tuberosity.

Medial Subcranial Structures

Anteriorly, the sphenoid sinus is related to the middle skull base. The anatomy of this is important in respect to transsphenoidal approaches to the pituitary and clivus. The pneumatization of the sphenoid is highly variable and can influence the type of approach used. Sellar and presellar pneumatization allows ready access to the pituitary fossa (13). As mentioned previously, the ICA, optic nerve, and sometimes even the nerve of the vidian canal indent the lateral wall of the sphenoid sinus and may even be dehiscent or contained within the sinus.

More posteriorly in the midline lies the nasopharynx. This is lined by pharyngobasilar fascia that is suspended from the

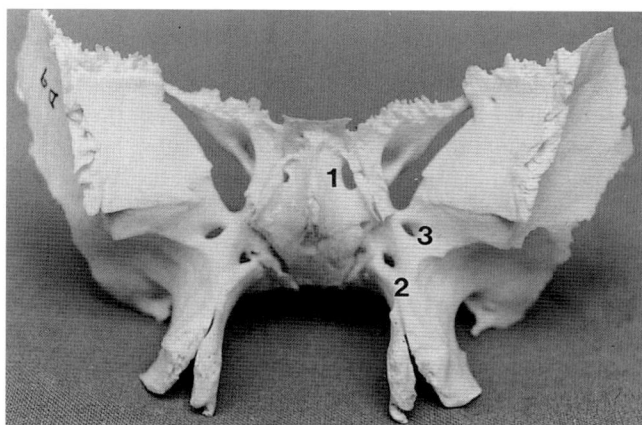

FIG. 20. Anterior face of sphenoid bone. *1,* Sphenoid ostium; *2,* vidian canal; *3,* foramen rotundum.

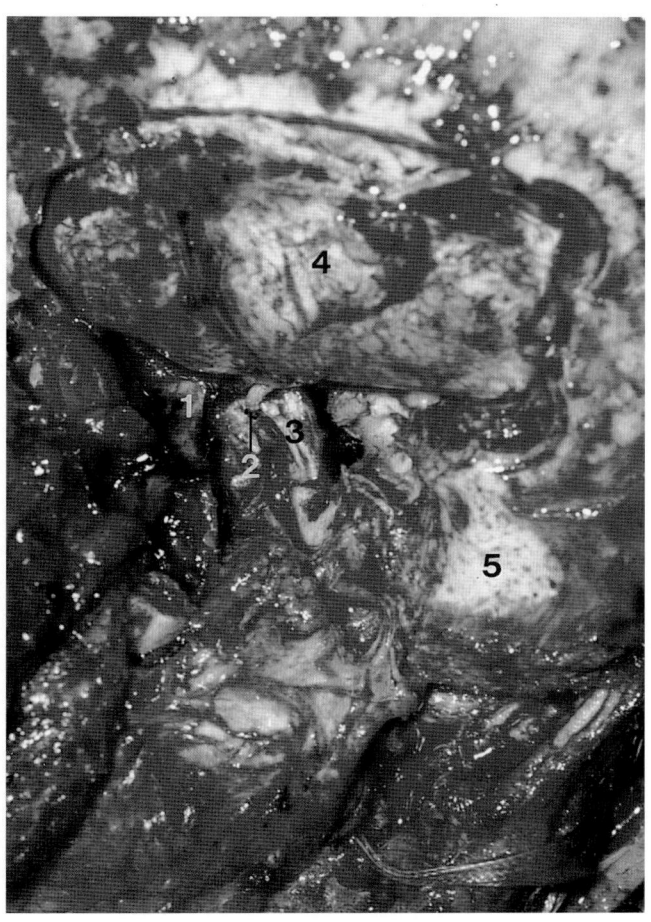

FIG. 19. Intraoperative photograph of left-sided deep infratemporal fossa dissection. *1,* Lateral pterygoid plate; *2,* middle meningeal artery (tied); *3,* mandibular division of trigeminal nerve; *4,* temporal lobe; *5,* remnant of glenoid fossa.

skull base and clivus. The clivus is formed by the basisphenoid and basiocciput, and directly posterior to this lies the vertebrobasilar artery and brainstem. The clivus is covered by dense periosteum, pharyngobasilar fascia, and mucosa. It is important to note that directly above the nasopharynx lies the foramen lacerum. This is plugged by fibrous tissue and cartilage, and directly above this lies the ICA in its canal, just before it enters the cavernous sinus.

The lateral wall of the nasopharynx is made up of mucosa, pharyngobasilar fascia, and the superior pharyngeal constrictor muscle. The gap between the superior constrictor and the skull base is termed the foramen of Morgagni. This is a potential route for nasopharyngeal tumor spread. The potential space is largely filled by the eustachian tube and the tensor and levator palati muscles.

POSTERIOR SKULL BASE

Osteology

The anterior wall of the posterior fossa is made up of the posterior surface of the petrous bone laterally and in the midline by the clivus. The clivus is a flat, trapezoidal bone formed by the synostosis of the basisphenoid and basiocciput. The floor and posterior and lateral walls are formed by the occipital bone. The roof is made up of the tentorium cerebelli.

The cranial surface of the occipital bone is deeply grooved by the cerebellar hemispheres. The internal occipital crest runs vertically from the foramen magnum to the internal occipital protuberance. The crest marks the line of attachment of the falx cerebelli, which contains the occipital sinus. On each side of the internal occipital protuberance lies a horizontal groove for the transverse sinus. Anteroinferiorly from this is the deep groove for the sigmoid sinus ending at the jugular foramen. A sulcus for the inferior petrosal sinus lies between the clivus and the petrous apex anteriorly.

Foramina of the Posterior Fossa

On the posterior surface of the petrous temporal bone are two foramina. The first is the porus acusticus or opening of the IAC, which transmits the vestibulocochlear and facial nerves, nervus intermedius, and branches of the anterior inferior cerebellar artery (AICA) to the inner ear. The second is the vestibular aqueduct, lying posteroinferiorly to the IAC. It transmits the endolymphatic duct.

Below these two foramina lies the jugular foramen. This is formed by the occipital bone posteriorly and the sharp posteroinferior border of the petrous bone (processus jugularis) anteriorly. Posteriorly, the jugular foramen contains the termination of the sigmoid sinus and the jugular bulb. In the anterior and middle portions of the foramen, cranial nerves IX, X, and XI run through a connective tissue septum. The glossopharyngeal nerve lies most anteromedially. In this segment the inferior petrosal sinus also enters the foramen. It usually passes between cranial nerves IX and X, but its relationship to the cranial nerves is highly variable. It may even enter the internal jugular vein below the skull base. A posterior meningeal branch of the ascending pharyngeal artery frequently enters through the jugular foramen.

The hypoglossal canal lies inferior and medial to the jugular foramen. This transmits cranial nerve XII, a meningeal branch of the ascending pharyngeal artery, and the hypoglossal venous plexus. Foramina also exist for the mastoid and condylar emissary veins.

The foramen magnum provides a wide communication between the posterior fossa and the vertebral canal. Through it passes the dura, medulla oblongata, the spinal branches of the accessory nerve, the vertebral arteries, the posterior spinal arteries, and the apical ligament of the dens and membrane tectoria. Around it are attached the atlantooccipital membranes.

Intracranial Contents of the Posterior Fossa

The dura mater of the posterior fossa and tentorium cerebelli encloses the superior petrosal, transverse, occipital, and straight sinuses. The straight sinus is formed by the great cerebral vein of Galen and the inferior sagittal sinus. The midbrain, pons, medulla, and cerebellum lie within the posterior fossa. Thus, all of the exit zones of the lower ten cranial nerves lie in the posterior fossa. Of these, only the oculomotor nerve does not exit through the dura of the posterior cranial fossa. It enters the dura of the middle fossa, in the roof of the cavernous sinus, lateral to the posterior clinoid process. Only cranial nerves VII to XII, however, actually exit the cranium through the posterior fossa. Cranial nerves VII and VIII and the nervus intermedius pass through the porus acusticus, nerves IX, X, and XI through the jugular foramen, and XII exits via the hypoglossal canal.

The main arteries in the posterior fossa originate from the vertebral arteries. These ascend ventral to the roots of cranial nerves IX, X, and XII. They usually give off the posterior inferior cerebellar arteries before joining to form the basilar artery at the lower border of the pons. The basilar artery gives rise to the AICA, which pass to the inferior surface of the cerebellum and come into close relationship with cranial nerves VII and VIII in the cerebellopontine angle. This relationship, and also that of the AICA to the internal auditory meatus, is highly variable, as described by Mazzoni and Hansen, and Kim et al. (14,15). The basilar artery then gives rise to the superior cerebellar arteries and the posterior cerebral arteries, which form the posterior axis of the circle of Willis. Other branches are the pontine and, occasionally, labyrinthine arteries.

Subcranial Relationships of the Posterior Skull Base

Posterolateral Structures

Knowledge of anatomy in this area is important for surgery involving tumors of the cerebellopontine angle and vascular tumors of the temporal bone, or in far lateral approaches to the foramen magnum region.

This region is protected by the mastoid tip and the strong suboccipital musculature. The sternocleidomastoid and the digastric muscles arise from and deep to the mastoid tip, respectively. The occipital artery runs posteriorly deep to the

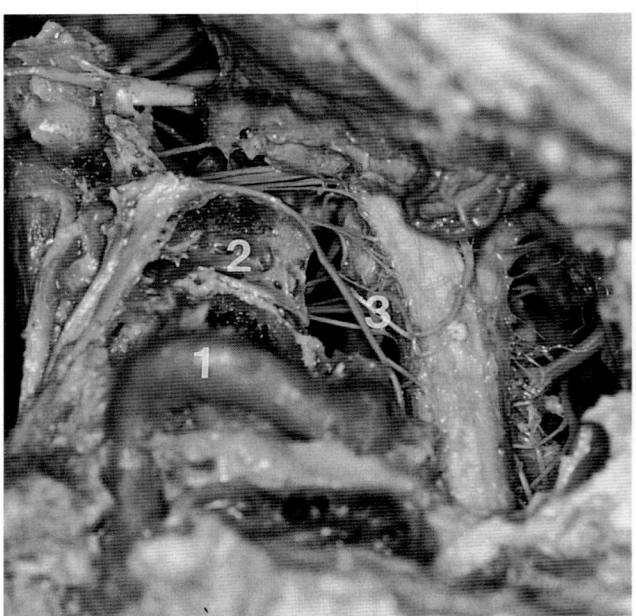

FIG. 21. Dissection of vertebral artery showing relationship to occipital condyle and brainstem. *1*, Vertebral artery; *2*, occipital condyle partly drilled; *3*, spinal root of accessory nerve.

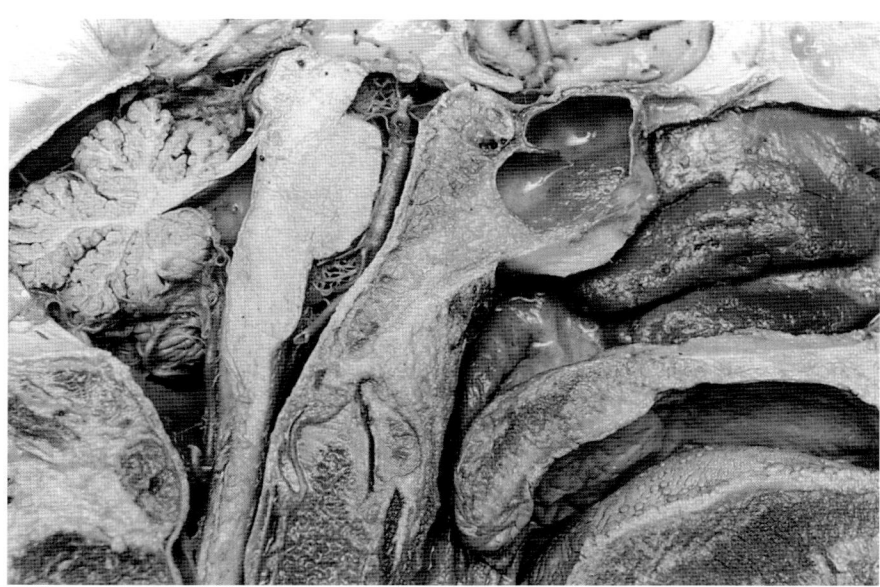

FIG. 22. Sagittal cadaver section showing relationship of clivus to basilar artery and pons.

mastoid tip. The splenius capitis and longissimus capitis lie deep to sternocleidomastoid. Posteriorly in the midline lies the trapezius and deep to this arises the semispinalis capitis. After these muscles are reflected off the superior nuchal line, the all-important suboccipital triangle is exposed. This triangle is bordered by the obliquus capitis superior and inferior and the rectus capitis posterior major. Within the triangle lie the dorsal ramus of the first cervical nerve and the vertebral artery with its venous plexus. The triangle is crossed by the great occipital nerve.

Dissection in this triangle allows mobilization of the vertebral artery and exposure of the occipital condyle, which can be drilled away to gain access to the foramen magnum and anterior brainstem.

Vertebral Artery

The vertebral artery arises from the subclavian artery and has four parts, cervical, foraminal, atlantic, and subarachnoid.

The cervical part runs up and backward between the longus colli and scalenus anterior to reach the transverse foramen of the sixth cervical vertebra.

The foraminal part of the artery ascends through the transverse foramina of the upper six cervical vertebrae, turning upward and laterally to enter the transverse foramen of the atlas. Its branches are to the spinal cord.

The atlantic part of the vertebral artery curves backward and medially behind the lateral mass of the atlas and onto the upper surface of the posterior arch of the atlas (Fig. 21). This portion is accessible through the suboccipital triangle and is surrounded by a plexus of veins. Branches from this part are to the suboccipital muscles. It then enters the subarachnoid space below the posterior atlantooccipital membrane.

The subarachnoid part of the vertebral artery has been considered with the posterior fossa. Branches are meningeal, posterior and anterior spinal, and the posterior inferior cerebellar artery.

Midline Posterior Skull Base

This area has partially been dealt with in the section on the middle fossa. It is important in approaches to the clivus, the basilar invagination of the odontoid process, and vertebrobasilar aneurysms.

The nasopharyngeal area is covered anteriorly by mucous membrane and dense periosteum overlying the clivus and upper cervical spine. Of particular concern are the atlantooccipital and atlantoaxial joints. The anterior arch of the atlas can be removed to expose the odontoid process. Deep to the clivus lies dura and the vertebrobasilar arterial system, with the brainstem immediately posterior (Fig. 22). Dissection too far laterally in the region of the lower clivus and occipital condyle may damage the hypoglossal nerve and, of more concern, the ICA.

REFERENCES

1. Ritter FN. *The paranasal sinuses: anatomy and surgical technique.* St. Louis: CV Mosby, 1978.
2. Neal GO. External ethmoidectomy. *Otolaryngol Clin North Am* 1985;18:55–60.
3. Van Alyea OE. In discussion of operation on the sphenoid. *Transactions of the American Academy of Ophthalmology and Otolaryngology* 1949;53:542–543.

4. Lang J. Structure and postnatal organization of heretofore uninvestigated and infrequent ossifications of the sella turcica region. *Acta Avat* 1977;99:121–139.
5. Lang J. The anterior and middle cranial fossae including the cavernous sinus and orbit. *Surgery of cranial base tumors*. New York: Raven Press, 1993:106–121.
6. Fisch U. Neurectomy of the vestibular nerve: surgical techniques, indications and results obtained in 70 cases. *Rev Laryngol Otol Rhinol (Bord)* 1969;11:661–672.
7. House WF. Surgical exposure of the internal auditory canal and its contents through the middle cranial fossa. *Laryngoscope* 1961;71:1363–1385.
8. Lang J. *Clinical anatomy of the head, neurocranium, orbit and craniocervical regions*. New York: Springer-Verlag New York, 1983.
9. Parkinson D. A surgical approach to the cavernous portion of the carotid artery: anatomical studies and case report. *J Neurosurg* 1965;23:473–482.
10. Pitanguy I, Ramos AS. The frontal branch of the facial nerve: the importance of its variations in face lifting. *Plast Reconstr Surg* 1966;38:352–356.
11. Liebman E, Webster RC, Berger AS, Dellavechia M. The frontalis nerve in the temporal brow lift. *Arch Otolaryngol* 1982;108:232–235.
12. Donald PJ. *Head and neck cancer: management of the difficult case*. Philadelphia: WB Saunders, 1983:284.
13. Hardy J, Maina G. Microsurgical anatomy in transphenoid hypophysectomy. *J Neurol Sci* 1977;21:151–153.
14. Mazzoni A, Hansen CC. Surgical anatomy of the arteries of the internal auditory canal. *Archives of Otolaryngology* 1970;91:128–135.
15. Kim HN, Kin YH, Park IY, Kim GR, Chung IH. Variability of the surgical anatomy of the neurovascular component of the cerebellopontine angle. *Annals of Otology, Rhinology, Laryngology* 1990;99:288–296.

BIBLIOGRAPHY

Hollinshead WH. *Anatomy for surgeons*. Vol 1. *The head and neck*. 3rd ed. Philadelphia: Harper and Row, 1982.
Gray's anatomy. 35th ed. Edinburgh: Langman, 1973.

CHAPTER 3

Pathology of Skull Base Tumors

Regina Gandour-Edwards, Silloo B. Kapadia, and Leon Barnes

INTRODUCTION

Histology

The complex diversity of tissues that interface the skull base contributes to the diagnostic challenge of skull base surgical pathology. Extracranially, the nasal cavity, nasopharynx, and paranasal sinuses are lined by squamous and respiratory mucosa as well as specialized olfactory epithelium. The submucosa includes numerous seromucinous salivary glands, blood and lymphatic vessels, peripheral nerves, and fibrous and adipose tissue. These mucosae and soft tissues are adherent to underlying bone and hyaline cartilage. Intracranially, the pituitary gland occupies a central position with surrounding meninges and intrinsic myelinated and nonmyelinated brain tissues. This extraordinary array of tissues gives rise to numerous pathologic lesions of diverse histologic differentiation.

Immunohistochemistry/Special Methodology

Lesions of the skull base are a challenge for both surgeon and pathologist and include several lesions that have similar or overlapping morphology. Modern pathologic techniques, including immunohistochemistry or electron microscopy, are commonly used for diagnosis. Immunohistochemistry has become a powerful tool for pathologic diagnosis and has proven particularly effective in the classification of the undifferentiated or small cell lesions of the skull base. It is important to appreciate, however, that no one antibody can determine whether a lesion is benign or malignant. Standard pathologic criteria of architecture, nuclear morphology, and mitotic rate remain the essential morphologic features for diagnosis. A general overview of the commonly used antibodies for immunohistochemical diagnosis is provided in Table 1.

The transfer of technology from basic research to clinical application is advancing rapidly. Molecular probes, including both *in situ* hybridization and polymerase chain reaction methodology, are being used, for example, in the study of Epstein-Barr virus in nasopharyngeal carcinoma (NPC). Current and future studies will use techniques such as DNA ploidy analysis and probes for biologic markers, including tumor suppressor genes, oncogenes, proliferation markers, and other, as yet unidentified entities.

To optimize diagnosis and patient care, it is essential that the surgeon and pathologist maintain a dialogue of mutual respect and vigilant communication. A preoperative or prebiopsy consultation with the pathologist ensures that the tissue is properly allocated and processed for special studies if indicated. Individual pathology laboratories have preferred media and fixatives for immunohistology, electron microscopy, flow cytometry, and so forth. Provision of the pertinent clinical history and precise anatomic location is mandatory.

Frozen-Section Diagnosis

Frozen-section diagnosis is uniquely challenging in skull base surgery. Frozen sections are sought for two general reasons, diagnosis or control of resection margins. Intraoperative frozen section is *not* the optimum technique for definitive initial diagnosis of an unknown process because of the potential for sampling error or interpretive error due to freezing artifact. An intraoperative consultation including frozen section or touch preparations may be indicated to ensure that adequate, representative tissue has been obtained for the diagnostic work-up.

To prevent intraoperative frozen-section discrepancies, we recommend thorough sampling and technically adequate sections (1). The pathologist, surgeon, and patient should

---

R. Gandour-Edwards, S.B. Kapadia: Department of Pathology, University of California, Davis Medical Center, Sacramento, California 95817.
L. Barnes: Department of Pathology, University of Pittsburgh, Pittsburgh, Pennsylvania 15213.

TABLE 1. *Common antibodies used in skull base pathology*

Antibody	Target tissues
Cytokeratins	Epithelial tissues (e.g., squamous and glandular mucosa, carcinomas)
Epithelial membrane antigen	Epithelial tissues, glands, poorly differentiated carcinomas
Vimentin	Mesenchymal tissues (e.g., connective tissue, muscle, sarcomas)
Human muscle actin	Smooth/skeletal muscle, rhabdomyosarcoma, leiomyoma
Leukocyte common antigen	Lymphocytes, plasma cells
L26	B-cell lymphocytes, B-cell lymphoma
UCHL-1	T-cell lymphocytes, T-cell lymphoma
S-100	Neural crest tissues (e.g., melanoma, olfactory neuroblastoma)
HMB 45	Melanoma
Chromogranin A	Neurosecretory granules (e.g., olfactory neuroblastoma)
CD68	Macrophages, histiocytes; malignant fibrous histiocytoma
Factor VIII, CD 31, *Ulex europaeus*	Endothelial cells (e.g., hemangioma, angiofibroma)
Synaptophysin	Major integral membrane protein of synaptic vesicles; paraganglioma, olfactory neuroblastoma
013	Ewing's sarcoma

also realize that, infrequently, a definitive diagnosis cannot be rendered and a deferral of diagnosis may be the most prudent interpretation.

EPITHELIAL TUMORS

Squamous Cell Carcinoma

Definition. Squamous cell carcinoma is a malignant tumor derived from squamous epithelia such as epidermis and the squamous mucosal lining of the upper respiratory tract. It is characterized by a disorganized, invasive growth of large epithelial cells with intercellular bridges and cytoplasmic keratin.

Clinical Features. Squamous cell carcinoma is the most common malignancy of the head and neck. Skull base involvement by squamous cell carcinoma has been reported from the sinonasal tract, oropharynx, and hypopharynx and from the skin of the scalp and external auditory canal (2–4). Squamous carcinoma can directly invade soft tissue and bone (as well as spread through lymphatic channels and by perineural extension through skull base foramina (Table 2).

Histopathology. Squamous cell carcinoma is graded into well, moderate, and poorly differentiated types by the degree of resemblance to normal squamous tissue. Specific criteria include definition of intercellular bridges, amount of keratinization, nuclear pleomorphism, mitotic rate, and degree of cell cohesion (sheets vs. small nests). Tumors that involve the skull base are typically moderately or poorly differentiated (Figs. 1–3).

Differential Diagnosis. Melanoma, a tumor noted for its protean manifestations, may present a pattern consisting of

TABLE 2. *Squamous cell carcinoma of the skull base: analysis of 21 consecutive cases from the Center for Skull Base Surgery, University of California, Davis Medical Center, 1990 to 1994*

Age/sex	Grade	Primary site	Skull base	Neural invasion
55/M	Moderate	Hypopharynx	Middle fossa	Yes
61/M	Poor	Auricle	Middle fossa	No
61/M	Moderate	Scalp	Occiput	Yes
65/F	Moderate	Frontal sinus	Anterior fossa	No
65/F	Moderate	External ear canal	Temporal bone	Yes
77/F	Moderate	External ear canal	Temporal bone	Yes
58/M	Moderate	Tonsilar fossa	Middle fossa	Yes
47/F	Moderate	External ear canal	Temporal bone	No
63/F	Poor	Tonsilar fossa	Temporal fossa	Yes
44/F	Moderate	Maxilla	Infratemporal fossa	No
57/M	Poor	Maxilla	Infratemporal fossa	Yes
63/F	Poor	Retromolar trigone	Infratemporal fossa	Yes
60/M	Moderate	Maxilla	Middle fossa	No
69/M	Poor	Frontal sinus	Middle fossa	Yes
72/M	Moderate	Oropharynx	Infratemporal fossa	No
53/M	Moderate	Auricle	Temporal bone	Yes
44/M	Poor	External ear canal	Temporal bone	No
60/M	Poor	Skin of face	Infratemporal fossa	Yes
51/M	Moderate	Ethmoid sinus	Middle fossa	No
62/M	Poor	Oropharynx	Middle fossa	No
44/M	Poor	Hypopharynx	Infratemporal fossa	Yes

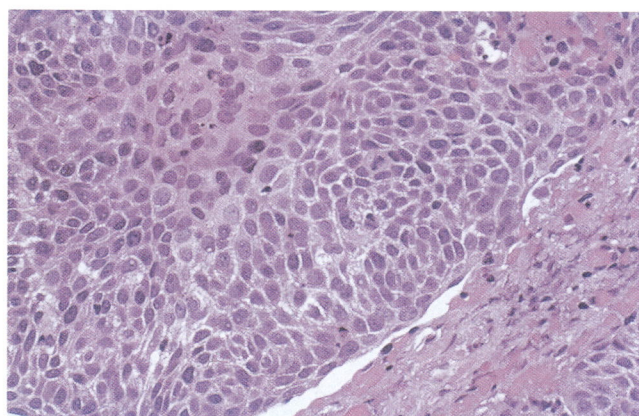

FIG. 1. Moderately differentiated squamous cell carcinoma. Cohesive nests of plump, polygonal cells are adjoined by intracellular bridges. Keratinization is not present in this section. (Hematoxylin and eosin, original magnification 400×.)

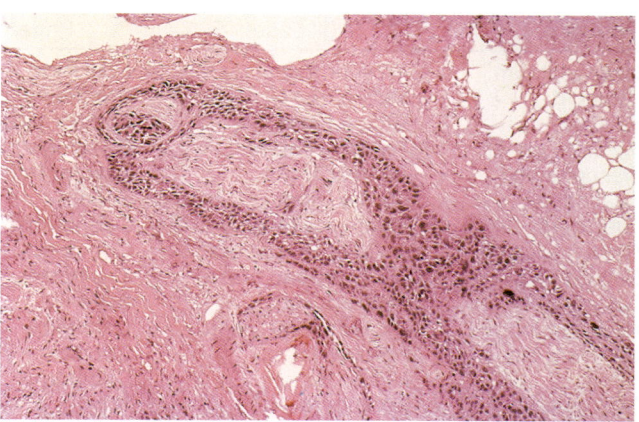

FIG. 3. Squamous cell carcinoma involving cranial nerve V at the supraorbital fissure. (Hematoxylin and eosin, original magnification 40×.)

sheets of plump, polygonal cells with abundant pink cytoplasm. Melanoma may be distinguished from squamous carcinoma by the absence of intercellular bridges. Less reliable features include the characteristic nuclear inclusions of melanoma and variably present cytoplasmic brown pigmentation. Immunohistochemistry is usually definitive in distinguishing these entities, with squamous cell carcinoma reactive to cytokeratin and melanoma reactive to S-100 and HMB-45. Benign reactive conditions that can mimic invasive squamous carcinoma include the squamous metaplasia and atypia of minor salivary ducts that can result from radiation therapy or necrotizing sialometaplasia.

Adenoid Cystic Carcinoma

Definition. Adenoid cystic carcinoma, a tumor of salivary origin, is composed of small, basal duct lining cells and myoepithelial cells arranged in a characteristic cribriform pattern.

Clinical Features. Adenoid cystic carcinoma is the most common malignant tumor of minor salivary glands and may occur in the sinuses and oral cavity as well as in major salivary glands. The disease is characterized by slow but relentless progression over years, with occasional late (after 10–15 years) recurrences and distant metastases. Adenoid cystic carcinoma characteristically spreads along perineural spaces, including those of the maxillary division of the trigeminal nerve, and may traverse the foramen ovale to the gasserian ganglion. Lymphatic spread is low (i.e., 13–16%); however, hematogenous metastasis is high (40%), with lung and bone representing the most common sites of distant spread (5). In our series of 18 adenoid cystic carcinomas, the tumors most commonly originated in the maxillary sinus and demonstrated a predilection for invasion of the middle cranial fossa (6) (Table 3).

Histopathology. Histologically, three patterns have been described: tubular, solid, and cribriform, and tumors are classified by which pattern dominates. The cribriform type is the most common and is considered the "classic" pattern. Nests of cells demonstrate multiple circular spaces filled with bluish, mucinous material or pink, hyalinized material (Fig. 4). The tubular–trabecular pattern consists of cells arranged in individual ducts or tubules, whereas the solid pattern, as expected from the name, has nests or sheets of basaloid cells with little cystic formation (Fig. 5).

Perzin et al. (7) found a correlation between these histologic patterns and survival rates as follows: tubular, 8 years; cribriform, 9 years; and solid, 5 years. Recurrence rates were tubular, 59%; cribriform, 89%; and solid, 100%. Neural invasion, in both perineural and intraneural patterns, is frequently observed and considered a diagnostic feature (Figs. 6, 7).

Differential Diagnosis. Polymorphous low-grade adenocarcinoma has a mixture of cuboidal and columnar cells with open vesicular chromatin and small nucleoli. A mixture of

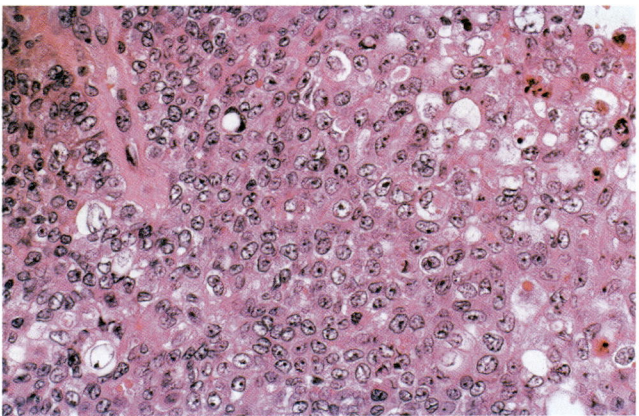

FIG. 2. Poorly differentiated squamous cell carcinoma. The tumor cells have markedly pleomorphic, vesicular nuclei with prominent nucleoli. Intracellular bridges are seen focally and no keratinization is present. (Hematoxylin and eosin, original magnification 400×.)

TABLE 3. *Adenoid cystic carcinoma involving the skull base: combined University of Pittsburgh, University of California, Davis, 1988 to 1993*

Primary	Skull base	Pattern	Neural involvement	Follow-up
Nasal septum	Anterior fossa	Cribriform	Yes	No evidence of disease
Ethmoid	Middle fossa	Cribriform	Yes	Died of metastatic disease
Ethmoid	Middle fossa	Tubular trabecular	Yes	No evidence of disease
Auditory canal	Temporal bone	Cribriform	Yes	Died of other causes
Nasopharynx	Anterior fossa	Tubular trabecular	Not observed	No evidence of disease
Oral cavity	Middle fossa	Solid	Yes	Died of disease
Oral cavity	Middle fossa	Cribriform	Yes	Died of other causes
Nasal septum	Anterior fossa	Cribriform	Not observed	No evidence of disease
Left parotid	Infratemporal fossa	Cribriform	Yes	Died of metastatic disease
Nasal cavity	Middle fossa	Solid	Yes	No evidence of disease
Maxillary sinus	Infratemporal fossa	Cribriform	Yes	Died of metastatic disease
Maxillary sinus	Anterior fossa	Cribriform	Yes	Unknown
Ethmoid	Middle fossa	Cribriform	Yes	No evidence of disease
Nasopharynx	Anterior fossa	Solid	Yes	Died of metastatic disease
Maxillary sinus	Temporal bone	Cribriform	Yes	Died of metastatic disease
Oral cavity	Infratemporal fossa	Tubular trabecular	Yes	Died of disease
Maxillary sinus	Anterior fossa	Cribriform	Not observed	Died of disease
Maxillary sinus	Middle fossa	Tubular trabecular	Yes	Unknown

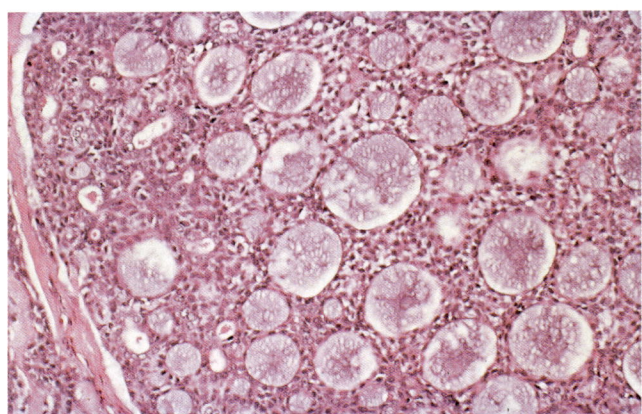

FIG. 4. Adenoid cystic carcinoma, classic cribriform pattern. The tumor cells are small, uniform, and basaloid with dense nuclei and no mitoses. Bluish mucin material fills the multiple small lumina. (Hematoxylin and eosin, original magnification 200×.)

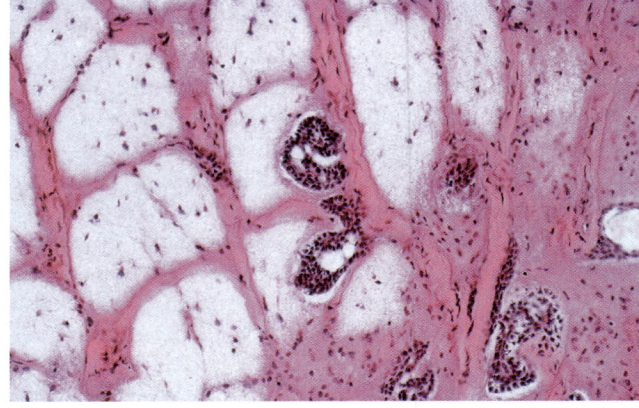

FIG. 6. Adenoid cystic carcinoma involving the optic nerve. Cribriform nests of tumor are present in perineural and intraneural invasive patterns. (Hematoxylin and eosin, original magnification 200×.)

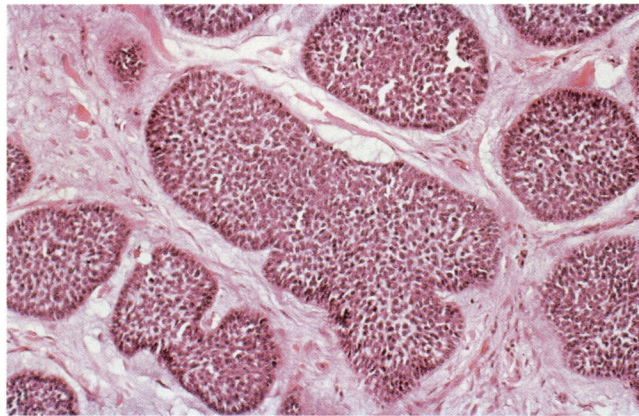

FIG. 5. Adenoid cystic carcinoma, solid pattern. The basaloid cells are present as solid nests with a peripheral palisading pattern. This pattern has been associated with a poorer prognosis. (Hematoxylin and eosin, original magnification 200×.)

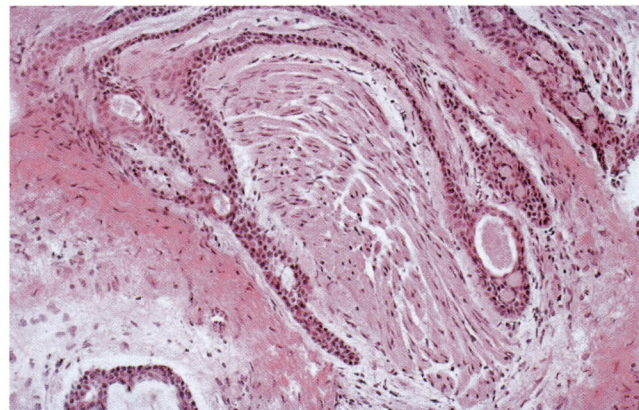

FIG. 7. Adenoid cystic carcinoma with perineural invasion of cranial nerve III. (Hematoxylin and eosin, original magnification 200×.)

patterns, including single-layer tubules, cribriform, tubular, trabecular, solid, papillary, and solitary cell "Indian file" types, is seen. Basal cell adenoma is an encapsulated benign growth of solid masses of basaloid cells with peripheral nuclear palisading. Mitoses usually are absent and no infiltrative pattern or neural involvement is seen.

Nasopharyngeal Carcinoma

Definition. Nasopharyngeal carcinoma (NPC) is a malignant tumor derived from the surface epithelium of the nasopharynx. It has a strong association with the Epstein-Barr virus and a worldwide distribution, but it is especially common among residents of Southeast Asia.

Clinical Features. Nasopharyngeal carcinoma occurs in all age groups (average, 45–50 years) and is more common in men by a ratio of 3 to 1 (8,9). It arises primarily on the lateral wall of the nasopharynx in the region of Rosenmüller's fossa and usually presents as serous otitis media, nasal obstruction, or epistaxis, or with asymptomatic enlargement of the cervical lymph nodes, especially those in the apex of the posterior cervical triangle (8–10).

Prognosis is related to clinical stage and histologic type. The best prognosis is associated with the undifferentiated type (60% 5-year survival) and the worse with the squamous cell variant (20% 5-year survival) (11).

Histopathology. In 1978, the World Health Organization proposed that NPC be divided into three types: squamous cell carcinoma, nonkeratinizing carcinoma, and undifferentiated carcinoma (12). In 1991, the classification was slightly modified (13) (Table 4).

The term "squamous cell carcinoma" is used for any NPC that shows evidence of squamous differentiation (e.g., intercellular bridges, keratinization), whereas "differentiated nonkeratinizing carcinoma" exhibits no evidence of keratin formation and resembles, for all practical purposes, transitional cell carcinoma of the urinary tract.

Undifferentiated carcinoma, previously known as lymphoepithelioma, is composed of cells with large vesicular nuclei, prominent nucleoli, and amphophilic cytoplasm (Fig. 8). It is also characteristically associated with a prominent component of lymphocytes.

Based on their appearance under the electron microscope, it is apparent that all of the aforementioned types of NPC are actually variants of squamous cell carcinoma. Those tumors

TABLE 4. *Classification of nasopharyngeal carcinoma*

World Health Organization (1978)
1. Squamous cell carcinoma
2. Nonkeratinizing carcinoma
3. Undifferentiated carcinoma

World Health Organization (1991)
1. Squamous cell carcinoma
2. Nonkeratinizing carcinoma
   A. Differentiated nonkeratinizing carcinoma
   B. Undifferentiated carcinoma

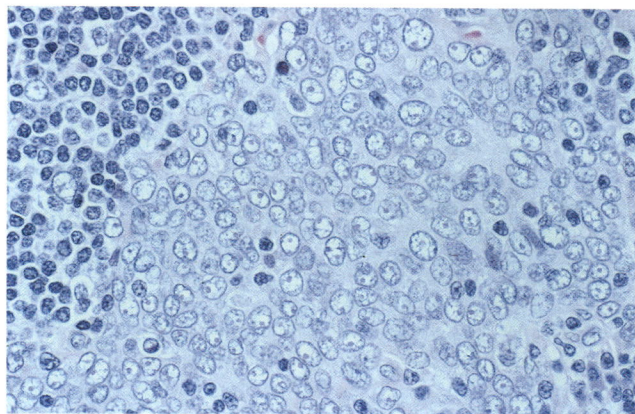

FIG. 8. Nasopharyngeal carcinoma, undifferentiated type. Note central aggregate of pale-staining cells with large, round, vesicular (clear) nuclei; prominent nucleoli; and amphophilic, poorly defined cytoplasm. A prominent component of lymphocytes is apparent in the background. (Hematoxylin and eosin, original magnification 400×.)

that show keratinization (squamous cell carcinoma), however, have the worst prognosis and are rarely associated with Epstein-Barr virus.

Differential Diagnosis. Nasopharyngeal carcinoma must be distinguished from malignant lymphoma. This is easily accomplished with the use of immunohistochemistry. NPC is positive for cytokeratin (Fig. 9) and negative for leukocyte common antigen, whereas lymphomas are positive for the latter and negative for cytokeratin.

Pituitary Adenoma

Definition. Most pituitary tumors are benign epithelial tumors or adenomas of the anterior lobe (8,14–16). Pituitary adenomas comprise 10% of all intracranial tumors. Small islands of primitive anterior lobe tissue may be sequestered

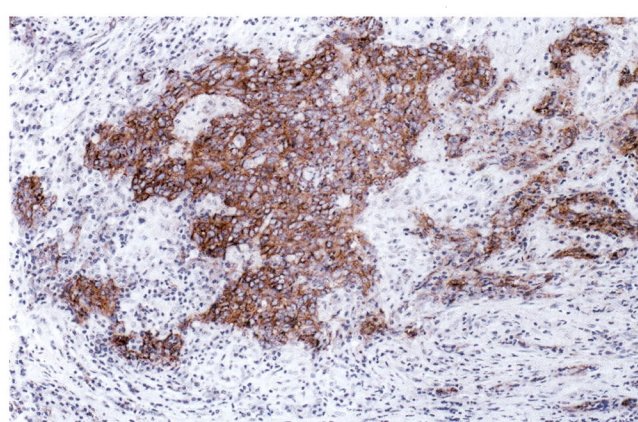

FIG. 9. Nasopharyngeal carcinoma, undifferentiated type. The tumor cells react strongly with cytokeratin, whereas background lymphocytes are nonreactive. (Immunoperoxidase stain, original magnification 100×.)

during migration and persist into adult life, where they may be found in the sphenoid bone, sella turcica outside the pituitary capsule, or nasopharynx (pharyngeal pituitary). Rarely, these remnants may give rise to true ectopic pituitary adenomas.

Clinical Features. Approximately 20% to 40% of pituitary adenomas are nonfunctioning (nonsecretory); the remainder are hormone producing. The functional status can be clinically assessed by hormonal assays. Nonfunctioning adenomas are often large and may grow beyond the confines of the sella, compressing the adjacent structures. Rarely, adenomas may invade the pituitary capsule and extend through the bone of the sella to involve the cavernous sinuses, sphenoid sinus, nasopharynx, or nasal cavity (invasive pituitary adenomas) (17). In biologic behavior, they rank between intrasellar adenomas and pituitary carcinoma. However, local invasion is insufficient to designate a pituitary tumor as carcinoma, the latter being defined by the presence of metastasis.

Histopathology. Pituitary adenomas may demonstrate a variety of growth patterns, including diffuse, papillary, festoon, or pleomorphic patterns (14–15). These patterns have no prognostic significance but are important in the differential diagnosis. Tumor cells may be eosinophilic, basophilic, or chromophobic, with round to oval nuclei and at times prominent nucleoli (Figs. 10, 11). There are no major histologic differences between invasive and noninvasive adenomas; hence, no conclusion regarding biologic behavior of pituitary adenomas can be drawn on the basis of histologic appearance alone. Invasive adenomas often may be cellular or pleomorphic or have more abundant mitoses (8,17).

The ultrastructural demonstration of neurosecretory granules or the immunophenotypic expression of neuroendocrine markers (neuron-specific enolase, synaptophysin, chromogranin) or pituitary hormonal markers may be essential for diagnosis. Nonfunctioning adenomas show no reactivity for pituitary hormones, but do show reactivity for neuroendocrine markers such as chromogranin, and neu-

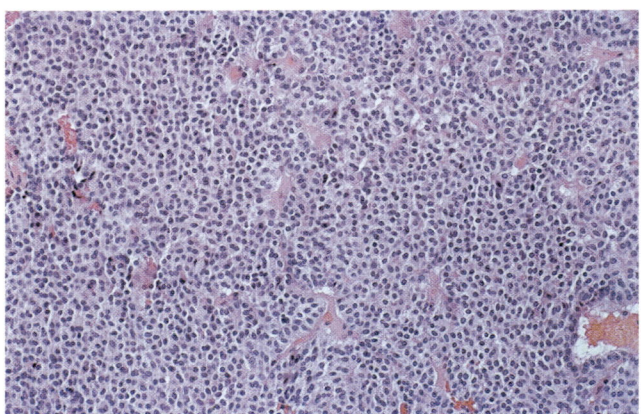

FIG. 10. Pituitary adenoma. The tumor is composed of sheets of uniform, round cells. (Hematoxylin and eosin, original magnification 200×.)

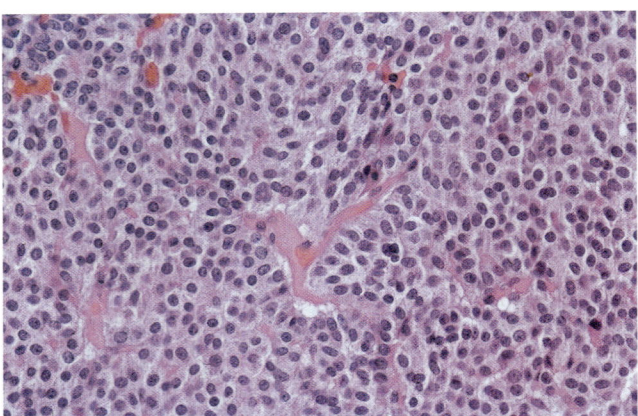

FIG. 11. Pituitary adenoma. Higher magnification shows uniform neoplastic cells with round nuclei and clear cytoplasm. (Hematoxylin and eosin, original magnification 400×.)

rosecretory granules are seen ultrastructurally. The estimated rate of gross invasion by pituitary adenomas of all types is 35% (17).

Differential Diagnosis. In addition to the histologic features, the demonstration of secretory products by electron microscopy or immunohistochemistry helps distinguish pituitary adenoma from other tumors at this site, such as chordoma, plasmacytoma, lymphoma, meningioma, carcinomas, or sarcomas of the skull base.

Histologic features are not reliable predictors of pituitary tumor recurrences or invasiveness. In a study using antibodies to PCNA and Ki-67, Gandour-Edwards et al. reported that compared with normal pituitary glands, the proliferative index of intrasellar and invasive pituitary adenomas was increased. However, these proliferation markers did not distinguish between invasive and noninvasive variants of pituitary adenoma (18).

MESENCHYMAL TUMORS

Inflammatory Pseudotumor

Definition. Inflammatory pseudotumor is a nonneoplastic, reactive chronic inflammation that presents as a mass lesion. It is a somewhat controversial entity that has been reported with a wide variety of histologic features and unpredictable behavior. The pulmonary lesion has been best characterized as a benign, nonneoplastic tumefaction. Reported inflammatory "pseudotumors" at other sites have on occasion, however, demonstrated recurrence and cytogenetic evidence supporting a neoplastic rather than inflammatory etiology, and have been better termed "inflammatory myofibroblastic tumors." The term "inflammatory pseudotumor" therefore should be used with caution and restricted to nonneoplastic lesions (19).

Clinical Features. True inflammatory pseudotumors are nonneoplastic lesions that occur most commonly in the lung.

Pseudotumors of the skull base occur most often as an extension of orbital disease. Primary lesions involving the clivus, sphenoid sinuses, infratemporal fossa, and temporal bone have also been reported. The lesions have a propensity to behave aggressively and frequently demonstrate bony erosion and cranial neuropathy (20).

Histopathology. Inflammatory pseudotumors are characterized by uniform, widely spaced fibroblasts with variable, dense collagen and small, uniform vessels with a mixed infiltrate of small lymphocytes, histiocytes, and plasma cells. Surrounding bone may exhibit erosion characterized by irregular islands of bone with osteoblastic and osteoclastic rimming. The density of the inflammatory infiltrate and of the collagen deposition is variable, with fewer inflammatory cells and increased fibrosis as the lesion ages (Fig. 12).

Differential Diagnosis. Inflammatory myofibroblastic tumors are distinguished by a cellular mixture of fibroblasts and myofibroblasts arranged in whorls and fascicles. A variable infiltrate of inflammatory cells is present, especially at the periphery, and mitoses are rare. Malignant fibrous histiocytoma is a densely cellular sarcoma with haphazard bundles of pleomorphic spindle cells and multinucleated giant cells. The mitotic rate is high and necrosis is common. Lymphoma is a cellular, monomorphic infiltrate of atypical lymphoid cells with a clonal pattern of reactivity on immunohistochemistry.

Fibrous Dysplasia

Definition. Fibrous dysplasia is a benign, fibroosseous process of bone that results in the replacement of normal bone with fibrous connective tissue and structurally weak fibrillar bone.

Clinical Features. Fibrous dysplasia may be monostotic (one bone) or polyostotic (several bones) and frequently involves the craniofacial complex. It is a self-limited process that starts in childhood, but because of slow growth may not

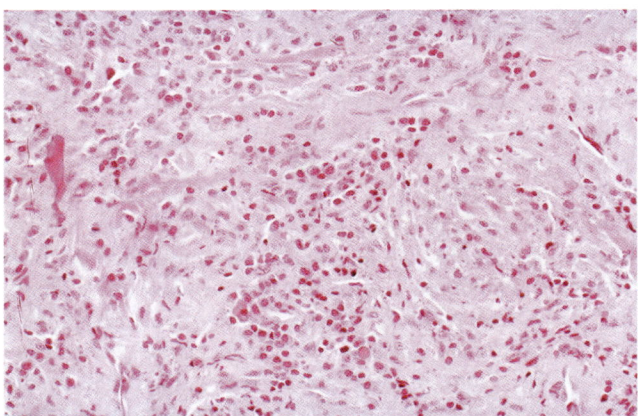

FIG. 12. Inflammatory pseudotumor. This clival lesion consisted of fibroblasts, myofibroblasts, and scattered lymphocytes, macrophages, and plasma cells. (Hematoxylin and eosin, original magnification 200×.)

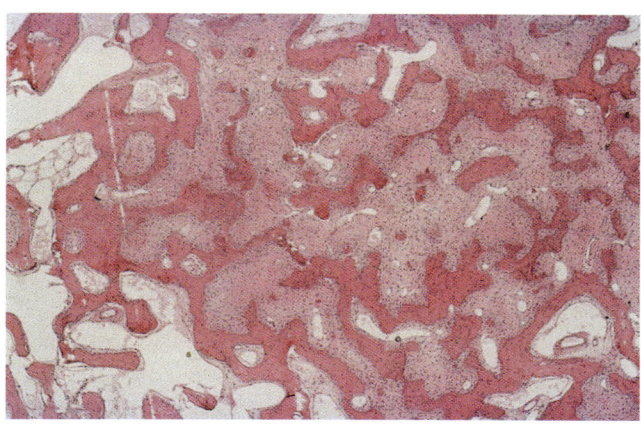

FIG. 13. Fibrous dysplasia. This low-power view illustrates the multiple irregular bony islands, forming "C"- and "Y"-shaped fragments in a fibrous stroma. (Hematoxylin and eosin, original magnification 40×.)

cause symptoms until adulthood. Albright's syndrome consists of polyostotic fibrous dysplasia, pigmented skin macules, and endocrine abnormalities, typically precocious puberty (21,22).

In the craniofacial area, fibrous dysplasia occurs most commonly in the calvarium and maxilla. Involvement of the skull base, orbits, sinuses, and cranial ostia has been well documented, however, and can result in significant morbidity (23). Monostotic fibrous dysplasia of the temporal bone may lead to cholesteatoma (24). Malignant transformation of fibrous dysplasia to osteosarcoma has been reported, particularly after radiation therapy (25).

Histopathology. Fibrous dysplasia consists of multiple, irregular, immature fibrillar or woven bony trabeculae surrounded by loose, uniform fibroblastic spindle cells. The trabeculae often have "C" or "Y" shapes and have been described as "Chinese characters." Osteoclasts are rarely observed and osteoblasts are seen infrequently (Figs. 13, 14).

The fibrous stroma is characterized by a lack of pleomorphism and mitotic figures.

Differential Diagnosis. Ossifying or cementoossifying fibroma is a neoplastic lesion with uniform trabeculae or oval islands of new bone or cementum sharply separated from the surrounding fibrous tissue. Prominent osteoblasts rim these bony formations, although osteoclasts are scant. Some believe that fibrous dysplasia and ossifying fibroma represent a histologic spectrum of similar or closely related lesions (26). Chronic osteomyelitis has irregular bony islands that blend into the adjacent bone. Osteoblastic and osteoclastic rimming is present as well as scattered inflammatory cells and areas of necrosis. Osteosarcoma is characterized by large cells with hyperchromatic, irregular nuclei and immature, randomly distributed osteoid.

Angiofibroma

Definition. Angiofibromas (AF) are histologically benign vascular tumors that have a propensity for local aggressive

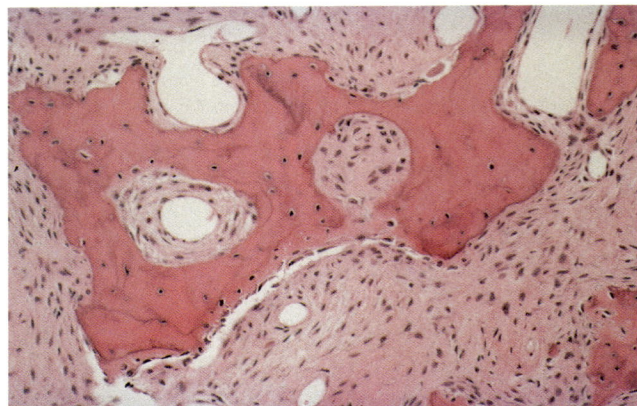

FIG. 14. Fibrous dysplasia. The higher-power view illustrates one irregular bony island with scant osteoblastic rimming. The stroma is composed of benign, moderately cellular fibroblasts. (Hematoxylin and eosin, original magnification 200×.)

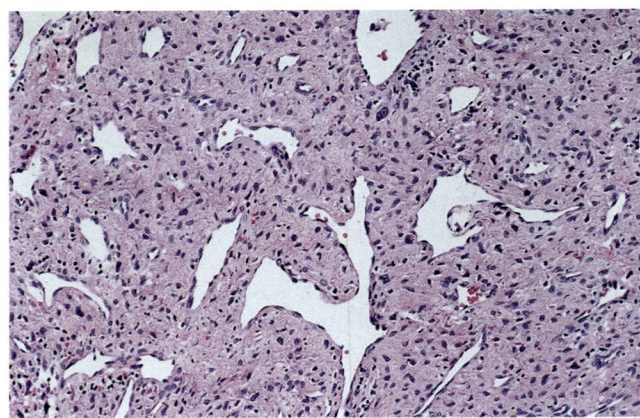

FIG. 16. Angiofibroma. Note the characteristic "staghorn"-shaped vascular channels and collagenous stroma containing stellate cells. (Hematoxylin and eosin, original magnification 400×.)

behavior and occur almost exclusively in male patients (8,27,28).

Clinical Features. Angiofibroma typically occur in male adolescents between 10 and 17 years of age (range, 1–60 years) (8). Their occurrence in women is questionable. They are rare tumors, estimated to comprise 0.5% of all head and neck neoplasms. The site of origin is the posterolateral nasal wall in the region of the sphenopalatine foramen. Initial manifestations include nasopharyngeal or nasal mass causing nasal obstruction and recurrent epistaxis. At diagnosis, approximately two thirds of patients have localized disease, and 20% have intracranial involvement (28). About 10% of AF recur after surgical resection. AF has no malignant potential. Rare sarcomatous transformation has been reported after massive doses of radiation.

Histopathology. On gross examination, AF are firm, rubbery, smooth, and coarsely nodular. The cut surface may show a spongy to firm, red-brown or gray-tan appearance. Histologically, AF is composed of vascular and stromal elements (Figs. 15, 16). The tumor is nonencapsulated. Interspersed in the fibrous stroma are slitlike or gaping vascular channels ("staghorn" shaped) of varying size, lined by a single layer of endothelial cells (15,16). The collagenous matrix contains round or stellate nuclei, the latter superficially resembling neurons. A fascia-like appearance to the stroma is imparted by the parallel arrangement of collagen fibers. Reactive stromal cells with nuclear hyperchromatism, binucleation, and occasional mitoses may be seen and should not be mistaken for malignant criteria. Inflammatory and mucoserous glands are rare or absent.

Ultrastructurally, round, electron-dense granules are found in the stromal cell nuclei and represent tightly bound RNA–protein complexes (29). Immunohistologic studies suggest that AF are composed of myofibroblastic and vascular elements. Stromal cells invariably express vimentin and, at times, muscle-specific antigen, but are negative for endothelial markers (factor VII-related antigen and *Ulex europaeus*) (27,30). Hormone receptor studies have shown the presence of androgen receptor proteins in stromal cells and some endothelial cells (31). Most AF are negative for estrogen receptors.

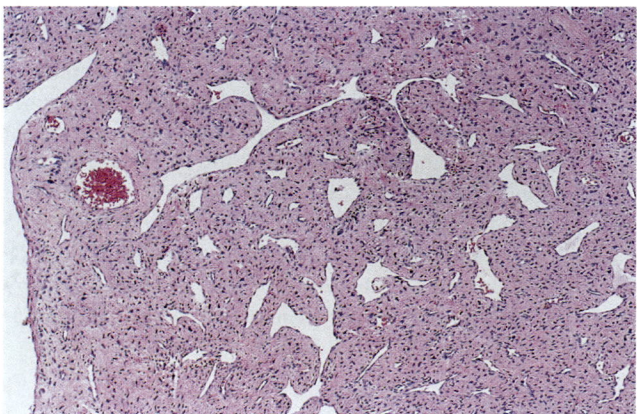

FIG. 15. Angiofibroma. Both the vascular and stromal components are illustrated. (Hematoxylin and eosin, original magnification 200×.)

Differential Diagnosis. Angiofibroma should be distinguished histologically from richly vascular, fibrosed inflammatory nasal polyps, lobular capillary hemangioma (so-called "pyogenic granuloma"), and sinonasal hemangiopericytoma (27). These lesions have a distinctive histologic appearance and lack the typical vascular channels and stromal characteristics of AF. Fibrosed nasal polyps are distinguished by the presence of prominent stromal edema, thickened epithelial basement membrane, eosinophils, and mucoserous glands. Pyogenic granuloma typically shows a lobular proliferation of capillaries and endothelial cells. Sinonasal hemangiopericytoma is characterized by round to short spindle cells intimately related to irregular vascular channels and a reticulin network surrounding individual tumor cells, as seen on special stains.

It is not possible to predict which of the AF will have a biologically aggressive local behavior on the basis of clinical or pathologic features. To determine if DNA ploidy can be used to predict tumor behavior, Barnes et al. studied 31 AF by flow cytometry (28). However, all of the tumors were DNA diploid, including those with recurrences or intracranial extension, suggesting that DNA ploidy is not useful in predicting local aggressiveness.

Meningioma

Definition. Meningiomas are generally benign tumors that arise from meningocytes of arachnoid granulations (8,32–34) They comprise approximately 15% of all intracranial tumors and 25% of intraspinal neoplasms.

Clinical Features. The mean age of patients is 45 years, with a female predominance (2–4:1). Meningiomas commonly occur in the parasagittal area along the dural sinuses, lateral cerebral convexities, sphenoid ridge, and areas of dural penetration by cranial nerves. Most develop within the neuraxis, but in 20% of cases extracranial extension may occur into the calvarium, skull base, orbit, middle ear, sinonasal passage, or parapharyngeal space. Extracranial meningiomas usually represent extension of a primary intracranial tumor, but occasionally they may originate from arachnoidal cells within the trunk or perineural sheath of cranial nerves near a neural foramen (35). Meningiomas are slow-growing tumors that compress rather than invade neural tissue. They may recur in 10% of cases, often within 5 years of therapy, because of incomplete excision or intrinsic biologic aggressiveness. When meningiomas occur in patients younger than 30 years of age or when they are multiple, the possibility of neurofibromatosis is raised.

Histopathology. Meningiomas are usually solitary, well demarcated, firm, gray-tan, smooth or lobulated tumors. They show a histologic diversity with four basic growth patterns: (a) syncytial (meningothelial), composed of whorls of meningothelial cells displaying round to oval nuclei containing rare intranuclear cytoplasmic inclusions, and pale pink cytoplasm with indistinct cell borders (Figs. 17, 18); (b) fibroblastic, showing interwoven fascicles of spindle-shaped cells and collagen fibers; (c) transitional, having features of both of the preceding types; and (d) "angioblastic," now considered to be a meningeal hemangiopericytoma (8,32–33). Psammoma bodies and a whorled pattern are seen in all types. These histologic patterns have no prognostic significance. Mitoses are rare or absent. In meningiomas, the presence of mitoses and local invasion of dura, bone, or extracranial soft tissue does not necessarily indicate malignancy; only the presence of metastasis is sufficient evidence of malignant behavior (32).

Differential Diagnosis. The histologic diversity of meningioma can present problems in differentiating it from

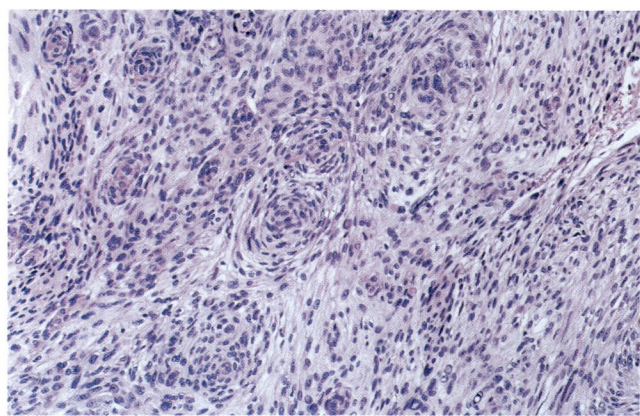

FIG. 17. Meningioma. The tumor is composed of spindle-shaped and whorled meningothelial cells. (Hematoxylin and eosin, original magnification 200×.)

other tumors, namely, schwannoma, hemangiopericytoma, paraganglioma, and metastatic carcinoma (8,32–34). Immunohistochemically, meningiomas exhibit a dual epithelial and mesenchymal differentiation with positivity for epithelial membrane antigen and vimentin, and in a lesser proportion of cases, for keratin and S-100 protein (34). Tumors cells are negative for desmin, neurofilament, synaptophysin, chromogranin, and glial fibrillary acidic protein. Progesterone receptors have been demonstrated in a high proportion of meningiomas.

The biologic behavior of meningioma is not always predictable from its histologic appearance. Although the presence of necrosis, brain invasion, or mitoses may indicate aggressive behavior, not all meningiomas that recur or metastasize have these features, and it is difficult to predict which of the tumors will behave aggressively. Cytogenetic studies have shown that loss of chromosome 22 (monosomy 22) represents the most common chromosomal abnormality (50–70%). In the remaining 30% of cases there is a normal

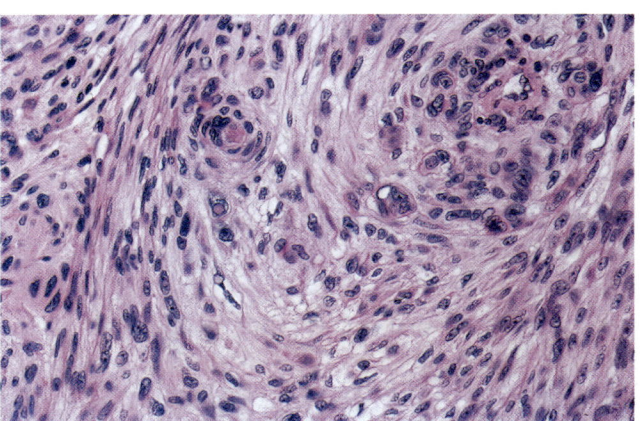

FIG. 18. Meningioma. Note the fibroblastic and whorled pattern of neoplastic cells with scattered intranuclear cytoplasmic inclusions. (Hematoxylin and eosin, original magnification 400×.)

karyotype (36). Structural changes of chromosome 1, along with numeric changes, may indicate aggressive tumor behavior. Studies have suggested that the proliferating fraction, using DNA content by digital cell image analysis and immunohistochemical staining for the proliferating cell nuclear antigen (PCNA) or Ki-67 nuclear antigen, may be useful in predicting biologic aggressiveness of the tumor (37).

Olfactory Neuroblastoma

Definition. Olfactory neuroblastoma is an uncommon neuroectodermal tumor that arises from the nasal olfactory epithelium. As such, it characteristically arises high in the nasal cavity and is attached to the cribriform plate.

Clinical Features. Olfactory neuroblastoma affects both sexes equally and occurs in all age groups (median, 40–50 years) (38,39). On physical examination, it presents as a unilateral red-gray or tan, polypoid growth attached high in the nasal cavity. Nasal obstruction and epistaxis are the most common symptoms. Others include anosmia, pain, proptosis, and visual disturbances. The tumor may remain confined to the nasal cavity, but with neglect, often extends secondarily into adjacent paranasal sinuses, orbits, or base of the skull.

Metastasis to cervical lymph nodes occurs in 10% to 30% of patients during the course of the disease and systemic metastasis (lung and bone) in 8% to 46% of cases (38–41). Local recurrences after initial therapy eventually develop in 30% to 40% of patients (38–40). Five- and 10-year survival rates of 70% to 80% and 60% to 70%, respectively, have been reported (38,39).

Histopathology. Microscopically, olfactory neuroblastomas are composed of small, round cells slightly larger than lymphocytes that grow in a lobular or diffuse pattern, or a combination of both. The nuclei are hyperchromatic with a uniform chromatin distribution (Figs. 19, 20). Nucleoli are inconspicuous, cytoplasm is sparse, and mitoses are rare.

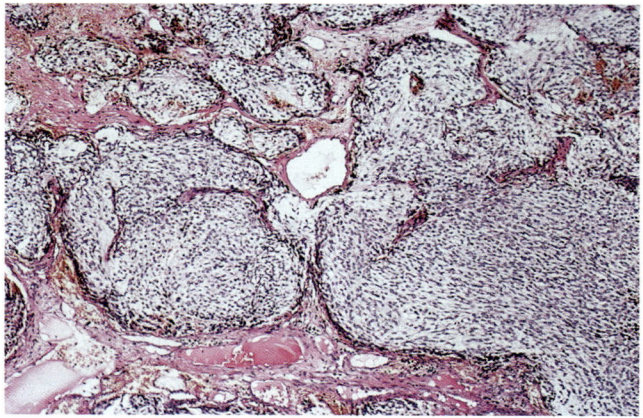

FIG. 19. Olfactory neuroblastoma. The lobular arrangement of tumor cells is characteristic. (Hematoxylin and eosin, original magnification 100×.)

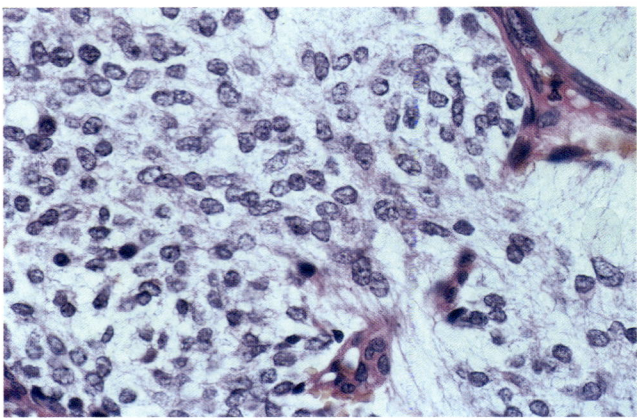

FIG. 20. Olfactory neuroblastoma. Note the small round cells and neurofibrillary background. (Hematoxylin and eosin, original magnification 400×.)

The stroma is highly vascular and often has a neurofibrillary appearance. Homer Wright and Flexner-Wintersteiner rosettes are additional features.

Ultrastructurally, olfactory neuroblastomas contain neurosecretory granules, neurotubules, and neurofilaments. On immunostaining, they are positive for synaptophysin and neuron-specific enolase, but only focally positive for S-100 protein (40,42). Some may also be positive for low–molecular-weight cytokeratin.

Olfactory neuroblastomas are sometimes graded histologically on a scale of I (well differentiated) to IV (poorly differentiated). Some have found this grading system to have prognostic significance, whereas others have not.

Differential Diagnosis. The differential diagnosis includes innumerable "small round cell" tumors that occur in the sinonasal tract (43). Among the more common ones are malignant lymphoma, rhabdomyosarcoma, undifferentiated carcinoma, and malignant melanoma. Most often, these tumors can be distinguished by the use of immunostains. Malignant lymphomas are positive for leukocyte common antigen, rhabdomyosarcomas for desmin and myoglobin, undifferentiated carcinomas for epithelial membrane antigen, and malignant melanoma for HMB-45. Olfactory neuroblastomas are negative for these markers.

Paraganglioma

Definition. Paragangliomas are a group of histologically similar neoplasms that arise from neuroectodermally derived paraganglionic cells associated with autonomic ganglia (7,43–46). The extraadrenal paraganglia can be classified into (a) branchomeric, which includes the jugulotympanic, carotid body, laryngeal, subclavian, and aortopulmonary paraganglia; (b) intravagal, at the level of the jugular or nodose ganglion; (c) aorticosympathetic; and (d) visceral–autonomic paraganglia (44).

Clinical Features. In the head and neck, carotid body tumors are the most common type (60%), followed by jugulotympanic and vagal tumors (45,46). Patients are usually between 40 and 60 years of age. Head and neck paragangliomas may be multifocal (10–20%), familial (10%), expressed as an autosomal dominant trait, or malignant (2–13%). Only rarely (2–3%) do paragangliomas at this site show manifestations of norepinephrine overproduction. Occasionally, paragangliomas may be a component of the multiple endocrine neoplasia syndrome.

Histopathology. Paragangliomas have a beefy, red-brown to gray-tan appearance. Histologically, paragangliomas may have a thin capsule and are composed of two cell types: chief cells, arranged in compact cell nests (*Zellballen*) (Fig. 21), and sustentacular or modified Schwann cells located peripheral to the chief cells (44–47). The chief cells have centrally located nuclei with finely stippled chromatin and a moderate amount of eosinophilic cytoplasm. Nuclear pleomorphism, necrosis, mitoses, and even vascular or neural invasion may be seen in benign paraganglioma and are not sufficient for a diagnosis of malignancy. Only the presence of metastasis, to sites such as the lymph nodes, lung, and bone, establishes a diagnosis of malignancy in these tumors. Immunohistochemical stains confirm the neuroendocrine nature of the chief cells with diffuse, strong positivity for neuron-specific enolase, synaptophysin (Fig. 22), and chromogranin, as well as other polypeptides, such as serotonin, leu-enkephalin, somatostatin, bombesin, and adrenocorticotropic hormone (46). The sustentacular cells may be positive for S-100 protein and glial fibrillary acidic protein, but are negative for neuroendocrine markers. An inverse relationship between tumor grade and sustentacular cell number has been observed. Ultrastructurally, chief cells contain small, dense core neurosecretory granules (100–200 nm), representing sites of catecholamine storage (16).

Differential Diagnosis. The typical histologic features and immunophenotype distinguish paraganglioma from other neoplasms with which it may be confused, including meningioma, nerve sheath tumor, hemangiopericytoma, adult rhabdomyoma, melanoma, or metastatic carcinoma

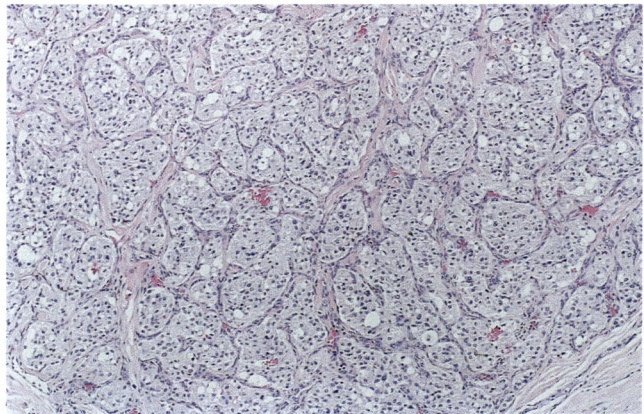

FIG. 21. Paraganglioma. The typical *Zellballen* pattern of chief cells is illustrated. (Hematoxylin and eosin, original magnification 200×.)

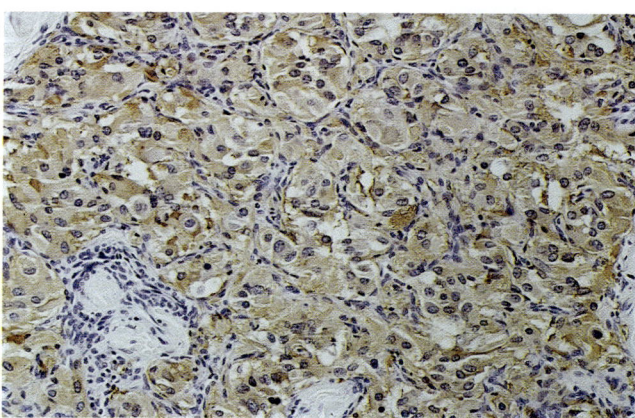

FIG. 22. Paraganglioma. Note the compact nests of chief cells with a moderate amount of cytoplasm that are strongly positive for synaptophysin. (Immunoperoxidase stain, original magnification 400×.)

(especially renal cell carcinoma). However, the diagnosis of paraganglioma may be made difficult by the presence of extensive fibrosis, which may mask the typical *Zellballen* pattern, or when chief cells are spindled, granular, or vacuolated. In difficult cases, the diagnosis can be confirmed by immunohistochemical or ultrastructural studies.

Unlike other neoplasms, the biologic behavior of paragangliomas cannot be predicted by the presence of atypical features. Studies of head and neck paragangliomas have shown that although DNA abnormalities are common, DNA ploidy using flow cytometry is of limited value in predicting prognosis and is not useful for assessing its malignant potential (45,46).

Rhabdomyosarcoma

Definition. Rhabdomyosarcoma is a malignancy of skeletal muscle cells (rhabdomyoblasts) with varying degrees of maturation and resemblance to normal skeletal muscle.

Clinical Features. Rhabdomyosarcoma is the most common soft tissue sarcoma in children and young adults as well as the most common soft tissue sarcoma of the head and neck.

The head and neck sites are divided into three broad groups: cranial parameningeal (50%), orbital (25%), and nonorbital–nonparameningeal (25%). The orbital tumors have the best prognosis, whereas parameningeal involvement is associated with the poorest outcome (48).

Parameningeal sites include the nasopharynx, paranasal sinuses, middle ear–mastoid, and pterygoid–infratemporal regions. Skull base involvement by tumor infiltration occurs commonly relatively early in the disease, with involvement of cranial nerves. Traditional thinking has viewed skull base involvement as a contraindication to surgery, and aggressive chemotherapy, radiation therapy, or both have been used, with overall survival rates of 57% reported in the Intergroup Rhabdomyosarcoma Study II (49). There is limited experi-

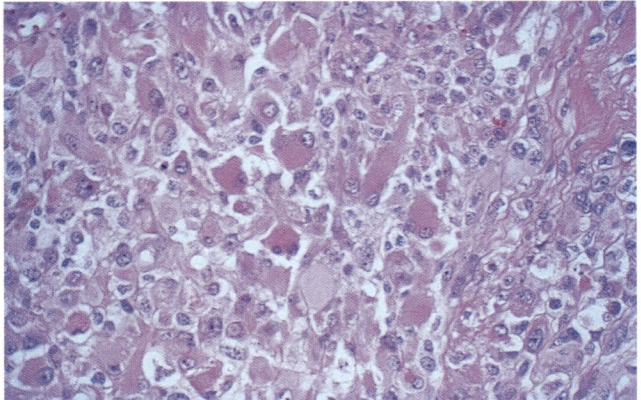

FIG. 23. Embryonal rhabdomyosarcoma. The tumor consists of large, irregular, polygonal and straplike cells with abundant pink cytoplasm and coarse, irregular nuclei. (Hematoxylin and eosin, original magnification 200×.)

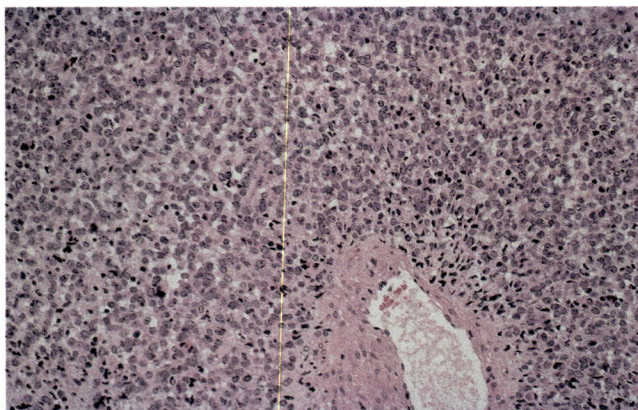

FIG. 25. Alveolar rhabdomyosarcoma. The alveolar variant of rhabdomyosarcoma is characterized by small, round cells with scant cytoplasm. (Hematoxylin and eosin, original magnification 200×.)

ence with skull base surgery for rhabdomyosarcoma in an adjuvant setting after chemotherapy or radiation therapy (50–53).

Prognosis is also linked to histologic type, with the alveolar variant having a less favorable course than the embryonal type at all stages. Rhabdomyosarcoma metastasizes to regional lymph nodes as well as hematogenously to bone, lung, and brain. Overall 5-year survival rates are stage I, 83%; stage II, 70%; stage III, 52%; and stage IV, 20% (49)

Histopathology. Three histologic subtypes are described: embryonal, alveolar, and pleomorphic (54). The embryonal variant is the most common, with sheets of large round and spindle cells with abundant eosinophilic cytoplasm called rhabdomyoblasts (Fig. 23). Cross-striations resembling those found in skeletal muscle fibers are often present. Mitoses and necrosis are commonly seen. Immunohistochemical reactivity for desmin, human muscle actin, and myo-

globin is seen. Electron microscopy reveals primitive bundles of actin and myosin filaments with Z banding (Fig. 24).

The alveolar subtype consists of poorly defined groups of single, small, dense, round cells with irregular nuclei and scant cytoplasm (Fig. 25). This histologic type is included in the poorly differentiated "small round blue cell tumors of childhood." An alveolar pattern with cell clusters resembling lung alveoli is variable, and the primitive cells may appear in solid sheets or trabecular nests. Mitoses and necrosis are common. Immunohistochemical stains are positive for desmin and human muscle actin. A characteristic translocation between chromosomes 2 and 13, the t(2;13)(q35;q14), is found in most alveolar rhabdomyosarcomas. The translocation involves the *PAX3* gene, which is involved in segmentation and neural tube differentiation in embryogenesis and is a candidate oncogene (55).

The pleomorphic histologic type is uncommon, particularly in the head and neck, and consists of large, multinucleate, pleomorphic cells with bizarre nuclear features.

Differential Diagnosis. Embryonal rhabdomyosarcoma may be distinguished from rhabdomyoma, its benign counterpart, by the presence of enlarged atypical nuclei and mitoses. Alveolar soft part sarcoma, a tumor of uncertain histogenesis, has uniform nuclei and characteristic ultrastructural rhomboid crystals. Granular cell tumor of Schwann cell derivation is characterized by large pink cells, but has uniform nuclei and shows reactivity with S-100. Alveolar rhabdomyosarcoma resembles several small round cell tumors, including lymphoma, Ewing's sarcoma, neuroendocrine carcinoma, and neuroblastoma. Morphologic and ultrastructural features as well as immunohistochemistry are used to distinguish these entities. Alveolar rhabdomyosarcoma typically does not form the thick–thin filaments seen in the embryonal type, but shows positivity for desmin or human muscle actin. A list of the characteristic differentiation-specific markers for the common round cell tumors is given in Table 1.

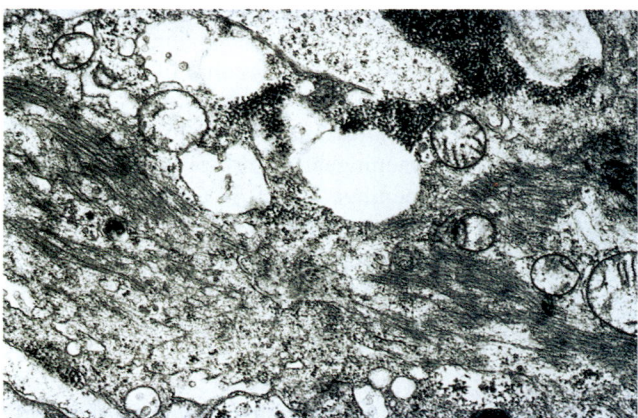

FIG. 24. Embryonal rhabdomyosarcoma. Rhabdomyoblast with dense bundles of thick (myosin) and thin (actin) myofilaments. (Electron micrograph, original magnification 30,000×.)

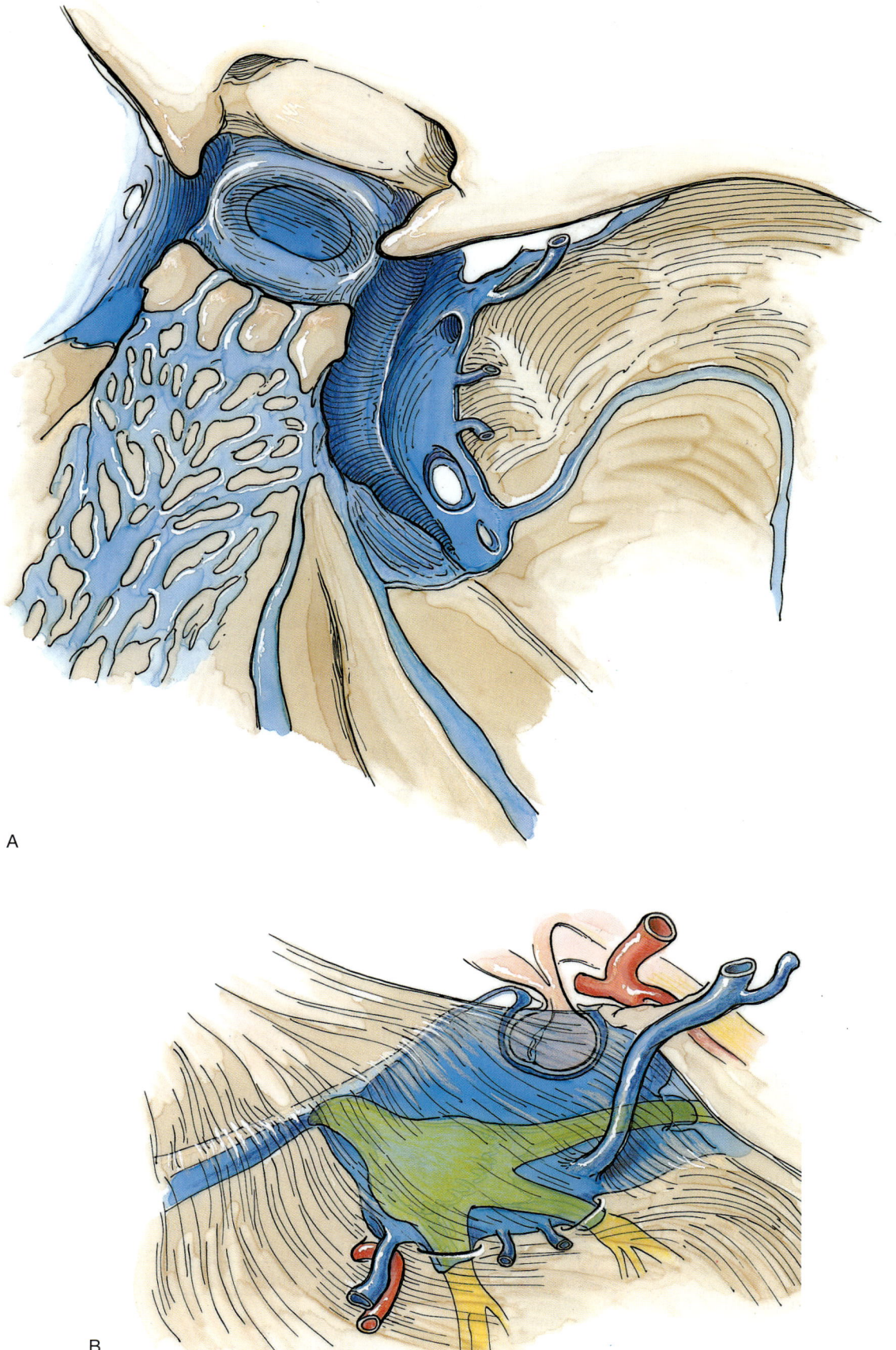

FIG. 24. The cavernous sinus. **A:** Oblique view showing connections to the opposing side through circular sinus and basilar plexus. **B:** Connections of cavernous sinus to cerebral vessels by bridging veins and extensions to superior orbital fissure and into foramen of trigeminal nerve.

TABLE 6. Two-year and 5-year survival rates of patients with cavernous sinus involvement

	A&W		DOD		DOC		AWD		Total	
	2	5	2	5	2	5	2	5	2	5
No.	13	5	3	8	4	5	2	2	22	20
Survival (%)	59.1	25	13.4	40	18.2	25	9.1	10	NA	NA

A&W, alive and well without disease; DOD, dead of local disease; DOC, dead of other causes (no local disease); AWD, alive with disease; NA, not applicable.

Independent of the debate, one fact is clear, and that is that surgery in the cavernous sinus is nightmarishly difficult. It is tucked away in the geographic center of the head, houses the major supply of blood to the ipsilateral cerebral hemisphere, and has cranial nerves II through VI traversing it or in close proximity.

In the authors' series of patients, 25 had cavernous sinus invasion. There are 2-year follow-ups on 22 and 5-year follow-ups on 20. The fate of these patients is described in Table 6. Survivorship obviously is related to the amount of the sinus involved. In an earlier study, seven patients who had no evidence of disease at 3-year follow-up had had an average of 24% of the sinus involved, and in the five of those seven who had recurrences in the sinus, the average involvement was 56%.

In light of the high local recurrence rate and the dismal survival of patients with extensive cavernous sinus involvement, the authors have redesigned their surgical attack in this area. With greater than 40% of the sinus involved, a complete removal of the sinus is done that includes complete removal of its lateral dural wall; resection of the carotid artery, which is replaced with an interposition graft; removal of the venous and venous sinus connections that are in the vicinity; and excision of all the bone in the proximity of the sinus. Although early signs are encouraging, only the test of time will prove the efficacy of this more radical approach.

METASTATIC DISEASE TO THE SKULL BASE

Approximately 1.2 million new cases of cancer were diagnosed in 1995. Prostate cancer was the most frequently diagnosed new cancer, followed by breast, lung, colorectal, and skin (melanoma). Over a half-million patients will die from cancer (18). A significant mortality factor is metastatic disease.

True metastasis is distinguished from secondary extension, which is a manifestation of local growth factors. Furthermore, metastasis can be divided into regional and distant types; common to each is secondary spread outside of the confines of the primary tumor.

A *single* skull base metastasis refers to an isolated lesion with no implication about the extent of cancer elsewhere in the body. The term *solitary* metastasis, on the other hand, describes the rare occurrence of an isolated lesion with no other evidence of metastatic cancer elsewhere in the body.

Skull base metastases have become a more recognized entity despite the lack of detailed studies on this phenomenon.

Incidence

The true incidence of skull base metastases is unknown; they are frequently included with cerebral metastasis data. The estimated overall incidence of brain metastasis is in the range of 12% to 35% of all cancer patients (19,20). Most authors state the incidence is underreported. In fact, many authors believe the incidence of metastatic brain tumors is higher than that of primary brain tumors (18,21,22).

The largest series dealing with skull base metastasis demonstrated breast, lung, prostate, and head and neck carcinomas as the most common malignancies (23). Table 7 illustrates the sources of the primary tumors in this series of 51 patients (23). Table 8 shows the sites of these metastases.

Skull base metastases tend to localize to certain areas. The middle fossa, jugular foramen, and parasellar sites are most frequently involved.

Specific Sites

The most detailed studies on skull base metastases were on those located in the orbit and temporal bone. Metastatic tumors to the temporal bone are uncommon and usually are seeded by the hematogenous route. Marrow-containing areas, most notably the petrous portion, may promote the development of metastatic lesions. The slow blood flow in the marrow acts as a filter mechanism, allowing tumor cells to propagate. The most common metastatic lesion in the temporal bone is breast carcinoma (24,25). Lung, prostate, and renal carcinomas are all well documented for their metastatic potential to the temporal bone (26).

Metastatic Orbital Malignancies

Malignant tumors metastatic to the orbit represent 3% to 5% of all solid orbital mass lesion (27–29). Font et al. (30),

TABLE 7. Primary sites of cancer in patients with metastasis to the base of the skull

Primary tumor	No. of cases
Breast	19
Lung	6
Prostate	6
Head and neck	8
Lymphoma	3
Renal	2
Miscellaneous	7

TABLE 8. *Metastases to skull base and location*

Primary tumor	Clival	Orbit	Parasellar	Middle fossa	Jugular foramen	Occipital condyle
Breast	0	3	3	7	2	4
Lung	0	1	1	2	1	1
Prostate	1	0	2	1	1	1
Head and neck	0	1	0	3	4	0
Lymphoma	0	0	1	1	0	1
Renal	0	1	0	0	1	0
Miscellaneous	0	0	1	2	1	2

in a study of 28 metastatic tumors to the orbit, demonstrated that 20% were breast carcinomas and 14% were lung cancers. Less common sites included kidney, prostate, testis, pancreas, and ileum.

Pathophysiology

Two major routes have been suggested for metastatic tumors to reach the brain and skull base. Blood-borne tumor emboli may reach the skull base through small arteries that freely anastomose and branch at the neural foramina. Tumor-derived factors enhance invasion of the thick arterial walls. In addition, Batson in 1940 (31) described the rich plexus of veins and anastomotic connections that allow intraabdominal neoplasms to propagate tumor emboli throughout the body. These veins are valveless and, with increased intraabdominal and intrathoracic pressure, blood is shunted through the vertebral, prevertebral, and epidural venous networks. This can allow tumor emboli to reach the skull base (Figs. 25–27).

Direct extension from adjacent regions such as paranasal sinuses, external ear, and nasopharynx, although not representing true metastasis, accounts for a significant proportion of secondary skull base neoplasms. The overall incidence of skull base invasion by sinonasal malignancies appears to be approximately 15% (32) (Fig. 28). There are different routes of extension, particularly along the muscles attached to the skull base, the fibrofatty spaces between these muscles, along neurovascular bundles, and through the foramina (33) (Fig. 29).

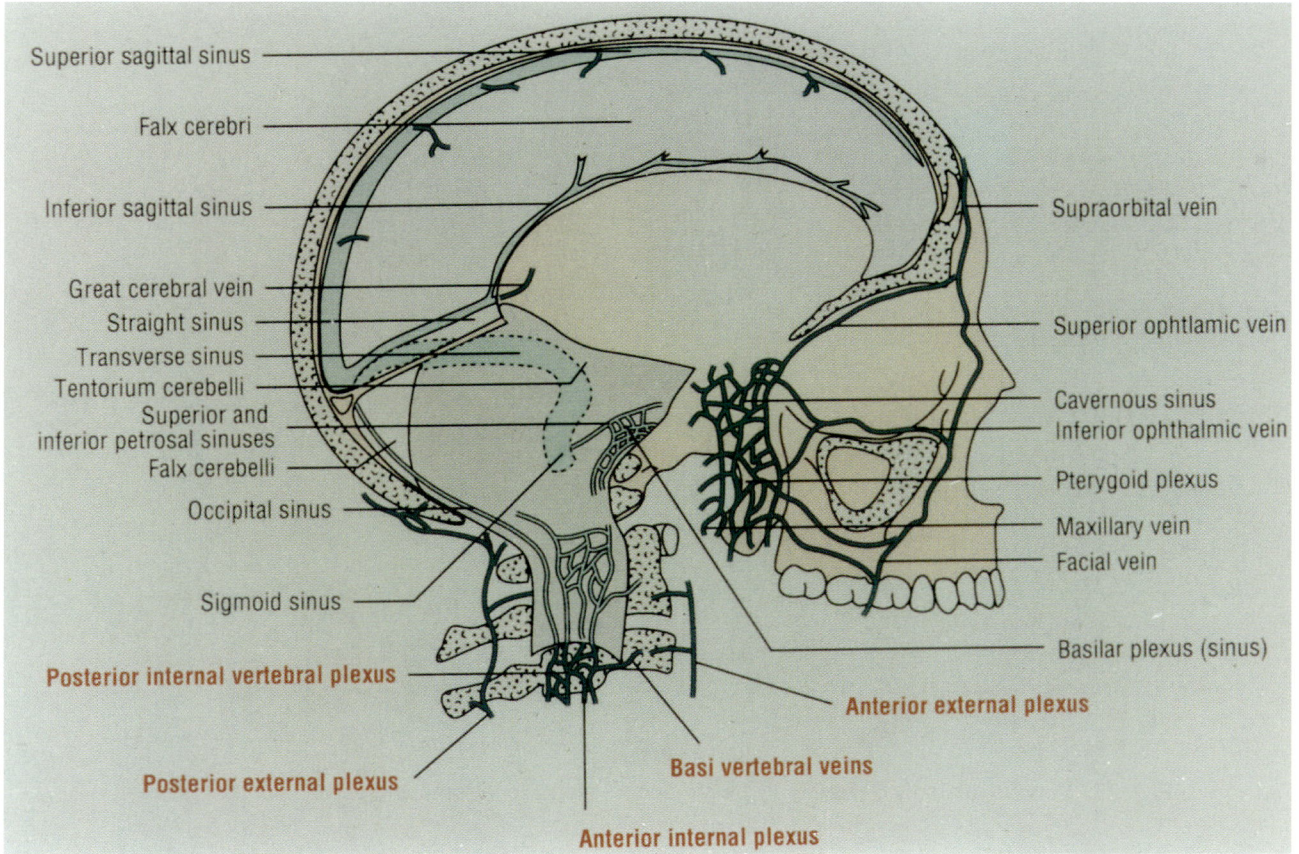

FIG. 25. Venous anatomy of vertebral column, skull, and skull base.

68 / Chapter 4

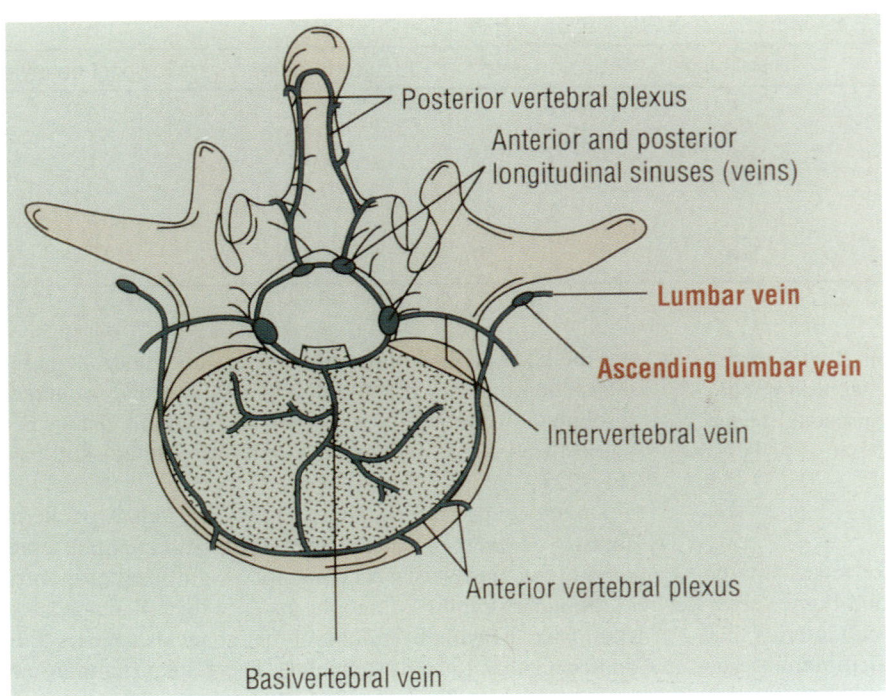

FIG. 26. Venous anatomy of vertebral body.

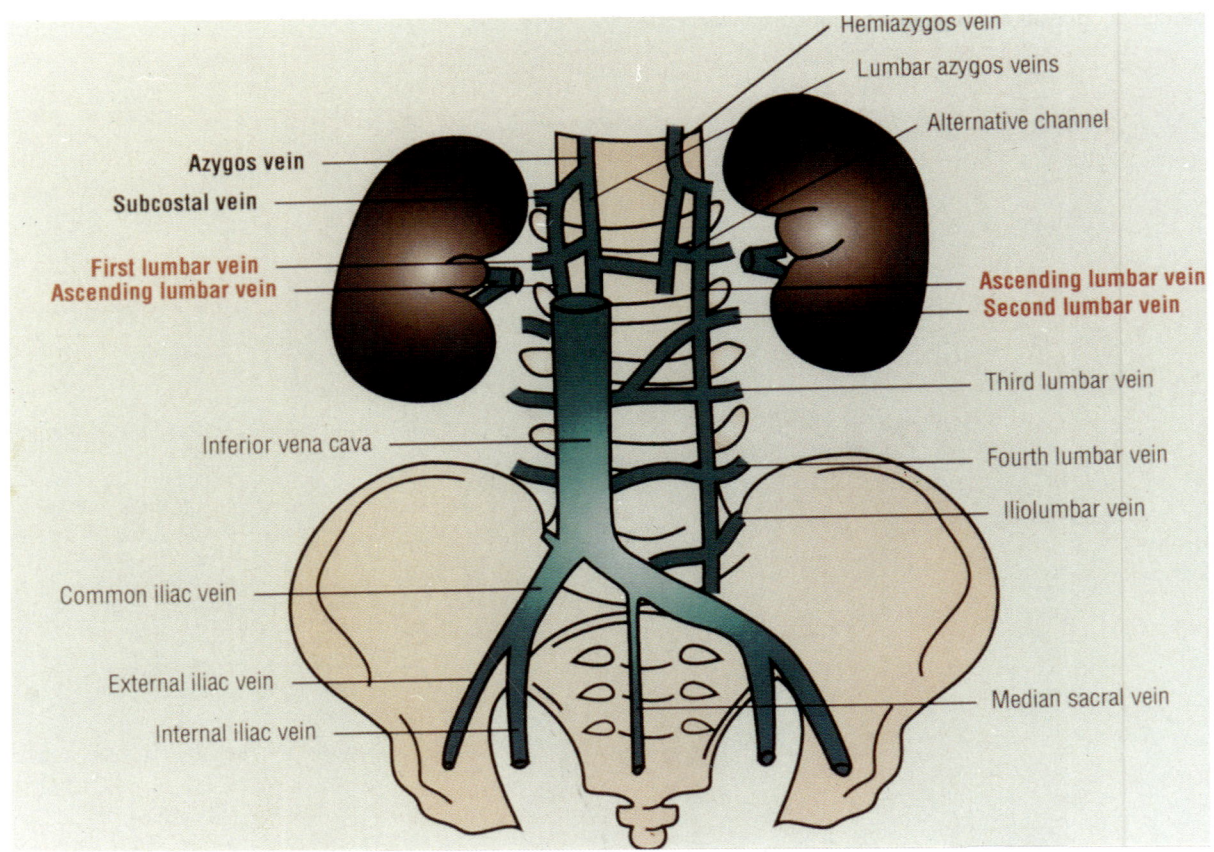

FIG. 27. Venous anatomy of vertebral column and relationship to renal and pelvic venous systems.

PATHOPHYSIOLOGY OF SKULL BASE MALIGNANCIES / 69

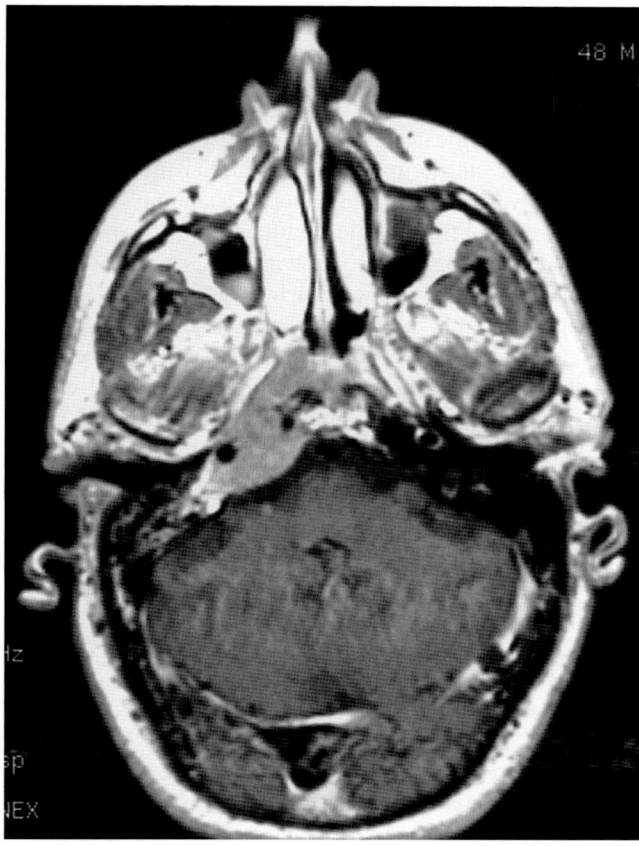

FIG. 28. Magnetic resonance image demonstrating nasopharyngeal carcinoma extending to right middle cranial fossa.

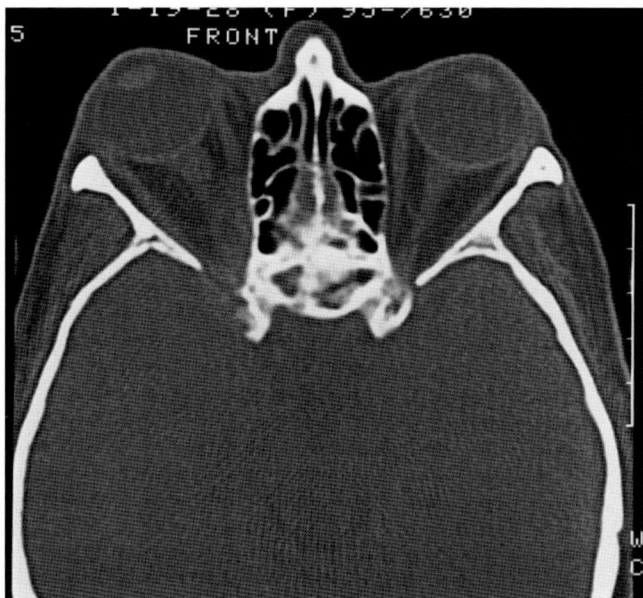

FIG. 29. Orbital computed tomography scan demonstrating perineural spread from supraorbital cutaneous squamous cell cancer to orbital apex and cavernous sinus.

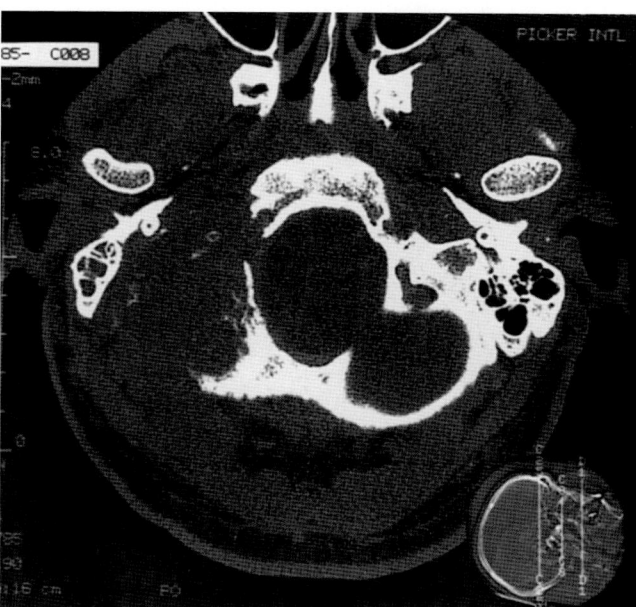

FIG. 30. Computed tomography scan of a patient presenting with dysarthria, demonstrating destructive mass of right jugular bulb involving temporal and occipital bones. A biopsy showed renal cell carcinoma.

Presenting Signs and Symptoms

Metastases to the skull base affect the neurovascular structures entering the foramina at the basicranium. Invasion of bone by metastatic primary tumor is the most common cause of pain in patients with cancer, and such pain usually precedes neurologic signs and symptoms by weeks (34). Greenberg et al. (23) described five clinical syndromes: orbital, parasellar, middle fossa, jugular foramen, and occipital condyle (Fig. 30). The current authors include a sixth—clival.

The orbital syndrome is characterized as progressive, dull, continuous pain in the supraorbital area of the affected eye. This is followed by diplopia and hypesthesia over the ophthalmic division of the trigeminal nerve. As the metastasis enlarges, proptosis and ophthalmoplegia result.

The parasellar syndrome is characterized as a unilateral frontal headache and ocular paresis without proptosis or visual loss. Other signs and symptoms, including pituitary dysfunction and hypesthesia, can occur.

The middle fossa syndrome is characterized by facial pain and paresthesia or numbness over the second and third divisions of the trigeminal nerve. When the tumor is on the anterior surface of the petrous ridge, the abducens nerve is likely to be affected at Dorello's canal. When the lesion involves the posterior surface, the facial and vestibulocochlear nerves can be affected.

The jugular foramen syndrome is characterized by paralysis of cranial nerves IX through XII with resultant hoarseness, dysphagia, atrophy of the sternocleidomastoid and upper trapezius muscles, as well as weakness of the palate.

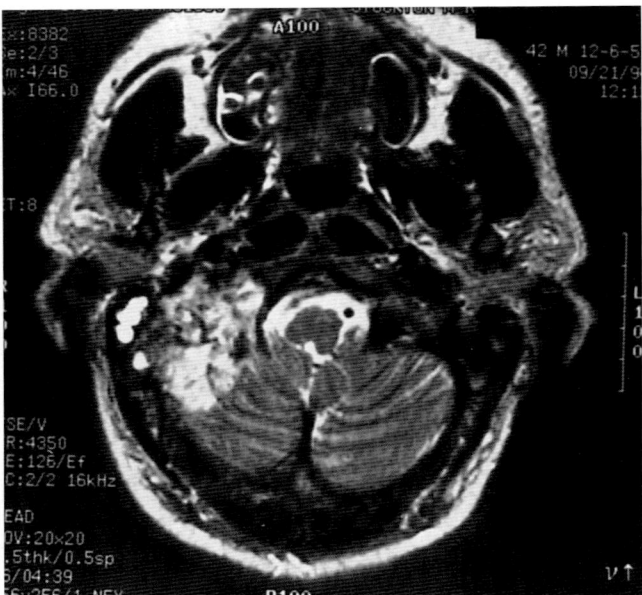

FIG. 31. T1-weighted, gadolinium-enhanced magnetic resonance image showing same renal cell carcinoma metastatic to the right jugular bulb as in Fig. 30.

Occipital or postauricular pain commonly occur, referred to the vertex (Fig. 31).

The occipital condyle syndrome is characterized by severe, unilateral occipital pain exacerbated with flexion of the neck and cranial nerve XII paralysis. Owing to the proximity of the jugular foramen, associated signs and symptoms may occur.

The clival syndrome is characterized by vertex headache exacerbated by head flexion. Lower cranial nerve dysfunction (VI–XII) begins unilaterally, but often becomes bilateral.

Diagnostic Assessment

Patients with skull base lesions that are radiographically suggestive of metastases but who have no known primary cancer need histologic confirmation. An extensive search for a primary is not undertaken until the diagnosis is confirmed. Once histologic study confirms metastasis, CT scans of the chest, abdomen, and pelvis may prove helpful for identifying the primary site. Likewise, sputum cytology and blood tests for more markers may aid in the diagnosis.

Patients with known cancer represent most of the patients with skull base metastases. The need for tissue diagnosis should be individualized according to the site, suspected type, and the prognosis and overall condition of the patient.

A search for leptomeningeal metastasis should be considered. Cytology is the most important examination, but high opening pressures and elevated protein can also be present. Tumor markers such as carcinoembryonic antigen and β-glucuronidase can be helpful once the initial diagnosis of leptomeningeal metastasis is made (35).

Radiologic Evaluation

Because of their insidious onset, skull base metastases are often difficult to identify initially on MRI or CT scan. Prostate and lung cancers may produce metastases that are either lytic or blastic in nature. Most other metastases produce only lytic lesions. Radionuclide scanning is the most sensitive method for detecting skull base metastasis (36).

Computed tomography scans with high spatial resolution, bone algorithm, and bone windowing are superior to MRI for delineating osseous destruction or sclerosis (Figs. 32, 33). MRI is superior to CT for delineating the soft tissue component of metastases and for determining invasion of cranial nerves, the underlying dura, leptomeninges, and brain (Figs. 34, 35). Gadolinium enhancement further increases sensitivity. Positron emission tomography may be useful for following or distinguishing between recurrent tumor and necrosis secondary to radiation therapy or chemotherapy, provided the initial evaluation shows increased fluorodeoxyglucose uptake (22).

Surgical Management and Recommendations for Treatment

It is evident from the surgical results of the 1990s that the resection of a single brain metastasis not only can improve a patient's neurologic condition, but can increase the rates of local control and survival (37,38). Patients with a single skull base metastasis are the most appropriate surgical candidates. However, Bindal et al. have demonstrated that at least with regard to brain metastasis, removal of multiple metastatic lesions is as effective as resection of single metastasis as long as each lesion is removed in its entirety (39).

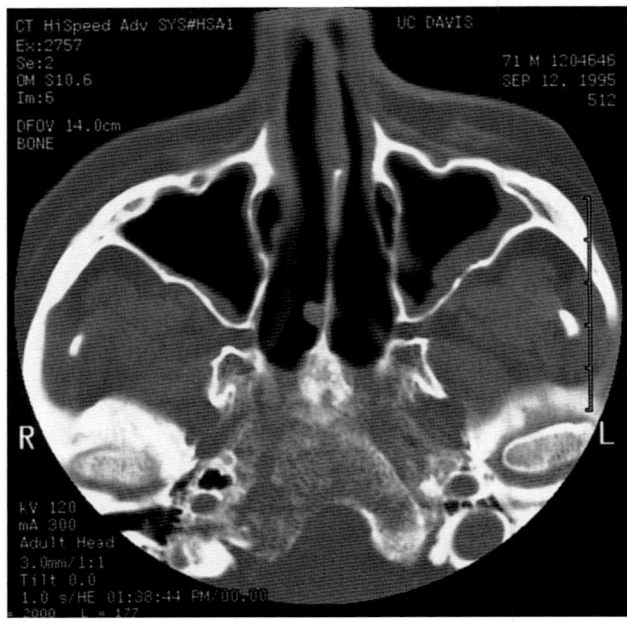

FIG. 32. Metastatic prostatic carcinoma of clivus.

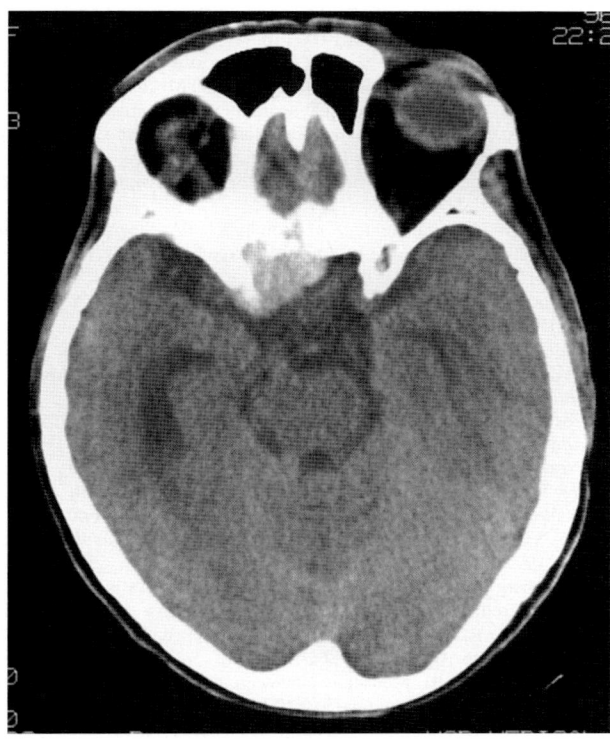

FIG. 33. Metastatic breast adenocarcinoma of right parasellar region.

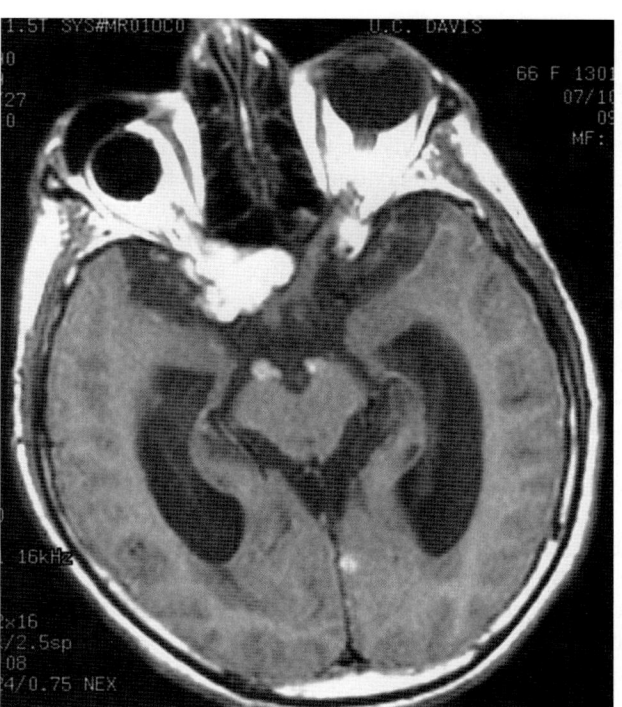

FIG. 35. Corresponding magnetic resonance image of metastatic breast adenocarcinoma (see Fig. 33) showing intracranial extension.

The resectability of each lesion should be assessed independently.

It is equally important to consider the tumor's radiosensitivity and chemosensitivity before proceeding with surgery. Small cell lung cancer, lymphoma, and germ cell tumors are particularly sensitive to radiation and chemotherapy. Therefore, radiation and chemotherapy protocols are indicated. On the other hand, melanoma, renal cell carcinoma, and sarcomas are radioresistant and surgical resection should be considered. Most other neoplasms are intermediately sensitive to radiation, and surgery combined with radiation therapy may be used.

Stereotactic radiosurgery remains a potential option, but no prospective, randomized trials have been performed. Additional concerns over side effects, including osteoradionecrosis, must be considered.

Not all patients with skull base metastases are candidates for surgical resection. Ultimately, ideal surgical candidates are selected carefully by analyzing the clinical status of the patient, pertinent radiographic studies, and the tumor's histologic characteristics. Based on the neurosurgical data, resection of skull base metastases seems promising. With recently developed skull base approaches and microsurgical techniques, it appears that gross total removal could approach the 90% resection capabilities quoted in the neurosurgical literature (40).

CONCLUSIONS

Epithelial and connective tissue malignancies adopt a fairly predictable method of invasion when making the transition from the upper aerodigestive tract and its supporting tissues to the intracranial space. Perineural spread is id-

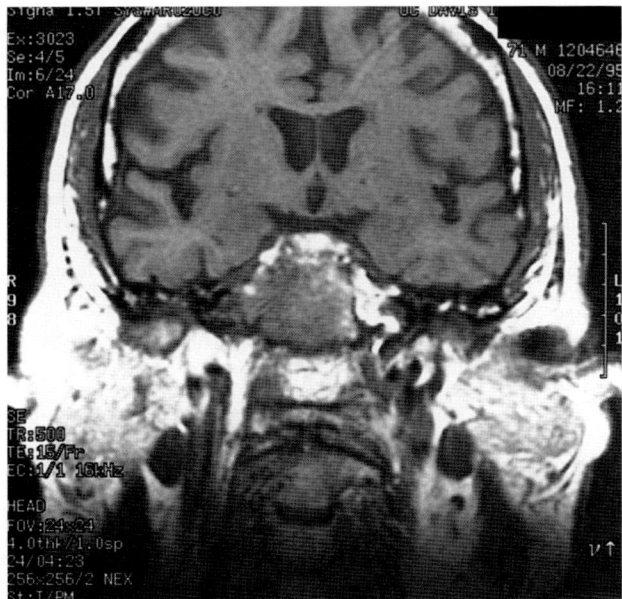

FIG. 34. Corresponding magnetic resonance image of prostatic cancer (see Fig. 32) showing proximity to middle fossa dura.

iosyncratic of certain tumors, and this avenue of tumor extension is one of the principal means of access of the cranial cavity. Dura provides a stout barrier to tumor spread, as does the periosteum lining the carotid canal. Brain invasion of these cancers proceeds in a fashion that is in stark contrast to the behavior of primary tumors. The presence of dural invasion does not adversely affect survival results compared with skull base tumors without such invasion. Resection of invaded brain is compatible with local tumor control in a significant percentage of patients.

Cavernous sinus and internal carotid artery involvement are unfavorable prognostic signs. Local control is difficult and second primaries as well as distant metastases are not uncommon. Nevertheless, cavernous sinus and internal carotid artery invasion are not incompatible with local control and cure.

An isolated skull base lesion may represent a distant metastasis from a primary at a remote site below the clavicles. Biopsy and careful histologic analysis are necessary to rule out such a phenomenon and prevent an extensive and unnecessary surgical procedure.

Skull base surgery is in evolution. Continued study of the pathophysiologic behavior of malignancies that invade both intracranial and extracranial compartments and the modification of surgery and adjunctive measures in light of these findings should improve the prognosis of this cohort of challenging and deserving patients.

REFERENCES

1. Lang J. *Clinical anatomy of the nose, nasal cavity and paranasal sinuses.* New York: Thieme Medical Publishers, 1989:121.
2. Larson DL, Rodin AE, Roberts DK, O'Steen WK, Rappaport AS, Lewis SR. Perineural lymphatics: myth or fact. *Am J Surg* 1996;112:488–492.
3. Rodin AE, Larson DL, Roberts DK. Nature of the perineural space invaded by prostate carcinoma. *Cancer* 1967;20:1772–1779.
4. Carter RL, Foster CS, Dinsdale EA. Perineural spread by squamous carcinomas of the head and neck: a morphological study using antiaxonal and antimyelin monoclonal antibodies. *J Clin Pathol* 1983;36:269–275.
5. Prassad S, Barnes L, Janecka I. Anatomy of the internal carotid artery. Presented at the Third Meeting of the North American Skull Base Society, Acapulco, Mexico, Feb. 16–20, 1992.
6. Tiedemann K. Cross sectional anatomy. In: Janecka IP, Tiedemann K, eds. *Skull base surgery: anatomy, biology and technology.* Philadelphia: Lippincott–Raven Publishers, 1997:118–119.
7. Chole RA. Differential osteoclast activation in endochondral and intramembranous bone. *Ann Otol Rhinol Laryngol* 1993;102:616–619.
8. Yoneda T, Mundy GR, Roodman GD. Induction of differentiation of the human promyelocytic HL-60 cells into cells with the osteoclastic phenotypes. *J Bone Miner Res* 1989;4:559.
9. Sabbatini M, Chavez J, Mundy GR, Bonewald L. Stimulation of tumor necrosis factor release for monocytic cells by the A-375 human melanoma via granulocyte-macrophage colony stimulating factor. *Cancer Res* 1990;50:2673–2678.
10. Kinney S, Woods BC. Malignancies of the external auditory canal. *Laryngoscope* 1987;97:158.
11. Donald PJ. The significance of invasion of key intracranial structures in skull base surgery for malignancy. Presented at the Triological Society Meeting, Scottsdale, Arizona, May, 1997.
12. Mohs FE. *Chemosurgery: microscopically controlled surgery for skin cancer.* Springfield, IL: Charles C Thomas Publisher, 1978.
13. Tromovitch TA, Stegman SJ. Microscopically controlled excision for skin tumors. *Arch Dermatol* 1974;110:231–232.
14. Krespi YP, Levine TM, Sisson GA. *Tumor surgery of the skull base.* AAO Instructional Program. Vol. 2. St. Louis: Mosby, 1989:279–288.
15. Sepehrnia A. True microsurgical anatomy of the human cavernous sinus. Presented at the Second International Skull Base Congress, San Diego, California, June 29–July 4, 1996.
16. Alencastro LC. The anterior loop of the carotid siphon. *Skull Base Surgery* 1991;1:73–77.
17. Alencastro LC. Commentary on Tromovitch TA, Stegman SJ. Microscopically controlled excision for skin tumors. *Arch Dermatol* 1974;110:231.
18. Wingo PA, Tong T, Bolden S. Cancer statistics, 1995, *CA Cancer J Clin* 1995;45:8–30.
19. Galicich JH, Arbit E, Wronski M. Metastatic brain tumors. In: Wilkins RH, Rengachary SS, eds. *Neurosurgery.* 2nd ed. New York: McGraw-Hill, 1996:807–821.
20. Posner JB, Chernik NL. Intracranial metastases from systemic cancer. *Adv Neurol* 1978;19:579–592.
21. Posner JB. *Neurologic complications of cancer.* Contemporary Neurology Series, Vol. 45. Philadelphia: FA Davis Co., 1995:3–14, 77–110.
22. Walker AE, Robins M, Weinfeld FD. Epidemiology of brain tumors: the National Survey of Intracranial Neoplasms. *Neurology* 1985;35:219–226.
23. Greenberg HS, Deck MDF, Vikram B, et al. Metastasis to the base of the skull: clinical findings in 43 patients. *Neurology* 1981;31:530–537.
24. Feinmesser R, Libson Y, Uziely B, Gay I. Metastatic carcinoma to the temporal bone. *Am J Otol* 1986;7:119–120.
25. Hill BA, Kohut RI. Metastatic adenocarcinoma of the temporal bone. *Archives of Otolaryngology* 1976;102:568–571.
26. Schuknecht H, Allam A, Murakami Y. Pathology of secondary malignant tumors of the temporal bone. *Ann Otol Rhinol Otolaryngol* 1968;77:5–22.
27. Henderson JW. *Orbital tumors.* 2nd ed. New York: Brian C. Decker, 1980:451–471.
28. Reese AB. Expanding lesions of the orbit (Bowman Lecture). *Transactions of the Ophthalmological Society of the United Kingdom* 1971;91:85–104.
29. Silva D. Orbital tumors. *Am J Ophthalmol* 1968;65:318–339.
30. Font RL, Ferry AP. Carcinoma metastatic to the eye and orbit: III. a clinicopathologic study of 28 cases metastatic to the orbit. *Cancer* 1976;38:1326–1335.
31. Batson O. The function of the vertebral veins and their role in the spread of metastases. *Ann Surg* 1940;112:138–149.
32. Weymuller E, Reardon E, Nash D. A comparison of treatment modalities in carcinoma of the maxillary antrum. *Archives of Otolaryngology* 1980;106:625–629.
33. Vignaud J, Pharabaz C, Mourag M. Tumors of the skull base. In: Portman M, ed. *Rhino-otological microsurgery of the skull base.* Edinburgh: Churchill Livingstone, 1995:40–65.
34. Raj PP, Phero JC. Pain control in cancer of the head and neck. In: Thawley W, Panje W, Batsakis J, et al, eds. *Comprehensive management of head and neck tumors.* Philadelphia: WB Saunders, 1987:42–68.
35. Chamberlain MC, Friedman HS. Leptomeningeal metastasis. In: Levin V, ed. *Cancer in the nervous system.* New York: Churchill Livingstone, 1996:281–290.
36. Schaefer P, Budzik R, Gonzalez G. Imaging of cerebral metastases in management of cerebral metastases. *Neurosurg Clin N Am* 1996;7:393–416.
37. Patchell RA, Tibbs PA, Walsh JW, et al. A randomized trial of surgery in the treatment of single metastases to the brain. *N Engl J Med* 1990;322:494–500.
38. Vecht CJ, Haaxma-Reiche H, Noordijk EM, et al. Treatment of single brain metastasis: radiotherapy alone or in combination with neurosurgery? *Ann Neurol* 1993;33:583–590.
39. Bindal AK, Bindal RK, Hess KR, et al. A comparison of surgery and radiosurgery in the treatment of brain metastasis. *J Neurosurg* 1995;82:355A(abst).
40. Arbit E, Wronski M. Clinical decision making in brain metastasis in management of cerebral metastasis. *Neurosurg Clin N Am* 1996;7:447–457.

CHAPTER 5

Presentation and Preparation of Patients with Skull Base Lesions

Paul J. Donald

Patients presenting with lesions of the skull base can be entirely asymptomatic or in horrible pain with an obviously large tumor and dysfunction of multiple cranial nerves. The asymptomatic patient may have a radiographic finding that was discovered during routine investigation of an unrelated problem, whereas the symptomatic patient not uncommonly has had extensive prior therapy and a persistent lesion.

Many of the subsequent chapters describe some presenting signs and symptoms of patients with skull base lesions; this chapter, with a few exceptions, is designed to present as exhaustively as possible the clinical picture that typifies patients who have lesions of areas involving the anterior, middle, and posterior cranial fossae or central compartment (Fig. 1).

PRESENTATION ACCORDING TO SITE

Symptoms arise according to functional disturbances of the system involved. Obviously, multiple systems may be compromised with more advanced disease processes. Often, a single presenting symptom alerts the patient to seek medical attention. Unfortunately, the symptom may be dismissed by the primary care physician, and not until further organ dysfunction has occurred is the practitioner spurred to either a more in-depth investigation or referral to the appropriate specialist. The insidious dangers posed by the scourge of managed care, especially its most heinous variety—capitation—include discouragement of expensive investigative procedures and specialist referral. As a result, in regions of the country where these systems have heavily intruded, more and more tumors and other disease processes are not being seen until they have reached an advanced stage.

P. J. Donald: Department of Otolaryngology—Head and Neck Surgery, and Center for Skull Base Surgery, University of California, Davis Medical Center, Sacramento, California 95817.

Facial Skin

With the avidity of so many people for the sun and the increasing danger posed by the diminished atmospheric protection to skin-damaging ultraviolet irradiation, cutaneous malignancy is becoming increasingly commonplace. Added to this is the popularity of tanning booths, which appear to appeal particularly to the young.

Basal cell carcinoma is the most frequent skin lesion observed. Fortunately, most of these tumors begin as an actinic keratosis and remain as such for a considerable time. However, many or most of these eventually progress to an invasive carcinoma. The early basal cell tumor is commonly very small and enlarges slowly over a period of years. Certain basal cell carcinomas are important for their implications for skull base surgery. These are the tumors in susceptible areas: those that have had multiple recurrences, sclerosing types, and neurotropic varieties. The most susceptible areas for skull base spread are the canthal areas of the eyes (Fig. 2), the nasal–facial groove, the external auditory canal, and postauricular skin (Fig. 3). Multiple recurrences speak to the aggressiveness and invasiveness of a specific tumor (see Fig. 3). Failures of well done Mohs resections are particularly worrisome. It is abundantly clear that basal cell carcinomas must be completely excised with histologically tumor-free margins (albeit narrow in Mohs resections). Opinions to the contrary are continuously refuted by the high frequency of local recurrence if total resection is not effected. Sclerosing basal cell carcinomas are characteristically aggressive and commonly recurrent. Such tumors often require a much wider resection than the nodular type (Fig. 4). When recurrent, they are especially difficult to encompass. They have a particular propensity to spread into the orbit and the anterior cranial fossa and from the ear to the middle cranial fossa. Some of these are multifocal, presenting a therapeutic dilemma that often defies solution (Fig. 5).

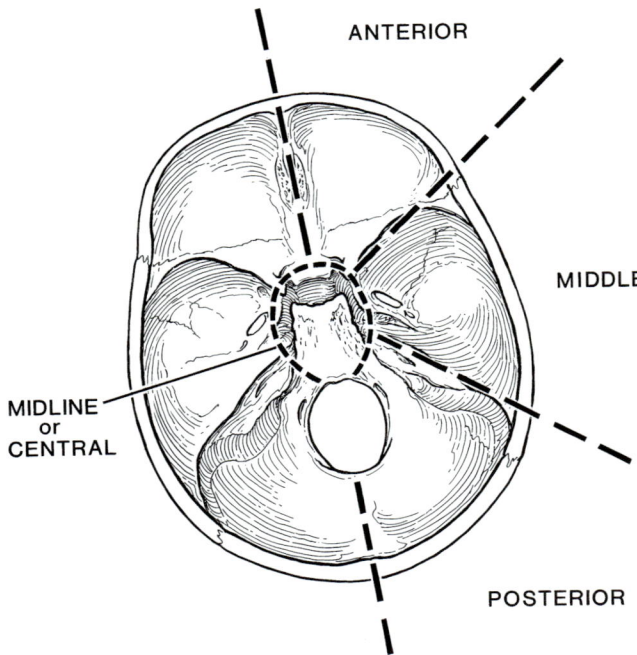

FIG. 1. Diagram outlining the various regions of cranial base surgery.

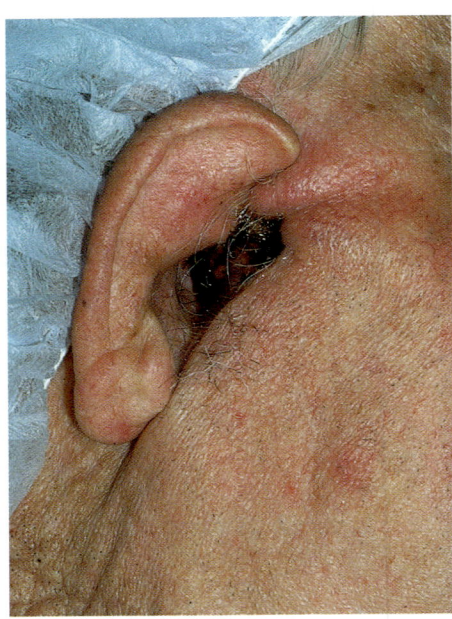

FIG. 3. Elderly patient with extensive basal cell carcinoma of the auricle after numerous prior resections requiring extensive temporal bone and skull base resection.

Neurotropism is a property not uncommonly seen in cutaneous neoplasms, and it is seen in squamous cell carcinoma, basal cell carcinoma, and malignant melanoma. Neurotropic basal cell cancers are not seen as commonly as the other two. Any facial numbness in a patient with a history of cutaneous malignancy must be carefully investigated for the possibility of neurotropic spread (Fig. 6). As in adenoid cystic carcinoma of glandular origin, there may be skip areas along nerves in the subcranial course of these lesions. Spread as far as the cavernous sinus can occur without clinical evidence of spread beyond the nerve sheath (Fig. 7).

In patients who have had orbital exenteration, rhinectomy, or temporal bone resection for skin cancer (especially if it is recurrent), it is important to keep the cavity open, covered only with a split-thickness skin graft, for at least 2 years. Major flap reconstruction obscures deep recurrences that can be effectively treated when small and superficial. Current investigative modalities such as computed tomography, magnetic resonance imaging, and positron emission tomography still do not provide sufficient information regarding early recurrence. Early detection is obscured by flaps as well as by postoperative and postradiation fibrosis (Fig. 8).

Nose and Paranasal Sinuses

Nose

Although malignancies can originate in the nasal skin and present with nasal symptoms, their gross appearance often detracts from the appreciation of the more subtle symptoms of nasal dysfunction. Nasal obstruction, epistaxis, and foul nasal drainage are the most common symptoms of intranasal and sinus tumors, whether benign or malignant. Pain is uncommon. The patient shown in Fig. 9 had symptoms of nasal obstruction for over 3 years and had been treated for allergic rhinitis until a palatal mass, bulging cheek, and proptosis alerted the treating physician to obtain a referral. Figure 10

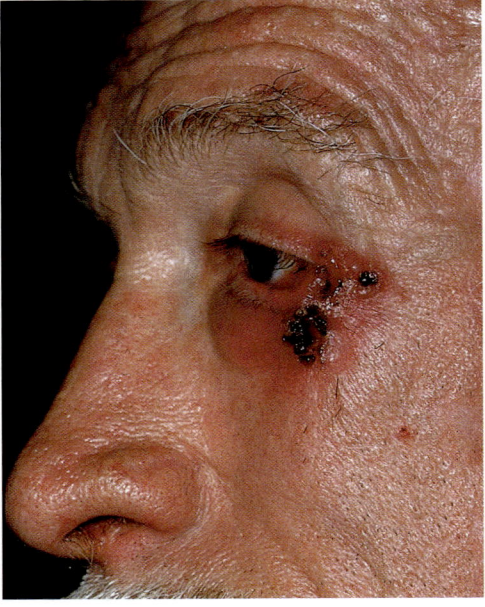

FIG. 2. Basal cell carcinoma of the lateral canthal skin. The patient eventually required orbital exenteration to effect complete tumor removal.

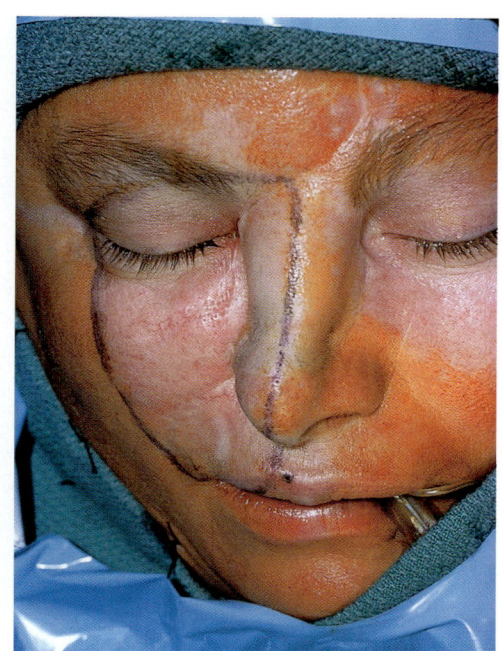
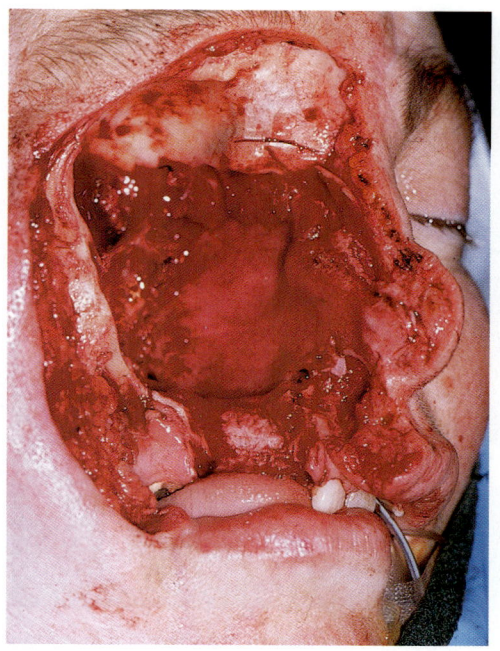

FIG. 4. A sclerosing basal cell carcinoma required a resection much wider than initially expected. **A:** Original tumor in cheek adjacent to nose, with resection outlined. **B:** Amount resected to achieve complete removal.

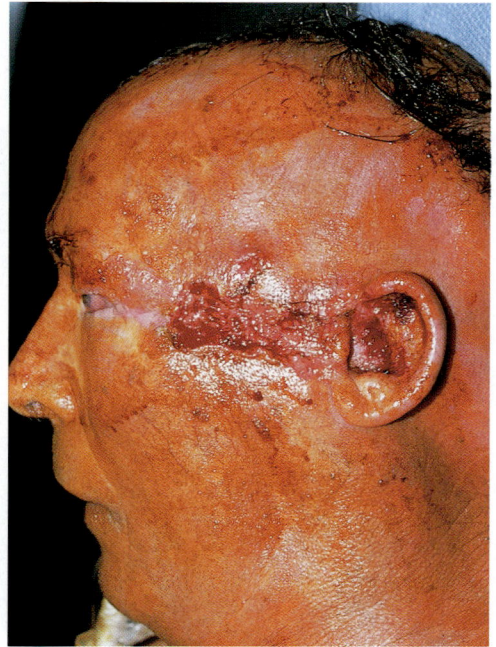

FIG. 5. Sixty-four-year-old patient with face covered in multiple basal cell carcinomas.

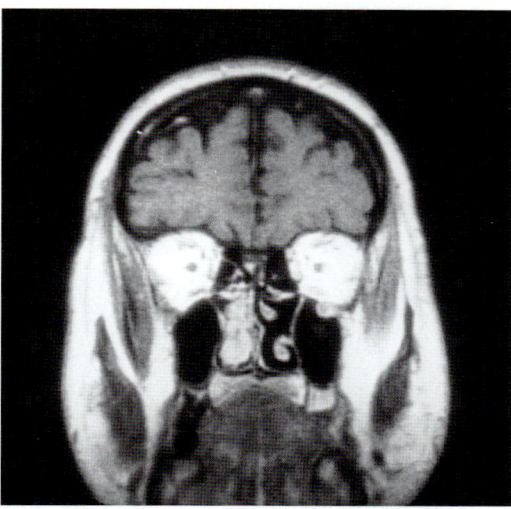

FIG. 6. Magnetic resonance image of a patient who had a carcinoma of the skin resected previously. He complained of numbness over his cheek. This coronal section shows enlargement and enhancement of the infraorbital nerve, characteristic of perineural spread.

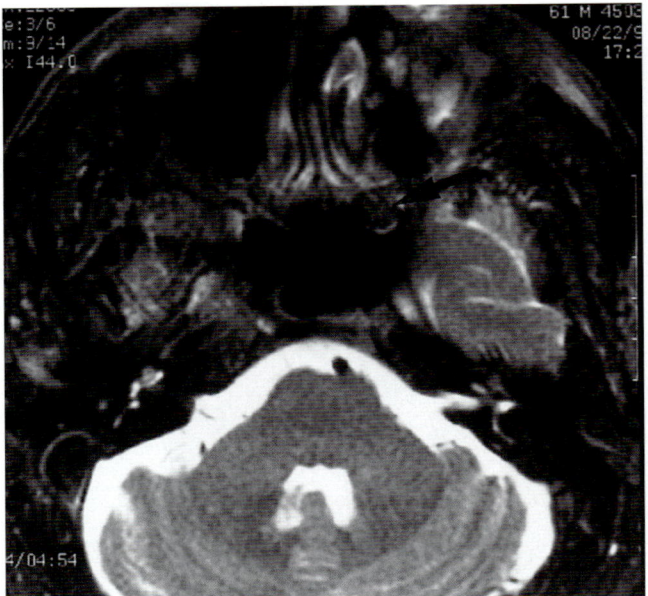

FIG. 7. Magnetic resonance image of cutaneous squamous cell carcinoma that invaded only the infraorbital nerve but remained confined by the perineural sheath and extended all the way to the cavernous sinus. Tumor in pterygomaxillary space indicated by *arrow*.

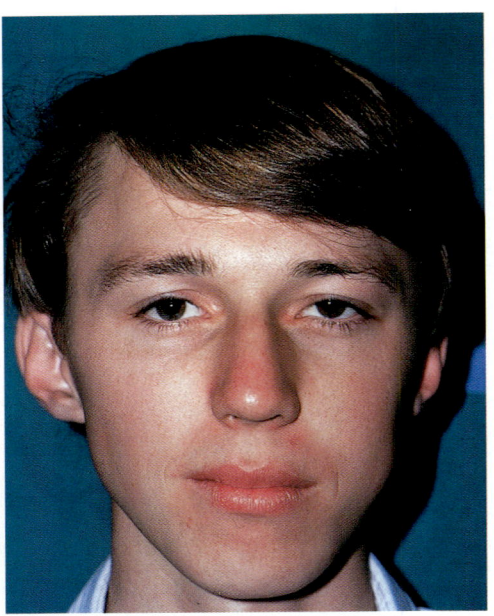

FIG. 9. Nineteen-year-old patient with a massive nasopharyngeal angiofibroma mistaken for allergy (see text). Note proptosis of left eye and bulging of left cheek and intracranial extension.

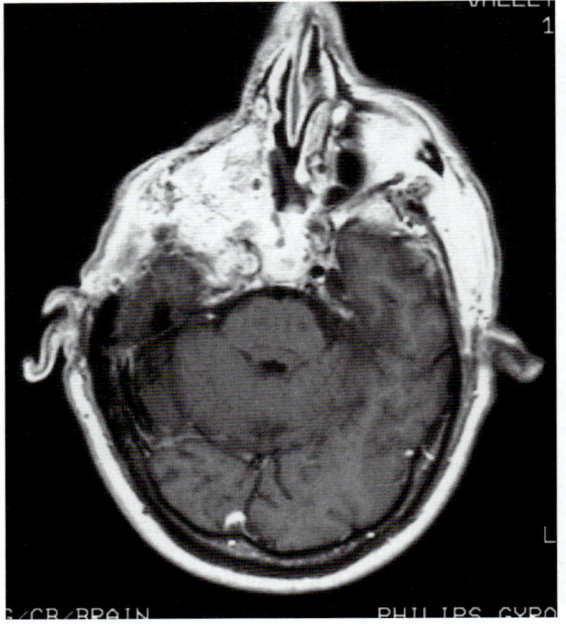
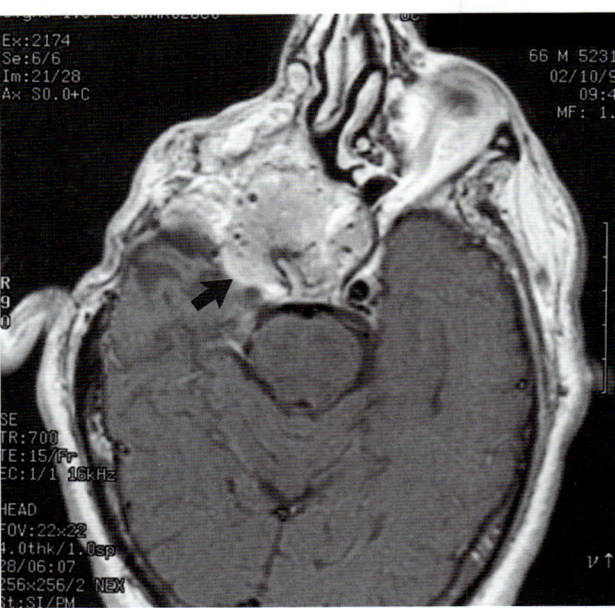

FIG. 8. Patient status postsurgery for tonsillar carcinoma who complained of pain in the infratemporal fossa. **A:** Axial magnetic resonance image showing no tumor in the infratemporal fossa, but area obscured by postradiation and postsurgical fibrosis and free flap reconstruction. **B:** Similar view taken 19 months later, finally demonstrating recurrent tumor.

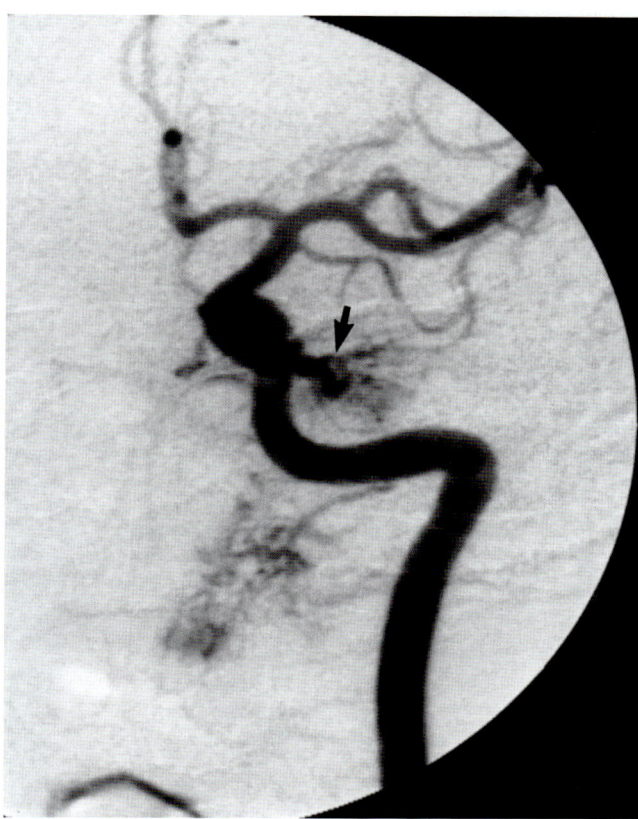

FIG. 10. Angiogram of 14-year-old boy with a large nasopharyngeal angiofibroma, showing feeding vessels from the internal carotid system. Arrow points to feeding vessels from cavernous internal carotid artery. (From Lyons BM, Donald PJ. Intracranial juvenile angiofibroma with intradural and cavernous sinus involvement. *Skull Base Surgery* 1992;2:87–91, with permission.)

shows the angiographic appearance of the nasopharyngeal angiofibroma that had spread to the cavernous sinus in the same patient. Complete tumor removal was effected by a combination extended transpalatal and middle fossa excision.

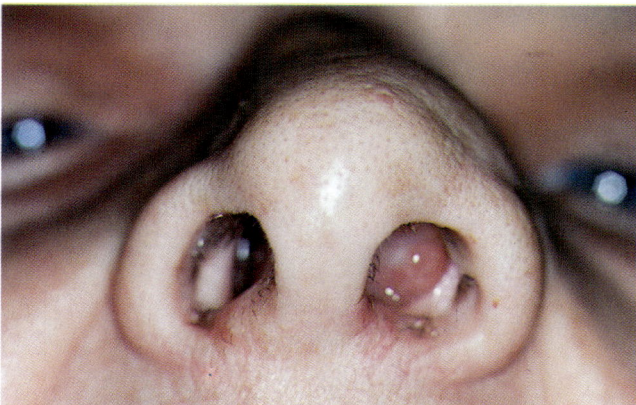

FIG. 11. Elderly woman with large squamous cell carcinoma of nasal cavity and maxillary and ethmoid sinuses presenting with an obvious intranasal mass that causes deformity of overlying soft tissues.

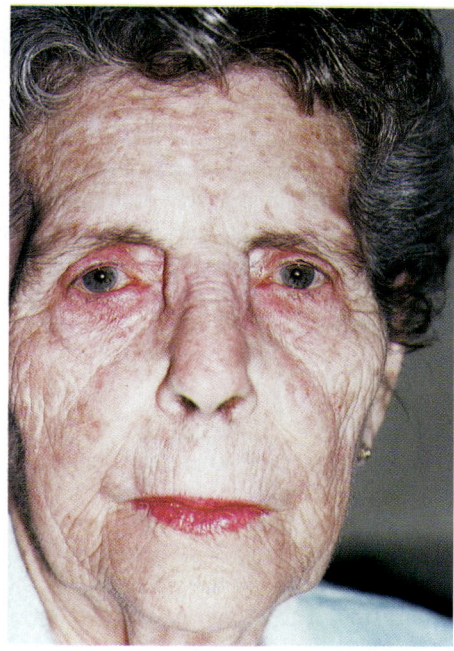

FIG. 12. Elderly woman with an impact tumor with esthesioneuroblastoma and squamous cell carcinoma that has eroded the nasal bones and expanded the overlying skin.

The nasal obstruction may be entirely painless and, if extending far anteriorly, not necessarily accompanied by nasal drainage. The mass may produce an external deformity. This deformity may be simply a mechanical swelling caused by displacement of soft tissue (Fig. 11) or erosion through the nasal bones with expansion of the overlying skin (Fig. 12). The symptom of anosmia usually accompanies the obstruction.

Epistaxis is the most common presenting symptom of nasal and paranasal sinus carcinoma. It may be intermittent and scant in amount, or massive and necessitate packing and hospitalization (Fig. 13). If scant, it usually is unilateral, but

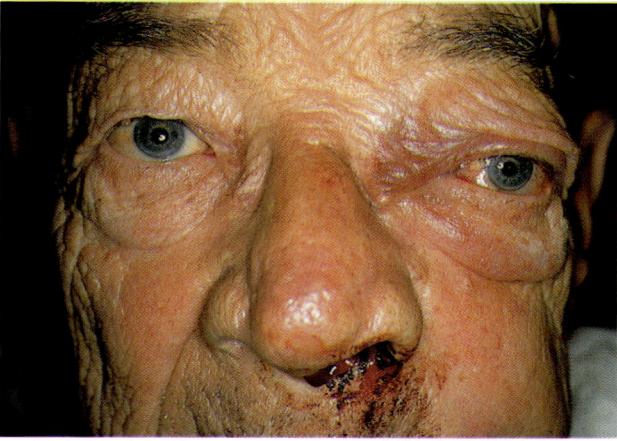

FIG. 13. Elderly man with a massive ethmoid carcinoma protruding from nostril and displacing the right eye, admitted for profuse epistaxis. Note displacement of globe.

if bilateral but still bleeding in small amounts, an extensive tumor penetrating the nasal septum would be suspected. Heavy bleeds are often bilateral and do not help in the diagnosis of sidedness of tumor. Foul smell often accompanies any epistaxis, but this symptom may arise from tumor necrosis or sinus obstruction with secondary purulent sinusitis. Indeed, the fever, facial pain, purulent drainage, and nasal obstruction may lead the unwary physician to a diagnosis of sinusitis, unmindful of the possible presenting obstruction by tumor. A careful nasal examination often reveals the presence of the obturating neoplasm.

Maxillary Sinus

Tumors of the maxillary sinus can present in multiple ways, depending on the wall of penetration. If the sinus is envisioned as a six-sided box, transgression of each wall presents with a distinctive array of symptoms (Fig. 14). Based on this paradigm, invasion of the sinus floor produces loosening or protrusion of teeth and palatal swelling (Fig. 15). Further extension may produce an ulcerating mass (Fig. 16). Teeth may be painful or numb. Similarly, the palate and gum may be hypesthetic or anesthetic. An ill-fitting denture is a common complaint in the edentulous patient. Invasion of the anterior wall of the sinus "box" leads to cheek swelling (Fig. 17) and, when more advanced, overlying skin ulceration

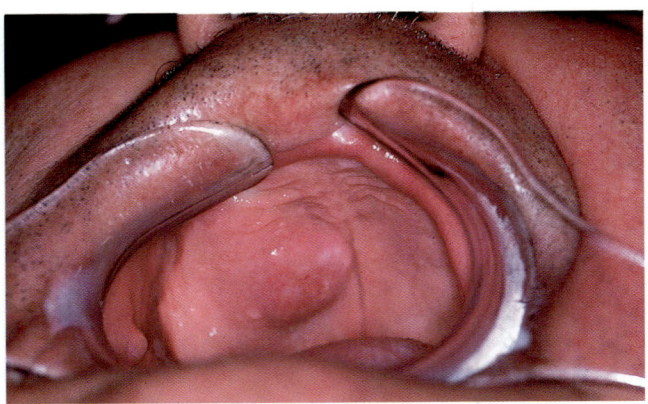

FIG. 15. Palatal swelling from squamous carcinoma of maxillary sinus.

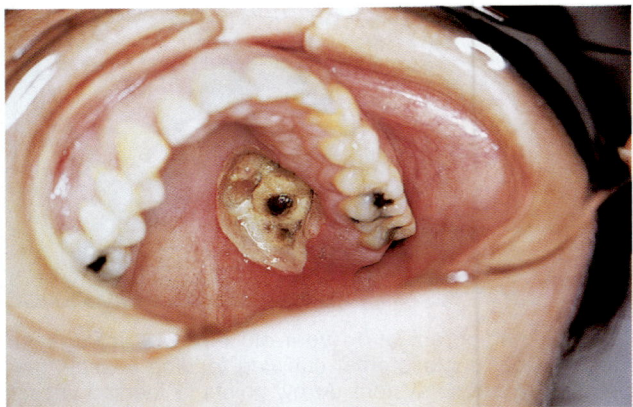

FIG. 16. Adenoid cystic carcinoma with ulceration of palate.

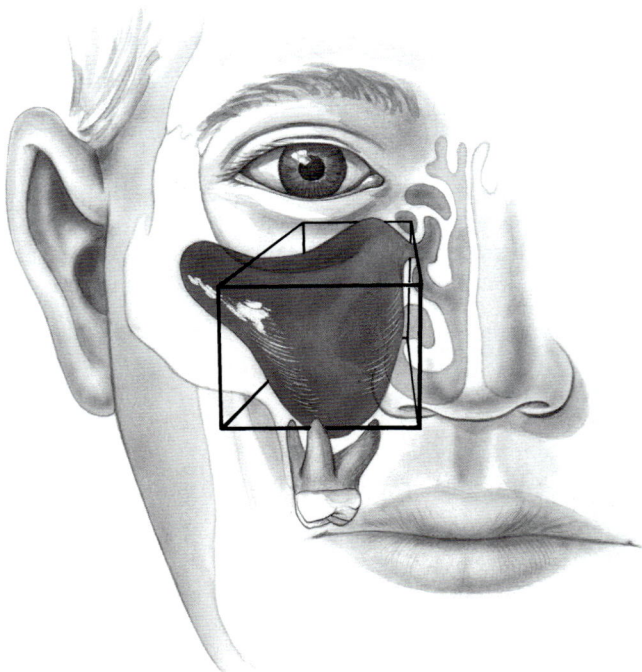

FIG. 14. Maxillary sinus with superimposed six-sided box paradigm. (From Donald PJ. Diagnosis of tumors of the paranasal sinuses and nasal cavity. In: Thawley SE, Panje WR, eds. *Comprehensive management of head and neck tumors.* Philadelphia: WB Saunders, 1987:304–326, with permission.)

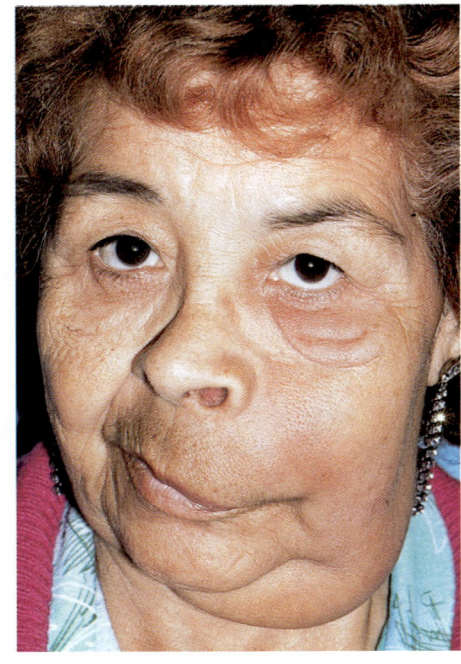

FIG. 17. Massive cheek swelling secondary to large tumor of the maxillary sinus.

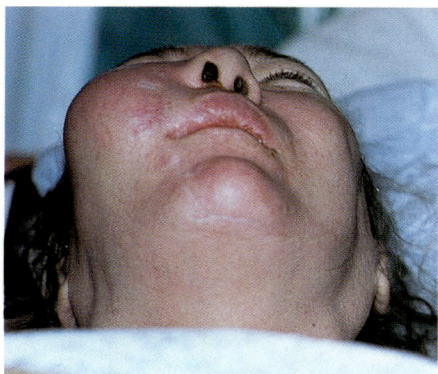

FIG. 18. Elderly woman with bulging and erythema of skin secondary to invasion from large squamous cell carcinoma of the maxillary antrum invading the skull base.

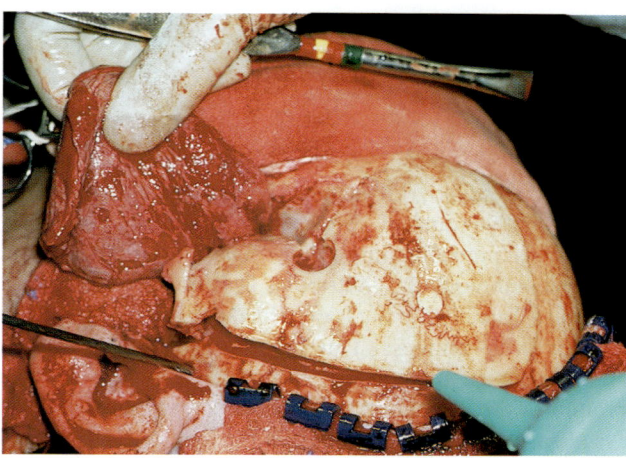

FIG. 20. Same patient as in Fig. 19. Tumor penetration through the lateral maxillary wall reaches the infratemporal fossa and from there to the foramen ovale. Again, no tumor seen at these sites in scans.

(Fig. 18). The proximity of the infraorbital nerve can lead to cheek anesthesia by direct invasion. Often this may be the single presenting symptom (Fig. 19). Lateral invasion of the sinus is often asymptomatic in the early stages. Then, as the infratemporal fossa is invaded, the patient complains of trismus when the muscles of mastication are invaded, especially the pterygoids and the insertions of the temporalis. Invasion of the mandibular division of the trigeminal nerve produces deep-seated pain in the fossa and numbness anterior to the ear and the scalp above through compromise of the auricular–temporal nerve (Fig. 20). Posterior wall penetration is another sign of an advanced lesion. Invasion of the pterygoid muscle origins produces trismus and involvement of the maxillary nerve, resulting in mid-facial pain and numbness.

Dry eye results from spread to the lacrimal nerve or the sphenopalatine ganglion; it is rarely complained of because concern is diverted by the severity of the other symptoms.

The final wall in the box paradigm is the roof, which comprises the orbital floor and medially is a part of the floor of the ethmoid labyrinth. Involvement of the orbit produces orbital displacement superiorly, proptosis, eye pain, diplopia, and painful movement of the eye (Fig. 21). The periorbita is quite resistant to tumor penetration and often the apex of the orbit is more involved than the anterior part, especially if tumor penetrates the posterior sinus wall as well as the roof. Diminished visual acuity, chemosis, and ocular motility disturbance imply penetration of periorbita and a poor prognosis for ocular sparing during subsequent surgery. Epiphora is the result of invasion of the lacrimal sac or nasal lacrimal duct. Sudden blindness is very uncommon and usually is the result of vascular occlusion rather than direct nerve invasion.

The intracranial invasive route of maxillary sinus cancers progresses through the ethmoid sinuses into the anterior cra-

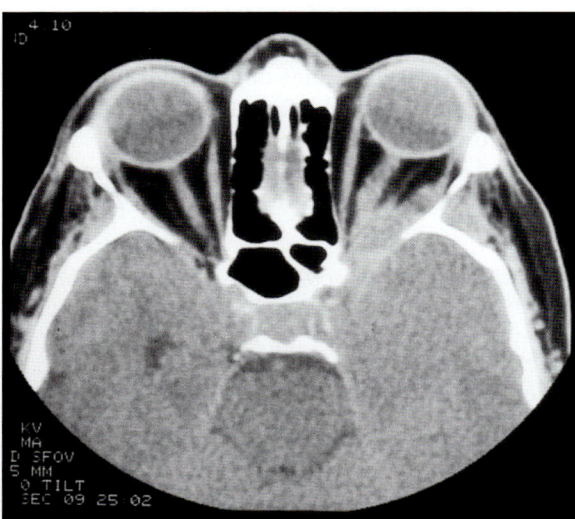

FIG. 19. Axial computed tomography scan of middle-aged woman with an adenoid cystic carcinoma of nasal septum, ethmoid sinuses, and orbital apex that invaded the infraorbital nerve and that was not apparent on scans. Patient presented with the solitary symptom of cheek numbness for 1 year.

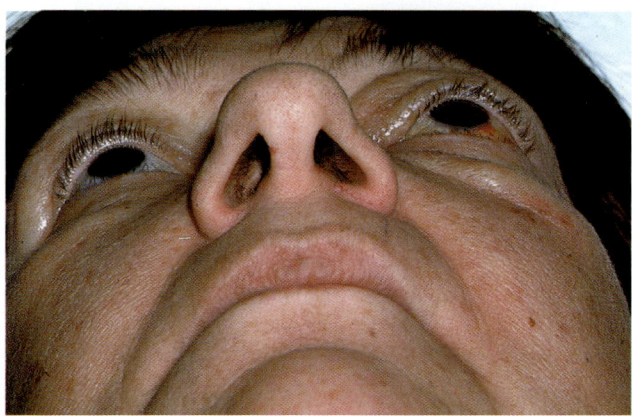

FIG. 21. Orbital displacement of maxillary carcinoma.

nial fossa, or from the pterygomaxillary space and the infratemporal fossa into the middle cranial fossa.

Ethmoid Sinus

The ethmoid labyrinth can be the *de novo* site of origin of tumors or the route of spread from maxillary sinus neoplasms (see preceding discussion). The roof of the ethmoid, the fovea ethmoidalis, contributes significantly to the anterior fossa floor. This bone is exceeded only by the lamina papyracea in its thinness. This latter bony component comprises much of the medial wall of the orbit, and orbital symptoms are common in tumors affecting this sinus. The eye is pushed laterally and out (see Fig. 13), but if the frontal sinus is also invaded, the eye may be displaced laterally and inferiorly. The ethmoid tumor, rather than invading the frontal sinus *per se*, often ends up obstructing the nasofrontal duct, producing an expanding mucocele. The mucocele, with its own distinctive bone-eroding characteristics (1), penetrates the orbital roof, displacing the globe downward and outward (Fig. 22). This is almost never accompanied by diplopia. Diplopia usually results from invasion of ocular muscles or their innervation. The exception is the rapidly growing neoplasm that produces marked displacement in a short time.

Epistaxis and foul nasal drainage are common. Pain in or behind the eye or in the bridge of the nose may be present and is often confused with ethmoid sinusitis.

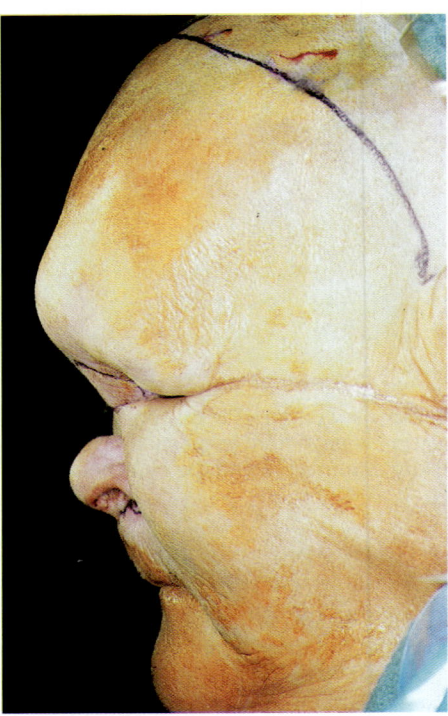

FIG. 23. Tumor of frontal sinus creating a bulge of the overlying skin. Coronal incision marked out for craniotomy portion of excision.

Frontal Sinus

Malignancies involving the frontal sinus are rare. Frontal and ethmoid mucoceles and mucopyoceles are much more prevalent and can result from ductal obstruction by benign or malignant tumors, as already mentioned. Extensive ethmoid tumors invading the frontal sinus are much more common than those lesions beginning as frontal sinus primaries. The tumors of this sinus have three direct routes of spread: anteriorly to the forehead skin, inferiorly into the orbit and nose, and posteriorly into the anterior cranial fossa.

Forehead extension is appreciated as a mass lesion bulging the soft tissues of the forehead (Fig. 23). Orbital in-

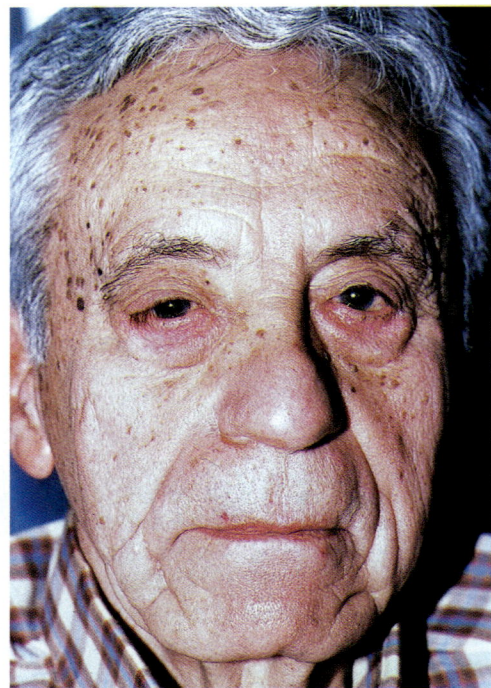

FIG. 22. Frontal sinus mucopyocele secondary to obstruction from inverting papilloma with intracranial penetration displacing globe downward and outward.

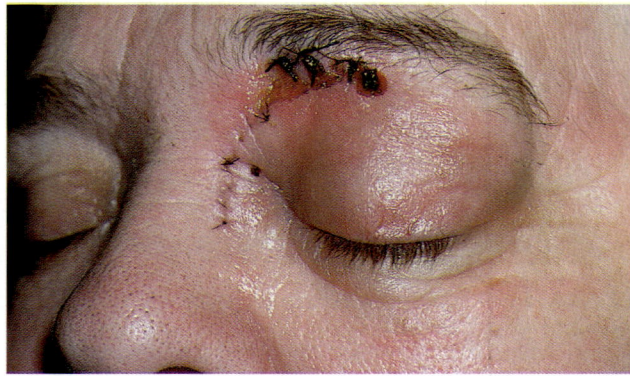

FIG. 24. Elderly woman with a frontal sinus squamous cell penetrating the upper eyelid.

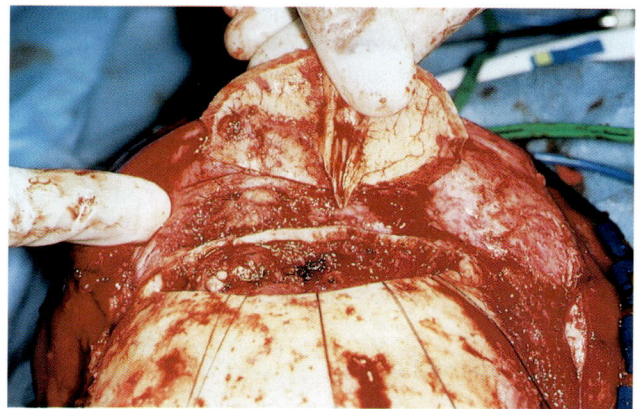

FIG. 25. Intraoperative photograph of same patient as in Fig. 24, showing penetration of the posterior frontal sinus wall and extensive involvement of anterior fossa dura.

vasion not only produces the downward and outward displacement already described, but tumor may penetrate the eyelid, producing an exophytic ulceration (Fig. 24). Posterior invasion penetrates the thin bone of the wall and infiltrates the adjacent dura (Fig. 25). Penetration to the frontal lobe of the brain or occlusion of the superior sagittal sinus is extremely rare (see Chapter 4).

Forehead and retroorbital pain are common symptoms. Numbness over the forehead indicates invasion of the supraorbital, supratrochlear, or frontal nerves.

Sphenoid Sinus

Slightly less rare than frontal sinus malignancies are primaries of the sphenoid sinus. Like the frontal sinus, the sphenoid is a common site of spread for malignancies from other sites. The posterior ethmoid sinuses, the maxillary sinuses (advanced tumors with posterior penetration; Fig. 26), and the nasopharynx are the usual primary sites. Pituitary tumors, lesions of the cavernous sinus, and clival tumors can spread to the sinus.

Sphenoid sinus mucoceles and mucopyoceles are often radiographically indistinguishable from solid tumors (Fig. 27). Symptoms are also similar, with headache, retroorbital pain, diplopia, and diminished vision the common presentations of both types of lesions. The characteristic sign of tumor, bone erosion, is not uncommon with chronic infections at this site.

Nasal examination, even aided by endoscopic inspection, may not reveal the presence of tumor. If the anterior wall has been breached and the sphenoethmoid recess entered, the endoscope will provide a view of the neoplasm.

The most common route of direct tumor spread is laterally into the cavernous sinus. In a capacious sinus, spread may be into the middle cranial fossa after crossing the orbital apex (Fig. 28; see also Chapter 4). It is curious that so few tumors breach the flimsy bone of the sella and invade the pituitary. The author has yet to see a patient with an advanced malignant tumor of the sphenoid sinus presenting with hypopituitarism.

Posterior wall penetration provides access to the posterior cranial fossa. The tough periosteum of the cranial side of the clivus interposes a strong barrier to further tumor penetration.

Central Invasion

Tumors of the nose and paranasal sinuses can directly invade any of the three cranial fossa floors. Often, intracranial invasion is entirely asymptomatic. A generalized headache, and especially one directed to a fossa of potential involvement, should alert the physician to intracranial spread and dural involvement. Increased intracranial pressure due to mass effect causes headache as well. This is uncommon and

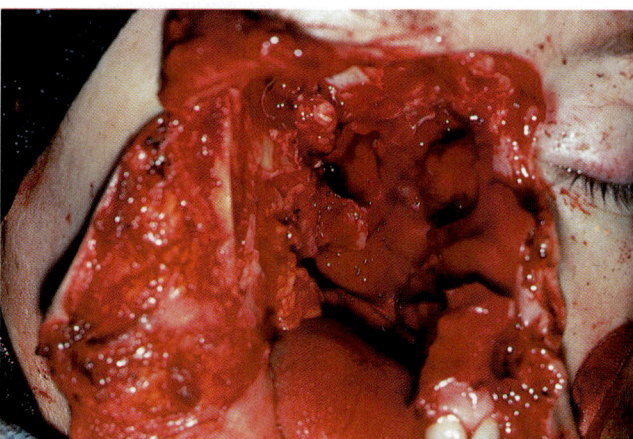

FIG. 26. Intraoperative photograph of young woman with squamous cell carcinoma of the maxillary sinus eroding the posterior sinus wall and involving the sphenoid sinus lateral wall.

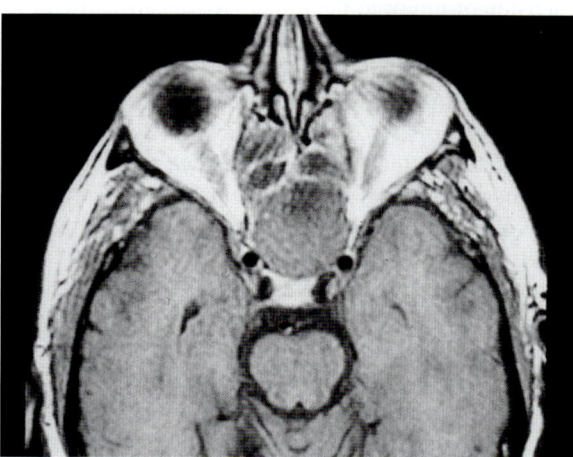

FIG. 27. Axial magnetic resonance image showing mass lesion filling the sphenoid sinus with extensive bone erosion. Distinction between mature mucopyocele and tumor cannot be made.

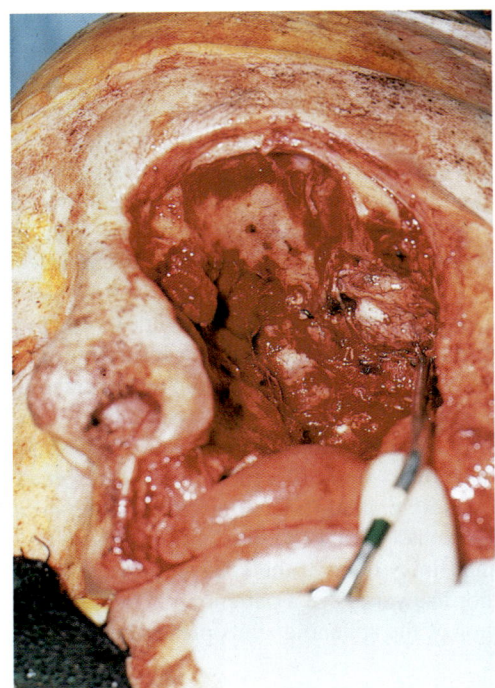

FIG. 28. Intraoperative photograph of patient with extensive maxillary, ethmoid, and sphenoid sinus carcinoma extending across the orbital apex and reaching into the middle cranial fossa and invading the temporal lobe.

usually means the tumor has breached the dura and invaded the brain.

Primary nasal and ethmoid tumors can invade the cribriform plate, and esthesioneuroblastomas usually take origin there. Erosion may cause a cerebrospinal fluid (CSF) leak, but this is extremely uncommon. Anosmia is common, but often secondary to nasal obstruction rather than invasion of the olfactory bulbs. Frontal lobe areas, being "silent," produce few to no symptoms if invaded.

Extension of tumor to the middle fossa is usually through the foramen ovale, the superior orbital fissure, the optic canal, the foramen rotundum, or the lateral wall of the sphenoid sinus. Tumor through the foramen ovale invades Meckel's cave and, if malignant, infiltrates the gasserian ganglion. Cancers that initially presented with mandibular nerve symptomatology then produce numbness and tingling over the cheek (maxillary branch) or forehead and eyelid (ophthalmic branch).

Foramen rotundum invasion compromises the maxillary nerve, producing the symptoms described previously. Rarely, the vidian canal is involved, and may be manifested by a dry eye due to compromise of the nerve of the pterygoid canal. Patients uncommonly complain of this symptom.

Superior orbital fissure invasion presents symptoms indistinguishable from those of cavernous sinus involvement. Careful inquiry may pick up an isolated III or IV nerve palsy. Isolated lateral rectus palsies can occur as tumors erode through the lateral sphenoid sinus wall into the cavernous sinus, picking off the nerve as it courses in the medial aspect of this venous sinus. Temporal lobe invasion is usually anterior, uncommonly seen, and most often asymptomatic. More advanced extension can produce seizures and even speech disturbance.

Erosion of the posterior wall of the sphenoid sinus can produce invasion of dura and a spontaneous CSF leak (see Chapter 26, Fig. 24). Superior spread can invade the optic nerves, creating a bitemporal homonomous hemianopsia or blindness. This is an extremely rare symptom.

Ear and Temporal Bone

The clinical presentations of the various neoplasms are well covered in the chapters devoted to lesions of the ear and temporal bone, especially those in Section IV, Midline Approaches. Malignancies of the pinna, retroauricular skin, and preauricular area that invade the skull base are tumors of substance. They are usually exophytic and deeply ulcerative (Fig. 29). They are painful, weeping (sometimes exuding a mixture of serum and CSF), prone to bleed with minor trauma, and unsightly. Some neglected lesions even present crawling with maggots (Fig. 30). Such tumors are so unsightly that one wonders why these patients would endure such an array of symptoms before visiting a physician. Often what brings these people in is the sudden onset of facial paralysis (Fig. 31). This is usually complete, but a careful topographic localization should be made regarding the extension of tumor to the geniculate ganglion with the production of dry eye.

Hearing loss is common and may be simply a conductive loss brought about by obstruction of the external auditory canal by the bulk of the tumor, ossicular erosion, or the dampening of ossicular movement by the presence of tumor

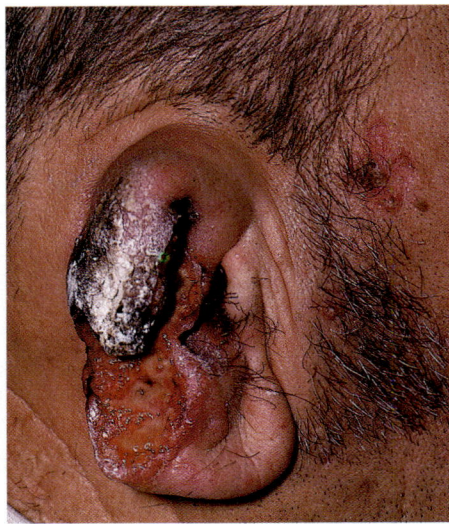

FIG. 29. Large squamous cell carcinoma beginning in skin of auricle.

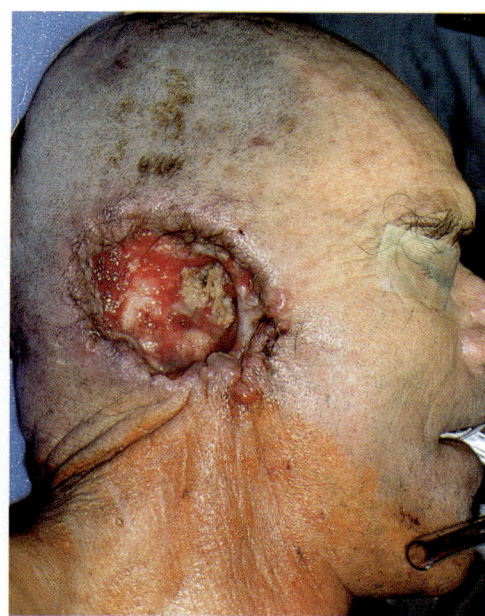

FIG. 30. Squamous cell carcinoma of the pinna in a reclusive middle-aged man. Tumor extended intracranially and into cervical muscles. Lesion was crawling with maggots at the time of presentation.

in the middle ear cleft. Erosion of the cochlea or invasion of the internal acoustic canal produces a sensorineural deafness. Involvement of the labyrinth produces vertigo. With malignancies involving the ear, this is unusual. In acoustic tumors, it is an important symptom, as is hearing loss, which

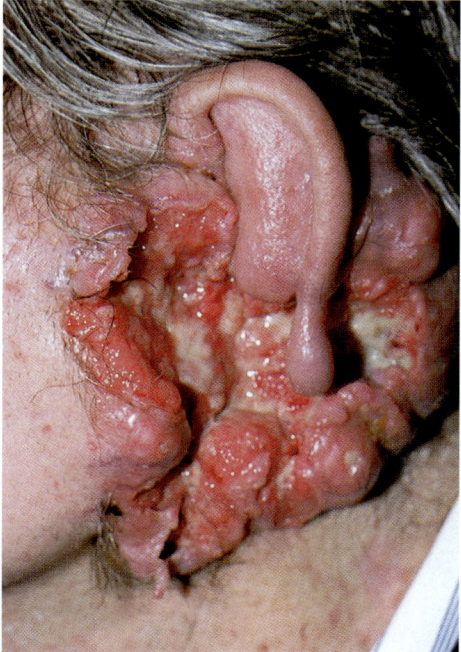

FIG. 31. Elderly man with a 10-year history of a basal cell carcinoma of the pinna who did not present until lesion caused a facial nerve paralysis.

is thoroughly covered in Chapter 23. Although true vertigo is uncommon, disequilibrium and a feeling of fullness and pressure are produced by tumor in the external auditory canal or middle ear and mastoid.

Erosion of tumor into the temporomandibular joint produces trismus. Auriculotemporal nerve involvement brings on numbness anterior to the ear and in the scalp above. If widespread in the occipital scalp, tumor invasion of the occipital nerve produces numbness from the nuchal line to the vertex. Tumor extension through the fissures of Santorini of the cartilaginous external auditory canal to the parotid gland often brings about facial nerve branch weakness, then branch paralysis, and finally paralysis of the main division of the entire nerve.

Spread of tumor to the jugular bulb may produce weakness or paralysis of cranial nerves IX, X, and XI with dysphagia, hoarseness, and shoulder weakness. Thrombosis of the jugular vein and sigmoid sinus is usually asymptomatic.

Nasopharynx

Nasopharyngeal lesions may begin in the mucosa, as in the case of nasopharyngeal carcinoma, or in the bone, as in chordoma. The most common benign tumor in the nasopharynx is juvenile nasopharyngeal angiofibroma, and squamous cell carcinoma is the most common of the malignant tumors. Masses in the nasopharynx obstruct nasal breathing and either obtund or impede the function of the eustachian tube. Angiofibromas tend to block the tube and the malignancies invade it. Next to the symptom of a mass in the neck, hearing loss from serous otitis media is the second most common presenting complaint of nasopharyngeal carcinoma. Rhinorrhea due to the lack of mucus clearance and epistaxis may be present, especially in angiofibroma. Bleeding from nasopharyngeal cancer is uncommon and usually runs down the back of the throat. Epistaxis from angiofibroma varies in severity from minor to catastrophic. Chordoma, chondromas, and chondrosarcomas of the clivus rarely protrude so far into the nasopharynx to produce this symptom.

Nasopharyngeal carcinoma has two avenues of direct access to the intracranial cavity: the foramen ovale and the foramen lacerum. The latter is close to the nasopharynx anterolaterally. The tumor penetrates the cartilage plug at the inferior end, then travels along the artery as it exits the temporal bone and enters the cavernous sinus (Fig. 32). In doing so, it invades the abducens nerve, producing a lateral rectus palsy—the third most common initial symptom of nasopharyngeal carcinoma. Moreover, the tumor may travel along the path of the internal carotid in its horizontal course through the petrosa. The mode of entry up the foramen ovale occurs as the tumor spreads laterally from the nasopharyngeal vault through the foramen of Morgagni from the fossa of Rosenmüller, then along the cartilaginous tube on the undersurface of the temporal bone. On reaching the foramen ovale, which is nearby, the tumor travels to Meckel's cave along the mandibular branch of cranial nerve V. Lower facial

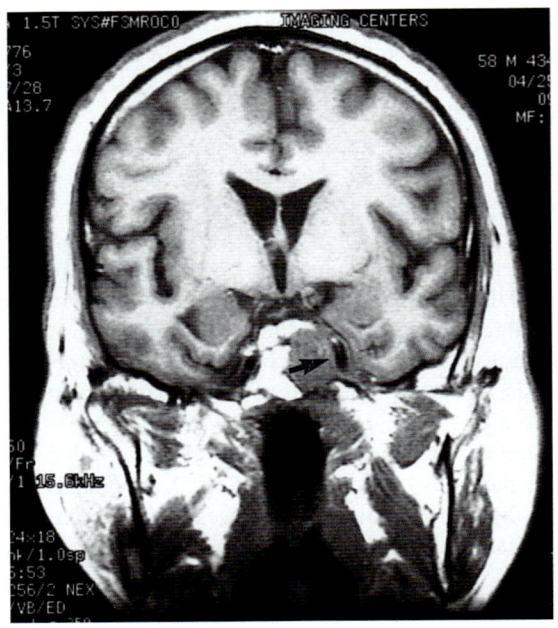

FIG. 32. Magnetic resonance image of middle-aged man with adenoid cystic carcinoma of the nasopharynx that invaded the foramen lacerum, then followed the intrapetrous and intracavernous course of the internal carotid artery. Arrow points to internal carotid artery surrounded by tumor.

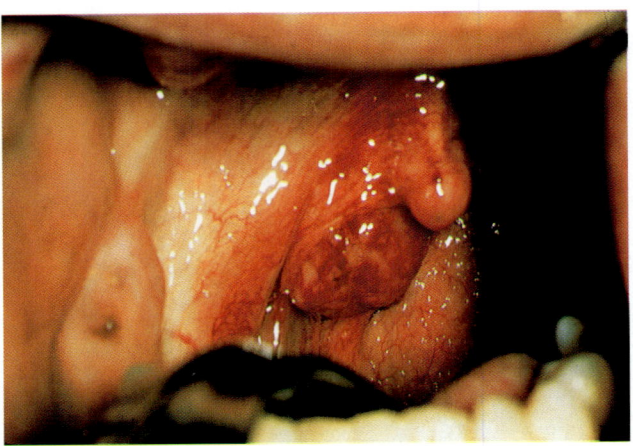

FIG. 33. Nasopharyngeal carcinoma prolapsing below the level of the right soft palate.

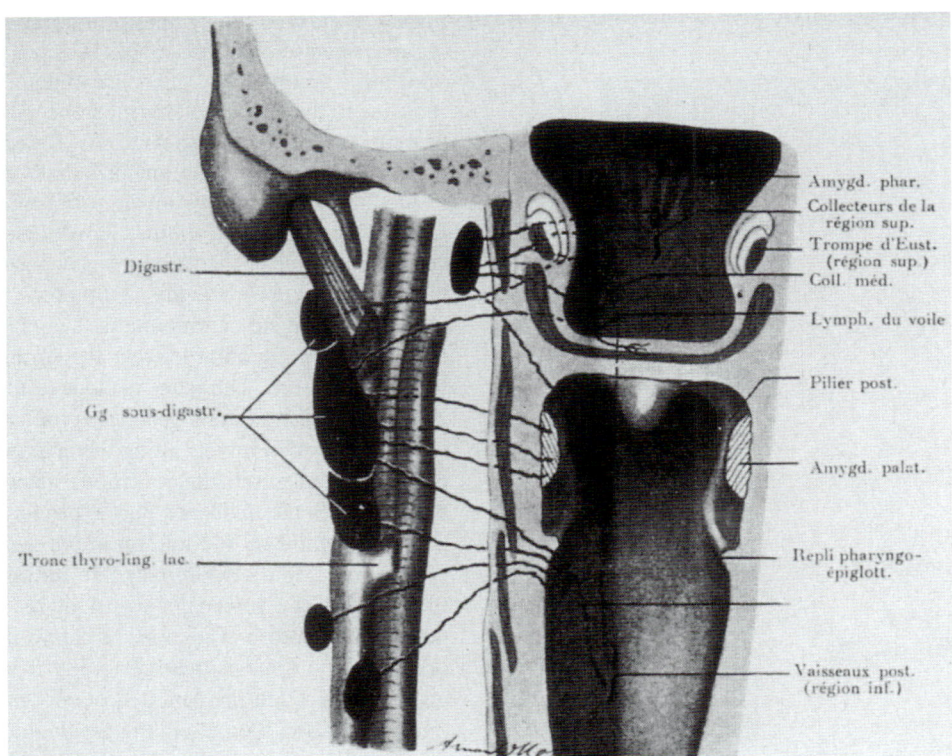

FIG. 34. The node of Rouviére adjacent to the jugular foramen. (From Rouviére H. *Anatomie des lymphatiques*. Libraries de l'académie de Médecine. Paris: Masson, 1932:109, with permission.)

hypesthesia, deep infratemporal pain, and masticatory weakness or trismus result.

Indirect visualization of the nasopharynx with a mirror or directly by endoscopy reveals the tumor. Occasionally the tumor is seen bulging the palate or prolapsing into the oropharynx (Fig. 33). Lesions primary to clival bone rarely produce symptoms of nasopharyngeal dysfunction. Posterior neck pain, pain over the mastoid tip, neck stiffness, and then signs of cord and brainstem compression, if the tumor begins to encroach on the brainstem and cord, may result. Symptoms of central involvement are described in detail in Chapters 22 and 26.

Oropharynx, Parotid Gland, and Upper Neck

These three entities are described together because the mode of spread of cancer to the intracranial compartment is so similar. The common route is through the infratemporal fossa and through the foramen ovale and even foramen spinosum. Superficial lobe parotid tumors and especially deep lobe malignancies invade through the foramen spinosum along the facial nerve. Oropharyngeal primaries, most commonly from the tonsillar area, tend to invade deeply through the superior constrictor muscle to the medial pterygoid and the inferior alveolar nerve as it enters the mandible. Neurotropic tumors by perineural spread make their retrograde course through the foramen ovale. Such invasion and spread to the pterygoid muscles cause trismus. Such spread may begin as distantly as the alveolar ridge or lip, extend to the mental nerve, make its way up the inferior alveolar to the mandibular branch of the trigeminal, and traverse the foramen ovale (see Chapter 15, Fig. 34).

Similar spread is seen with high cervical lymph nodes as they extend superiorly. Spread to the jugular foramen is not uncommon, producing IX, X, and XI nerve symptoms (the so-called "jugular foramen syndrome") and not infrequently symptoms from cranial nerve XII as it exits the hypoglossal canal close by. This is a particular peculiarity of lymph nodal metastasis from the nasopharynx to the node of Rouviére, which is the highest retropharyngeal lymph node in the neck (Fig. 34). Symptoms from the metastasis may precede any from the primary tumor.

THE INTERVIEW

Much of the process of patient intake and the patient's subsequent hospital course is covered in detail in Chapter 8. It is probably prudent quickly to review the usual procedure that the typical patient with a skull base lesion goes through during the first visits to the host of consultants comprising the cranial base team.

The patient is often apprehensive, having frequently undergone multiple therapies and considered by many previous consultants to be inoperable and incurable. This is particularly germane to the head and neck oncologic patient who has usually already undergone chemotherapy, radiation therapy, and surgery. This also applies to the neurosurgical patient who may have undergone multiple less-than-complete operations (e.g., for meningioma or chordoma) and now has neurologic compromise as a result of regrowth of residual neoplasm.

A thorough history and complete examination then ensue, including a thorough head and neck and complete neurologic assessment. Meticulous examination of all cranial nerves is especially important.

A careful review of past medical records, operative reports, radiographs, and special tests is conducted, which does not always entirely agree with the referring physician's verbally presented summary that preceded the consultation. Attention is specifically directed toward the pathology report, and histologic slides should be reviewed by the designated skull base pathologist to confirm the accuracy of diagnosis. Similarly, the outside films are reviewed by the team neuroradiologist and the appropriateness of further studies is determined.

At the conclusion of the history and physical examination, the examining physician makes a tentative assessment of the case and the possibilities for subsequent treatment. Sometimes, a definitive statement regarding the nature of approach and degree of resection can be done at this first visit, but most often these decisions are contingent to some degree on the findings of more refined testing and therefore delayed until these results are in.

For those patients who are treatable, either by surgery alone or in combination with adjunctive measures (which make up the vast majority of those seen), there is often a great sense of relief in the patient and family. To be suddenly reassigned from the ranks of the hopelessly incurable to the status of possibly or probably resectable is a source of enormous joy. Soon after, the appreciation of the compromise of some functions and the possibility of complications integral to the proposed surgery serves to dampen some of this initial enthusiasm. It is essential for the surgeon realistically and dispassionately to detail to the patient and family the key elements of surgery, the risks, the potential benefits, and the possible complications. Most patients wish a complete explanation of all the facts surrounding the surgery and its consequences. Realistic expectations must be transmitted to the patient, but, when appropriate, should be suffused with an air of optimism. Undue dwelling on the possible complications (although it is essential to outline them sufficiently) only adds to the fear and apprehension from which the patient already suffers. Morbid preoccupation with these details for the sake of a sense of medicolegal security for the physician can do enormous harm to the confidence and sense of well-being in a patient already committed to surgery. In our modern, litigious society, this is a very difficult element to manage. The message is that adequate but not necessarily excessive information be transmitted to the patient and family.

Next comes the time for questions. Often, during the first visit, this takes as long as the assessment. Posing the questions does much to dissipate the anxiety built up during the physician's explanation phase. Sometimes the content of the question is of marginal relevance. The ventilating process is, however, of great benefit to the patient. The physician's answer is most beneficial when it is couched in a sympathetic and friendly tone and given in language the patient can understand. A hard, clinical, detached demeanor simply aggravates the apprehension and does little to dispel the patient's fear. The questioning also provides the physician with an opportunity to judge how realistic the patient is about his or her disease and therapeutic expectations.

One of the principal issues often raised is that of quality of life. Many times, the question arises without a clear understanding of its implications. Especially for the cancer patient, an understanding that the current day they are experiencing will probably be the best day of the rest of their life if further treatment is withheld brings a perspective that usually has not occurred to them. Predicted deficits of function and appearance must be weighed against the prospect of a deforming, agonizing, painful death from cancer.

This interview is only the first step in the total assessment of the patient. All the consultants involved in the patient's care participate in the process.

The essential role of the skull base surgery team coordinator now comes into play. The coordinator orchestrates all the consultations with the various members of the surgical team, schedules computed tomography, magnetic resonance imaging, positron emission tomography, and angiography, obtains outside radiographs and pathology specimens, and schedules and coordinates the skull base surgery team pretreatment conference. The coordinator forms an important connection with the medical insurance companies and even, at times, arranges accommodations for patients' families.

TABLE 1. *Skull base surgery team members*

Head and neck surgeon
Neurologic surgeon
Otologist/neurotologist
Plastic surgeon
Neuroradiologist
Pathologist
Ophthalmologist
Skull base surgery operating room nurse coordinator
Skull base surgery clinical coordinator
Head and neck oncologic clinical nurse specialist

All the various team members (Table 1) contribute valuable input to the management of these difficult and complex patients. The conference provides a forum for free discussion and, once all input is considered, the final formulation of the operational plan for definitive treatment.

The patient is now ready for surgical treatment. A final meeting with the intake physician, who is usually either a head and neck, plastic, or neurosurgeon, provides an opportunity for final questions and the signing of the consent form.

Constant contact with the patient and family before and during surgery and in the recovery phase provides the continuity they require through this difficult ordeal.

REFERENCE

1. Fenton WH Jr, Donald PJ, Carlton W III. Pressure exerted by mucoceles in the frontal sinus: an experimental study in the cat. *Arch Otolaryngol Head Neck Surg* 1990;116:836–840.

CHAPTER 6

Imaging of the Skull Base

Alfred L. Weber and Hugh D. Curtin

The skull base represents a bony partition between the intracranial cavity and facial structures, including the orbits, nasal cavity, paranasal sinuses, and nasopharynx. Multiple foramina within the skull base and fissures transmit nerves and vessels that are also pathways for spread of disease processes.

Endoscopic inspection provides some information concerning lesions adjacent to the skull base, but involvement of the skull base can be assessed only by radiologic means, principally by computed tomography (CT) and magnetic resonance imaging (MRI) (1,2).

Imaging characteristics are important in the preoperative assessment of anatomic location and extent of skull base lesions. Especially with the advent of newer skull base surgical techniques, the lesion's precise location and definition of its extent and relationship to vascular structures and cranial nerves have assumed great importance (3,4).

This chapter summarizes the radiologic techniques and their indications for evaluation of the skull base, along with the most important findings of various lesions.

COMPUTED TOMOGRAPHY AND MAGNETIC RESONANCE IMAGING: TECHNIQUES AND GENERAL DIAGNOSTIC CRITERIA

Computed Tomography

Computed tomography is the method of choice for assessment of bony structures, foramina, fissures, and canals (carotid) and for evaluation of calcifications. Likewise, CT is optimal for assessment of the paranasal sinuses, nasal cavities, pharynx, and infiltrative orbital lesions. The examination is carried out using 3- to 5-mm axial and coronal sections with a bone and soft tissue window algorithm.

The disadvantages consist mainly of the inadequate display of the intracranial structures, such as dura, meninges, and brain. Furthermore, CT does not allow direct acquisition of sagittal images, which provide optimal demonstration of lesions in the sagittal and immediate parasagittal planes. These structures include the sella, clivus, foramen magnum, cribriform plate area, and nasopharynx. Reconstructed sagittal images (from 1- to 2-mm axial sections) may be applied in cases where MRI is unavailable. On CT, tumor is usually isodense with muscle, whereas secretions in an obstructed sinus cavity have low attenuation values (water density). However, secretions with a high protein content are isodense with muscle and cannot be differentiated from tumor. After the introduction of iodinated contrast material, the mucosal lining of a sinus cavity enhances, along with variable enhancement of tumor but no enhancement of secretions.

Magnetic Resonance Imaging

Magnetic resonance imaging has been the most important development in the assessment of skull base lesions. MRI superbly demonstrates the intracranial contents (dura, meninges, and brain), and lesion conspicuity is considerably improved after the introduction of gadolinium (gadopentetate meglumine).

The examination is performed in the axial, coronal, and sagittal planes with 3-mm sections. All signal intensities (T1- and T2-weighted, and proton-density images) are used for evaluation of the anatomy (T1-weighted images) and lesion characterization (T2-weighted images). Gadopentetate with fat suppression is mandatory for defining intracranial tumor extension and differentiation of cystic from solid lesions. Gradient-echo images and magnetic resonance angiography define the vascular anatomy in relation to tumors and cysts and may also depict hypervascularity of lesions (angiofibroma).

The cortical bone of the skull base is indicated by a signal void. Some bony structures have a medullary cavity, which contains fatty marrow and can be differentiated from the cortex by signal differences. The clivus has a fat-con-

---

A. L. Weber, H. D. Curtin: Department of Radiology, Harvard Medical School and Massachusetts Eye and Ear Infirmary, Boston, Massachusetts 02114.

taining marrow cavity that is characterized by high signal intensity on the T1-weighted images. Tumor is usually of intermediate signal intensity and obliterates the marrow spaces with replacement of the high-intensity fat. If invasion of the cortex is present, the signal void of the cortex is interrupted or irregular. If the bone marrow has not been replaced with fat, however, as in a young child, differentiation is more difficult.

Tumor can usually be separated from muscle and fat using a combination of short TR (relaxation time) and short TE (excitation time)(T1-weighted images), long TR and short TE (proton-density images), and long TR and long TE (T2-weighted images). The tumor usually has the same signal intensity as muscle on short TR sequences, but the long TR sequences differentiate the usually higher-intensity tumor from the medium-intensity muscle. If tumor invades fatty planes, the normal high–signal-intensity fat on the short TR sequences is obliterated by the more intermediate signal intensity of the tumor. This is relevant in the evaluation of the pterygoid fossa, parapharyngeal space adjacent to the base of the skull, and exit foramina of the cranial nerves (foramina rotundum, ovale, and spinosum, and the stylomastoid foramen), which all contain fatty tissue.

Perineural tumor spread obliterates the fat at the extracranial opening of the foramina (5,6). With the introduction of gadolinium, lesion detection and conspicuity are increased (7). Fat suppression techniques with contrast enhancement have been used to define tumor extent optimally in the region below the skull base (8,9). This perineural spread may originate from tumors arising in the nasopharynx, paranasal sinuses, face, orbit, palate, oral cavity, and other areas that receive branches from the trigeminal nerve. Carcinomas of the oral cavity with mandibular invasion spread along V3 to the foramen ovale, and carcinomas from the parotid extend to the stylomastoid foramen (6).

Invasion of the cavernous sinus is best evaluated with MRI (10). The cavernous sinus is composed of a tangle of small veins and venous sinusoids adjacent to the sella. The cavernous sinus is traversed by cranial nerves III, IV, and VI, and the V1 segment of the fifth nerve. Meckel's cave, which contains cerebrospinal fluid (CSF) and the gasserian ganglion of the fifth nerve, is posterior to the cavernous sinus and located at the lateral aspect of the petrous pyramid. Tumor can reach the cavernous sinus by direct extension or by spread along the nerves (nerve V most commonly) that traverse the sinus and Meckel's cave (11). If tumor reaches Meckel's cave, the high signal of the CSF on T2-weighted images is usually replaced.

Before gadolinium introduction, tumor may be difficult to delineate within the cavernous sinus because of signal characteristics similar to those of surrounding tissues. The tumor, after introduction of gadolinium and contrast enhancement, is characterized by a filling defect in the enhanced cavernous sinus. Tumor involvement may cause increased bowing of the lateral wall of the sinus, which is best seen on axial and coronal images. Tumor contiguous to Meckel's cave may compress the normal oval or triangular high-signal CSF space or completely obliterate Meckel's cave (10).

Carotid artery evaluation at the base of skull is an important consideration before surgical intervention. The carotid artery is well seen on conventional spin-echo sequences as a signal void passing through the skull base. With MRI, areas of contact between tumor and the carotid artery can be defined. Involvement of the carotid artery is indicated by narrowing of the lumen. Luminal narrowing may also indicate invasion of the arterial wall itself. For evaluation of bony details of the carotid canal and the adjacent petrous bone, however, CT is mandatory.

When tumor is located in the paranasal sinuses, the signal void of air is replaced by the most common intermediate signal intensity of the tumor (12). Inflammatory tissue and fluid can usually be optimally separated from the tumor margin with the T2-weighted image (13,14). Mucosal edema and fluid have a high signal intensity on the long TR sequences (T2-weighted image). Tumors may be relatively bright, but seldom is the intensity as pronounced as that of the secretions and edema in an obstructed sinus cavity.

Simple sinus obstruction with edema and retained fluid displays a low or intermediate signal intensity on T1- and a high signal on the T2-weighted images. If the protein content of secretions in the sinus cavity increases, the signal may be bright on both short and long TR images. However, if a further increase in protein occurs, with loss of water, a decrease in signal intensity occurs on the T1- and T2-weighted images (15,16). If this is pronounced, the viscous sinus secretions may mimic air in the sinus cavity. Hemorrhage as a concomitant finding in tumors has signal intensities characteristic for blood degradation products, usually reflected by high signal intensity on T1- and T2-weighted images from methemoglobin.

COMPUTED TOMOGRAPHY AND MAGNETIC RESONANCE IMAGING FINDINGS OF LESIONS OF THE SKULL BASE

The skull base can be divided into three anatomic areas: (a) the anterior skull base, which includes the floor of the anterior cranial fossa, including the orbital roofs, the cribriform region, and the roof of the ethmoid sinuses; (b) the central region, which includes the clivus, sella, planum sphenoidale, cavernous sinus, and, more laterally, the greater and lesser wings of the sphenoid bone; and (c) the posterior and posterolateral region, which is made up of the temporal bone, jugular fossa, and foramen magnum (17).

Location

Anterior Skull Base Lesions

A variety of different lesions are encountered in the anterior skull base (18) (Table 1). The various types of meningocele or meningoencephaloceles may occur in the frontal sinus, cribriform plate area, ethmoid sinuses, and sphenoid sinus (19) (Fig. 1), or extend laterally through the lamina pa-

TABLE 1. *Anterior skull base lesions*

Meningoencephaloceles
Mucoceles
Benign tumors and tumor-like conditions
   Polyps
   Inverted papilloma
   Langherhans' cell histiocytosis
   Giant cell granuloma
Malignant tumors from paranasal sinuses and nasal cavity
   Carcinomas
   Esthesioneuroblastoma
   Lymphoma
   Plasmacytoma
   Melanoma
   Malignant fibrous histiocytoma
   Sarcomas

pyracea into the orbit (20–22). More anteriorly, lesions extend into the upper nasal cavity or ethmoid sinuses. MRI is the method of choice in the analysis of these lesions (23,24).

These lesions reveal characteristic signal intensities that are displayed as CSF or brain; moreover, they can be traced from the paranasal sinuses and nasal cavity into the cranial cavity by way of bony defects. Evaluation of the presence and size of a bony defect is best accomplished with CT. Benign lesions, including mucoceles, of the sinonasal cavities can affect the skull base. Mucoceles of the frontal, ethmoid, and sphenoid sinuses may expand and extend intracranially (25). Rarely, nasal polyps have been reported to protrude

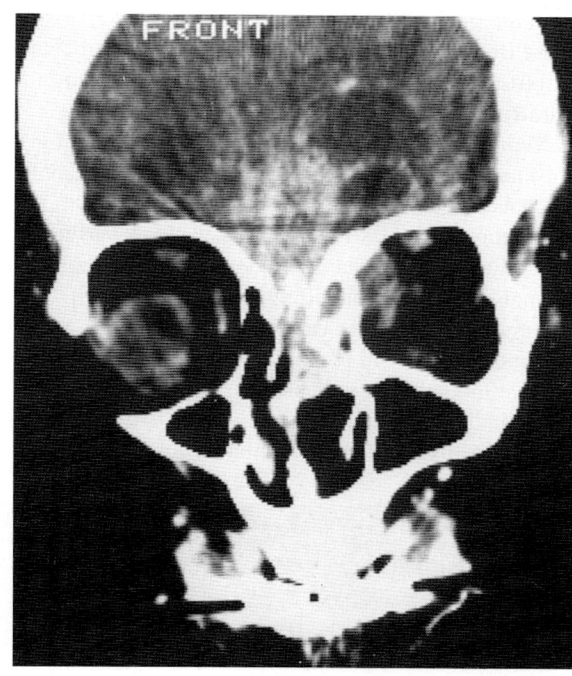

FIG. 2. Esthesioneuroblastoma of the upper nasal cavity and left ethmoid sinus with invasion of the left orbit and intracranial cavity. Coronal contrast-enhanced computed tomography scan through the mid-cribriform plate area demonstrates an enhancing mass in the upper nasal cavity and left ethmoid sinus with invasion of the left orbit and the intracranial cavity. The intracranial mass reveals moderate enhancement and cystic degeneration of tumor inferiorly and laterally on the left.

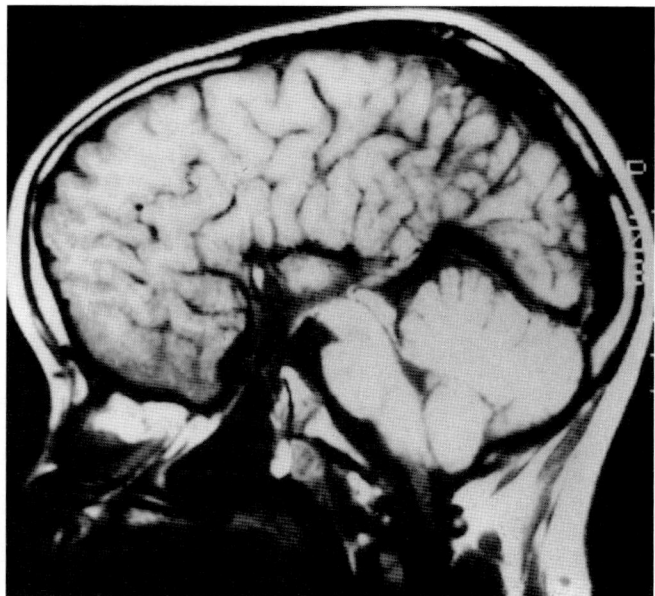
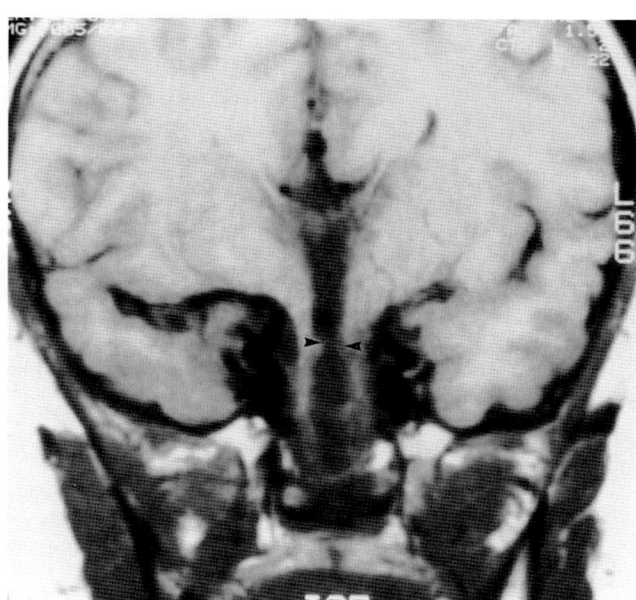

FIG. 1. Meningocele of the sella and sphenoid sinus with extension into the pharynx and posterior nasal cavity. **A:** Sagittal T1-weighted magnetic resonance image (MRI) demonstrates a sharply defined, low-intensity structure extending from the anterior–inferior third ventricle through the sella into the anterior nasopharynx and posterior left nasal cavity. The low signal intensity is consistent with cerebrospinal fluid. **B:** Coronal T1-weighted MRI shows the stalk of the meningocele connected to the floor of the third ventricle (*arrowheads*).

through the floor of the anterior cranial fossa (12,13). Osteomas and fibroosseous lesions may protrude into the anterior cranial fossa (most commonly from the frontal, ethmoid, and sphenoid sinuses) (26).

Malignant tumors arising in the sinuses, including nasal cavities and orbits, may extend into the anterior cranial cavity, such as carcinomas (80% of malignant sinus tumors), olfactory neuroblastomas (27,28) (Fig. 2), and various other, less common tumors, such as adenocarcinoma, plasmacytoma, melanoma, and rhabdomyosarcoma (12). MRI fails to differentiate between the various histopathologic subtypes. Most tumors are low in signal intensity on T1-weighted images, have moderate to increased signal intensity on the T2-weighted images, and enhance moderately to markedly on the T1-weighted images after gadolinium introduction (Fig. 3).

In some melanomas, the diagnosis may be suggested by bright signal on the T1-weighted image and low signal on the T2-weighted image. Tumor-like conditions, including Langerhans' cell histiocytosis and giant cell granuloma, may invade the skull base (29). They reveal low signal intensity on T1-weighted images and high signal intensity on T2-weighted images, and enhance intensely with contrast administration.

Extensions of mucoceles and benign and malignant lesions from the paranasal sinuses and nasal cavities into the anterior cranial fossa are best evaluated with MRI using coronal and sagittal images in conjunction with axial images and gadolinium administration (18) (Figs. 4, 5). Demonstration of the proximity of the tumor to the optic nerve or the optic canal is of considerable importance in the preoperative assessment.

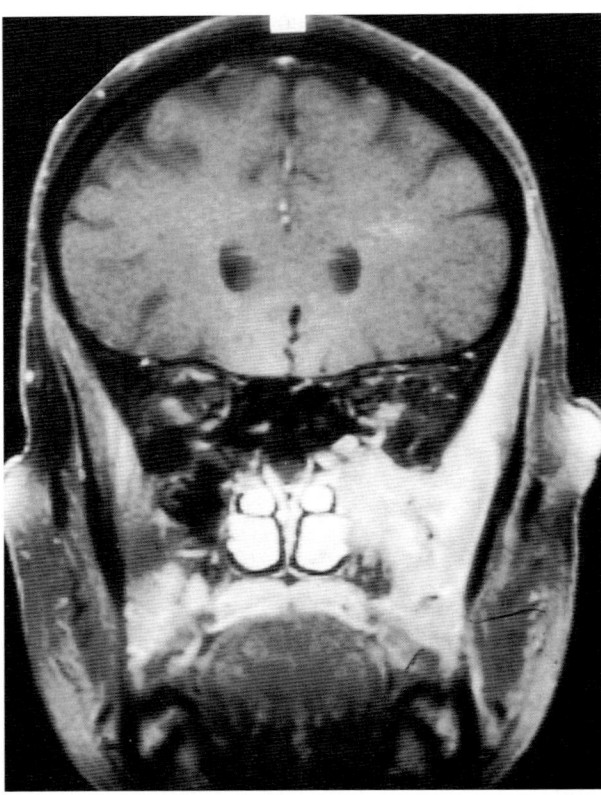
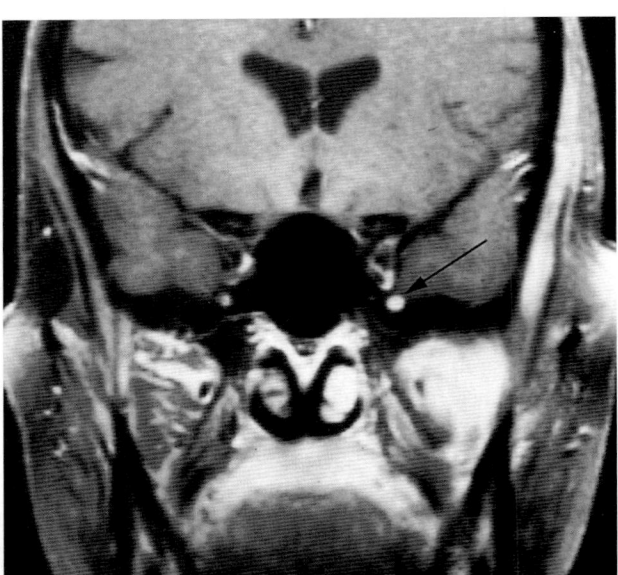
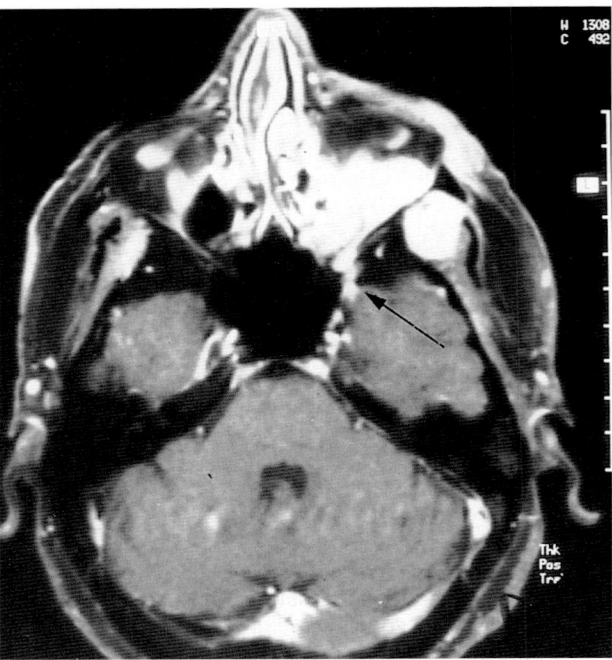

FIG. 3. Carcinoma of the antrum with perineural extension. **A:** Coronal T1-weighted magnetic resonance image (MRI) after contrast infusion shows a markedly enhancing tumor mass in the left maxillary antrum. **B:** Coronal postcontrast T1-weighted MRI demonstrates enhancing tumor in the left foremen rotundum (*arrow*). **C:** Postgadolinium axial T1-weighted MRI shows tumor in the maxillary nerve at the foramen rotundum (*arrow*). Also note enhancing tumor in the left maxillary antrum with extension into the area of the left pterygopalatine fossa.

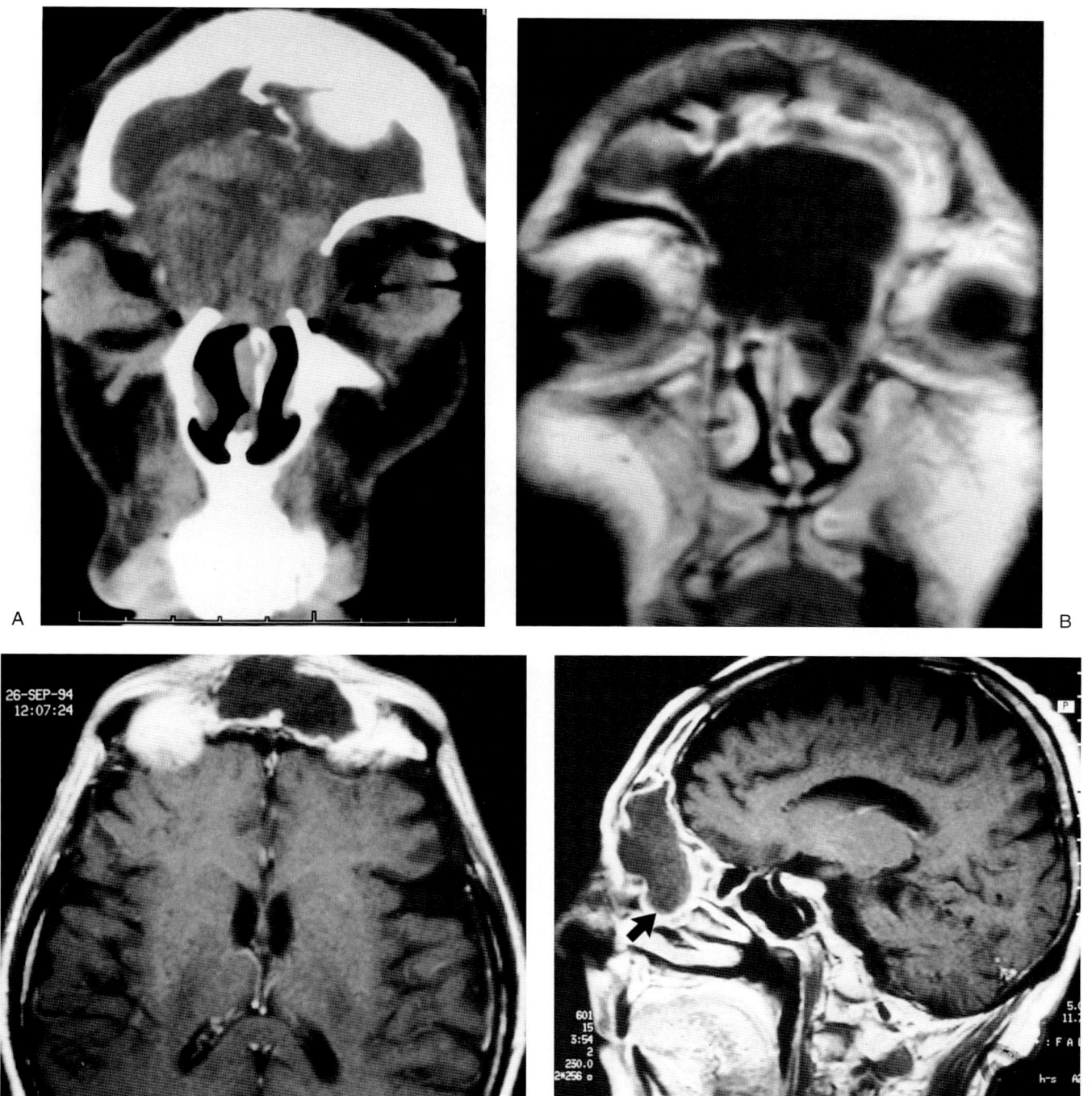

FIG. 4. Frontal sinus mucocele with intracranial extension. **A:** Coronal computed tomography scan through the anterior intracranial cavity reveals an isodense, slightly heterogeneous mass lesion in the upper nasal cavities and both ethmoid sinuses, with bulging into both orbits and the anterior intracranial cavity. There is the suggestion of slight linear calcification at the superior aspect of the mucocele. **B:** Postcontrast coronal T1-weighted magnetic resonance image (MRI) through the anterior cranial fossa shows the mucocele to be nonenhancing and of low signal intensity. **C:** Postcontrast axial T1-weighted MRI through the frontal sinus demonstrates a nonenhancing, fluid-filled mucocele. Lateral and medial to the mucocele is enhancing polypoid tissue penetrating through the posterior frontal sinus wall into the extradural space. **D:** Postcontrast lateral T1-weighted MRI through the mid-frontal sinus shows expansion of the sinus cavity secondary to a fluid-filled, nonenhancing mucocele. There is inferior bulging from the frontal sinus into the adjacent nasal cavity (*arrow*). Note enhancement of the wall of the mucocele.

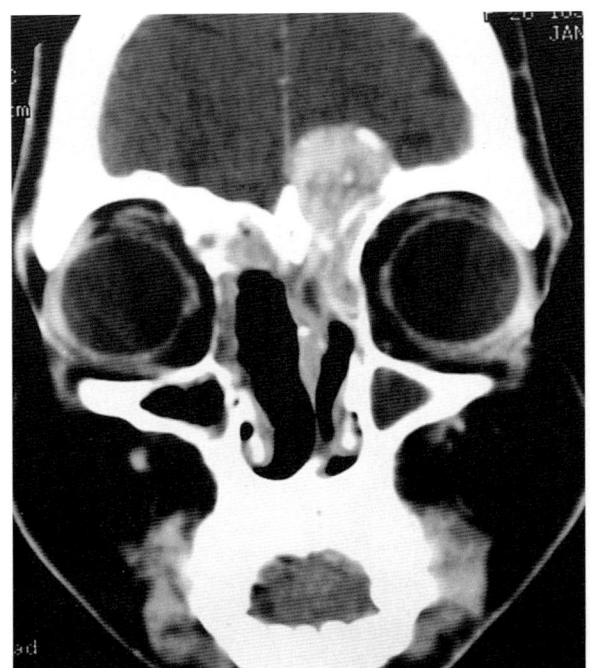
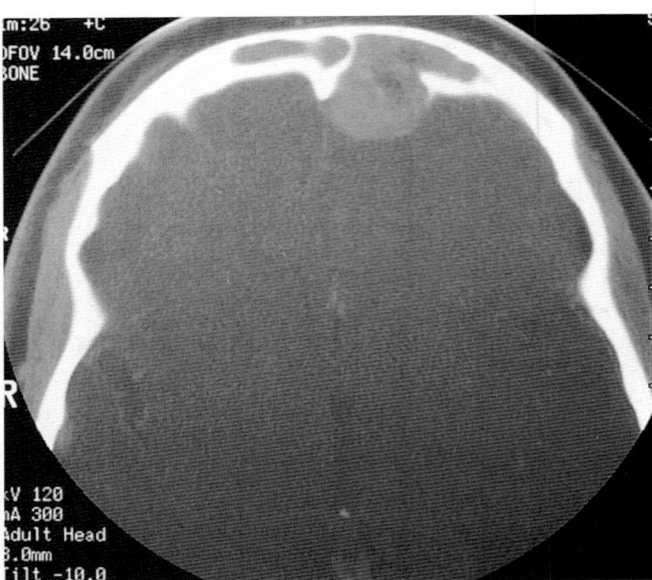

FIG. 5. Polypoid tissue of the paranasal sinuses extending through the roof of the left ethmoid sinus into the anterior cranial cavity. **A:** Postcontrast coronal computed tomography (CT) scan through the midnasal fossa demonstrates polypoid tissue in the upper nasal cavities and ethmoid sinuses with extension through the roof of the ethmoid sinus into the left anterior intracranial cavity. Note surgical defects in both nasal cavities from previous polypectomies. **B:** Axial CT scan through the frontal sinus shows extension of polypoid tissue from the sinus cavity through a defect on the left into the anterior cranial cavity.

Central Skull Base Lesions

A large group of diverse lesions is encountered in the central skull base (Table 2). Meningiomas are one of the more common neoplasms occurring in the central skull base, chiefly located in the lesser and greater wings of the sphenoid bone (30). A meningioma can arise in the dura covering the intracranial surface of the skull base or from dural sleeves, following some of the cranial nerves. The signal characteristics of meningiomas vary, but these lesions are often isointense with brain on both T1- and T2-weighted images (31). After contrast administration, meningiomas enhance, often intensely and homogeneously. The enhancement may extend along the dura beyond the edge of the main tumor mass (dural tail sign). Hyperostosis, if extensive, can be evaluated by MRI, but CT is more accurate in the assessment of minor degrees of hyperostosis. Calcifications may be present in meningiomas (20% of cases) and are detected, if of sufficient size, by absence of signal. Small calcifications, however, are often undetectable by MRI and are visualized by CT.

Lesions in the sella often are represented by pituitary adenomas, which most commonly extend into the suprasellar cistern and laterally into the cavernous sinus, but may extend into the sphenoid sinus and infrequently extend through the skull base into the nasopharynx (32,33).

Neuromas arising from cranial nerve V present as parasellar tumors and may straddle the incisura with components in the middle and posterior fossae (34–36) (Fig. 6). They are characterized by low signal intensity on T1-weighted images (see Fig. 6B), high signal intensity on T2-weighted images (see Fig. 6A), and marked enhancement after gadolinium administration (see Fig. 6C). They may display cystic degenerative areas, that fail to enhance, imparting a heterogeneous appearance to the tumor matrix. Craniopharyngiomas are usually suprasellar in location but may erode and extend into the sella, clivus, and rarely, into the nasopharynx (33). They are heterogeneous in appearance, caused by a variable combination of cystic and solid areas, with the inclusion of calcification in 80% of cases.

TABLE 2. *Central skull base lesions*

Epidermoid cyst
Cholesterol cyst
Neurogenic tumors
  Schwannoma
  Neurofibroma
Meningioma
Chordoma
Chondrosarcoma
Carcinoma of nasopharynx invading skull base
Metastases
Multiple myeloma, including plasmacytoma

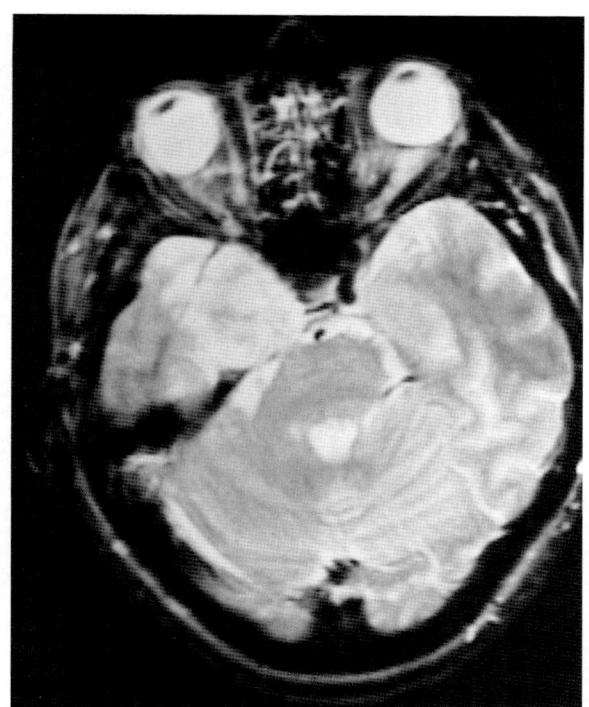
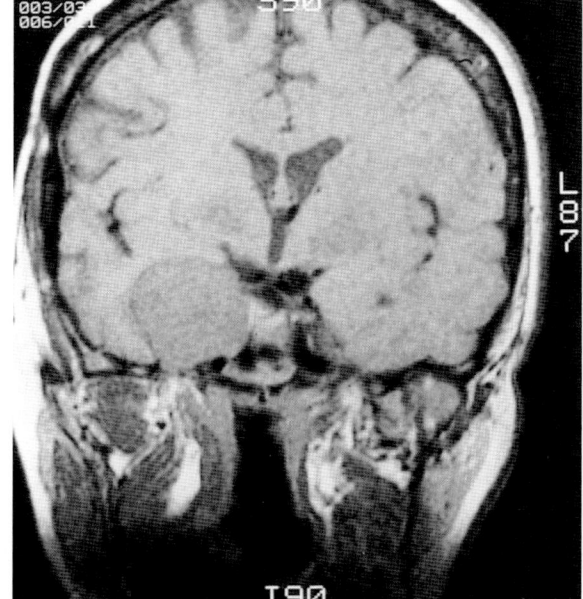
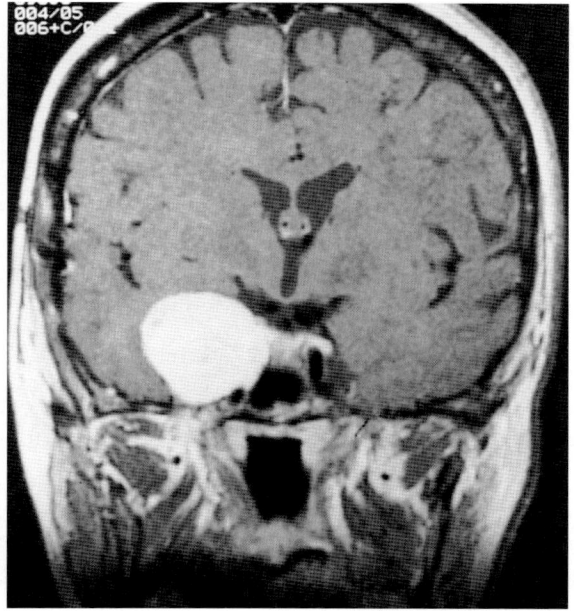

FIG. 6. Trigeminal neuroma of the right gasserian ganglion with extension into the right middle cranial fossa. **A:** Axial T2-weighted magnetic resonance image (MRI) through the middle cranial fossa shows a well defined, high–signal-intensity tumor in the right cavernous sinus and middle cranial fossa with extension through the right incisura into the prepontine cistern. **B:** Coronal T1-weighted MRI demonstrates the sharply defined, homogeneous low–signal-intensity tumor in the region of right Meckel's cave. **C:** Postcontrast coronal T1-weighted MRI demonstrates marked enhancement of the neuroma.

The aggressive angiolipoma, originating in soft tissue, rarely invades the skull base. The density or signal characteristics are reflected by fatty tissue with fibrous strands and increased vascularity (37–40) (Fig. 7).

The most common primary tumors originating in the middle cranial fossa are chondrosarcomas and chordomas (41–44). Chordomas arise from remnants of the notochord, usually in the clivus. If large, they may extend over a significant distance intracranially or into the paranasal sinuses, nasopharynx, and foramen magnum (Fig. 8). Chordomas have low signal intensity on T1-weighted images (see Fig. 8A) and high signal intensity on T2-weighted images, and display marked contrast enhancement after injection of gadolinium (44,45) (see Fig. 8B,C). Most chordomas are heterogeneous in signal intensity, with occasional components of high signal intensity on T1-weighted images that are secondary to blood degradation products (see Fig. 8A, arrow). Low signal intensity within the lesion on T1- and T2-weighted images may represent sequestrations of cortical bone or areas of calcification. Calcification of chordomas is

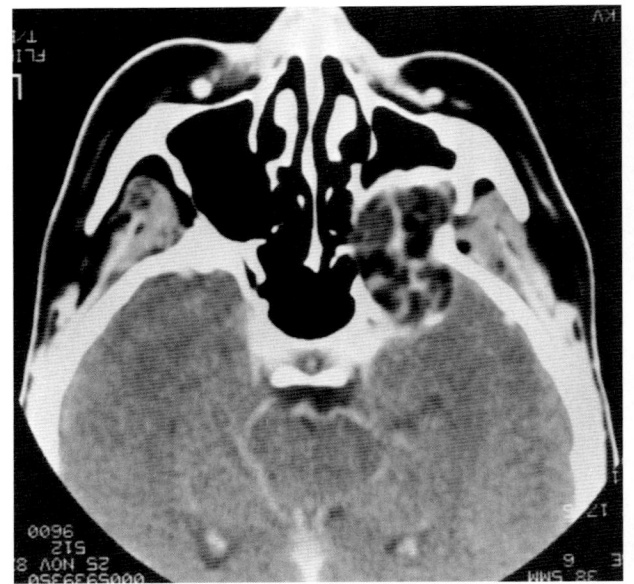
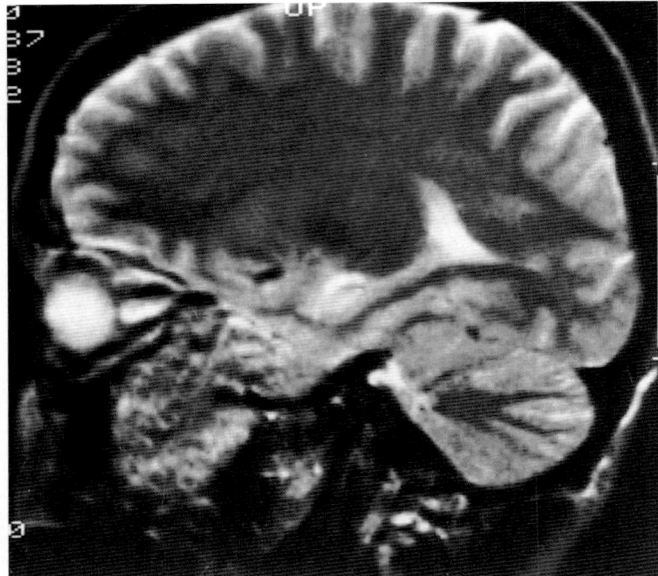
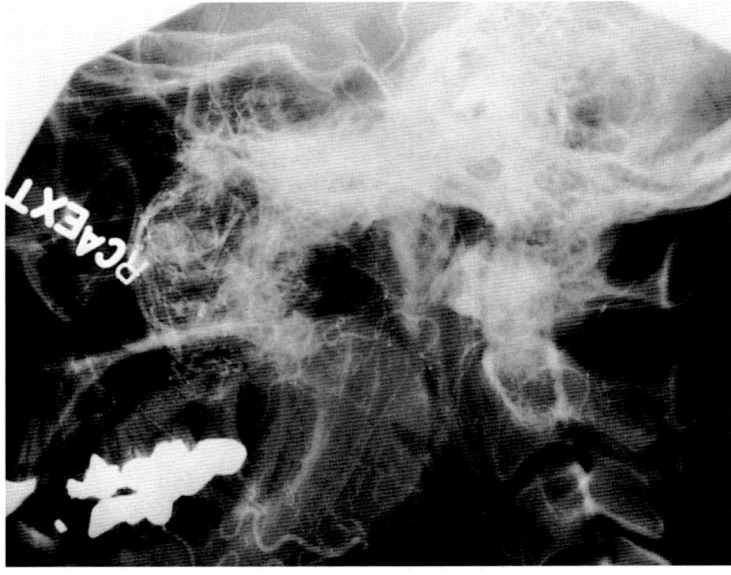

FIG. 7. Angiolipoma. **A:** Axial computed tomography study shows a low-density mass in a defect of the left middle cranial fossa floor with extension into the middle cranial fossa and pterygopalatine fossa. The low-density areas are consistent with fat. They are traversed by linear higher-density areas within the fatty tissue. **B:** Sagittal T2-weighted magnetic resonance image demonstrates multiple tubular flow voids in the tumor. **C:** Sagittal conventional angiogram shows marked hypervascularity of the tumor.

uncommon. Chordomas are located in the clivus, but in one third of cases grow laterally and then simulate the location of chondrosarcomas.

Chondrosarcomas usually originate more laterally in the petroclival fissure. These tumors may contain calcification, which may not be obvious on MR but can easily be discerned on CT. On CT, they demonstrate cystic bone destruction (Fig. 9A). Calcifications are often increased after proton beam therapy (41). Chondrosarcomas have low signal on T1-weighted images (see Fig. 9B) and a bright signal on T2-weighted images (46). They usually reveal marked heterogeneous enhancement after gadolinium introduction (see Fig. 9C,D; Fig. 10). The signal intensities and enhancement patterns of chondrosarcomas are similar to those of chordomas (43).

Lesions of the nasopharynx not infrequently erode into the central skull base, frequently through the foramen lacerum with subsequent extension into the cavernous sinus (47,48). The foramen lacerum represents the line of least resistance. Intracranial extension may also occur by perineural spread

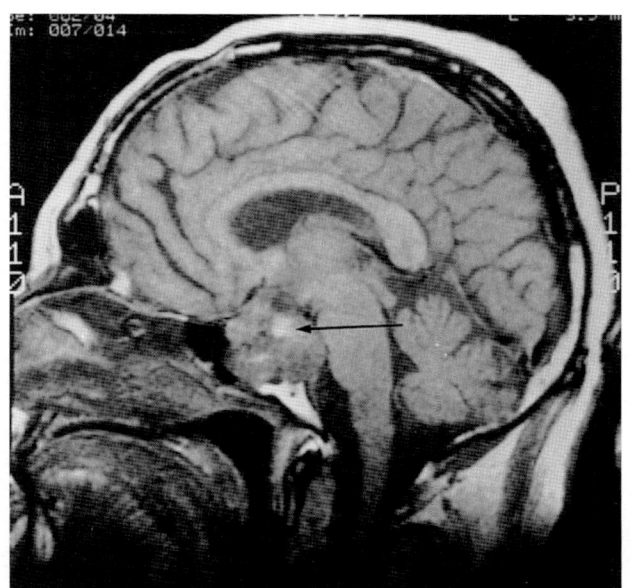
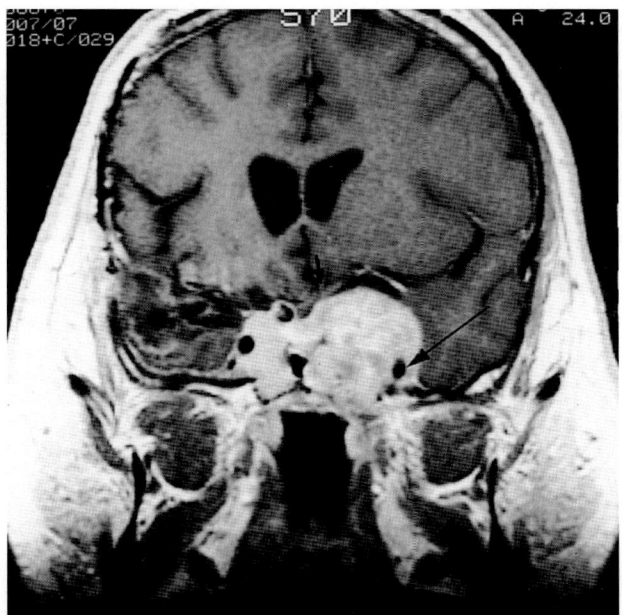
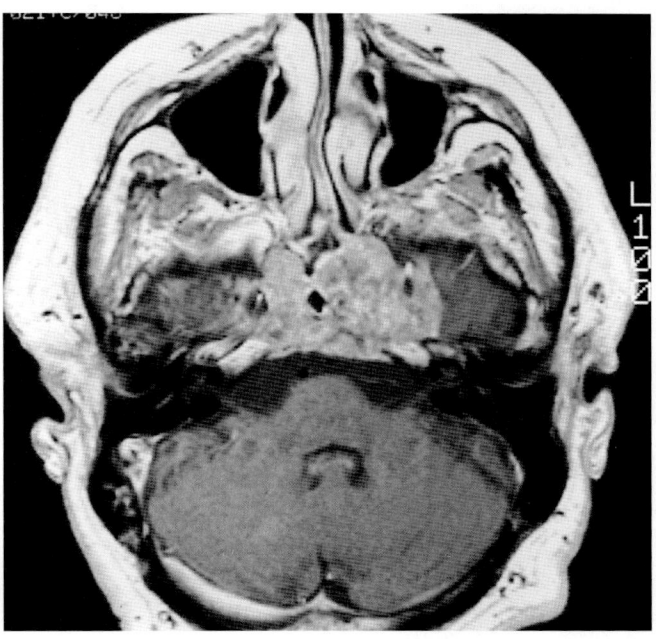

FIG. 8. Chordoma in the clivus with destruction of the sella turcica. **A:** Sagittal T1-weighted magnetic resonance image (MRI) demonstrates a destructive, heterogeneous mass lesion in the middle and upper clivus with high-intensity blood (*arrow*). There is associated destruction of the sella turcica. Note tumor extension into the prepontine cistern with flattening of the anterior border of the pons, suprasellar cistern, and posterior half of the sphenoid sinus. **B:** Contrast-enhanced coronal T1-weighted MRI demonstrates marked enhancement of the chordoma in the areas described. Note superior displacement of the chiasm, which is oriented obliquely (*arrow*). Also note engulfment and displacement of the left cavernous carotid artery (*arrow*) and some encirclement and lateral and superior displacement of the right cavernous carotid arteries. **C:** Postcontrast axial T1-weighted MRI shows the lateral extension of the enhancing chordoma. Note erosion of both petrous apices.

(see Fig. 3). The most common tumor implicated in perineural extension is the adenoid cystic carcinoma. Perineural spread can also occur in squamous cell carcinoma and lymphomas (7). Tumors around the nerves are usually low or intermediate in signal intensity on T1-weighted images and may be bright on T2-weighted images. Obliteration of fat around the nerves occurs at the exit foramina on T1-weighted images. Frequently, enhancement of the tumor can be seen within and at the foramina after gadolinium infusion with fat suppression (47) (see Fig. 3). Tumor extension along the nerves (most commonly V1, V2, or V3) is reflected by a thickened, enhancing, cordlike structure (see Fig. 3).

Metastases and *multiple myelomas*, including plasmacytoma, not infrequently are located in the central skull base (49). In most cases, the primary tumor is evident clinically, but occasionally the tumor may manifest first in the skull base. No specific features are recognized on CT and MRI in most cases, except for metastases from carcinoma of the prostate, which is characterized by diffuse or localized sclerosis. CT with bone algorithm is mandatory to demonstrate minor bone changes, either lytic destruction or sclerosis.

Epidermoid and *cholesterol cysts* occur in the skull base, usually at the petrous apex and adjacent clivus. They are characterized by a sharply marginated, spherical or ovoid bony defect involving the clivus, middle cranial fossa, and

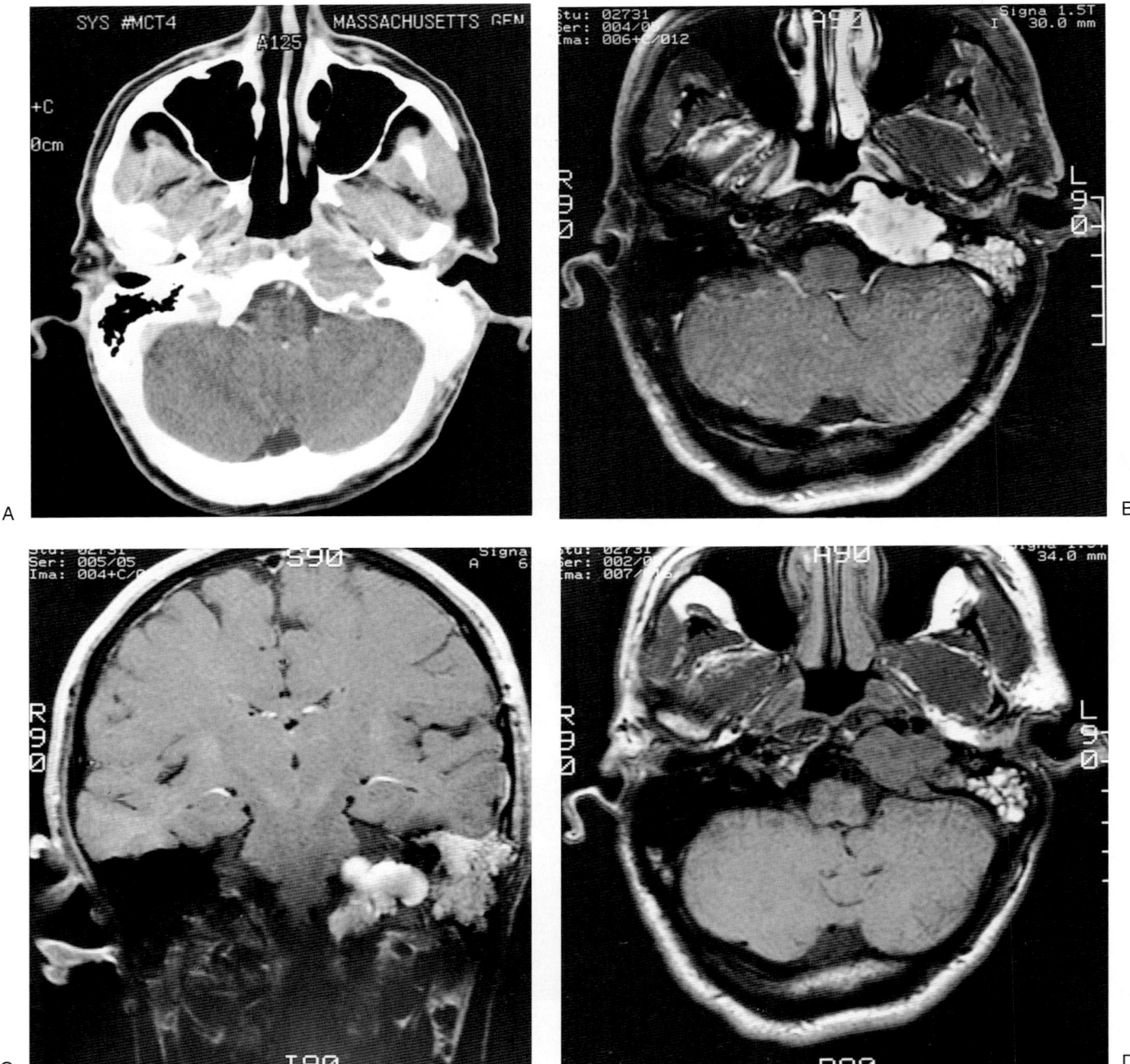

FIG. 9. Chondrosarcoma of the left petrous apex. **A:** Axial computed tomography scan through the temporal bones demonstrates an isodense tumor mass in the destroyed left petrous apex. **B:** Contrast-enhanced axial T1-weighted magnetic resonance image (MRI) shows marked enhancement of the tumor. The scattered, low–signal-intensity areas are consistent with areas of calcification. **C:** Coronal T1-weighted MRI shows the enhancing tumor mass in the petrous apex with inferior extension into the uppermost portion of the parapharyngeal space. **D:** Axial T1-weighted MRI through the temporal bones demonstrates the homogeneous, fairly well defined tumor in the left petrous apex. Note increased signal intensity in the left mastoid from retained secretions secondary to eustachian tube obstruction.

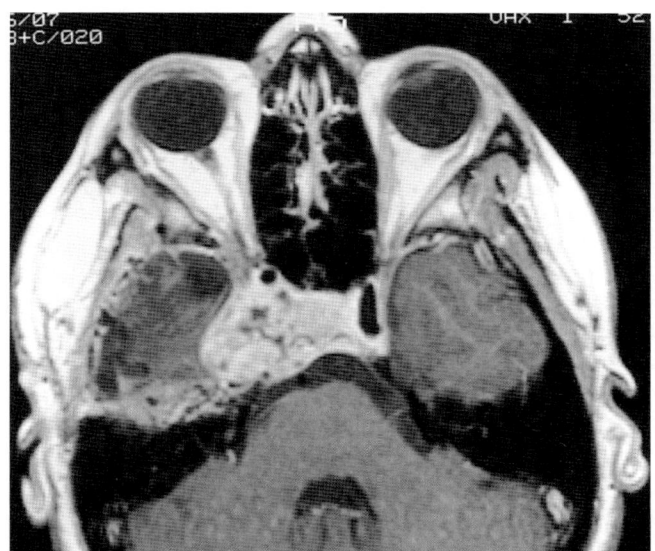 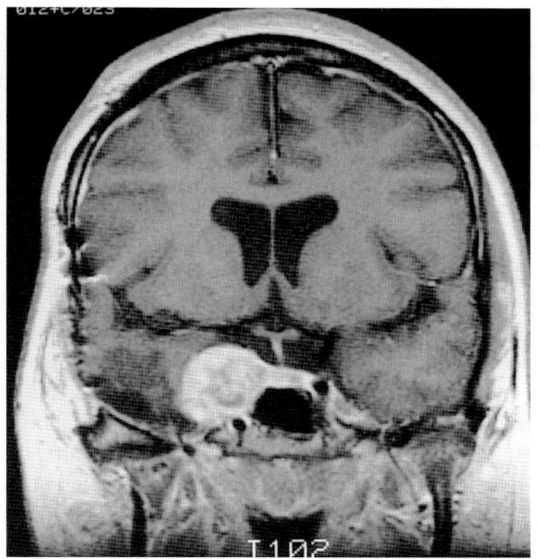

FIG. 10. Chondrosarcoma of the right cavernous sinus and adjacent middle cranial fossa. **A:** Axial T1-weighted magnetic resonance image (MRI) after gadolinium introduction shows marked enhancement of the tumor in the right cavernous sinus with extension into the adjacent middle cranial fossa. Note linear, low–signal-intensity areas within the tumor, indicating calcification. **B:** Postcontrast coronal T1-weighted MRI demonstrates the enhancing tumor mass in the right cavernous sinus and the right middle cranial fossa.

petrous apex. They may also encroach on the sphenoid sinus, as indicated by a defect in the bony wall and an intraluminal soft tissue density. On preinfusion CT scans, epidermoids and cholesterol cysts manifest as lesions isodense with brain. On CT, as well as MRI, they may reveal a slight ringlike area of enhancement that corresponds to the pseudocapsule of the cysts. On MRI, the epidermoid has a low signal intensity on T1- and high signal intensity on T2-weighted images (50), whereas the cholesterol cyst demonstrates high signal intensity on T1- and T2-weighted images (51,52) (Fig. 11).

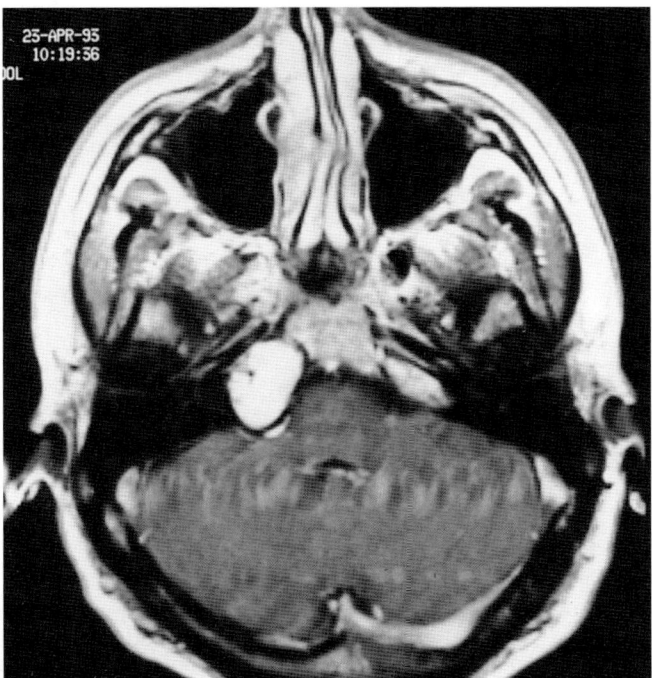 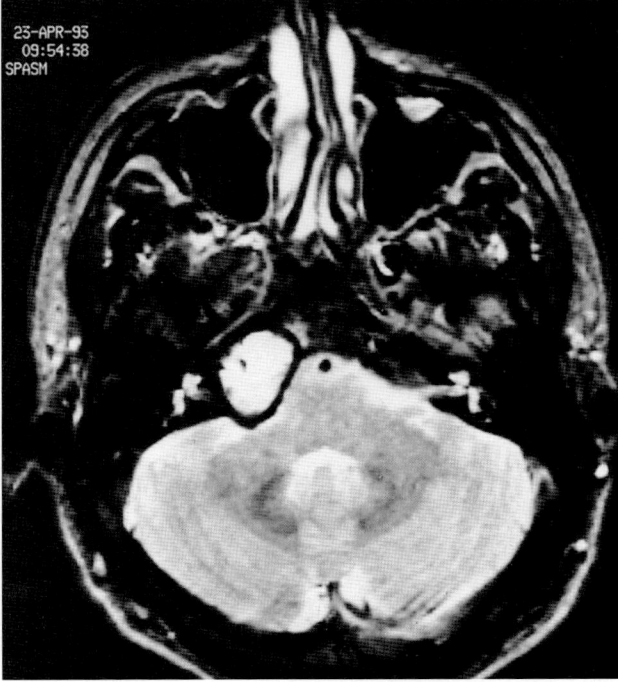

FIG. 11. Cholesterol cyst. **A:** Postcontrast axial T1-weighted magnetic resonance image (MRI) reveals a high-intensity, nonenhancing cyst in the right petrous space. **B:** The cyst is of high signal intensity on axial T2-weighted MRI.

Osteomyelitis

Osteomyelitis of the skull base is most commonly caused by malignant external otitis (53–56). This infectious process originates in the external auditory canal and, if unchecked because of a delay in diagnosis or inadequate treatment, extends to the nasopharynx, paranasopharyngeal space, and adjacent skull base. The disease is encountered in patients with diabetes and immunocompromised patients infected with *Pseudomonas aeruginosa*, the causative organism in most cases. On CT, there is evidence of lytic bone destruction often associated with a soft tissue mass in the lateral nasopharynx. On MRI, the inflammatory tissue displays low signal intensity on T1-weighted images, high signal intensity on T2-weighted images, and a variable degree of enhancement after gadolinium introduction. Other causes of osteomyelitis of the skull base include fungus disease (aspergillosis, mucormycosis), and there are cases with unknown etiologies. Other than a soft tissue mass with bone destruction, these lesions have no specific imaging features.

Posterior Skull Base Lesions

Tumors of the posterior skull base can be categorized according to site of origin as (a) cerebellopontine (CP) angle lesions, (b) jugular fossa tumors, and (c) foramen magnum lesions (Table 3).

The *CP angle lesions* comprise, in order of frequency, acoustic neuroma (70–80%), meningioma (10%), and miscellaneous pathologic processes, including epidermoid cysts, arachnoid cysts, metastases, and ependymoma of the fourth ventricle with lateral extension. MRI with gadopentetate is the optimal modality to define the origin and characterize this diverse group of lesions (57). In 95% of cases, acoustic neuroma arises in the internal auditory canal and either remains within the canal or, more commonly, extends from the canal into the CP angle cistern (Fig. 12). After the

TABLE 3. *Posterior skull base lesions*

Cerebellopontine angle lesions
Acoustic neurinoma
Meningioma
Tumors of temporal bone:
    Malignant lesions
    Carcinoma
    Endolymphatic sac tumor
    Facial nerve neurinoma
Epidermoid cyst
Arachnoid cyst
Vascular lesions
Metastatic disease
Ependymoma originating in fourth ventricle or cerebellum
Jugular fossa tumors
Glomus jugulare tumor
Neurogenic tumors
Chondrosarcoma
Meningioma
Foramen magnum lesions
Intradural extramedullary
    Meningioma
    Neurogenic tumors
Extradural
    Bone lesions
        Metastases
        Chordoma
    Inflammatory and miscellaneous lesions
        Rheumatoid arthritis
        Synovial cyst

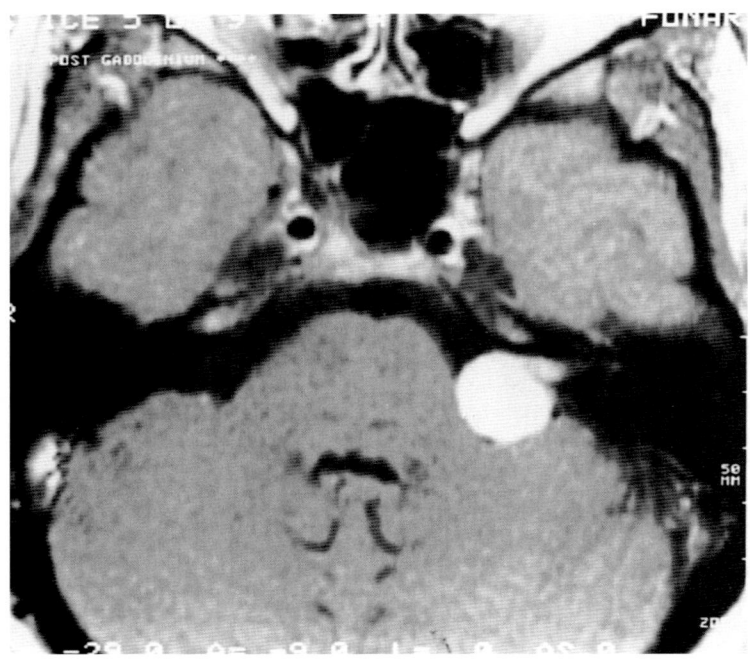

FIG. 12. Acoustic neuroma in left cerebellopontine angle. Postcontrast axial T1-weighted magnetic resonance image through the temporal bone demonstrates a left acoustic neuroma encroaching on the cerebellum and pons. Note marked enhancement and intracanalicular and extracanalicular extension.

administration of gadolinium there is marked enhancement, associated in a smaller percentage of cases with cystic degeneration or adjacent arachnoid cysts (see Fig. 12). Large lesions may indent the adjacent brainstem or cerebellum with contralateral displacement.

Facial nerve neuromas most commonly originate from the facial nerve at the geniculate ganglion (Fig. 13), but may arise at other locations in the temporal bone. Large tumors may extend into the middle or posterior intracranial cavity (58). Their imaging findings parallel those of acoustic neuromas (see Fig. 13).

The *meningioma* usually has a broad-based attachment to the medial posterior surface of the petrous bone anterior or posterior to the internal auditory canal. Meningiomas enhance diffusely and intensely after the introduction of gadolinium (Fig. 14). In a small percentage of cases, there may be slight extension of the meningioma into the internal auditory canal (57).

Epidermoid cysts in the CP angle have a low signal intensity on T1-weighted images, increased signal intensity on T2-weighted images, and a slightly greater signal intensity compared with CSF on proton-density images (50). Epidermoid cysts frequently have frondlike projections from the margin and insinuate into the adjacent structures, especially in the prepontine cistern.

Arachnoid cysts have the same signal intensities as CSF and are differentiated from a dilated subarachnoid space by the presence of a thin wall and a variable degree of mass effect on adjacent structures (59).

Metastatic lesions comprise a diverse group of primary tumors (most commonly bronchogenic carcinoma in men and carcinoma of the breast in women). They may be localized to

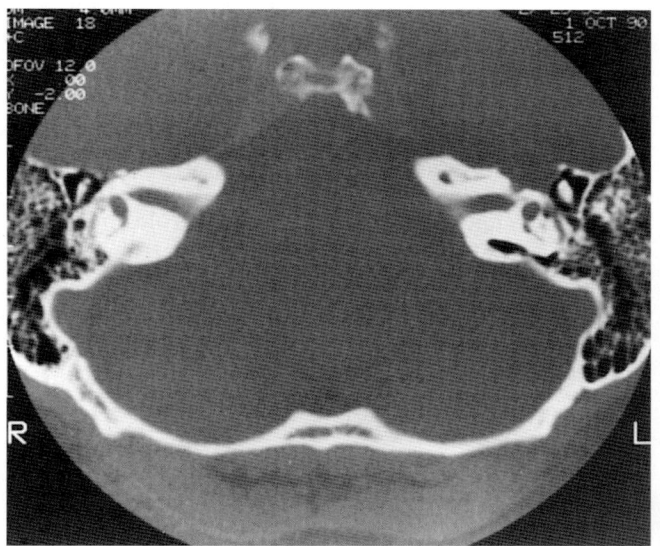

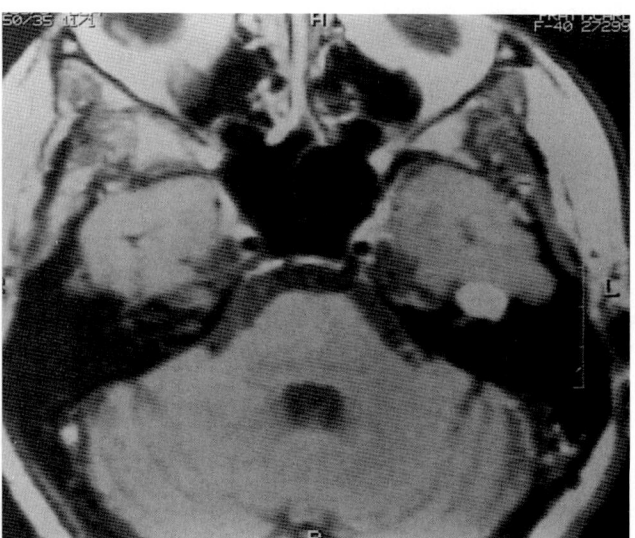

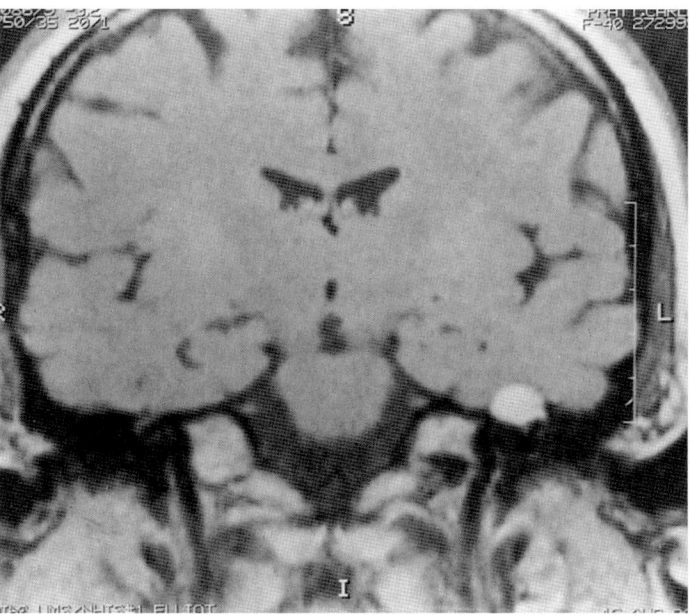

FIG. 13. Neuroma of the geniculate ganglion. **A:** Axial computed tomography scan (bone window setting) through the temporal bone shows a saucer-shaped, sharply defined defect in the geniculate ganglion area of the left temporal bone. **B:** Postcontrast axial T1-weighted magnetic resonance image (MRI) through the temporal bone shows a sharply defined, homogeneous, enhancing tumor mass in the geniculate ganglion consistent with a neuroma. **C:** Postcontrast coronal T1-weighted MRI through the temporal bone demonstrates an enhancing mass in the region of the left geniculate ganglion.

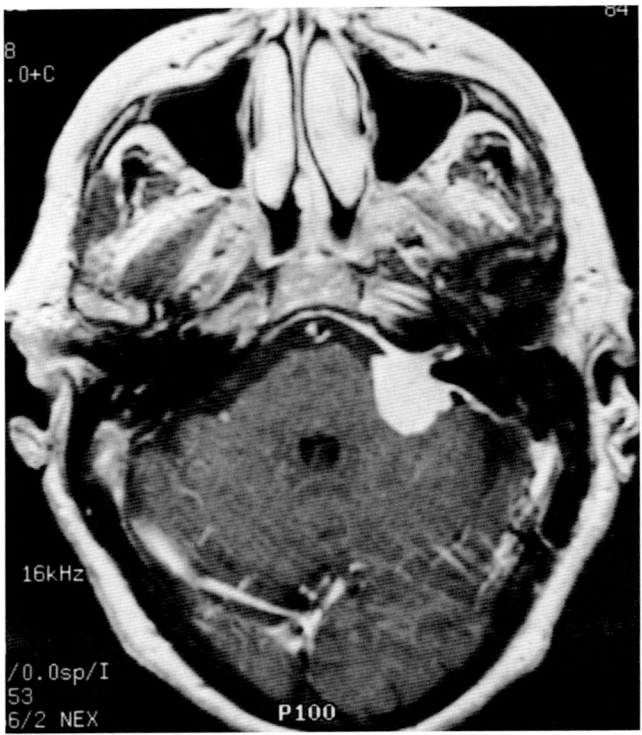

FIG. 14. Meningioma of the left cerebellopontine (CP) angle. Postcontrast axial T1-weighted magnetic resonance image demonstrates a markedly enhancing, broad-based meningioma in the left CP angle cistern. Note enhancement of the adjacent dura and minimal extension into the internal auditory canal.

the CP angle cistern and have also been reported to invade the internal auditory canal.

Ependymomas arising in the fourth ventricle have a tendency to spread laterally through the foramen of Luschka and manifest as a mass in the CP angle cistern. They are usually low in signal intensity on T1-weighted images and show increased signal intensity on T2-weighted images, with heterogeneous enhancement after introduction of gadolinium. They may reveal areas of necrosis which are nonenhancing and in areas of calcification.

Jugular Fossa Tumors

The most common tumor of the jugular fossa is the *glomus jugulare tumor*. This lesion causes enlargement of the jugular foramen with irregular bone destruction, which is best delineated by CT with bone window settings (60) (Fig. 15A). The lesion frequently extends inferiorly into the upper neck but may also extend into the posterior fossa, including the CP angle cistern, if of sufficient size. The tumor most frequently extends into the middle ear cavity and can be detected as a pinkish, pulsating mass in the middle ear on otoscopic examination. The tumor may reveal multiple, tubular, undulating signal voids reflecting the increased vascularity of this lesion (61) (see Fig. 15B). The lesions are hypointense on T1-weighted images and hyperintense on T2-weighted images (62) (see Fig. 15B). There is usually marked enhancement after introduction of gadolinium. Coronal images are especially useful for demonstrating the

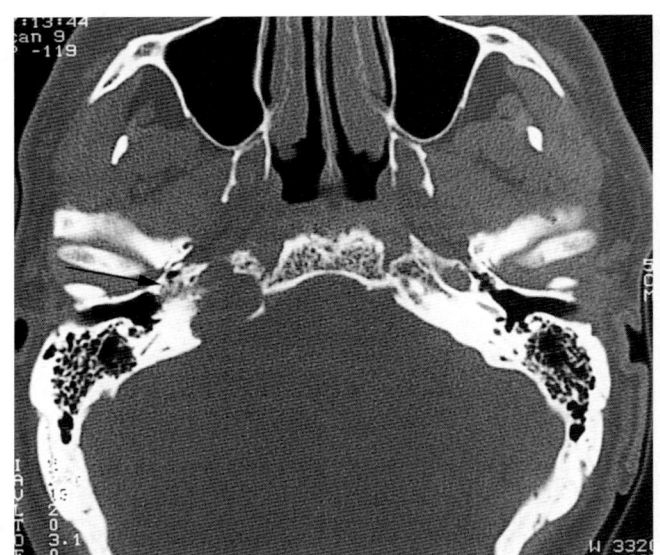
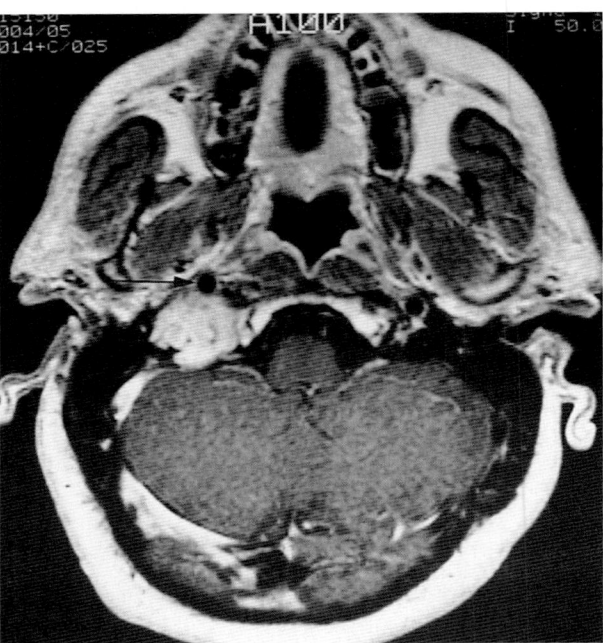

FIG. 15. Glomus tumor of the right jugular fossa. **A:** Axial computed tomography scan (bone window setting) through the temporal bone reveals enlargement and erosion of the right jugular fossa. Note small area of soft tissue density, indicating tumor extension into the hypotympanum (*arrow*). **B:** Postcontrast axial T1-weighted magnetic resonance image shows marked enhancement of the tumor in the right jugular fossa. Note anterior displacement of the internal carotid artery (*arrow*). Hypovascularity is reflected by low–signal-intensity tubular structures within the mass.

superoinferior extent of the lesion, especially the CP angle component.

The second most common tumors of the jugular fossa are the *neurofibroma* and *neurilemoma*. These lesions usually are accompanied by sharply defined bony expansion of the jugular fossa (61) (Fig. 16A,B). Large lesions may extend into the CP angle cistern and simulate an acoustic neuroma, especially if they are near the internal auditory canal. Coronal images are indicated in the differential diagnosis (63). Neurilemomas show marked enhancement, occasionally with areas of cystic degeneration (see Fig. 16C,D). The neurofibroma enhances to a variable degree after gadolinium introduction.

There are a variety of less common lesions that arise in the

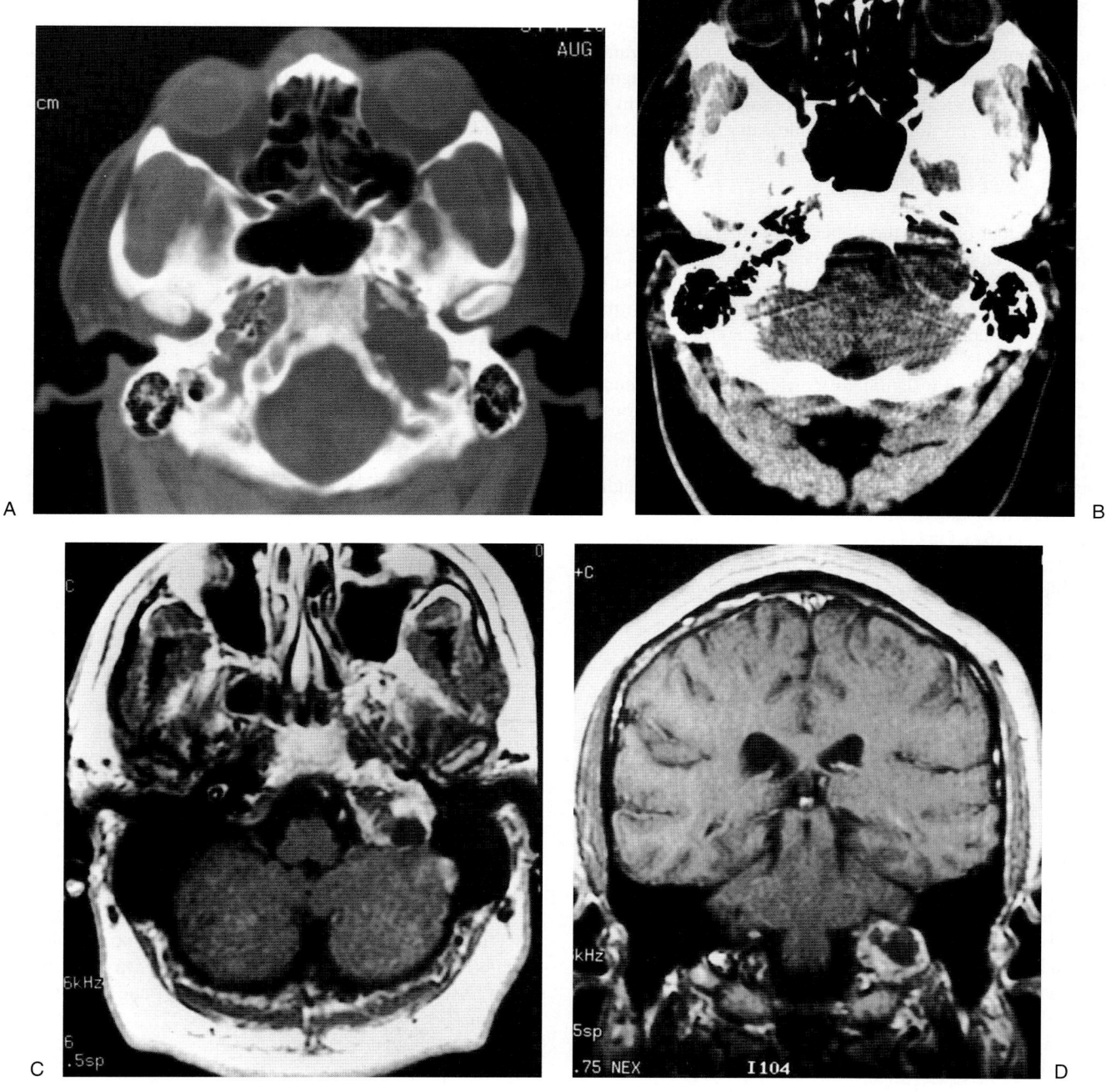

FIG. 16. Neuroma of the left jugular fossa. **A:** Axial computed tomography (CT) scan demonstrates a large, lytic, bony defect in the area of the left jugular fossa with extension to the left middle cranial fossa. **B:** Axial CT scan (soft tissue window) shows an isodense mass in the lytic defect. **C:** Postcontrast axial T1-weighted magnetic resonance image (MRI) demonstrates heterogeneous enhancement of the left jugular fossa neuroma. Note cystic–degenerative, nonenhancing areas in the tumor. **D:** Coronal T1-weighted MRI shows an enhancing tumor with central areas of cystic degeneration.

jugular fossa, such as hemangiopericytoma (61), which has enhancement and intensity characteristics similar to those of the glomus jugulare tumor. Meningiomas may arise in the jugular fossa and have the same radiologic characteristics as reported elsewhere (64). Chondrosarcomas rarely arise from the jugular fossa and have imaging features similar to those described previously (65). Metastases also may involve the jugular fossa and are characterized as a soft tissue mass with bone destruction or sclerosis.

Multiple lesions occur in the area of the area of the *foramen magnum*. Most frequently they represent meningiomas or neurogenic tumors that arise from the dura of the foramen magnum or from nerve roots that exit the foramen magnum or the upper cervical spine (11). Tumors that arise in the clivus, such as chordoma and chondrosarcoma, may extend into the foramen magnum, causing displacement of the medulla or upper cervical spinal cord (44). Their radiologic characteristics have been previously described.

Lesions that arise in the upper cervical spine, especially from the C1 and C2 vertebrae, may also extend into the foramen magnum. The most common lesions arising from the bony structures represent metastases and, rarely, primary bone lesions such as chordoma, Ewing's sarcoma, and chondrosarcoma (11).

Tumefactions of inflammatory origin, especially rheumatoid arthritis, may cause changes, including pannus formation with secondary encroachment on the foramen magnum (66). Synovial cysts have been reported to arise from the joint between the atlas and odontoid process with secondary extension into the foramen magnum and upper cervical spinal canal (67). On CT, they are well defined and of low attenuation, whereas on MRI, they are hypointense on T1-weighted images and hyperintense on T2-weighted images.

Diffuse Lesions of the Skull Base

Various disease entities may affect the skull base diffusely (Table 4). Among these, metastases are the most common lesions.

Metastases in the skull base are common in advanced disease and are frequently asymptomatic. They may be lytic (breast, lung, thyroid, hypernephroma, and multiple myeloma, including plasmacytoma) or sclerotic (prostate) or mixed (breast). CT is the preferred radiologic method to demonstrate these bony lesions because the soft tissue component may be small and the bony abnormality inconspicuous on MRI.

Bone dysplasias constitute different entities, including fibrous dysplasia, Paget's disease, osteopetrosis (68,69), and metaphyseal and diaphyseal dysplasias (70,71). Fibrous dysplasia is usually localized (monostotic variety) and most commonly involves the sphenoid bone. On CT, the bone is expanded and appears sclerotic and cystic, reflected histologically by osteoid and fibrotic bundles, respectively. MRI is characterized by low signal intensity on T1- and T2-weighted images (72). Because of hypervascularity, there is

TABLE 4. *Diffuse lesions of the skull base*

Fibrous dysplasia
Paget's disease
Metaphyseal and diaphyseal dysplasias
Osteopetrosis
Metastatic disease, including multiple myeloma

bleeding into bone, followed by cavity formation. Blood degradation products (methemoglobin) cause increased signal intensity on T1- and T2-weighted images in the signal void of bone. There is moderate enhancement after introduction of gadolinium (73). In Paget's disease, there is usually associated involvement of the skull table. The imaging features are described as a "cotton wool" appearance produced by radiolucent and radiodense areas associated with bony expansion. Metaphyseal and diaphyseal dysplasia and osteopetrosis involve the skull table and skull base as well as the central and appendicular skeleton. A diffuse, variable sclerosis affects the base of the skull along with the skull table. The findings in the axial and peripheral skeleton allow differentiation of these entities.

SUMMARY AND CONCLUSIONS

Computed tomography and MRI are the principal methods for evaluation of skull base lesions. CT in the axial and coronal planes optimally demonstrates bone detail and defines areas of calcification. Its major disadvantage is its inability to image intracranial structures, including brain, aura, and meninges, and their relationship to various pathologic entities.

Magnetic resonance imaging is the preferred modality to investigate the soft tissue component of skull base lesions. When MRI is used with gadolinium administration and fat suppression, the location and extent of various primary and secondary tumors can be precisely mapped out.

Their signal characteristics and enhancement patterns allow tumors to be differentiated from cysts. The origin and components of a meningocele or meningoencephalocele are clearly depicted on MRI. Moreover, by defining the location (anterior, middle, or posterior cranial fossae), margin, and signal characteristics of mass lesions, a preliminary or definitive diagnosis can be established. MRI and CT findings enable the surgeon to select a drainage (cysts) or biopsy site, or plan a surgical approach for partial or complete resection of the lesion. Vital structures (i.e., nerves, arteries, veins) can be identified and surgically extirpated or preserved, depending on the size, location, and nature of the lesion.

REFERENCES

1. Curtin HD, Hirsch WJ. Base of the skull. In: Atlas SW, ed. *MRI of the brain and spine.* New York: Raven Press, 1991:669–701.
2. Ginsberg LE. Neoplastic diseases affecting the central skull base: CT and MR imaging. *AJR Am J Roentgenol* 1992;159:581–589.

3. Janecka IP. Surgical approaches to the skull base. *Neuroimaging Clin N Am* 1994;4:639–656.
4. Janecka IP, Sen C, Sekhar LN, et al. Cranial base surgery: results in 183 patients. *Otolaryngol Head Neck Surg* 1994;110 539–546.
5. Curtin HD, Williams R, Johnson J. CT of the perineural tumor extension–pterygopalatine fossa. *AJR Am J Roentgenol* 1985;144:163–169.
6. Curtin HD, Wolfe P, Snyderman N. Facial nerve between the stylomastoid foramen and parotid: CT imaging. *Radiology* 1983;149:165–169.
7. Laine FJ, Braun IF, Jensen, et al. Perineural tumor extension through the foramen ovale: evaluation with MR imaging. *Radiology* 1990;174:65–71.
8. Tien RD. Fat suppression MR imaging in neuroradiology: techniques and clinical application. *AJR Am J Roentgenol* 1992;158:369–379.
9. Tien RD, Hesselink JR, Chu PK, et al. Improved detection and delineation of head and neck lesions with fat suppression spin-echo MR imaging. *AJNR Am J Neuroradiol* 1991;12:19–24.
10. Hirsch WL, et al. Comparison of MR imaging, CT, and angiography in the evaluation of enlarged cavernous sinus. *AJNR Am J Neuroradiol* 1988;9:907–915.
11. Johnson MH, Smoker WRK. Lesions of the craniovertebral junction. *Neuroimaging Clin N Am* 1994;4:599–618.
12. Som PM, Dillon WP, Sze G, et al. Benign and malignant sinonasal lesions with intracranial extension: differentiation with MR imaging. *Radiology* 1989;172:763–766.
13. Som PM, Curtin HD. Inflammatory lesions and tumors of the nasal cavities and paranasal sinuses with skull base involvement. *Neuroimaging Clin N Am* 1994;4:499–514.
14. Som PM, Shapiro MD, Biller HF, et al. Sinonasal tumors and inflammatory tissues: differentiation with MR imaging. *Radiology* 1988;167:803–808.
15. Dillon WP, Som PM, Fullerton GD. Hypointense MR signal in chronically inspissated sinonasal secretions. *Radiology* 1990;174:73–78.
16. Som PM, Dillon WP, Fullerton GD, et al. Chronically obstructed sinonasal secretions: observations on T1- and T2-shortening. *Radiology* 1989;172:515–520.
17. Lustrin ES, Robertson RL, Tilak S. Normal anatomy of the skull base. *Neuroimaging Clin N Am* 1994;4:465–478.
18. Paling MR, Block BC, Levine PA, et al. Tumor invasion of the anterior skull base: a comparison of MR and CT studies. *J Comput Assist Tomogr* 1984;8:944–952.
19. Pollack JA, Newton TH, Hoyt WF. Transsphenoidal and transethmoidal encephaloceles. *Radiology* 1968;90:442–453.
20. Byrd SE, Harwood-Nash DC, Fitz CR, et al. Computed tomography in the evaluation of encephaloceles in infants and children. *J Comput Assist Tomogr* 1978;2:81–87.
21. David DJ, Proudman TW. Cephaloceles: classification, pathology, and management. *World J Surg* 1989;13:349–357.
22. Nager GT. Cephaloceles. *Laryngoscope* 1987;97:77–84.
23. Koch BL, Ball WS Jr. Congenital malformations causing skull base changes. *Neuroimaging Clin N Am* 1994;4:479–498.
24. Naidich TP, Altman NR, Braffman BH, et al. Cephaloceles and related malformations. *AJNR Am J Neuroradiol* 1992;13:655–690.
25. Osborn AG, Johnson L, Roberts TS. Sphenoidal mucoceles with intracranial extension. *J Comput Assist Tomogr* 1979;3:335–338.
26. Som PM, Lidov M. The benign fibro-osseous lesion: its association with paranasal sinus mucoceles and its MR characteristics. *J Comput Assist Tomogr* 1992;16:871–876.
27. Li C, Yousem DM, Hayden RE, et al. Olfactory neuroblastoma: MR evaluation. *AJNR Am J Neuroradiol* 1993;14:1167–1171.
28. Som PM, Lidov M, Brandwein M, Catalano P, Biller HF. Sinonasal esthesioneuroblastoma with intracranial extension: observations on marginal tumor cysts as a diagnostic MRI finding. *AJNR Am J Neuroradiol* 1994 15(7):1259–1262.
29. Cunningham MJ, Curtin HD, Butkiewicz BL. Histiocytosis of the temporal bone: CT findings. *J Comput Assist Tomogr* 1988;12:70–74.
30. Aoki S, Sasaki Y, Machida T, et al. Contrast-enhanced MR images in patients with meningioma: importance of enhancement of the dura adjacent to the tumor. *AJNR Am J Neuroradiol* 1990;11:935–990.
31. Elster AD, Challa VR, Gilbert TH, et al. Meningiomas: MR and histopathological features. *Radiology* 1989;170:857–862.
32. Felsberg GH, Tien RD. Sellar and parasellar lesions involving the skull base. *Neuroimaging Clin N Am* 1994;4:543–560
33. Zimmerman RA. Imaging of intrasellar, suprasellar, and parasellar tumors. *Semin Roentgenol* 1990;25:174.
34. McCormick PC, Bello JA, Post KD. Trigeminal schwannomas. *J Neurosurg* 1988;69:850.
35. Pollack IF, Sekhar LN, Jannetta PJ, et al. Neurilemmomas of the trigeminal nerve. *J Neurosurg* 1989;70:737.
36. Yuh WTC, Wright DC, Barloon TJ, et al. MR imaging of primary tumors of trigeminal nerve and Meckel's cave. *AJR Am J Roentgenol* 1988;151:577.
37. Chew FS, Hudson TM, Hawkins IF. Radiology of infiltrating angiolipoma. *AJR Am J Roentgenol* 1980;135:781–787.
38. Matsuoka Y, Kurose K, Nakagawa O, Katsuyama J. Magnetic resonance imaging of infiltrating angiolipoma of the neck. *Surg Neurol* 1988;29:62–66.
39. Takeuchi J, Handa H, Keyaki A, et al. Intracranial angiolipoma. *Surg Neurol* 1988;29:62–66.
40. Wilkins PR, Hoddinott C, Hourihan MD, et al. Intracranial angiolipoma. *J Neurol Neurosurg Psychiatry* 1987;50:1057–1059.
41. Brown E, Hug EB, Weber AL, Munzenrider J. Chondrosarcoma and other chondromatous lesions arising from the base of skull. *Neuroimaging Clin N Am* 1994;4:529–541.
42. Oot RF. The role of MR and CT in evaluating clival chordomas and chondrosarcomas. *AJNR Am J Neuroradiol* 1988;9:715–727.
43. Weber AL, Brown EW, Hug EB, Liebsch NJ. Cartilaginous tumors and chordomas of the cranial base. *Otolaryngol Clin North Am* 1995;28:453–471.
44. Weber AL, Liebsch N, Sanchez R, Sweriduk S. Chordomas of the skull base. *Neuroimaging Clin N Am* 1994;4:515–527.
45. Meyers SP, Hirsch WL Jr, Curtin HD, et al. Chordomas of the skull base: MR features. *AJNR Am J Neuroradiol* 1992;13:1627–1636.
46. Meyers SP, Hirsch WL Jr, Curtin HD, et al. Chondrosarcomas of the skull base: MR imaging features. *Radiology* 1992;184:103–108.
47. Braun IF. MRI of the nasopharynx. *Radiol Clin North Am* 1989;27:315.
48. Sham JST, Cheung YK, Choy D, et al. Nasopharyngeal carcinoma: CT evaluation of patterns of tumor spread. *AJNR Am J Neuroradiol* 1991;12:265.
49. Greenberg HS, Deck MGF, Vikram B, et al. Metastasis to the base of skull: clinical findings in 43 patients. *Neurology* 1981;31:530–537.
50. Mafee ME, Kumar A, Heffner DK. Epidermoid cyst (cholesteatoma) and cholesterol granuloma of the temporal bone and epidermoid cysts affecting the brain. *Neuroimaging Clin N Am* 1994;4:561–578.
51. Gherin SG, Brackman DE, Lo W. Cholesterol granuloma of the petrous apex. *Laryngoscope* 1985;85:659–664.
52. Lo WWM, Solti-Bohman LG, Brackmann DE, et al. Cholesterol granuloma of the petrous apex. *Radiology* 1984;153:705–711.
53. Chandler JR. Malignant external otitis and osteomyelitis of the base of the skull. *Am J Otol* 1989;10:108–110.
54. Chandler JR, Grobman L, Quencer R, Serafine A. Osteomyelitis of the skull base. *Laryngoscope* 1977;86:417–428.
55. Gherin SG, Brackman DE, Bradley WG. Magnetic resonance imaging and computerized tomography in malignant external otitis. *Laryngoscope* 1986;96:542–548.
56. Gold S, Som PM, Lucente FE, et al. Radiographic findings in progressive necrotizing "malignant" external otitis. *Laryngoscope* 1984;94:363–366.
57. Weber AL. Magnetic resonance imaging and computed tomography of the internal auditory canal and cerebellopontine angle. *Isr J Med Sci* 1992;28:173–182.
58. Horn KL, Crumley RL, Schindley RA. Facial neurilemmomas. *Laryngoscope* 1981;91:1326–1331.
59. Weiner SN, Pearlstein AE, Eiber A. MR imaging of intracranial arachnoid cysts. *J Comput Assist Tomogr* 1987;11:236.
60. Lo WWM, Solti-Bohman LG. High resolution CT in the evaluation of glomus tumors of the temporal bone. *Radiology* 1984;150:737–742.
61. Weber AL, McKenna MJ. Radiologic evaluation of the jugular foramen: anatomy, vascular variants, anomalies, and tumors. *Neuroimaging Clin N Am* 1994;4:579–598.
62. Olsen WL, Dillon WP, Kelly W, et al. MR imaging of paragangliomas. *AJR Am J Roentgenol* 1987;148:701–704.

63. Sasaki T, Takakura K. Twelve cases of jugular foramen neurinoma. *Skull Base Surgery* 1991;1:152–160.
64. Molony TB, Brackman DE, Lo WWM. Meningiomas of the jugular foramen. *Otolaryngol Head Neck Surg* 1992;106:761–765.
65. Harvey SA, Wiet RJ, Kazan R. Chondrosarcoma of the jugular foramen. *Am J Otol* 1994;13:257–263.
66. Castor WR, Miller JDR, Russell AS, et al. Computed tomography of the craniocervical junction in rheumatoid arthritis. *J Comput Assist Tomogr* 1983;7:31–36.
67. Choe W, Walot I, Schlesinger C, et al. Synovial cyst of dens causing spinal cord compression: case report. *Paraplegia* 1993;31:803–807.
68. Bartynski WS, Barnes PD, Wallman JK. Cranial CT of autosomal recessive osteopetrosis. *AJNR Am J Neuroradiol* 1989;10:543–550.
69. Lori-Cortex R, Quesada-Calvo E, Cordero-Chaverri C. Osteopetrosis in children. *J Pediatr* 1977;91:43–47.
70. Kaforti JK, Kleinhaus U, Naveh Y. Progressive diaphyseal dysplasia (Camurati-Engelmann): radiographic follow-up and CT findings. *Radiology* 1987;164:777–782.
71. Naveh Y, Kaftori JK, Alon U, et al. Progressive diaphyseal dysplasia: genetics and clinical and radiologic manifestations. *Pediatrics* 1984;74:399–405.
72. Casselman JW, DeJonge I, Neyt L, et al. MRI in craniofacial fibrous dysplasia. *Neuroradiology* 1993;35:234–237.
73. Maeda M, Kimura H, Tsuchida C, et al. MR imaging of monostotic fibrous dysplasia of the clivus: a case report. *Acta Radiol* 1993;34:527–528.

CHAPTER 7

Carotid Artery Assessment and Interventional Radiologic Procedures Before Skull Base Surgery

William R. Nemzek

CAROTID ARTERY ASSESSMENT IN PATIENTS WITH SKULL BASE LESIONS

A multispecialty team approach, combining the talents of the neurosurgeon, otolaryngologist, plastic surgeon, and pathologist, has overcome the technical obstacles to performing successful skull base surgery. Extensive, complex lesions once considered inoperable can be completely extirpated (1). One formidable barrier remains. What should be done with the carotid artery if it is involved by a skull base lesion? Permanent occlusion of the internal carotid artery may be necessary to treat skull-based neoplasms and cavernous sinus and petrous carotid aneurysms and carotid–cavernous fistulas (2–4). Stroke is still a major risk in these patients. Without preoperative testing, abrupt internal carotid occlusion results in a stroke rate of 26% and a mortality rate of 12% (3). Can a group of patients be identified preoperatively who can safely tolerate carotid sacrifice, as opposed to those who must have carotid revascularization and bypass procedures?

Physiology of Regional Cerebral Blood Flow

Average normal cerebral blood flow (CBF) is 50 to 55 ± 12 ml/100 g/minute. There is about four times more flow to gray matter compared with white matter. Normal CBF is about 80 ml/100 g/minute to gray matter and 20 ml/100 g/minute to white matter (5,6).

Neuronal conductivity ceases and loss of consciousness ensues if CBF falls below 15 to 20 ml/100 g/minute (7–9).

Irreversible cellular damage occurs when CBF decreases below 6 to 8 ml/100 g/minute (9). The depth and duration of ischemia profoundly affects resultant brain injury. The brain may tolerate CBF of 12 to 15 ml/100 g/minute for 2 hours before infarction occurs (9,10). However, CBF of 2 to 3 ml/100 g/minute may be tolerated for only a few minutes before irreversible damage occurs (11).

Cerebral blood flow is directly coupled to metabolism, so increased metabolic activity is associated with a rapid local increase in CBF. Anesthesia, barbiturate coma, and hypothermia decrease cerebral metabolism and lower blood flow to the brain (12). The partial pressure of carbon dioxide (P_{CO_2}) also has a potent effect on CBF. CBF varies by 3% per mm Hg CO_2. A P_{CO_2} greater than 60 mm Hg causes maximal vasodilation, whereas a P_{CO_2} less than 20 mm Hg is associated with severe vasoconstriction (5). Therefore, P_{CO_2} must be monitored during CBF measurements.

Autoregulation refers to a proportional change in vascular resistance to maintain constant CBF despite a changing cerebral perfusion pressure. CBF normally remains constant at mean arterial pressures between 60 to 150 mm Hg. Injecting 1 g of acetazolamide (a carbonic anhydrase inhibitor) intravenously increases CBF by 30% to 40% after 20 minutes. Failure to increase flow means that the vessels are maximally dilated and lack functional reserve (5).

Preoperative Evaluation

Magnetic resonance scanning is the best method to evaluate the extent of a neoplasm and demonstrate the course of the carotid artery through the tumor. Magnetic resonance angiography is helpful for assessing patency of the major vessels and their relationship to lesions involving the skull base. Magnetic resonance angiography, however, does not surpass

---

W. R. Nemzek: Department of Radiology, Division of Diagnostic Radiology, University of California, Davis Medical Center, Sacramento, California 95817.

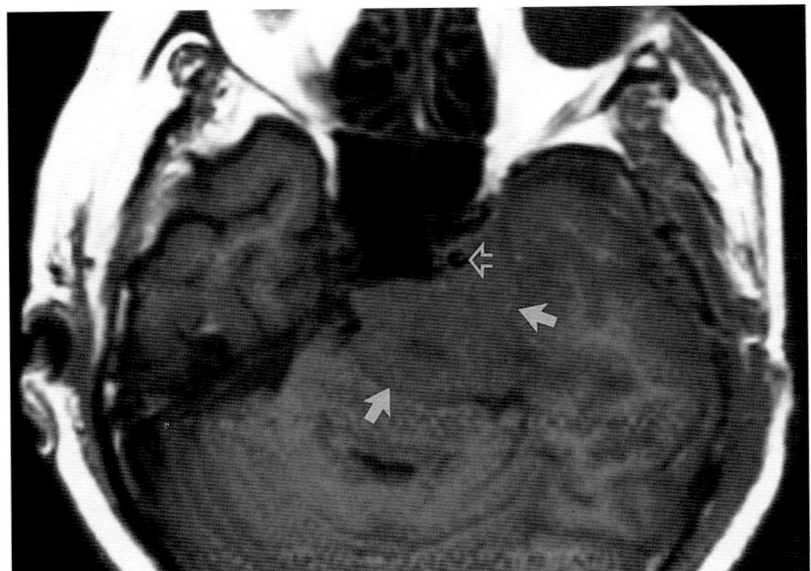
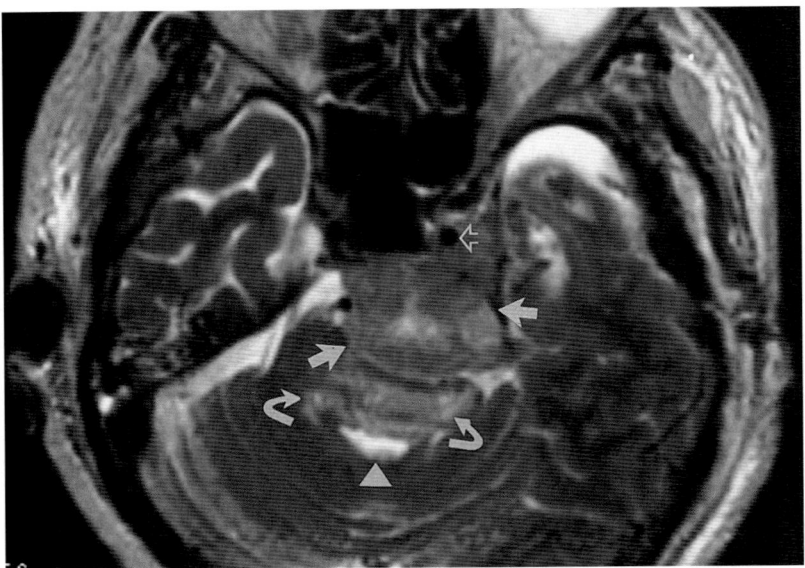
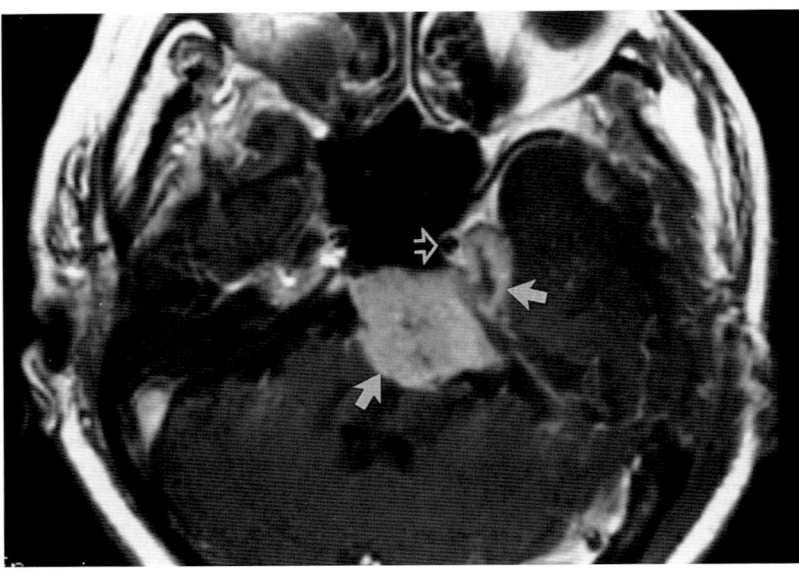

FIG. 1. Clival meningioma, recurrent, in a 72-year-old woman. **A:** T1-weighted (T1W) axial magnetic resonance image (MRI). **B:** T2-weighted (T2W) axial MRI. **C:** T1W axial MRI after gadolinium enhancement. The meningioma is isointense with gray matter on the T1W and slightly hyperintense on T2W images, with marked enhancement after gadolinium. The lesion arises from the clivus and extends into the prepontine and cerebellopontine angle cistern and Meckel's cave (*arrows*). Note encasement of internal carotid artery in the cavernous sinus (*open arrow*). In **(B)**, there is edema of the adjacent pons (*curved arrows*) on the T2W image. There is posterior displacement of the fourth ventricle (*arrowhead*). In **(C)** (slightly inferior to **[A]** and **[B]**), the enhancing meningioma abuts the internal carotid artery (*open arrow*).

conventional angiography in demonstrating small vessel detail (13). Much the same information about the major vessels and their relationship with the lesion can be gleaned from standard, cross-sectional magnetic resonance imaging (MRI) with proton-density and T2-weighted images (Fig. 1). Large vessels appear as absent signal (flow voids). Magnetic resonance venography is an excellent modality to exclude sigmoid sinus thrombosis (13).

If the carotid artery appears invaded by tumor, cerebral angiography and temporary balloon test occlusion (BTO) are performed.

Evolution of Preoperative Carotid Occlusion

In 1911, Matas described manual compression of the internal carotid artery as a method to assess risk for carotid occlusion (14). This test was unreliable because of the difficulty of obtaining complete internal carotid artery occlusion to exclude the external carotid artery and to avoid confounding vasovagal responses (3). Contralateral carotid arteriography with ipsilateral carotid compression provides anatomic assessment of anterior communicating artery patency, but it fails to provide information about functional reserve (15).

The measurement of *stump pressure* in the occluded carotid artery to determine carotid flow reserve is quite unreliable. Temporary shunt placement has been advocated for stump pressures below 20 to 70 mm Hg. Stump pressures vary widely in patients with normal and decreased regional CBF. Measurement of stump pressure is inaccurate in predicting delayed neurologic compromise (4,15,16). Continuous electroencephalographic monitoring during surgery is a measure of adequate CBF (17). The sensitivity is poor because major impairment of brain perfusion may be necessary to cause an electroencephalographic abnormality (18).

Intraoperative occlusion of the internal carotid artery under direct vision was replaced by BTO with local anesthesia.

Balloon Test Occlusion

Temporary trial occlusion of the internal carotid artery has been used to identify those patients with no flow reserve who are at very high risk for neurologic sequelae if the carotid is permanently occluded. A bilateral carotid and a vertebral arteriogram are performed, using the femoral artery approach, to assess the relation of the vessels to the lesion and to evaluate the collateral circulation through the circle of Willis. Contraindications to performing BTO include severe stenosis or occlusion of the contralateral carotid artery (15), or a vascular anomaly such as an isolated middle cerebral artery or an embryonic carotid basilar anastomosis (Fig. 2). This group of patients require bypass surgery if the carotid must be sacrificed, and no further diagnostic evaluation is needed.

If there are no anatomic contraindications, then BTO is performed. The patient is anticoagulated with 5,000 to 7,000 units of intravenous heparin (6). A 5-Fr double-lumen Swan-

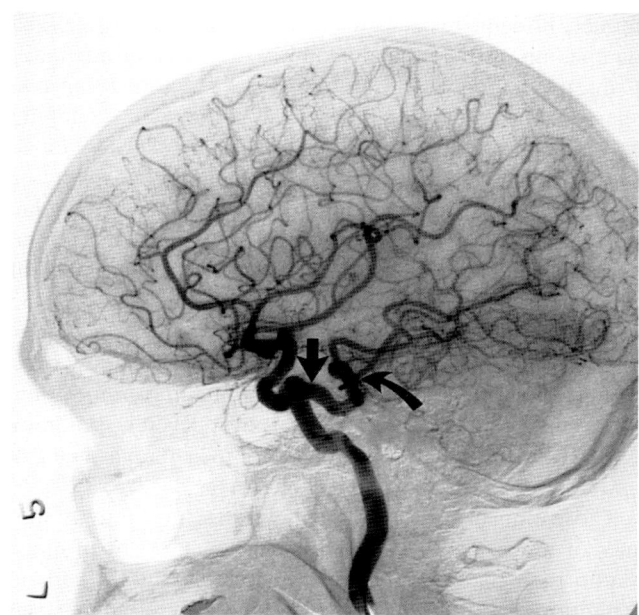

FIG. 2. Persistent trigeminal artery (*arrow*), a fetal carotid–basilar anastomosis, connects the cavernous internal carotid artery with the basilar artery (*curved arrow*).

Ganz catheter is passed through a 6-Fr introducer sheath, and the balloon catheter is flow-directed into the internal carotid to the level of C1 or C2. A 0.018-in. exchange guide wire may also be used to place the Swan-Ganz catheter in very tortuous vessels. The Swan-Ganz catheter is most commonly used because of its ease of introduction, its double-lumen configuration, which allows alternating pressure measurements and infusion of heparinized saline into the occluded internal carotid artery, and its relatively low cost (6). As an alternative, a single-lumen, nondetachable silicone balloon catheter manufactured by Interventional Therapeutics Corporation (ITC-NDSB [1509]) can be used. This is a very supple, 2-Fr polyethylene catheter that can be used in very tortuous vessels. Limitations of this system include the use of a larger guiding catheter (7.3-Fr minimum size) and a single-lumen configuration, which precludes infusion of heparinized saline and pressure measurements in the occluded internal carotid artery (6). Micro Interventional Systems has introduced a 5.4-Fr, double-lumen silicone balloon-tipped catheter with a large inner diameter (0.042 in.) that accepts standard 0.038-in. guide wires.

If there is significant atherosclerotic disease at the common carotid artery bifurcation, then trial occlusion of the common carotid artery is elected. A baseline neurologic evaluation is performed, testing both hemispheres for motor function (cranial nerves, pronator drift, grip, foot flexion and extension, finger to nose), sensation, and higher cortical function (name, place, counting). The pressure in the carotid is monitored through the double-lumen catheter, distal to the balloon, before, during, and after balloon occlusion. The balloon is inflated with 0.1 to 0.2 ml of dilute contrast material (7) Adequate occlusion can be determined by maximal dampening of the preocclusion arterial waveform (Fig. 3). Contour change of the balloon from a round to an oval shape, as the balloon coapts the wall of the artery, is another method of judging vessel occlusion. Care must be taken not to overinflate the balloon and damage the intima. Monitoring arterial pressure waveforms is probably a safer method of determining optimal balloon inflation (6). Contrast can also be injected through the end hole to confirm a static column of contrast in the occluded carotid artery, but this is not necessary.

Heparinized saline must be infused slowly to allow retrograde flow of blood to perfuse the ophthalmic artery. Rapid saline infusion can produce the ocular ischemic syndrome (19). The patient may then experience ipsilateral orbital pain and progressive uniocular visual loss.

Close clinical monitoring continues for the 15 to 20 minutes of test occlusion. If there is any change in neurologic status, the balloon is immediately deflated and the catheter withdrawn. No further testing is done. These patients presumably have CBF less than 20 ml/100 g/minute (3–5).

Immediate neurologic deficits during BTO occur in 5% to 10% of patients. These deficits usually occur within 1 to 3 minutes of balloon inflation, often within seconds. Neurologic deficits rapidly resolve on balloon deflation (3,17).

Tests of Cerebral Blood Flow Reserve

It is evident that BTO with clinical monitoring alone will miss a significant number of patients with inadequate flow reserves (20,21). Patients who tolerate clinical BTO need additional testing of the adequacy of collateral flow to avoid delayed neurologic complications. Ten to 20% of patients who safely tolerate 20 minutes of BTO of the carotid suffer delayed neurologic sequelae if the carotid artery is permanently occluded (3,4,20,22–24). These patients are particularly at risk if episodes of hypotension, anemia, hypoxemia, or hypoglycemia occur after surgery.

Better evaluation of collateral flow may be obtained by measuring CBF (23). Angiography with only clinical BTO and no other tests of CBF reserve resulted in a postoperative neurologic complication rate of 43% after carotid artery sacrifice (20). In one study, the postoperative neurologic complication rate fell to 0% after the addition of technetium-99m (^{99m}Tc) hexamethylpropyleneamine oxime (HMPAO) single photon emission computed tomography (SPECT) to the BTO study (21). Therefore, temporary test occlusion of the carotid artery and clinical neurologic evaluation must always be accompanied by CBF measurements.

Ideally, the measurement of CBF should be easy to perform, simple to interpret, and provide quantitative data correlating with physiologic thresholds for function and survival (5). Unfortunately, the ideal test does not exist.

Based on the Fick principle, nitrous oxide, an inert, lipid-soluble gas, was originally used to measure flow. The Fick principle states that the quantity of gas taken up in a tissue per unit time is equal to the quantity entering the tissue in the arterial blood minus the quantity leaving in the venous blood. Kety and Schmidt calculated the average CBF by knowing the time course of the change in the inert gas concentration in the arterial blood entering the brain and in the venous blood leaving it, as well as the partition coefficient. This assumes that blood flow is in a steady state during the study and is not affected by the tracer. Substituting radioactive ^{133}Xe allowed the use of external scintillation counting to measure the tracer in the brain. Xenon computed tomography (CT) uses nonradioactive Xe gas as a contrast agent during serial CT scanning (25).

Stable Xe is radiodense with an atomic number of 54 and a k-edge similar to iodine. Xe is a chemically inert noble gas that is highly lipid soluble and, after inhalation, moves rapidly from the blood pool to cross the blood–brain barrier and enter the brain. The concentration of Xe is an indicator of tissue perfusion (26). Although 80% Xe is an anesthetic similar to nitrous oxide, most people tolerate 33% Xe concentration with few sensory disturbances other than a mild euphoria (27). Thirty-three percent Xe has a CT density of about 10 Hounsfield units (5).

A routine CBF study can be accomplished in 30 to 40 min-

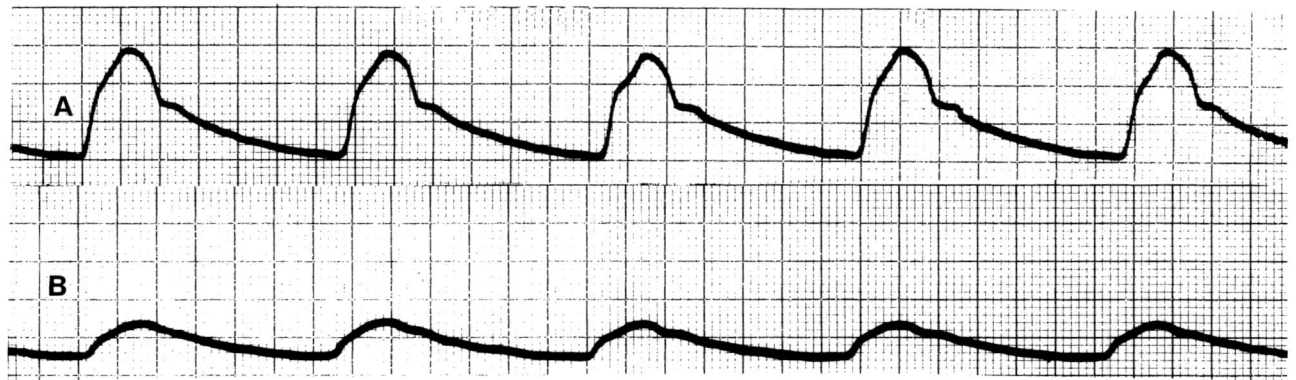

FIG. 3. Internal carotid artery pressure, measured distal to the occlusion balloon, through the end-hole of the balloon occlusion catheter. **A:** Preocclusion pressure of 151/39, mean 109 mm Hg. **B:** Occlusion pressure with balloon inflated of 89/52, mean 63 mm Hg. Note maximal dampening of arterial waveform.

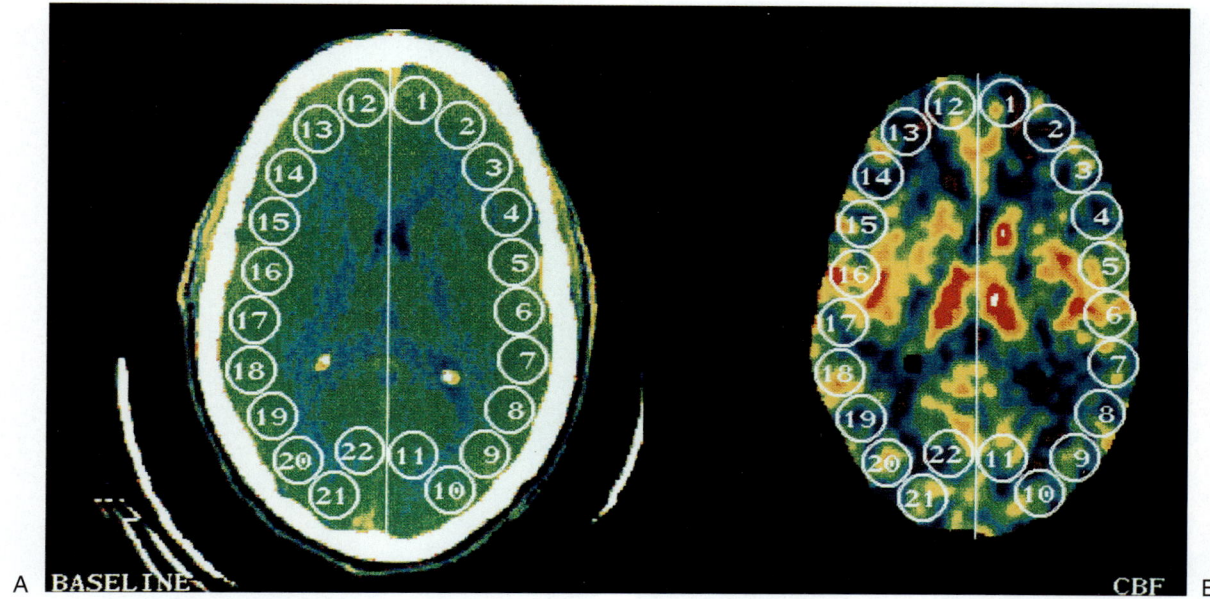

FIG. 4. Normal Xe computed tomography regional cerebral blood flow study. Scan at level of lateral ventricles and foramen of Monro. **A:** Baseline study with regions of interest placed over cortex. **B:** After Xe inhalation, a color regional blood flow map is obtained. The brighter colors (yellow and red) correspond to higher blood flow in the cortex and basal ganglia.

utes and can be repeated in 20 minutes. The concentration of arterial Xe is indirectly measured by the end-tidal concentration using a thermal conductivity analyzer. CT images are obtained during 4 to 5 minutes of Xe inhalation, which is sufficiently rapid not to allow any pharmacologic effects of Xe to alter flow dynamics. Baseline images are subtracted from contrast-enhanced xenon images (3,5) (Fig. 4). The data obtained are used to solve the modified Kety equation (2,5):

$$\Delta CT(t) = f\int_0^t \Delta Ca(u)e^{-f/\lambda(t-u)}du$$

where f is flow, λ is the tissue partition coefficient, and $f = k\lambda$. Each computed tomography (CT) voxel is defined as a series of changes in CT enhancement values as a function of time, $\Delta CT(t)$. $\Delta Ca(u)$ is the arterial concentration of xenon indirectly determined from the thermoconductivity detector recording of xenon end-tidal values.

Two axial levels are chosen for Xe CT CBF analysis. Contiguous 2-cm regions of interest are placed over the cortical mantle at the level of the foramen of Monro and at the top of the ventricular system. A quantitative value for each region of interest is determined, with special attention given to border zone territories between the anterior, middle, and posterior cerebral arteries (3). *Adequate CBF is defined as greater than 30 ml/100 g/minute* (5,7,17) (Fig. 5).

Regional CBF may also be evaluated with SPECT using [99mTc] HMPAO (26). HMPAO is injected intravenously during test occlusion of the carotid artery. [99mTc] HMPAO is a lipophilic tracer that freely crosses the blood–brain barrier. [99mTc] HMPAO has an extraction fraction of 0.75 (28). Once inside the brain tissue, the compound is rapidly converted to a hydrophilic form and is retained for several hours to allow imaging. The uptake of [99mTc] HMPAO is maximum within 10 minutes after intravenous injection (29). HMPAO is regionally distributed in proportion to local CBF (30,31) (Fig. 6).

When areas of regional brain perfusion in opposite hemispheres are compared, a 10% difference is considered to be a positive study (29). HMPAO SPECT provides only an assessment of asymmetry between cerebral hemispheres, and not quantitative CBF data. Some claim that SPECT may be overly sensitive and lacks adequate specificity (32). Occasionally, CBF may rise on the occluded or unoccluded side, producing asymmetries of normal or even elevated CBF. Without quantitative data, these CBF levels may be given unwarranted significance (3,33,34). The advantage of SPECT is that it is easy to perform and uses readily available technology that provides regional perfusion information (30).

Positron emission tomography depicts quantitative regional CBF and metabolism. It requires an on-site cyclotron plus the supporting technology, thereby limiting its availability.

Limitations of Preoperative Balloon Test Occlusion and Testing of Cerebral Blood Flow

Even in patients identified as safe for abrupt carotid occlusion by preoperative testing, delayed ischemic complications develop in 3% to 22% (6,34). This dilemma has caused many surgeons to forgo preoperative quantitative CBF anal-

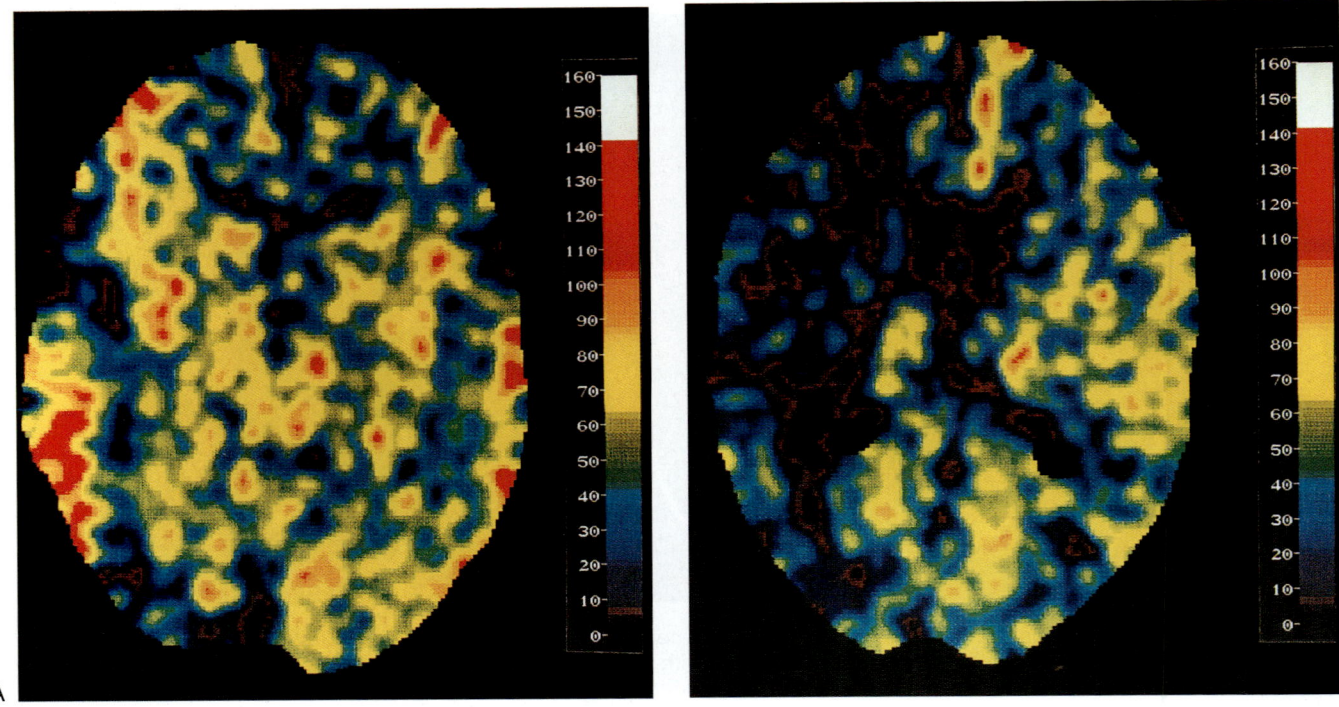

FIG. 5. A: Preocclusion baseline Xe computed tomography cerebral blood flow study showing normal symmetric cerebral blood flow. **B:** Balloon test occlusion of right internal carotid artery for 15 minutes. Even though the patient remained asymptomatic, with a negative neurologic examination, there is a significant decrease in blood flow in the territory of the right middle cerebral artery, right anterior border zone, and the right anterior cerebral artery. (Reproduced with permission from ref. 3.)

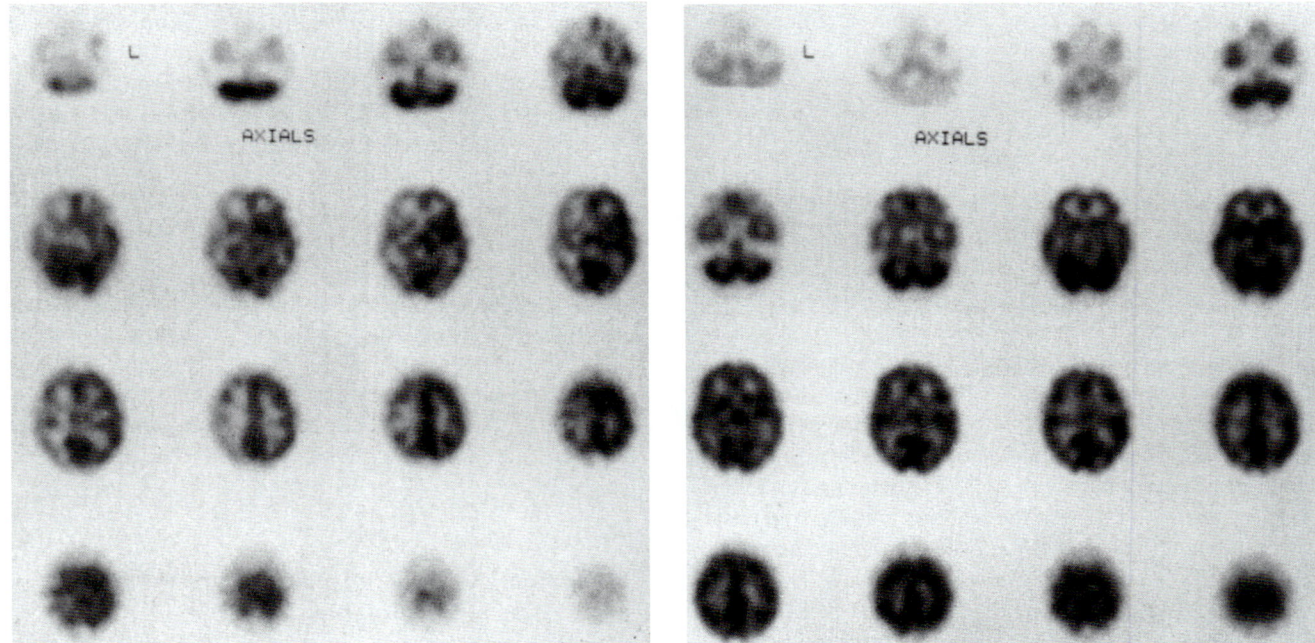

FIG. 6. ^{99m}Tc HMPAO single photon emission computed tomography scan. The axial images are displayed from skull base to vertex. **A:** During balloon test occlusion of the right internal carotid artery, there is decreased perfusion of the right cerebral hemisphere. **B:** A baseline study performed the next day shows normal symmetric perfusion. (Reproduced with permission from ref. 29.)

ysis, and to determine the need for shunting based on clinical and physiologic criteria of cerebral ischemia (17).

Even if the elusive goal of perfect testing for CBF is attained, other delayed conditions compromising CBF cannot be predicted. Critics of preoperative assessment of the carotid with BTO and CBF mapping claim that these tests can never completely define that subset of patients requiring revascularization. Tests of CBF cannot measure all the confounding variables (34–36).

The first and foremost unpredictable complication after carotid artery sacrifice is *embolization* arising from thrombus in the occluded supraclinoid segment of the internal carotid artery (6,35). Opponents site several other limitations of BTO, including (a) BTO is performed under ideal conditions that do not truly test the patient during additional ischemic challenge such as hypotension, vasospasm, and radiation-induced vasculopathy (4); (b) regional CBF measurements are technically challenging and time consuming (35); and (c) the risk of complication from BTO alone varies from 0% to 8.3% (6,34).

In the largest series, comprising 500 BTO procedures (6), 3.2% had complications. Asymptomatic complications were seen in 1.6%, including dissection (1.2%), pseudoaneurysm formation (0.2%), and embolism (0.2%). Neurologic deficits that persisted beyond the test period were also seen in 1.6%; these were either transient (1.2%) or permanent (0.4%). In one series, approximately 50% of asymptomatic patients with a positive SPECT scan after BTO had a positive MRI scan. This suggests that patients sustain residual focal subclinical ischemia due to the test occlusion (31). The neurologic complication rate after diagnostic cerebral angiography ranges from 1.3% to 2.6%, which is similar to the neurologic complication rate from BTO (6,37,38).

Some surgeons have abandoned internal carotid artery occlusion, claiming that it is never totally safe (36,39). Delayed ischemic neurologic complications may occur several years after carotid artery ligation (24,40–43). The natural history of carotid occlusion without revascularization in young patients is unknown (44). Aneurysm formation after carotid ligation has been described as a potential complication (45). Opponents of BTO advocate liberal revascularizaton and preservation of the carotid whenever possible (34,44).

Conclusions

1. Balloon test occlusion of the internal carotid artery with only clinical neurologic monitoring is an inadequate evaluation of cerebrovascular reserve. BTO should always be accompanied by CBF studies, such as Xe CT or SPECT.
2. Preoperative assessment assists decision making by indicating inadequate CBF reserves.
3. Causes of stroke after carotid occlusion include marginal perfusion due to inadequate collateral circulation and embolization of clot from the occluded segment of carotid artery.
4. BTO with CBF studies predict many, but not all, delayed neurologic sequelae after carotid artery sacrifice.

INTERVENTIONAL RADIOLOGIC PROCEDURES

Fine-Needle Aspiration Biopsy

Technique

Computed tomography- or MRI-guided fine-needle aspiration biopsy (FNAB) is a potent diagnostic tool in the evaluation of head and neck disease. Deep or nonpalpable lesions that would otherwise require an open surgical biopsy sampling procedure are made accessible with imaging guidance (46). FNAB is especially valuable in areas of anatomic distortion secondary to surgery or radiation (47).

Fine-needle aspiration biopsy is performed in an outpatient setting. The procedure is carefully explained to the patient. Intravenous sedation and analgesia are given with midazolam (Versed) and fentanyl. Lidocaine is used for local anesthesia.

Stainless steel needles are unsuitable for MRI because of high magnetic susceptibility and the creation of large artifacts. MRI-compatible needles have been developed that have a higher nickel content than stainless steel (48–50). Nickel stabilizes iron in a nonmagnetic form and reduces the magnetic susceptibility artifact of stainless steel (51). The advantages of MRI guidance include imaging in any plane, which makes it easy to follow the needle by imaging in a plane orthogonal to the path of the needle. MRI also has superior soft tissue contrast resolution (48).

Twenty-two- to 26-gauge needles are used for FNAB. To avoid multiple needle insertions, a coaxial needle system can be used. A 19-gauge/22-gauge combination can be used, but for areas such as the head and neck, where critical, complex anatomy is contained in a compact space, smaller needles are preferred to minimize risk to neural and vascular structures. Another benefit of a smaller needle is improved patient comfort. Lufkin and Layfield (52) describe a smaller coaxial needle system using a standard 22-gauge MRI-compatible needle that accepts a 26-gauge needle. The smaller 26-gauge needle should be chosen so the tip extends 5 to 10 mm beyond the tip of the larger 22-gauge needle. A small amount of curve is formed in the tip of the smaller needle. Once the 22-gauge needle is positioned at the margin of the lesion, no further imaging is necessary. The 26-gauge needle is inserted and multiple aspirations are performed with varying tip angulations and depths until adequate cells are obtained for cytologic diagnosis (52).

Approach

The approach depends on the area to be sampled (46,48,53–55).

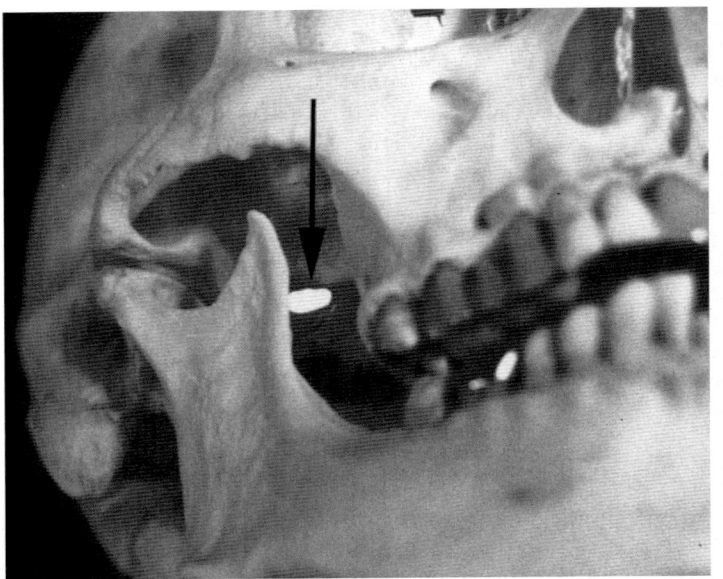
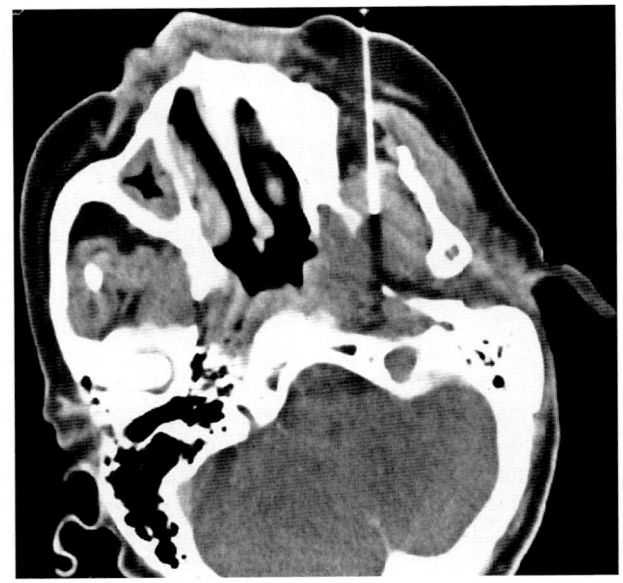
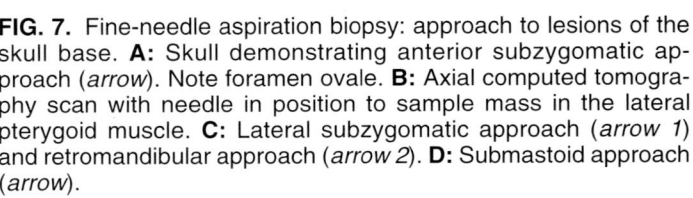
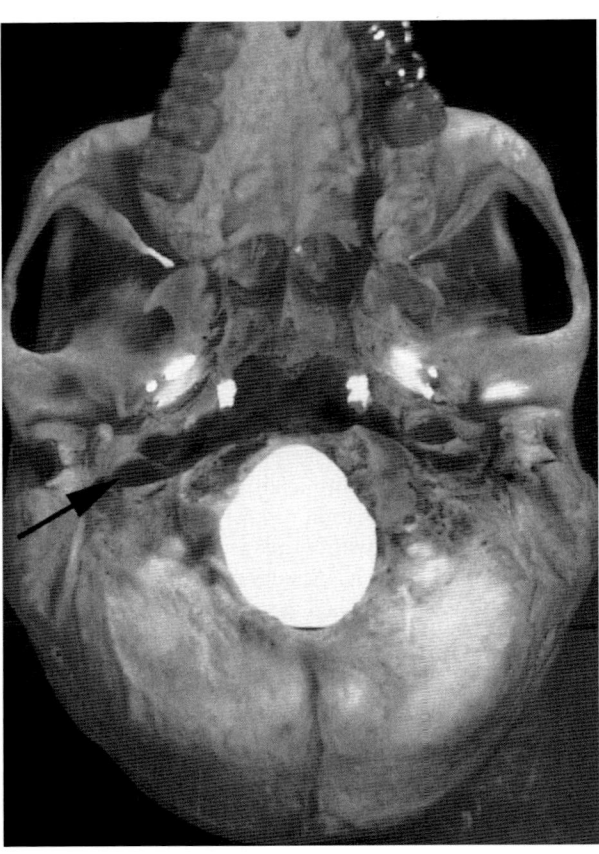

FIG. 7. Fine-needle aspiration biopsy: approach to lesions of the skull base. **A:** Skull demonstrating anterior subzygomatic approach (*arrow*). Note foramen ovale. **B:** Axial computed tomography scan with needle in position to sample mass in the lateral pterygoid muscle. **C:** Lateral subzygomatic approach (*arrow 1*) and retromandibular approach (*arrow 2*). **D:** Submastoid approach (*arrow*).

Anterior Subzygomatic

This approach is best for lesions in the region of the foramen ovale, parapharyngeal space, and infratemporal fossa (46,55) (Fig. 7A,B). The needle is inserted inferior to the malar eminence of the zygomatic bone parallel to the lateral wall of the maxilla. The neck should be slightly extended with a small pad placed beneath the shoulders. The head is rotated 15 to 20 degrees away from the side of the lesion. This opens a direct line from the anterior face to the foramen ovale, which does not cross vital structures. Care must be taken to avoid injury to the carotid artery and the cavernous sinus.

Lateral Subzygomatic

This approach is best for paranasopharyngeal and infratemporal fossa lesions (48) (see Fig. 7). The needle is inserted inferior to temporal zygomatic process and superior to the coronoid notch of the mandible.

Retromandibular

This path is used for paraesophageal, parotid, and masticator space lesions (see Fig. 7C). The needle is placed posterior to the mandibular ramus.

Submastoid

Skull base disease (e.g., jugular foramen lesions) may be sampled using the submastoid approach (see Fig. 7D). The needle is inserted at the inferior mastoid tip, angled cranially, and directed in a rostrad direction.

Therapeutic Techniques: Preoperative Embolization of Vascular Lesions

The goal of preoperative embolization is to decrease tumor vascularity and facilitate surgical removal (56). Embolization may also be performed for palliation and has the advantage of being readily repeatable. Embolization of the *external carotid artery* should not be undertaken lightly. There is potentially dangerous flow to the central nervous system, cranial nerves, and orbit. Risks include stroke and cranial nerve palsies and blindness (57,58). A thorough understanding of neurovascular anatomy and the important "dangerous" anastomoses is critical (58–60) (Tables 1–5).

The *ascending pharyngeal artery* supplies the pharynx, base of skull, posterior fossa, and cranial nerves IX, X, XI, and XII. There are also normal anastomoses between the ascending pharyngeal and the vertebral and internal carotid arteries (59).

The *middle meningeal artery* supplies the skull base and dura and cranial nerve VII. There are also important anasto-

TABLE 1. *Anastomoses of the ascending pharyngeal artery*

Communicates with	By way of
Occipital artery	C-1/C-2 collaterals
Vertebral artery	Odontoid and spinomuscular branches
Middle meningeal	
Meningohypophyseal trunk	Clival branches
Inferolateral trunk	
Distal internal maxillary artery	
Petrous internal carotid artery	Persistent mandibular (mandibulovidian) artery

Modified with permission, from ref. 4.

TABLE 2. *Anastomoses of the internal maxillary artery*

Communicates with	By way of
Ophthalmic artery (orbit)	Anterior and posterior ethmoidal branches (ophthalmic artery) Orbital branch middle meningeal Anterior deep temporal Infraorbital Sphenopalatine
Cavernous ICA	Inferolateral trunk Artery of the foramen rotundum Accessory meningeal artery Vidian artery
Petrous ICA	Persistent mandibular (mandibulovidian) artery

ICA, internal carotid artery.

TABLE 3. *Anastomoses of the occipital artery*

Communicates with	By way of
Vertebral artery	C-1/C-2 collaterals Costocervical, thyrocervical trunks

TABLE 4. *Anastomoses of the middle meningeal artery*

Communicates with	By way of
Ophthalmic artery	Anomalous-origin ophthalmic artery Lacrimal artery
Cavernous internal carotid artery	Falx and meningeal branches of ethmoidal arteries from ophthalmic artery

TABLE 5. *Causes of extracranial vertebral artery aneurysms*

Dissecting hematoma
Fibromuscular dysplasia
Collagen diseases (Ehler-Danlos syndrome)
Neurofibromatosis
Atherosclerosis
Trauma
Radionecrosis

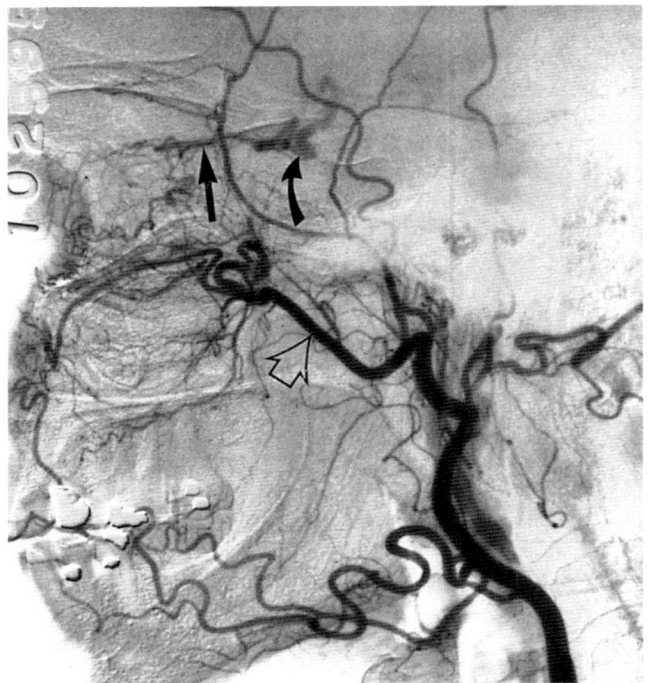

FIG. 8. Common carotid arteriogram (lateral projection) showing near-occlusion of the internal carotid artery. Note retrograde filling of the carotid siphon (*curved arrow*) from the ophthalmic artery (*arrow*), which opacifies through branches of the internal maxillary artery (*open arrow*).

moses with the ophthalmic artery and the cavernous internal carotid (59).

The distal *internal maxillary artery* may supply the eye by anterior deep temporal, infraorbital, and sphenopalatine branches (59) (Figs. 8, 9).

There is a consistent anastomosis between the *occipital artery* and the vertebral artery (Fig. 10).

These anastomoses may fail to appear on the initial arteriogram, but this does not mean they do not exist (58). As embolization progresses, distal perfusion decreases and the hemodynamic balance and flow patterns change, opening potentially dangerous collaterals (57,58).

The goal of embolization dictates the type of embolic agent (Table 6). Gelfoam is absorbable and is considered a temporary embolic agent, whereas coils, polyvinyl alcohol, and tissue adhesives are permanent. Therapeutic embolization is palliative but rarely curative. It must be remembered that collateral vessels will form and occluded vessels will recanalize, even after treatment with so called "permanent" embolic materials (61–64). Recanalization occurs slowly over weeks and months and should not be of clinical concern if embolization is performed several hours or days before surgery (61).

Alcohol and small particulate emboli, such as Gelfoam or polyvinyl alcohol particles, penetrate deeply distal to the point at which a surgical ligature may be applied. Liquid and small emboli produce optimal devascularization because they destroy the nidus and penetrate beyond where collateral flow may resupply the lesion (58). These are the most dangerous of the embolic agents because the liquids and small particles may reach tiny anastomoses with major intracranial vessels or arteries supplying cranial nerves. The result is the potential for disastrous complications, such as stroke and cranial nerve palsies. Large emboli, such as detachable balloons and wire coils, achieve proximal occlusion similar to surgical ligation. Proximal occlusion may be ineffective because of recruitment of collateral vessels to supply the lesion. Proximal occlusion also blocks access to the lesion if additional embolization therapy is necessary (57).

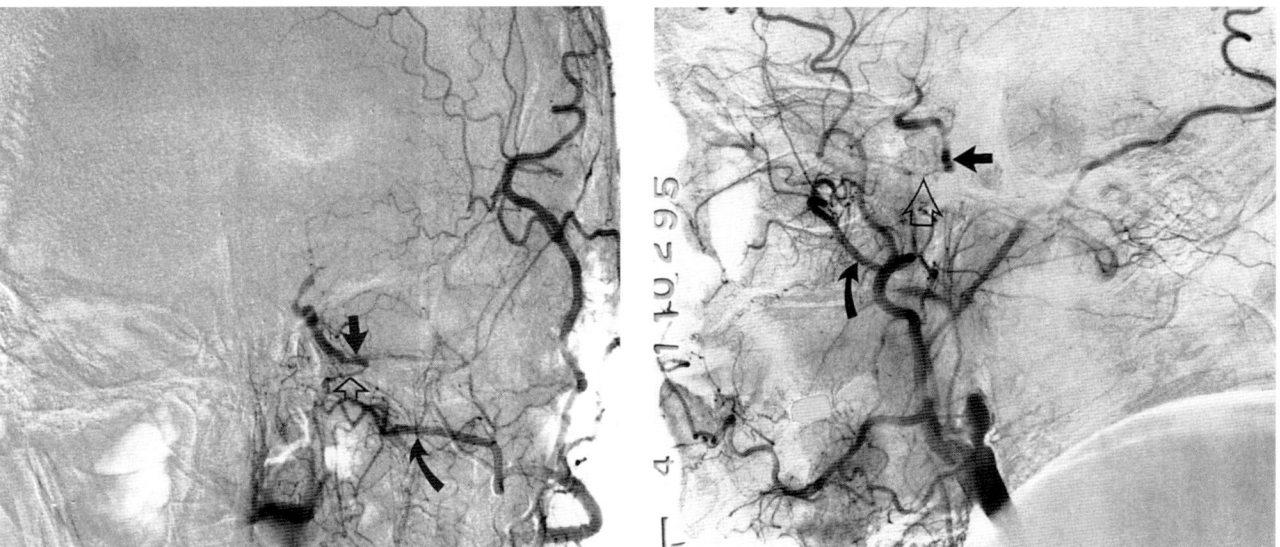

FIG. 9. Left common carotid arteriogram, anteroposterior (**A**) and lateral (**B**) projections. There is occlusion of the internal carotid artery. Note filling of the distal internal carotid (*arrow*) from the vidian branch of the mandibular artery (*open arrow*), which is filled by branches of the internal maxillary artery (*curved arrow*).

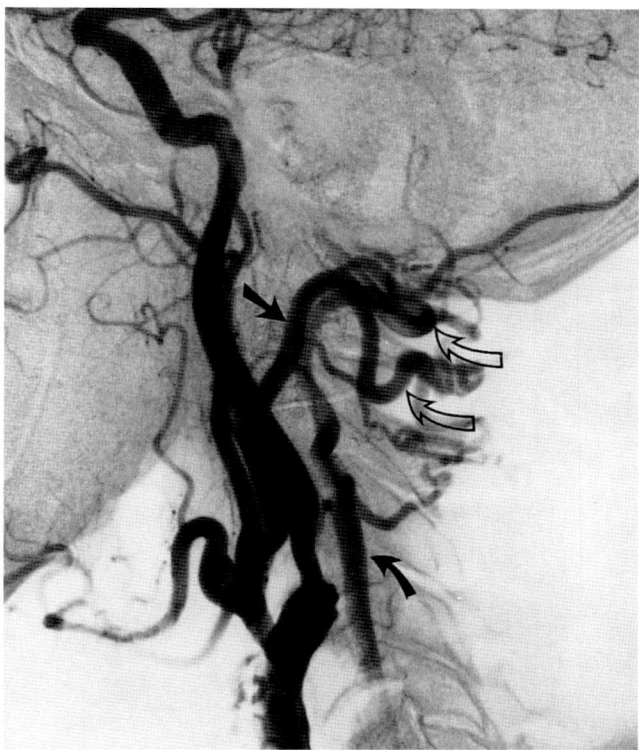

FIG. 10. Common carotid arteriogram (lateral projection) showing occlusion of the vertebral artery (*curved arrow*), which fills from C1-2 collaterals (*open arrows*) by way of the occipital artery (*arrow*).

When embolization involves branches of the external carotid artery, 2 in. of nitroglycerin ointment (Nitro-paste) is applied cutaneously before the procedure to prevent vasospasm (65).

Before embolization, provocative testing of the arterial feeder must be performed with 25 to 50 mg of cardiac lidocaine to discover the cranial nerve blood supply (57,66). If lidocaine injection produces a cranial nerve deficit, then the vessel cannot be safely embolized with Gelfoam powder or liquid agents (57). Larger particles may be used to produce a more proximal occlusion and allow recruitment of collateral vessels (67). Protection of normal vascular territories may be accomplished by using a large piece of Gelfoam or polyvinyl alcohol sponge to occlude a "dangerous anastomosis" to prevent emboli from entering the unwanted normal artery (67,68). Amytal testing (50 mg) is used if there is potential supply to intracranial structures.

Embolic material may be introduced by catheter or by direct puncture. Most vascular lesions of the head and neck are supplied by branches of the external carotid artery. Once the tumor has invaded the skull base, blood supply may be recruited from internal carotid or vertebral artery branches that would be difficult or impossible to approach safely with small catheters. Direct percutaneous, transoral, or transnasal puncture of these lesions under general anesthesia makes them amenable to treatment with liquid embolic agents, such as alcohol or N-butyl cyanoacrylate (NBCA) (69).

Complete surgical removal of *meningiomas* can be facilitated by preoperative tumor devascularization (56). Most meningiomas at the convexity are extremely vascular, whereas fewer than half of those at the skull base are vascular enough to warrant embolization (67). Angiographic evaluation includes study of both internal and external carotid arteries. The convexity meningiomas are supplied by ipsilateral and contralateral middle meningeal arteries. If there is extension to the falx, the anterior falx artery arising from the ophthalmic is involved. Meningiomas of the skull base are supplied by the ascending pharyngeal, occipital, and posterior auricular arteries, the posterior meningeal branch of the vertebral artery, and the posterior clival and tentorial branches of the cavernous internal carotid artery (67). Meningiomas may recruit pial blood supply from cerebral branches of the internal carotid artery.

Preoperative embolization of *juvenile nasopharyngeal angiofibromas* can reduce intraoperative blood loss. After combined embolization and surgery, tumor recurrence is reduced, probably because of more complete removal of a devascularized tumor (57).

Both internal maxillary arteries should be studied. There may also be supply from ipsilateral and contralateral accessory meningeal, ascending pharyngeal, and ascending palatine arteries. Angiography of both internal carotid arteries is necessary to define potential supply from the cavernous carotid, ethmoid, and mandibular arteries (57,68).

For *paragangliomas* originating in the temporal bone (Fig. 11), ipsilateral internal carotid, vertebral, and external carotid arteries should be evaluated. External carotid supply may arise from the posterior auricular, occipital, and ascending pharyngeal arteries (57). Intracranial extension of paragangliomas may be supplied by branches of the posterior inferior cerebellar artery or anterior inferior cerebellar branches of the vertebrobasilar system (70). For cervical lesions, the ipsilateral internal carotid, vertebral, and external carotid arteries are examined. Potential external carotid supply includes the facial, lingual, superior thyroid, ascending cervical, and both ascending pharyngeal arteries. *Carotid body* tumors are also supplied by the artery of the carotid body (57,70).

TABLE 6. *Embolic agents*

Liquid
  95% Ethanol
  Tissue adhesives (e.g., *N*-butyl cyanoacrylate)
Small particulate emboli
  Gelfoam powder
  Gelfoam particles
  Polyvinyl alcohol
Large particulate emboli
  Suture
  Coils (stainless steel, platinum)
  Detachable balloons

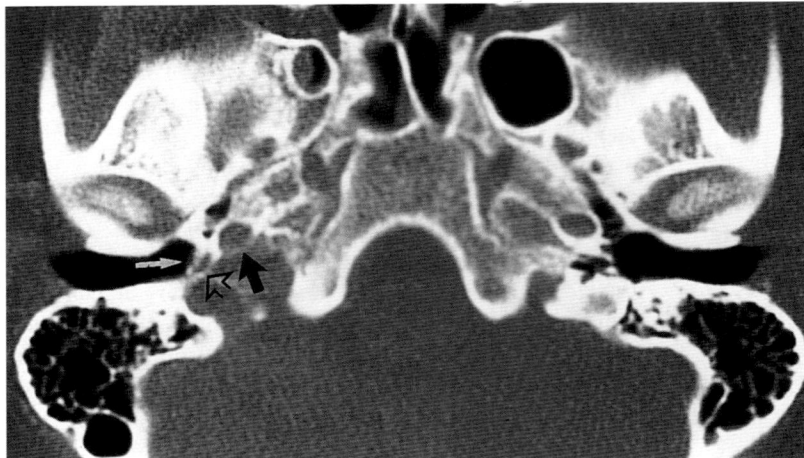
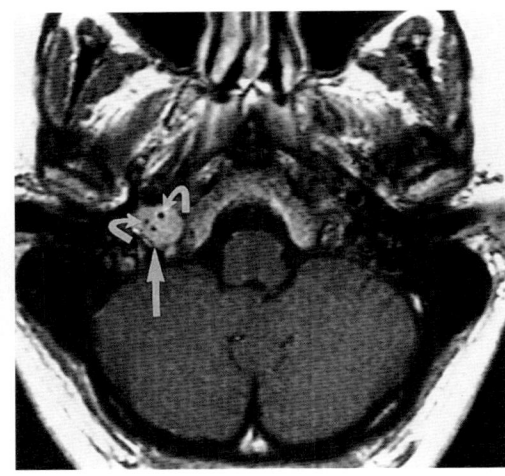
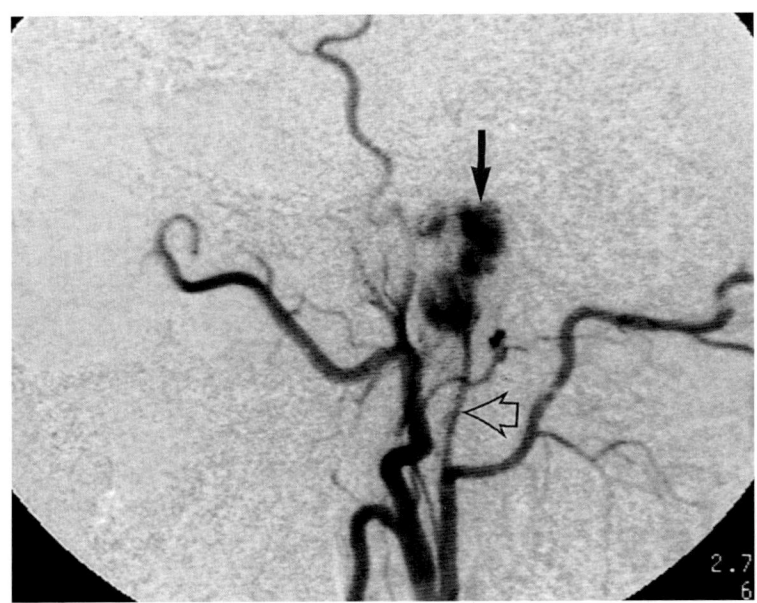
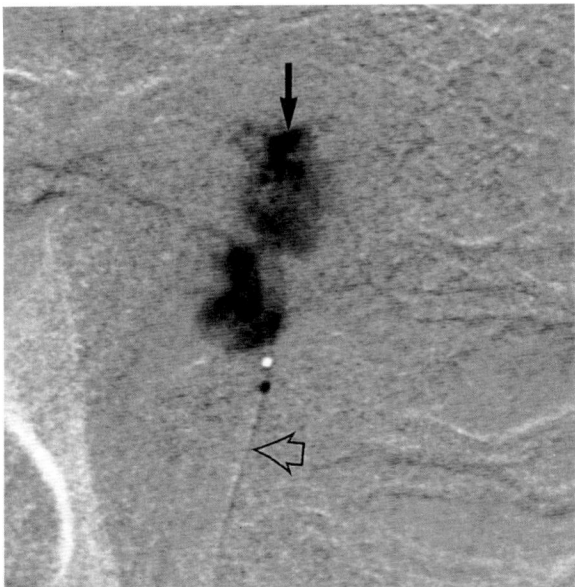

FIG. 11. Glomus jugulotympanicum. **A:** Axial computed tomography scan. There is erosion of the caroticojugular spine (*arrow*) and the lateral wall of the jugular fossa (*open arrow*), with extension of the mass into the middle ear (*white arrow*). **B:** Axial T1-weighted magnetic resonance image with gadolinium enhancement. There is an enhancing mass in the right jugular fossa (*arrow*). The signal voids (*curved arrows*) represent enlarged feeding arteries. **C:** External carotid arteriogram (lateral projection). There is a hypervascular tumor (*arrow*) fed by the ascending pharyngeal artery (*open arrow*). **D:** A Tracker catheter (*open arrow*) has been advanced into the ascending pharyngeal artery before embolization of the glomus tumor (*arrow*).

Conclusion

Preoperative embolization facilitates surgery by decreasing blood loss and allowing more complete removal of devascularized tumor. Thorough knowledge of neurovascular anatomy is necessary for safe, effective endovascular therapy.

ACKNOWLEDGMENT

The author thanks Kathy Sommers for invaluable assistance in preparing the manuscript.

REFERENCES

1. Donald PJ. Management of the internal carotid artery in skull base operations. *West J Med* 1993;159:70–71.
2. Andrews JC, Valavanis A, Fisch U. Management of the internal carotid artery in surgery of the skull base. *Laryngoscope* 1989;99:1224–1229.
3. Linskey ME, Jungreis CA, Yonas H, et al. Stroke risk after abrupt internal carotid artery sacrifice: accuracy of preoperative assessment with balloon test occlusion and stable xenon-enhanced CT. *AJNR Am J Neuroradiol* 1994;15:829–843.
4. DeVries EJ, Sekhar LN, Horton JA, et al. A new method to predict safe resection of the internal carotid artery. *Laryngoscope* 1990;100:85–88.
5. Yonas H, Gur D, Johnson DW, Latchaw RE. Xenon/CT cerebral blood flow analysis. In: Lathcaw RE, ed. *MR and CT imaging of the head, neck and spine.* 2nd ed. St. Louis: Mosby–Year Book, 1991:109–128.

6. Mathis JM, Barr JD, Jungreis CA, et al. Temporary balloon test occlusion of the internal carotid artery: experience in 500 cases. *AJNR Am J Neuroradiol* 1995;16:749–754.
7. Mathis JM, Barr JD, Jungreis CA, Horton JA. Physical characteristics of balloon catheter systems used in temporary cerebral artery occlusion. *AJNR Am J Neuroradiol* 1994;15:1831–1836.
8. Sundt TM Jr, Sharbrough FW, Anderson RE, et al. Cerebral blood flow measurements and electroencephalograms during carotid endarterectomy. *J Neurosurg* 1974;41:310–320.
9. Astrup J, Symon L, Branston NM, et al. Cortical evoked potential and extracellular K^+ and H^+ at critical levels of brain ischemia. *Stroke* 1977;8:51–57.
10. Morawetz RB, DeGirolami U, Ojeamann RG, et al. Cerebral blood flow determination by hydrogen clearance during middle cerebral artery occlusion in unanesthetized monkeys. *Stroke* 1978;9:143–149.
11. Jones TH, Morawetz RB, Crowell RM, et al. Thresholds of focal cerebral ischemia in awake monkeys. *J Neurosurg* 1981;54:773–782.
12. Sekhar LN. The work-up and management of the internal carotid artery in neoplastic and vascular lesions of the cranial skull base. In: *Sacramento skull base surgery symposium: a multidisciplinary approach.* Course syllabus, University of California, Davis. June 25–30, 1995: 76–80.
13. Rodgers GK, Applegate L, De la Cruz A, Lo W. Magnetic resonance angiography: analysis of vascular lesions of the temporal bone and skull base. *Am J Otol* 1993;14:56–62.
14. Mattas R. testing the efficiency of collateral circulation as a preliminary to the occlusion of the great surgical arteries. *Ann Surg* 1911;53:1–43.
15. Tarr RW, Jungreis CA, Horton JA, et al. Complications of preoperative balloon test occlusion of the internal carotid arteries: experience in 300 cases. *Skull Base Surgery* 1991;1:240–244.
16. Kelly JJ, Callow AD, O'Donnell TF, et al. Failure of carotid artery stump pressures: its incidence as a predictor for temporary shunt during carotid endarterectomy. *Arch Surg* 1979;114:1361–1366.
17. Steed DL, Webster MW, DeVries EJ, et al. Clinical observations on the effect of carotid artery occlusion on cerebral blood flow mapped by xenon computed tomography and its correlation with carotid artery back pressure. *Vasc Surg* 1990;11:38–44.
18. Askienazy S, Lebtahi R, Meder JF. SPECT HMPAO and balloon test occlusion: interest in predicting tolerance prior to permanent cerebral artery occlusion. *J Nucl Med* 1993;34:1243–1245.
19. Russell EJ, Goldberg K, Oskin J, Darling C, Melen O. Ocular ischemic syndrome during carotid balloon occlusion testing. *AJNR Am J Neuroradiol* 1994;15:258–262.
20. McIvor NP, Willinsky RA, TerBrugge KA, Rutka JA, Freeman JL. Validity of test occlusion studies prior to carotid artery sacrifice. *Head Neck* 1994;16:11–16.
21. Nayak UK, Donald PJ, Stevens D. Internal carotid artery resection for invasion of malignant tumors. *Arch Otolaryngol Head Neck Surg* 1995;121:1029–1033.
22. Nishioka H. Report on the Cooperative Study of Intracranial Aneurysms and Subarachnoid Hemorrhage, section VIII, part 1: results of the treatment of intracranial aneurysms by occlusion of the carotid artery in the neck. *J Neurosurg* 1966;24:660–682.
23. Eckard DA, Purdy PD, Bonte FJ. Temporary balloon occlusion of the carotid artery combined with brain flow imaging as a test to predict tolerance prior to permanent carotid sacrifice. *AJNR Am J Neuroradiol* 1992;13:1565–1569.
24. Linskey ME, Sekhar LN, Horton JA, Hirsch WL, Yonas H. Aneurysms of the intracavernous carotid artery: a multidisciplinary approach to treatment. *J Neurosurg* 1991;75:525–534.
25. Yonas H, Gur D, Good BC, et al. Stable xenon CT blood flow mapping for evaluation of patients with extracranial–intracranial bypass surgery. *J Neurosurg* 1985;62:324–333.
26. Gur D, Good WF, Wolfson SK, Yonas H, Shabason L. In vivo mapping of local cerebral flow by xenon-enhanced computed tomography. *Science* 1982;215:1267–1268.
27. Yonas H, Darby JM, Marks EC, Durham SR, Maxwell C. CBF measured by Xe-CT: approach to analysis and normal values. *J Cereb Blood Flow Metab* 1991;11:716–725.
28. Nakano S, Kinoshita K, Jinnouchi S, Hoshi H, Watanabe K. Comparative study of regional cerebral flow images by SPECT using xenon-133, iodine-123 IMP, and technetium-99m HM-PAO. *J Nucl Med* 1989;30:157–164.
29. Peterman SB, Taylor A, Hoffman JC. Improved detection of cerebral hypoperfusion with internal carotid balloon test occlusion and 99m Tc-HMPAO cerebral perfusion SPECT imaging. *AJNR Am J Neuroradiol* 1991;12:1035–1041.
30. Monsein LH, Jeffrey PJ, van Heerden BB, et al. Assessing adequacy of collateral circulation during balloon test occlusion of the internal carotid artery with 99m Tc-HMPAO SPECT. *AJNR Am J Neuroradiol* 1991;12:1045–1051.
31. Simonson TM, Ryals TJ, Yuh WTC, Farrar GP, Rezai K, Hoffman HT. MR imaging and HMPAO in conjunction with balloon test occlusion. *AJR Am J Roentgenol* 1992;159:1063–1068.
32. Yonas H, Linsky M, Johnson DW, et al. Internal carotid balloon test occlusion does require quantitative CBF. *AJNR Am J Neuroradiol* 1992;13:1147–1152.
33. Witt JP, Yonas H, Jungeis C. Cerebral blood flow response pattern during balloon test occlusion of the internal carotid artery. *AJNR Am J Neuroradiol* 1994;15:847–857.
34. Origitano TC, Al-Mefty O, Leonetti JP, DeMonte F, Reichman OH. Vascular considerations and complications in cranial base surgery. *Neurosurgery* 1994;35:351–363.
35. Eskridge JM. Xenon-enhanced CT: past and present. *AJNR Am J Neuroradiol* 1994;15:845–846.
36. Sekhar LN, Patel SJ. Permanent occlusion of the internal carotid artery during skull base surgery: is it really safe? *Am J Otol* 1993;14:421–422.
37. Dion JE, Gates PC, Fox AJ, Barnett HJM, Blom RJ. Clinical events ollowing neuroangiography: a prospective study. *Stroke* 1987;18:997–1004.
38. Ernest F, Forbes G, Sandok BA, et al. Complications of cerebral angiography: prospective assessment of risk. *AJR Am J Roentgenol* 1984;142:247–253.
39. Spetzler RF, Fukushima T, Martin N, Zabramski JM. Petrous carotid-to-intradural carotid saphenous vein graft for intracavernous giant aneurysm, tumor, and occlusive cerebrovascular disease. *J Neurosurg* 1990;73:496–501.
40. Roski RA, Spetzler RF, Nulsen FE. Late complications of carotid ligation in the treatment of intracranial aneurysms. *J Neurosurg* 1981;54:583–587.
41. Barnett HJ. Delayed ischemic episodes distal to occlusion of major cerebral arteries. *Neurology* 1978;28:769–774.
42. Oldershaw JB, Voris HC. Internal carotid artery ligation, a follow up study. *Neurology* 1966;16:937–938.
43. Winn HR, Richardson AE, Jane JA. Late morbidity and mortality of common carotid ligation for posterior communicating aneurysms. *J Neurosurg* 1977;47:727–736.
44. Sekhar LN, Sen CN, Jho HD. Saphenous vein graft bypass of the internal carotid artery. *J Neurosurg* 1990;72:35–41.
45. Dyste GN, Beck DW. De Novo aneurysm formation following carotid ligation: case report and review of the literature. *Neurosurgery* 1989;24:88–92.
46. Barakos JA, Dillon WP. Lesions of the foramen ovale: CT-guided fine-needle aspiration. *Radiology* 1992;182:573–575.
47. Abemayor E, Ljung BM, Larsson S, Ward PH, Hanafee W. CT-directed fine needle aspiration biopsies of masses in the head and neck. *Laryngoscope* 1985;95:1382–1386.
48. Duckwiler G, Lufkin RB, Teresi L, et al. Head and neck lesions: MR-guided aspiration biopsy. *Radiology* 1989;170:519–522.
49. Lufkin R, Teresi L, Hanafee W. New needle for MR-guided aspiration cytology of the head and neck. *AJR Am J Roentgenol* 149;380–382.
50. Hathout G, Lufkin RB, Jabour B, Andrews J, Castro D. MR-guided aspiration cytology in the head and neck at high field strength. *J Magn Reson Imaging* 1992;2:93–94.
51. Mueller PR, Stark DD, Simeone JF, et al. MR-guided aspiration biopsy: needle design and clinical trials. *Radiology* 1986;161:605–609.
52. Lufkin R, Layfield L. Coaxial needle system of MR- and CT-guided aspiration cytology. *J Comput Assist Tomogr* 1989;13:1105–1107.
53. Dresel SH, Mackey JK, Lufkin RB, et al. Meckel cave lesions: percutaneous fine-needle-aspiration biopsy cytology. *Radiology* 1991;179:579–581.
54. Ljung BME, Larsson SG, Hanafee W. Computed tomography-guided aspiration cytologic examination in head and neck lesions. *Archives of Otolaryngology* 1984;110:604–607.
55. Yousem DM, Sack MJ, Scanlan, KA. Biopsy of parapharyngeal space lesions. *Radiology* 1994;193:619–622.
56. Manelfe C, Lasjaunias P, Ruscalleda J. Preoperative embolization of intracranial meningiomas. *AJNR Am J Neuroradiol* 1986;7:963–972.

57. Kagetsu NJ, Berenstein A, Choi S. Interventional radiology of the extracranial head and neck. *Cardiovasc Intervent Radiol* 1991;14:325–333.
58. Russell EJ. Functional angiography of the head and neck. *AJNR Am J Neuroradiol* 1986;7:927–936.
59. Eskridge JM. Interventional neuroradiology. *Radiology* 1989;172:991–1006.
60. Lasjaunias P, Berenstein A. Dangerous vessels. In: *Surgical neuroangiography, vol. 1: functional anatomy of craniofacial arteries.* Berlin, Heidelberg: Springer-Verlag, 1987:239–244.
61. Davidson GS, Terbrugge KG. Histologic long-term follow-up after embolization with polyvinyl alcohol particles. *AJNR Am J Neuroradiol* 1995;16:843–846.
62. Mathis JA, Barr JD, Horton JA, et al. The efficiency of particulate embolization combined with stereotactic radiosurgery for treatment of large arteriovenous malformations of the brain. *AJNR Am J Neuroradiol* 1995;16:299–306.
63. Germano IM, Davis RL, Wilson CB, Hieshima GB. Histopathological follow-up study of 66 cerebral arteriovenous malformations after therapeutic embolization with polyvinyl alcohol. *J Neurosurg* 1992;76:607–614.
64. Purdy PD, Batjer HH, Risser RC, Samson D. Arteriovenous malformations of the brain: choosing embolic materials to enhance safety and ease of excision. *J Neurosurg* 1992;77:217–222.
65. Erba M, Jungreis CA, Horton JA. Nitropaste for prevention and relief of vascular spasm. *AJNR Am J Neuroradiol* 1989;10:155–156.
66. Horton JA, Kerber CW. Lidocaine injection into external carotid branches: provocative test to preserve cranial nerve function in therapeutic embolization. *AJNR Am J Neuroradiol* 1986;7:105–108.
67. Halbach VV, Hieshima GB, Higashida RT, David CF. Endovascular therapy of head and neck tumors. In: Vinuela F, Halbach V, Dion J, eds. *Interventional neuroradiology: endovascular therapy of the central nervous system.* Raven Press: New York, 1992:17–28.
68. Davis KR. Embolization of epistaxis and juvenile nasopharyngeal angiofibromas. *AJNR Am J Neuroradiol* 1986;7:953–962.
69. Casasco A, Herbreteau D, Houdart E, et al. Devascularizaton of craniofacial tumors by percutaneous tumor puncture. *AJNR Am J Neuroradiol* 1994;15:1233–1239.
70. Valavanis A. Preoperative embolization of the head and neck: indications, patient selection, goals, and precautions. *AJNR Am J Neuroradiol* 1986;7:943–952.

CHAPTER 8

Nursing Care of Skull Base Surgery Patients

Ann E. F. Sievers and Denise Borcyckowski

CARING FOR THE PATIENT WITH A SKULL BASE LESION

An entire new combined discipline of otolaryngologic and neurosurgical nursing has developed with the advent of skull base surgery. This discipline combines the most advanced and dedicated aspects of both nursing practice professions. Those who choose to practice in this setting are working on an exciting and very challenging forefront of medical practice and nursing intervention.

Patients with skull base tumors, whether benign or malignant, present with unique problems because of tumor involvement of the brain, cranial nerves, and facial structures. Deformity of appearance and alterations in function are major deficits that can occur with such tumors and the surgical procedures that correct them. With the patient at the center and as the driving force of the process, the team approach is the only possible way to deliver comprehensive care (1).

The skull base team meets regularly and frequently to present each patient and to develop team consensus and a plan of care. The skull base team comprises specialists from many different disciplines. Physicians include specialists from departments of otolaryngology, neurosurgery, plastic surgery, pathology, both neurovascular and interventional radiology, nuclear medicine, anesthesiology, and their accompanying residents and fellows. Representatives of the nursing profession include clinical nurse specialists in both otolaryngology and neurosurgery, operating room clinicians, intensive care unit staff, otolaryngology staff nurses, clinic triage, nursing discharge planners, and home care staff. Multidisciplinary professional staff members include social service workers, nutritionists, physical therapists, speech pathologists, discharge planners, and home health liaison staff.

One of the pivotal roles in the skull base team is the team coordinator. This role consists not only of team coordination, but of compiling patient information and supporting team research. The skull base team coordinator is responsible for the inner workings of the team as well as interaction with the patient and family (Table 1).

The coordinator must be chosen carefully for his or her ability to coordinate multiple schedules and deal with stressful and complicated situations gracefully. This role requires a true professional. Coordination and communication with insurance agencies are essential functions in the environment of managed care programs. This insurance interface allows the patient to concentrate on his or her medical care and not the financial morass that often can add such significant stress to an already difficult situation. To secure funding is imperative before beginning testing, evaluation, and contraction for evaluation and intervention. By attending to these functions, the coordinator enables the skull base team, patient, and the family to concentrate on the most important aspect, the care of the patient.

Funding and insurance coverage of skull base surgery and evaluation is only beginning to be understood and accepted by insurance companies. The roles of the team are to interface with the insurance carriers and elucidate the complexity of skull base surgery, to educate them about the enormity of skull base surgery, and to ensure their cooperation and their acceptance of their responsibilities for patient coverage. The skull base team should develop an information book, a treatment algorithm, and a plan of care as standard information for insurance companies. The packet could include physician qualifications, research results, length of estimated hospitalizations, as well as hospital and professional charges.

Preparation and Patient Education

The skull base surgical team has an enormous task of planning not only for the surgical procedure and care plan, but for informing and educating the patient. Patient education and obtaining informed legal consent are two very different processes. Patient education is the ongoing process of learning,

---

A. E. F. Sievers, D. Borcyckowski: Departments of Patient Care Services and Otolaryngology—Head and Neck Surgery, University of California, Davis Medical Center, Sacramento, California 95817.

TABLE 1. *Skull base team coordinator responsibilities*

Surgical scheduling
Team meetings
Preoperative test coordination
    Specialized tests: computed tomography, magnetic resonance imaging, magnetic resonance angiography, balloon test occlusion, single-photon emission computed tomography, positron emission tomographys, biopsy
Team information
Total quality assurance (TQA)
Policy and procedures
Patient and family schedule coordination
Insurance authorization
Research, data collection and coordination
Postoperative clinic scheduling
Postoperative repeat testing

---

for the patient and family, about the patient's diagnosis and care. This is a huge process for those who have a life-threatening illness. It becomes incumbent on the skull base team members to recognize that learning under stress is suboptimal, but that learning about the plan of care is absolutely necessary to the patient's survival and cooperation with therapy. Translation of medical terms into "the common vernacular" enables better communication regarding illness and therapy. The authors often tell patients that this is an odyssey into a foreign land that they do not want to take, and that it includes learning a foreign language, "the medical language," again not because they choose to do so. The role of the skull base coordinator and the clinical nurse specialist is to translate information and be the ongoing simultaneous translators for the patient and family.

If the medical team is sensitive to these issues, the patient's and family's odyssey turns from a nightmare into a positive journey with much support, caring, and guidance. The most important issues to discuss are those related to survival and the unique facets of skull base surgery the patient faces during recovery. Patients often ask why they got cancer, and a frank discussion related to the known issues may allay the fears of other family members. Molecular epidemiology suggests that the effects of environmental exposure and poor nutrition can be exacerbated in certain groups by inborn differences in the internal processing of carcinogens (2). Patients and family need to discuss their individual fears of cancer and of the upcoming surgery. The issues are, but are not limited to, tracheostomy, alteration in method of nutrition (oral vs. enteral), disfigurement, balance disorders, and changes from normal activities of daily living. It is the lack of information related to their life changes, and the diagnosis of tumor, that often makes patients and their families unable to cope with the rigors of skull base surgery and recovery.

Informed Consent

Informed consent is a mandated legal process to attempt to ensure that patients understand and consent to medical care. Obtaining informed consent gives another opportunity to the skull base team to interact with the patient in the information process. If the patient is properly educated, signing the consent is often an anticlimax because trust and a cooperative tenor have developed over time. If a good cooperative relationship is not present, then this signing can often be *the* most stressful time. Patients have described signing the consent as "so what," "no problem," "I already knew everything anyway," to "this was the most terrifying time" and "I felt like I was signing my life away to someone else."

The establishment of cooperative trust between the skull base team and the patient and family occurs over time. Unfortunately, this is a period where the passage of time is stressful, and often painful. With the urgency of surgery looming, the skull base team must make every attempt to educate and inform at the earliest time available.

The Role of the Clinical Nurse Specialist

The clinical nurse specialist serves as one of the clinical coordinators of the multidisciplinary team, an advocate for the patient, and clinical nursing expert through the entire process. The traditional roles of the clinical nurse specialist include clinical expert, educator of both staff and patient, community liaison, researcher, and multidisciplinary team member. The clinical nurse specialist provides continuity of care from initial contact, to discharge to home, and return to the clinic. With the skull base team coordinator, the clinical specialist acts as case manager to streamline the medical system and as an advocate for the patient. This involves an interface with insurance providers, family, clinical nursing staff, and medical teams. The clinical specialist is the nursing clinical expert for staff nurses both in-house and for home nursing intervention.

Multidisciplinary Team

The multidisciplinary team (Table 2) meets twice a week, once on Tuesdays to review inpatient care needs and plans and again at the end of the week, usually on Fridays, to coordinate with the otolaryngology tumor board, meet new patients, and plan for the following week. The Tuesday meetings include all inpatient care planning needs regarding medication, ambulation, coping, pain management, family meetings, wound care and healing, cognition, airway care,

TABLE 2. *Multidisciplinary team members*

Clinical nurse specialist	Home health liaison
Skull base coordinator	Hospice (as needed)
Licensed clinical social worker	Staff nurses
Dietician	Administrative staff nurses
Physical therapist	Occupational therapists (as needed)
Speech pathologist	Physical medicine and rehabilitation team
Discharge planner	Dysphagia team (as needed)

nutrition, neurologic status, consultant reports, and in-house plan of care for educating patient and family for discharge.

In this forum, the team and staff conceptualize and develop teaching plans and formulate discharge plans. The team discusses psychosocial issues specifically regarding coping strategies, psychological adaptation, and behavior of both patient and family. They address staff issues and formulate plans for intervention. This organized group functions as a team to treat patients, but also as a peer review group and internal support group. When constantly faced with patients whose diagnosis is of such gravity, it is important for the team to be introspective and support each other.

At the Friday team meeting, in conjunction with the tumor board and clinic, the multidisciplinary team meets new patients and formulate their plan of care with the physicians. The team evaluates former patients for ongoing needs, including wound care, nutrition, coping, pain management, home care, and insurance status. Symptom control and home health problems often take precedence. The team communicates with the home health nurses, and home health plans are revised after team evaluation of the patient.

One of the critical purposes of the team meeting during tumor board is to evaluate new skull base patients who are presented at tumor clinic and discussed at tumor board. This is often the first time that a patient hears his or her diagnosis and its implications. This is also the first time the patient meets the team that will be caring for him or her throughout the hospitalization. Many patients often are unaware of the large numbers of professional staff required to care for them. In this initial meeting the beginnings of trust, education, and coping develop. Each patient receives a handbook describing the team, each member, and his or her role in the patient's care. These handbooks give patients and their families reference information, phone numbers, and contact information for use throughout hospitalization and home care.

The formal skull base team meeting occurs monthly or more often as is required by patient numbers and requirements for planning. This team meeting is primarily for medical decision making, care planning, and surgical operative planning. It is a time for the team to discuss issues of care, appropriate therapy, and coordination of surgical interventions, and the meeting provides the medical multidisciplinary team an opportunity critically to evaluate the preoperative testing results and finalize their plans. In the team meeting, both the skull base team coordinator and the operating room clinicians participate in the operative planning. This enables all parties to communicate better their requirements for care of each individual patient.

PREOPERATIVE NURSING CARE

Preoperative nursing care can be divided into two parts. Part I includes planning, organization, materials management, and research, and part II includes the provision of direct patient care. Part I consists of the behind-the-scenes planning that *must* make part II seamless for the patient and his or her family. Part I ensures that the collaborative care pathway is used properly and fully. A collaborative path allows for leveling of all personnel involved in the care of the patient, and also ensures that each discipline is aware of the other professional processes and plans of care.

In part II, the patient and family should see and experience team coordination without flaws or problems. In today's very complex medical systems and changes in insurance coverage, the health care system should work for the patient, not in spite of, or instead of, the patient's insurance coverage. Collaborative paths, patient information books, care plans, standing orders, and team meetings provide fundamental guidelines for the skull base team. These tools allow the practitioner to use time more efficiently to individualize the patient's immediate care needs.

Preoperative Testing

Preoperative testing for evaluation and suitability can be exhausting and can present a daunting prospect for patient and family. Nursing care is based on knowledgeable intervention with the patient regarding each test and procedure. Early identification of risk factors for postoperative pulmonary complications is extremely important. Six major risk factors have been identified as having a significant association with postoperative pulmonary complications. It is significant to have two or more of these risk factors present: (a) age 60 years or older, (b) impaired preoperative cognitive function, (c) smoking history within the past 8 weeks, (d) body mass index of 27 or greater, (e) history of cancer, and (f) any incision that was either above the umbilicus, or both above and below the umbilicus (3).

Preparation for the experience, adequate sedation (if required), and pain management may allow a person to undergo a computed tomography (CT) scan, magnetic resonance imaging, magnetic resonance angiography, or balloon test occlusion (BTO) without stress or fear. Confinement in the magnetic resonance or CT scanner is often very unsettling to many people, so the explanation of the duration and extent of the test allows the patient to understand and cooperate better with the examination. Communicating with radiology technicians regarding the person's particular concerns, such as claustrophobia, can often change the test from a frightening experience to one that is understandable and manageable. Sedation is contraindicated only if the patient has airway problems and cannot lie flat; these particular people may require significant sedation and therefore need closer observation by nursing or anesthesia staff to be able to complete the study.

When the team anticipates that the extent of surgery may include resection of the carotid artery, a BTO with single photon emission computed tomography (SPECT) scans before and after the test are necessary to evaluate the integrity of cerebral contralateral blood flow. These suitability studies themselves pose risks of stroke, and therefore require full explanations to the patient and family. The radiologist who will be conducting the study obtains consent from the patient.

The BTO is a sophisticated test involving the insertion of a balloon catheter (often a Swan-Ganz catheter) into the carotid system by the groin approach. The catheter is inserted into the involved carotid artery for an initial angiogram of the involved vessels and assessment of the integrity of collateral flow through the circle of Willis.

The second part of the test consists of inflating the catheter balloon to occlude the carotid internal artery. The patient is continually evaluated for any neurologic signs, such as eye pain, change in vision or speech, and loss of motor function or sensation to the extremities. If such signs appear, the balloon is deflated and the test suspended. The post-SPECT scan is done after 20 minutes of carotid occlusion. The nursing care of these patients focuses on site observation for arterial leaks, neurologic sequelae, and pain and stress management. BTO is an outpatient procedure, but patients are observed for 12 hours for insertion site bleeding or hematoma.

A pre-SPECT scan is a radionuclide study to evaluate the person's brain activity at normal carotid flow before balloon occlusion. The post-SPECT scan is done immediately after the BTO with the catheter balloon inflated to evaluate the blood flow from the opposite side of the brain to the brain tissue of the occluded side. This test ascertains opposite carotid flow adequacy if the involved carotid is resected. It also helps to determine whether a carotid resection is even possible and whether vein grafting replacement is a viable option.

If the patient requires a vascularized free flap for reconstruction, ultrasound mapping of the donor site is critical to define to the surgical team the position of the donor vessel and flow rates. This is not a painful procedure because it uses ultrasound technology, but the patient still must be adequately informed before the testing. The patient usually can have this procedure as an outpatient because it requires no medication or sedation.

With head and neck cancer, the initial tissue mapping study of the tumor often is a panendoscopy and tumor mapping. This is still done with skull base patients, but not as often as previously. A biopsy is critical for tissue diagnosis and planning but often takes a different direction than the traditional panendoscopy for head and neck cancer. This may be an infratemporal approach or an oral approach through the palate or posterior pharyngeal wall. The goals are still the same, to obtain tissue for diagnosis and to plan the operative procedure. Unlike in head and neck cancer patients, this procedure may be omitted because the location of the tumor necessitates a more extensive surgery, and all is completed at the time of definitive surgical resection. The skull base team pathologist is in the operating room to diagnose the histologic type of tumor and the status of surgical margins. At this juncture, the surgeon needs to apprise the family of the plan of care, given the histologic type of the tumor. Support, understanding, and information from the clinical specialist and team coordinator make the waiting less difficult for the family. Continual updates provide on important link for the family to their family member in the operating room.

Pain Management

The issue of pain control is often the crux of nursing and medical intervention and can become one of the most difficult issues of care if not addressed promptly and efficiently. Many patients present with unremitting pain. It is incumbent on the team to address the patients' needs and prescribe adequate analgesia. This may often include the use of a pain management consultant to supplement the team's care. High doses of morphine and morphine derivatives are used along with such medications as amitriptyline (Elavil) or carbamazepine (Tegretol) to address the neuropathic pain of cancer nerve invasion. Fentanyl (Duragesic) patches are used for basal rate drug administration, and concentrated morphine sulfate (Roxinol) for breakthrough pain, if required. MS Contin, a sustained-release morphine, is another medication that can be used if the patient is able to take oral fluids and foods. This extended-release medication can produce a steady-state drug level. Given two, three, or four times a day, MS Contin can give patients consistent relief from pain. Extensive teaching and continual reevaluation are the hallmarks of pain management. Pain is what the patient says it is, and the care team should be able to respond to the needs with medication and with ongoing assessment of physical and psychological symptoms.

When patients have been on high doses of pain management before surgery, it is imperative that the anesthesiologist be aware of what dose and administration schedule the person requires. This is critical to balance anesthesia and to address basal rates of pain medication after surgery to prevent drug withdrawal, as well as the postoperative pain requirements.

After discharge, if acute pain that cannot be related to the surgical procedure continues for long periods, and the requirements for medication escalate, the possibility of infection or recurrent tumor must be entertained. This then introduces the possibility of recurrent cancer, another surgery, or, even worse, the possibility of unresectable disease. If the disease is unresectable, team intervention at this time directs the patient and family to hospice and supportive care.

Understanding, planning, and documenting the effectiveness of pain management is a critical issue for the nurse to address. As the patient transitions from hospital to home, there must be good communication between in-hospital staff and clinic staff regarding pain relief measures. Assistance from the pain management team is invaluable for the patient and family. The Agency for Health Care Policy and Research guidelines on pain management, published in 1994, is a helpful document that should be included in all care plans and standards of therapy regarding the management of both acute and chronic pain (4).

Nutrition

Nutritional evaluation by a registered dietitian early on in the preoperative process accomplishes three goals in the care of the patient: (a) it establishes a current health status; (b) it establishes a plan of care throughout the hospitalization; and (c) it allows for early nutritional intervention, if required, to begin to correct defined problems. Initial evaluation begins with weight and height and the calculation of the body mass index (BMI). The equation for BMI is weight (in kilograms) divided by height (in meters) squared (kg/m^2). A healthy index is 18 to 25 (3). A BMI of 27 or greater carries nearly three times the risk of pulmonary complications. The patient is also assessed for other risk factors, in these cases a skull base tumor, as well as other comorbid conditions (e.g., obesity, diabetes, cardiovascular diseases, gastrointestinal disturbances, osteoarthritis). The net weight gain or loss over the last year should be assessed as well as current weight versus usual weight. Significant changes in weight alert the clinician to an overall change in the patient's nutritional health status. Because of the length of skull base surgical procedures, patients who are severely underweight are at risk for pressure sore–ulcer development. Many pressure ulcers that may begin during surgery do not actually appear until 1 to 4 days after an operation (5). Early intervention and alleviation of pressure areas during the surgery may prevent such complications (6).

When data collection is complete, a nutritional treatment plan is individualized and therapy begun. Nutritional support must supply essential nutrients for growth, wound repair, immune competence, and organ function. In the absence of adequate nutrition support, protein catabolism and malnutrition can decrease organ mass and impair the function of major organ and body systems such as skeletal and respiratory muscles, liver, kidneys, heart, gastrointestinal tract, endocrine system, and immune system. Malnutrition is directly associated with morbidity and mortality (7).

Usual levels of caloric replenishment should range around 35 kcal/kg/day. The choice of enteral feeding, if necessary, is based on the nutritionist's experience with formula and the patient's response to the individual formula chosen. Patients with malnutrition and severe stress benefit most from early nutritional support (7). There are many good formulas that meet and exceed American Dietetic Association requirements. Some feedings have high caloric density, with and without fiber, and all have varying levels of osmolality. Repletion should be begun slowly to prevent refeeding syndrome in the severely malnourished. The patient's tolerance determines caloric and osmolality advancement. The choice of continuous versus bolus feeding again is determined by tolerance. Enteral feeding by bolus is usually better tolerated by outpatients, who tend to be more active. Immediately after surgery, continuous feeding is initially better tolerated, with a switch to bolus as the patient recovers. Bolus feeding can be administered in a standard three-meal and snack fashion, mimicking normal eating habits. As an example, a normal-weight woman of average nutritional requirements might tolerate 360 ml of Osmolite HN every 6 hours with 50 ml of free water flushes. A man may require more volume, such as Sustacal HC or Ensure Plus at seven cans per day, two cans at breakfast, two cans at lunch, two cans at dinner, and one can in the evening with 50- to 100-ml free water flushes after each "meal." Administer extra water if the patient's insensible water loss is significant, as with artificial airways or large amounts of oral suctioning. Free water replacement is approximately 27 to 32 ml/kg body weight; 22 ml/kg is a minimum. A general rule is 1 ml of water replaced for each 1 ml of formula delivered. This is predicated on the caloric density and osmolality of the formula and the patient's requirements and general health status. Consultation with a clinical dietitian familiar with repletion ensures that the patient's needs are being addressed properly. All patients should be on aspiration precautions and a reflux regimen. Nasogastric placement must be accurate.

Skull base patients often have significant cranial nerve deficits, some because of tumor invasion and some because of the surgical resection. Before surgery, if any swallowing dysfunction is identified, measures should be instituted to ensure safe nutrition by the oral or enteral route. After surgery, a complete swallowing evaluation is initiated to ensure that oral nutrition is safe. If the patient shows *any* signs of aspiration or inability to meet nutritional goals, enteral nutrition is begun. Early identification of nutritional problems leads to earlier intervention and an improved chance at increasing body levels of protein and albumin. It is not efficacious to push oral nutrition and further stress the patient if there is any indication of swallow dysfunction or vocal fold dysfunction. Identification of the cause of aspiration and prevention of an aspiration pneumonia are imperative. Swallow therapy is begun as soon as the patient can follow directions and after a dynamic swallow study, so that a safe rehabilitation program can be exactly defined. As the patient improves, safe oral nutrition can be combined with enteral nutrition, and then a weaning process from the enteral nutrition is begun. The patient should be on calorie counts, have nutritional counseling, and be under observation for aspiration pneumonia.

A swallowing rehabilitation program may include such tasks as chin tuck, head turning, gravity assist, breath holding, and double swallowing. These measures must be defined by a radiographic study to ensure success in oral nutrition.

Social Service and Psychiatry

Social service intervention in the preoperative period adds an important psychosocial dimension to the total patient evaluation. Before surgery, the social service representative completes a full family and patient evaluation. Social service addresses issues of coping, adaptation, and family support, provides for the support of patients and families, and helps improve their ability to manage the illness. Discussions may include such topics as feasibility of the surgery and predicting outcomes related to quality-of-life issues and length of hospitalization (8). Details of insurance and finance can be openly discussed at this time. The patient's alcohol and drug history often are more clearly reported to the nurse and social worker than the physician. The complement of social service and nursing evaluation adds to the multidimensional care of the patient and family.

Social service intervention also aids the nursing staff in dealing with the issues of disfigurement and adaptation in skull base patients. Frequent nursing staff debriefings are very helpful in assisting the staff to be both compassionate and objective, and at the same time deal with their own human feelings toward their patients. Social service has been of invaluable assistance to the skull base team in addressing both staff and patient needs.

If, after social service evaluation, it is deemed necessary to obtain a formal psychiatric evaluation, the social worker then collaborates with psychiatry. Psychiatry is of assistance in medication administration, dealing with loss, and true psychiatric diagnosis. The psychiatric department has become an adjunct to the skull base team in difficult patients and family situations.

INTRAOPERATIVE NURSING CARE

PERIOPERATIVE NURSING CONSIDERATIONS

Preoperative Assessment

The Planning Stage

Clinic

Seeing the patient in the clinic or on admission to the hospital the night before surgery allows the operating room (OR) nurse to begin the preoperative teaching, answer questions the patient may have forgotten or was afraid to ask the surgeon about the operative procedure, meet the family, and assess any special needs the patient may have. This is an opportunity for the patient to express any fears he or she may have about the pending operation and affords the nurse the opportunity to reassure the patient and incorporate this information into the intraoperative plan. Seeing and interviewing the patient also provides information concerning any special physical needs of the patient which may be important when considering positioning and padding intraoperatively. It also gives the patient and family a sense that the patient will be received in the OR by someone familiar to them; someone who knows something about them instead of a stranger wearing a shower cap and a mask.

Skull Base Conference

During skull base conference, the treatment options are discussed, x-rays and scans are viewed, and the surgical plan is outlined and discussed. These sessions are attended by the head and neck surgeon, the neurosurgeon, the radiologist, the pathologist, the plastic surgeon, the fellows and residents, the skull base coordinator, and the OR nurse. It is essential for the OR nurse to be part of this process. The hallmark of OR nursing is the ability to anticipate the needs of both the surgeons and the patient accurately. In order to do so, it is necessary to understand the entire operative plan. Important information to be gained is the location of the tumor, insight into the pathology of the tumor (and any special requests of the pathologist), the surgical approach (anterior vs. middle fossa or posterior fossa), any reconstruction plans (grafts or flaps), and any necessary implants. It is also important to know how many teams will be involved and whether or not they plan to work simultaneously. The OR nurse can communicate this information to the rest of the OR team in order to adjust personnel and equipment accordingly.

Intraoperative Assessment

Equipment

Understanding the plan makes gathering the necessary equipment in advance much easier. The following items are fairly standard equipment for skull base surgery:

1. Bovie machines × 2 (in case more than one team operates simultaneously).
2. Irrigating bipolar machine (for neurosurgery). Regular bipolar machine [for plastic surgery and ear, nose, and throat (ENT)].
3. Suction canisters (sufficient for 2 teams).
4. Suction regulators × 2 for neurology.
5. Rolling, padded stools for seating (during microscopic work or drilling of temporal bone).
6. Mayfield headrest(pins or horseshoe).
7. Suture carts for all appropriate services (i.e., plastic surgery, neurosurgery, ENT).
8. Microscope and TV monitor.
9. Eggcrate mattress, pillows, elbow and heel pads, bean bag and any other necessary positioning supplies.
10. K thermia machine and blanket.
11. Appropriate OR tables to accommodate ENT and neurosurgery instrument sets and drills as well as extra tables for free flap and skin grafts as necessary.
12. Sequential compression stockings.
13. Nitrogen tanks and hoses for power equipment (there should be at least 2 separate supplies).
14. Electric shaver and multiple razors.

Intraoperative Planning

Another reason it is important to know the plan is to enable the OR nurse to gather and open the proper drapes and instruments in advance. There are many variations and possibilities and it is best to be as prepared as possible. Some considerations for the nurses are as follows:

1. What approach have the surgeons decided upon? The three most common are the anterior cranial fossa, middle cranial fossa, and posterior fossa approaches.

2. If the anterior cranial fossa approach is elected, will the surgeons need endoscopic equipment in conjunction with the standard open equipment? If so, the telescope will require sterilization by means of the steris method or a process other than a quick soak in Cidex. Using a sterile scope rather than one that has merely been decontaminated minimizes the contamination hazards associated with communication of the instrument with cerebrospinal fluid (CSF), the dura, or the brain.

3. If the middle cranial fossa approach is elected, will the surgeon need to drill the temporal bone or work on the inner ear or ear canal? Will plates and screws be required to replace bone flaps or to replace the zygoma, if it must be removed for exposure?

4. If the posterior fossa approach is elected, will the patient need to be placed in the lateral position ? Is the pin headrest necessary instead of the horseshoe?

5. What about reconstruction? Will a free flap be required or will a local flap be sufficient? If a free flap is required, from what area will it be harvested? There are multiple possibilities, including a rectus free flap from the abdomen, a forearm free flap, a latissimus free flap, or a fibula free flap if soft tissue and bone are needed. Hip grafts are also possible as are a number of other free flaps. This information is critical not only for draping, but also for prepping, positioning and instrumentation needs. Another question when reconstruction is necessary is whether it will be necessary to re-prep and re-drape as opposed to prepping and draping everything at the outset. If it is necessary to re-drape and re-prep and possibly reposition, how will this be accomplished without compromising the sterility of the surgical wound and the sterile field? If these issues are not addressed and resolved in advance, then confusion, undue consumption of time, energy, and resources will result and patient care will be compromised.

6. Another question to consider regarding reconstruction is, will a saphenous vein graft be required? If the tumor involves the carotid artery, either extracranially or intracranially, the carotid may have to be bypassed. If so, it is important to know who will be harvesting the vein and to have a separate sterile setup for the harvest.

7. What about implants? Will it be necessary to patch or replace the dura? Will the jaw require reconstruction? Will bone in the skull need to be replaced or reinforced? Will the patient need a gold weight for their eye if there is facial nerve involvement? There are many options to consider and it is important for the nurse to anticipate and discuss the possibilities with the surgeons, and ensure that the necessary equipment is available, especially since, more often than not, such items are required late in the evening or at night when the usual resources are not available.

Sterile Supplies and Instrumentation

Basic Pack. This pack should contain basins, suction tubing, lap tapes, 4 × 8 sponges, needle magnet, trash bag and pitcher.

Neuro Pack or Equivalent. This pack should contain extra suction tubing, an irrigation pouch, cottonoids, bone wax, surgicel, bulb irrigators × 2, a neuro split sheet, bipolar cord, and bipolar forceps. These items can be combined in a custom pack or opened individually.

Extra Basic Packs. The number of extra basic packs required depends upon which procedures are planned. An extra pack will be needed for the free flap donor portion of the case if a free flap is planned. An extra pack will be needed if a saphenous vein needs to be harvested. Because the primary surgical procedure may involve the sinuses or oral cavity, it is important to be mindful of clean contaminated setups versus sterile setups. Also, because tumor is present in the primary surgical site, it is important to keep the primary setup separate from all donor or harvest setups to prevent possible tumor contamination of an otherwise healthy tissue site. Extra bovie pencils, suction tubings, irrigation tubing, and sponges should be opened accordingly.

Instrumentation. Standard instrumentation for skull base cases should include an instrument tray that contains a combination of basic ENT elevators, sinus instruments, facial fracture instruments, and neuro craniotomy instruments. Neuro micro instrument sets should be part of a standard setup and a drill (i.e., Midas Rex) that includes burrs, saws and drill bits, to perform multiple functions. Other instrument trays may be required depending on which procedures are planned. A second set of power equipment may be needed if bone is to be harvested (such as in fibula free flap), and a dermatome may be needed for skin grafting. A basic plastic set will be required as well as plastic micro instrumentation if a free flap is anticipated. Vascular clamps should be available if they are not included as part of the standard set. Also, depending on the approach, ear instruments may be required.

Positioning

Positioning depends upon which approach is planned and what kind of reconstruction is anticipated. The standard and most common position will be supine on a mayfield horseshoe headrest. The following issues should be considered:

1. If the mayfield horseshoe headrest is utilized, it is imperative that it either be equipped with gel pads or that the circulating nurse double pad the horseshoe with eggcrate and webril or some other material that provides adequate cushioning for the patient's head. Many of these cases can last 18 to 24 hours, so adequate padding is essential. Also, if the patient's head must be turned intraoperatively for long periods of time, it is important to be sure that undue pressure is not placed upon the ear on the opposite side, causing tissue compromise.

2. The OR table should be arranged so that the surgeons may be seated as necessary with room to accommodate their knees. This may require turning the bed around and putting the head where the feet are ordinarily positioned; it depends

upon the individual bed types in each institution. The microscope will be in use at some point and the surgeons may need to be seated. An eggcrate mattress or gel mattress pads should be used to add extra support and padding. A K thermia blanket should be placed on top of this padding to provide an important source of heat for the patient, since much of the patient's body may be prepped. Sheets can then be placed over the K thermia making certain that the draw sheet has plenty of length on both sides as both arms are frequently tucked.

3. The arms and heels require extra padding with eggcrate-like material. If the arms are tucked, be sure to pad them well, especially protecting the ulnar nerve near the elbow. Also, be sure that IV connectors, tubing, and blood pressure cuff tubing are not lying against the skin. These items may require padding with small pieces of foam or gauze. The arms can then be tucked by using the draw sheet and placing protective sleds over the tucked arms and secured under the mattress, not under the patient. It is also important to place a pillow under the knees to relieve pressure to the lower back. Be sure to pad the heels well.

Prepping

It is important to be aware of all the reconstruction possibilities prior to prepping. If all the preps can be done initially, it saves money and time in terms of draping and effort. This also avoids possible wound contamination when re-prepping and re-draping. However, sometimes this is not practical. The preps should be discussed with the surgeons (all services) in order to formulate a final plan. Prior to initiating the prep, the heat in the room is increased and the K thermia machine is activated to warm the patient. If large areas are to be prepped, the patient can lose heat rapidly, making it difficult to compensate for heat loss later. The prep sets should also be warmed slightly in order to remove the chill. This can be accomplished by placing the prep sets in the warmer before the patient is brought into the room. Before beginning the preps, it is important for the circulating nurse to have adequate assistance in the event there are multiple preps, and to be sure that the scrub nurse is ready for draping with all of the appropriate supplies.

Draping

Draping can be an enormous challenge, depending upon the number of surgical procedures to be performed. Again, it is important to stress the necessity for teamwork in discussing the draping plan. All team members should be aware of the plan to facilitate a unified approach. Basic draping begins with the use of a small sheet folded in half with two towels over it. These are placed under the patient's head and over the mayfield horseshoe. (If pins are utilized, this step is eliminated.) One of the towels is then brought up over the patient's head, turban style, and fastened with a towel clip. If the entire head must remain exposed, the turban is eliminated. All areas of the body that have been prepped are then squared off with sterile towels and either stapled or sewn to the patient to prevent gaps in the towels which would compromise sterility. A large reinforced split sheet is then placed over the entire body with the tails of the split fastened around the patient's head. A suction tubing is attached to the irrigation pouch and the pouch is attached to the drapes at the head after which the suction tubing is passed to the circulator who then connects it to a suction canister. If any extremity, such as an arm or a leg, is prepped, an impervious stockinette is used to drape the extremity and sterile sheets are placed beneath it. Thereafter, holes can be cut in the large split sheet to expose other areas such as the abdomen, the thigh, or the chest, which have been prepped and squared off with towels. This allows these areas to be available and sterile, while remaining covered and protected until it is necessary to expose them. It is important to remember to achieve adequate coverage while remaining able to expose all areas that are prepped without compromising sterility. This can be difficult when areas need to be covered for the initial part of the case and uncovered later when another team begins to operate. It is a judgment call whether it is easier and safer to drape everything initially or in stages. This will be decided as a team.

Sequence of Events

Arrival of the OR Team

The scrub and circulating nurse begin the case by entering the OR suite and assessing the need for equipment and supplies. If possible, it is wise to leave a list on the preceding day of all necessary items to be placed in the OR so that when the team arrives in the morning they can begin setting up immediately. Because these cases can be very lengthy, good early preparation ensures an efficient and timely start and incision time.

Once the team has checked the OR suite and determined what equipment and supplies are still required, it is important to elevate the heat in the room to 80°. This is important not only for the initial comfort of the patient upon entry into the OR suite but also to prevent hypothermia during the intraoperative phase. Hypothermia can cause changes in the behavior of anesthetic agents and can delay metabolism, thereby impeding a patient's emergence from anesthesia. As many areas of the body may be exposed during prepping and line placement, it is important from the outset to help regulate the patient's temperature throughout the entire perioperative phase. Raising the temperature in the room, using a warming blanket beneath the patient, and placing warm blankets over the patient until prepping begins will help to accomplish this. At this point, the remaining equipment and supplies can be gathered and placed in the OR suite and the circulator and scrub person can prepare to open sterile supplies.

The circulator can now prepare the OR table for the patient while the scrub person is opening the sterile packages and instrument trays. The OR table should be well padded with an eggcrate mattress over the table pads unless gel table pads are used as standard equipment. A K thermia blanket should then be placed over the eggcrate mattress or gel pads. Thereafter, a sheet is placed over the warming blanket and a second sheet is placed as a draw sheet, being careful to leave the sides of the draw sheet with plenty of length as this sheet will assist in tucking and securing the patient's arms. (See positioning, above.) This is a good time to pad the mayfield headrest with a foam donut if the headrest is not equipped with gel pads on the frame. The warming blanket should be turned on to warm the sheets and the prep sets can be placed in the warmer. If the surgeons will be seated for any part of the case, it is important to be sure they will have adequate room to place their knees under the OR table. In order to accommodate their legs, the OR table may need to be adjusted placing the headpiece at the foot of the table, making it the head of the table, eliminating obstructions underneath where the patient's upper body will be. Depending upon the type of OR tables available in each institution, this may or may not be necessary. The important thing to remember is to facilitate the smooth and orderly progress of the case without compromising the safety and comfort of the patient. If the bed must be adjusted, be sure that padding is sufficient and that the lumbar spine region has adequate support. In our institution, a board is placed under the OR table pads, within the gap in the frame that is created when the bed is turned. This board is then padded with foam to make it the same height and thickness under the pad as the rest of the frame.

Greeting the Patient

Once the above steps have been accomplished, the circulating nurse can visit the patient in the preoperating room and begin the process of checking the patient's chart. Usually, by this time the anesthesia personnel have arrived and have begun to check over the anesthesia equipment and to prepare the medications and lines to begin the case. This is a good opportunity for the circulating nurse to have a few minutes alone with the patient and family.

One of the advantages of attending the skull base conferences is that the patient's history is familiar to the circulating nurse. This leaves more time to spend reassuring the patient and answering any last minute questions the patient or family may have. The circulator should introduce him or herself to the patient at this time, even if they may have met previously, because people appear unfamiliar when dressed in green scrub clothes and a hat. After the introduction, the nurse checks the patient's identification band for the correct spelling of the patient's name, the medical record number, and the patient's date of birth. This is a very important step as this information must be consistent with the medical records and the blood bank order sheets.

Once patient identification is completed, the nurse can review the preoperative checklist to obtain all the necessary information. The nurse must ensure that the patient has had nothing to eat or drink after midnight the night before, unless there is a physician's order allowing the patient to take the medications they usually take at home (i.e., antihypertensive or cardiac medications) with a small sip of water. Any allergies to medications will be noted, and if preoperative antibiotics are ordered but have not yet been given, the nurse can alert the preoperating room staff to administer them. The operative consent is checked to be sure the patient has consented to all of the procedures that are planned. At this time, the nurse can ask the patient which surgical procedures will be performed to allow the patient to state the procedures in their own words. This assists in identifying any misconceptions or misunderstandings the patient may have. Once the consent is verified, the nurse examines the chart for the informed consent note from the surgeon stating that all the risks and benefits of surgery have been explained and the patient wishes to proceed. Next, the lab work is checked and any abnormal or questionable values are noted and discussed with anesthesia and the surgeons. Routine lab work includes a complete blood count (CBC), Chem 20, prothrombin time (PT), partial prothrombin time (PTT), and urinalysis. Availability of blood and blood products is also checked at this time. Other lab work may have been ordered as well, depending upon other medical conditions the patient may have. It is important at this time to check on x-rays, CT scans, and MRI scans, not only for a report in the chart, but also to ensure the availability of the films in the OR suite. After the check-in process has been completed, the nurse explains to any family members who are present the location of the waiting room and lets them know that the skull base coordinator will check on them every few hours and provide them with updates on the progress of the surgical procedures and the condition of the patient. This helps alleviate much of the anxiety the family members are experiencing.

Setting Up the Case

The circulating nurse can now return to the OR suite to assist the scrub person in opening any remaining sterile supplies. Once this is accomplished, the scrub nurse can perform the surgical scrub at the scrub sink and the circulator can assist the scrub nurse in gowning. The circulator can then open any remaining sterile supplies that required sterile personnel receive, such as items too large or packaged in such a way that delivery to the sterile surgical field requires assistance.

While the scrub nurse is setting up and arranging the sterile field, the circulating nurse prepares the paperwork for pathology and frozen sections.

Once the scrub nurse has cleared an area on the sterile field for sterile cups (which are diligently labeled by the scrub nurse), the circulating nurse can deliver the medications to the sterile field. Most commonly, the medications are thrombin, gelfoam, xylocaine with epinephrine, methylene blue, bacitracin, and surgicel.

If there is time before the patient arrives and the scrub nurse is ready, a count can be performed at this time. Otherwise, the count can be performed later while lines are being placed—provided the count is completed before any incision is made. Items to be counted are laps, raytecs (4 × 8s), needles, cottonoids, and dura hooks, at minimum. Instruments are not usually counted.

The Arrival of the Patient

By now anesthesia personnel have interviewed the patient, prepared their equipment, and are ready to bring the patient into the OR suite. The circulating nurse assists in transferring the patient to the OR bed, places a pillow under the patient's knees, and places a warm blanket over the patient. The safety strap is secured over the patient's thighs just above the knees, the arm boards are connected to the OR bed, and the patient's arms are placed comfortably at the patient's side. The nurse then assists the anesthesia provider in placing the blood pressure cuff, electrocardiogram (EKG) leads, and pulse oximeter on the patient for monitoring purposes.

NOTE: KEEP IN MIND THAT THE FOLLOWING STEPS MAY OCCUR IN SEQUENCE, SIMULTANEOUSLY, OR IN A DIFFERENT ORDER. THE IMPORTANT THING IS THAT EVERYONE WORKS AS A TEAM SO THAT THE CASE FLOWS WITHOUT INTERRUPTION AND THERE ARE NO UNNECESSARY DELAYS.

Induction of the patient can now begin. The circulator stands by the bedside and is immediately available to assist by administering cricoid pressure if necessary or by helping to secure the endotracheal tube once it is placed. The nurse will also provide emotional support to the patient as the anesthetics are being administered, by reassuring the patient and touching the patient's arm or holding a hand. This is a simple but very important role for the circulating nurse because the patient is probably most anxious at this time. It is important that the surgeon be present at the time of induction in case there are any difficulties in maintaining the patient's airway. The scrub nurse will also be standing by and will be prepared to assist in performing an emergency tracheostomy on the rare occasion that it is needed.

Once the anesthesia provider is satisfied with the tube placement and has appropriately secured the endotracheal tube, the bed can be rotated 180° so the head of the bed is where the foot of the bed was and the foot of the bed is in front of the anesthesia provider. This is done to give the surgeons access to the entire patient. The anesthesia provider will have extensions on the breathing circuit and also on all of the intravenous (IV) tubing. It is much easier to turn the bed before all the lines have been placed so that there is less likelihood of tangling lines. If possible, it is easiest to disconnect the EKG leads, blood pressure cuff, and pulse oximeter very briefly until the turn is made. They can be replaced immediately once the turn is complete.

The anesthesia provider can now begin to place the intraoperative lines. An arterial line, two large bore IV lines and a peripherally inserted catheter (PIC) line or long arm central venous pressure (CVP) line are placed. Communication between all the members of the team is important so that the anesthesia provider understands which areas of the body are to be prepped into the sterile field. This information will determine where the lines are to be placed.

While the anesthesia provider is placing the lines, the surgeon is injecting the neck at the site where the tracheostomy is to be performed with 1% xylocaine with epinephrine 1:100,000 as local infiltration to reduce intraoperative bleeding at the site. At this time, the circulating nurse and scrub nurse can complete the operative count if this has not already been done. The scrub nurse will have a separate setup for the tracheostomy and will also have a primary back table with ENT supplies and another table with neurological supplies, and perhaps, later in the intraoperative phase, there will be other setups made available for free flap or saphenous vein harvesting. Although many of these procedures and setups may begin as separate entities, the count is done as one procedure with additional counted items being added as the case progresses. This is much easier during the closing counts as everything will eventually be combined. Several closing counts may be necessary depending upon how many procedures are performed.

The temperature foley is placed and TED stockings and pneumatic sleeves are placed if the legs are not to be prepped into the sterile field. If the thighs are to be prepped into the field for skin grafting or saphenous vein harvesting, the pneumatic sleeves and TED stockings can be placed on the lower legs up to the knees. If the anesthesia provider has completed line placement, the arms are padded and tucked as described earlier in the section on positioning. If line placement has not been completed, the arm boards are lowered so anesthesia personnel can continue placing lines while the circulating nurse begins the prep for the tracheostomy.

The grounding pad is placed on whichever thigh will not be prepped into the sterile field. If both thighs are to be prepped, the grounding pad is placed on the buttocks. If more than one bovie will be needed, an additional grounding pad will be placed on the other buttock. The position of the grounding pads will have to be reevaluated after placement of the lumbar drain as the patient will be turned to a lateral position for drain placement and then back to supine and the grounding pads may become dislodged and require replacement.

Intraoperative Procedure

The circulating nurse removes a prep tray from the warmer and preps the patient's neck for tracheostomy while the surgeons are performing the surgical hand scrub. Once the prep is completed and the surgeons are gowned and gloved by the scrub nurse, the patient is draped for tracheostomy. Four towels are placed around the neck in a squared fashion leaving the anterior neck available for incision. Towel clips are used to secure the towels and a large split or U sheet is placed over the patient with the tails of the sheet forming around the patient's head. The scrub nurse then hands the cautery cord and suction tubing to the circulator who connects them to the appropriate equipment. The tracheostomy is performed as a separate procedure from the main portion of the case. An anode tube is placed in the tracheal stoma and sewn to the patient's chest with an O-silk suture to prevent the tube from being dislodged during the remaining portions of the case. Before the patient is transferred to the postanesthesia recovery room (PAR), the anode tube is replaced with a tracheostomy tube.

When the surgeons place the anode tube in the trachea, the circulating nurse summons the neurosurgeon to place the lumbar drain. The neurosurgeon will then be arriving while the tracheostomy is being completed, thereby eliminating any delays in the case. If neurosurgeon is unavailable or delayed, the anesthesia provider can place the lumbar drain.

A sterile towel is placed over the site of the tracheostomy and kept in place to keep the tracheostomy site as clean as possible until the final prep. The scrub nurse and circulating nurse perform a sponge and needle count once the tracheostomy is completed. The sponges are arranged in a sponge counting bag and remain in the OR suite as they are part of the entire count. The needles are placed in a needle magnet and saved for the same reason. These items may be counted and removed from the OR suite and a separate count can be performed for the remaining operative procedure if everyone agrees to do it that way. The problem with counting in this manner is that when the initial team of nurses has gone home, questions may arise and confusion may result if there is an incorrect count. We have found it more efficient to keep everything together so there is no question about which procedures were included in the count and which were not. This approach has worked well for us. The drapes are then removed and the team prepares for insertion of the lumbar drain.

The patient is then placed in the lateral position with pillows between the knees. The knees and head are bent toward the chest to flex the lumbar spine to facilitate placing the lumbar drain. The scrub nurse changes gown and gloves and prepares a small sterile setup for the lumbar drain placement. This includes a bayonet forcep, scissors, a needle holder, and a sponge forcep. Two small bowls are placed on this table, one containing sterile saline and the other containing betadine solution. A package of 4 × 4s or fluffs, O-silk, strands, and a 3-0 nylon suture are placed, as well as the lumbar drain and external drainage kit. The neurosurgeon gently washes the patient's back with the betadine solution and places the lumbar drain in the lumbar space using sterile technique. The drain is then connected to the external drainage kit fastened with an O-silk strand and handed to the anesthesia provider. The anesthesia provider checks to ensure that the drain is closed, and then fastens the drainage bag to an IV pole where it is readily accessible when and if the neurosurgeon asks the anesthesia provider to open the drain and drain CSF into the bag during the neurosurgical portion of the procedure. The surgeon then sews the drain to the patient's skin with 3-0 nylon suture and places an op site over the insertion site. The drain is then loosely coiled and taped to the patient's back. After the drain is placed, the patient is returned to the supine position with a pillow placed under the knees. It is important for the circulating nurse to remain with the patient during this procedure to ensure proper positioning and protect the patient from falling. It is also important to keep the patient covered as much as possible with warm blankets.

Once the lumbar drain has been placed and the patient is returned to the supine position, the circulating nurse can reevaluate the position of the grounding pads and replace them if necessary. The circulating nurse and the surgeons can then begin shaving the head and any other portion of the body that will be included in the sterile field, such as the legs or the abdomen. Also, at this time another surgeon can be placing frost stitches in the eyelids. This is done with a 4-0 silk suture on a small G-3 needle using a 10 french robinson catheter as a bumper to sew the eyelids together. This protects the corneas from abrasion and irritation during the long hours to follow. The eyelids are lightly prepped first with betadine solution being very careful not to allow any betadine inside the eyes. Betadine swabs work very well for this. If any betadine does enter the eyes it can be rinsed out immediately with balanced salt solution. The needle holder and suture scissors used for the frost stitches are sterile and provided by the scrub nurse. The surgeon uses sterile gloves while inserting the frost stitches.

The Mayfield headrest is now fastened to the OR table and the patient's head is placed on the headrest. If the patient's head is to be turned to the side for the majority of the case, care is taken to be sure undue pressure is not placed on the downward ear. The Mayfield horseshoe is well-padded as described earlier and is adjusted so that the patient's head fits comfortably with no areas of pressure. Positioning is completed as described earlier in the section on positioning and the circulating nurse removes the remaining prep sets from the warmer and begins to prep all the appropriate anatomy for the procedures to follow.

The surgeons return to the scrub sink for the final surgical scrub. Meanwhile, the scrub nurse has been busily setting up the rest of the surgical field. The scrub nurse separates items for a skin graft onto a small prep table and covers the table to protect it from contamination until the supplies are needed. The gelfoam is cut into pieces and added to the thrombin. Surgicel is cut into strips, labeled, and placed in a towel for easy access. Before the circulating nurse dons gloves for the prepping, the scrub nurse asks for any other needed supplies such as extra gloves or gowns for the surgeons who are scrubbing.

Once the surgeons are gowned and gloved, the draping begins. As described earlier, draping can be a challenge. Everyone must work as a team. The circulator remains available to assist with the draping and to ensure that strict aseptic technique is followed and adequate coverage is obtained with no breaks in sterile technique. Drapes around the head and neck are secured with staples and 2-0 silk sutures. This allows the head to be turned repeatedly without creating gaps in the sterile drapes. A fluid pouch is used at the head to catch blood and irrigation fluid and this is connected to suction. The remaining drapes are stapled and the prepped areas of the body that will not be operated on immediately are covered with a sterile towel for both warmth and protection. The circulator connects the bovie, bipolar, and suction and the bipolar pedal is covered and placed in close proximity to the primary surgeon. The circulator assesses the OR field to be sure everything is in place and in working order before beginning documentation and charges.

Once the procedure is underway, it is the responsibility of the scrub nurse to anticipate the needs of the surgical team for instrumentation and suture and to communicate with the circulating nurse when supplies will be needed that are not already part of the sterile setup. The scrub nurse and circulating nurse work together in anticipating when it is time to connect the power equipment, drape the microscope, or set up another sterile field for a reconstruction procedure or harvesting of tissue. The circulator may have to communicate to the nurse in charge of coordinating the staff the need for a second scrub nurse if another team of surgeons wishes to work simultaneously.

The circulating nurse is the primary coordinator of all that happens in the OR suite. He or she is the facilitator and the link between all the surgical teams and anesthesia providers. The circulating nurse is the patient advocate, assisting the entire team in providing safe and optimum care to the skull base patients, as well as being the link between other departments and the surgical suite, such as pathology, blood bank, and x-ray. It is crucial for the circulator to be aware of all the aspects of the case in order to anticipate the needs of the scrub nurse, surgeons, and anesthesia provider. This requires being aware of blood loss and communicating with anesthesia personnel by displaying the sponges where they can easily be seen and placing the suction canisters within direct vision of the anesthesia provider. The circulator also assists the surgeons in the placement of foot pedals, sitting stools, microscopes, headlights, and other equipment. He or she also will answer pagers, screen information and calls that can be handled by personnel outside of the operating room. It is also necessary to anticipate the needs of the scrub nurse for extra suture, sponges, irrigation fluid or medications.

One of the most critical roles of the circulating nurse is the responsibility of recording, collecting, and labelling the tissue specimens for frozen section and sending them to pathology in a timely fashion. Good communication between the surgeons, the scrub nurse, and the circulator is imperative. There can be as many as 100 or more specimens taken during the course of the case. It is therefore very important that everyone work together. The surgeon calls out the name of the specimen clearly to the circulator and the scrub nurse. The scrub nurse collects the specimen in a small sterile container (small paper souffle cups can be used for this). The circulator communicates to the scrub nurse which letter to label the specimen(i.e., A,B,C,D, etc.) The scrub nurse then writes only that letter on the paper cup with the specimen. The circulator writes the letter and the name of the specimen on the pathology sheet, repeating the name of the specimen to the surgeon as it is being written so the surgeon can clarify if the circulator has heard the name incorrectly or is unsure of what the specimen is. The reason the circulator writes the information rather than both the circulator and the scrub nurse is to avoid confusion. If only one person writes the name of the specimen, less opportunity for error is presented. Also, the scrub nurse is very busy collecting the specimens from the surgeons and continuing to hand instruments to the surgical team. It is critical, however, for the circulator and the scrub nurse to be working in complete harmony and to be on the same letter at the same time. If there is any confusion or doubt, it is the responsibility of the circulator to alert the surgeons and stop the case until clarification is obtained.

Accuracy of the frozen sections helps to determine the extent of the tumor whereas inaccuracy may result in major complications. Sometimes many specimens are taken at the same time and sometimes just a few are taken. In either case, the circulator writes the names of all of the specimens on the pathology sheet, labels the specimen containers, and then collects the specimens from the scrub nurse. At no time should a specimen be placed in an unlabeled specimen cup. As the circulator collects the specimen from the scrub nurse, the letter is spoken aloud by both the scrub nurse and the circulator to verify that specimen A is being delivered to the cup labeled specimen A and that B is in specimen cup B and so forth throughout the alphabet. When the letter Z is reached, the specimens are then labeled AA, BB, CC, etc., until ZZ is reached and then AAA, BBB, CCC, etc., until all specimens are collected. As each group of specimens is collected, that group is sent fresh (not in formalin) to pathology accompanied by the patient's chart. As pathology calls to state which specimens are positive and which are negative for tumor, the circulator marks a plus or minus sign in the margin of the appropriate specimen on the pathology sheet thereby creating a list to which reference may be made upon request by the surgeon.

At approximately 4-hour intervals, the circulating nurse will give a report to the skull base coordinator and the clinical nurse specialist on the progress of the surgery. The skull base coordinator can then relay this information to the family. Because these cases can be so lengthy, it is important for the family to receive periodic information so that they feel included, and so they can understand that progress is being made and even though the wait may be long, they will be kept aware of the stages of the operation.

It is very important that during the case, the circulating nurse is careful to keep track of the discarded sponges and to display them so that the anesthesia provider can assess blood loss. Keeping track on a regular basis and displaying the sponges also helps later when closing counts need to be performed. It is much easier to perform a closing count when the sponges have been accounted for periodically, rather than waiting, as it becomes very busy towards the end of the case and more mistakes are made when there is confusion and personnel are hurrying. It is of equal importance for the scrub nurse to pay close attention throughout the case to the location of sponges, needles, and cottonoids as well as instrumentation. The scrub nurse should be counting privately at frequent intervals and should enlist the help of the circulator and the surgeons if an item cannot be accounted for. This will save a lot of time at the end of the case.

As the case progresses, it is important for the circulating nurse to continue to plan and organize for the remainder of the case. Before being relieved by a new team at the end of the shift, the primary circulator should verify and obtain an intensive care unit (ICU) bed, give the PAR a report regarding when they can expect the patient (even if it will be hours later) so they can adjust their staffing, and obtain any other equipment or supplies that may be needed later in the case. The circulating nurse then gives the oncoming team a full and detailed report. Information included in report is as follows:

The patient's history and diagnosis.
All of the planned procedures, including the procedures already performed, procedures pending, and the present status of the case.
Any allergies the patient may have.
Transfusion status. How many units of blood have been transfused, how many units are remaining in the blood bank, and whether or not there are other blood products available such as platelets, fresh frozen plasma or cryoprecipitate for fibrin glue.
What family members are waiting and where they are waiting and what information they have been given to date.
How much irrigation has been used on the field.
The status of the frozen sections and any other specimens.
The location of the grounding pads and which areas of the body have been prepped.
The potential use of special implants and the location of the implants if they are not already present in the OR suite. (i.e., dura substitute, plates and screws, etc.)
Anything unusual about the sponge and needle count. If it is possible a sponge and needle count should be performed by one member of the oncoming shift and a member of the shift that is leaving. Most of the time this is difficult to do since there may be more than one procedure being performed and sponges or cottonoids may be packed in a wound. This is another reason why it is so important for the primary scrub nurse and circulator to be counting on an ongoing basis during the case.
Once a full report is given, all questions are answered and both teams are comfortable, the circulating nurse checks all the documentation and charges to be sure that everything is up to date.

Closure of the Case

As with the beginning of the case, the end of the case inevitably produces a flurry of activity with many functions being performed simultaneously. The anesthesia provider is busy preparing for the patient's emergence from anesthesia, the circulating nurse and scrub nurse are performing closing counts, and the surgeons are asking for suture and assistance in closing the wounds. At least two closing counts are performed; one count as closure is beginning and the other count as the skin is being closed. If the count is incorrect, the circulating nurse and the scrub nurse make every attempt to locate the missing item or items. The scrub nurse checks the field and enlists the help of the surgeons to check the wound. The circulating nurse checks all the sponge buckets and, if necessary, checks the linen and trash bags to ensure that a sponge or needle was not inadvertently thrown into the wrong container. If the missing item or items are still not located, an x-ray is taken to be sure the item has not been retained in the wound. An incorrect count is less likely if the team has been keeping track and counting throughout the case. However, multiple teams can be involved and this makes the process more difficult.

The circulating nurse must also call a report to the PAR at least 30 minutes before the end of the case. Transfusion status, the location of any drains or packing, allergies, line placement, and the procedures performed are all part of the report, as well as the status of the patient's condition. If a ventilator will be needed to assist the patient's breathing postoperatively, the settings are given to the PAR nurse at this time. It is also important to let the PAR nurse know where the family is waiting. The anesthesia provider will also give report to the PAR nurse regarding fluid replacement, medications and drips, and the anesthetic agents delivered during the procedure. This is usually done upon the patient's arrival to the PAR.

Once the wounds are closed, the counts are completed and the dressings are placed on the surgical sites. The drapes are carefully removed to avoid displacing any drains. A warm blanket is placed over the patient and the OR bed is slowly and carefully returned to its original position with the head of the bed directly in front of the anesthesia provider. This requires careful team work as there are lines, drains, etc., that must be kept in place. If there is adequate help and the anesthesia provider is comfortable with it, the OR bed can stay in the operative position, and emergence from anesthesia can proceed without turning the bed. This, however, requires extra personnel so that the anesthesia provider can be at the patient's head to manage the airway and another provider can be at the anesthesia machine managing the oxygen and the ambu bag.

After the patient has emerged from anesthesia and the tracheostomy tube is connected to the transport oxygen supply, the patient can be transferred onto the ICU bed. The pulse oximeter, arterial line, and EKG leads are connected to a transport monitor and the patient is taken to the PAR accompanied by the circulating nurse, the anesthesia provider, and the surgeon. The ICU bed is utilized rather than a gurney to avoid transferring the patient onto a bed twice. When the patient is transferred from PAR to ICU, they will already be settled in their bed.

On arrival to the PAR, the circulating nurse assists the PAR nurse in transferring the monitoring lines from the transport monitor to the PAR monitor. Oxygen is transferred from the transport tank to the PAR supply or the ventilator, whichever is appropriate. It is important for the OR nurse to stand by and assist when necessary until the patient is settled and an initial set of vital signs is taken. Any additional information necessary for the postoperative care of the patient can be shared at this time and any questions the PAR nurse may have about the procedure can be answered. It may also be necessary to keep the patient warm with a Bair Hugger machine or some other external device to maintain a constant normal temperature. The OR nurse can assist with this as well.

Postoperative Phase

At some point in the postoperative recovery period, the team of OR nurses should pay a visit to the patient. It is very rewarding to see the patient's progress and to discuss the intraoperative course with the nurses who are responsible for the patient's postoperative care. This provides necessary continuity for the patients and can be an excellent mechanism for continued quality improvement.

It is important for the perioperative nurse and the preoperative and postoperative nurses to work together as a team. Each nurse plays an important role in the care of the skull base patient. Each contributes their special expertise and assists in providing a truly collaborative and integrated approach to this very complex group of patients. This is a very challenging and rewarding area of nursing and one that is changing and growing every day.

POSTOPERATIVE NURSING CARE IN THE INTENSIVE CARE UNIT

Postoperative care of the skull base surgery patient is one of the most challenging roles in nursing today. The combination of intensive care expertise in otolaryngology and neurosurgical nursing demands the dedication of a very specialized group of nurses. The designation of one intensive care unit to care for these patients is critical to the consistency and performance of any group of staff. For the patient undergoing skull base surgery, nurses who are specially trained provide the optimal care for a smooth recovery and prevention of complications. Subtle changes often herald later, more significant problems. Educated nursing staff who work closely with the surgical staff can anticipate problems in such a way that leads to effective and early solutions.

The ICU has standard orders for skull base patients that have been written in concert with the surgical staff. These orders allow for more efficient care and a significant time savings, as well as the standardization of orders that would normally take an exceptional amount of physician time to write. All orders can be individualized for the specific patient's needs, and are driven by the type of surgical procedure and the patient's response. Diagnosis, surgical procedure, and reconstruction are well defined so the nurse has a full understanding of the patient's nursing requirements. The intensive care unit flow sheets are also standardized to provide consistency in documentation in an ICU setting. As with the standard orders, each flow sheet is individualized as necessary to document the specific patient's needs and responses.

Neurologic Monitoring

Foremost in the monitoring of neurologic status is a check on neurologic vital signs every 1/2 to 1 hour in the immediate postoperative period. These signs include cognitive functioning, pupillary response, hand grasps, extremity movement, and reflexes. Cognitive functioning also is assessed by asking the patient to write (if he or she is literate). Alteration in syntax, fluency, or spelling may be indicative of postoperative deficits. The Glasgow Coma Scale is invaluable in objective management. Most patients who have had a dural entry have an epidural drain placed during the operative procedure. This epidural catheter is placed to decompress the brain and allow for careful monitoring of CSF pressure in the ventricular system. Intracranial pressure (ICP) is the pressure that is exerted by the volume of the intracranial components, namely, brain tissue, blood, and CSF. Brain tissue comprises 80%, blood 10%, and CSF 10% of the intracranial volume. According to the Monro-Kellie doctrine, the intracranial components inside the closed compartment of the skull and meninges exert a certain normal pressure, known as ICP. If any one of the components increases, there is an increase in ICP. The danger is the possible destruction of the components by such an increase in pressure (9), ultimately resulting in brain herniation if not treated. Early detection of increasing ICP allows us to react early to such problems by making volume adjustments with the external catheter, to stop bleeding, or to give medications and change ventilation pressures (10).

Nursing care includes elevation of the head of the bed to about 30 degrees. The ventricular drainage system should be kept at the level of the external ear canal, which corresponds internally to the foramen of Monro. Placement at this level equalizes drainage within the ventricular system. Neurologic monitoring includes assessment of level of consciousness, lethargy, unequal pupils, or response to light. Change in sensation to pinprick, abnormal reflex responses, or change in ability to move extremities may signal an immediate problem. Changes in heart rate and respiration may signal neurologic as well as cardiovascular changes. Headache, specifically increasing head pain, should be considered a serious symptom of increasing intracranial pressure, meningitis (chemical or mechanical), or infection.

The epidural catheter is considered sterile because of the increased risk of infectious meningitis with its use. Most skull base patients may have a wound that has traversed the facial structures and the dura, inducing a chemical meningitis from blood in the spinal fluid. Dressing changes are done under sterile conditions, including gown, gloves, and mask. Great care must be taken to avoid inadvertent removal of the drain during dressing changes, changes in the patient's position, and transfer from bed to gurney or chair.

The nurse observes the patient for a CSF leak by inspection of nasal drainage, clear drainage through the incision, any fluctuant area near the incision, salty taste in the mouth, or clear fluid leak from the external ear canal. With anterior cranial fossa resections, CSF leaks may be more obvious after the nasal packing is removed. The *halo test* is a test to ascertain if CSF is part of the fluid that collects at the leaking site. A drop of fluid is placed on a clean cloth or dressing. The serum stays in the center and the CSF creates a halo around the center circle. A CSF leak may respond to a slight increase in ventricular drainage through the epidural catheter to decompress the ventricular system. CSF leaks are treated with additional antibiotic therapy for infection prophylaxis. A leak can be detected by a CT study using metrizamide contrast, and if it does not respond to conservative therapy, surgical closure is required.

Artificial Airway

A tracheostomy decompresses the surgical site from increased pressures that are generated by coughing, sneezing, or similar increases in airway pressures. In addition, it provides a means for assisted ventilation, if necessary, as well as a means of ensuring pulmonary toilet. During skull base surgery, the entry through the cranial vault often breaches the dura, which consequently requires repair. Air in the cranial vault is called pneumocephaly. Such trapped air can compress the brain and cause alteration in the patient's level of consciousness. The upper respiratory tract is in direct contact with the skull base during the surgical procedure, although through advances in reconstruction a tissue barrier is established at the completion of surgery. A tracheostomy can decompress the upper aerodigestive tract and prevent complications. For anterior cranial vault surgeries, the tracheostomy is often left in place until the surgical packing is removed at about day 7 to 10. At that time, the integrity of the repair is evaluated, and if no CSF leaks are found, the tracheostomy can be downsized, capped, and removed. This presupposes that all other routine parameters for weaning and decanulation are met.

Reconstruction: Flaps and Grafts

Cranial base surgery creates large defects, and reconstruction is undertaken at the completion of tumor resection. Pericranium and osseous–myocutaneous flaps are often used to fill the defect. Surgical therapy in general, and specifically craniofacial skeletal surgery, is undergoing a transformation from traditional surgery to surgical tissue engineering. Tissue engineering is a paradigm for surgical therapy that uses computer-aided presurgical planning, cosmetically innovative approach techniques, tissue-integrating biomaterials, and cellular and cytokine therapy to achieve the therapeutic goal. Although adoption of this paradigm is in the early phases, continued progress in molecular medicine and macromedicine will ultimately lead to broad acceptance (11).

The reconstruction flaps commonly used are the pectoralis major myocutaneous, scapular, radial, fibular, and rectus abdominis free flaps, as well as skeletal reconstruction. These flaps require a microvascular anastomosis to an artery and a vein to survive. Nursing care of the patient with such a flap centers on preserving this microvascular reconstruction of blood supply to the flap tissue. Any decrease in blood flow created by low blood pressure or pressure on the anastomotic vessels could place the reconstructed flap vessels, both venous and arterial, in jeopardy. Maintenance of blood flow to the flap, frequent monitoring with Doppler signals, and judicious administration of blood products, albumin, and fluid all maximize blood flow during the early postoperative period. It is critical to check capillary refill with Doppler findings. Flaps often look pale in the first 12 hours after surgery, during the period of general rewarming and gradually improving vascularization of the flap. Capillary refill should be brisk and color must be maintained. Changes should be reported and discussed immediately to ascertain if the flap requires any immediate surgical intervention.

Carotid Resection

Patients who require a carotid resection during skull base surgery are at very high risk of stroke. With the advent of BTO and SPECT scanning, the skull base surgical team is better able to predict the outcomes and make the resection safer for those patients requiring a carotid resection at the time of surgery. The incidence of stroke after carotid resection has dramatically decreased because of improved surgical techniques, better preoperative evaluation, and better patient selection. But the patient is still at risk and strokes can occur, and not necessarily perioperatively.

Nursing care of patients who undergo a carotid resection during skull base surgery is predicated on intense observation, documentation of neurologic signs, and prevention of hypotension. The patient requires rigorous neurologic testing. Obvious motor weakness in extremities is a hallmark sign. Facial nerve paralysis may or may not be indicative of stroke, depending on the surgical approach and the location of the tumor. The facial nerve may have been sacrificed during the procedure. It is incumbent on nursing staff to know the cranial nerves and understand the surgical procedures and which cranial nerves are involved in each of the resections. The more subtle signs and symptoms of aphasia (expressive and receptive) are very difficult to identify in the early postoperative period, but these subtle signs can explain why patients do not "cooperate" with instructions. "Yes" and "no" questions may be simple for the nurse, but give no insight into the cognitive component of the patient's neurologic status. Incorporating the family in discussions may assist in the evaluation; the family knows the patient better than the staff and may be able to detect subtle differences in response or personality.

CASE STUDY

A 56-year-old man underwent radiation therapy for a right tonsilar squamous cell cancer in 1984. He represented in 1995 with a recurrence that encased his right carotid artery and coursed into the skull base along the mandibular branch of the trigeminal nerve, through the foramen ovale. At the surgical resection, it was found that the carotid could be preserved and the tumor fully resected with clear margins. The postoperative course was relatively uneventful, with the exception of major wound breakdown at the surgical site. This poor wound healing was due to the previous radiation therapy to the area, and low serum protein and albumin. Subsequently the carotid artery became exposed in the open wound. After a very long hospitalization, the patient went home with the carotid covered with granulation tissue that appeared pink and healthy. Nursing care in the hospital had included meticulous dressing changes every 4 hours with wet to dry dressings. The patient and his wife had been trained in wound care. The nursing staff had discussed what to do if the carotid were to bleed, and what, if any, intervention should be undertaken. Both the patient and wife were adamant about intervention, and they were educated how to treat a carotid bleed at home. They understood that even with quick action and pressure on the carotid, survival was uncertain.

The patient was home for 18 days. He was readmitted to our hospital after an episode of bright red blood spurting from his neck wound in the area of the carotid artery. Direct pressure over the carotid artery by the patient's wife had controlled the bleeding until he could be transported to the hospital. The patient came in by helicopter from 60 miles away, with his wife maintaining pressure on the carotid artery. On admission examination, the previously healed granulation tissue was clearly disrupted and the carotid was again exposed. The patient and family consented to a carotid resection, without the benefit of BTO and SPECT scanning. The surgery was undertaken immediately.

After surgery, the patient awoke moving all extremities and appeared alert and responsive, showing no clinical signs of a stroke. He knew the routines and cooperated with care. He was unable to speak because of his tracheostomy. On postoperative days 2 and 3 he was out of bed to a chair, nodding "yes" and "no" to questions. His wife mentioned that she felt he was depressed because he was not writing notes as he had before. A more thorough evaluation elucidated that he was not writing because he was unable. He had suffered a stroke that rendered him aphasic in both writing and speech. There appeared to be no motor function deficits. He was able to complete usual hospital routines because he was aware of and remembered his last hospitalization. His speech could be fully tested only later because of the tracheostomy in the early postoperative period. During surgery or in the immediate postoperative period, the patient had an episode of hypoperfusion to the brain because of the diminished flow after carotid resection. The aphasia was his only obvious outward symptom.

Although an unusual example, this case serves to demonstrate how subtle some of the neurologic symptoms of stroke are after carotid resection. The patient underwent extensive rehabilitation and he is now able to communicate fairly well. At over 3 years after this incident, he still demonstrates no outward, physical signs of a stroke other than aphasia, and with therapy the aphasia is improving.

Wound Care

The wound care of skull base patients is determined by the extent of the resection and the reconstruction. Immediately after surgery in the ICU, wound care focuses on flap viability, suture line care, and suction drain care. No pressure dressing, tape, or respiratory equipment is placed over the reconstruction flap or its pedicle.

The surgeon places suction drains in very specific positions to drain a respective anatomic area of the resection. It is important to secure the drains in place in addition to placing stay sutures. Stomahesive or a similar skin barrier is placed on the skin, and elastoplast secures the drain to the Stomahesive (Fig. 1). Even if Silastic drains are used, they should be stripped every 2 to 4 hours to ensure that clots are not obstructing them and permitting the accumulation of fluid/serum under the reconstruction flap. The drain suction is usually set at 100 mm Hg suction pressure. The determining factor in drain removal is an output volume that has fallen to less than approximately 30 ml in a 24-hour period. After drain removal, a pressure dressing is placed over the reconstruction to seal the flaps to the underlying tissue.

Home Care Planning

As the patient progresses from the intensive care unit to acute care to a homegoing goal-oriented program, the nursing care focus must be in parallel. Preparation of a patient and family for home care is a progressive teaching process that must begin early in the interaction of the patient with the health care system.

As with most patients, the step from hospital to home is usually a good progression, but not without stress. The task of coping with the rigors of skull base surgery and the resultant disfigurement and body image changes can be overwhelming. It is well proven (12) that those patients who have fewer overall illnesses and are younger are better able to adapt and cope (13). The older the patient, the more comor-

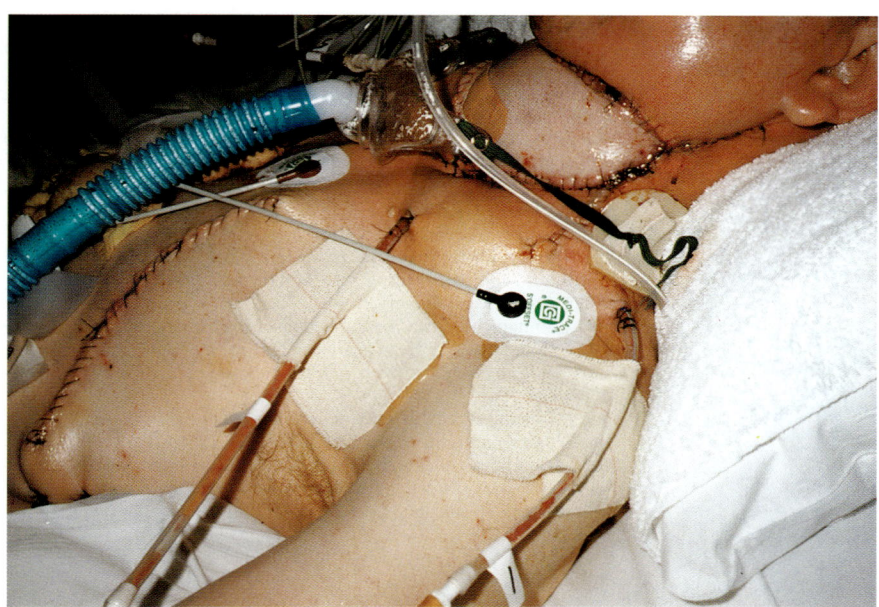

Fig. 1. Stomahesive skin protector and elastoplast tape secure the surgical drains following skull base, head and neck surgery.

bid illnesses, the harder it becomes to rebound after yet another serious illness and surgical procedure. The home care focus should be on independence with attention to goals of rehabilitation. These goals must be set before discharge by the multidisciplinary team in the hospital. It is incumbent on the team to transmit these goals to the home health team for continuation in the home setting.

The nurse's role in this adaptation process is to help patients effectively use what resources they have and use them to their best effect. Patients and families must be familiar with their care needs well before the day they are discharged. Teaching of home-oriented self-care activities of daily living, enteral feeding, and wound and tracheostomy care should become part of the patient's routine before discharge. As much as possible, no significant changes should be made immediately before discharge; such changes only add confusion for the patient and family. Written information regarding medications, specific wound care instructions, and enteral feedings should be thoroughly reviewed with the patient, family, and caregivers. Follow-up clinic appointments, emergency numbers, and resources should be given to the patient in writing before discharge.

The principles of geriatric medicine are important to include for the older patient population. The major goal is to return to safe independence in their previous environment. Elderly sleep–wake cycles may be easily disrupted by medication and ongoing nursing care requirements.

If possible, home management of enteral feedings and wound and tracheostomy care should be scheduled to allow for uninterrupted sleep for both patient and family. Sleep deprivation often leads to failure of the home plan, requiring rehospitalization or admittance to a skilled nursing facility.

Home health nurses who are assigned to skull base patients are often very unfamiliar with their care needs, so the patient's written material may also help the home health nurse to understand better the care needs of the patient. Close contact with the clinical nurse specialist and the skull base coordinator should make the patient's transition from hospital to home smoother.

CONCLUSION

Care of the patient undergoing skull base surgery involves complex, advanced nursing care. As medical knowledge advances, so must the nursing professional respond with new methods of therapy. Such surgical advances are a challenge with each new patient, and stretch and expand the expertise of each nurse. Nursing must respond with science-based practice to the advances in surgical resection of skull base tumors.

It is the nurse who cares for patients, makes them feel better, tends to their wounds, and ministers to healing. Coping, cognition, pain management, and wound care are all issues and tasks that the patient must endure during recovery. It is the highly skilled nurse who will be at the patient's bedside, whether it be the operating room table, hospital bed, bedroom at home, or in the clinic, caring for the person.

REFERENCES

1. Donald PJ. Combined middle fossa/infratemporal fossa surgery. *AORN J* 1992;55:480–489.
2. Perera F. Uncovering new clues to cancer risk. *Sci Am* 1996;276(5): 54–62.
3. Brooks-Brunn J. Protecting the lungs. *Reflections, Sigma Theta Tau International* 1997;23(1):16.
4. Agency for Health Care Policy and Research. *Clinical practice guidelines on management of cancer pain.* AHCPR publication no. 94-0595. Rockville, MD: U.S. Department of Health and Human Services, Agency for Health Care Policy and Research, 1994.
5. Vermillion C. Operating room acquired pressure ulcers. *Decubitus* 1990;3(1):26–30.

6. Papantonio C. Sacral ulcers following cardiac surgery: incidence and risks. *Advances in Wound Care* 1995;7(2):24–36.
7. Zaloga G. *Enteral nutrition in hospitalized patients: a summary.* Ross Products Division publication A6382. Abbott Park, IL: Abbott Laboratories, 1995:44–51.
8. Dropkin MJ. Coping with disfigurement/dysfunction and length of hospital stay. *ORL–Head and Neck Nursing* 1997;15(1):22–26.
9. Cummings R. Understanding external ventricular drainage. *Journal of Neuroscience Nursing* 1992;24:84–87.
10. Clevenger V. Nursing management of lumbar drains. *Journal of Neuroscience Nursing* 1990;22:227–229.
11. Friedman C, Costantino P. General concepts in craniofacial skeletal augmentation and replacement. *Otolaryngol Clin North Am* 1994;27:847–857.
12. Dropkin MJ. Coping with disfigurement and dysfunction after head and neck cancer surgery: a conceptual framework. *Semin Oncol Nurs* 1989;15:213–219.
13. Mulgrew B, Dropkin MJ. Coping with craniofacial resection: a case study. *ORL Nursing* 1991;Summer:8–18..

BIBLIOGRAPHY

American Association of Neuroscience Nurses. *Standards of practice.* Chicago: American Association of Neuroscience Nurses, 1997.

Association of Operating Room Nurses, Inc. *AORN core curriculum.* Denver: Association of Operating Room Nurses, Inc., 1991.

Association of Operating Room Nurses, Inc. *1991 AORN standards and recommended practices for perioperative nursing.* Denver: Association of Operating Room Nurses, Inc., 1991.

Cammermeyer M, eds. *Core curriculum for neuroscience nursing.* 3rd ed., update. American Association of Neuroscience Nurses, 1996.

Cavenee W, White R. (1995) The genetic basis of cancer. *Sci Am* 1995;275(3):72–79.

Dennison D. Thermal regulation of patients during the perioperative period. *AORN J* 1995;61:827–831.

Donald PJ. *Craniofacial surgery for head and neck cancer.* American Academy of Otolaryngology Head and Neck Surgery instructional course no. 2434. Alexandria, VA: American Academy of Otolaryngology Head and Neck Surgery, 1989.

Harris L, Huntoon M, eds. *Core curriculum.* New Smyrna Beach, FL: Society of Otolaryngology Head and Neck Nurses, 1997.

Lazarus RS. *Psychological stress and the coping process.* New York: McGraw-Hill, 1966.

Rennie J, Rusting R, eds. *What you need to know about cancer: Scientific American special issue.* 1996;276(9):56–167.

Society of Otorhinolaryngology Head and Neck Nursing Standards of Practice Committee. *Guidelines for otorhinolaryngology nursing practice.* New Smyrna Beach, FL: Society of Otorhinolaryngology and Head–Neck Nurses, 1996.

CHAPTER 9

Intraoperative Neurophysiologic Monitoring

State of the Art

Robert J. Sclabassi, Jeffrey R. Balzer, and Donald N. Krieger

Cranial base surgery poses significant risk to the functioning of the cranial nerves, the brainstem, and the cerebral hemispheres. This risk is due both to problems associated with maintaining adequate blood supply to the brainstem and cerebral hemispheres and to the effect of various operative maneuvers aimed at, for example, adequately exposing and removing tumors. These risks may be reduced if appropriate information concerning the relationships between surgical manipulations and their impact on the functioning of the patient's central nervous system (CNS) is available to the surgeon. To provide information of this type, aimed at reducing both the probability and severity of injury to the neural tissue, methodologies have been developed and are being used to obtain and evaluate multimodal neurophysiologic measures in real time, during surgery to the cranial base.

Intraoperative neurophysiologic monitoring provides a real-time control loop around a system composed of the surgeon and the patient. The goals of this control loop are both the reduction of morbidity and a dynamic assessment of structure–function relationships of the patient's nervous system. These objectives are accomplished by making specific and sensitive measurements that reflect the interactions between the surgeon's intraoperative manipulations and the functioning of the patient's CNS. These goals require obtaining real-time measurements of CNS function that can be closely correlated with operative manipulations. To achieve these goals within a time frame that is of value to the progress of the operation, multiple channels of data need to be acquired, processed, and displayed rapidly.

This chapter reviews the intraoperative monitoring approach the authors use to provide multimodality neurophysiologic monitoring during cranial base surgery. In particular, a detailed description of the authors' overall approach to this complex monitoring problem is presented. The technical approaches to the acquisition and interpretation of these neurophysiologic measures are then presented. Finally, the implications of this approach for the successful performance of cranial base surgery are discussed.

APPROACH

The surgeon needs information about the functional status of the nervous system during surgery to adapt surgical strategy so as to minimize morbidity. Immediate knowledge of the physiologic effect of each surgical manipulation is an irreplaceable help in the pursuit of aggressive surgical techniques, such as those involved in operating at the cranial base (1). Thus, the objective of intraoperative monitoring during cranial base tumor cases is to help the surgeon reduce morbidity, and when it is necessary to produce morbidity, to do so in a controlled fashion—that is, to provide information about what is being done and what its consequences might be.

It has long been appreciated that the patient's physiologic status is dynamic, and that during surgery rapid and life-threatening changes may occur. This realization has led to sophisticated patient monitoring by anesthesiologists in which extensive physiologic monitoring is routinely used to maintain the homeostasis in the patient (2). This monitoring may be thought of as putting a control loop around the anesthesiologist and the patient for the purposes of life support. Some information is available from these procedures that also reflects the stress on the CNS, such as changes in heart rate related to both brainstem and vagal stimulation. However, the comparative ability to evaluate the nervous system by either clinical means or by the commonly used physio-

R. J. Sclabassi, J. Balzer, D. Krieger: Center for Neurophysiology, Children's Hospital of Pittsburgh, Pittsburgh, Pennsylvania 15213.

logic monitoring tools available to the anesthesiologist is limited during surgery.

These limitations in the ability to assess nervous system function have led to the development of neurophysiologic intraoperative monitoring techniques that add another dimension to the assessment of patient status during surgery. Intraoperative neurophysiologic monitoring also can be thought of as establishing a real-time control loop—this time between the surgeon and the patient (Fig. 1). The primary goals are to reduce morbidity and dynamically assess structure–function relationships of the patient's nervous system during surgical manipulation. This dynamic assessment can guide a surgeon by providing specific, sensitive measurements that reflect operative maneuvers and their impact on the patient's CNS functioning. These goals require real-time measures of the CNS functions that can be closely correlated to operative manipulations within a time frame valuable to the progress of the operation. Thus, multiple types of neurophysiologic data must be acquired, processed, and displayed in real time.

The various neurophysiologic measures described in this chapter provide objective measures of nervous system function and have significant potential for providing ongoing and relevant information about the status of the CNS. Neurophysiologic measures have value in many types of operative procedures (3–5); however, the ones described in this chapter are most useful in cranial base surgery, which involves particularly complex and lengthy surgical procedures.

Depending on the surgical procedure, the authors routinely measure electrical activity dependent on the functioning of the brainstem [brainstem auditory evoked potentials (BAEPs) and brainstem somatosensory evoked potentials (BSEPs)], the cortex [the electroencephalogram (EEG), median nerve somatosensory evoked potentials (MSPs), and visual evoked potentials (VEPs)], and electromyograms (EMGs) from muscles innervated by cranial nerves II, III, IV, V, VI, VII, VIII, X, XI, and XII. It is imperative that the measures used are both specific to the neural tissue being manipulated and sensitive to changes in the functioning of the neural tissue produced by the surgical manipulations. Many of these measures are obtained, displayed, and interpreted simultaneously, permitting a multidimensional assessment of the integrity of the neural structures at risk. In addition, many of these measures provide information not only about function itself but also about variables that indirectly affect function, such as blood flow, hypoxia, and hypotension.

An additional important aspect necessary for successful intraoperative monitoring is the planning and execution of surgical procedures in such a way that the neurophysiologists are in close communication with all other members of the surgical team, including surgeons, neuroanesthesiologists, and neuroradiologists. This preoperative and intraoperative communication between the members of the surgical team ensures that the appropriate neurophysiologic measures are used during the case, that the neuroanesthesiologist is prepared to switch anesthetic technique in support of the requirements imposed by each technique, and that the significance of observed changes is appreciated by all members of the operative team.

The authors' conceptual approach requires that the neurophysiologist understand the nature of the patient's disease, the operative strategy of the surgeon, and the anesthesiolo-

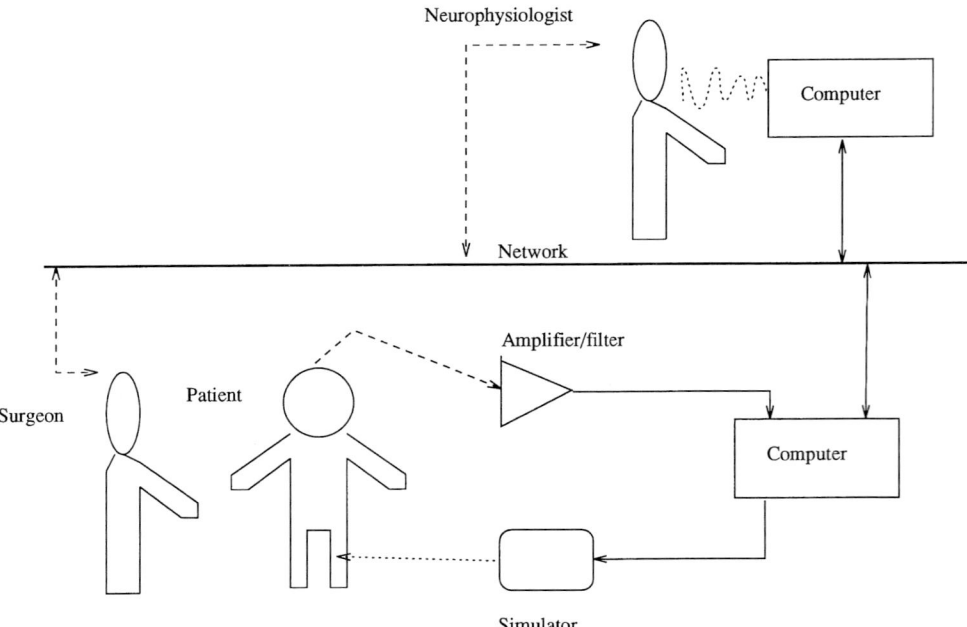

FIG. 1. Neurophysiologic monitoring establishes a control loop around the surgeon and the patient to reduce morbidity. The neurophysiologist may continuously interpret the monitored data, either in the operating room or remotely.

gist's approach to the management of that particular patient. It requires that the surgeon understand the level of information that the neurophysiologist can provide as the operative procedure is evolving, and it requires that the neuroanesthesiologist understand the effects of the pharmacologic manipulations on the monitoring tools available to the neurophysiologist. Thus, the keystone of the authors' approach to intraoperative monitoring is the close and continuous interchange of information between all the members of the surgical team.

Attention to detail begins before the patient is taken to the operating room. It is the authors' policy that all patients for whom intraoperative monitoring is ordered undergo preoperative neurophysiologic studies to determine baseline responses. The reasons for this are many, and include introducing the neurophysiologic monitoring concept to the patient, ensuring that the neurophysiologist understands the nature of the case to be monitored, ensuring that the peculiarities of the patient's responses are understood before arrival in the operating room, and determining the existence of unsuspected secondary lesions. Moreover, it is not uncommon for patients with large skull base lesions to present with very abnormal neurophysiologic responses. Knowledge of these abnormalities before the patient arrives in the operating room allows for a better assessment once operating room baselines are obtained. This approach has the support of the surgeons, who write specific orders for every patient who is to be evaluated and monitored.

The neurophysiologists participate in preoperative discussions concerning patient management, and also attend and participate in the surgical complications conferences. Thus, the neurophysiologist has a detailed understanding of each patient and his or her unique monitoring requirements before the surgical case, as well as an appreciation for the outcome of the case and for the role that intraoperative monitoring may have played in that outcome. This close coordination between the neurophysiologist and the surgeon not only ensures the most appropriate and highest-quality intraoperative monitoring, but facilitates the evolution of improved monitoring techniques to provide better the types of information the surgeons need and desire.

The neurophysiologists must communicate with the surgeon and the neuroanesthesiologist concerning the anesthetic requirements before the start of the case to ensure that no conflicts exist over the required anesthetic approach. For example, when will the use of paralytic or potent inhalation agents interfere with neurophysiologic monitoring? Many of the monitoring procedures requested by surgeons place competing and complex demands on the anesthesiologists. Thus, a variety of anesthesia techniques may be used at different times during a single operative procedure to enable the appropriate neurophysiologic measures to be taken when needed.

Based on this information and on anticipation of what may happen, the appropriate subset of monitoring tools from the total armamentarium must be selected before the beginning of the case. For example, if an injury to a carotid artery occurs during tumor resection and the surgeon wishes to place the patient under pentobarbital protection, the neurophysiologists must be prepared to provide a measure of burst suppression from both ongoing EEG activity and somatosensory evoked potentials (SEPs). Thus, the need for EEGs must have been anticipated before the draping of the patient. Finally, at some point before the actual beginning of surgery, the surgical team must be informed about the quality of the recordings: that is, how consistent or variable they are, and how they compare with baseline preoperative studies.

Pertinent information during the case is entered into the computer record and is appended to the operative data. These notes provide a permanent record of the case and can alert the neurophysiologist observing a case remotely of any significant changes. In addition, a continuous log sheet with the time of each saved response, stimulating sites, and any additional information relevant to the operation is maintained.

NEUROPHYSIOLOGIC METHODOLOGY

Neurophysiologic recording during cranial base procedures can rapidly become quite complex. It is not unusual to monitor as many as five different neurophysiologic variables simultaneously: for example, EEGs, BAEPs and BSEPs, MSPs, and EMGs recorded from multiple cranial nerves. This requires a well organized and theoretically parsimonious approach to monitoring. In addition, the recording of high-quality neurophysiologic data depends on the appropriate utilization of technology. In particular, attention must be paid to the electrode properties, amplifiers, and the equipment used for acquiring and displaying the data.

Electrode Properties

Where possible, all scalp electrodes are placed according to the International 10/20 system of electrode placement (6). Recording electrodes are placed symmetrically to provide for control recordings from the side contralateral to the surgery, even when electrodes may not be positioned in the standard recording sites. The patient is prepared for monitoring by measuring the head according to the 10/20 system and marking it appropriately for the desired electrode placement. This system, originally devised for EEG recordings, specifies the position of 21 evenly spaced locations on the scalp, with the sites determined as 10% or 20% of the separations between definitive bony landmarks. If possible, this is accomplished in the operating room holding area because this permits more accurate and rapid placement of electrodes in the operating room.

All recordings are performed using subdermal needle electrodes. Electrodes that are not in the operative field but that are on the scalp and not accessible during surgery, are either sutured or stapled in place. Electrodes on the face, which are placed for recording EMG activity, are taped in place. Electrodes in the operative field are placed by the surgeons using sterile technique, usually early in the procedure. The electrodes are checked for impedance values and are accepted if the impedance is less than 10,000 ohms. If electrodes fail the impedance test and all connections are intact, the faulty electrodes are identified and replaced. In all cases, every effort is made to reduce noise and artifact to obtain a robust and consistent potential. This is particularly important in measuring small signals in the electrically noisy environment of the operating room.

Needle electrodes also may be used as electrical stimulating electrodes, and the application techniques are the same in these instances as for recording purposes.

Monitoring System

The authors and others have been actively researching the development of distributed computer networks for the acquisition, integration, and assessment of neurophysiologic data for several years (7–11). This work has resulted in the development of a distributed computer system (NeuroNet) that has been extensively used at the Center for Clinical Neurophysiology of the University of Pittsburgh Medical Center (UPMC) and a number of other teaching hospitals not associated with UPMC. The system provides real-time and non–real-time capabilities, along with extensive facilities for supporting data distribution and communication remotely from the operating room. Most important, the system supports the acquisition and processing of multiple data types, simultaneously, and in real time. Thus, NeuroNet is a fully integrated system that transparently combines the collection, processing, and presentation of real-time data sources, including all of the physiologic monitoring functions, with non–real-time functions and extensive on-line database information.

Figure 2 presents a control flow diagram of the system with the major system components identified. The user station is any host that can support NeuroNet functions, ranging from workstations to personal computers. NeuroDisplay (Fig. 3) is a user interface screen and constitutes the front end to NeuroNet. NeuroDisplay is based on X-window's and Motif. The real-time application software supports those tasks that require guaranteed low-latency end-to-end performance, such as acquisition, processing, and display of neurophysiologic data. The non–real-time application software supports tasks that require average throughput and maximum average delay, such as file transfers and text-based e-mail.

Workstations are mounted in instrumentation racks and configured with appropriate electronics to support various data acquisition tasks, including EEGs, EMGs, and multimodality evoked potentials. Multiple units may be used in parallel on the same case if the number of variables to be monitored is greater than the capacity of a single system. The data being acquired on these systems are transparently accessible, in real time, across local area networks for review, analysis, and consultation.

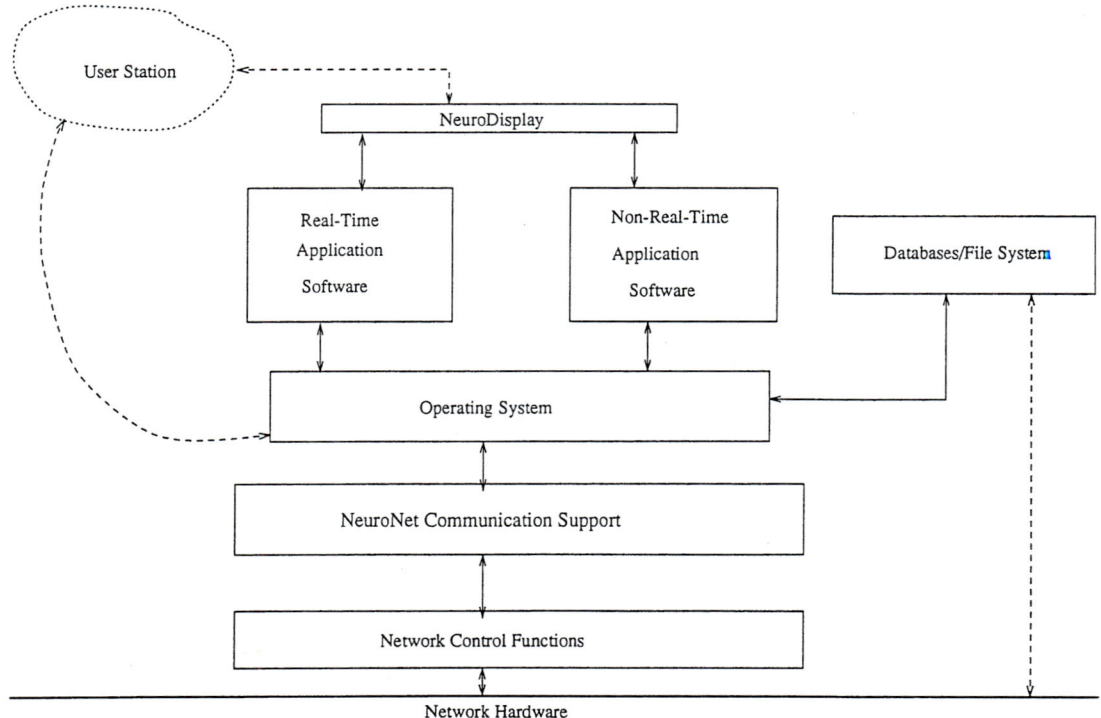

FIG. 2. Schematic representation of the NeuroNet control flow.

Below this layer are the system support modules. They include an operating system layer, a database/file system level, a communication support layer, and a network control layer. The communication support layer encapsulates the communication control structure, whereas network control functions provide the lowest-level access to the underlying network. The databases act as the integrating agent for all the data acquired and manipulated through the system.

NeuroNet permits simultaneous data collection and on-screen viewing of multiple modalities, each with user-determined observation intervals, collection rates, and stimulus rates that can be independently displayed and processed in real time on any other system on the network.

All NeuroNet software is integrated; that is, there is no concept of separate packages for each type of data collection. This provides maximum capability for collecting and analyzing combinations of different data types. The EEG capabilities include compressed spectral arrays on all available channels, digital filtering of EEG, and real-time spectral computations on the incoming data with arbitrary-length spectral averages. The EMG capabilities are the same. The evoked potential capabilities include multimodality data collection with individually controllable stimulation rates, sampling rates, observation intervals, digital filters, feature marking, baseline selection, noise estimation, and even/odd averaging. The system provides real-time remote viewing of all acquired data; multiway communication across local area networks, either digital audio or text; and unified user interfaces for local and remote systems that requires familiarity with only one user interface.

Instrumentation racks perform a number of functions, including stimulus control and generation, data acquisition, signal processing, and data display. Each workstation has a high-resolution (1,024 × 1,280 pixel), 24-bit color monitor. Data acquisition is accomplished through a custom-designed data acquisition system. This unit includes a 12-bit analog–digital (A/D) converter with a 16-channel multiplexer that can be expanded to 64 channels, and is used for acquir-

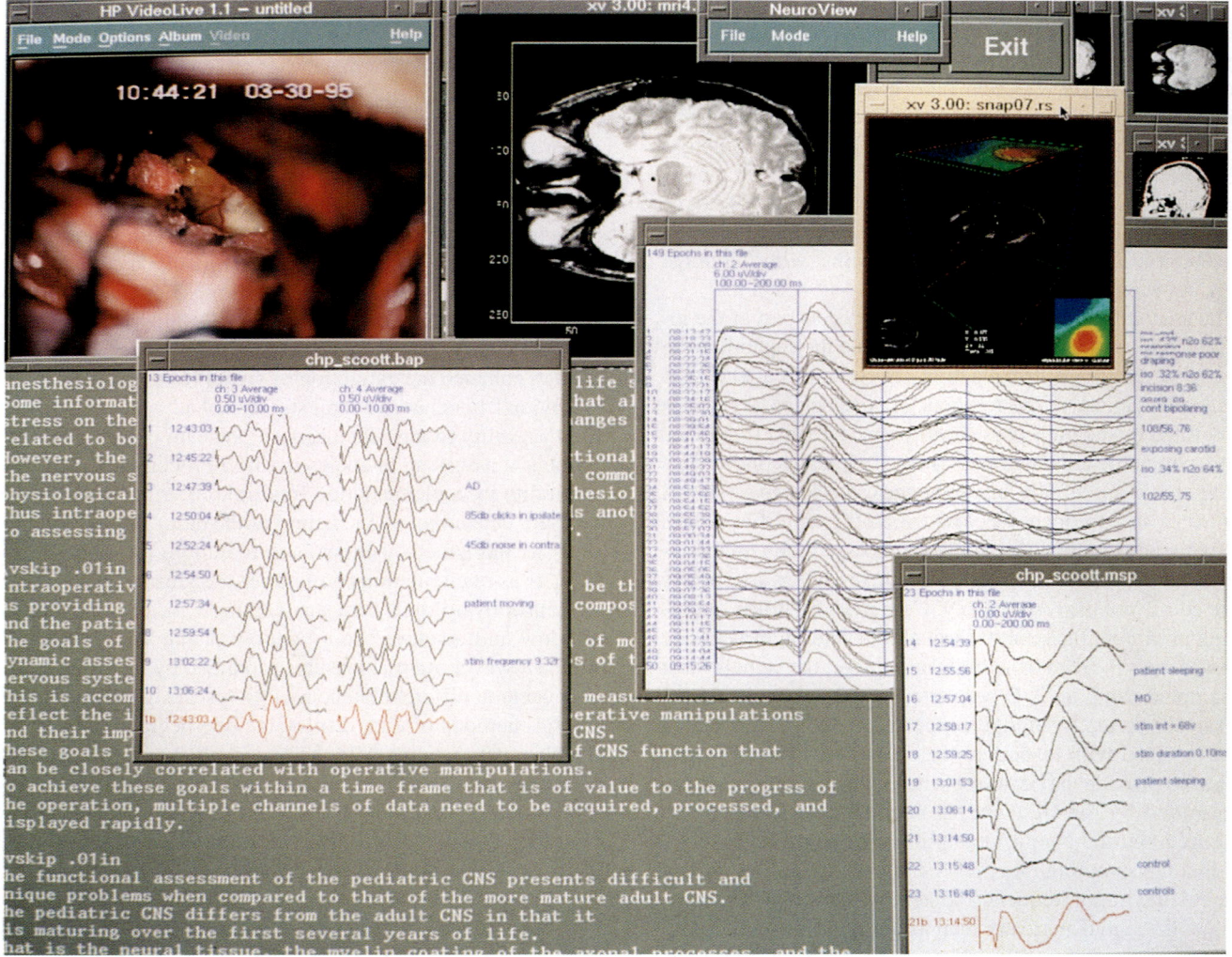

FIG. 3. Remote NeuroDisplay windows showing data from the operating room along with imaging data available to the neurophysiologist.

ing physiologic data from the anesthesiology monitors simultaneously with the neurophysiologic data. All data manipulations are handled by calls to the NDF (Neuro Data File) library.

Signal Acquisition and Processing

Neurophysiologic signals are most commonly amplified using differential amplifiers. This differencing has the effect of eliminating identical (in-phase) signal components that might be present at each recording electrode (presumably noise), and retaining the signals that are different (out-of-phase) and presumably produced by different physiologic generators. Apart from brain activity, bioelectric activity originating from muscles in the head, neck, and generators in the eyes and heart is present and is likely to be much greater in amplitude than the evoked potential of interest. Also present at the scalp are relatively large induced voltages of extraneous origin arising from electrical equipment. Any potentials that are picked up equally at both electrodes (common-mode or in-phase signals) are canceled out, and only the voltages developed between the two electrodes (out-of-phase signals) are separated and preferentially amplified. The common-mode rejection ratio governs the amplifiers' efficiency in discriminating between the local potentials of interest and these other, usually larger, interference potentials, picked up at both input electrodes. Differential amplifiers used in neurophysiologic investigations typically have common-mode rejection ratios greater that 80 dB (10,000:1). These amplifiers also have adjustable gains, with the range being between 20,000 and 500,000.

The analog filtering capabilities, provided as part of the input preamplifiers and amplifiers, determine the capabilities to remove or reduce electrical activity at certain frequencies in the recorded signals. The frequency response characteristics are defined by the high-pass cutoff point (i.e., that frequency above which the amplifier passes the frequency components of the signal essentially unattenuated), the low-pass cutoff point (i.e., that frequency below which the amplifier passes the frequency components of the signal essentially unattenuated), and the rate of attenuation occurring below and above these cutoff points, respectively. Care must be given to providing minimum phase shift through the filtering process.

To process the data on a digital computer, the signals must be sampled using an A/D converter, which has a maximum peak-to-peak input voltage range (e.g., 10 V) and which must be sized with respect to the characteristics of the amplifiers to provide maximum sensitivity. The sampling rate is determined by the frequency content of the signal being measured and the Nyquist sampling criterion, which specifies that the sampling rate must be at least two times greater than the maximum frequency content of the signal. The sampling of the signal at greater than the Nyquist rate avoids signal distortion produced by aliasing due to a too-low sampling rate.

Evoked potentials are typically a fraction of the size of the spontaneous brain activity appearing in the background EEG, and about one thousandth the size of the other physiologic and extraneous potentials with which they are intermixed. The most effective method for extracting the signal of interest from the noise, after amplifying the signal with differential amplifiers, is to use signal averaging, which is in effect a cross-correlation between a point-process defined by the occurrence of the stimuli and the recorded evoked activity (i.e., an optimal filter; Fig. 4). In averaging, the signal component at each point is coherent and adds directly, whereas the background and noise components tend to be statistically independent and summate in a more-or-less root-mean-square fashion.

The usefulness of averaging as a signal extraction technique depends on the assumption that the observed data are stationary, that is, the data are not changing rapidly in time. This assumption reinforces the need to acquire data as rapidly as possible for any single average. The authors have been investigating techniques for estimating time-varying evoked potentials (12), which allow evoked potentials to be extracted from nonstationary data. In addition to the classic averaging techniques, a number of modified averaging techniques have been developed and found to be useful. These include odd/even averaging (where two responses are computed for each data channel, one from the even number stimuli, the other from the odd numbered stimuli), moving averaging (which allows a sliding average to be computed), averaging to bursting trains (which allows high-frequency response properties to studied), random train stimulation (which allows nonlinear properties and system interactions to be characterized) (13), and noise estimation by plus/minus averaging (which allows the residual noise on a response to be estimated). The latter is extremely useful when a patient has particularly severe disease. Digital filters also may be used to enhance the extraction of signal from noise.

Digital filters have several significant advantages, including the ability to introduce zero or constant phase shift (important in assessing latencies in different components), and flexibility in implementation (multiple filtering routines can be used, depending on the nature of the data). These calculations are implemented either as convolutions (9), regressions (12), or as manipulations on Fourier transforms (14).

Neurophysiologic data are captured in an observation window and displayed in a window of the same length of time. However, many measures produced by the same stimulus occur at different latencies with respect to that stimulus. Useful methods of data display include being able to tailor the observation window to the expected latency of the interesting component of the response. For example, far-field potentials typically occur within 20 milliseconds (msec) of the stimulus, whereas near-field potentials occur within the first 100 msec of the stimulus presentation. Thus, the optimal observation of these different components is facilitated by the capability to specify different observation windows for different waves of interest being observed at the same time.

NeuroNet has an extensive package for evoked potential data collection and presentation to the user. All modalities

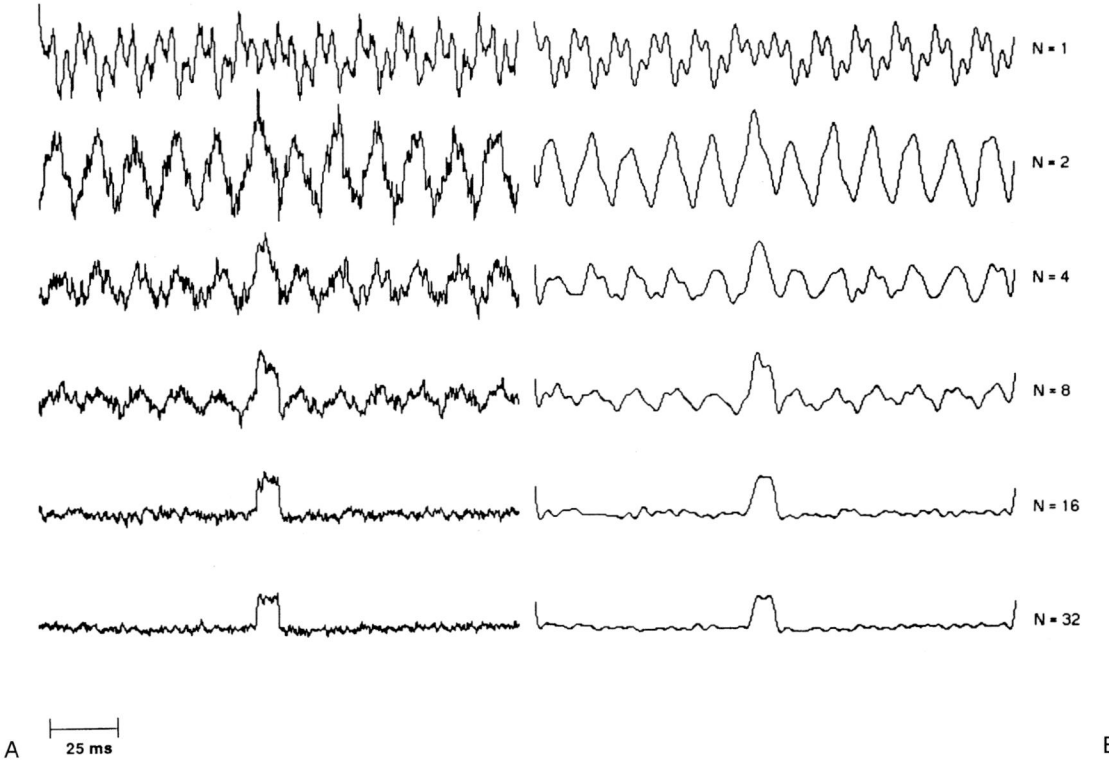

FIG. 4. Examples of **(A)** averaged and **(B)** digitally filtered average, demonstrating the capabilities of both averaging and digital filtering to extract signals from noise.

may be collected individually or mixed simultaneously (Fig. 5).

Data trending over time is flexible in that each channel of each modality may be independently displayed and controlled. Examples of processing available for all signals include digital filtering, standard averaging, odd/even averaging, noise estimation, and peak marking (both time and amplitude).

All stimulators must be precisely synchronized with the averaging process. This is accomplished either by triggering the stimulator from the computer or by triggering the computer data acquisition from the stimulator. The interstimulus intervals may be randomized to minimize contamination with phase-locked or quasiperiodic noise. SEPs are usually produced by electrical stimulators producing a shock through the skin. Both constant-current and constant-voltage stimulators are used. However, from the equivalent circuit perspective, there is no difference between these modes of stimulation.

Baseline responses are obtained before draping the patient and compared with the preoperative evaluation. Significant differences must be accounted for because signal deterioration may be due to patient positioning. The baseline responses are displayed as a background display on the computer monitor so that differences may be automatically calculated and displayed. A waterfall display window is used to follow the patterns of the change over a period of time during the case. New responses are automatically updated to this display as they are saved from the current data display. Thus, the waterfall display provides a comparative record of the patient's data and facilitates the process of identifying significant changes in activity.

The user may enter comments at any time during data collection and may store and retrieve comments from a list of predefined comments for quick annotation of a currently collected record through a pop-up window. Baseline data may be displayed for any waveform (both in the real-time displays and in trended displays). The baselines may be retrieved from any channel of any data file, thereby permitting the inclusion of baselines from preoperative studies. Artifact rejection is also fully user controlled. The user may define two time windows per channel for artifact rejection. Furthermore, the amplitude rejection criterion is user settable, along with a "spike allowance" parameter that permits a percentage of the data to exceed the artifact rejection limits without rejecting the trial.

Neuroanesthetic Considerations

It is well known that the type of anesthesia and the patient's blood pressure, cerebral blood flow, body temperature, hematocrit, and blood gas tensions all affect the functioning of the patient's CNS and thus the intraoperatively observed neurophysiologic measures (15).

Throughout the surgical procedures, close communication

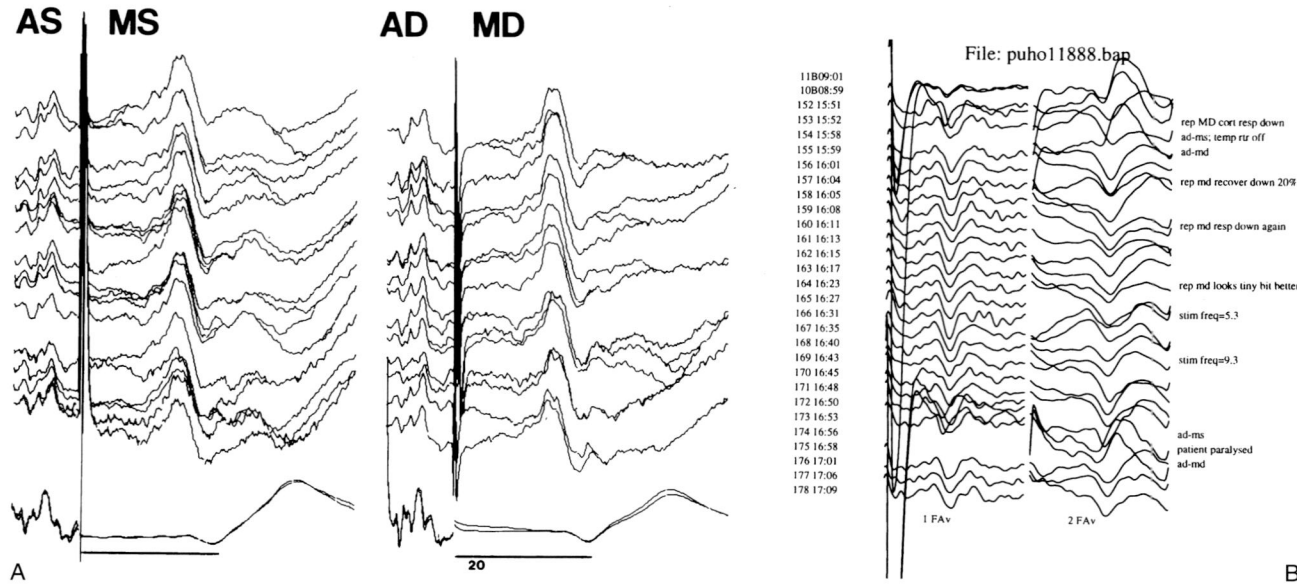

FIG. 5. Multimodality evoked potential showing **(A)** left and right (AS and AD) auditory brainstem potentials and left and right (MS and MD) median nerve potentials along with **(B)** median nerve for field and cortical potentials, all recorded simultaneously.

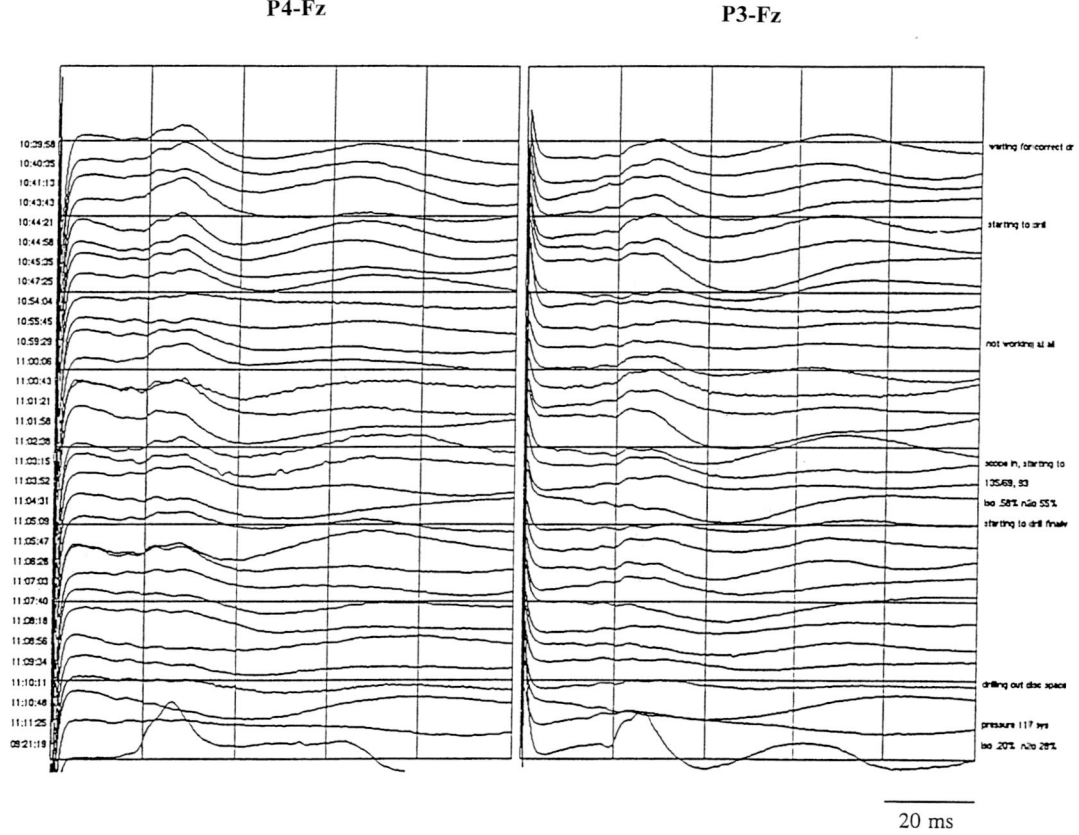

FIG. 6. Somatosensory evoked potential recordings in response to left (P_4–F_z) and right (P_3–F_z) median nerve stimulation, where P_4–F_z is over the right cortex and P_3–F_z is over the left cortex. Baseline recordings appear as the last trace at the bottom of the figure. During cervical discectomy, systolic blood pressure progressively decreases and a consequent bilateral loss in cortical amplitude is noted.

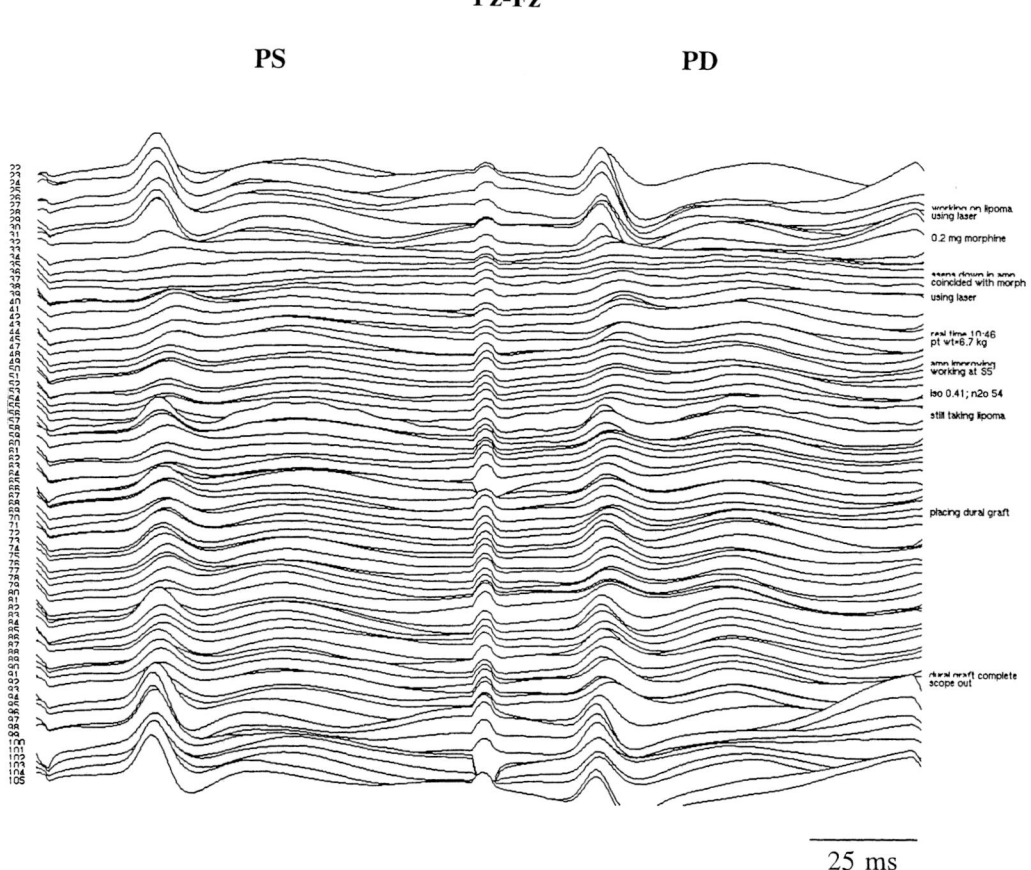

FIG. 7. Somatosensory evoked potential recordings in response to left (PS) and right (PD) peroneal nerve stimulation. Immediately after administration of a morphine bolus, responses were observed to decrease bilaterally and remain reduced for approximately 15 to 20 minutes. The bilateral loss in amplitude was not coincident with surgical manipulation, and no postoperative morbidity was observed.

is maintained with the neuroanesthesiologist regarding any changes in blood pressure, temperature, heart rate, or muscle tone, because changes in any of these variables may alter the responses (Fig. 6).

Cranial base tumor procedures are typically performed using isoflurane or a modified balanced narcotic procedure (16). However, muscle relaxants are rarely used because the monitoring of EMG activity related to cranial nerve function is a major factor in the successful outcome of these cases.

The neuroanesthesiologist typically uses constant-infusion techniques to minimize the use of inhalation agents and to maintain as constant as possible a baseline level of functioning. The neurophysiologist notes whenever a medication bolus is given in anticipation of decrements in response quality (Fig. 7).

NEUROPHYSIOLOGIC MEASURES

The neurophysiologic measures routinely used by the authors provide a functional map of much of the entire neuraxis. These include the EEG, an unstimulated measure of cortical function suitable for providing information concerning the degree of cortical activation related to either metabolic process (e.g., hypoxia) or to pharmacologic manipulation (e.g., pentobarbital-induced burst suppression to protect the patient's cortical function) (17); the MSPs and VEPs, which provide additional measures of cortical function specific to certain pathways and vasculature; the BAEPs and BSEPs, which provide information about the functioning of the brainstem, again specific to certain pathways (18); and, finally, EMGs produced by muscles innervated by the various cranial nerves, which provide information about both the cranial nerves themselves and their underlying brainstem nuclei (19).

Electroencephalogram

The functioning of the cerebral cortex is extremely sensitive to changes in arterial oxygenation and insufficient cerebral blood flow or an inadequate partial pressure of oxygen;

this sensitivity is rapidly reflected in the EEG (20). Oxidative metabolism supplies the energy for maintenance of the membrane potential of nerve cells, and because the EEG depends directly on the transmembrane potentials of neurons, it reflects disturbances of cerebral metabolism such as hypoxia. Some factors that may contribute to ischemic events in cranial base tumor patients are decreased oxygen-carrying capacity due to hypovolemia or decreased cerebral perfusion pressure due to factors associated with decreased systemic arterial pressure, increased intracranial pressure, or mechanical obstruction of cerebral vessels (21).

The major use the authors have seen in monitoring EEG during cranial base cases has been related to clamping and bypassing of the internal carotid artery in patients who have failed a preoperative blood flow study. This is usually related to the repair of a tear to the internal carotid artery that can be associated with the removal of tumor from the cavernous sinus. To control bleeding during a repair of this type, proximal and distal control of the internal artery is required, potentially reducing blood flow to the brain. Associated with this decreased availability of blood may be hypoxia caused by an inability of the remaining members of the vasculature adequately to perfuse the brain. The second most useful application of EEG monitoring in these cases has been to help define the occurrence of embolic phenomena, which again are characterized by decreased blood flow and therefore potentially an ischemic event. In both of these situations, EEG monitoring can be useful both to identify the presence of an

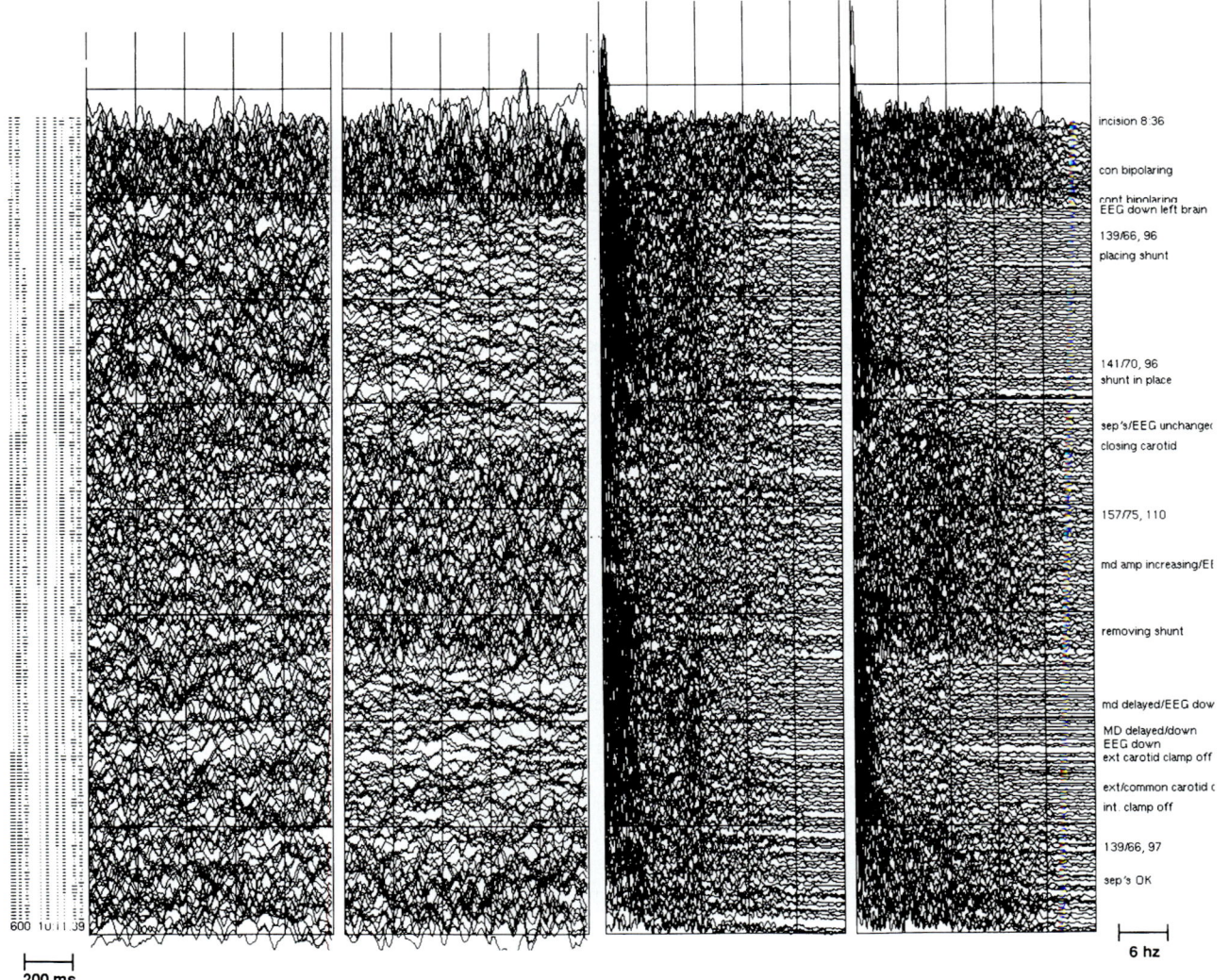

FIG. 8. Continuous two-channel electroencephalographic (EEG) recordings. **A:** Raw bihemispheric EEG recorded continuously. **B:** The same EEG displayed as a compressed spectral array (CSA).

insult and to define the degree of burst suppression if barbiturate brain protection is instituted. The EEG also may be helpful in identifying the locus of damage when compared with the data obtained from the other modalities.

The authors routinely provide at least two channels of continuous EEG monitoring during cranial base cases. This minimal configuration is thought to be adequate because the problems of concern are not related to precise focality, but rather are of global or hemispheric importance. The electrode configuration used is P_3/F_3 and P_4/F_4, which provides two parasagittal planes, one on the operative side, and the other contralateral to the operative side, providing a continuous comparative control. This electrode configuration may be simplified to P_3/F_z and P_4/F_z, if the desired frontal sites are not available. These same electrodes may also be used to obtain cortical SEPs; the dual function served permits a reduction in the number of electrodes used during the procedure. Because the authors routinely use these same electrodes to monitor the median nerve SEPs, the bandpass of the amplifiers is set to that which is appropriate for these measures; specifically, the high-pass filter is set at 1 Hz and the low-pass filter is set at 1,000 Hz. The gain is set between 10,000 and 50,000, depending on the level of cerebral activity demonstrated by the anesthetized patient.

The EEG is observed both as the ongoing, unprocessed signal and in a Fourier-transformed representation (Fig. 8). The raw EEG is observed continuously on an oscilloscope, provided on each rack, and also may be observed on the workstation screen. The oscilloscope is set to provide a 0.1 second/division sweep speed to provide a rapid visual estimate of the continuous frequency. The Fourier-transformed data may be displayed as either a compressed spectral array or as a density spectral array, depending on the preference of the neurophysiologist. In either case, both the instantaneous frequency and the spectral edge may be estimated and overlaid on the displays. Because the signals on which the spectra are being computed have significantly higher frequency content than that normally of interest in the EEG, the spectral coefficients above an arbitrary value, typically 30 Hz, may be suppressed. Figure 8A presents an example of the EEG obtained before and during clamping of the internal carotid artery, whereas Fig. 8B shows the compressed spectral array computed on the same data. Note the preservation of EEG on the nonclamped side and the loss of amplitude and shift to the delta range on the clamped side.

The typical pattern seen in these measures during cerebral hypoperfusion is a reduction or loss in high-frequency activity and the appearance of large amplitude slow waves in the

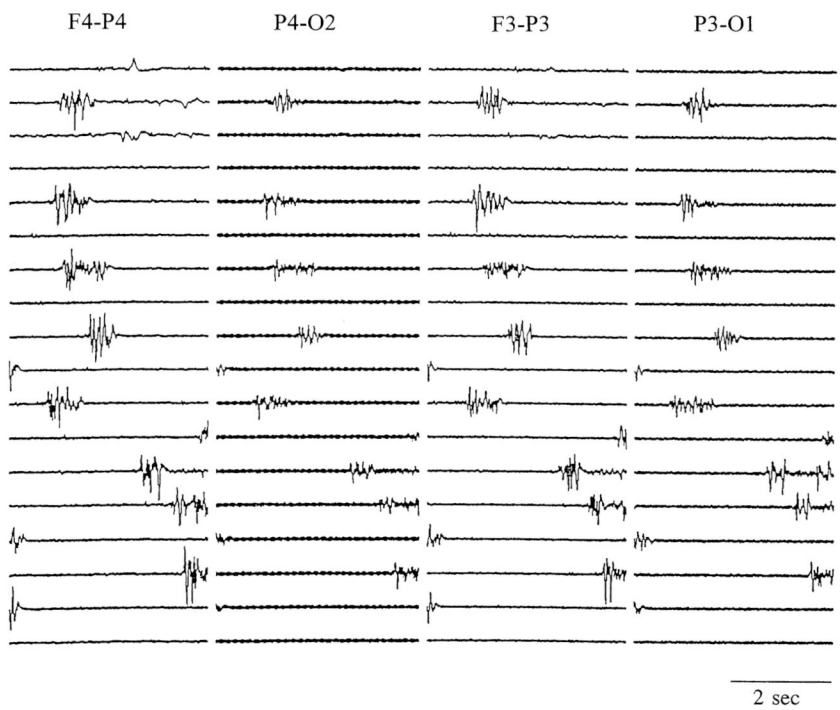

FIG. 9. Continuous four-channel bihemispheric electroencephalographic recordings. In this example, a continuous barbiturate infusion resulted in approximately 80% burst suppression in the patient.

delta range (1–4 Hz). The authors have even seen decreases in cerebral blood flow produced by radiographically verified cerebral emboli. The EEG appearances of any ischemic or hypoxic events are similar, and differentiation between the various putative causative factors is made by being particularly attentive to the clinical situation; for example, blood pressure, electrocardiography, oxygen saturation, administered drugs, and surgical manipulations may all have an observable effect. Other concurrent factors that may alter the EEG are changes in depth of anesthesia, temperature changes, and changes in CO_2 content. These factors may be recognized by their relatively slow onset, lasting for several minutes, in contrast to the changes of ischemia, which usually occur within seconds. One must keep in mind that there are situations where the EEG may be acutely depressed on injection of an anesthetic that rapidly passes the blood–brain barrier. Such situations may be found in high-dose opioid anesthesia, where fentanyl induces an immediate and marked reduction of fast-frequency activity in the EEG, with an increase in low-frequency, high-amplitude activity in the delta range (21).

The EEG may be used to titrate the level of burst suppression, as shown in Fig. 9. Note the waxing and waning of the bursts as produced by barbiturates typically administered by bolus. While titrating the level of burst suppression, the authors routinely turn off the spectral analysis and use only the raw EEG.

A simple, but useful summary of possible changes is that decreased frequency with increased amplitude (22) implies an ischemic event to the cortex. Widespread frequency slowing and decreased amplitude usually implies brainstem ischemia (23), whereas ischemic events affecting the thalamus and the internal capsule produce unremarkable changes in the EEG (22) but can produce significant changes in SEPs.

Somatosensory System

Median nerve SEPs are used to aid in determining the functional integrity of the somatosensory cortex and the ascending somatosensory system, primarily in the region of the brainstem and forebrain. These potentials are useful both in preventing or reducing surgical morbidity during procedures that pose potential harm to the upper cervical cord and in assessing the level of hypoxia in cortical tissue (24).

Stimulation of the median nerve elicits a series of potentials that ascend from the stimulus site to the somatosensory cortex (Fig. 10). Typically, the most peripheral recording site is Erb's point, which is above the clavicle, lateral to the insertion of the sternocleidomastoid muscle. A negative potential with a latency of 9 to 10 msec can be recorded at Erb's point and is probably generated by the branches of the brachial plexus. An electrode at cervical C_7 records a complex wave at 11 to 14 msec that consists of a small negative peak at 11 msec, a larger negative peak at 12 to 13 msec, and a positive peak at approximately 14 msec. The N_{11}, $N_{12/13}$, and P_{14} peaks are probably generated at the dorsal root entry

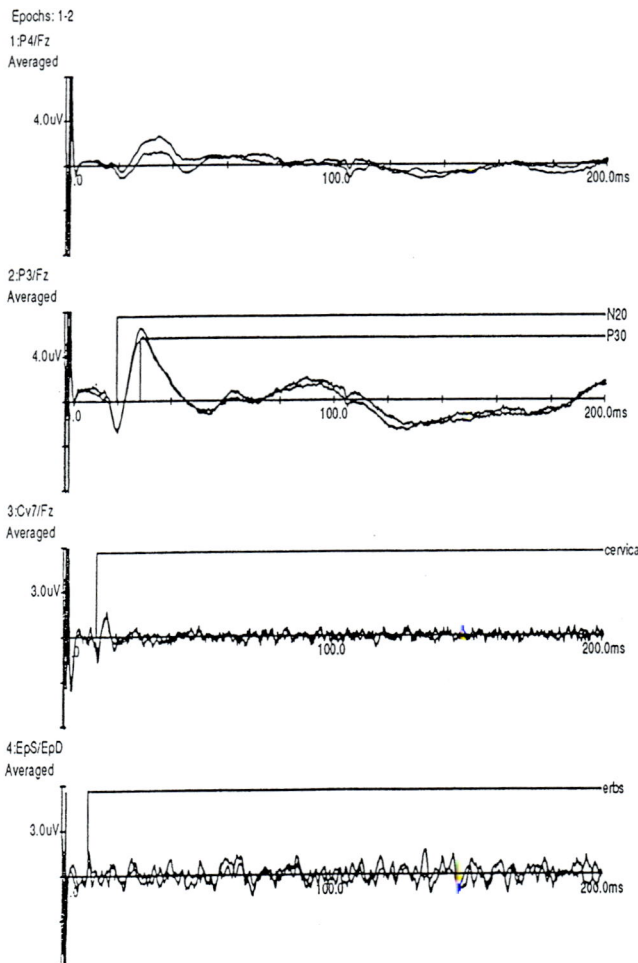

FIG. 10. Multiple-site somatosensory evoked potential recordings in response to median nerve stimulation. Responses are recorded from both somatosensory cortices (C_1 and C_2), the brainstem (C_3), and the brachial plexus (C_4) simultaneously. A characteristic N_{20}/P_{30} complex is recorded from the cortical channels bilaterally.

of the cervical spinal cord (N_{11}), the uppermost region of cervical spinal cord ($N_{12/13}$), and in the medial lemniscus of the brainstem (P_{14}) (25). Two negative peaks at 18 and 20 msec are easily seen at P_3 and P_4 parietal recording sites. These two negative peaks may appear as one negative complex in the operating room. The N_{20} wave is generated in the primary somatosensory cortex along the posterior bank of the central fissure (26). At longer latencies (approximately 25–100 msec), additional positive (P_{30}) and negative peaks are seen. These waves are generated by secondary somatosensory areas in the parietal lobe, and by cortical association areas (27). The authors normally monitor the P_{14} (medial lemniscal activity) and the cortical N_{20} activity to assess conduction and P_{30} to assess cortical perfusion.

The recording and stimulating electrodes are applied after the patient's intubation, but before final positioning. The stimulating electrodes are needle electrodes and are applied subdermally, above the median nerve at the wrist, with the leads firmly taped to the patient's extremities to secure them during positioning. After final positioning, a forehead ground electrode and P_3, P_4, F_3, and F_4 recording electrodes are applied in their optimal positions, if possible. The P_3 and P_4 recording electrodes should be placed 2 cm posterior and 7 cm lateral to C_z on the left (P_3) and right (P_4) scalp, respectively. The F_3 and F_4 recording electrodes are placed 3 cm anterior and 7 cm lateral to C_z. Again, these positions are optimal; however, many times the planned incision does not allow these positions to be used. In those cases, the authors attempt to place the electrodes as close as possible to recording sites. In some cases, these electrodes are placed using sterile technique by the surgeon, in the operative field, after the incision is completed.

The stimulus intensity is usually preset at 30 V and adjusted as necessary to maximize the response, while producing minimal patient movement. If right and left median nerve responses are being observed concurrently, then the two stimuli are separated by 100 msec and a pulse width of 100 microseconds is used.

Ideally, baseline responses are obtained individually for each recording condition, before the draping of the patient, to alleviate any technical difficulties before the beginning of surgery. If MSPs are acquired by themselves, usually 128 stimuli are used to elicit each averaged response; however, on some patients stable responses are seen with numbers of stimuli as low as 32. A stimulus rate of 3.43 typically is used. These data are compared with the preoperative evaluation and used as baseline data throughout the case.

The N_{20} and P_{30} waves are sensitive to certain types of anesthetics. Barbiturates and inhalation anesthetics (e.g., isoflurane, ethrane, and halothane) markedly decrease the amplitude of the cortically generated activity, including N_{20}, in a dose-dependent, but individualized manner (Fig. 11). Of the inhalation anesthetics, isoflurane produces the weakest effects on cortical activity. Thus, in those cases in which a balanced narcotic technique may not be used because of the need to measure EMG activity, isoflurane is used as the anesthetic. Balanced anesthetic (a combination of nitrous oxide, a muscle relaxant, and a minor tranquilizer) is a much preferred method for recording MSPs by themselves. In cases in which isoflurane is used to supplement another form of anesthesia, a concentration of under 0.4% end tidal produces minimal effects on the cortical somatosensory activity in adults; however, these effects are very individualized, and even low levels of inhalation agents may reduce the amplitudes of cortically generated activity in some patients (28).

Temperature changes significantly influence the SEP latency. For each degree Celsius of local cooling, the nerve conduction velocity decreases by about 2.5 m/second. During long operations of this type, a drop in temperature around the nerve being stimulated or in the brain tissue itself can result in a progressive increase in N_{20} latency that is unrelated to

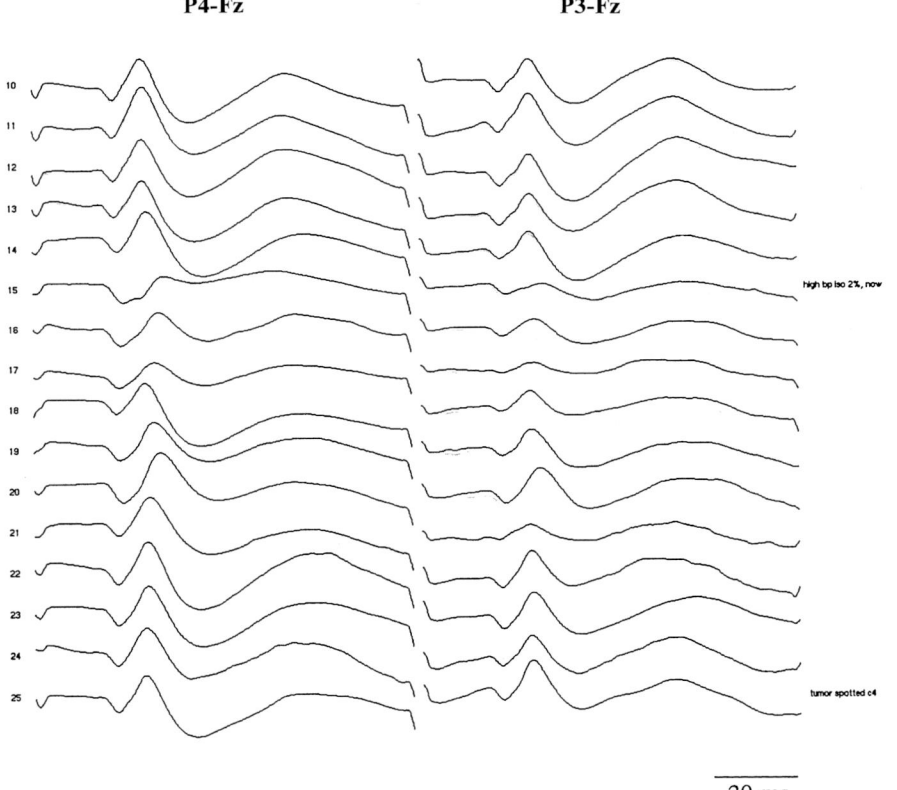

FIG. 11. Somatosensory evoked potential recordings in response to left (P_4–F_z) and right (P_3–F_z) median nerve stimulation. During cervical tumor exposure, isoflurane is increased to 2.0%. Note that just after increasing isoflurane, a significant bilateral reduction in cortical amplitude is observed. On reduction of isoflurane, responses returned to baseline amplitudes.

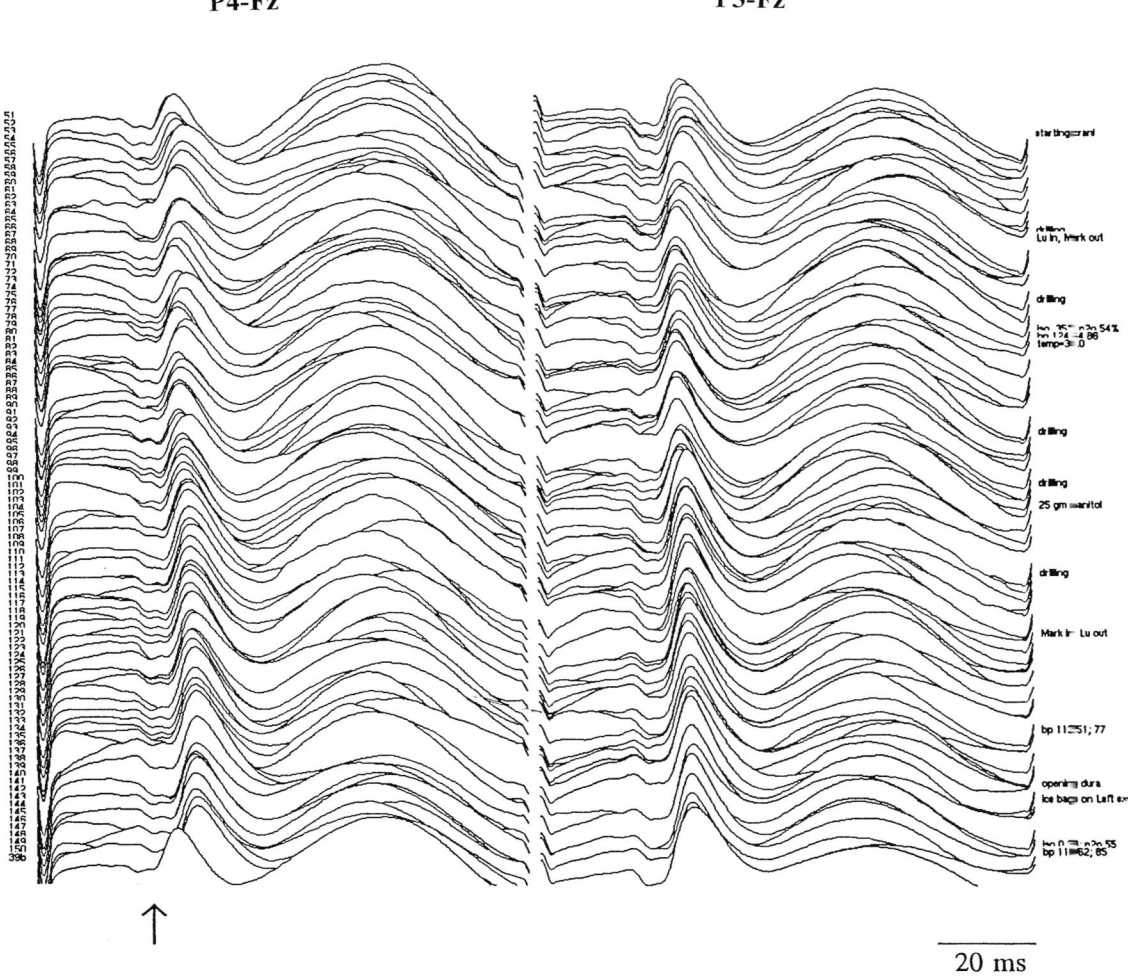

FIG. 12. Somatosensory evoked potential recordings in response to left (P_4–F_z) and right (P_3–F_z) median nerve stimulation. Baseline potentials are displayed as the last trace at the bottom of the figure. In an attempt to cool this patient, ice bags were placed on the left (exposed) brachial plexus during intracranial aneurysm surgery. Note with the passage of time the trace in response to left median nerve stimulation becomes increasingly delayed (*arrow*), while the contralateral response remains on baseline.

surgical manipulation (Fig. 12). Latencies also may be transiently affected when the surgeon irrigates with physiologic saline at cooler temperatures; thus, it is recommended that warm saline be used for irrigation. These potentially confounding effects reinforce the usefulness of bilateral recordings to delineate surgically induced changes, which should be observed on the operative side, versus global changes in temperature, which should cause a bilateral change.

For the cortical responses, the amplitude and latency of the N_{20}/P_{30} complex are of primary concern. In general, a decrease of more than 50% in amplitude or an increase of more than 10% in latency is considered to be significant and communicated to the surgeon. Another response is taken as soon as possible to confirm the stability of the change. The neurophysiologist consults with the anesthesiologist to determine if a change in blood pressure, level of anesthesia, or type of anesthesia could have contributed to the observed changes in the amplitude or latency of the evoked potential. In the case when the potentials are completely lost, the neurophysiologist immediately reports the loss and then checks to ensure that all electrodes and their connections are intact.

Significant changes compared with preoperative studies may be seen in MSPs related to patient positioning (Fig. 13). These changes should be corrected for by repositioning the patient before the beginning of surgery because they may reflect pressure being placed on the brachial plexus, brainstem, or spinal cord as a result of improper positioning of the patient.

Significant changes in the MSPs also may be noted due to emboli lodging, for example, in the mouth of the middle

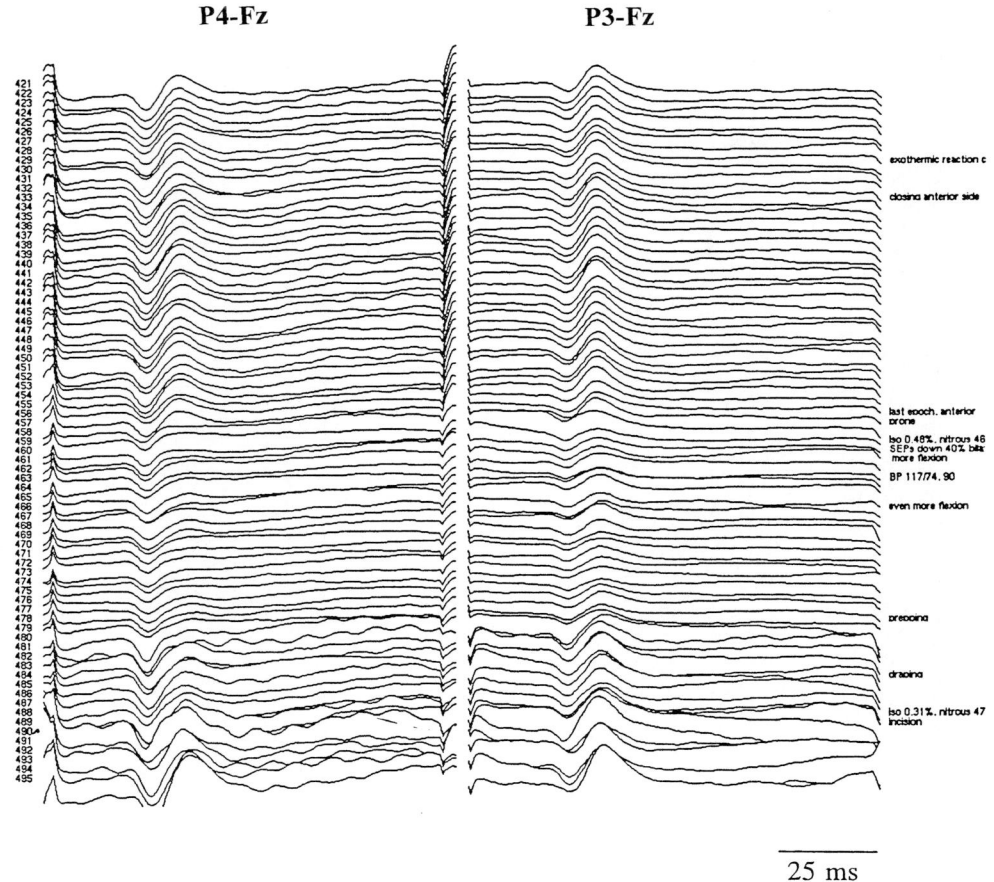

FIG. 13. Somatosensory evoked potential recordings in response to left (P_4–F_z) and right (P_3–F_z) median nerve stimulation. During positioning (minimal extension) of the neck, responses were observed to decrease bilaterally significantly. When the neck was subsequently flexed, responses slowly returned to baseline.

cerebral artery (Fig. 14). These changes are usually reflected in deterioration on the P_{30} amplitude, as seen in Fig. 15, and may be corrected through intraoperative lysis of the clot (29).

As mentioned previously, the authors routinely record simultaneous EEGs and MSPs, and many times these measures will change together (see Fig. 15). However, the authors have also observed many instances in which one has changed and not the other. A significant change in either modality must be treated with respect.

The authors also have found it useful to record the P_{14} BSEPs, using the same vertex-to-mastoid electrodes used to obtain the BAEPs. This allows the BSEPs to be recorded simultaneously with the BAEPs, and the cortical SEPs (MSPs). The somatosensory short-latency potentials behave similarly to those from the auditory system and are unaffected by most anesthetic manipulation.

The BSEPs are useful in providing another wave generated in the brainstem, and the authors have seen changes in the BSEPs and not the BAEPs, and conversely in the BAEPs and not the BSEPs. In addition, changes in the cortical SEPs and not the BSEPs provide additional localizing information.

Auditory System

Monitoring the function of cranial nerve VIII is useful in preserving hearing and the functional integrity of nerve VIII and of the brainstem.

The classic BAEP consists of a minimum of five and a maximum of seven peaks (Fig. 16). The first five peaks, Jewett waves I through V, are the principal peaks used in clinical practice, and waves I, III, and V are the principal waves used in operative monitoring. All occur with 10 msec of a brief click or tone presentation. Wave I is generated in the auditory portion of cranial nerve VIII. Its latency is approximately 1.5 to 2.1 msec in a normal adult. Wave I is present

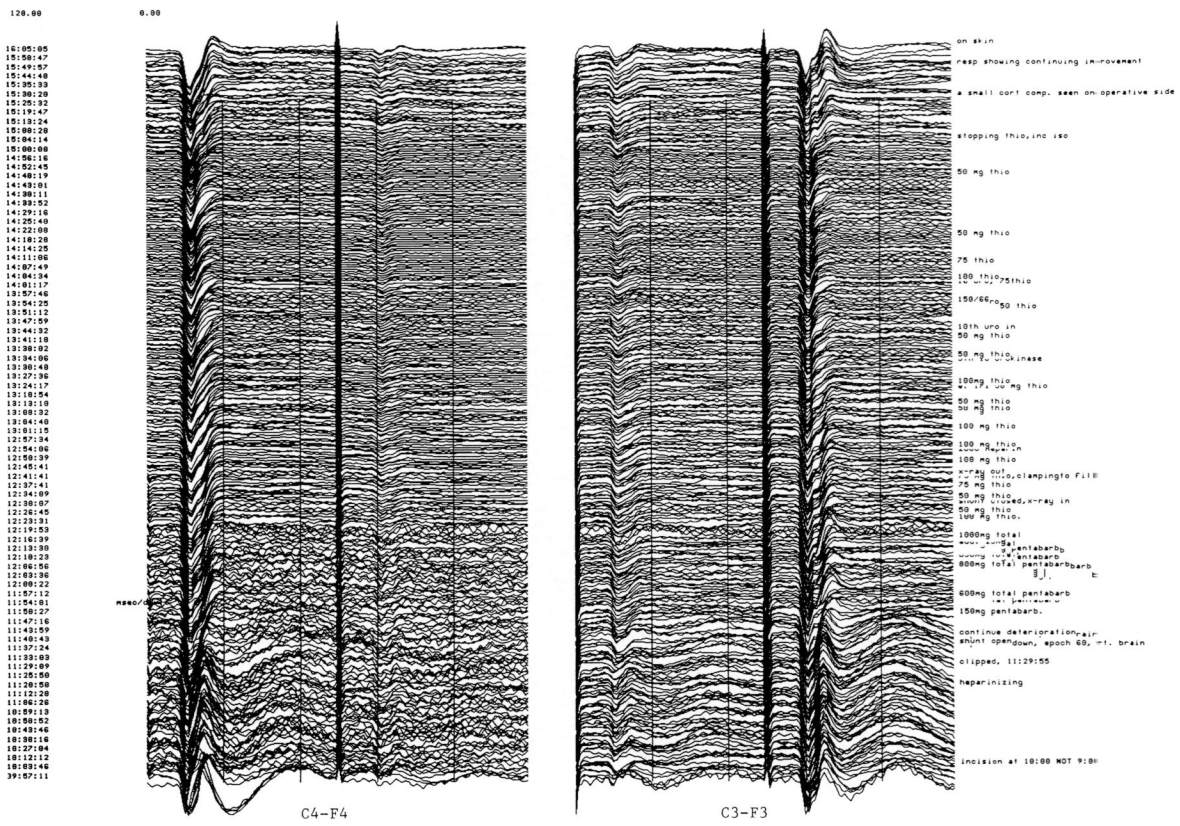

FIG. 14. Bilateral median nerve evoked potentials obtained simultaneously from C_4/F_4 and C_3/F_3 to left and right median nerve stimulator. An embolus was thrown to the right middle cerebral artery. The P_{30} wave immediately changed. The patient was placed in barbiturate coma, the physiologic situation was then confirmed by intraoperative angiography, and the embolus dissolved with urokinase. The evoked potentials returned to baseline and the patient awoke without deficit.

on the ipsilateral side to the stimulus but is not usually seen on the contralateral side. Wave II is generated bilaterally at or near the cochlear nucleus. The latency between waves I and II is approximately 0.8 to 1.0 msec. The amplitude of wave II on the contralateral side may be greater than on the ipsilateral side. Wave III is generated bilaterally from the lower pons near the superior olive and trapezoid body. The latency between waves I and III is approximately 2.0 to 2.3 msec in a normal adult. Wave III may be smaller on the contralateral side than on the ipsilateral side. Waves IV and V are probably generated in the upper pons or lower midbrain, near the lateral lemniscus or possibly near the inferior colliculus (30). In ipsilateral recordings, waves IV and V may fuse into a complex that can vary between two identifiable components with a common base to a single wave with a tall, wide peak. On the contralateral side, the peaks tend to be more easily identified. Wave V tends to be the most robust peak and is typically the last to disappear when stimulus intensity is reduced. In addition, there tends to be a large negative-going wave after wave V, which aids the neurophysiologist in identifying wave V.

The BAEP is stimulated using one of several techniques, depending on the surgical procedure involved and, thus, whether the auricle is retracted and other considerations. Most often, the authors use miniature, open-air, high-fidelity earphones (i.e., those commonly used with personal tape players or radios) that rest in the concha of the ear. The earphones, along with the recording electrodes, are applied after the patient's intubation, before final positioning of the patient. After verifying that the earphones are working, they are securely taped in the ears with transparent tape so that they may remain visible. At the same time, the taping must be adequate to prevent fluids from getting to the earphones and into the ear canal, which might cause device failure or a conductive hearing loss, respectively. After final patient positioning, the vertex (C_z) and ear recording electrodes are placed. The contralateral ear electrode is placed over the mastoid (M_n) and the electrode for the operative side is

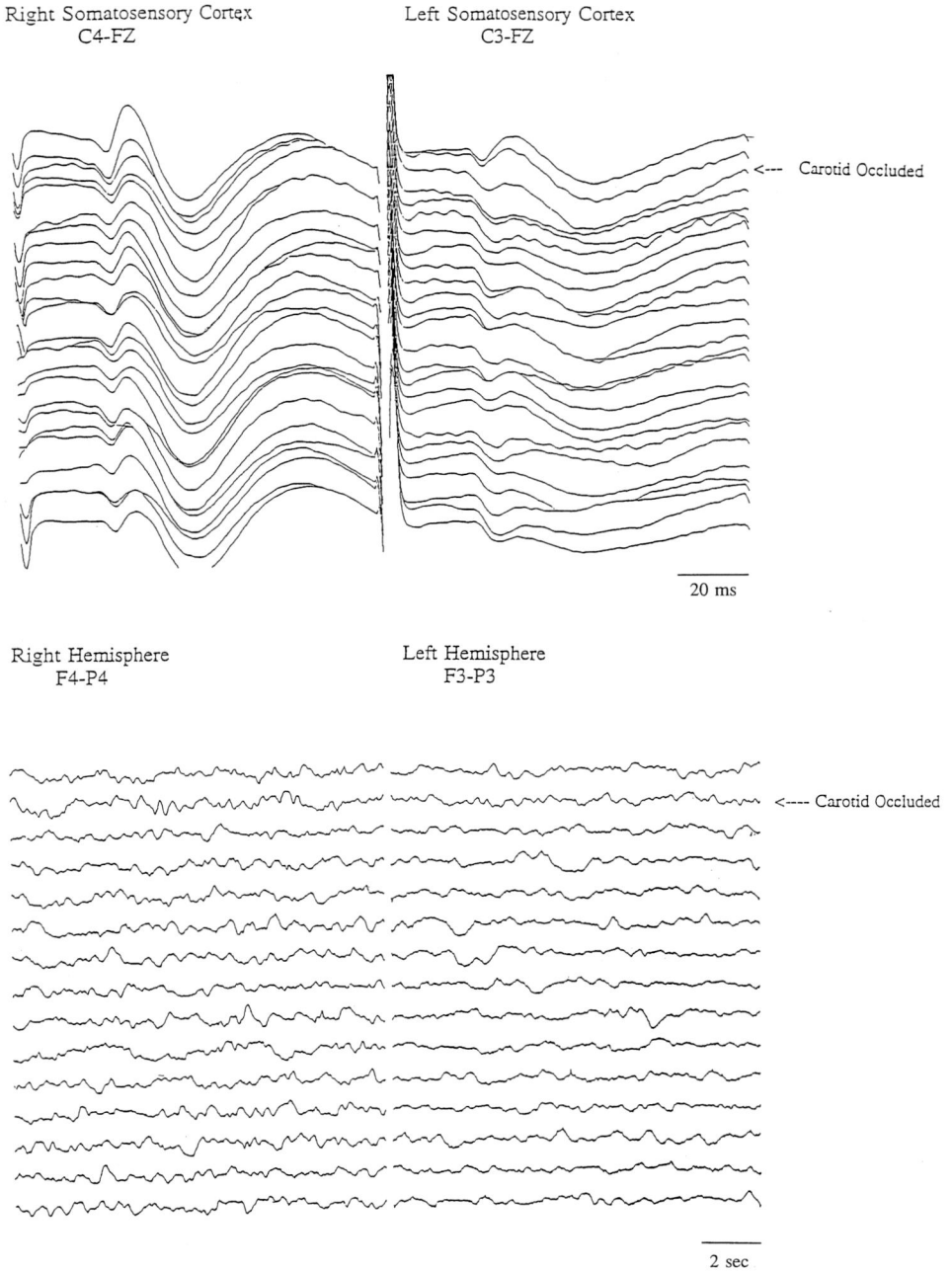

FIG. 15. Simultaneous somatosensory evoked potential (SEP) and electroencephalographic (EEG) recordings during a left carotid endarterectomy. Note that a significant decrease in cortical amplitude of the SEP recordings and a slowing and decrease in amplitude of EEG occur with occlusion of the internal carotid artery on the operative side.

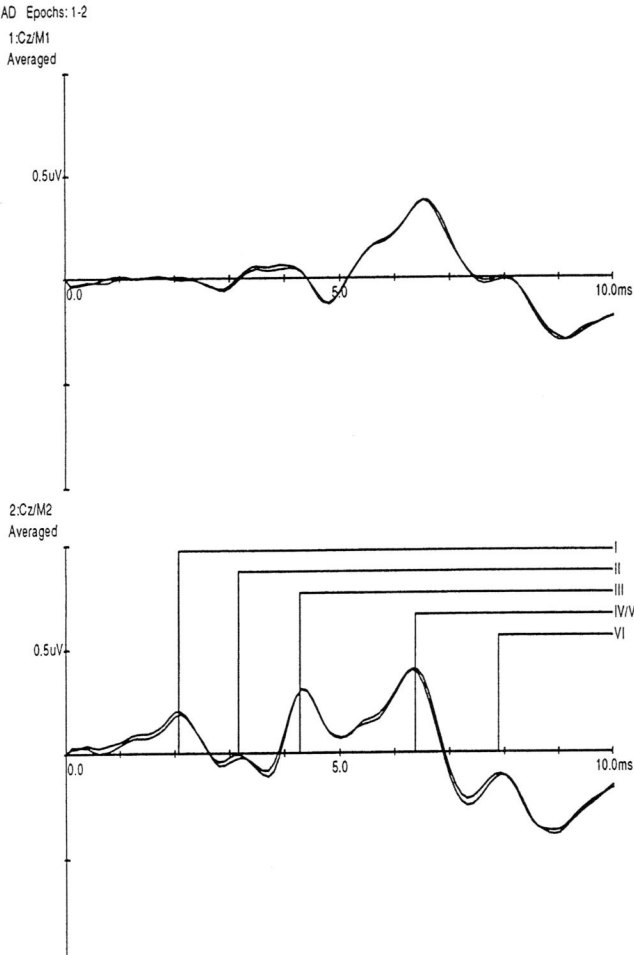

FIG. 16. Brainstem auditory evoked potentials recorded in response to click stimulation of the right ear (AD). Note that responses are recorded bilaterally and that a characteristic wave I, II, III and IV/V complex is recorded from the right side.

placed in the pinna of the earlobe (A_m). In some cases, it is not possible to place a nonsterile ipsilateral stimulating earphone and recording electrode because of the planned surgical incision. In such cases, the authors have placed sterile stimulating earphones or, in some situations, have monitored only the contralateral responses, which still provides valuable information concerning the status of the brainstem.

For a wide variety of cranial base tumors monitored, the intensity level of the click is set to approximately 70 dB nHL. However, when the patient is known to have a hearing loss, or a given patient's responses are not well defined, higher-intensity levels may be required. In such cases, an intensity level of 85 dB nHL is typical. Rarefaction and compression clicks are applied in an alternating fashion to minimize the apparent stimulus artifact. The stimulus rate is usually set between 9.3 and 19.3 Hz because of the well-known effects of higher stimulus rates on response latencies

(31). The interstimulus intervals may be randomized to minimize contamination with phase-locked or quasiperiodic noise.

Baseline responses for each ear are acquired before the beginning of surgery. Usually, 1,024 stimulus presentations are used for the baseline data; however, the number of stimuli may be adjusted to as few as 256 depending on the quality of the responses. These data are compared with the preoperative evaluation and used as baselines throughout the case.

Waves I to V are relatively resistant to sedative medication and general anesthetics. Thus these responses place no constraints on the anesthesiologist. However, they are sensitive to temperature changes, with absolute and interpeak latencies increasing by approximately 0.20 msec/1°C.

The latency of wave V is the primary concern in intraoperative monitoring of the BAEPs, because this is the most robust and easily identifiable of the waves in this response. In general, any repeatable or systematic change in the latency of wave V that exceeds 0.3 msec is reported to the surgeon. However, clear changes in the morphology, even with latency shifts less than 0.3 msec, are noted. The next sample is taken as soon as possible to confirm the stability of the change. In the case that the potentials are completely lost, the neurophysiologist reports the loss and then immediately checks to ensure that both the stimulating system and the recording electrodes are intact.

The BAEPs are affected by retraction on the cerebellum, retraction on the frontal poles, and decreases in blood pressure. Figure 17 illustrates clear changes in both the latency and amplitude of wave V related to retraction on the cerebellum. Usually only minor amplitude changes occur if the latency increase is less than 0.5 msec; however, with latency changes on the order of 1 msec, the amplitude of wave V usually decreases by at least 50%. In this case, wave V disappeared entirely when the increase in latency was greater than 1 msec. However, with removal of the retractor, the wave began to return and had returned in its entirety by the end of the case.

Direct recording of compound action potentials (CAPs) from cranial nerve VIII is also useful both for distinguishing between the vestibular and cochlear portions of the nerve and for reducing the likelihood of injury to the nerve (32). This is easily done during the removal of acoustic neuromas, where the CAPs can be recorded by placing a wick electrode on the exposed nerve. The CAPs may be recorded using the same parameters as the BAEPs; however, there is no need to average the responses.

Visual System

Visual evoked potentials are used to aid in determining the functional integrity of the visual system, primarily in the region of the optic nerves, optic chiasm, and optic radiations. The recorded activity is generated either at the retina (electroretinogram; Fig. 18) or at the cortex.

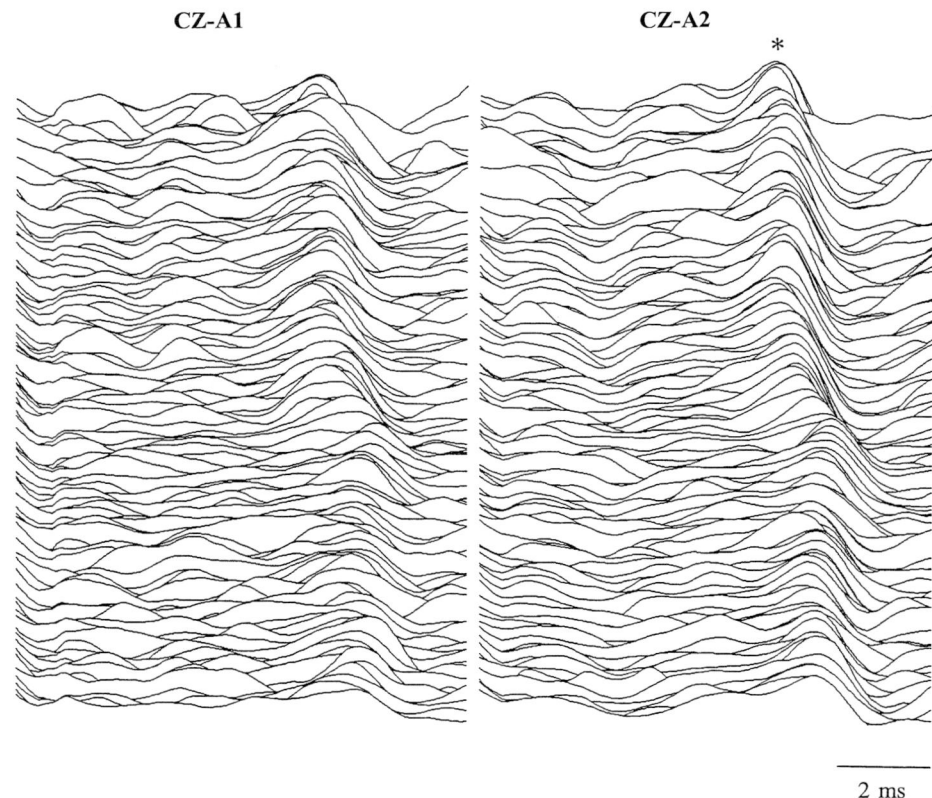

FIG. 17. Brainstem auditory evoked potentials recorded in response to click stimulation of the right ear (C_z–A_2). With retraction of the right cerebellar hemisphere, wave V (*asterisk*) is observed to increase significantly in latency with some decrease in amplitude. A latency shift and subsequent loss of wave V has been shown to be predictive of postoperative hearing deficits.

Stimulation of the visual system using a bright flash is not recommended for diagnostic purposes because of intersubject variability (33), except in selected situations; however, in the operating room, this is a very helpful and effective technique. Four waves are typically seen in the VEP: P_{60}, which is thought to be generated in subcortical structures; and N_{70}, P_{100}, and N_{120}, which are all thought to be generated in the primary visual cortex (34).

For intraoperative stimulation of the visual system, the authors use a fiberoptics system that is positioned directly under the eye, but not on the globe, and securely taped in place. This fiberoptics system was developed to allow VEPs to be obtained when a full bifrontal flap was used. The fiberoptic cables were designed to be mounted on the flash stimulator driven by a Grass photic stimulator (P22), and this stimulator is then set at maximum intensity. Recording electrodes are placed at O_1 and O_2, both referenced to C_z.

The stimulus rate used for the visual data is 1.3 Hz and the observation window is 200 msec. A bandwidth of 1 to 100 Hz and a gain of 20,000 are used. Baseline responses are obtained individually for each recording condition during the surgical preparation period so that any technical difficulties can be alleviated before the beginning of surgery. If the VEPs are acquired by themselves, usually 128 stimuli are used to elicit each averaged potential. These data are compared with the preoperative data and used as baseline data throughout the case (Fig. 19)

Electromyographic Evaluation of Cranial Nerve Function

Cranial nerve function is monitored continuously during skull base surgery for two reasons: first, to establish the location and orientation of the cranial nerves in the operative field; and second, to preserve functioning in the cranial nerves and their related brainstem nuclei (35).

The major observed variables are the EMGs from the appropriate muscle group innervated by the cranial nerves of interest. The cranial nerves, along with the associated muscle groups, that are usually monitored using EMG techniques are the facial nerve (VII), and the orbicularis oculi, oricularis oris, and the mentalis muscles innervated by the zygomatic branch, the buccal branch, and the mandibular branch, respectively; the abducens nerve (VI) and the lateral

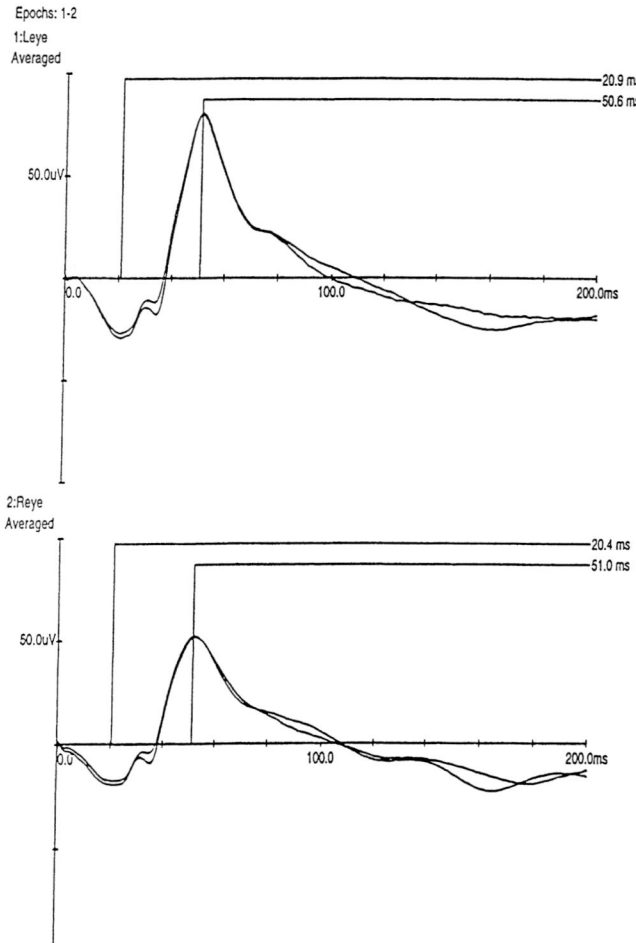

FIG. 18. Electroretinogram in response to left eye (C₁) and right eye (C₂) stimulation. Characteristic negative (~20 msec) and positive (~50 msec) waves are recorded from both channels using contact electrodes positioned on the cornea.

rectus muscle; the trigeminal nerve (V) and the masseter muscle; the trochlear nerve (IV) and the superior oblique muscle; and the oculomotor nerve (III) and the medial and inferior rectus and inferior oblique muscles of the eye. When appropriate, the functioning of the glossopharyngeal (IX), vagus (X), spinal accessory (XI), and hypoglossal (XII) nerves are monitored by placing electrodes in the stylopharyngeus, the cricothyroid, the trapezius, and the intrinsic muscles of the tongue, respectively. In general, the cranial nerves ipsilateral to the operative side are monitored; however, when appropriate, bilateral activity is monitored.

Three different types of electrodes are used to record the EMGs. These are fine-wire electrodes, which have the highest impedance and the narrowest field of view; subdermal needles, which have an intermediate impedance and a larger field of view; and disk surface electrodes, which have the lowest impedance and the largest field of view (by field of view is meant the integrated level of electrical activity). The authors' recording techniques are essentially the same for all cranial nerves and all muscle groups. Subdermal platinum needle electrodes are used in bipolar recording configurations; that is, all recordings are done between a pair of electrodes inserted into the same muscle group. There is one exception to the bipolar recording technique in which the authors occasionally record transfacially between the orbicularis oculi and the mentalis muscles to reduce the number of channels allocated to monitoring cranial nerve VII. Bipolar recordings are used to minimize confusion regarding which cranial nerve or branch of a cranial nerve is producing the observed EMG. The electrodes are normally placed before the start of the procedure; however, occasionally electrodes are placed in a sterile field by the surgeons. The EMG electrodes are held in place with tape and benzoin. The authors favor the needle electrodes over the fine-wire and disk electrodes because of the signal characteristics they provide and their ease of application and maintenance.

The amplifier bandpass is set from 10 to 1,000 Hz, and a gain of 5,000 to 20,000 is routinely used. Unstimulated EMG activity from up to eight channels is monitored continuously throughout the case. This ongoing activity is continuously monitored on an oscilloscope, and any episode of interesting activity may be saved into a computer file.

Most important, the sound from all channels of activity is monitored continuously. The authors' system has the capability to amplify the activity on eight channels simultaneously and drive an audio system with this amplified signal. This system has gauges that measure the relative amounts of activity on each channel, allowing the channel with the most activity to be isolated and listened to by itself, if so desired. In addition, the system has circuits capable of suppressing the artifactual sounds related to bipolaring and stimulating. The importance of the audio system in identifying the level of activity in the muscle groups cannot be overstressed. These signals are listened to continuously for evaluation of nerve function both by the neurophysiologists and by the surgeons.

Four categories of EMG activity are observed: (a) no activity, which in an intact nerve is the best situation, but which also may be the case when a nerve has been sharply dissected; (b) irritation activity, which sounds like soft, intermittent flutter and is consistent with working near the nerve; (c) injury activity, which sound like a continuous, nonaccelerating tapping and which can be an indicator of permanent injury to the cranial nerve; and (d) a "killed-end" response, which sounds like an accelerating firing pattern and is an unequivocal indicator of nerve injury (36) (Fig. 20). It is important to note that a sharply cut nerve may produce only a brief burst of activity, and thus monitoring cannot be expected to replace extreme caution when working near the cranial nerves.

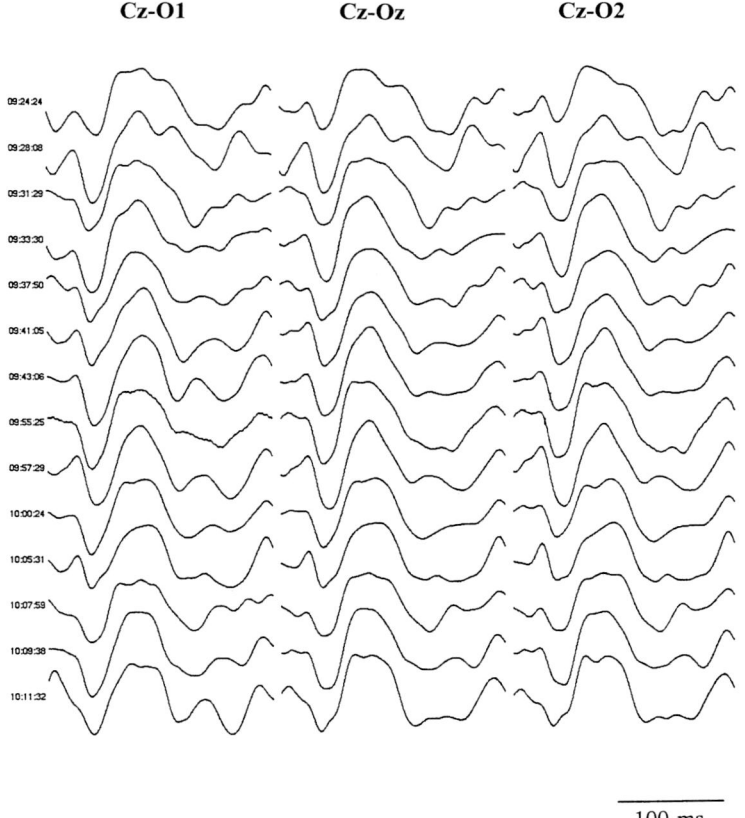

FIG. 19. Visual evoked potentials in response to flash stimulation of the right eye during suprasellar tumor resection. Responses are recorded simultaneously from three channels encompassing the left, midline, and right visual cortices. A characteristic negative/positive complex can be observed on all channels.

Besides these signals of interest, various electrical artifacts must be identified and ignored. These include high-frequency electrode pops, activity related to electrode manipulation, static from surgical instruments, and activity produced by irrigation.

In addition to monitoring the ongoing EMG activity related to the various cranial nerves, the cranial nerves also may be electrically stimulated. This usually is done to determine the location of the nerve in the operative field because many times the nerve is enveloped by tumor and may not be directly observable, or to determine the functional integrity of the nerve (37). The most common example of this procedure is the direct stimulation of cranial nerve VII (Fig. 21). The authors use Grass S44 or S88 stimulators to control the stimulus rate, pulse duration, stimulus intensity, and switching of the sound system. A stimulus isolation transformer is used to drive a monopolar stimulating electrode. The stimulating electrode is a low-impedance ($\leq$ 1,000 ohms) electrode, with the shaft insulated to, but not including, the tip. These devices are capable of producing currents as high a 15 mA, requiring care in their use. The return path for the stimulating current is provided by a metal electrode inserted into the adjacent muscle mass. The stimulus used is a constant voltage, with a pulse frequency of 10 Hz, and a pulse width of 100 microseconds. The voltage amplitude is typically varied between 0.1 and 1 V. In some situation in which very precise localization of the nerve is required, bipolar stimulating electrodes are used. However, most of the time the stimulating effort is directed toward determining if the nerve is located near to where the surgeon is currently working.

When cranial nerve VII is stimulated, activity on all three branches usually is observed on the oscilloscope. The parameters typically measured for the stimulated cranial nerve VII EMGs are the voltage threshold required to produce the evoked response of 0.3 to 0.5 V, the latency to onset of 8 to 10 msec, and a peak-to-peak voltage of 1.0 to 2.0 mV (38) (Fig. 22). These threshold parameters are measured at the beginning and end of the case, and whenever appropriate during the case. It is also important to distinguish between proximal and distal stimulation of the cranial nerve. Excellent thresholds voltages ($\leq$ 0.3 V) obtained distally on a cranial nerve are not predictive of excellent nerve function after surgery, whereas the same results obtained by stimulating the nerve proximally usually are.

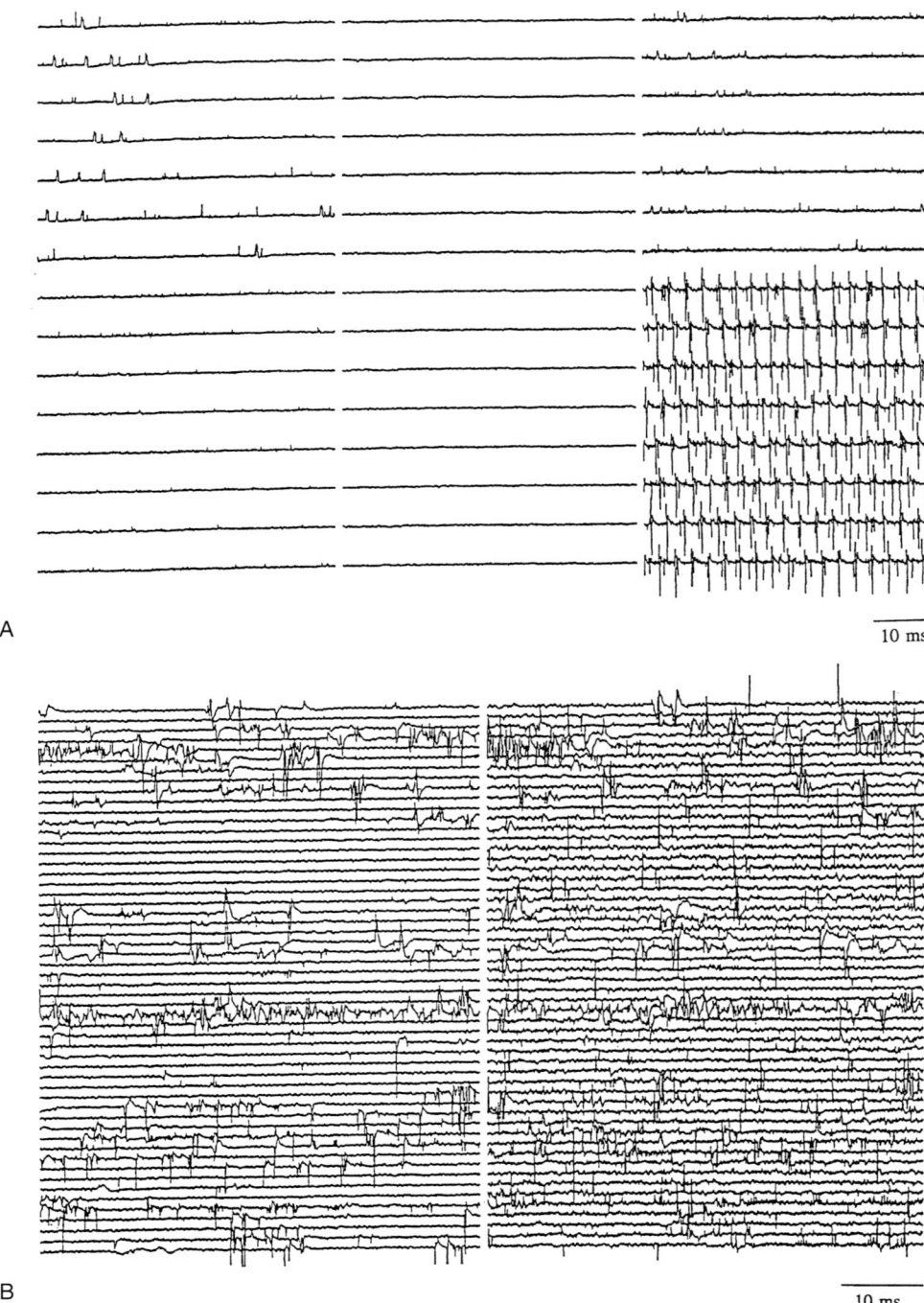

FIG. 20. Spontaneous intraoperative electromyographic (EMG) activity recorded from three branches of cranial nerve VII **(A)** and the cranial nerves III (*left*) and IV (*right*) **(B)** during posterior fossa tumor resection. In **(A)**, spontaneous sustained trains of EMG activity are recorded from the mentalis branch of cranial nerve VII. In **(B)**, spontaneous burst activity is observed from both cranial nerves III and IV.

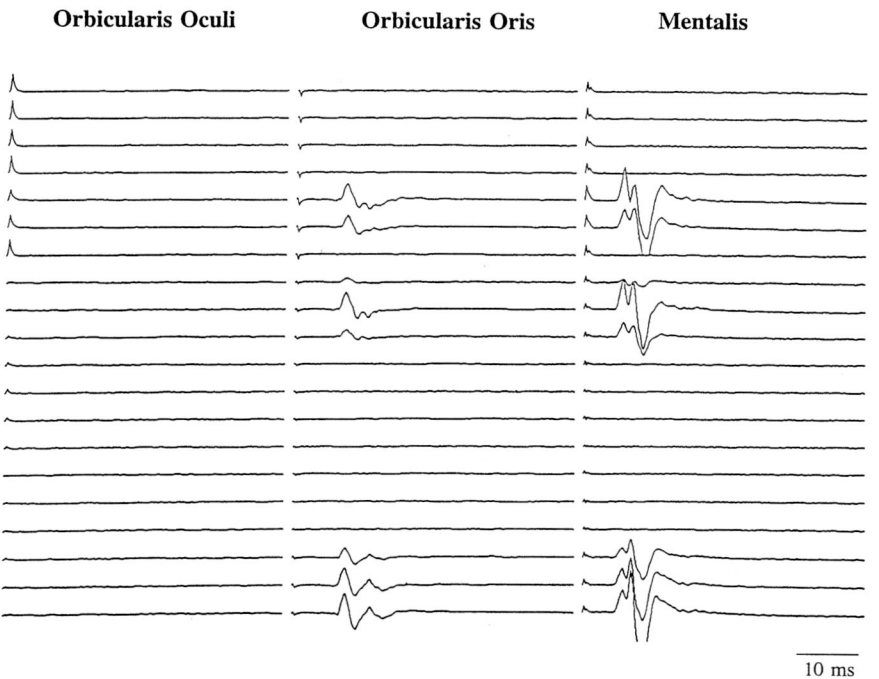

FIG. 21. Evoked intraoperative electromyographic (EMG) activity recorded from three branches of cranial nerve VII during removal of an acoustic neuroma. A monopolar stimulating electrode is used to evoke EMG activity. Stimulation is attained by placing the stimulator directly on cranial nerve VII.

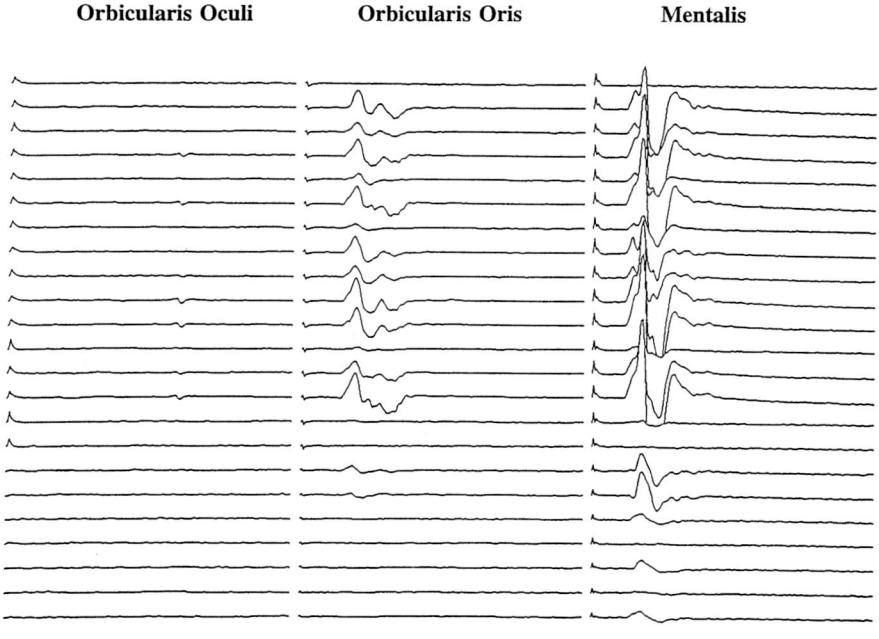

FIG. 22. Evoked intraoperative electromyographic (EMG) activity recorded from three branches of cranial nerve VII during removal of a cerebellopontine angle meningioma. Stimulation of cranial nerve VII can result in the recording of evoked activity from all branches of the nerve.

SUMMARY

This chapter reviews the authors' approach to the intraoperative monitoring of neurophysiologic function during cranial base surgery. The commonly accepted principal goal of intraoperative monitoring is to prevent morbidity, and at a certain level this is true; however, the more fundamental goal of intraoperative monitoring is to provide the surgical team with information that allows them to accomplish the desired operative objective with as optimal a surgical strategy as possible, while having a clear idea of what surgical morbidity is being induced along the way. This latter goal is particularly important in cases in which the degree of difficulty is high and it is virtually impossible to prevent morbidity.

Essentially, the authors place a real-time feedback control loop around the dynamic, changing system comprising the surgeon and the patient. This requires a strong commitment to the concept that the patient's CNS is highly sensitive to the operative manipulations of the surgeon and that appropriately observed variables may predict lesions about to develop. This information permits the surgeon dynamically to modify his or her approach to the operation and thereby minimize the degree of morbidity induced in the patient.

Based on these considerations and viewpoints, the neurophysiologists, who support the intraoperative monitoring service for the Cranial Base Tumor Center at UPMC, have evolved an integrated approach to the problem of assessing the dynamic functional status of the patient's nervous system and of providing this information to the rest of the surgical team in as relevant and clear a fashion as possible. This approach is based on the combined experience of monitoring more than 300 cranial base surgical resections to date.

Neurophysiologic monitoring differs from and is complementary to that provided by the anesthesiologist in fundamental ways, and it is important to recognize and appreciate the distinctions. The monitoring performed by the anesthesiologist is aimed at maintaining the patient's homeostasis. That is, the anesthesiologist wishes to preserve the life of the patient and is focused on those measures that provide information concerning this most fundamental issue.

The use of evoked potentials in the evaluation and monitoring of patients with actual or potential neurologic deficits provides a set of objective measures of nervous system function that are more specific and reliable than previously used methods of nervous system monitoring (1). EMG measures are also highly specific and reliable. The EEG measures are also highly reliable; however, they are routinely used to assess more global factors than the EMGs.

Many apparently benign surgical manipulations may have significant effects on the neural responses and resultant clinical condition. For example, retraction of structures that are close to, or within, the pathway being monitored, noise and vibration from drilling, and heat diffusion from lasers, all affect the underlying neural tissue and the neurophysiologic responses.

Stringent time constraints exist in intraoperative monitoring of neurophysiologic function, and damage to the CNS may occur rapidly, over seconds. This constraint has inspired the development of methods for extracting and analyzing evoked potential, EMG, and EEG waveforms rapidly and efficiently. A corollary of the increased sensitivity required to decrease the monitoring time is a higher rate of individually false-positive measures. These are usually rapidly identified as such and produce no disruption in the flow of the case.

In support of the intraoperative monitoring of these measures, the authors have developed a distributed computer system, NeuroNet, specifically configured to support the considerations discussed in this chapter. This system provides both off-line and real-time signal processing and data review capabilities, and it addresses many of the problems associated with the acquisition, processing, and display of multivariate neurophysiologic data in these complex cases.

Monitoring of these measures in the operating room uses computationally based techniques and presents a significant step forward in reducing patient morbidity due to surgery. Previously, the integrity of the CNS could be examined only clinically, when the patient recovered from anesthesia; however, the measures described in this chapter provide an immediate assessment of the effects of surgery on the nervous system, with implications for modifying surgical techniques.

ACKNOWLEDGMENTS

The authors acknowledge the collaboration of their colleagues over the years: in particular, Laligam Sekhar, Chandra Sen, Donald Wright, Ivo Janecka, Carl Snyderman, Barry Hirsch, Steve Cass, Andrew Kofke, Mark Bloom, James Krugh, Matt Caldwell, Steve Whitehurst, Pedro Vera, Don Weiss, and John Durrant.

REFERENCES

1. Villani RM. Forward. In: Grundy BL, Villani RM, eds. *Evoked potentials: intraoperative and ICU monitoring.* New York: Springer-Verlag, 1989:v.
2. Gerson GR. *Monitoring during anesthesia.* Boston: Little, Brown and Company, 1981.
3. Desmedt JE. *Neuromonitoring in surgery.* New York: Elsevier Science, 1989.
4. Loftus CM, Traynelis VC. *Intraoperative monitoring techniques in neurosurgery.* New York: McGraw-Hill, 1994.
5. Moller AR. *Intraoperative neurophysiological monitoring.* Luxembourgh: Harwood Academic, 1995.
6. Tyner FS, Knott JR, Mayer WB. *Fundamentals of EEG technology, Vol. I: basic concepts and methods.* New York: Raven Press, 1983.
7. Sclabassi RJ, Lofink RM, Doyle EL. NeuroNet: a distributed microprocessor network for clinical neurophysiology. In: Geisow MJ, Barret AN, eds. *Microcomputers in medicine.* New York: Elsevier Science, 1987:283–303.
8. Krieger DN, Lofink RM, Doyle EL, Burk G, Sclabassi RJ. NeuroNet: implementation of an integrated clinical neurophysiology system. *Medical Instrumentation* 1987;21:296–303.
9. Krieger DN, Burk G, Sclabassi RJ. NeuroNet: a distributed real-time system for monitoring neurophysiological function in the medical environment. *Computer* 1991;24(3):45–55.
10. Simon R, Krieger DN, Znati T, Lofink R, Sclabassi RJ. MultiMedia MedNet: a medical collaboration and consultation system. *Computer* 1995;28(5):65–73.

11. Sclabassi RJ, Krieger DN, Simon R, Gross G. NeuroNet: collaborative intraoperative guidance and control. *IEEE Computer Graphics and Applications* 1996;16(1):39–45.
12. Krieger DN, Sclabassi RJ. Time varying evoked potentials. *J Med Eng Technol* 1994;18(3):96–100.
13. Sclabassi RJ, Risch H, Hinman CL, Kroin JS, Enns N, Namerow NS. Complex pattern evoked somatosensory responses in the study of multiple sclerosis. *Proceedings of the IEEE* 1977;65:626–633.
14. Sclabassi RJ, Harper RM. Laboratory computers in neurophysiology. *Proceedings of the IEEE* 1973;61:1602–1614.
15. Grundy BL. Intraoperative monitoring of sensory-evoked potentials. *Anesthesiology* 1983;58:72–87.
16. Domino KB. Anesthesia for cranial base tumor operations. In: Sekhar LN, Schramm VL, eds. *Tumors of the cranial base: diagnosis and treatment*. Mount Kisko, NY: Futura Publishing, 1987:107–122.
17. Niedermeyer E, Lopes da Silva F. *Electroencephalography*. Baltimore: Urban and Schwarzenberg, 1987.
18. Regan D. *Human brain electrophysiology: evoked potentials and evoked magnetic fields in science and medicine*. New York: Elsevier Science, 1989.
19. Kamura J. *Electrodiagnosis in diseases of nerve and muscle*. Philadelphia: FA Davis Co, 1983.
20. Meyer JS, Marx PW. The pathogenesis of EEG changes during cerebral anoxia. In: Van der Drift JHA, ed. *Cardiac and vascular diseases/handbook of electroencephalography and clinical neurophysiology*. Amsterdam: Elsevier Science, 1972:14(Appendix):5–11.
21. Freye E. *Cerebral monitoring in the operating room and the intensive care unit*. Boston: Kluwer Academic Publishers, 1990.
22. Van der Drift JHA. The EEG in cerebro-vascular disease. In: Vinken PJ, Bruyn GW, eds. *Handbook of clinical neurology*. Vol. II. Amsterdam: Elsevier Science, 1972:267–291.
23. Roger J, Roger A, Gastaut H. Electro-clinical correlation in 36 cases of vascular syndromes of brainstem. *Electroencephalogr Clin Neurophysiol* 1954;6:164(abst).
24. Gentili F, Lougheed WM, Yamashiro K, Corrado C. Monitoring of sensory evoked potentials during surgery of skull base tumors. *Can J Neurol Sci* 1985;12:336–340.
25. Desmedt JE, Cheron G. Central somatosensory conduction in man: neural generators and interpeak latencies in the far-field components recorded from neck and right or left scalp and earlobes. *Electroencephalogr Clin Neurophysiol* 1980;50:382–403.
26. Allison T. Developmental and aging changes in human evoked potentials. In: Barber C, Blum T, Nodar R, eds. *Evoked potentials III*. Boston: Butterworth, 1987:72–90.
27. Goff WR, Williamson PD, Vangilder JC, Allison T, Fisher TC. Neural origins of long latency evoked potentials recorded from the depths and from the cortical surface of the brain in man. *Progress in Clinical Neurophysiology* 1980;2:126–145.
28. Samra SK. Effect of isoflurane on human median nerve evoked potentials. In: Ducker TB, Brown RH, eds. *Neurophysiology and standards of spinal cord monitoring*. New York: Springer-Verlag, 1988:147–156.
29. Barr JD, Horowitz MB, Mathis JM, Sclabassi RJ, Yonas H. Intraoperative urokinase infusion for embolic stroke during carotid endarterectomy. *Neurosurgery* 1995;36:606–611.
30. Buchwald JS, Haung CM. Far-field acoustic responses: origins in the cat. *Science* 1975;189:382–384.
31. van Olphen AF, Rodenberg M, Verwey C. Influence of stimulus repetition rate on brainstem evoked responses in man. *Audiology* 1979;18:388–394.
32. Moller AR, Jannetta PJ. Auditory evoked potentials recorded from the cochlear nucleus and its vicinity in man. *J Neurosurg* 1983;59:493–499.
33. Ciganek L. The EEG response to light stimulus in man. *Electroencephalogr Clin Neurophysiol* 1961;13:165–172.
34. Kraut MA, Arezzo JC, Vaughan HG. Intracortical generators of the flash VEP in monkeys. *Electroencephalogr Clin Neurophysiol* 1985;62:300–312.
35. Moller AR. Electrophysiological monitoring of cranial nerves in operations in the skull base. In: Sekhar LN, Schramm VL, eds. *Tumors of the cranial base: diagnosis and treatment*. Mount Kisko, NY: Futura Publishing, 1987:123–134.
36. Prass RL, Kinney SE, Hardy RW, Hahn JF, Luders H. Acoustic (loudspeaker) facial EMG monitoring: II. use of evoked EMG activity during acoustic neuroma resection. *Otolaryngol Head Neck Surg* 1987;97:541–551.
37. Daube JR, Harper CM. Surgical monitoring of cranial and peripheral nerves. In: Desmedt JE, ed. *Neuromonitoring in surgery*. Amsterdam: Elsevier Science, 1989:115–138.
38. Harner SG, Daube JR, Beatty CW, Ebersold MJ. Intraoperative monitoring of the facial nerve. *Laryngoscope* 1988;98:209–212.

SECTION II
Anterior Fossa Approaches

# CHAPTER 10

Transfacial Approach

Paul J. Donald

Of all the various approaches to skull base surgery, those to lesions involving the anterior cranial fossa have the greatest variety of techniques. This is in part because the anterior approaches have been in existence for the longest time. The basic goal of any procedure should be to provide the simplest technique that will provide optimal exposure so that all tumor can be safely excised, producing the minimal amount of deformity. When the lesion is malignant, surgery must be designed to excise the entire tumor with a margin of healthy tissue. Anything less guarantees a high incidence of local recurrence, even with adjunctive postoperative irradiation.

Most surgical procedures for excision of malignancies describe removal of the tumor *en bloc*. This is unarguably not only the classic method of cancer removal, but the most prudent method of ensuring tumor-free margins. However, in some areas at the skull base, it is highly impractical or impossible to perform a total *en bloc* resection. The major impediments are the obscuring effect created by large, bulky tumors of the deepest or most posterior aspects of the neoplasm, especially that portion that invades the skull base. In addition, the unnecessary sacrifice of uninvolved facial soft tissue that may have significant functional or aesthetic value can be avoided if a modified piecemeal resection is used. The objections to piecemeal resection are (a) the concern that there will be tumor spillage with malignant implantations in the tumor bed, and (b) the danger of leaving residual tumor at the margins. The techniques described here are in reality modified *en bloc* rather than piecemeal approaches. An *en bloc* resection is done whenever feasible, but if it is not, the tumor may be debulked initially to visualize where the resection margins are to be. Moreover, it may be necessary to remove about 90% of the tumor *en bloc* and then remove the deep portion, sometimes with the intracranial component as a second block.

Any form of piecemeal resection imposes the significant burden of responsibility on the surgeon of ensuring that *eventually* tumor-free margins are obtained. The close cooperation of the pathologist is essential in this regard. Numerous frozen sections are required, often late at night. The presence of a dedicated head and neck/skull base pathologist goes a long way toward achieving this goal. At the end of the resection, copious lavage of the wound with sterile water clears the area of residual, loose, "floating" tumor cells. Assiduous attention to the maintenance of tumor-free margins with meticulous visual inspection coupled with multiple frozen sections has enabled the author's surgical team to use a modified *en bloc* technique with a minimal number of local recurrences. Although this in a way violates one of the basic tenets of oncologic surgery, it is successful in complete tumor removal and avoidance of local recurrence. Slavish adherence to the *en bloc* principle will often result in the unnecessary removal of vital tissues. Moreover, it may create a mind set precluding the resection of lesions that appear to be inoperable by virtue of the fact that removal is not feasible using the *en bloc* principle.

INDICATIONS

The tumors most commonly requiring combined anterior craniofacial surgery usually begin in the nose or sinuses. Many of these tumors, to a greater or lesser degree, are malignant. Inverting papilloma (Fig. 1) is an example of a transitional type of tumor that is locally invasive, does not metastasize, but must be resected aggressively to avoid recurrence. Esthesioneuroblastoma varies from a very indolent to a highly aggressive tumor (Fig. 2). Most tumors of nasal or paranasal sinus origin are squamous cell or adenocarcinomas of the maxillary or ethmoid sinuses. Aggressive neurotropic cutaneous malignancies present a frightening scenario in which a small, seemingly innocuous basal cell or squamous cell carcinoma of the skin can travel the length of a cutaneous sensory nerve, such as the infraorbital, and gain access to the intracranial cavity (Fig. 3).

P. J. Donald: Department of Otolaryngology–Head and Neck Surgery, and Center for Skull Base Surgery, University of California, Davis Medical Center, Sacramento, California 95817.

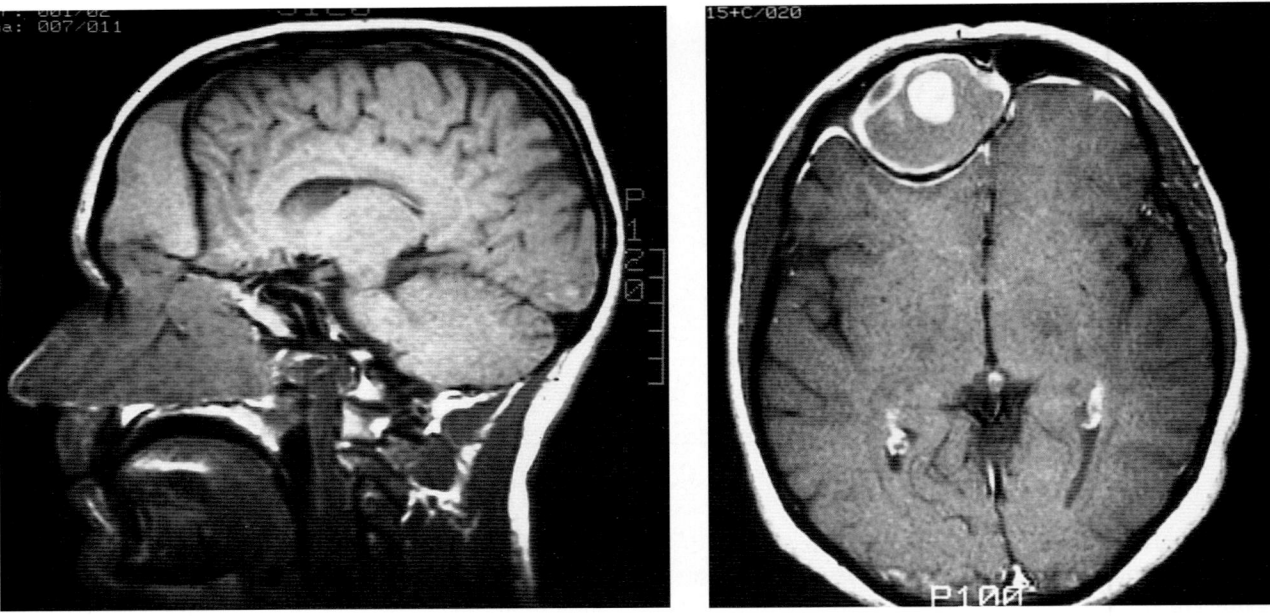

FIG. 1. T1-weighted magnetic resonance images showing an inverting papilloma that had extensively invaded the anterior cranial fossa but remained intradural and extradural. **A:** Sagittal view. **B:** Axial view.

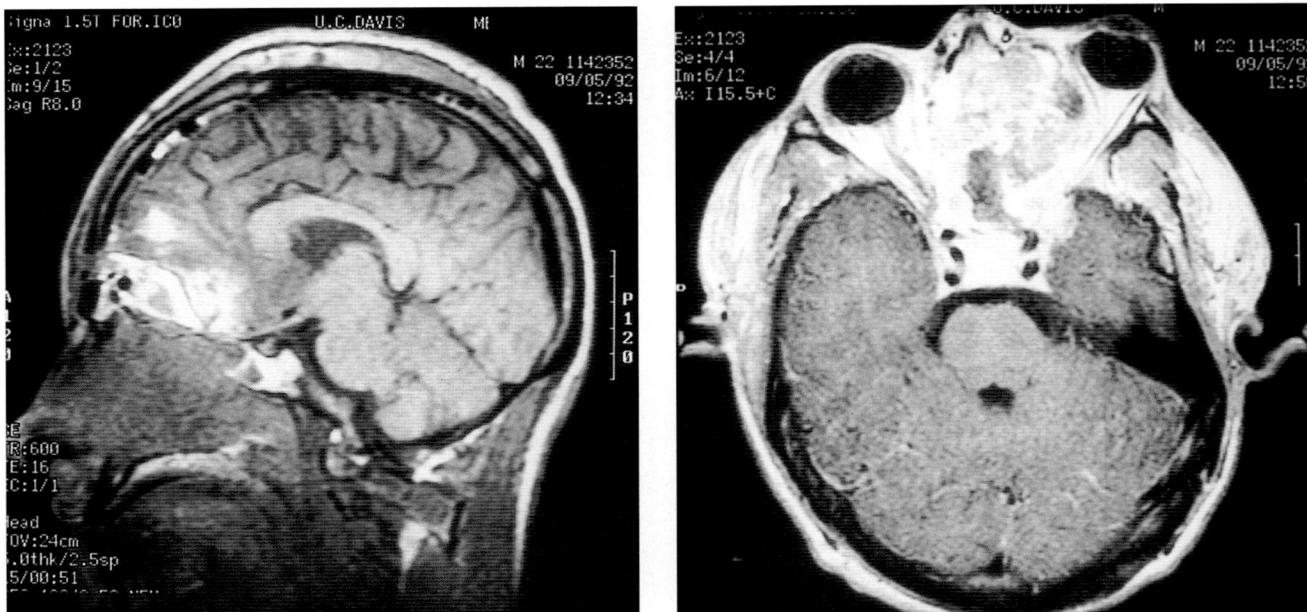

FIG. 2. T1-weighted magnetic resonance images of patient with highly aggressive esthesioneuroblastoma. He had bilateral cervical lymph nodal metastases and extensive intracranial and intracerebral invasion. Despite extensive skull base surgery, he died within 6 months of meningeal carcinomatosis. **A:** Sagittal view. **B:** Axial view.

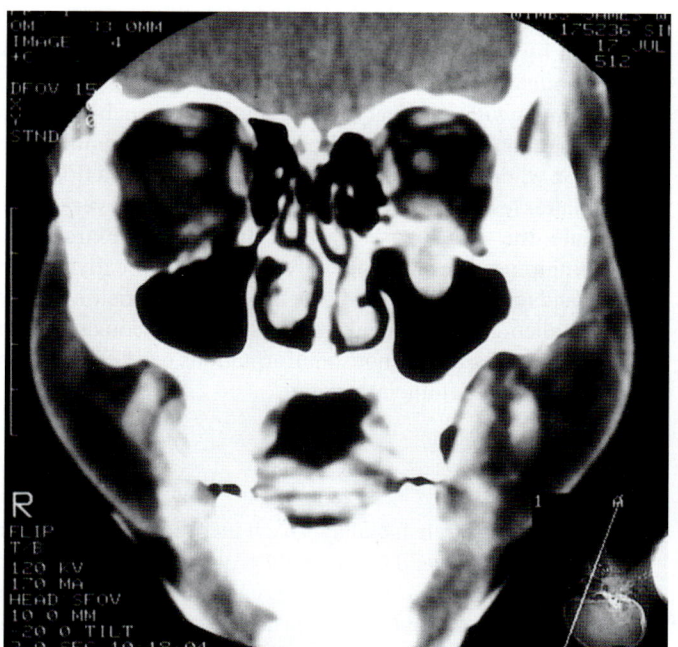
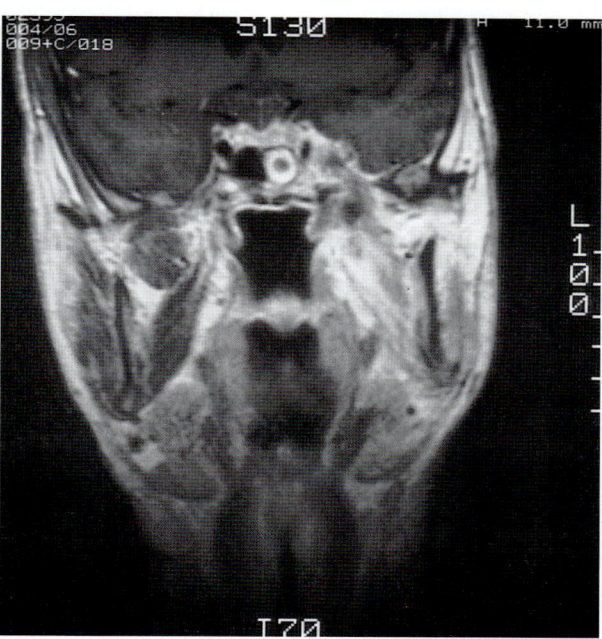

FIG. 3. T1-weighted coronal magnetic resonance images showing apparently innocuous actinically activated squamous cell carcinoma of the facial skin that invaded the infraorbital nerve to the gasserian ganglion. **A:** Tumor along left infraorbital nerve. **B:** Spread to cavernous sinus and middle fossa, 1 year after initial resection.

The most common mode of anterior cranial fossa spread is from the ethmoid sinuses through the ethmoid fovea to the undersurface of the dura over the gyrus rectus of the frontal lobe (Fig. 4). Tumors of the nasal vault, such as esthesioneuroblastoma, can proceed directly through the cribriform plate or along the filaments of the fila olfactoria. Tumors penetrating the orbit and invading the eye can proceed through the orbital roof into the anterior fossa or travel along the optic nerve to the middle cranial fossa. Primary tumors of the frontal sinus are rare (Fig. 5). Those originating in the anterior ethmoid and frontoethmoid cells have a propensity to invade superiorly through the frontal sinus floor and then posteriorly through that sinus' posterior wall.

The decision to use craniofacial surgery to resect a lesion of the paranasal sinuses is not always easy. Malignant tumors that show a clear line of separation on computed tomography (CT) and magnetic resonance imaging (MRI) between tumor and the bone of the anterior cranial base are clearly not candidates for this procedure. Conversely, those with obvious bone erosion at this site should have the operation. The problem patients are those in whom tumor abuts the bone as visualized on CT and MRI, but who have no evidence of bone erosion. Despite this lack of evidence of intracranial intrusion, highly malignant tumors should have the combined intracranial/extracranial approach because these studies are not yet refined enough to show early bone invasion. Benign tumors usually do not require such aggressive treatment. Tumors such as inverting papilloma and esthesioneuroblastoma stand to benefit significantly from the combined approach. Local recurrences, and thus the potential for future significant morbidity and even mortality, can be avoided by combination surgery. Occult invasion may not be appreciated despite the sophistication of current scanning techniques.

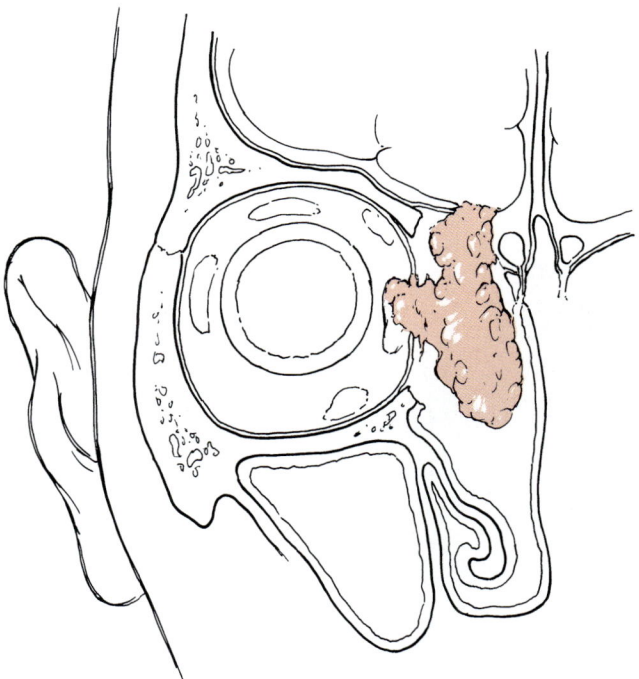

FIG. 4. Spread of tumor from the ethmoid sinus through the ethmoid fovea to the dura over the gyrus rectus.

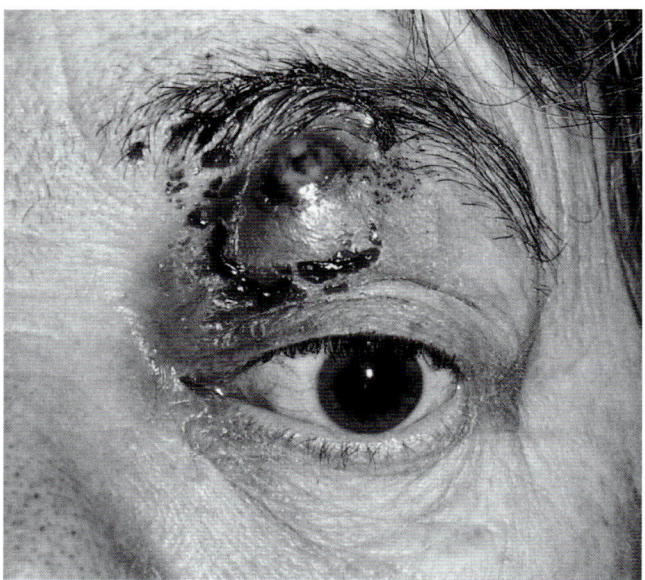

FIG. 5. Patient with a primary squamous cell carcinoma of the frontal sinus with extensive invasion through the posterior frontal sinus wall, into the dura. Frontal view of patient shows tumor penetration through upper eyelid.

The issue of ocular sacrifice presents an agonizing dilemma. Routine orbital exenteration for invasion of malignant tumors into the periorbita or even through the bony orbital walls is commonplace. The work of Perry et al. (1) and Mann et al. (2) raises the possibility that orbital exenteration may not always be indicated when the orbit is invaded by malignancy. For tumors of less aggressive malignant behavior such as well differentiated fibrosarcoma and esthesioneuroblastoma, the eye can often be saved, even with extensive resection of periorbita, orbital fat, and even oculomotor muscles (Fig. 6). The preservation of the eye when the periorbita is invaded by a highly malignant tumor is, the author believes, ill advised but currently remains controversial. Invasion of fat, ocular muscles, or the nerve sheath by any malignancy is a clearly definitive indication for orbital exenteration.

Tumors with a primary intracranial origin such as meningioma, chordoma, or chondrosarcoma require combined resection when they clearly violate the anterior fossa floor. The two latter lesions take origin in bone and by their very nature violate the skull base barrier. Intracranial/extracranial meningiomas are histologically benign but locally aggressive and impossible to eradicate unless total excision is done. Purely benign intracranial lesions such as osteomas, fibrous dysplasia, or arteriovenous malformations can be better controlled with craniofacial surgery.

TECHNIQUE

The anterior transfacial approach incorporates a combination of transfacial and transcranial procedures. The facial approach consists of a graduated greater exposure depending on the extent of disease. The basic excision is done through a lateral rhinotomy approach coupled with a low craniotomy. The lateral rhinotomy incision may be extended into a Weber-Fergusson incision if a more extensive maxillary excision is required. Most ethmoid and orbital tumors are easily managed through the lateral rhinotomy.

Lateral Rhinotomy—Denker—Medial Maxillectomy

The incision begins in the medial one third of the brow. It is carried in the inferior hairs of the eyebrow and inclined in the direction of the hair follicles. Although a complaint of "split brow" appearance is occasionally made, the usual result in the author's experience is of an excellent cosmetic result with the scar well hidden by the brow hairs. The incision is carried through a point midway between the midline of the nose and the caruncle of the eye (Fig. 7). It continues slightly on the nasal side of the nasal-facial groove, and is carried

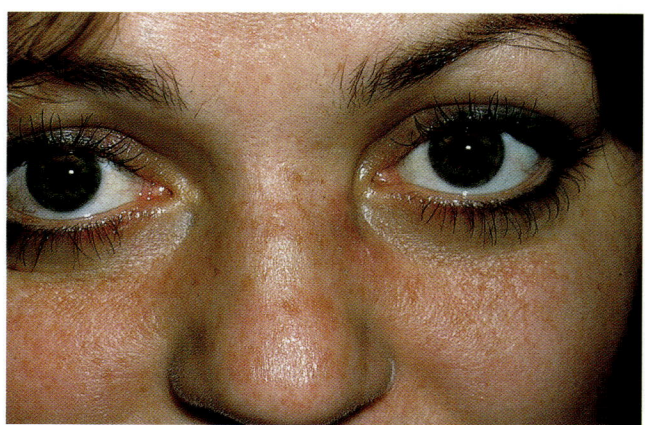 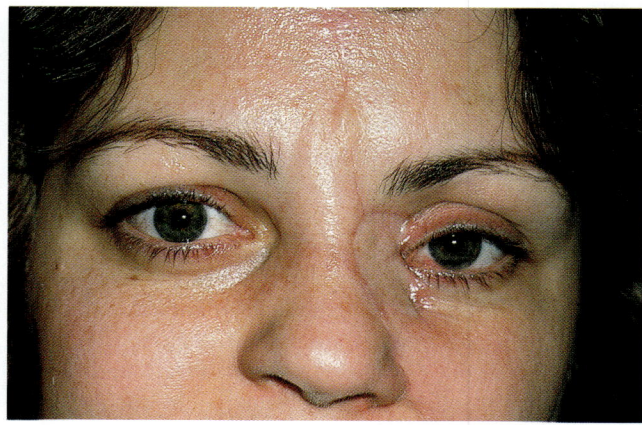

FIG. 6. Young woman with a low-grade fibrosarcoma of the skin of the inner canthus of the orbit, invading the anterior ethmoids. **A:** Preoperative frontal view of patient. **B:** Patient without recurrence 1 year after globe-sparing surgery in which the periorbita, periorbital fat, and medial rectus muscle were taken. She has now been tumor free for 10 years.

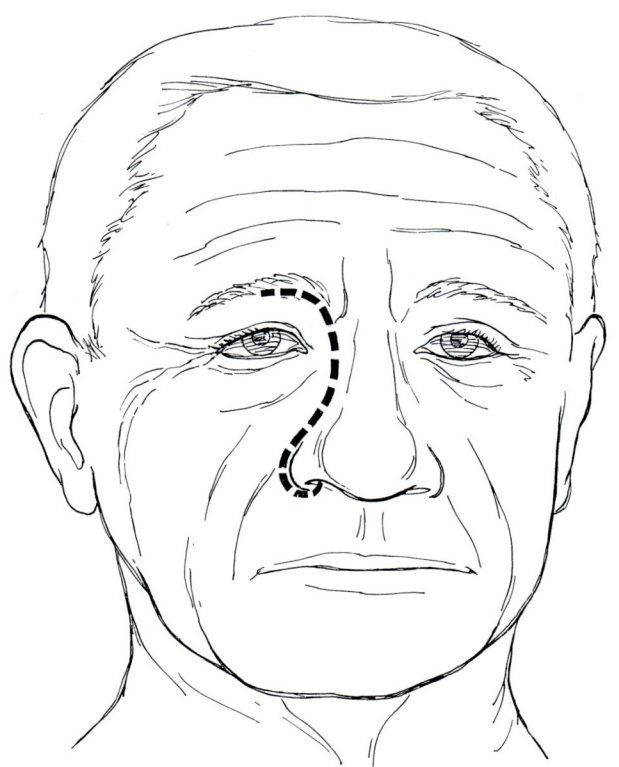

FIG. 7. Lateral rhinotomy skin incision.

around the nasal ala and into the floor of the nose. The incision medial to the eye is deepened with a small hemostat and the angular vessels exposed. These are clamped, cut, and ligated or coagulated with the bipolar cautery. The incision is carried through the periosteum and the nasal mucosa cut up to the pyriform rim. Elevation of the maxillary periosteum is done over the maxillary face, initially preserving the infraorbital nerve.

A curved osteotome used for rhinoplasty is placed low on the pyriform rim (Fig. 8). It is driven in a laterally inclined curvilinear manner through the frontal process of the maxilla and carried to a level adjacent to the infraorbital nerve. It is then inclined medially toward the nasal dorsum. This cut should cross the nasal dorsum below the level of the nasal process of the frontal bone, allowing for an easy greenstick fracture medially. If the osteotomy unluckily courses above this point, it is wise to back-cut the bone inferiorly for ease of fracture. The 1.1-mm blade (B5) of the Midas Rex drill provides an easy-to-use alternative to the osteotome. The mucosa is incised separately along the osteotomy line and carried up to the septum. The lateral nasal fragment is greenstick fractured medially by placing a broad, flat osteotome against its mucosal surface and then gently twisting the instrument medially (Fig. 9). An anchor suture placed subcutaneously in the fractured fragment is attached to a Kelly clamp and hung over the opposite side of the face.

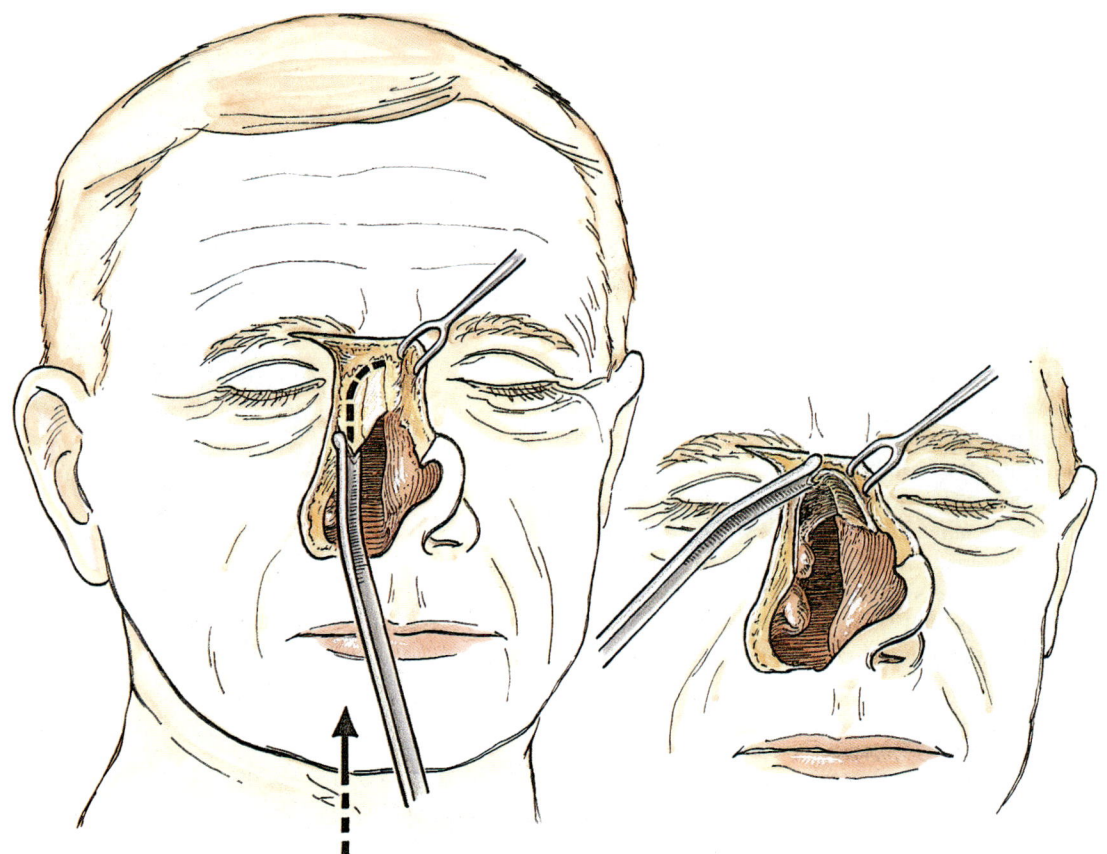

FIG. 8. Curved osteotome used to create bony lateral rhinotomy incision.

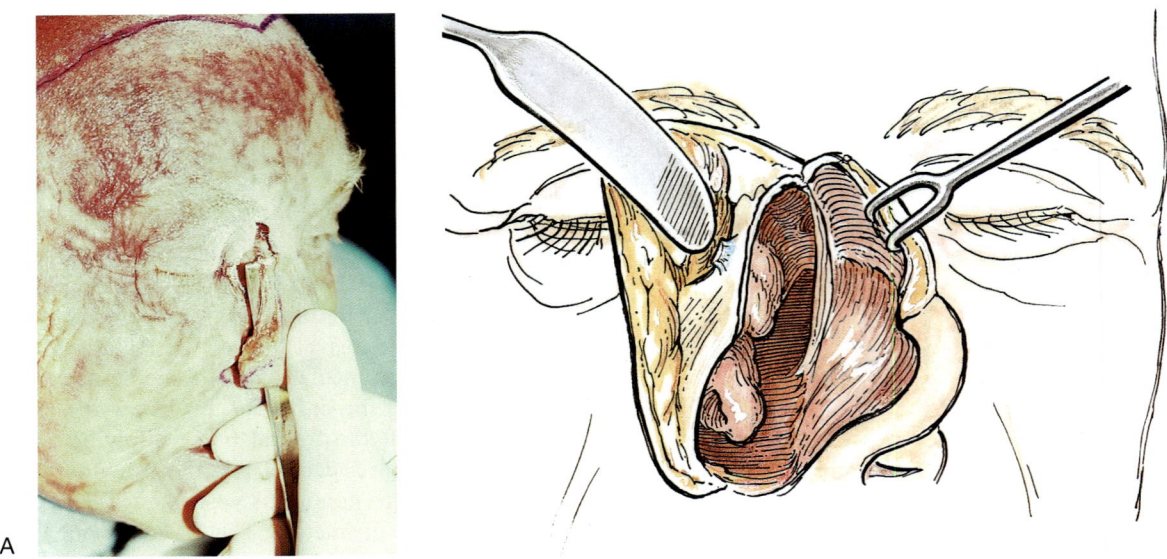

FIG. 9. The lateral nasal wall is outfractured with a broad, flat osteotome. **A:** Illustrated in cadaver. **B:** Drawing of completed rhinotomy.

The medial orbital periosteum and medial canthal tendon are elevated by sharp dissection, maintaining vigilance for the first sign of tumor. An external ethmoidectomy is done in the usual fashion until the point of tumor involvement. Healthy air cells are removed around the periphery of the tumor as much as possible (Fig. 10). Care is taken to cease dissection at the point at which tumor invades the globe. The periphery of the tumor is followed up to the point where it erodes or abuts the anterior fossa floor. If the tumor is so massive that this delineation is difficult and landmarks are obscure, then the tumor should be debulked. A rim of clearly visible tumor is left behind so that it can be encircled at the time of final, definitive *en bloc* removal. If the lacrimal sac and ducts are invaded by aggressive malignancies, the eye usually needs to be excised. Eye preservation is predicated on the malignant character of the lesion.

The ethmoidectomy is carried to the anterior face of the sphenoid. The excision of the ethmoid cells helps in establishing the superior cut for the medial maxillectomy. Orbital involvement by tumor and penetration of the ethmoid contribution to the orbital roof can be assessed.

The Denker procedure now proceeds by excision of the junction between the anterior and medial walls of the maxillary sinus with a Kerrison rongeur. This exposes the inferior portion of the maxillary sinus, allowing a clear view of its medial wall and the orbital floor. If tumor does not involve the infraorbital nerve, a small collar of bone is preserved around it (Fig. 11).

As an alternative to the Denker operation, an anterior wall ostectomy as described by Bagatella and Mazzoni (3) can be done. An area of bone including the pyriform rim and anterior maxillary wall is removed with a cutting tool such as the Midas Rex and preserved for later reconstruction (Fig. 12). This has become the author's procedure of preference.

The medial maxillectomy is done by driving a small osteotome along the floor of the nose through the bone of the inferior meatus from the pyriform rim to the posterior maxillary wall (Fig. 13). The anterior bone incision has already been completed with the anterior maxillary wall resection

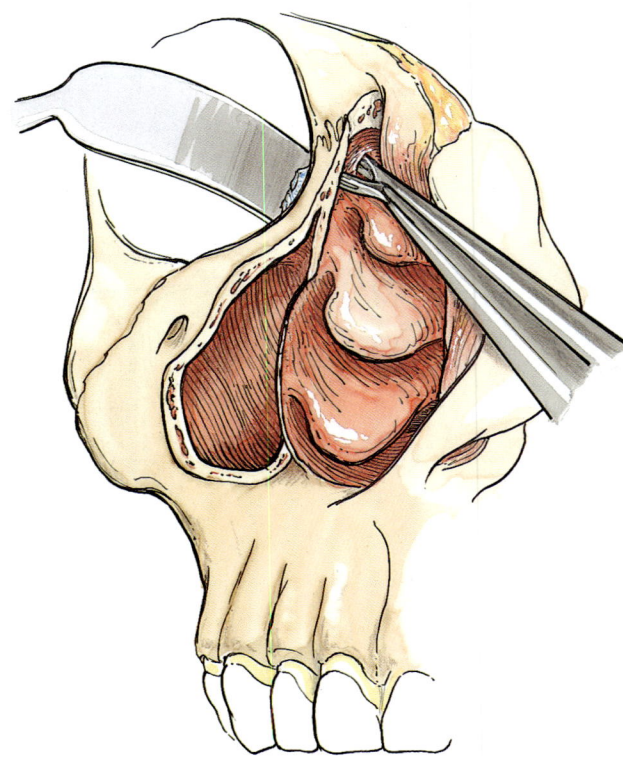

FIG. 10. External ethmoidectomy dissected up to point of orbital invasion and invasion of anterior cranial fossa floor.

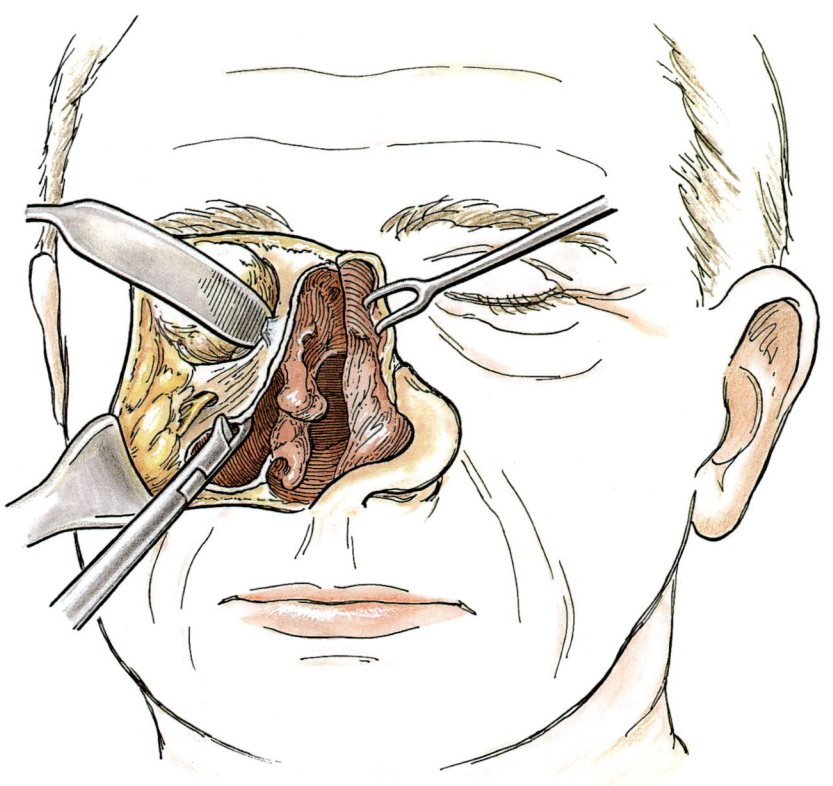

FIG. 11. Denker procedure done to expose the maxillary sinus and set the stage for medial maxillectomy.

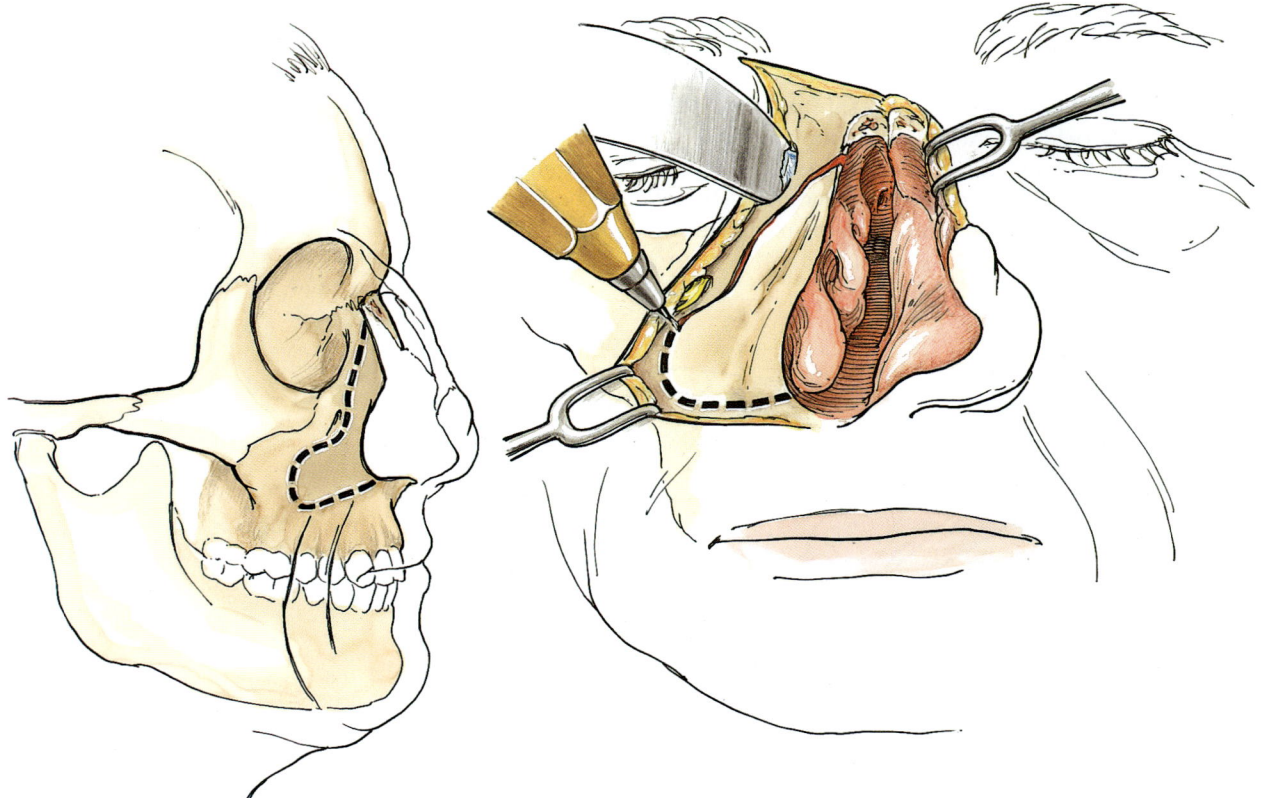

FIG. 12. Anterior wall ostectomy done as alternative to Denker procedure, allowing preservation of bone flap with return at the end of operation.

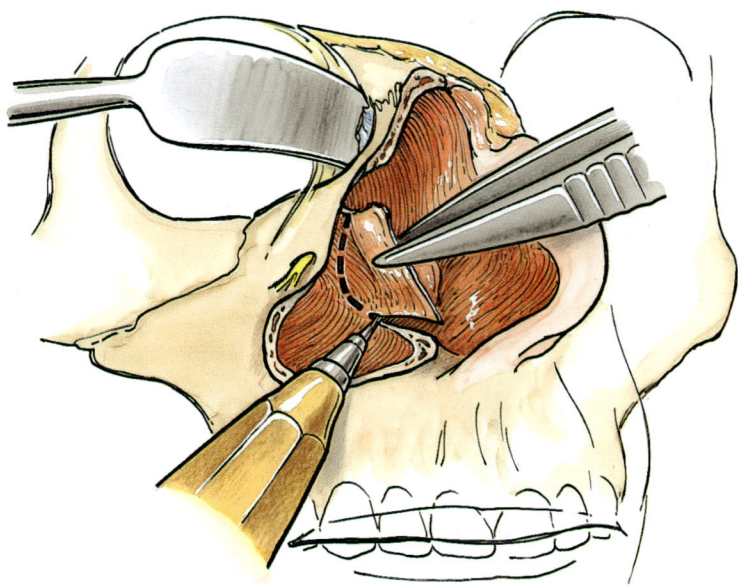

FIG. 13. Medial maxillectomy.

and the external ethmoidectomy. A connection is made through the medial orbital floor, sparing the lacrimal fossa or including it, depending on the exigencies of tumor. If a more posterior extent of tumor becomes apparent when the medial maxillary wall is removed, this must be addressed by carrying the resection into the sphenoid sinus or pterygomaxillary space. This is discussed in the next section.

A superior cut is made close to the anterior fossa floor, usually cutting directly across tumor. Although most surgeons shudder at this maneuver, it is safe providing that eventually a wide-field resection of the tumor-bearing area is carried out, including a margin of healthy tissue, with careful assurance of tumor-free margins. The final step in the excision is to cut the posterior attachment of the medial maxillary wall. A curved scissors is introduced through the inferior cut along the floor of the nose. It is directed superiorly and a separation of the medial from the posterior wall begun (Fig. 14). A careful incision separating the medial from posterior wall is often difficult to impossible to achieve, so a large grasping forceps like the Luc forceps is used to avulse this medial wall. Any posterior remnants are removed with the Blakesly and Takahashi forceps.

Now that the lateral rhinotomy, anterior maxillotomy, external ethmoidectomy, and medial maxillectomy have been done, an excellent exposure of residual tumor has been accomplished (Fig. 15). Residual subcranial tumor that will not be included in the craniotomy block must be resected with visual and frozen-section control. Tumor extending to the in-

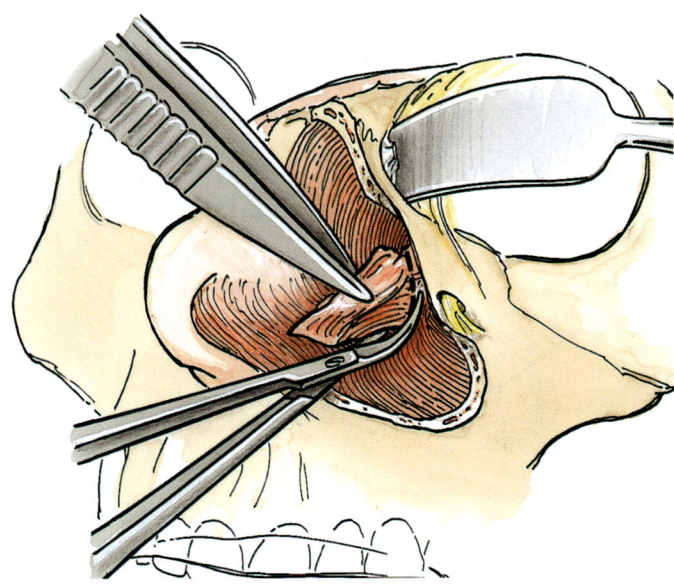

FIG. 14. Final cut with curved scissors made through the posterior aspect of the medial maxillary wall.

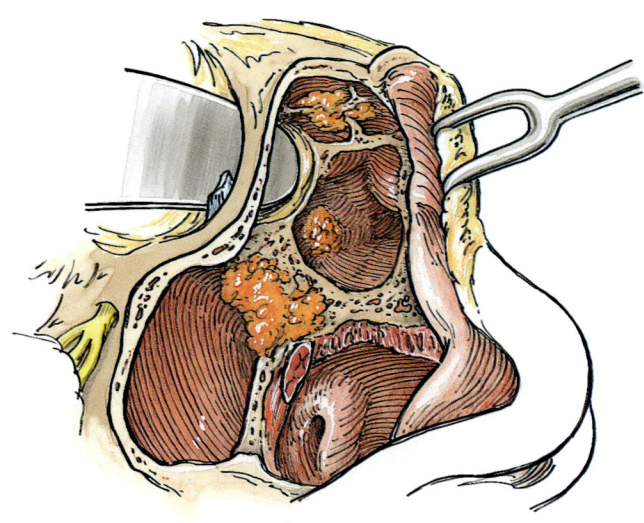

FIG. 15. Initial tumor block removed, with only tumor penetrating anterior cranial fossa floor and posterior maxilla remaining.

ferior half of the maxilla often mandates a full maxillectomy and is covered later in this chapter.

Involvement of the sphenoid sinus, anterior clivus, and posterior maxillary wall can be managed easily with this approach. The posterior maxillary wall is removed with a cutting bur, exposing the pterygomaxillary space and the greater palatine canal (Fig. 16). At this point, the internal maxillary artery, the maxillary nerve, the sphenopalatine ganglion, and some fat that invests these structures are exposed. Tumor is removed and involved structures are assessed. The pterygoid plates are removed with the cutting bur and pterygoid muscle involvement evaluated. Once these muscles are invaded, an additional approach is developed to resect them with a wide margin or to remove them com-

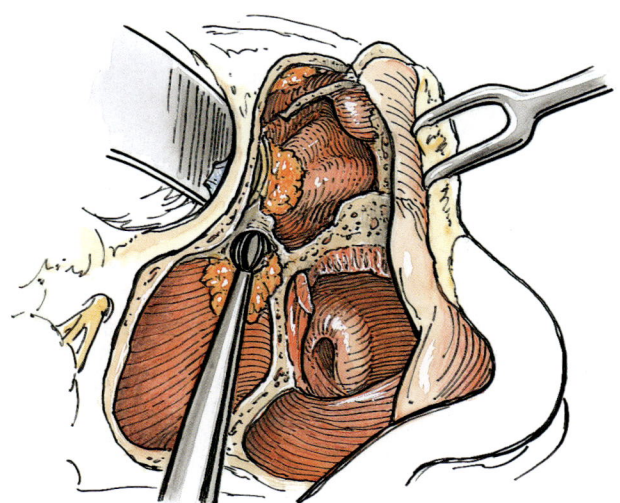

FIG. 16. Posterior wall maxillectomy done with cutting bur.

pletely, including their attachments to the mandible. (This is covered more completely in Chapter 15, on the Extended Transfacial Subcranial Approach.) Invasion of tumor superiorly at this point can be simply managed by drilling the origin of the pterygoid plates and the thick, substantial sphenoid bone that subtends them (Fig. 17). Delineation of involved bone from that which is tumor free is relatively easy. If doubt exists, curettage of marrow with frozen-section analysis is a useful guide, keeping in mind that only cancellous bone involvement can be adequately assessed.

The sphenoid sinus and its floor, the anterior portion of the sphenoid contribution to the clivus, are easily removed with the drill (Fig. 18). The sphenoid rostrum is similarly removed in its entirety, exposing the anatomy of the lateral sinus wall. Tumor involvement of the lateral wall is removed with the bur. Only limited cavernous sinus invasion can be adequately and safely managed though this approach (Fig. 19). The cavernous sinus dura and perhaps a small amount of the sinus proper is safely excised, but the exposure is limited. Bone drilling posteriorly can be carried down to the pontine dura if necessary.

Further dissection laterally is limited by the optic canal in the patient with an intact eye. Removal of bone from the medial aspect of the optic canal in a seeing eye must be done with extreme caution to avoid trauma to the sheath and the ocular vascular supply. When the eye is removed, a much wider view is permitted with more facile exposure of the inferior orbital fissure and foramen rotundum, vidian canal, superior orbital fissure, and optic canal. Further dissection leads to the middle fossa and is covered in Chapter 16.

Orbital Exenteration

General Considerations and Indications

Of all the organs that require excision during head and neck surgery, the eye carries with it the most profound emotional and aesthetic implications. Most patients balk to some degree at the idea of exenterating the orbit, and the idea of bilateral resection with the prospect of total blindness is anathema to most. It is surprising that despite the many successes of so many completely blind people in our society, which is common knowledge, many patients would rather face certain death than contemplate the loss of their sight. The role of the skull base surgeon is to present to the patient his or her therapeutic options and what the anticipated losses and impairments might be. Only the patient can decide in view of his or her own sense of values whether to proceed.

Decisions regarding eye preservation based on known and anticipated tumor pathophysiology have already been discussed. The guidelines set up by the studies of Perry et al. (1), Mann et al. (2), and Carrau et al. (4) must be tempered in the face of highly malignant tumors such as squamous cell carcinoma, adenoid cystic carcinoma, and malignant melanoma. Local control of disease is key to long-term patient survival.

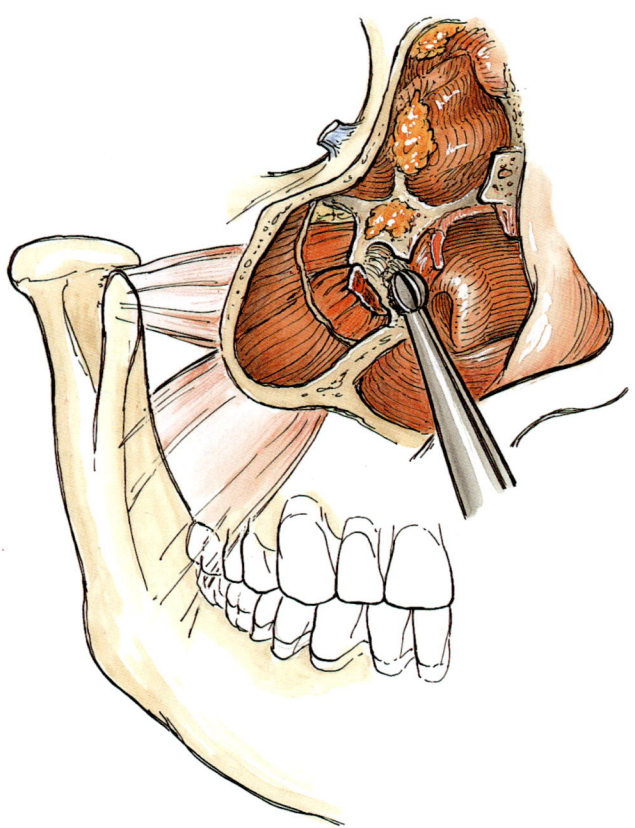

FIG. 17. Management of pterygoid plate and sphenoid body tumor invasion by resection with the cutting bur.

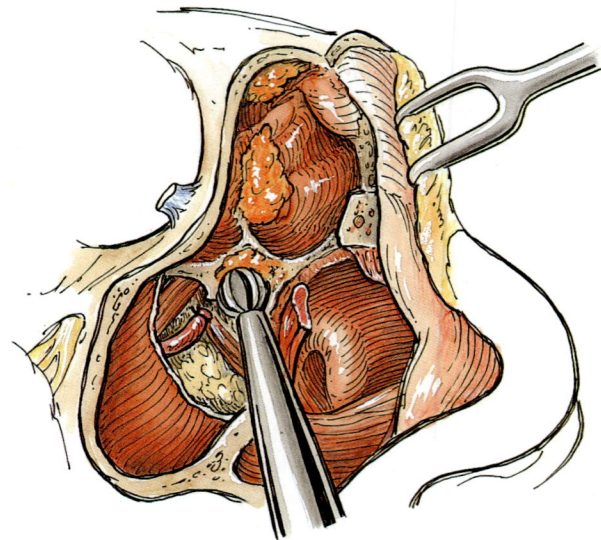

FIG. 18. Removal of anterior wall and floor of sphenoid sinus, and heavy bone of the base of the sphenoid removed until tumor exenteration complete.

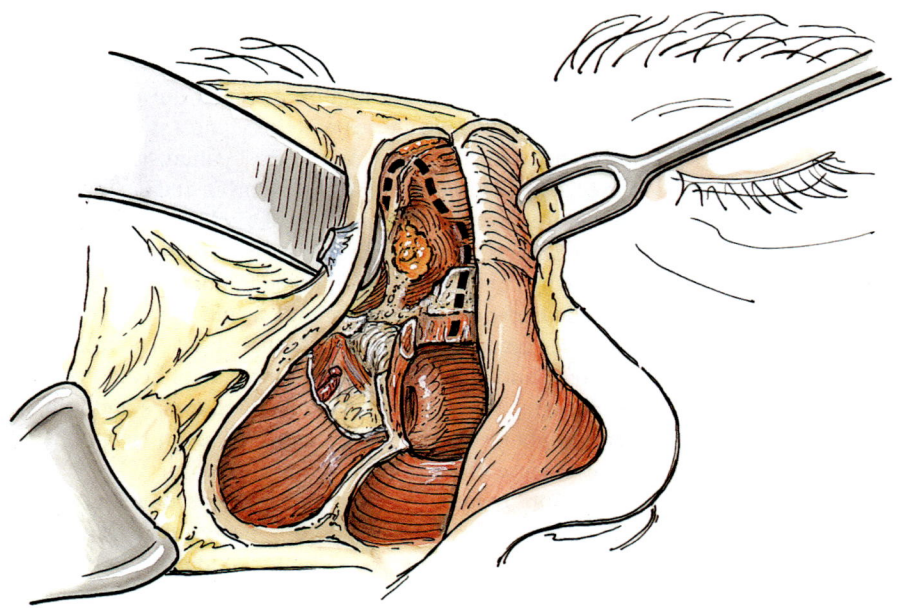

FIG. 19. Resection of sphenoid sinus and lateral sphenoid sinus wall outlined. Minimal cavernous sinus invasion can be managed through this route.

Orbital exenteration includes in these cases the periorbita as well as some or all of the bony walls. The medial wall, the lamina papyracea, the floor, and the maxillary roof are almost always resected. Violation of the orbital roof by tumor is managed in the intracranial portion of the excision. Lateral extension into the infratemporal fossa is decidedly rare and easily managed. Tumor penetration at the orbital apex is the most challenging exigency in management. The superior aspect of the apex above and lateral to the optic canal is at the posterior limit of the anterior cranial fossa floor. The lateral wall in the posterior orbit faces the anterior reach of the middle cranial fossa; more anteriorly, it is related to the infratemporal fossa. The region of the apex contains the optic canal, the superior orbital fissure superolaterally (leading inferiorly to the foramen rotundum), and medially the thickened posterior extent of the lamina papyracea. Extending inferolaterally from the foramen rotundum is the inferior orbital fissure. Related to the medial wall are the posterior ethmoid cells, the cell of Onodi (if present), and the sphenoid sinus (see Chapter 2 for more on anatomy).

Inclusion of the lids in the resection is another important consideration. Proximity of tumor makes their inclusion mandatory. In the absence of involvement, decision making centers around the potential for rehabilitation and the opportunity for postoperative inspection of the cavity for possible complications, as well as the ability to detect any early local recurrence during the follow-up period. Because of the disappointment accompanying inadequate aesthetic rehabilitation of the eye and the ease of both cavity cleansing and inspection, the author's surgical team usually sacrifices the eyelids. Aesthetic rehabilitation is done with an onlay prosthesis, often anchored by interosseous implants.

Technique

Although the lids are sacrificed, as much periorbital skin as possible is preserved for use in cavity lining. Before incision, a 3-0 silk tarsorrhaphy suture is placed for easy traction. The secret of conducting a clean exenteration is preserving the integrity of the periorbita, thus staying outside the periorbital fat. Within the limits of sound oncologic judgment, an incision is made outside the limits of the tarsal plates, but not through the septum orbitale (Fig. 20). Dissection between skin and orbicularis oculi is carried up to the orbital rims (Fig. 21). With lid skin involvement, incision through periorbital skin directly down to the bone of orbital rim is done in a circumferential manner (Fig. 22). Much of the periosteal elevation is easy, but there are three major points of tethering: the trochlea and the medial and lateral canthal tendons. Dissection into the trochlear fossa in the anterosuperior aspect of the orbit will prize out the trochlea and its attachment to the superior oblique muscle tendon. Sharp incision at the canthal tendons, especially the lateral, is necessary to free the periorbita. Dissection with an elevator is done with ease until the area of the infraorbital fissure where,

again, more vigor is required to complete the freeing of tissue to the apex.

A right-angled clamp is placed around the soft tissues of the orbital apex and the area transected with right-angled scissors (Fig. 23). Hemostasis is secured with a 3-0 silk suture ligature. Depending on tumor extent, a greater amount of orbital apical tissue may need to be resected. The first application of the clamp usually encompasses the tissue just anterior to the annulus of Zinn. This fibrous ring is tightly attached to the bone encircling the optic nerve. Firm dissection is required to free this origin of the ocular muscles. Once the globe is removed, the ophthalmic artery is now more easily identifiable. A second echelon of orbital tissue around the optic nerve is now removed (Fig. 24). All that is left now is the optic nerve stump and ophthalmic artery as they exit the optic canal and the stump ends of the cranial nerves and the ophthalmic vein in the superior orbital fissure. A margin of healthy, uninvolved tissue may require a burring away of the optic canal (Fig. 25). This bone is quite thick, but often thins out as it transverses the superolateral wall of the sphenoid sinus. This dissection can be carried out all the way to the optic chiasm (Fig. 26). In general, only microscopic involvement of the nerve with tumor limited to the nerve sheath can be managed by this maneuver. Gross tumor involvement usually requires the addition of intracranial exposure.

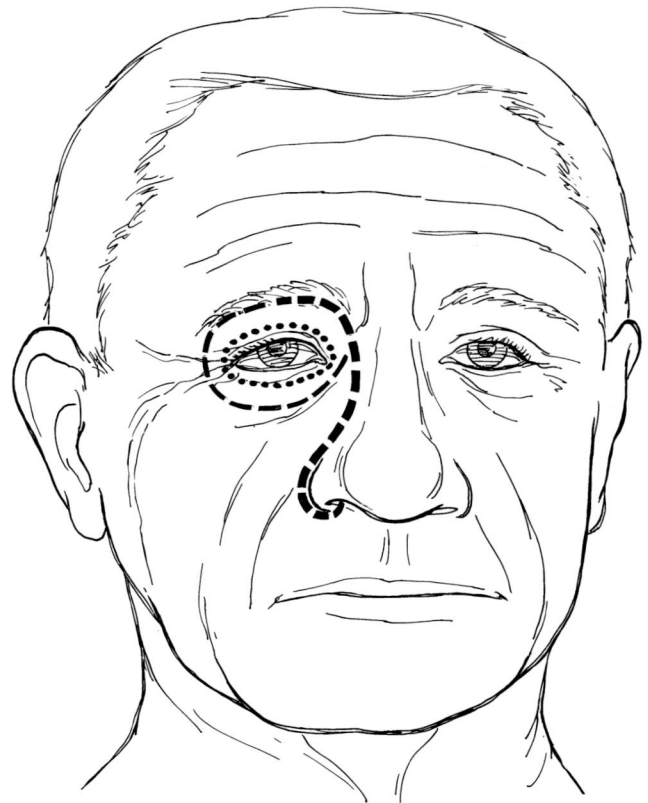

FIG. 20. Periorbital skin incision.

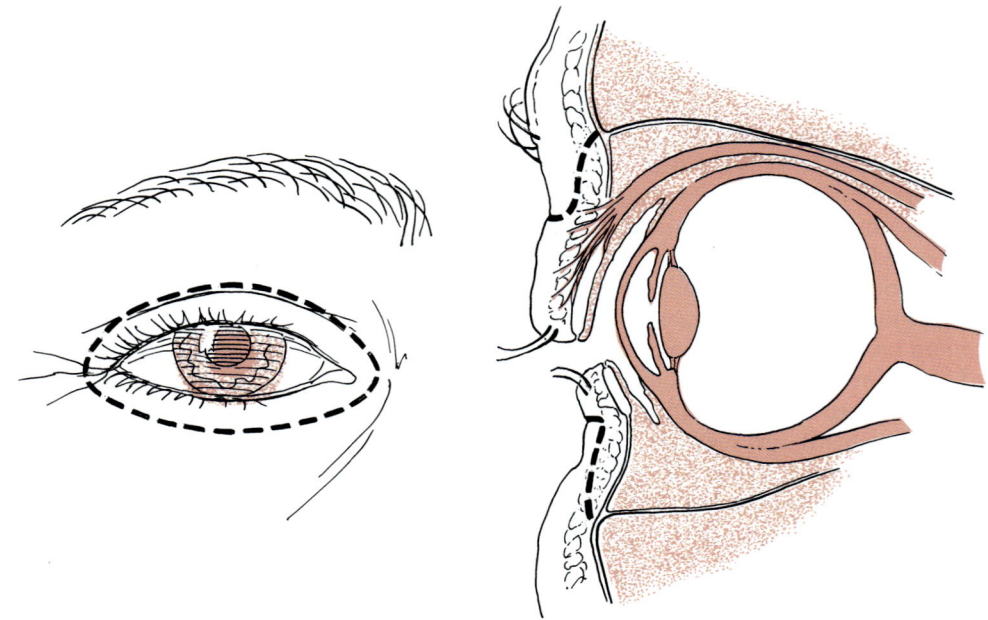

FIG. 21. Dissection between lid skin and orbicularis oculi up to the periorbital rims.

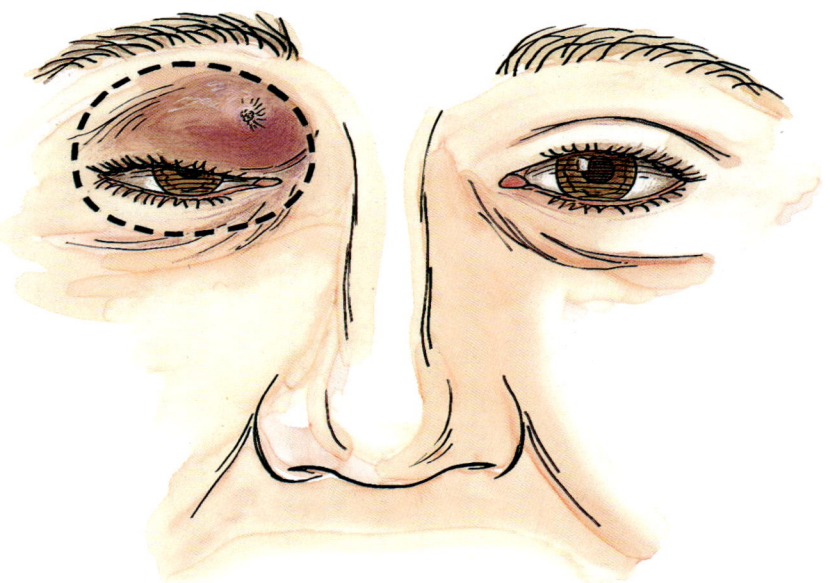

FIG. 22. Wide margin of lid skin resected around tumor penetrating upper eyelid.

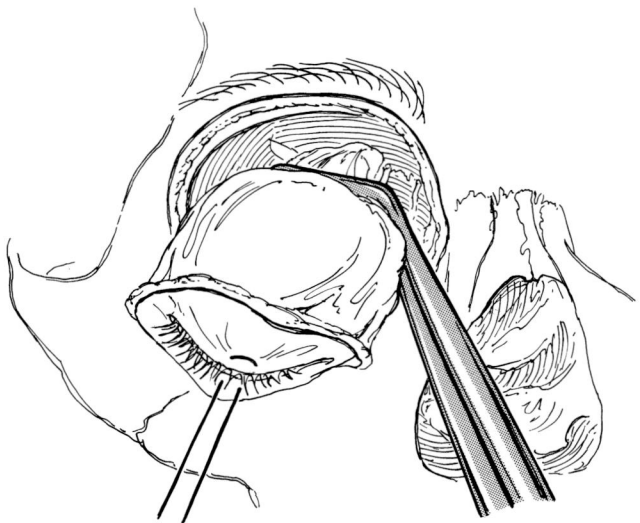

FIG. 23. Right-angled clamp placed around soft tissues of orbital apex, which are transected with right-angled scissors.

Similarly, tumor extension through the superior orbital fissure requires craniotomy that provides access to the middle fossa. Extension along the vidian nerve mandates drilling the sphenoid bone surrounding it, leading to the foramen lacerum and the region of the petrous apex, thus further mandating an intracranial approach to the middle fossa and the potential need for management of the internal carotid artery. Infraorbital nerve involvement mandates a drilling out of the foramen rotundum and amputation of the nerve at the level of the dura, then a frozen-section check for tumor. If even a scant deposit of tumor is found at this site, an intracranial exploration of Meckel's cave is required.

Maxillectomy

Tumor invasion of the maxillary sinus infrastructure (Fig. 27), that is, that part of the sinus below Ohngren's line, necessitates maxillectomy. This usually takes the form of an "inferior maxillectomy," in which the eye and usually the floor of the orbit can be spared. However, the maxillectomy must be tailored to tumor extent. It is not uncommon for the nasal septum, facial soft tissues, orbital contents, and even facial skin to be involved with tumor in these advanced cases. Tumors above Ohngren's line, that is, involving the posterosuperior maxilla, carried in the past a dire prognosis (5–7). Invasion of the orbit is common. Extension through the posterior maxillary wall, with involvement of the pterygomaxillary space and infratemporal fossa, were considered by many experts to be signs of inoperability. Until the report of Ketcham et al. (8), patients with extension into the intracranial space were adjudged doomed to die of their disease. Tumors that are primary in the maxilla have commonly attained considerable size by the time they have invaded the

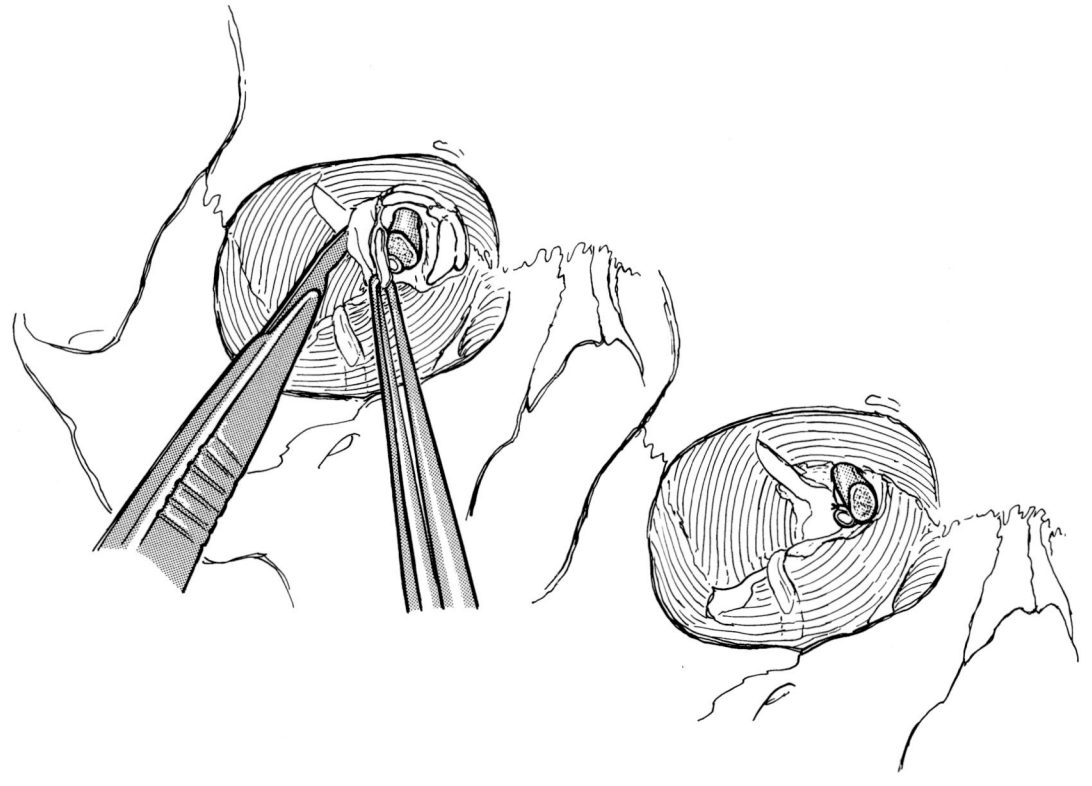

FIG. 24. Second echelon of orbital apex tissue resected to establish resection margin.

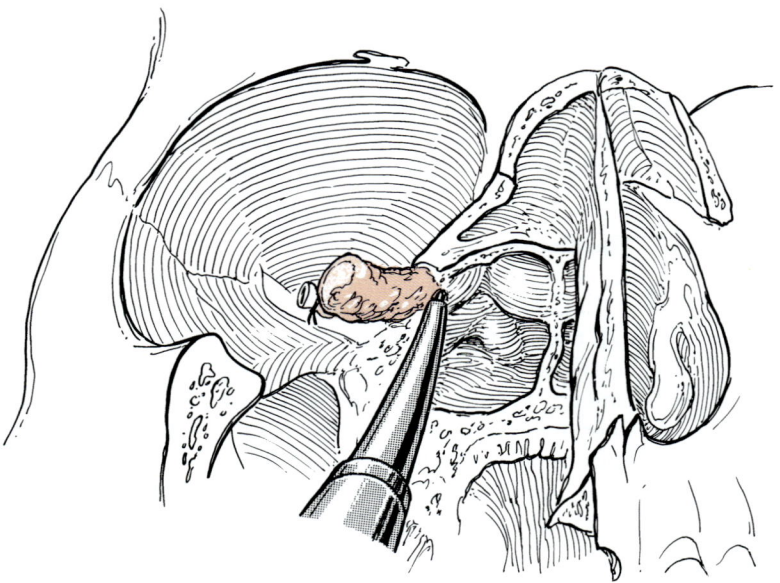

FIG. 25. Resection of optic canal with cutting bur to attain a tumor-free margin along optic nerve.

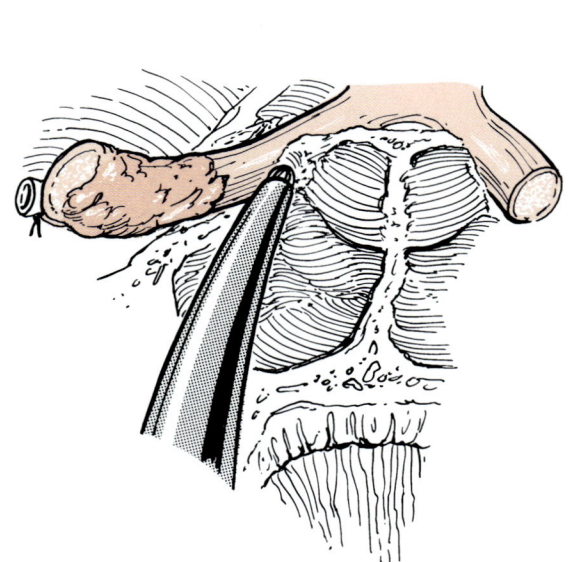

FIG. 26. Dissection along the optic nerve can be carried to the optic chiasm.

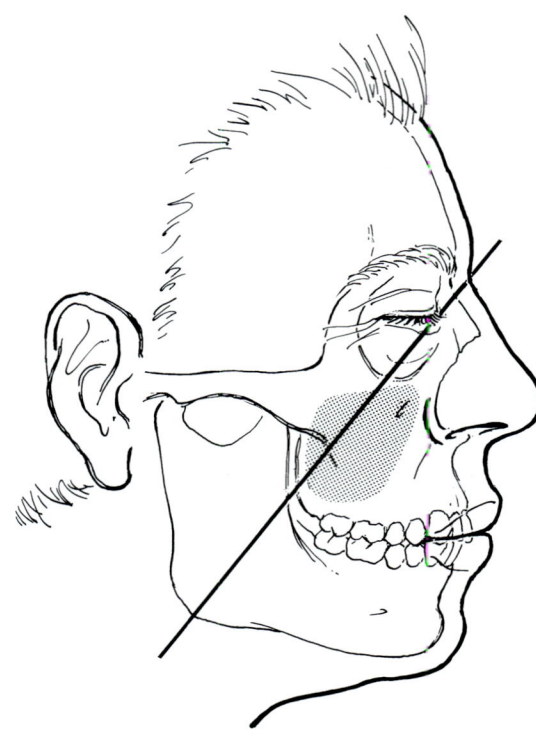

FIG. 27. Ohngren's line dividing the maxillary sinus into an infrastructure and superstructure. From a lateral view, the line runs from the medial canthus to the mandibular angle.

intracranial space. When tumor originates in the ethmoid block, the tumor may invade the superior maxilla and spare the palatal portion, and commonly invades the anterior cranial fossa. Superior maxillectomy then substantially preserves function and aesthetics.

In most cases, a complete maxillectomy is required. The Weber-Fergusson incision is used and the superior part is not unlike the lateral rhinotomy incision, except that an incision encircling the eye is made if an orbital exenteration is to be done, or a single limb extending under the lid if the eye is to be spared (Fig. 28). A dart in the nasal sill (I.P. Janecka, *personal communication*, 1994) and another in the upper lip, preserving the sucking tubercle of the vermilion, helps to prevent later scar contracture. Extending the vertical component of the incision down the philtral crest also helps to improve aesthetics. The incision is carried along the gingival-buccal sulcus, skirting any tumor penetration by a margin of at least 2 cm of healthy mucosal tissue. The cut curves around the maxillary tuberosity and stays close to the teeth on the palatal side unless tumor has extended into palatal mucosa. The 2-cm rule is used if such is the case, namely that the malignancy must be skirted by a 2-cm rim of healthy tissue.

The cut through the maxillary alveolar bone is either through the socket of the canine tooth or that of the lateral incisor. The involved tooth is extracted, taking care to preserve an intact lamina dura around the adjacent remaining tooth. This is essential because this will be the anchor for an eventual maxillofacial prosthesis.

The exposure of the nasal part, the ethmoidectomy, and maxillotomy are done in a manner similar to that described for the lateral rhinotomy. The exception is the antrostomy portion, which should be sufficient only to view the interior of the sinus. Although valuable clues to tumor extent are provided by the preoperative radiographic examination, precise appreciation of tumor extent can be achieved only through direct inspection. The antrostomy provides such an opportunity.

When tumor does not breach the walls of the sinus, a subperiosteal dissection of soft tissue is done over the anterior and lateral extent of the maxilla. When skin and soft tissue are invaded, the previously described requisite 2-cm margin is included, attached to the main specimen (Fig. 29). When the orbit is uninvolved, an uncommon occurrence in malignant tumors of the superior maxilla, a dissection of the periorbita from the orbital floor is done, exposing the bone to the level of posterior margin of the maxillary sinus. An attempt is made to preserve the attachments of both canthal tendons and the integrity of the lacrimal sac and fossa. These exigencies, especially the latter, are dictated by tumor extent. The palatal bone is separated from its overlying mucoperiosteum up to the midline. The muscles of the soft palate are cut away from the posterior margin of the hard palate. If the septum and nasal floor are free of tumor, a mucosal incision in the nasal floor is made from the pyriform rim to the junction of hard and soft palate. Tumor in the septum or floor requires septectomy and incision through the opposing nasal floor. Alveolar ridge excision is correspondingly tailored to tumor extent.

The bony cuts are now inscribed with a power saw or the Midas Rex blade. The cuts are outlined in Fig. 30. The lateral orbital rim, zygomatic eminence, and palate are incised. The superior medial cut connects the lateral rhinotomy cut to the ethmoidectomy. Obviously, the intracranial extension of tumor is exposed by now, and in extensive tumors, the neoplasm is cut across at this point. Smaller, more easily encompassed tumors are circumscribed in preparation for the

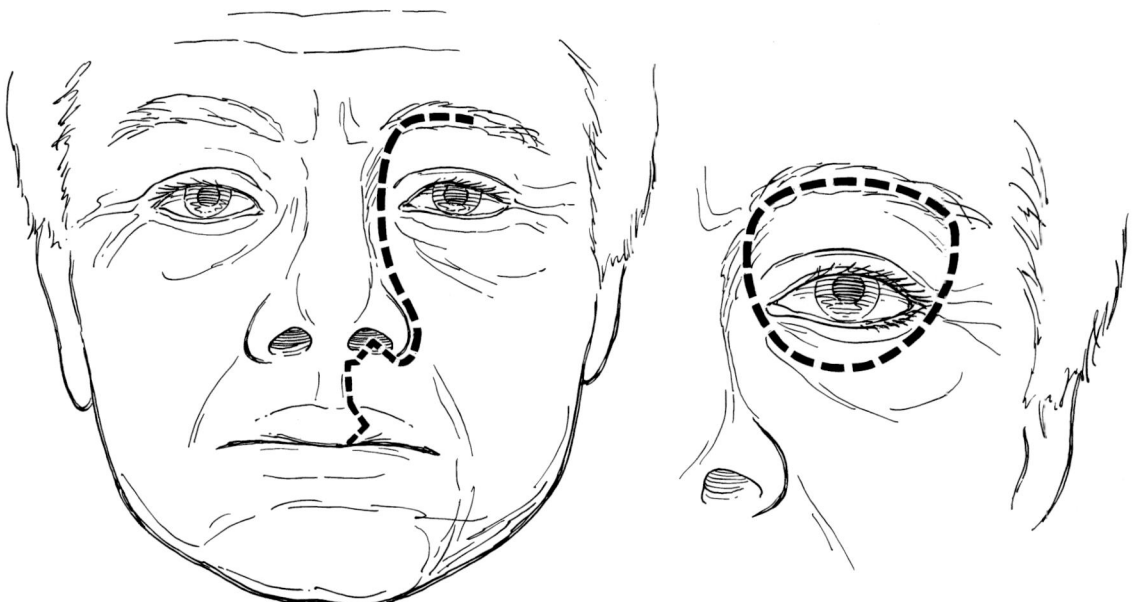

FIG. 28. Weber-Fergusson incision. Note darts in nasal sill and surrounding sucking tubercle of upper lip. (From Donald PJ, Gluckman JL, Rice DH, eds. *The sinuses.* New York: Raven Press, 1995:468.)

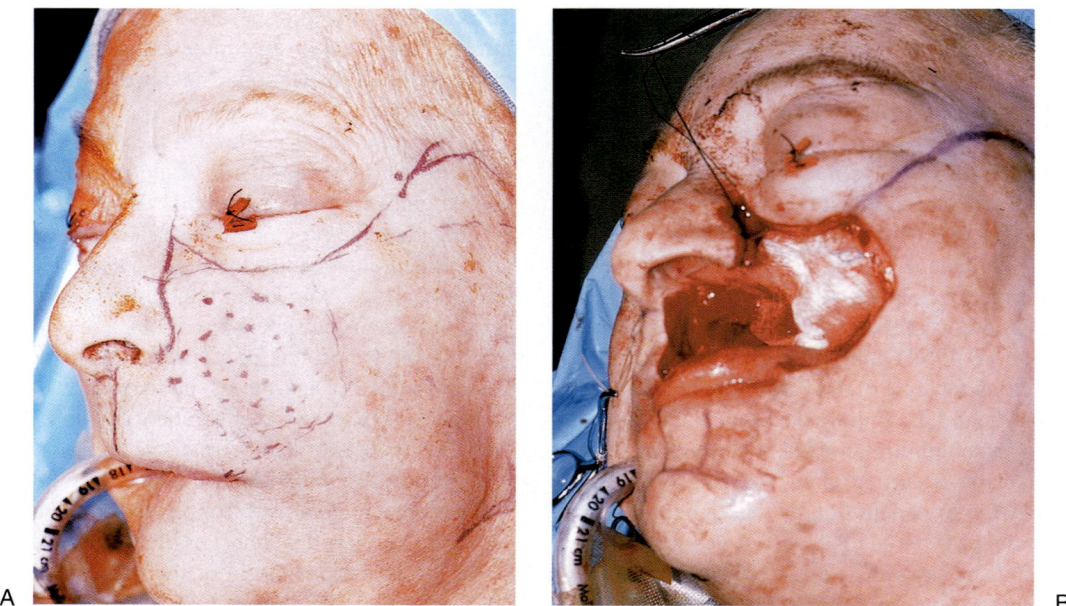

FIG. 29. Margin of healthy soft tissue including skin removed to ensure complete tumor exenteration. **A:** Weber-Fergusson incision drawn. Area of skin infiltration is outlined. **B:** Tumor resected. Cervicofacial rotation flap is outlined for reconstruction.

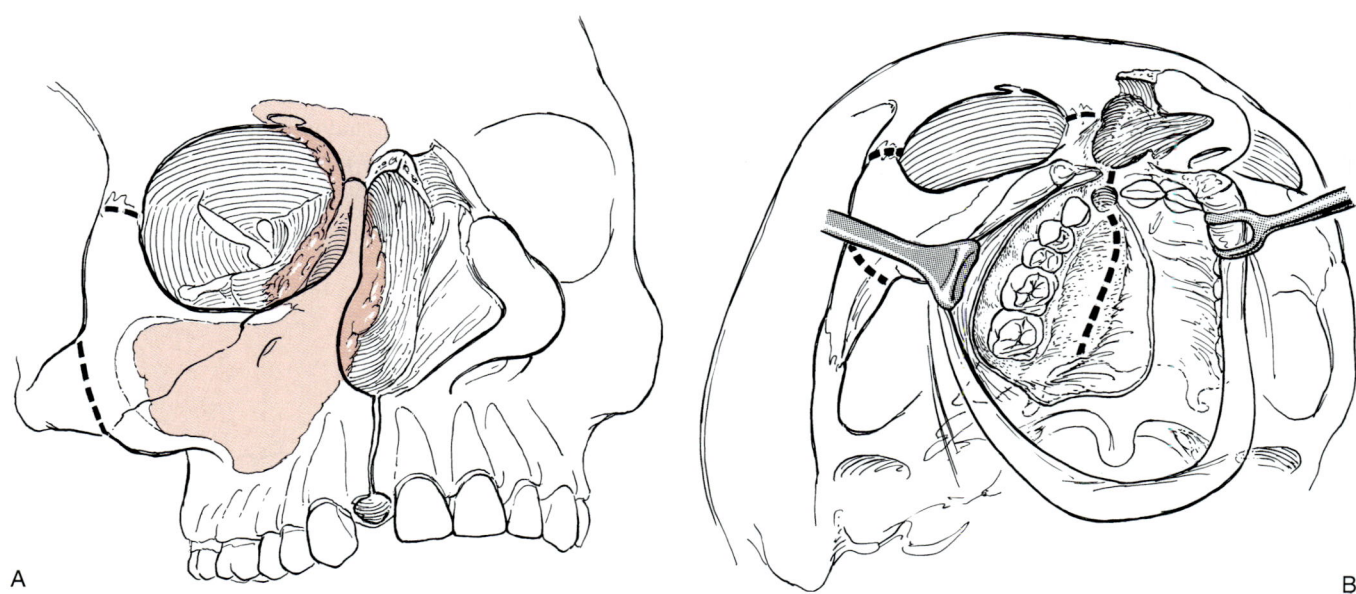

FIG. 30. Bony cuts for total maxillectomy. **A:** Through lateral orbital rim, zygomatic buttress, alveolar ridge, and nasal floor (ethmoid and nasal cut already done by lateral rhinotomy). **B:** Through palate, preserving as much palatal mucoperiosteum as possible.

intracranial exposure. In most cases, the tumor is transected at the ethmoid level. If only minor invasion of the zygomatic recess exists, the malar eminence can be preserved and the interior of the body of the zygoma excised with a drill, preserving a shell of overlying bone (Fig. 31) and thus maintaining the important aesthetics of this prominent facial feature. The lateral orbital wall is incised posteriorly as high up and as far posteriorly as dictated by tumor extent.

As the palate is cut, care is taken to preserve as much length as possible of the mucoperiosteal flap. This flap will

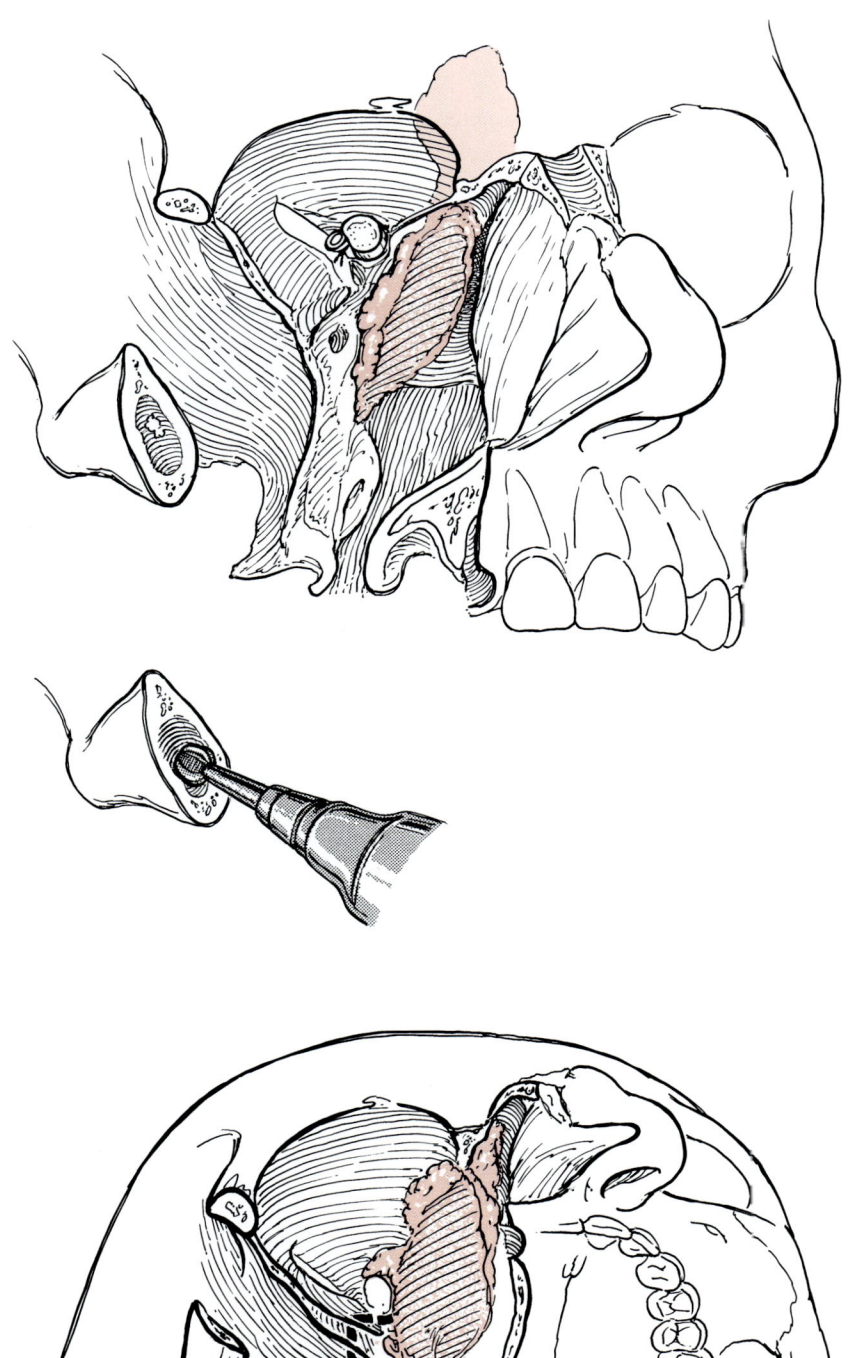

FIG. 31. Minimal tumor involvement of zygomatic recess removed with the cutting bur.

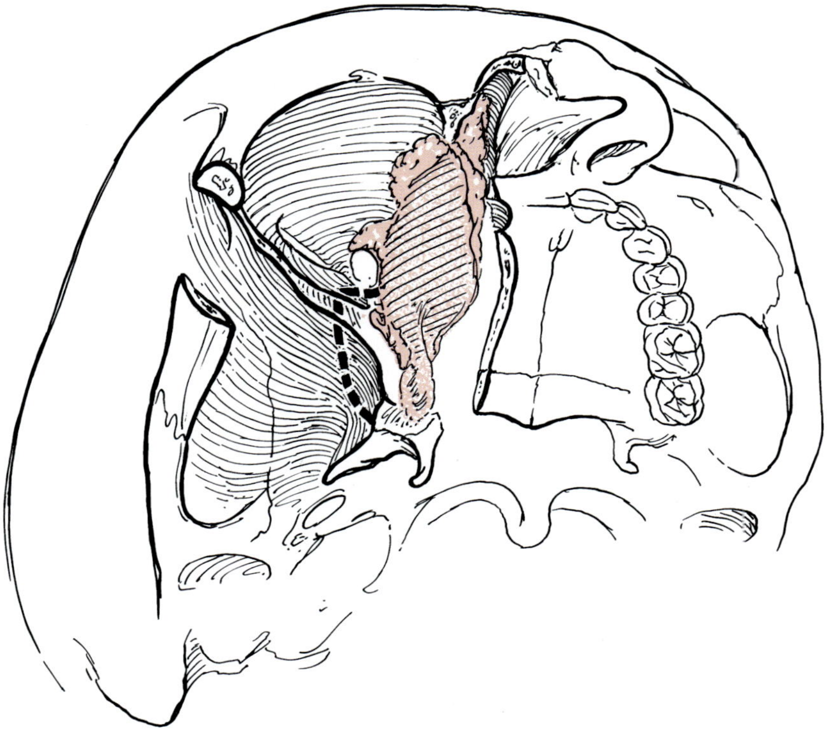

FIG. 32. Residual triangular piece of bone, remnant of maxillectomy. Tumor remains and can be removed with cutting bur.

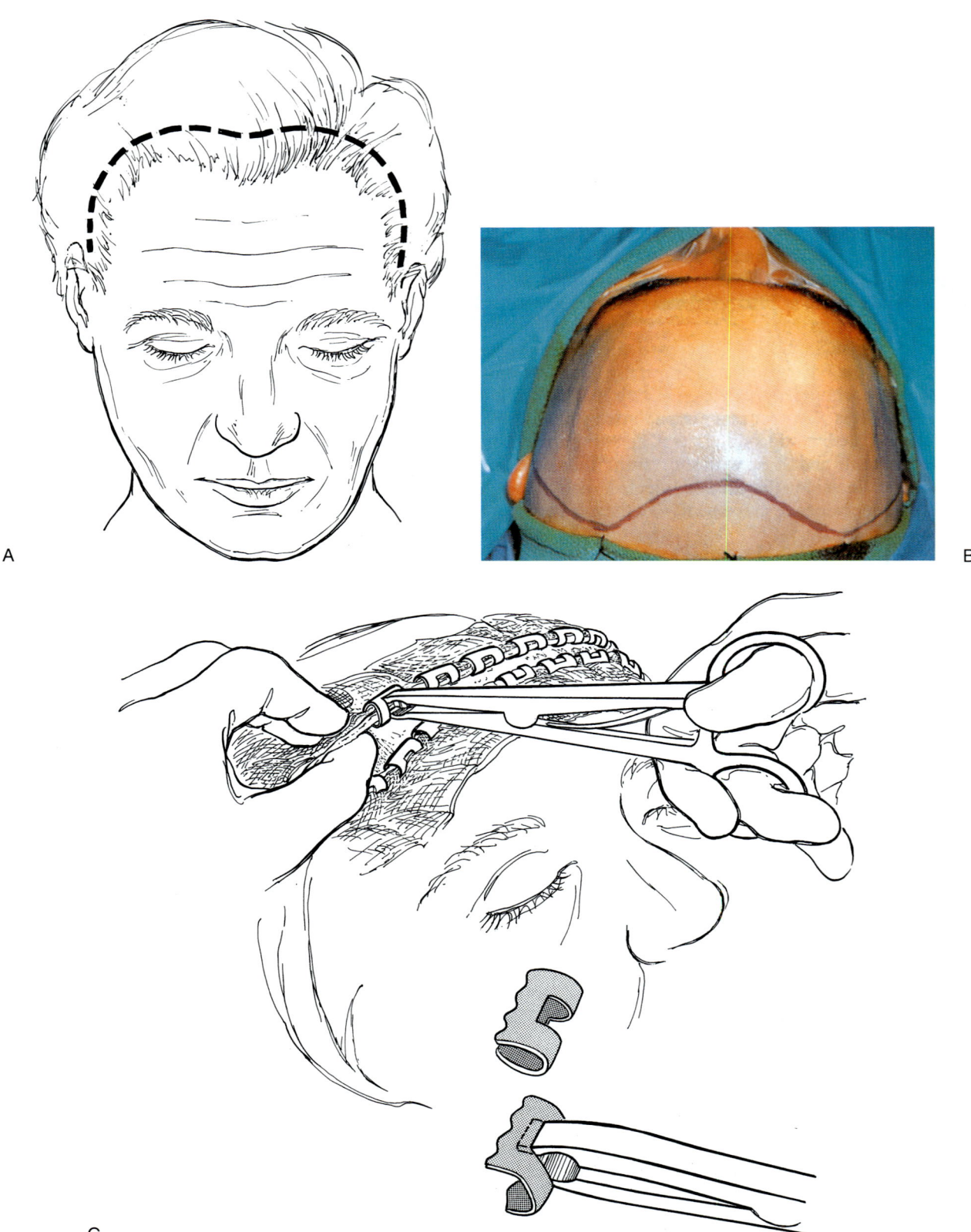

FIG. 33. A: Bicoronal scalp incision. **B:** Coronal incision marked out. **C:** Flap turned with Rainey clips in place. The flap edge is folded over by 4 × 4s and the clips applied. Inset shows clip and clip applier. (From Donald PJ, Gluckman JL, Rice DH, eds. *The sinuses*. New York: Raven Press, 1995:219–220.)

be used later to cover the cut edge of palatal and alveolar bone. This provides a durable epithelial covering that resists the trauma of the maxillary prosthesis used in subsequent rehabilitation (see Fig. 30B).

The last bony incision that finally mobilizes the maxilla is the posterior cut that separates the sinus from the pterygoid plates. A curved osteotome is placed between the maxillary tuberosity and the base of the plates. Sharp blows with a mallet or separation with a power cutting tool will separate these structures. Scissors are used to remove all remaining soft tissue attachments and the maxilla is removed.

What remains now is a small, triangular area on the posterior maxillary wall that comprises a small portion of maxillary sinus and the anterior, vertically disposed junction of the pterygoid plates on the ascending process of the palatine bone (see Fig. 16; Fig. 32). Superiorly, the floor of the orbit will have fractured at the site where it joins the posterior wall of the maxilla, near the orbital apex, during the maxillary extraction because of the thinness of this plate. The amputated stump of the infraorbital nerve is readily apparent and is an important structure to follow in the neurotropic tumors so often encountered in skull base surgery.

It can be appreciated now that with the exception of some debulking in large tumors and the cutting across of the intracranial and immediately extracranial component, the maxilla and its contained tumor are removed in one block. The intracranial portion can be outlined both from below and above and removed in a second block. In smaller tumors, the entire lesion can be removed in a single piece, with the intracranial and extracranial parts remaining connected and the *en bloc* principle preserved. This is desirable but not essential for total safe tumor removal.

In some cases, after the subcranial removal has been effected with the maxillectomy, there are tumor remnants at the orbital apex, the sphenoid sinus, and the root of the pterygoid plates. Their removal is accomplished as described in the previous section. All that now remains is the craniotomy.

Craniotomy

The craniotomy is tailored according to the extent of involvement of the anterior fossa floor, the subcranial tumor location, and the degree of dural or frontal lobe invasion. A bicoronal scalp incision is made, running 2 to 3 cm behind the hairline (Fig. 33). The incision is extended to the level of the root of the auricular helices and carried to the level of, but not through, the pericranium. The scalp is elevated posterior to the incision to provide access for the creation of a generous pericranial flap. Hemostatic clips, such as Rainey clips, are placed at the scalp edges for hemostasis. The flap is elevated in the subgaleal plane down to the brows, then to the lateral orbital walls laterally and just below the nasal glabella medially. A semicircular cuff of temporalis fascia is included in the flap to avoid injury to the ramus frontalis of the facial nerve (Fig. 34).

A large flap of pericranial tissue is created that will be used for later reconstruction (Fig. 35). Great care is exer-

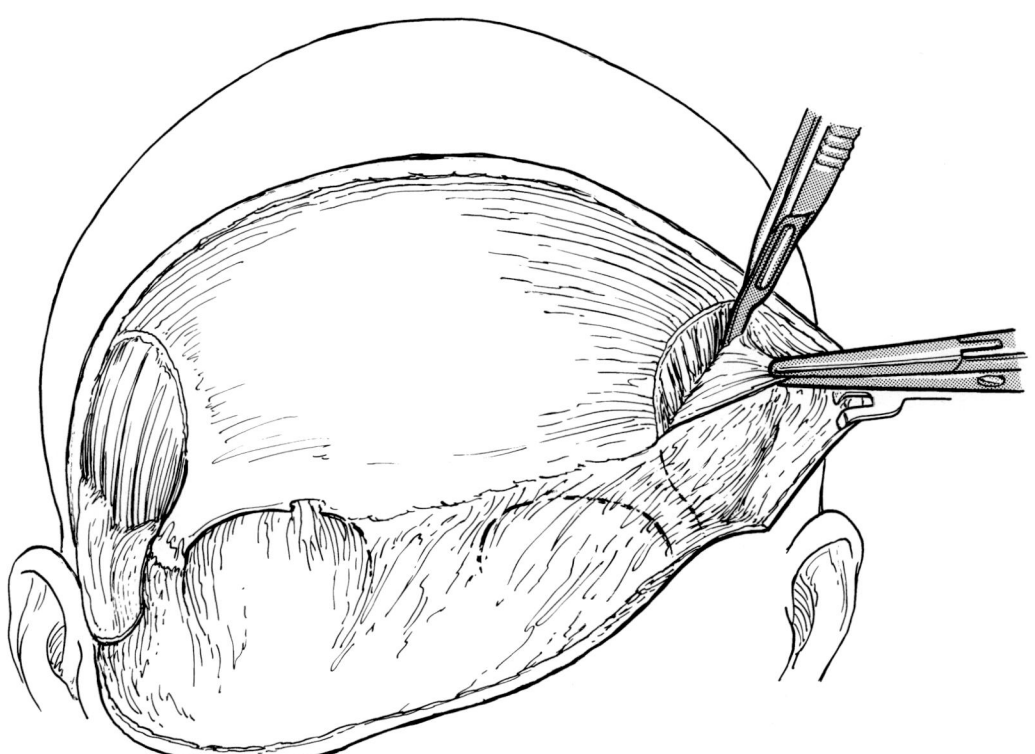

FIG. 34. A semilunar cuff of temporalis fascia is included in the skin flap.

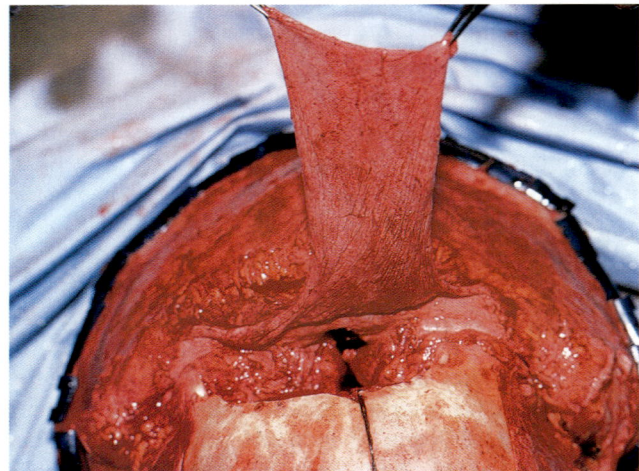

FIG. 35. Pericranial flap.

cised to keep it moist and protected during the operation to preserve its viability.

The superior orbital rim is exposed consonant with the width of the proposed craniotomy. The width, height, and position relative to the orbits are dictated by tumor factors. A variety of bone flaps have been designed to accommodate this. The flap design must take into account how far posteriorly the tumor extends. As dissection proceeds over the brows, the supratrochlear and supraorbital neurovascular bundles are exposed. Great care is taken to preserve them. Often, the supraorbital nerve emanates from a small bony canal. The canal wall adjacent to the orbital cavity is often merely composed of a small bar of bone, easily removed with a rongeur. If tumor penetrates the roof of the posterior ethmoid cells or the planum sphenoidale, intracranial exposure must accommodate dural elevation almost to the sphenoid ridge. Exposure must enable the placement of dural sutures once resection is complete because the necessity of providing a watertight closure is an absolute mandate in these cases to prevent cerebrospinal fluid leak and the possibility of infection. Bringing the craniotomy down to or even

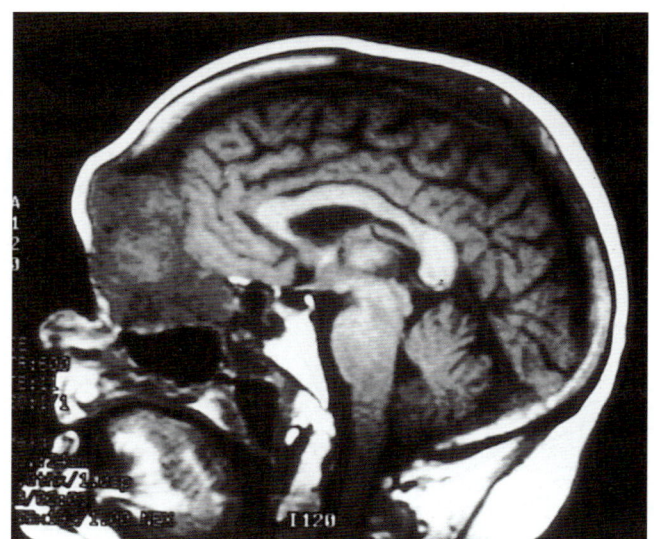
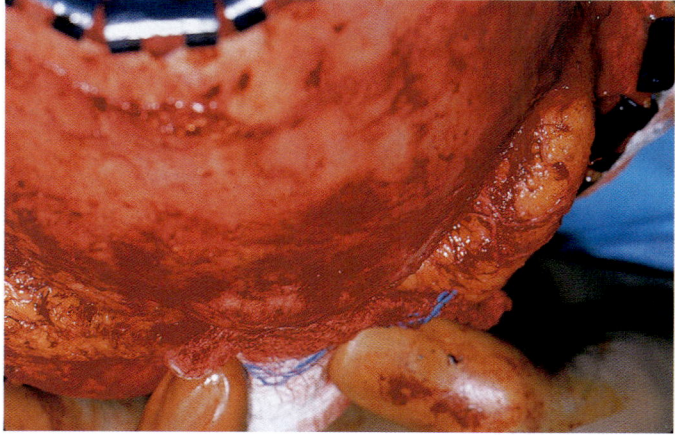
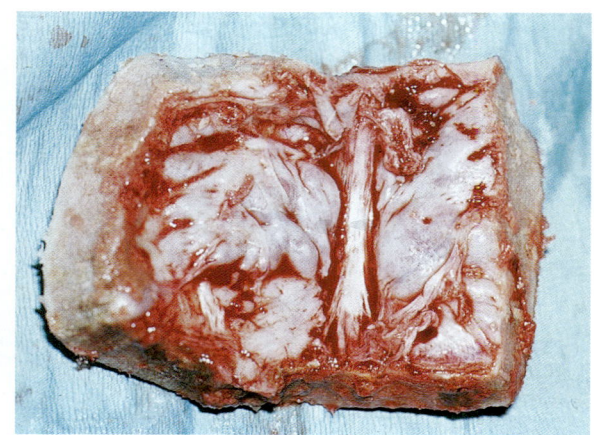

FIG. 36. Calvarial invasion by tumor. **A:** Lateral magnetic resonance image showing bony invasion. **B:** Intraoperative photograph showing calvarial bulging from tumor invasion. **C:** Operative specimen showing tumor in dura and bone.

including the orbital rims and roof may be necessary to enable the visualization of the posterior limits of tumor. There may be dural involvement over the anterior convexity of the frontal lobes or in the falx. Even the superior sagittal sinus may be invaded. Occasionally, the anterior calvarium is transgressed by tumor and requires resection (Fig. 36). Adequate exposure to remove cancer in the frontal lobe requires a more extensive craniotomy. A number of different craniotomies to accommodate anterior skull base resection are illustrated in Fig. 37.

Many tumors have minimal intracranial penetration, and these are often anteriorly located. A limited, but adequate, exposure can be achieved through the frontal sinus, especially if it is capacious enough. This is accomplished by applying a template of the sinus configuration cut out of a 5-foot Caldwell-view radiograph. This procedure is similar to that done for the osteoplastic flap and fat obliteration of the frontal sinus for inflammatory disease. The shape of the sinus is outlined with methylene blue and a nonsiliconized needle. A series of holes done with a small penetrating bur

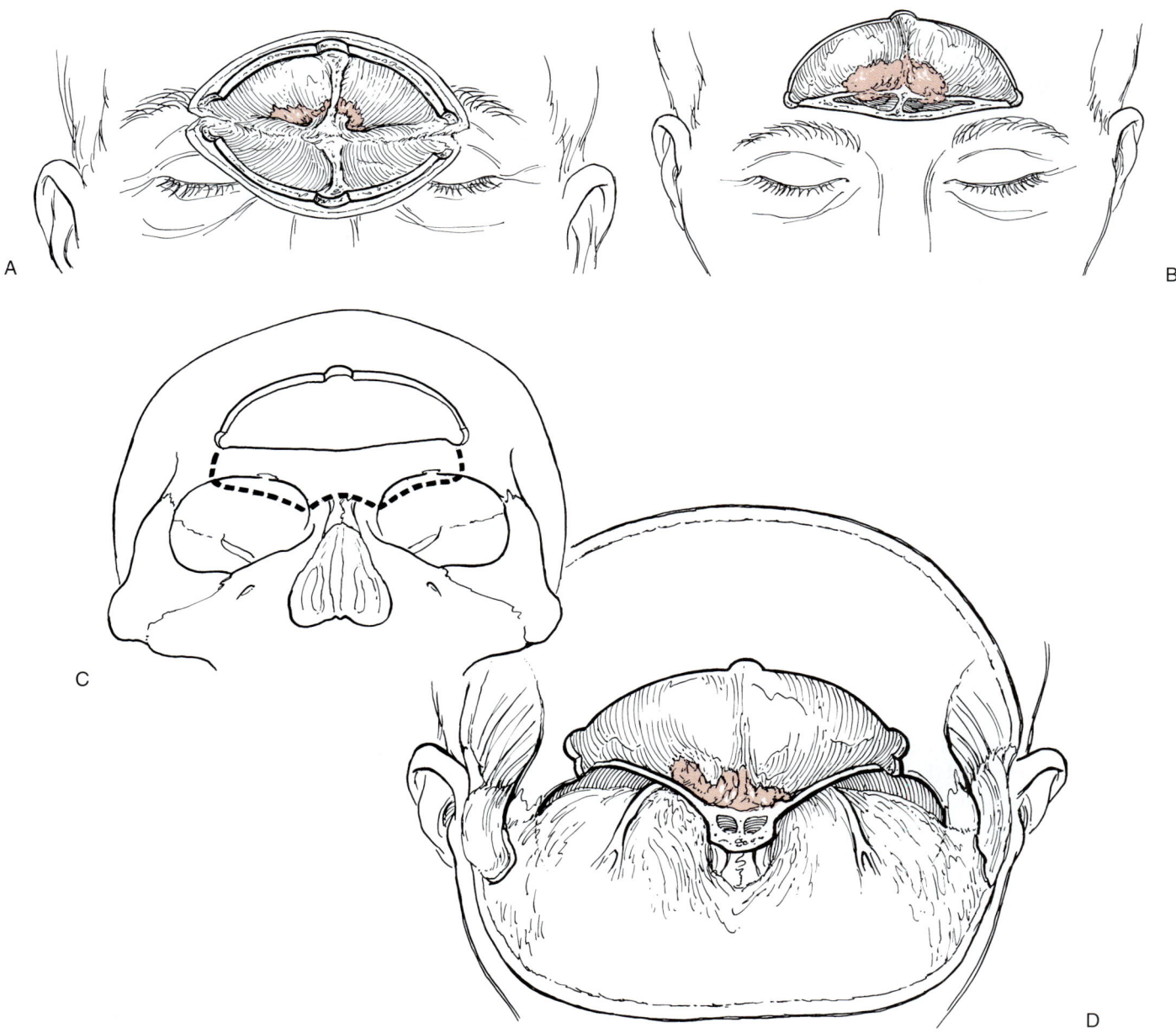

FIG. 37. Craniotomies designed for various anterior skull base exposures. **A:** Osteoplastic flap. **B:** Standard low craniotomy preserving the brow. **C:** Low craniotomy including supraorbital bandeau. **D:** Exposure after craniotomy in **(C)**.

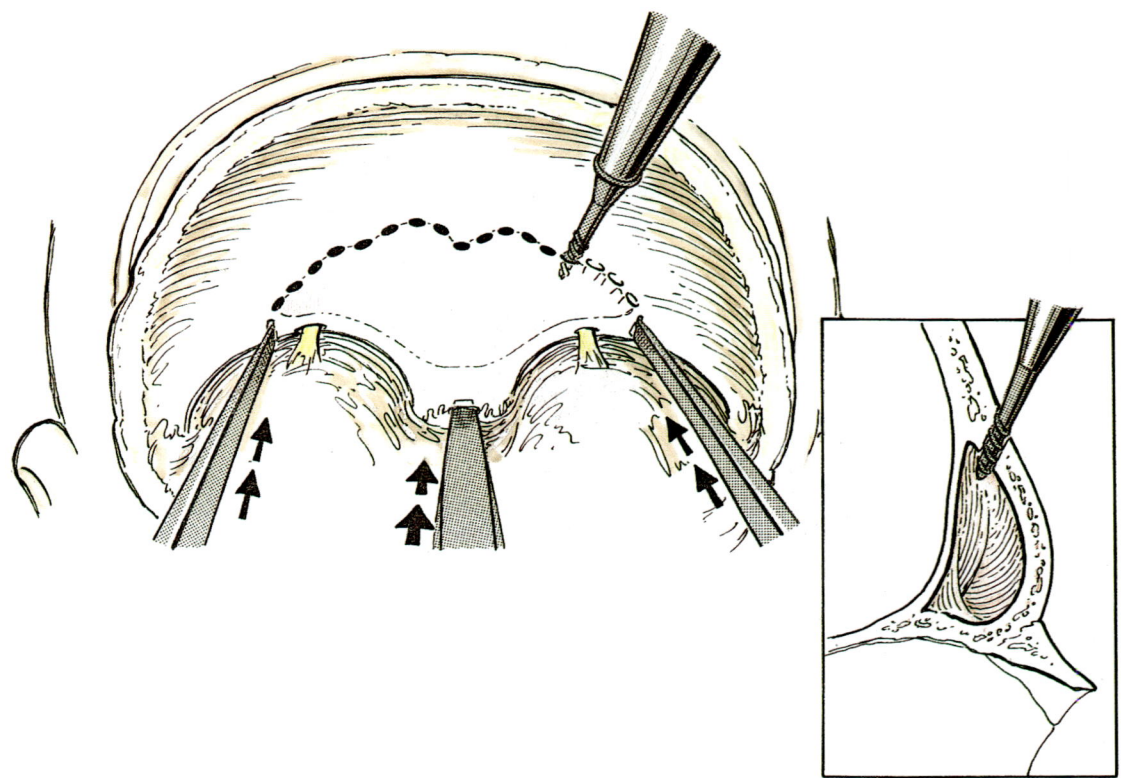

FIG. 38. Osteoplastic flap outlined.

follow this inscribed outline (Fig. 38). These are connected with a small osteotome, the Midas Rex blade, or the footed craniotomy tool. Both the bur holes and the osteotome are angled to create an oblique cut to prevent later prolapse of the flap when it is restored at the conclusion of the case. The intersinus septum is transected with a broad, flat osteotome and the osteoplastic flap fractured forward. The flap will be greenstick fractured over the anterior roofs of the orbits and through the root of the nose. Osteotome cuts judiciously placed at the lateral extremities of the frontal sinus and through the root of the nose facilitate this down-fracturing of the flap. The interior of the frontal sinus is now exposed and all mucosa is removed (Fig. 39). It is essential to bur away a thin layer of the bone of the flap's inner side to remove all mucosal remnants at the completion of tumor removal.

The posterior wall and floor of the sinus are removed. Sometimes tumor penetrates the floor, and this is included in the resected block (see Fig. 39B). Care is taken to elevate and protect dura as the removal of the posterior wall proceeds. The frontal sinus floor, which in some instances is quite extensive, is removed as well as the frontonasal ducts. With the exception of the anterior wall, the sinus has been entirely eliminated. When near the midline, it is important to remember that the superior sagittal sinus takes origin in the foramen cecum, just in front of the crista galli. The sagittal sinus arises from here as the termination of the dorsal nasal vein, then ascends along the frontal spine of the posterior frontal sinus wall. Fortunately, the vessel is of little substance near its origin and does not achieve significant size until it reaches the top of the sinus. This, however, is not true in patients with a capacious frontal sinus. Careful dissection preserves its integrity.

In those cases in which a particularly low entrance into the anterior fossa is desired, a low craniotomy combined with resection of the brow in the form of a cranial bandeau is done (see Fig. 37C). A dissection of the periorbita over the orbital roof and detachment of the trochlea provides excellent access to the horizontal portion of the osteotomy (Fig. 40).

In most cases in the author's experience, a modest low craniotomy as outlined in Fig. 37B is used. This transects the frontal sinus in most cases and requires its cranialization at the termination of the procedure.

In the elderly, dural elevation is done very carefully because of its brittleness in this age group. Delineation of dural invasion by tumor is indicated from below but is definitively established from above. Dural entry is made about 1 cm beyond known involvement by neoplasm. Brain retraction is kept to an absolute minimum. Brain slackness is provided by cerebrospinal fluid drainage through a lumbar drain and may be augmented by hypocapnia or diuretics. Usually the head

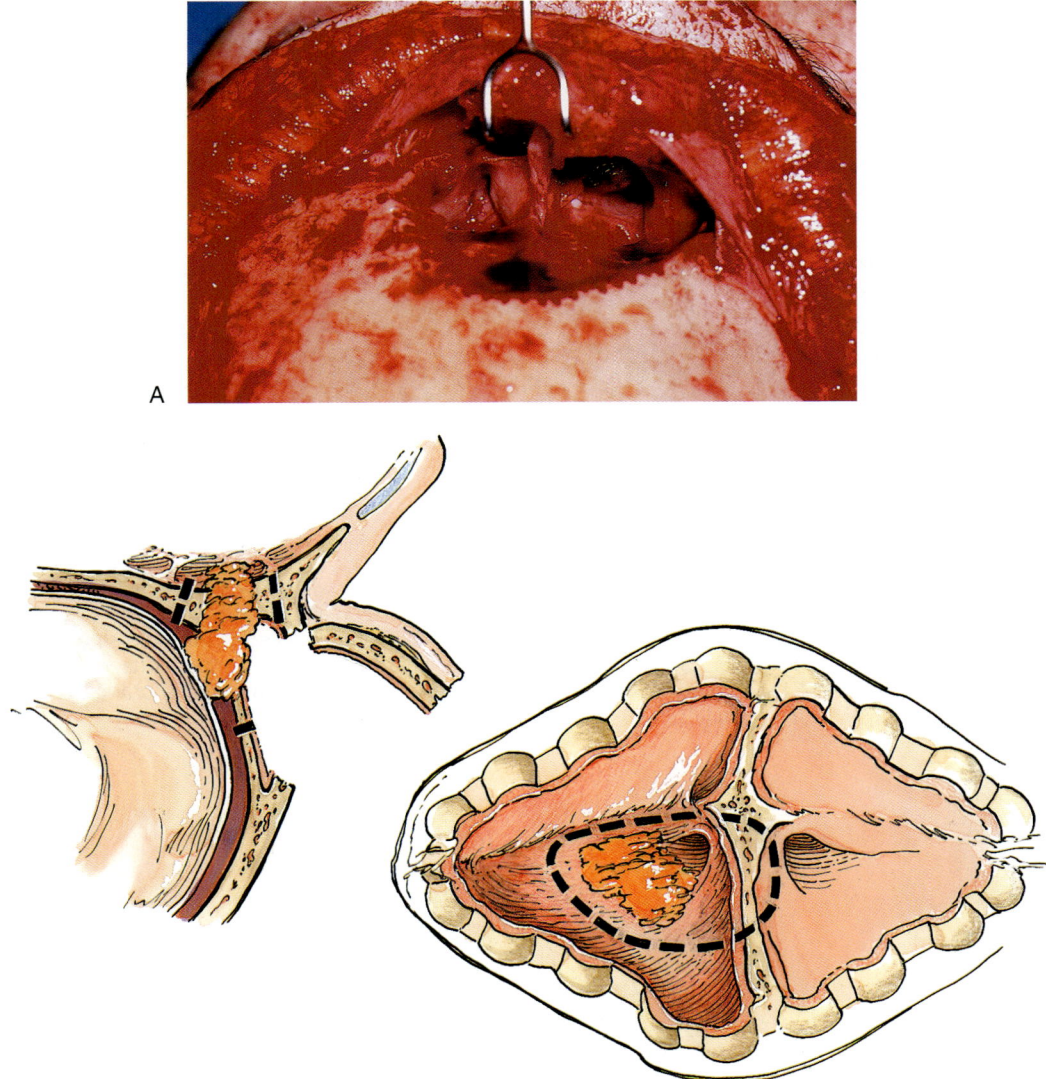

FIG. 39. Osteoplastic flap opened. Tumor is seen penetrating through the floor. **A:** Tumor seen through the floor of the frontal sinus in a patient with carcinoma of the ethmoid sinuses. **B:** Diagram outlining excised bone that will be removed with tumor.

and neck surgeon identifies the margin of healthy bone surrounding the tumor from below, whereas the overlying dura margin is established by the neurosurgeon by direct inspection. He or she places the osteotome and begins to cut the bone, or does so with a cutting bur or blade, while the neurosurgeon protects the brain with a retractor (Fig. 41). Any areas of tumor penetration of brain are skirted, with this part of the resection delayed to comprise the final step in the procedure. When the lesion has finally been encompassed by a margin of healthy tissue, the lesion is pushed from above down through the facial exposure (Fig. 42). Liberal use of frozen-section analysis establishes integrity of dural margins first, and, if involved, areas of invaded brain. It is essential to conduct a complete examination of the exenteration cavity on both the intracranial and extracranial aspects to be sure the tumor has been totally encompassed by the resection.

The amount of brain removal is determined by the neurosurgeon. The technique of brain removal differs somewhat from the standard approach for malignant neoplasms primary to brain substance. Malignancies of the head and neck tend to invade brain substance by a pushing margin, rather than by the diffuse extension that hallmarks the usual spread of central malignancies (see Chapter 4). A 5- to 1-mm margin of healthy tissue usually skirts the microscopic extent of disease. Tumor removal is done with sharp dissection and bipolar cautery rather than suction.

Gross total removal of tumor is not acceptable; only microscopically confirmed, tumor-free margins suffice. The

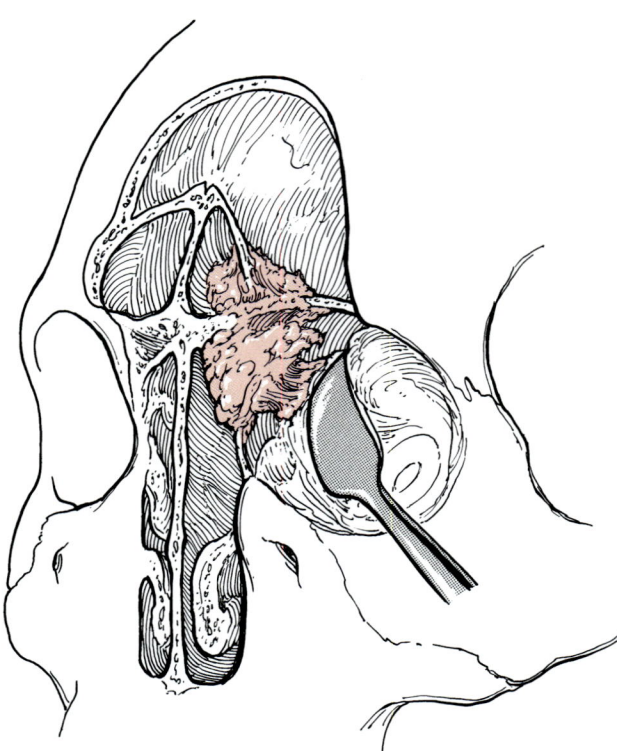

FIG. 40. Tumor arising in ethmoid sinus, penetrating the posterior wall and floor of frontal sinus, exposed by the combination of a low craniotomy and a cranial bandeau that includes the brows.

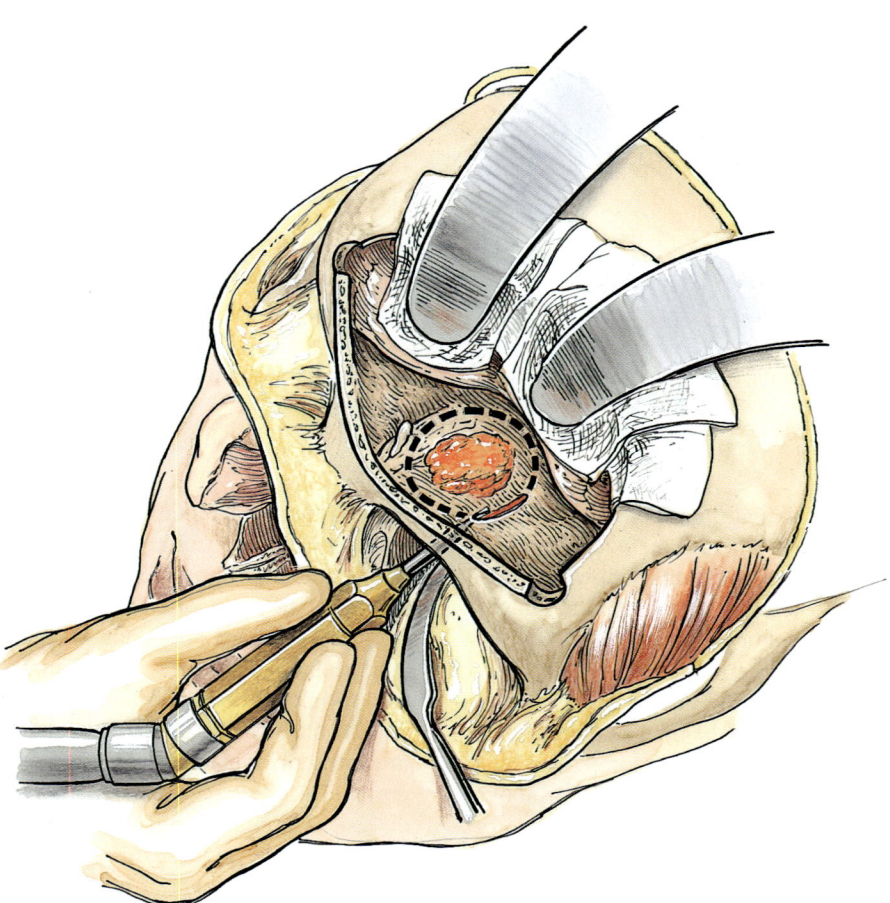

FIG. 41. The neurosurgeon protects the brain from above while the head and neck surgeon outlines the amount of bone resection from below.

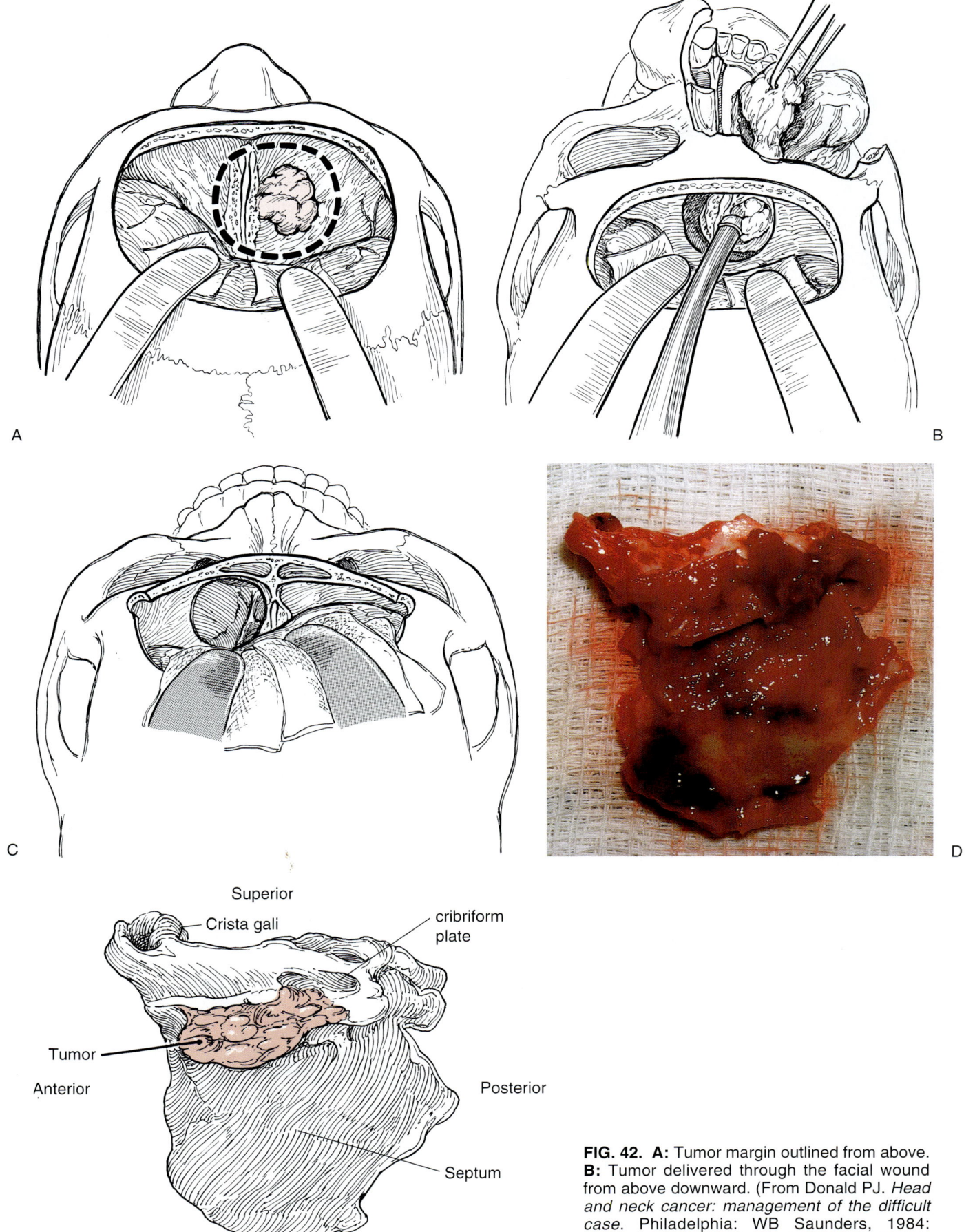

FIG. 42. **A:** Tumor margin outlined from above. **B:** Tumor delivered through the facial wound from above downward. (From Donald PJ. *Head and neck cancer: management of the difficult case.* Philadelphia: WB Saunders, 1984: 192–193.) **C:** Defect in cranial floor. **D:** *En bloc* specimen. **E:** Diagram of specimen.

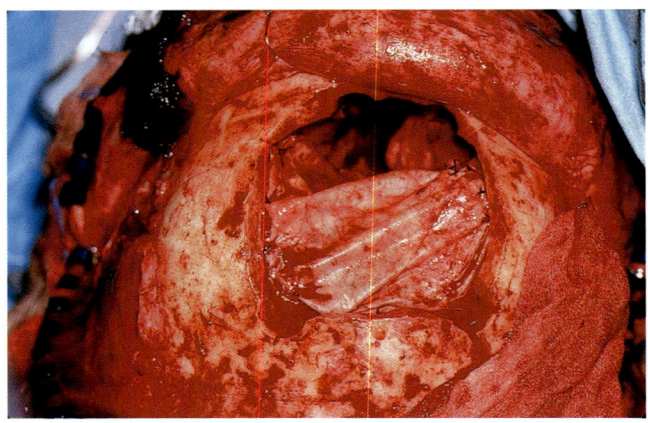

FIG. 43. Lyophilized dural patch used to replace extensive dural area of involvement over frontal lobe.

cavities are liberally lavaged with sterile water and closure begun.

RECONSTRUCTION

Intracranial reconstruction is done first. Hemostasis is meticulously secured before dural closure is initiated. Most of the patients in the author's series were closed with a dural closure, the intracranial interposition of a pericranial flap, and a split-thickness skin graft placed from below to line the cavity.

Dural graft tissue is either natural or homograft material; fascia lata harvested from the thigh or temporal fascia obtained from the region deep to the bicoronal scalp flap is most desirable. Lyophilized homograft dura or bovine pericardium is frequently used for large defects (Fig. 43). The tragic appearance of Jacob-Creutzfeldt disease in a few patients who received lyophilized dural grafts in Europe has not been seen in North America. The fear of this dreaded disease has dissuaded a number of surgeons on this continent from using this material.

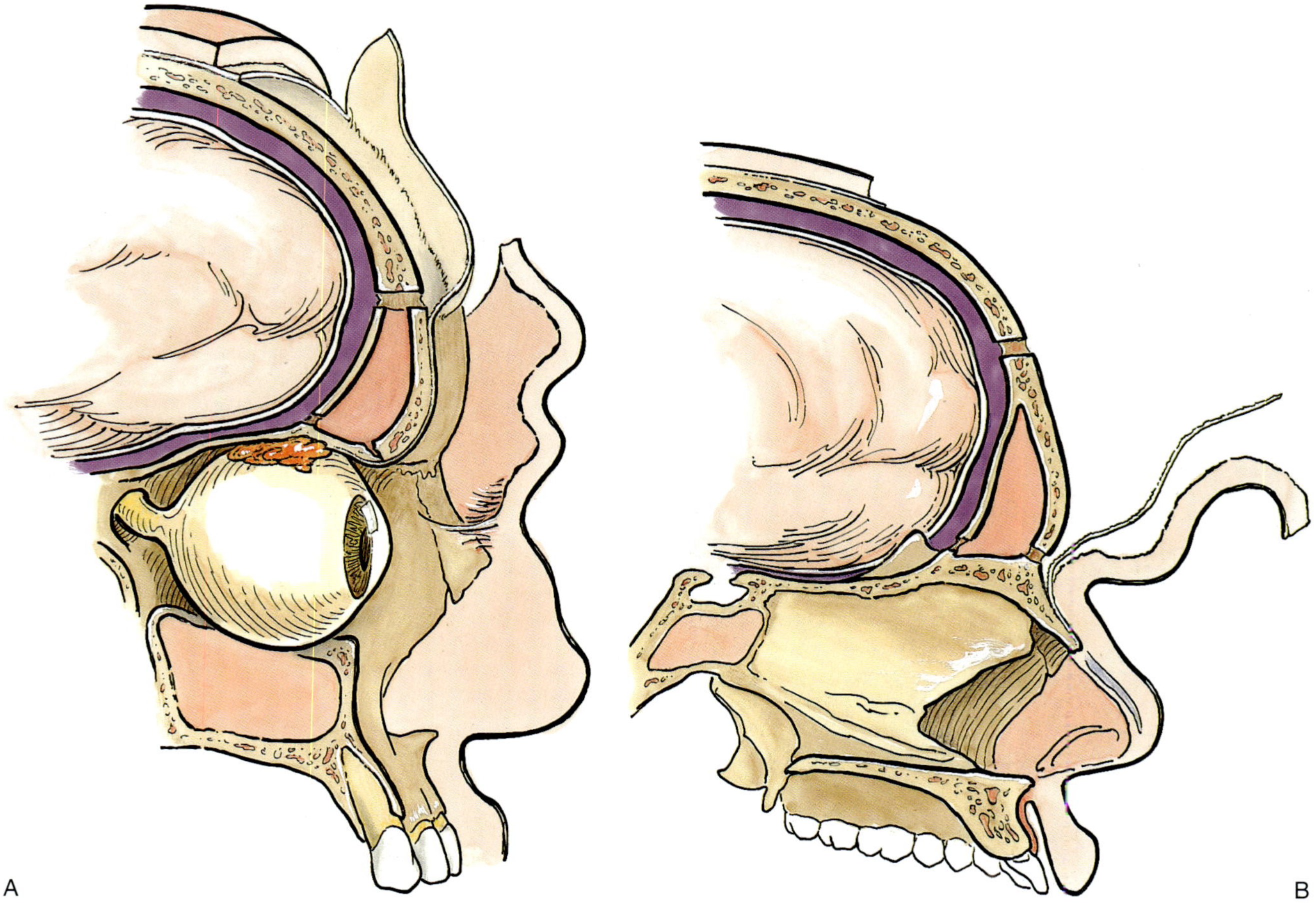

FIG. 44. Pericranial flap. **A:** Osteoplastic flap is used in a capacious frontal sinus, giving limited but adequate anterior cranial fossa extension. **B:** Sagittal view. Coronal scalp flap and pericranial flap are elevated. Bone flap is outlined. (From Donald PJ, Gluckman JL, Rice DH, eds. *The sinuses*. New York: Raven Press, 1995:466–467.)

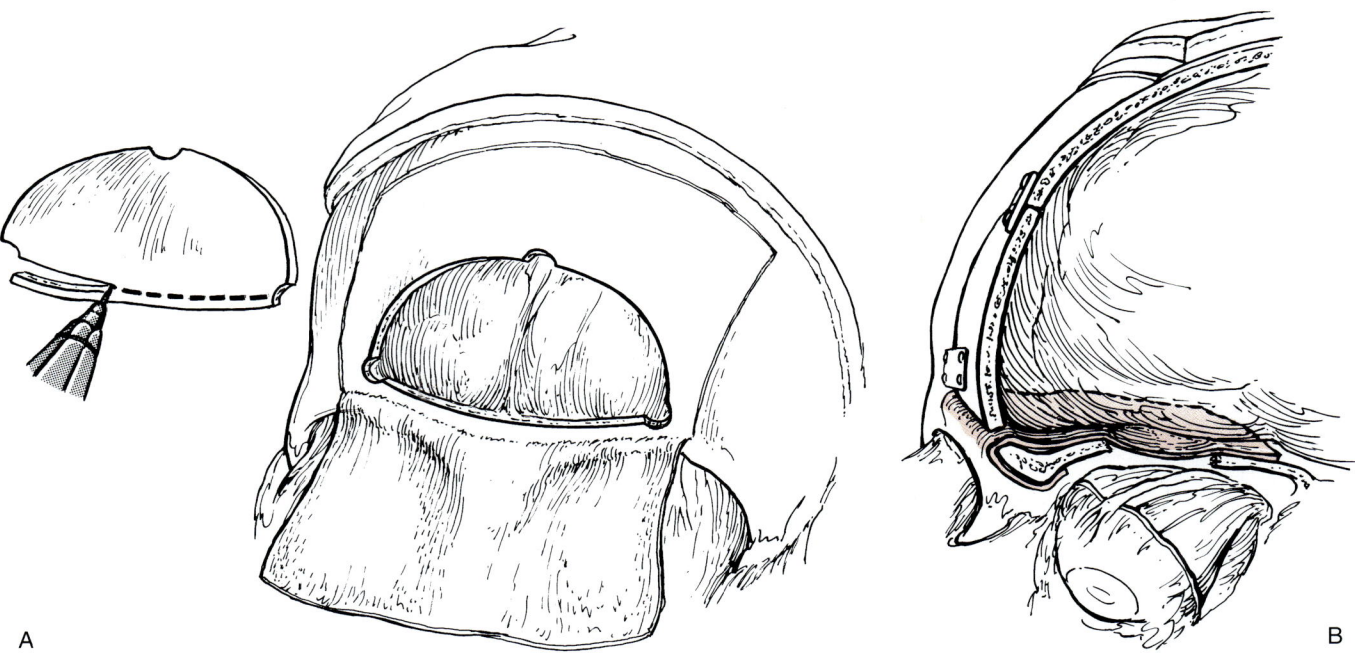

FIG. 45. The pericranial flap is placed intracranially. **A:** A slot of bone is removed from the inferior edge of craniotomy flap to accommodate the pedicle. **B:** Pericranial flap is placed intracranially over the area of skull base defect.

The secret to the avoidance of postoperative complications in anterior skull base surgery is the insurance of a watertight dural closure. Sutures between the dura and graft are often tacked to the calvarium in aid of this goal. Posteriorly, sutures are sometimes difficult to place, especially near the sphenoid wing and under the chiasm. The use of fibrin glue may help in anchoring the dura at this site.

The keystone structure in anterior fossa floor reconstruction is a viable flap of pericranium. It is usually pedicled on the supraorbital and supratrochlear arteries (see Fig. 35; Fig. 44). Jackson and colleagues (9) suggest that inclusion of the galea with the pericranium ensures a richer and more predictable blood supply. Their very convincing research, however, is not supported by the experience of most surgeons doing craniofacial surgery. It would appear prudent to use the compound flap in those patients who are at risk for vascular compromise, such as those patients who have a history of prior radiation or in cases in which a long flap must survive on a unilateral pedicle. It is essential to ensure the viability of the flap by keeping it moist during surgery using irrigation with physiologic solution or covering the flap with a wet sponge. Preserving the pericranium on the coronal scalp until required in the reconstruction also helps in this regard.

The pericranial or compound pericranial–galeal flap is folded over the inferiorly cut edge of the craniotomy and placed across the defect in the anterior fossa floor (Fig. 45). Sometimes a narrow strip of bone is removed inferiorly so as not to squeeze the flap and compromise its vascular pedicle. The distal end is tamped between the cranial floor bone and the overlying dura. It may be secured with sutures through the bone or anchored with fibrin glue. The important point to stress is that the flap is placed intracranially, not extracranially.

The cranial bone flap is anchored into place, usually with plates, and the bur holes effaced with a titanium bur hole cover (Fig. 46). Any retained facial bone fragments, such as the maxillary ostectomy (Fig. 47), are fixed into position with miniplates and microplates.

Epithelial lining to the cavity can be accomplished by pedicled flaps, free flaps, and split-thickness skin grafts, or by simply leaving the pericranium uncovered and allowing reepithelialization with sinus mucosa (Fig. 48). Pedicled

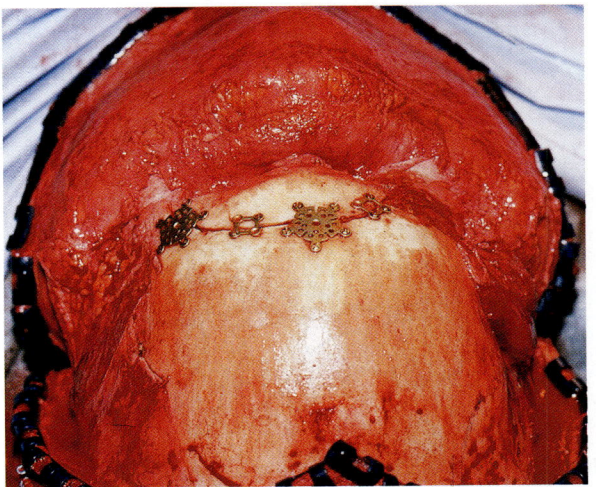

FIG. 46. The craniotomy flap is fixed *in situ* by square plates and the bur holes effaced by bur hole covers.

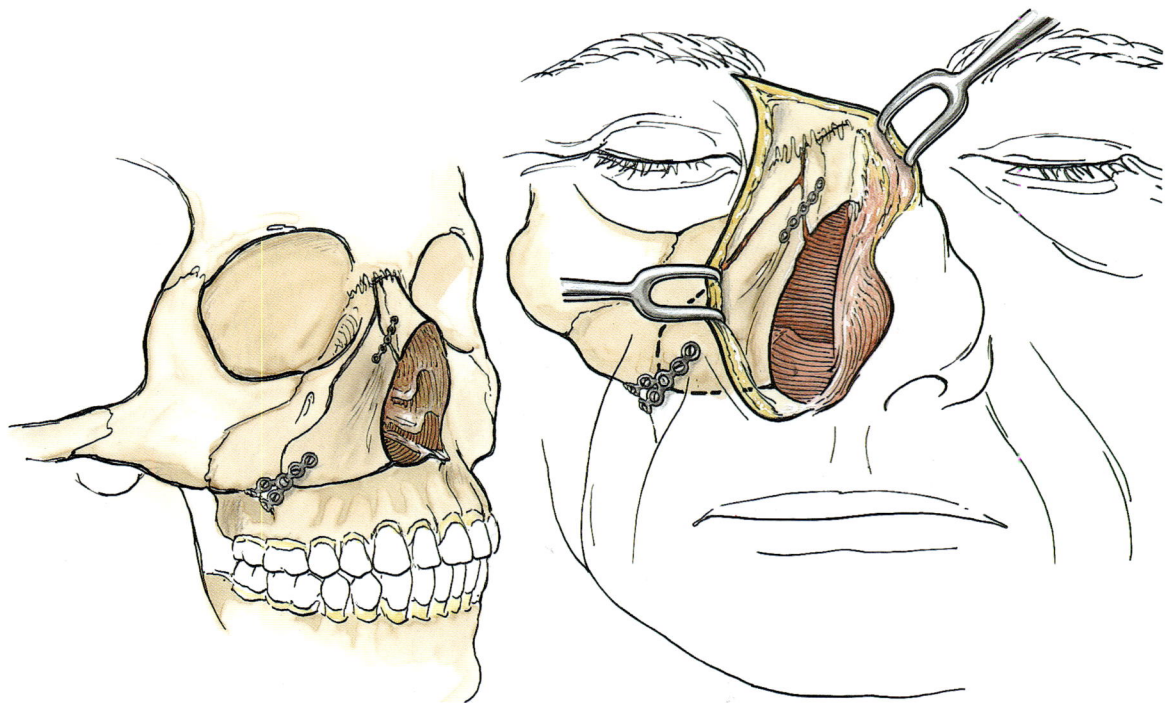

FIG. 47. The maxillary ostectomy segment is restored and fixed by miniplates and microplates.

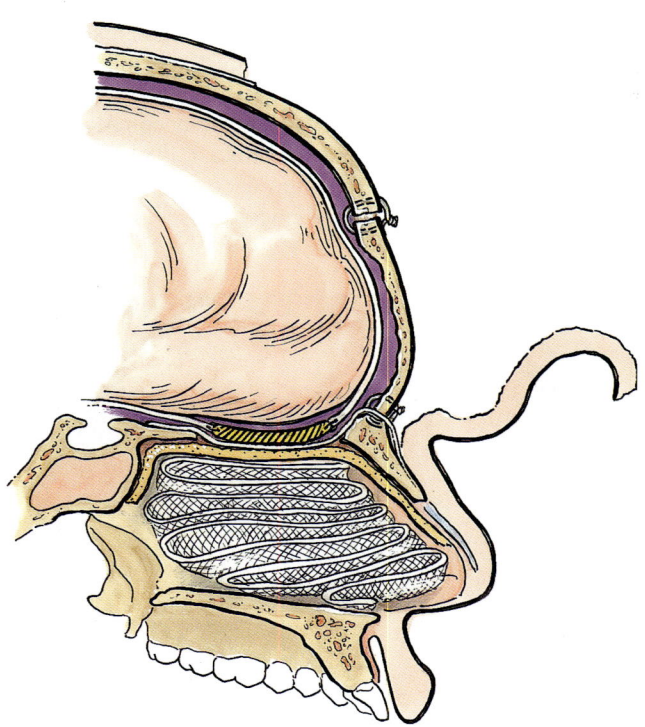

FIG. 48. The pericranial flap is in place, the defect covered by split-thickness skin grafts, and the cavity packed. (From Donald PJ, Gluckman JL, Rice DH, eds. *The sinuses*. New York: Raven Press, 1995:470.)

flaps and free vascularized flaps are usually unnecessary in the reconstruction. Moreover, they may preclude the detection of possible early recurrence of tumor. MRI and CT follow-up to diagnose such recurrences in these patients has been disappointing because early disease is often confused with postoperative and postradiation changes. They may, however, present the only viable solution in those cases in which there has been extensive prior radiation therapy and the residual tissues have poor vascularity.

The split-thickness skin graft most often provides a rapidly healing, durable cavity liner that can stand up to the demands of a weight-bearing prosthesis. The graft is held in place by medicated gauze packing material.

Before the placement of the pack in the cavity, attention must be drawn to the lacrimal system in those eyes that have escaped exenteration. During the medial wall maxillectomy, the nasolacrimal duct is amputated not too far from the lacrimal sac. The cut edges of the duct are sewn to any available adjacent soft tissue to evert this mucosa-lined tract. The newly markedly foreshortened duct is stented open with the instillation of a fine silastic cannula inserted into both of the lacrimal canaliculi and loosely tied in the cavity. If necessary, only one canaliculus is sufficient to maintain patency of the system.

The packing in the cavity is removed at 1 week under general anesthesia. An anesthetic is used to obviate pain and facilitate the best inspection possible of the newly healed cavity. Twice daily, gentle irrigations with a warm saline solution are done to remove debris and promote healing.

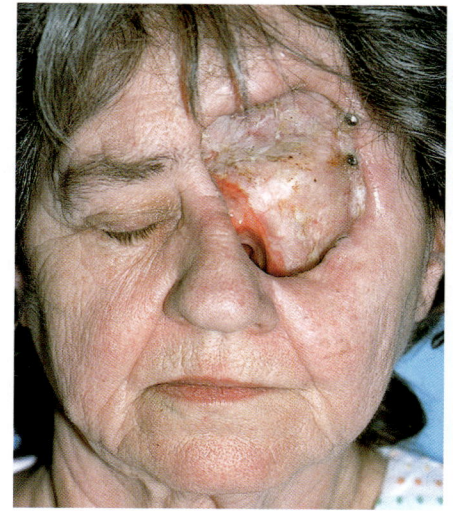
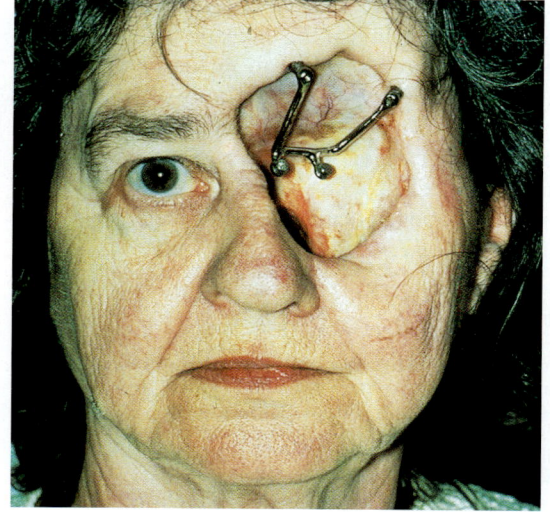
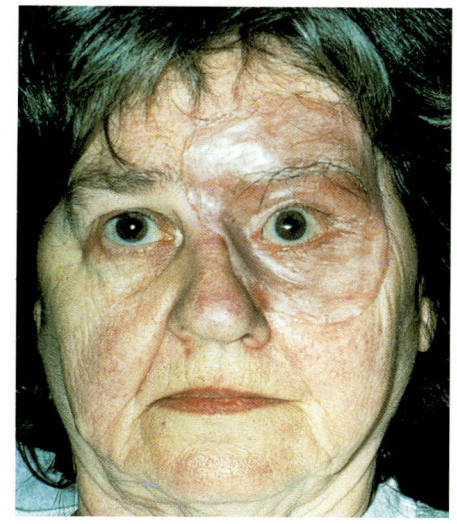

FIG. 49. Prosthetic rehabilitation required for the coverage of skull base defects is aided by the use of osseointegrated implants consisting of interconnecting bars and magnets. **A:** Large defect in patient after resection of large frontoethmoid tumor invading calvarial bone and dura. Osseointegrated implants are placed. **B:** Connecting bars and magnets attached. **C:** Prosthesis in place.

The lacrimal stent is left in place for about 12 weeks to ensure an effective drainage of tears and the prevention of troublesome epiphora.

The cavity is carefully monitored monthly to rule out early local recurrence.

Placement of a prosthesis is delayed until the cavity is healed and the skin graft matured, usually about 3 months or more. When there is substantial loss of facial skin and in some cases in which an ocular prosthesis will not be adequately retained, the use of osseous integrated implants helps. Titanium fixtures are strategically placed in bone and then, once integrated, each is mounted with an abutment cylinder. Magnets are incorporated into the abutment and these, in addition to an integrated connecting bar system, provide solid anchoring for the maxillofacial prosthesis (Fig. 49). The biggest drawback to this rehabilitation system is the time necessary for osseointegration to take place. In the unirradiated facial bones, 3 to 6 months is required between the first and second stages (implant placement until application of the abutment cylinder). In the irradiated cases in which bone healing is markedly prolonged, a delay of 12 months is not uncommon. The second drawback is cost. Reimbursement is sometimes difficult because insurance companies choose to label such techniques as cosmetic in nature rather than functionally restorative.

Complications are detailed in Chapters 29 and 30 and are not repeated here.

RESULTS

The first favorable results of skull base surgery were published by Ketcham et al. (8). They described the results of resecting malignancies that invaded the anterior cranial fossa, usually taking origin in the nasal cavities or paranasal sinuses. Their 45% tumor-free 5-year survival rate established cranial base surgery as a reasonable approach to highly aggressive sinonasal cancers. Tumor-free survival statistics have currently improved to about 65% (10). It is important to remember that without this therapy, most of these patients would have died from their disease. The improved survival rate is even more remarkable in that the indications for anterior skull base surgery have expanded to include patients with extensive dural invasion and even brain involvement. Bohrer et al. (11) have shown that there is no statistically significant difference in the survival between patients with or without dural invasion.

The results in the resection of benign tumors are much better than in malignant disease.

REFERENCES

1. Perry C, Levine PA, William BR, Cantrell RW. Preservation of the eye in paranasal sinus cancer surgery. *Arch Otolaryngol Head Neck Surg* 1988;114:632–634.
2. Mann W, Rareshide E, Schildwächter A. Nasennebenhöhlentumor mit orbitaler Beteiligung. *Laryngorhinootologie* 1989;68:667–670.
3. Bagatella F, Mazzoni A. Microsurgery in juvenile nasopharyngeal angiofibroma: a lateronasal approach with nasomaxillary pedicle flap. *Skull Base Surgery* 1995;5:219–226.
4. Carrau RL, Segas J, Nuss DW, Johnson JT, Janecka IP. Orbital invasion by squamous cell carcinomas arising in the sinonasal tract: outcome after selective orbital preservation. Presented at the Joint Annual Meeting of German and North American Skull Base Societies, Lake Buena Vista, Florida, February 13, 1994.
5. Ohngren LG. Malignant tumors of the maxilloethmoidal region: a clinical study with special reference to the treatment with electrocautery and irradiation. *Acta Otolaryngol Suppl (Stockh)* 1933;19:1–476.
6. Sisson GA, Johnson NE, Amiri CS. Cancer of the maxillary sinus: clinical classification and management. *Annals Otol Rhinol Laryngol* 1963;72:1050.
7. Jesse RH, Butler JJ, Healy JE Jr, Fletcher GH, Chau PM. Paranasal sinuses and nasal cavity. In: Maccomb WS, Fletcher GH, eds. *Cancer of the head and neck*. Baltimore: Williams & Wilkins, 1967:329–356.
8. Ketcham AS, Wilkins RH, Van Buren JM, Smith RR. A combined intracranial facial approach to the paranasal sinuses. *Am J Surg* 1963;106:698–703.
9. Fukuta K, Potparic Z, Sugihara T, Rachmiel A, Forte RA, Jackson IT. A cadaver investigation of the blood supply of the gabal frontalis flap. *Plast Reconstr Surg* 1994;94:794–800.
10. Schramm VL. Anterior craniofacial resection. In: Sekhar LN, Schramm VL, eds. *Tumors of the cranial base*. Mount Kisco, NY: Futura Publishing Co., 1987:265–278.
11. Bohrer PS, Donald PJ, á Wengen DF, Boggan JE, Stevenson T. The significance of dural and cerebral invasion by skull base malignancies. In: Mazzoni A, Sanna M, eds. *Proceedings of the First European Skull Base Society*. Amsterdam: Kugler Publications, 1995:133–138

CHAPTER 11

Facial Degloving Approach

João J. Maniglia and Ricardo Ramina

Facial degloving can be defined as a surgical approach to midface structures that leaves no visible incisions and scars on the face. The name itself means a subperiosteal dissection that degloves the soft tissue, exposing the midface bone and cavities to surgical exploration and ablation (Fig. 1).

Caldwell and Luc in the early 20th century used ipsilateral sublabial incision and subperiosteal dissection for the treatment of sinusitis. Converse (1) used it in the 1950s for facial contour for benign lesions. Dencker and Kahler (2) went further and removed the medial bony facial pillar in a radical treatment for sinusitis. Portmann and Retrouvery (3) were the first to describe facial degloving for a maxillectomy as treatment for cancer, and gave credit to Sibileau for the original idea.

Those unilateral approaches cannot, however, be considered as true facial degloving. Roe and Joseph in the late 19th century established the incisions and subperiosteal/subperichondral dissections for rhinoplasty without external incisions. Williams (4) used rhinoplasty incisions combined with external facial incisions for treatment of intranasal tumors. The Caldwell-Luc approach and rhinoplasty techniques were widely used by ear–nose–throat–head and neck surgeons, the former for the treatment of sinusitis and the latter for aesthetic and functional nasal repair. Casson et al. (5) reported on the use of rhinoplasty and vestibular incisions combined with bilateral subperiosteal dissection of the maxilla, firmly establishing the concept of mid-facial degloving (Fig. 2).

It is fair to say that many surgeons in the 1960s and 1970s successfully used the degloving procedure for treatment of a variety of lesions (e.g., fractures, benign and malignant tumors) for many years, without officially publishing any papers. Among the surgeons who published in the 1980s, there are Allen and Siegel (6), Conley and Price (7), Maniglia (8), Price et al. (9), and possibly many others.

The next development in facial degloving came with the publication by Mikko Paavolainen et al. (10) of a procedure using lateral osteotomies and septal transection, elevating the whole nasal pyramid with degloving. In the authors' opinion, this degloving variation should only be used in the treatment of malignant tumors.

Oncologic head and neck surgeons still prefer to use the Weber-Fergusson paranasal incision procedure and its modifications (Fig. 3). The authors see many advantages to the use of the degloving technique, which gives wider bilateral exposure from the septum to the mandible and from the orbit and skull base to the hard palate. There are no visible scars, and reconstruction is very simple with very little morbidity for the patient.

The first author learned the technique from A. Maniglia in the late 1960s, having used degloving technique only for paranasal and nasal fossa tumors. The authors extended its use to removal of extensive nasopharyngeal angiofibromas and clivus tumors, and, in combination with anterior and middle fossa craniotomy, for clival tumors and a variety of benign and malignant tumors of the anterior and middle skull base.

After degloving of soft tissues is performed, there are still the bony structures of the midface with which to contend. Bone resection is variable depending on the site and extension of the particular lesion being treated. The anterior wall of the maxilla can be removed and the antrum used as access to the pterygopalatine fossa, cavum, and sphenoid sinus. By removing the middle pillar of the maxillary bone and the medial antral wall, intranasal and ethmoid tumors can be approached, with the possibility of performing partial maxillectomy (Fig. 4). If the posterior pillar of the maxillary antrum and the pterygoid plates are removed, there is a wide approach to the nasopharynx and clivus (Fig. 5). Resection of the lateral pillar gives wide access to the temporal and infratemporal fossae and paralateropharyngeal space.

Type I Lefort osteotomies can be performed, allowing an ample bilateral approach to the cavum, clivus, and sphenoid

---

J. J. Maniglia: Department of Otolaryngology, Universidade Federal do Paraná, Curitiba 80440-080, Brazil.

R. Ramina: Skull Base Surgery Foundation, Curitiba 80240, Brazil.

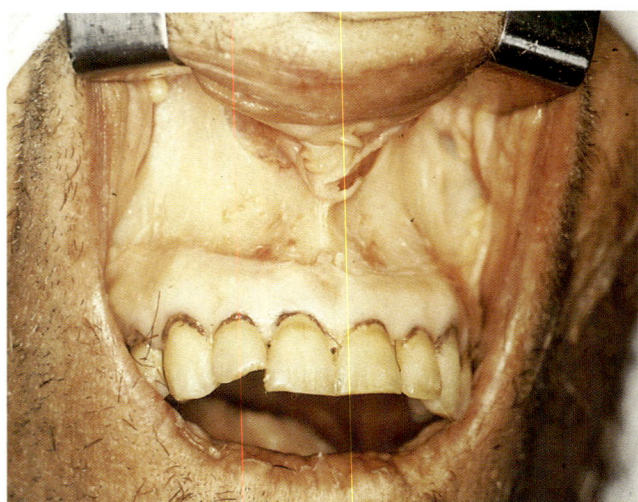

FIG. 1. Cadaver dissection: bilateral sublabial incision and periosteal displacement.

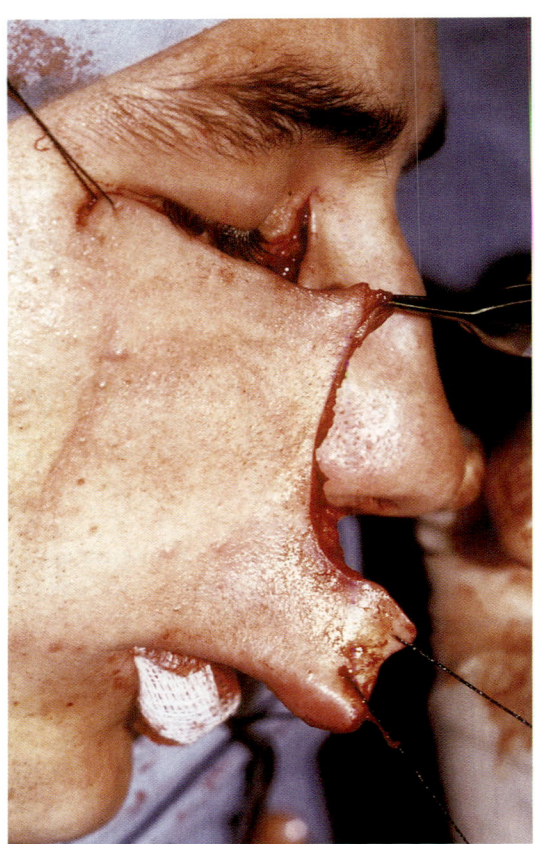

FIG. 3. Modified Weber-Fergusson incision.

sinus in the midline. If the lesion requires it, the mid-facial bone can be split; the lesion is removed and the midface reassembled using miniplates.

In the authors' experience, the most frequent indication for degloving and a transmaxillary approach is for the surgical treatment of juvenile nasopharyngeal angiofibromas with lateral extensions. The authors usually remove the anterior wall of the maxilla and the middle and lateral pillars, preserving the inferior turbinate and membranous nasolacrimal duct (Fig. 6). A wide approach is obtained and bony reconstruction usually is not necessary. This is the authors' favorite surgical procedure for removal of juvenile nasopharyngeal angiofibromas with intracranial extension. Occasionally, the authors have performed procedures in

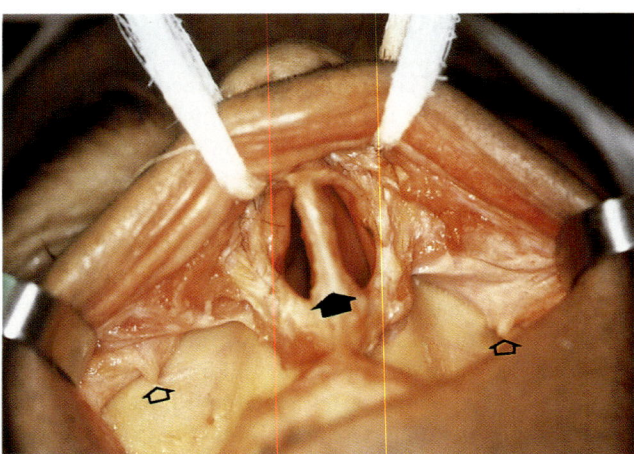

FIG. 2. Cadaver dissection: complete degloving. *Empty arrows* indicate infraorbital nerve and *full arrow* shows the nasal septum.

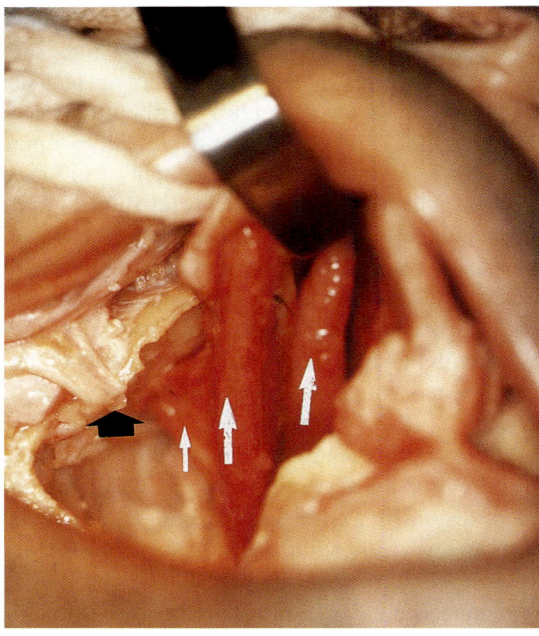

FIG. 4. Cadaver dissection showing infraorbital foramen and nerve (*black arrow*) and membranous nasolacrimal duct (*thin white arrow*), and inferior and middle turbinate (*large white arrows*).

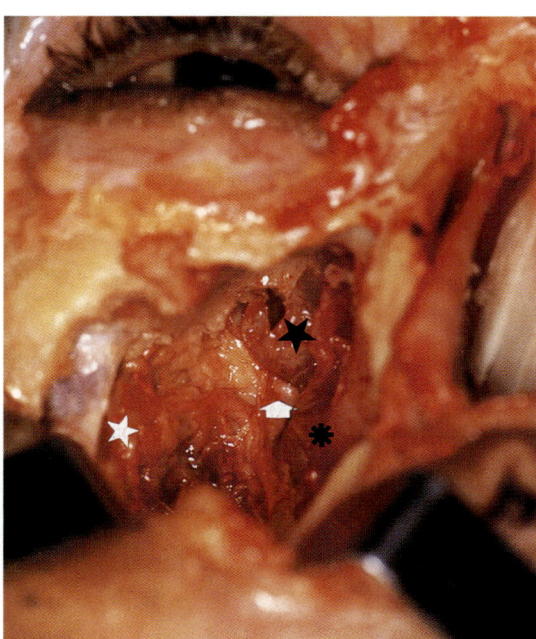

FIG. 5. Cadaver dissection showing infratemporal fossa (*white star*) and sphenoid sinus (*black star*), pterygopalatine artery (*white arrow*), and cavum (*asterisk*).

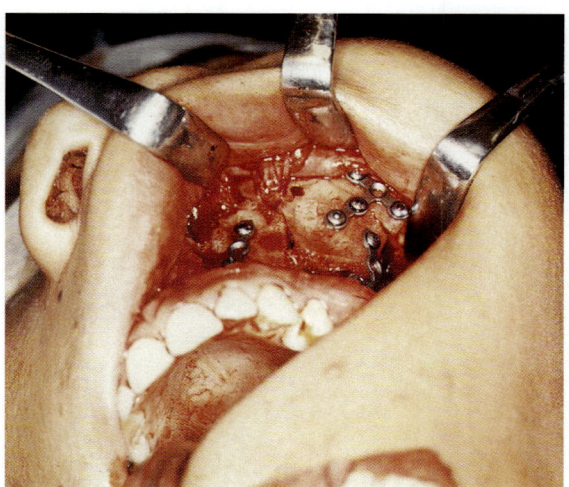

FIG. 7. Reconstruction of anterior maxillary wall with miniplates.

which the anterior wall of the maxilla connected with the middle and lateral pillars are preserved; these fragments are stabilized with miniplates (Fig. 7). However, the authors have seen no advantage in preserving these structures as far as long-term facial growth is concerned.

Degloving and a transfacial approach can be used with external ethmoidectomies, frontoethmoidectomies, and craniotomies, and to remove a wide variety of anterior and middle cranial base tumors.

SURGICAL TECHNIQUE

General Preparation

The patient is in the supine position with 30 degrees of head elevation. Orotracheal intubation and general anesthesia are started and the tube is fixed on the contralateral maxillary or mandibular premolars with dental floss.

Incisions and Subperiosteal Elevation

After administration of lidocaine 2% plus epinephrine 1:100,000 is infiltrated, rhinoplasty incisions (intercartilaginous and transfixion) and bilateral sublabial incisions are performed (Fig. 8).

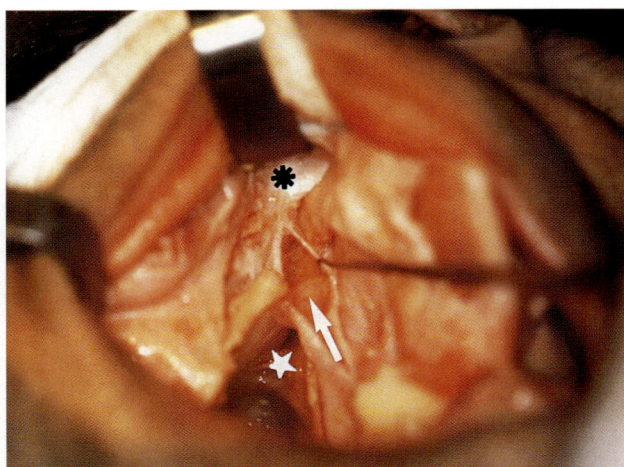

FIG. 6. Cadaver dissection. Hook shows opened membranous nasolacrimal duct (*white arrow*), and behind it the maxillary ostium (*white star*). Asterisk indicates the lacrimal sac.

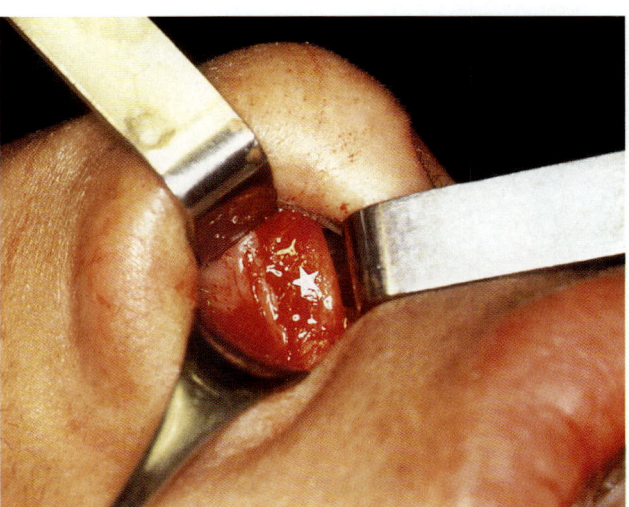

FIG. 8. Surgery: transfixion and intercartilaginous incisions. *Star* indicates caudal nasal septum.

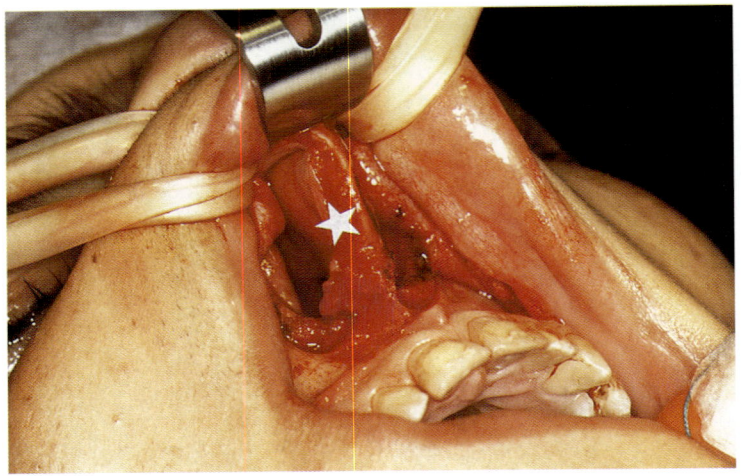

FIG. 9. Surgery: transfixion and intercartilaginous bilateral sublabial and vestibular incisions. *Star* indicates caudal nasal septum.

The soft tissues of the nose are elevated from the bony–cartilaginous framework, and the cheek is elevated from the anterior maxillary wall up to the infraorbital foramen on both sides. The pyriform aperture mucosa is incised, and the soft tissues of the nose and cheek can be widely displaced toward the glabella and held by two large Penrose drains fixed on head drapes (Fig. 9).

Medial to the infraorbital foramen, the soft tissue can be displaced up to the anterior orbital crest and lacrimal sac. Lateral to the infraorbital foramen, a portion of the zygomatic bone can be removed after severing the masseter muscle insertion if access to the temporal fossa is contemplated. If there is inferior extension of tumor to the paralateropharyngeal space, the posterior aspect of the sublabial incision may be extended to the anterior tonsil pillar in the retromolar space. If desired, the anterior attachment of the inferior turbinate and the soft tissue lacrimal duct to the vestibular skin can be kept, displacing it for surgery and replacing it at the end of the procedure.

Bone Resection

Bone resection is planned along the walls of the maxillary antrum. If preservation is attempted, reconstruction with miniplates can guarantee a sophisticated anatomic rearrangement.

Transmaxillary Approach

A degloving operation is not necessary to do a transmaxillary ethmoidectomy–sphenoidectomy. If more intranasal space is needed for removal of midline disease with mini-

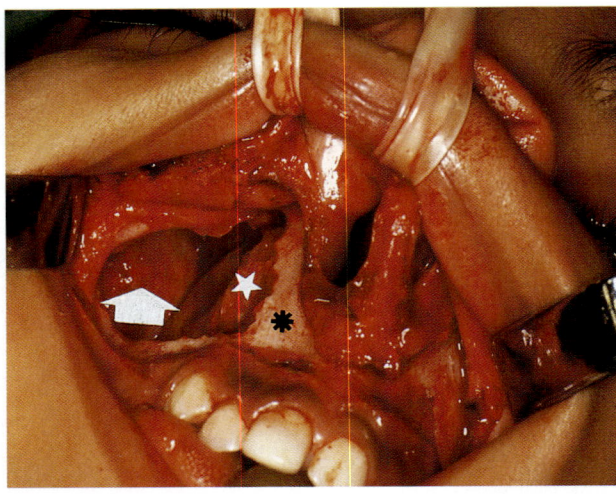

FIG. 10. Surgery: degloving/transmaxillary approach; maxillary antrum with bony nasolacrimal duct (*star*) and juvenile nasopharyngeal angiofibroma inside maxillary sinus (*white arrow*). *Asterisk* indicates medial pillar.

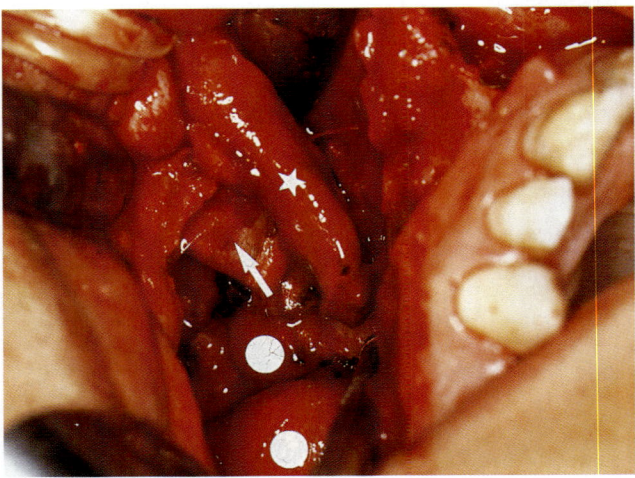

FIG. 11. Surgery: inferior turbinate (*star*) with attached membranous nasolacrimal duct (*arrow*) and juvenile nasopharyngeal angiofibroma (*balls*).

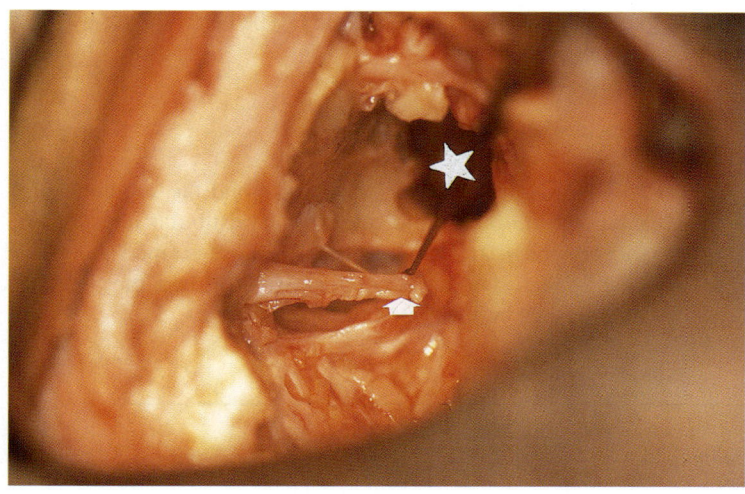

FIG. 12. Cadaver dissection: pterygopalatine fossa with artery (in hook; *arrow*) passing in the rostrum of the sphenoid sinus (*star*).

mal lateral extension, the medial pillar can be removed (as in the the Dencker operation). After removal of the anterior wall of the maxillary antrum, a horizontal bony bulge (inferior turbinate bone) and a vertical bulge (bony nasolacrimal duct) are visible on the medial wall (Fig. 10). Between them lies the maxillary sinus ostium and posterior ethmoid cells. After appropriate bone removal, the mucosa of the inferior meatus can be incised, leaving the soft nasolacrimal duct attached to the inferior turbinate, which can be displaced medially or anteriorly after incision of the inferior turbinate at its tail (Fig. 11).

The orbital rim portion of the infraorbital foramen and anterior lacrimal crest can be removed, allowing displacement of the infraorbital nerve and lacrimal sac superiorly along with the mid-facial degloving. In this way, intranasal, transethmoidal, transsphenoidal, and cavum resection of tumor can be accomplished.

Advancing posteriorly, the surgeon can remove the posterior (medial) pillar of the maxillary antrum, gaining access to the pterygopalatine foramen with its arteries. If the posterior wall of the maxillary antrum is removed, the pterygopalatine fossa is reached, where the vascular pedicle of a juvenile nasopharyngeal angiofibroma can be ligated (Fig. 12).

Extended Transmaxillary Approach

If necessary, an extended transmaxillary approach can be performed by removing the lateral facial pillar, gaining access to the temporal fossa, infratemporal and paralateropharyngeal space, and the floor of the middle cranial base and the cavernous sinus. The authors usually combine a bilateral degloving with an ipsilateral transmaxillary approach. If necessary, a bilateral bone approach with Lefort I osteotomies or mid-facial splitting can be done.

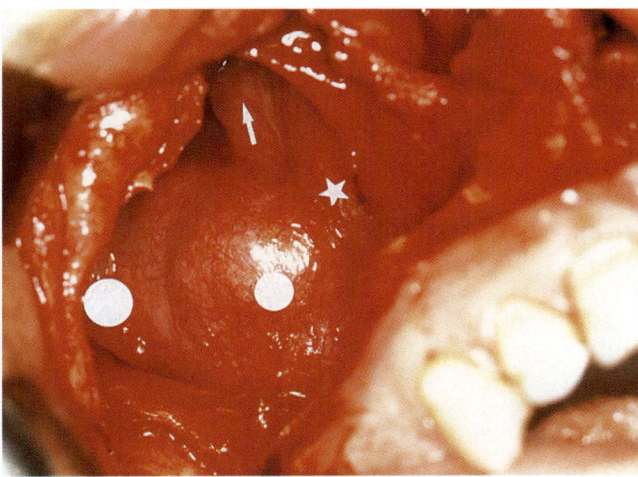

FIG. 13. Surgery: exposure of large juvenile nasopharyngeal angiofibroma (*balls*), showing membranous nasolacrimal duct (*arrow*) and inferior turbinate (*star*).

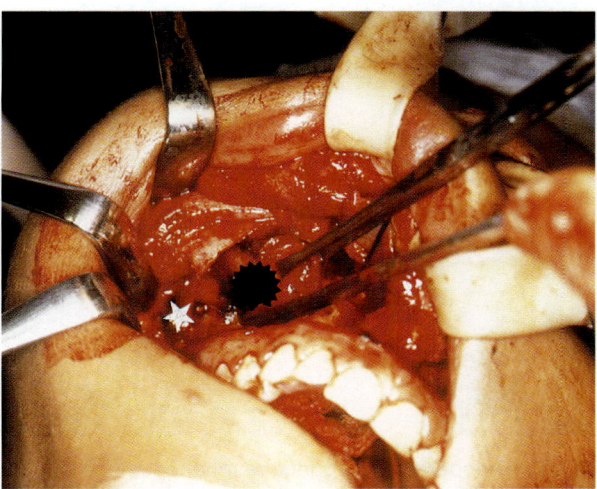

FIG. 14. Surgery: after pedicle coagulation and section (*star*), tumor removal is begun (*serrated ball*).

In general, the authors save more complicated approaches for deeper and bigger tumors (e.g., chordomas or chondrosarcomas of the clivus).

Tumor Resection

Preoperative embolization is helpful in preventing excessive tumor bleeding in surgery of large tumors.

After securing its vascular pedicles, the tumor is removed (Figs. 13, 14). Bleeding is controlled with Gelfoam, Surgicel, and light anterior and posterior nasal packings. Soft tissue is replaced. If desired, bone can be held in place by wires or miniplates.

Closure of Incisions

The authors close the transfixion and the sublabial incisions with 3-0 chromic catgut. The vestibular incisions are closed with 4-0 chromic catgut. The nose is taped and a light cast applied. Nasal packings are removed on the third day and the cast on the fifth day.

CASE 1

A 14-year-old boy presented with a large juvenile nasopharyngeal angiofibroma involving the cavum, sphenoid sinus, infratemporal space, and temporal fossa, with intracranial invasion (Fig. 15). The tumor was removed through a degloving procedure and transmaxillary approach (Figs. 16–18).

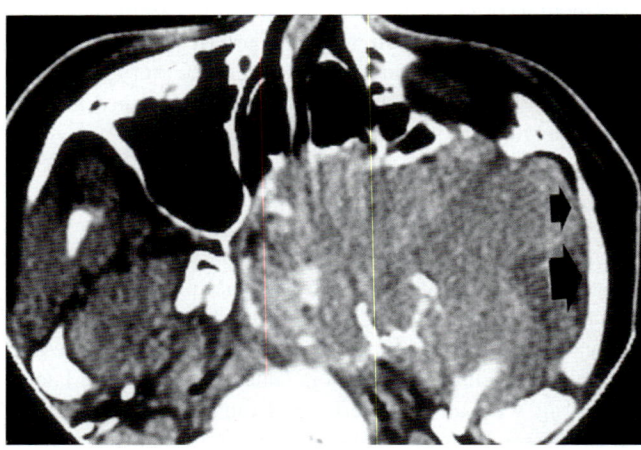

FIG. 15. Computed tomography scan of patient from case 1. *Arrows* indicate tumor in temporal fossa.

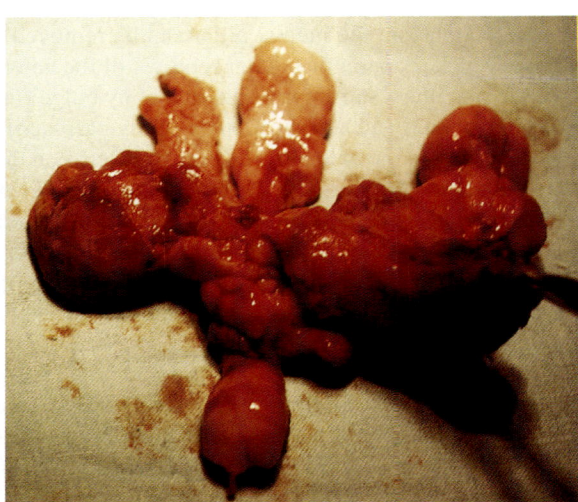

FIG. 16. Surgical specimen of juvenile nasopharyngeal angiofibroma removed from patient from case 1, with its various extensions.

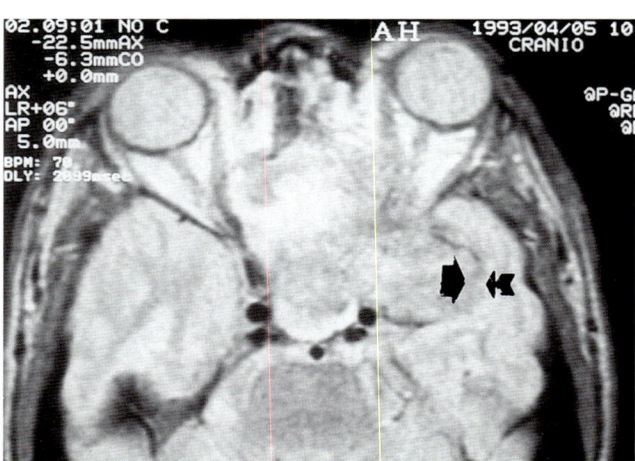

FIG. 17. Preoperative magnetic resonance image of patient from case 1. *Arrows* indicate extradural temporal lobe compression.

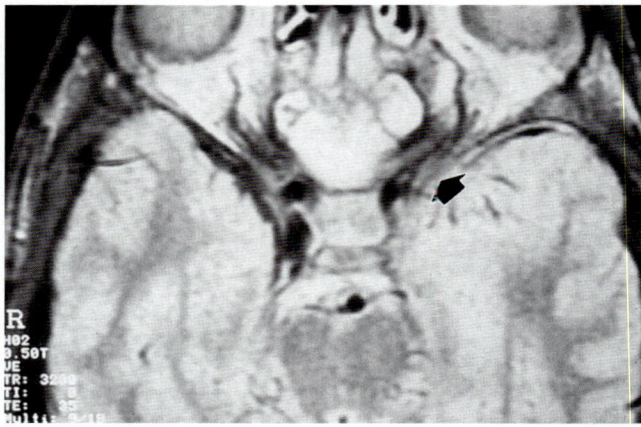

FIG. 18. Postoperative magnetic resonance image of patient from case 1, showing no brain compression. *Arrow* indicates normal brain position after lesion removal.

COMBINED SURGERY

The degloving/transmaxillary procedure can be combined with other approaches if the lesion extends toward the orbit, frontal sinus, or anterior or medial cranial base. To protect the orbit, optic nerve, cribriform plate, superior orbital fissure, and dura mater, safe landmarks are needed.

CASE 2

A 20-year-old white man presented with nasal obstruction. There was a large osteoma in the right nasal fossa and maxillary, ethmoid, and sphenoid sinuses, with orbital compression (Fig. 19). The os-

External Ethmoidectomy with Degloving

Ethmoid–sphenoid osteomas can be removed using periorbital and ethmoid neurovascular pedicles as landmarks to protect the periorbita and optic nerve. The remaining tumor is easily removed using degloving and a transmaxillary approach.

teoma was removed by an external ethmoidectomy–sphenoidectomy using a degloving procedure and a transmaxillary approach (Figs. 20–22).

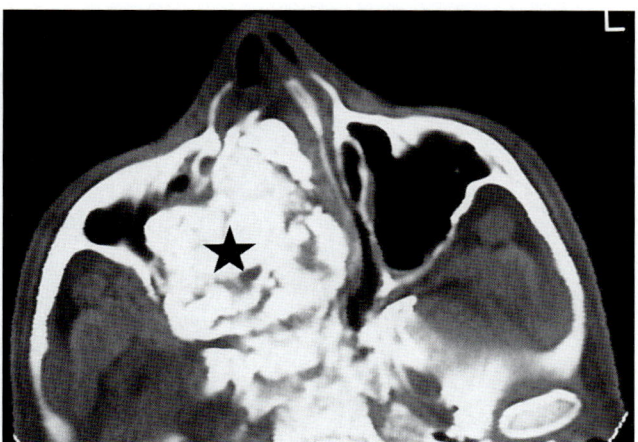

FIG. 19. Case 2. Axial computed tomography scan of large osteoma of right nasal fossa and ethmoid, sphenoid and maxillary sinuses (*star*).

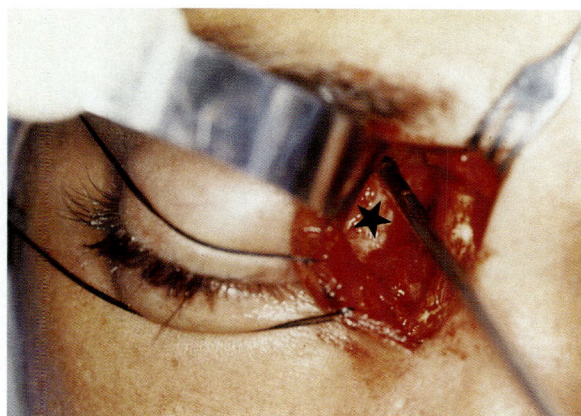

FIG. 20. Case 2. External ethmoidectomy–sphenoidectomy with orbital decompression and tumor removal (*star*).

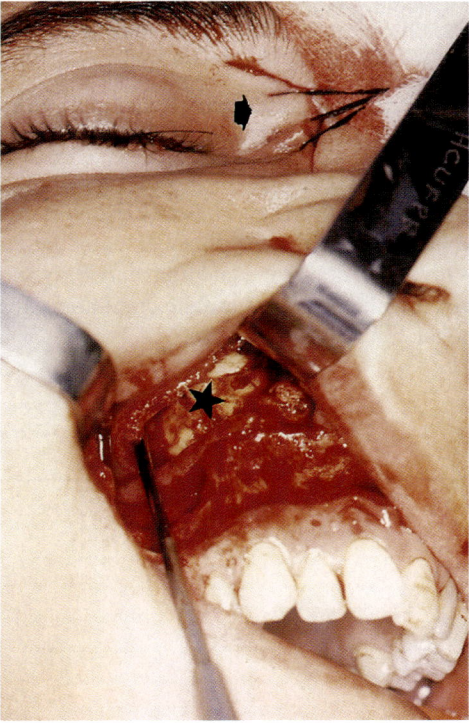

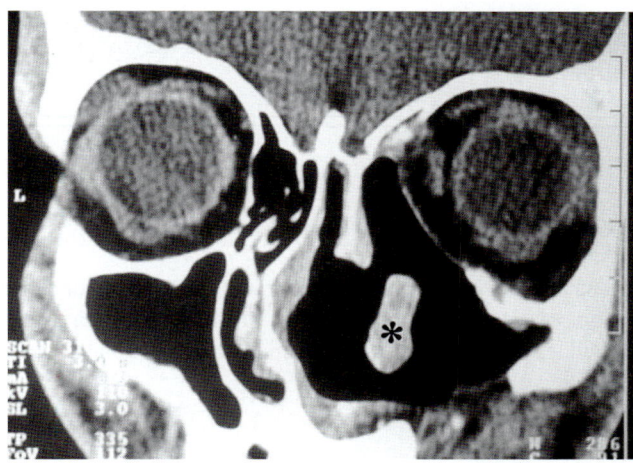

FIG. 22. Case 2. Postoperative coronal computed tomography scan; note inferior turbinate (*asterisk*).

FIG. 21. Case 2. Combined degloving and removal of remaining paranasal sinus osteoma (*star*); note inner canthus incision (*arrow*).

External Frontoethmoidectomy with Degloving

Extensive, recurrent inverted papilloma can be totally removed with preservation of orbital structures and the cribriform plate and the opportunity of reconstructing the frontonasal duct.

CASE 3

A 45-year-old white man had an inverted papilloma removed from his left maxillary sinus by another physician. He subsequently had intranasal recurrence, frontal sinusitis, and a left orbital fistula (Fig. 23).

Magnetic resonance imaging revealed frontal sinus involvement with an abscess draining into the orbit (Fig. 24). An external frontoethmoidectomy associated with a degloving/transmaxillary approach was used to remove the tumor and treat the frontal sinus infection.

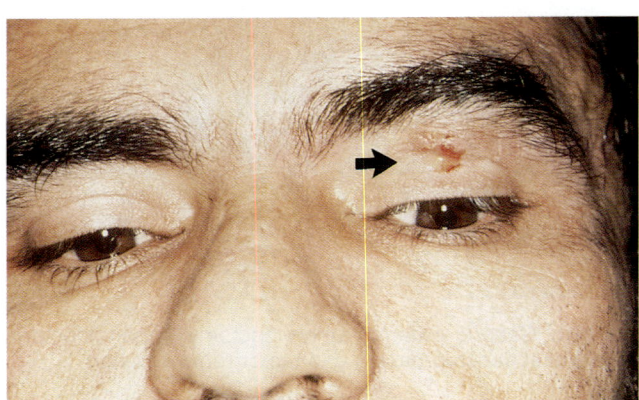

FIG. 23. Case 3. Patient with recurrent inverted papilloma, frontal sinus invasion, and chronic sinusitis with orbital fistula (*arrow*).

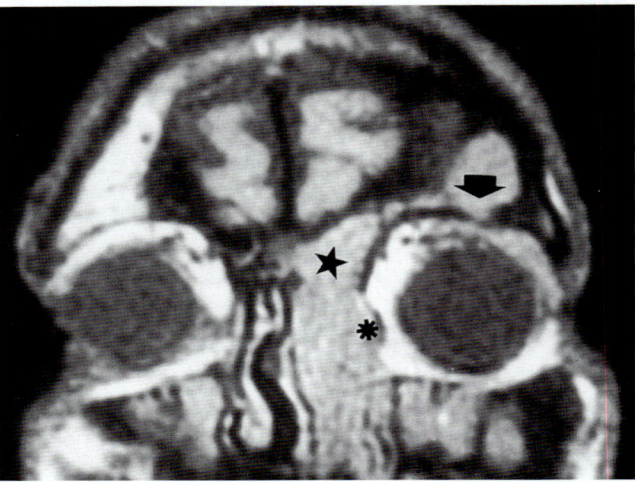

FIG. 24. Case 3. Magnetic resonance image showing papilloma invasion of frontal sinus (*star*), lamina papyracea erosion (*asterisk*), and orbital fistula (*arrow*).

Anterior Craniotomy and Degloving

The authors use an anterior subcranial approach alone that encompasses one or both superior orbital rims, with a low glabellar cut and frontal sinus cranialization, to ablate osteomas, chondrosarcomas, high clivus chordomas, and esthesioneuroblastomas. If the maxillary sinus or lateral orbital fissure is involved, degloving and transmaxillary surgery can be combined with anterior or middle craniotomy for safe tumor removal.

CASE 4

A 30-year-old white woman presented with a history of loss of vision in the right eye and proptosis with nasal obstruction. Visual evoked potential examination showed signs of optic nerve involvement. Computed tomography demonstrated osteoma of the sphenoid and maxillary sinuses (Fig. 25), and magnetic resonance imaging showed middle fossa invasion (Fig. 26). A subcranial craniotomy and degloving procedure were necessary for total tumor removal and orbit and optic nerve decompression with vision improvement (Figs. 27, 28).

CASE 4 (Continued)

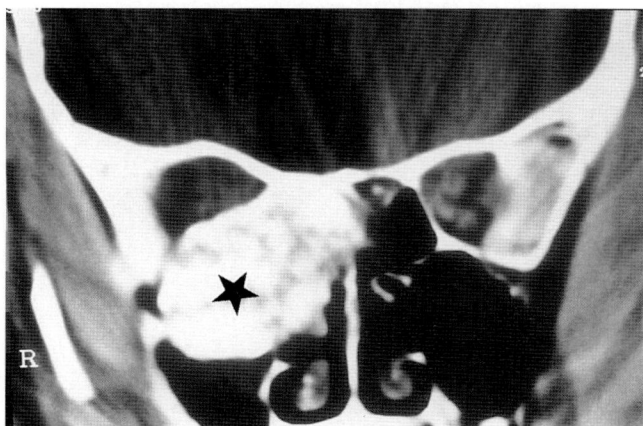

FIG. 25. Case 4. Large osteoma (*star*) involving maxillary sinus, orbit, and right nasal fossa.

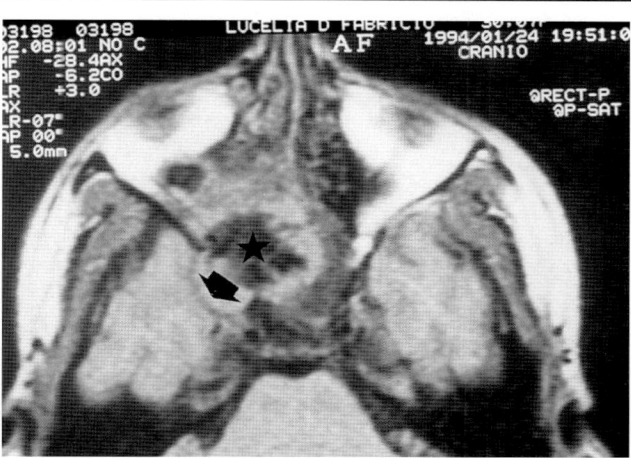

FIG. 26. Case 4. Magnetic resonance image showing middle fossa invasion (*arrow*) by osteoma (*star*).

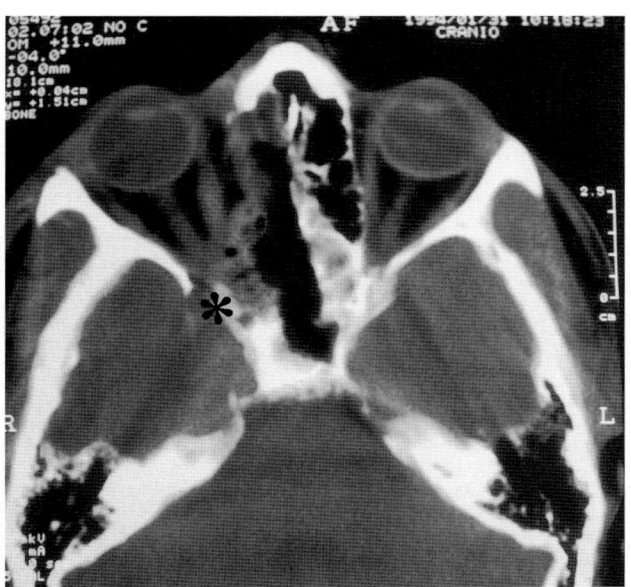

FIG. 27. Case 4. Axial computed tomography scan after surgical removal of osteoma. The *asterisk* indicates the previous site of osteoma.

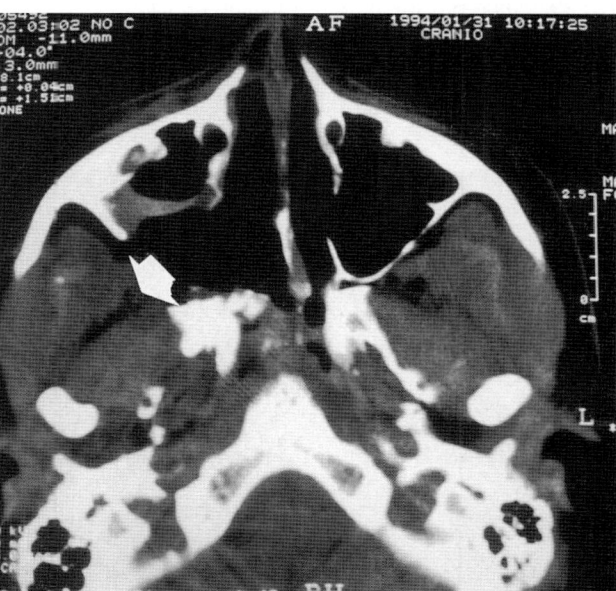

FIG. 28. Case 4. Postoperative axial computed tomography scan showing complete osteoma removal. *Arrow* indicates bone defect in infratemporal fossa.

CASE 5

A 49-year-old white man presented with an inverted papilloma of the left nasal fossa and paranasal sinuses and a history of multiple Caldwell-Luc operations. He had undergone bilateral external frontal surgery, a left Weber-Fergusson incision, and sinus surgery in Boston, Massachusetts, with persistence of tumor and a left dacryocystitis (Fig. 29). Magnetic resonance imaging showed bilateral frontal sinus papilloma, meningioma (Fig. 30), residual nasal fossa papilloma, chondroma of the sphenoid sinus, and brainstem hemangioma (Figs. 31, 32). A subfrontal craniotomy and degloving/transmaxillary approach with frontal sinus cranialization allowed total tumor removal, except for the brainstem lesion (Figs. 33, 34). A dacryocystorhinostomy corrected the lacrimal drainage obstruction in a second operation.

CASE 5 (Continued)

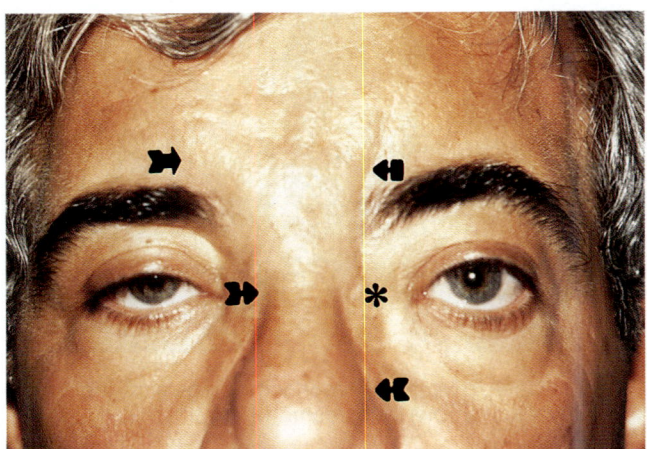

FIG. 29. Case 5. Patient after multiple pansinus operations (bilateral Weber-Fergusson and frontoethmoidectomies) with residual inverted papilloma and dacryocystitis (*asterisk*). *Arrows* indicate facial scars.

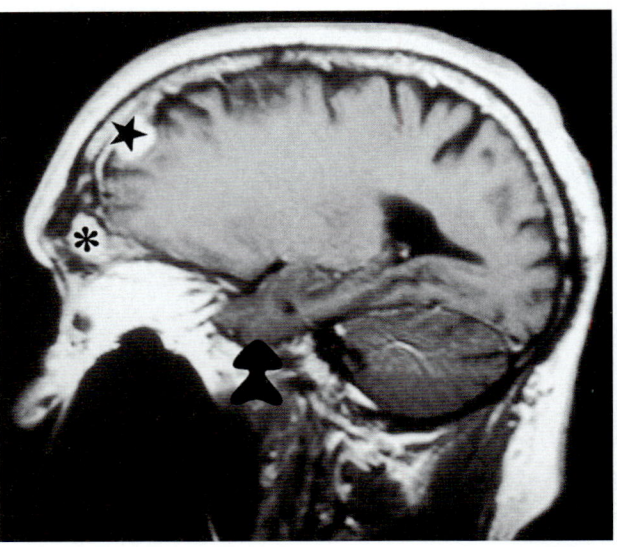

FIG. 30. Case 5. Recurrent inverted papilloma of nasal fossa and frontal sinus (*asterisk*), frontal meningioma (*star*), and chondroma of sphenoid sinus (*arrow*).

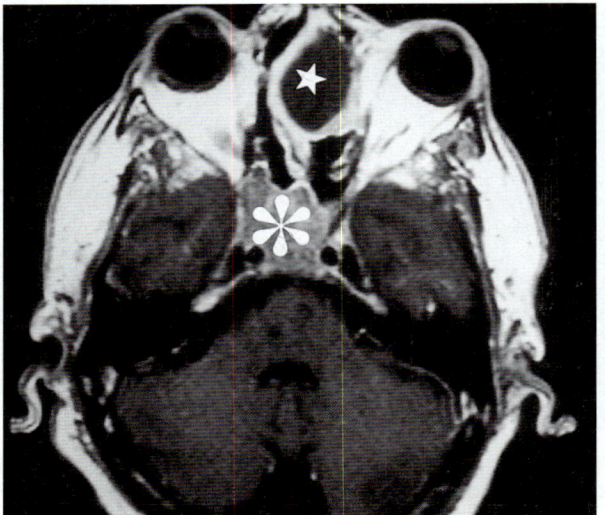

FIG. 31. Case 5. Cystic lesion of intranasal fossa—recurrent inverted papilloma (*star*). Chondroma (*asterisk*) in sphenoid sinus.

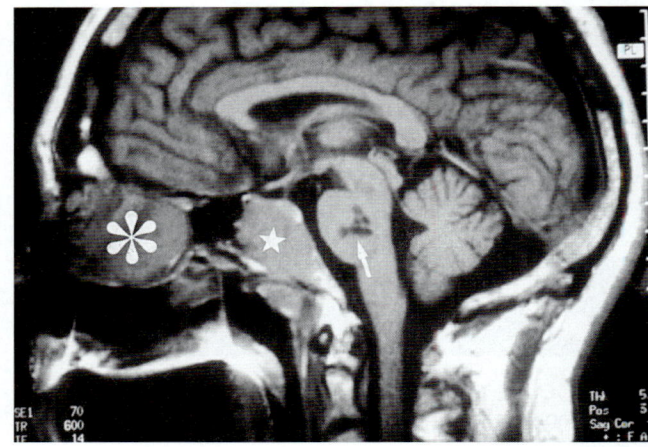

FIG. 32. Case 5. Inverted papilloma in cystic bony wall (*asterisk*) with frontal sinus involvement, chondroma of the sphenoid sinus (*star*), and asymptomatic angioma of the brainstem (*arrow*).

CASE 5 (Continued)

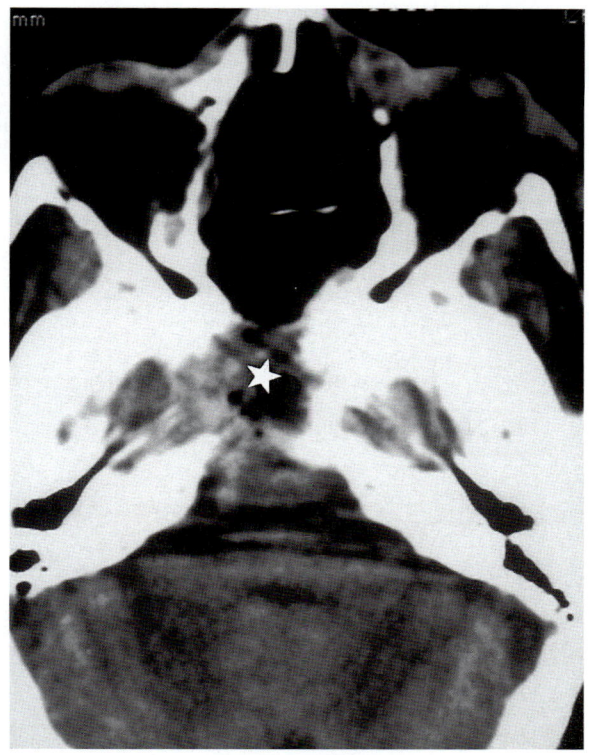

FIG. 33. Case 5. Postoperative axial computed tomography scan after total tumor removal. *Star* indicates sphenoid sinus.

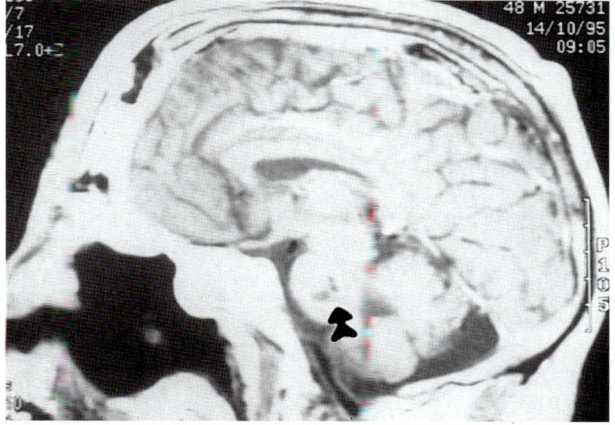

FIG. 34. Case 5. Sagittal postoperative magnetic resonance image showing removal of frontal bone meningioma, inverted papilloma, and sphenoid sinus chondroma. Note persistence of brainstem angioma (*arrow*).

CASE MATERIAL

The authors have used the degloving procedure/transmaxillary approach, alone or combined with other procedures, for a variety of lesions:

Juvenile nasopharyngeal angiofibroma	41
Inverted papilloma	7
Osteoma	8
Fibrous dysplasia	6
Osler-Weber-Rendue (septal dermoplasty)	2
Septal tumors	
Neurogenic tumor	1
Hemangiopericytoma	1
Malignant fibromatosis	1
Trigeminal neuroma	3
Clival chordoma	1
Chondroma	1
Clival chondrosarcoma	6
Aneurysmatic bone cyst	1
Clival giant cell tumor	1
Branchial hypertrophic myositis of masticator muscles	1
Aesthesioneuroblastoma	3

CONCLUSION

The degloving/transmaxillary approach to lesions of midface structures, the orbits, and the anterior and middle cranial base, alone or in combination with other procedures, is highly satisfactory to surgeon and patient alike.

It carries a very small morbidity and no visible scars for the patient. For the surgeon, it allows a bilateral midface approach with comfortable surgery even with large bleeding tumors (e.g., juvenile nasopharyngeal angiofibroma) or extensive and deeply located tumors.

Access to the anterior and middle cranial base (by degloving alone or in surgical combinations) can be readily accomplished with safe tumor removal and reconstruction.

This procedure has been successfully used in the authors' clinic for removal of large juvenile nasopharyngeal angiofibromas with invasion of the middle fossa and cavernous sinus. In the authors' opinion, in such cases there is no need for craniotomy because most of the lesions are extradural.

Even for ablation of selected malignant tumors, it is the authors' opinion that the head and neck oncologist could use this approach more frequently.

REFERENCES

1. Converse JM. Restoration of facial contour by bone grafts introduced through the oral cavity. *Plast Reconstr Surg* 1950;6:295.
2. Denker A, Kahler O. *Handbuch der Hals Nasen Ohren Heilkunde*. Berlin: Springer-Verlag, 1926.
3. Portmann G, Retrouvery H. *Le cancer du nez*. Paris: Gaston Doin et cie, 1927.
4. Williams RI. Utilization of rhinoplastic technique: hemilateral rhinotomy for the removal of intranasal tumors. *Laryngoscope* 1957;67:796–814.
5. Casson PR, Bonano PC, Converse JM. The midface degloving procedure. *Plast Reconstr Surg* 1974;53:102–113.
6. Allen G, Siegel G. The sublabial approach for extensive nasal and sinus resection. *Laryngoscope* 1981;91:1635–1639.
7. Conley J, Price J. Sublabial approach to the nasal and nasopharyngeal cavities. *Am J Surg* 1979;138:615–618.
8. Maniglia AJ. Indication and techniques in midfacial degloving: a 15 years experience. *Arch Otolaryngol Head Neck Surg* 1986;112:750–752.
9. Price J, Holliday M, Kennedy D, Johns ME, Richtsmeier WJ, Mattox DE. The versatile midface degloving approach. *Laryngoscope* 1988;98:291–295.
10. Paavolainen M, Malmberg H. Sublabial approach to the nasal and paranasal cavities using nasal pyramid osteotomy and septal transection. *Laryngoscope* 1986;96:106–108.

CHAPTER 12

Extended Unilateral Maxillotomy Approach

Edwin W. Cocke, Jr. and Jon H. Robertson

In this chapter, a technique for surgical exposure of the extracranial skull base for the removal of craniocervical lesions from the roof of the sphenoid to the fourth cervical vertebra and between the carotid canals is described in detail. Additional techniques and modifications of the original technique first described by the authors in 1990 are included. The authors' experience with 30 patients, from which the techniques have been refined, is discussed. Compared with the authors' earlier experiences, the complication and morbidity rates have diminished. A brief history is provided, and indications, preoperative and postoperative management, technique, complications, advantages, disadvantages, and comments identifying specific patient management are discussed.

The successful management of patients with skull base lesions depends on a thorough knowledge of the regional anatomy and the biologic nature of the conditions that may involve the area, as well as the accuracy of the diagnosis, the anatomic extent of the disease, and an understanding of a multitude of treatment modalities that may be expected to provide maximum relief for these patients. A multidisciplinary approach is commendable. The authors' team consists of a neurosurgeon, an otolaryngology–head and neck surgeon, an oral surgeon, and an anesthesiologist.

The authors describe an extended maxillotomy technique for skull base exposure that has proved satisfactory in their supervision of 30 patients. Techniques for improved patient care and improvements of the authors' surgical technique, permitting exposure from the roof of the sphenoid to the fourth or fifth cervical vertebra and reported in 1990 (1), are described. These improvements have resulted in additional skull base exposure and access for dural closure, facilitation of maxillary osteotomies, improved cosmesis, and a reduction in patient morbidity. Additional surgical options and expansion of the procedure, as well as the indications, advantages, disadvantages, and complications of the procedure, are discussed.

HISTORY

The original bilateral horizontal maxillary osteotomy technique was described by von Langenbeck in 1859 (2,3). He presented a case report in the medical literature in 1861 using the same technique to remove "fibroids of the pterygopalatine fossa." Cheever (4) is given credit for using in 1867 the same approach for the removal of a tumor in the nasopharynx in two patients. One patient had an incomplete unilateral horizontal maxillary osteotomy for removal of an angiofibroma; the other had an incomplete bilateral horizontal maxillary osteotomy for removal of a tumor that was not histologically diagnosed (5).

In 1893, Lanz (6) gave an account of an operation developed earlier by Kocher. The upper lip was divided in the midline as well as the maxilla. This was his palatal osteomyotomy contribution to von Langenbeck's bilateral horizontal maxillotomy, and represents an osteotomy in two sections. In 1898, Partsch (7) reported a technique for temporary mobilization of the upper jaw and eliminated Kocher's lip-splitting incision. In 1901, LeFort (8) classified facial fractures, including the LeFort I midface fracture. This fracture was described as passing through the nasal pyriform aperture transversely, the inferior meatus, the canine fossa to below the buttress of the zygoma, and along the antral wall to the pterygomaxillary fissure. It passed through the lower third of the pterygoid plates and separated the tooth-bearing upper maxilla from the cranial base. Loewe in 1902 (9) outlined a historical summary of the surgical techniques involving the superior maxilla. The basic concept of temporary mobilization and inferior displacement of the upper maxilla for the removal of a nasopharyngeal polyp was described by Pincus in 1907 (10). In 1927, Martin Wassmund performed a LeFort I

E. W. Cocke, Jr.: Department of Otolaryngology, Head and Neck Surgery, The University of Tennessee, Memphis, The Health Science Center, Memphis, Tennessee 38103.

J. H. Robertson: Department of Neurosurgery, The University of Tennessee, Memphis, The Health Science Center, and Semmes-Murphey Clinic, Memphis, Tennessee 38103.

osteotomy for correction of malocclusion, and reported the operation in the medical literature in 1935 (11). Numerous other authors have made contributions to this subject since 1934, including Axhausen in 1934 (12), Steinkamm in 1938 (13), Gillies and Rowe in 1954 (14), Dingman and Harding in 1951 (15), Cupar in 1952 (16), Obwegeser in 1962 to 1970 (17), Hogeman and Willmar in 1967 (18), and Pfeifer in 1969 (19). These historical events are beautifully described by Drommer in "The History of the LeFort I Osteotomy" (20). He makes the observation that the LeFort I osteotomy was reported 130 years before his (Drommer's) publication, and 80 years elapsed before it became a part of the surgical treatment of skeletal facial deformities, including management of the patient with cleft palate.

At the beginning of their experience in 1986, the authors were called on by a neurosurgeon to expose the skull base in a patient whose chordoma of the skull base had been incompletely removed on two previous occasions by conservative procedures. A subtotal maxillectomy through a Weber-Fergusson skin incision was carried out, along with removal of the lateral nasal wall, ethmoidectomy, and posterior nasal septectomy. After removal of the chordoma, the subsequent palatal defect was closed with an appropriate obturator. The skull base exposure was quite adequate. In selected patients with advanced disease, the surgeon still might consider it as the procedure of choice.

The authors conceived that perhaps the same surgical exposure could be obtained by mobilizing the homolateral maxilla below the level of the inferior orbital nerve and retracting the maxilla while preserving the nerve. They were concerned that the blood supply to the maxilla might be compromised, and designed a technique to preserve the attachment of the mucoperiosteum of the entire hard palate to the bone. The authors subsequently discontinued their efforts to maintain this attachment when it became obvious that it was perforated in the midline on numerous occasions, and the hard palate survived presumably from the blood supply it received only from its soft palate connection. The angiographic and radioactive microsphere studies, respectively, of Bell et al. (21–23) and Nelson et al. (24), and the clinical information obtained by Lanigan, an orthognathic surgeon, and his team (25), added to the authors' knowledge of the blood supply to the maxilla. As a result of these experiences, the authors now approach the skull base through a unilateral horizontal maxillary osteotomy with a modified LeFort I exposure (maxillotomy) that does not include a midline soft palate myotomy. The maxilla is divided through the middle meatus. The Weber-Fergusson incision has been discontinued except when the oral commissure is very small or the teeth too long. The upper lip is then divided in the midline. The incision may be extended laterally to beyond the nasal alar. The authors approach the maxilla through the sublabial transoral degloving technique (26–29) to expose not only the extracranial central and lateral compartments of the skull base, but the infratemporal fossa. This exposes the craniocervical region from the roof of the sphenoid sinus to the fourth or fifth cervical vertebra, between the eustachian tubes, carotid canals, hypoglossal canals, and condyles of the occipital bone that are adjacent to the anterior and lateral margins of the foramen magnum. This exposure is accomplished by dividing the lateral margin of the nasal pyriform aperture, removing the entire lateral wall of the nose above the middle meatus, the ethmoid and sphenoid sinuses, the posterior half of the nasal septum, sometimes the coronoid process of the mandible, and the pterygoid plates, without disturbing the cranial end of the ascending process of the maxilla. The maxilla with the lower half of the body of the zygoma is retracted inferiorly, medially, or laterally to gain adequate skull base exposure. Additional extension of the procedure with cervical spine exposure requires division and retraction of the soft tissues lateral to the palatine tonsil and its tongue base attachment. In the depths of this defect is the prevertebral fascia. The tonsil, anterior and posterior tonsillar pillars, superior constrictor muscle, soft palate, and maxilla are retracted toward the midline. As the degloving exposure is advanced, almost the entire zygoma may be exposed, and it can be temporarily removed and replaced. The bony foramen about the infraorbital nerve may be microfragmented and the nerve mobilized from its infraorbital canal, retracted, and elevated with the degloved soft tissues to a higher level. With preservation of the adjacent orbital periosteum, additional orbital floor may be divided, and the soft tissue retracted for additional exposure.

Gigli saw division of the maxilla continues to play a major role in the authors' technique. Other options for division of the maxilla have been developed.

The bilateral horizontal maxillary osteotomy with preservation of the soft palate and with a LeFort I exposure has been the procedure of choice for many skull base surgeons. The surgical literature includes reports by Wood and Stell in 1984 (30) and Archer et al. in 1987 (31). Belmont in 1988 (32) was concerned that the blood supply to the osteotomized maxilla would not be adequate. Additional experience with the bilateral osteotomy was reported by Uttley et al. (33) and Brown in 1989 (34), and Morril et al. in 1993 (35). The bilateral horizontal maxillary osteotomy with complete division of the maxilla and the soft palate in the midline has been described by Sasaki et al. (36) and Sandor et al. (37) in 1990, James and Crockard (38) and Anand et al. (39) in 1991, and O'Reilly et al. in 1993 (40). In 1990, the authors' team reported their experience with three patients with chordomas of the clivus (1). The tumors were resected by subtotal maxillectomy in two patients and a unilateral horizontal maxillary osteotomy in one patient. In the latter patient, the soft palate and the mucoperiosteum of the hard palate bilaterally remained intact. In 1993, Catalano et al. (41) reported a three-fourths horizontal maxillary osteotomy with preservation of the hard palate mucoperiosteum and the soft palate attachments.

Since 1990, the authors' approach in 30 patients for the removal of skull base tumors has been through a unilateral horizontal maxillary osteotomy (maxillotomy) with preservation of the soft palate attachment to the maxilla. The blood supply to the maxilla has been adequate even when the maxilla with its mucoperiosteum is divided in the midline. The maxilla and soft palate also survive if the soft palate is divided laterally beyond the anterior tonsillar pillar and tonsil, with division of the superior pharyngeal constrictor muscle, retraction of the retropharyngeal tissues, and exposure of the prevertebral fascia. With this additional exposure, the surgeon must be prepared to accept a unilateral motor weakness of the adjacent soft palate.

INDICATIONS

Numerous techniques have been described to manage lesions involving the skull base. The appropriate procedure for each patient varies, as well as the objective that is to be accomplished. This objective depends on several factors, including familiarity and experience with these techniques as well as knowledge of the regional anatomy, the location, extent, size, and consistency of the tumor, and the histologic diagnosis. An understanding of the natural history of the specific disease process may influence the surgeon's decision only to biopsy the tumor or to withhold treatment in the face of an asymptomatic, slow-growing neoplasm, one that has invaded the carotid artery, or one that is refractory to radiation therapy and unresectable.

Limited access rarely permits total excision. Extracranial tumors of the middle and posterior cranial fossae require extracranial procedures. Midline skull base tumors, most lateral compartment tumors, and clival tumors involving the dura require a maxillotomy. In the authors' opinion, it is unlikely that a tumor that crosses the midline can be resected through a lateral approach, as described by Fisch et al. (42). Tumors involving bone are rarely completely removed.

The extended maxillotomy was originally designed for the removal of chordomas at the skull base. Craniospinal lesions treated by mid–skull-base approaches are listed in Table 1.

A full review of the advantages of the maxillotomy is presented later, but these advantages suggest that the indications for this operation may be extended. For these and other reasons, the extended maxillotomy may be selected as the procedure of choice.

It is rare for this approach to be selected for the correction of bony abnormalities of the skull base. Although it produces excellent exposure, more conservative procedures are preferred.

The unilateral horizontal maxillotomy (extended maxillotomy) is an excellent approach for conditions that extend between the roof of the sphenoid and the fourth cervical vertebra, between the eustachian tubes, carotid arteries, petrooccipital fissures, hypoglossal foramina, and the occipital condyles. Most frequently, the surgical procedure is performed on the side corresponding to the tumor. In rare instances, the contralateral maxilla is mobilized and retracted inferiorly for maximum exposure of lesions that primarily involve the contralateral occipital condyle and hypoglossal foramen and nerve. This approach takes advantage of a surgical exposure that permits manipulation of instruments and the operating microscope to work at an extreme angle, in contrast to the usual anteroposterior working relationship. If the extent of the disease can be anticipated, treatment may be designed for incomplete removal and palliation only, or for cure with an attempt to remove the tumor completely. Complete extirpation is rarely, if ever, accomplished. Postoperative radiation therapy may be advantageous if the tumor has been incompletely removed and is radiosensitive.

The best results are obtained when the tumor is benign, well encapsulated, exophytic, noninfiltrative, slow growing, has a pushing border, and is extradural. The clival dura may

TABLE 1. *Craniospinal lesions treated by mid-skull base approaches*

Benign tumors
Angiofibroma
Chondroma
Chordoma
Craniopharyngioma
Fibrous dysplasia
Hemangioma
Hemangiopericytoma
Lymphangioma
Meningioma
Neurilemoma
Neurofibroma
Ossifying fibroma
Osteoblastoma
Osteochondroma
Osteoclastoma
Osteoma
Paraganglioma
Pericytoma
Pituitary adenoma
Schwannoma
Teratogenic cyst (brainstem)
Malignant tumors
Acinic cell adenocarcinoma
Adenocarcinoma
Adenoid cystic carcinoma
Carcinoma
Chondrosarcoma
Chordoma
Epidermoid (x-ray resistant)
Fibrous histiocytoma
Olfactory neuroblastoma
Plasmacytoma
Rhabdomyosarcoma
Sarcoma
Other lesions
Aneurysm
Arthritis (rheumatoid)
Atlantoaxial dislocation
Basilar impression
Craniospinal malformation
Fracture with dislocation (odontoid)
Meningocele

or may not be involved, but if so, it is easily removed without damage to a compressed brainstem. A complete clival craniectomy is usually required along with limited removal of the extracranial disease. Benign tumors involving the middle and lateral compartments of the skull base, as well as the infratemporal fossa, lend themselves more frequently to complete removal. The improvement in cure rates is directly related to the completeness of removal and extent of the resection at the time of the first operation. Secondary procedures are more hazardous. The complication rate is increased and the survival rate is reduced. The extended maxillotomy may be repeated for the removal of residual disease.

The poorest results are obtained when the tumor is malignant, without a capsule, aggressive, infiltrative, and invading the multiple foramina and crevices at the skull base. In most instances, these tumors cannot be completely removed with a good margin of normal tissue without seriously threatening the life of the patient.[1] These infiltrative tumors may occur as a result of radiation failure. In other instances, the patient may be given postoperative therapy for a primary tumor that may have been incompletely removed.[2]

This approach offers excellent access for reconstruction of the surgical defect. Nasal septal and temporalis muscle flaps are frequently rotated to cover dural defects. These may be unnecessary when the dural defect is closed watertight with interrupted sutures or with a sutured fascial graft and reinforced with bilateral nasoseptal mucoperiosteal flaps.

PREOPERATIVE MANAGEMENT

Before surgery, the patient is thoroughly evaluated by state-of-the-art techniques to determine his or her general physical condition, the diagnosis, and the anatomic extent of the disease. This frequently requires high-resolution computed tomography and magnetic resonance imaging scans with contrast and, in rare instances, an arteriogram. Not only may the surgeon have the opportunity to study the adequacy of carotid arterial function, but he or she may also consider whether embolization of a part of this system would be advantageous to reduce the degree of operative blood loss. These findings are presented to the surgeons and anesthesiologists involved so that a carefully planned approach may be developed.

Unless the patient is preoperatively dependent on a tracheostomy, percutaneous esophageal gastrostomy, or a nasogastric feeding tube, the authors have discontinued their use except in rare instances.

Antibiotic coverage consists of a cephalosporin and an aminoglycoside that are administered the day of surgery.

In the operating room, the head and neck are washed with an antiseptic soap and cleansed with alcohol. Table 2 lists

---
[1] **Editor's note:** *These cases are not perhaps suitable for a purely subcranial approach and will be more effectively resected by some of the other intracranial/extracranial approaches described in this book.*
[2] **Editor's note:** *This may provide palliation, but rarely a cure.*

TABLE 2. *Equipment for preoperative preparation of operative sites*

1. Head light
2. Betadine soap
3. Alcohol
4. Sponges
5. Cottonoid tapes (small and large)
    a. Vaseline
    b. Dry
6. Bayonet forceps
7. Nasal specula (three lengths)
8. Solution on cottonoid to nose for nasal mucous membrane shrinkage
    a. 4% Cocaine and 1% Neo-synephrine solution
9. Nasal injection
    a. 1% Lidocaine with 1:100,000 adrenaline
    b. 10-ml syringe
    c. 25-gauge 2-in. needle
    d. 25-gauge spinal needle
    e. Tonsil needle
10. Mouth retractors
    a. Jennings
    b. McIver
    c. Metal tongue blade
11. Suction
    a. Yankauer
    b. Neurosurgical
12. Retractors
    a. Richardson
        i. Wide
        ii. Narrow
    b. Senturia (palate)
    c. Love (palate)
13. For temporary tarsorrhaphy
    a. 6/0 Ethicon nylon
    b. Needle holder, small
    c. Tissue forceps and scissors
14. Vaselinized cottonoid sutured to lips
    a. #1 Silk with needle
15. To shave scalp, abdomen, and thigh in selected patients
    a. Razor
    b. Electric clipper
16. For myringotomy and insertion of pressure ventilating tube
    a. Operating microscope ×300 lens
    b. Shepard tube
    c. Ear suction
    d. Forceps
    e. Myringotomy knife

Equipment for sterile set-up
1. Betadine
2. Alcohol
3. Sponge
4. Towels
5. Drapes for head, abdomen, and thigh
6. Transparent drapes
    a. Face
    b. Microscope
    c. With irrigating container

equipment that should be available before surgery to prepare the operative sites. Table 3 lists selective surgical equipment that should be available for each operation and should be checked before surgery.

TABLE 3. *Selected operating instruments*

1. Rhinoplasty and septoplasty instruments
   a. Pierce elevator, button knife, Joseph knife
   b. Nasal scissors
2. Paranasal sinus instruments
3. Tonsil instruments
4. Retractors
   a. Richardson
      i. Broad
      ii. Small
      iii. Narrow
   b. Deaver, narrow
5. Mouth retractors
   a. Jennings
   b. McIver
   c. Senturia
   d. Love
   e. Crockard
   f. Leylar
   g. Fish hooks
   h. Small and large rake
6. Cottonoids (all sizes)
7. For bleeding
   a. Bipolar cautery
   b. Bovie cautery
   c. Stick ties (3-0 chromic)
   d. Surgicel
   e. Gelfoam soaked in thrombin
   f. Wax for bone
   g. Clips, small, and applicator
   h. Adrenal water (half-and-half)
8. Suctions
   a. Small and large Yankauer
   b. Neurosurgery (suction, irrigation, ultrasonic aspirator)
   c. Electrosuction
9. Knives
   a. Bard-Parker
   b. Electro (Shaw)
10. Red rubber catheter
11. Rongeurs
    a. Double action (large)
    b. Kerrison
    c. Needle-nose
    d. Kofler
12. Forceps
    a. Bayonet
    b. Brunning
    c. Sphenoid
    d. Tissue
    e. Pituitary (pullers)
13. Drill
    a. Midas with points, high-speed
14. Wire carrier
    a. Orthopedic
    b. Tuohy needle #14 (prepared before operation and ready for use)
       i. Medicine glass
    c. 9-in. curved broad ligament clamp
    d. Curved, sharp-pointed large thyroid ligature carrier
15. Wire #22 and cutter
16. Urethral sound #22 and smaller
17. Saws
    a. Four new Gigli saws (noncurled)
    b. Reciprocating
    c. Stryker with small blade
18. Suture
    a. 2-0 Vicryl
    b. 3-0 Chromic gut
    c. 4-0 Plain on Keith needle (pc 3), short, long needles
19. Chisels
    a. Straight
    b. Curved
    c. Narrow
    d. Broad
    e. Mastoid gouge
20. Dressing
    a. Nasal splint
21. Ice in glove (2)
    a. Apply during and after operation
22. Elevators
    a. Narrow
    b. Large
    c. Lempert
    d. Sharp
    e. Blunt
23. Hooks
    a. Nasal
       i. Single
       ii. Double
       iii. Sharp
       iv. Blunt
    b. Fibroid hook, single
    c. Fish hooks
24. Miniplates
25. Dermatome
26. For abdominal fat removal
    a. Rake retractor
27. Laser, CO_2
28. Operating microscope
    a. ×400 lens for neurosurgery
29. Scissors
    a. Curved Mayo
    b. Suture
    c. Dissection
       i. For nose
       ii. For abdominal fat
30. Neurosurgical instruments
    a. Nerve stimulator
    b. Fluoroscope with C-arm attachment

A 1% lidocaine solution containing 1:100,000 epinephrine is injected into the area to be operated on after shrinkage of the nasal mucous membranes with cottonoid strips saturated with 4% cocaine and 1% phenylephrine hydrochloride (Neo-Synephrine). Special attention is given to injecting the lining of the interior of the nose, each greater palatine canal, the hard palate mucoperiosteum, the anterior and posterior ethmoid arteries, the posterior and lateral nasopharyngeal walls, and the soft tissues of the cheek, pterygoid region, and the lines of incision.

If a temporalis muscle flap for reconstruction of the skull base is anticipated, the homolateral scalp is shaved. This area, as well as the face, neck, abdomen, and homolateral thigh, is shaved and cleansed with povidone–iodine (Betadine) and dried with alcohol preparatory to harvesting abdominal fat or a split-thickness skin graft for reconstruction.

A bilateral temporary tarsorrhaphy is performed and an indwelling urethral catheter is inserted.

The patient is given general anesthesia. An oral endotracheal tube is introduced and made to exit from the contralateral side of the mouth, and is sutured into place.

Appropriate drapes are applied, and a large vaselinized cottonoid strip is made to cover the entire lip surface. It is sutured in place to protect this area from injury that could develop from instruments used for electrocoagulation and retraction. Automatic compression stockings are applied.

In the event trauma to the eustachian tube is anticipated, a homolateral myringotomy and insertion of a pressure ventilating tube through the tympanic membrane is accomplished.

TECHNIQUE

The superior maxilla is exposed by a degloving technique. In the authors' experience, this technique has replaced the Weber-Fergusson incision. Not only is this surgical exposure just as satisfactory as the latter incision, but facial scarring is eliminated. It may be necessary to divide the upper lip to the alar crease in exceptional cases when the oral commissure is very small or when the teeth are exceptionally long.

Nasal Exposure

Exposure of the interior of the nose is by a standard rhinoplasty technique. One or both nasal cavities may be exposed, depending on the extent of the degloving incision. Usually the exposure is bilateral (Fig. 1).

A complete transfixation incision is used. This incision is extended inferiorly to the nasal floor and is continued through its lateral wall anterior to the bony pyriform aperture. Care is taken to leave a few millimeters of redundant mucous membrane anterior to the bony nasal floor and pyriform aperture to assist in subsequent closure of the defect.

An intercartilaginous incision is extended to join the initial incisions, resulting in a complete circumferential anterior

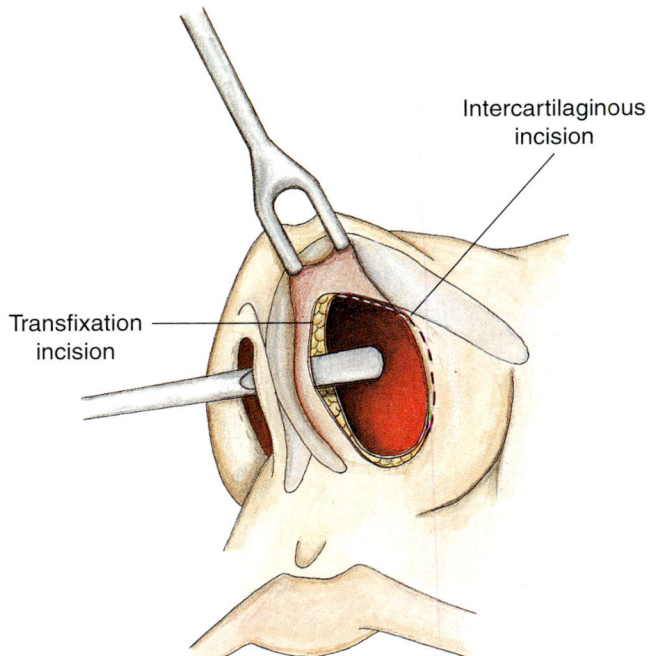

FIG. 1. Bilateral circumferential intranasal incisions.

intranasal incision. Through these incisions, the skin and subcutaneous tissues on the nasal dorsum may be unilaterally or bilaterally elevated to the nasofrontal suture. The periosteum remains attached to the bone and is not elevated.

Hard Palate Exposure

A vertical incision in the anteroposterior direction is made through the mucoperiosteum of the hard palate several millimeters to the contralateral side of the midline from the junction of the hard and soft palate to the interdental space between the central incisor teeth. The adjacent mucoperiosteum is elevated a few millimeters on each side of the incision to permit ease in subsequent closure (Fig. 2).

Through this incision, at the junction of the hard and soft palate on the homolateral side of the midline, the soft tissues are detached from the posterior margin of the hard palate to gain entrance into the nasopharynx. This defect should be large enough only to manipulate one arm of the lower Gigli saw into position.

Construction of Intranasal Flap

The mucoperiosteum of the posterior half of the nasal floor on the side of the lesion is elevated, including the dorsal lining of the soft palate. This is extended laterally to elevate the mucoperiosteum from the lateral wall of the nose to the level of the attachment of the inferior turbinate in its posterior half (Fig. 3A). The mucoperiosteum is divided hori-

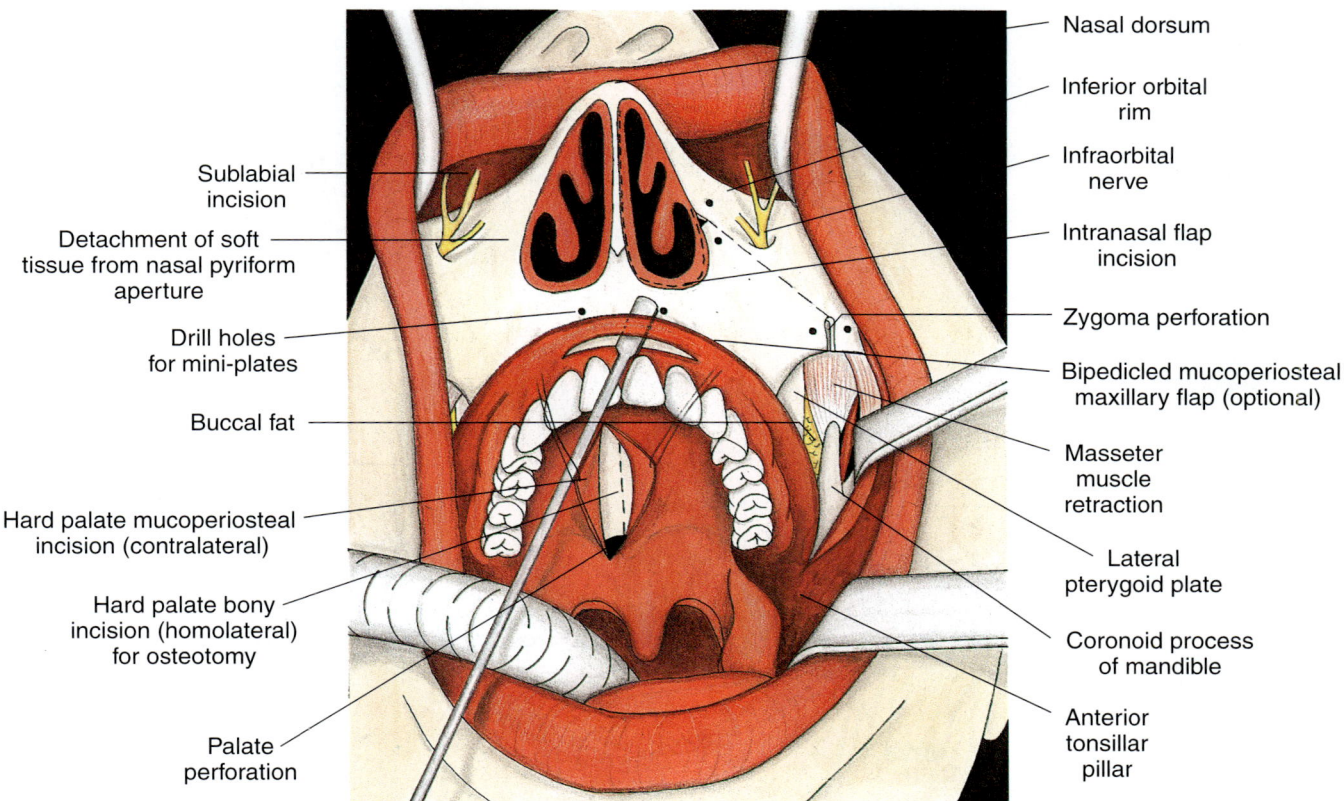

FIG. 2. A degloving technique is used for homolateral and bilateral exposure of the anterior maxilla, nose, masseter muscle, coronoid process of the mandible, lateral pterygoid plate, and zygoma. Construction of the bipedicled maxillary mucoperiosteal flap is optional. The mucoperiosteum of the hard palate is divided vertically in an anteroposterior direction on the contralateral side of the midline. A palate perforation into the nasopharynx is created to accommodate the lower Gigli saw.

zontally in the inferior meatus on the lateral wall of the nose from its incision site anteriorly to its posterior extent immediately below the attachment of the inferior turbinate. This dissection is extended medially to elevate the mucoperiosteum from the homolateral nasal floor and nasal septum (see Fig. 3).

The anterior septal mucoperichondrium and cartilage are allowed to remain attached to the maxillary crest, nasal spine, septal cartilage, and the distal margin of the nasal bone. This will avoid a saddle nasal deformity should the cartilage support be removed. To accomplish this, a vertical incision is made at the junction of the perpendicular plate of the ethmoid and the posterior margin of the septal cartilage from the cribriform plate superiorly to the nasal floor and the lateral nasal wall in the inferior meatus inferiorly. Posterior to this incision, the adjacent vomer and the perpendicular plate of the ethmoid are removed to the anterior face of the sphenoid. The contralateral septal soft tissues may also be preserved. The remainder of the cartilaginous nasal septum remains attached to the maxillary crest and adjacent nasal spine anteriorly.

The primary superior attachment of the intranasal flap is at the level of the cribriform plate. This attachment is divided transversely beneath the cribriform plate from its anterior to its posterior extent so that subsequently the flap may be elevated from the anterior wall of the sphenoid and rotated posteriorly. It remains pedicled to the soft tissue at the lateral margin of the sphenoid. The flap is designed to cover a subsequent sphenoclival defect where the dura has been closed. The adjacent clival defect may have been packed with fat, muscle, or bone. The surgeon may elect not to use this intranasal flap, which consists of mucoperiosteum originating from the lateral wall of the nose in the inferior meatus, the floor of the nose, the adjacent posterior nasal septum, and the anterior face of the sphenoid. A similar septal flap may be constructed from the opposite side of the septum to supplement coverage of the sphenoclival defect.

Anterior Maxillary Exposure

The gingivobuccal gutter is exposed and a transverse sublabial incision is made high in its apex through its oral mucoperiosteum from a point 2 cm lateral to the midline, to the homolateral retromolar region and into the anterior tonsillar pillar well lateral to the palatine tonsil (see Fig. 2).

Another 3-cm transverse mucoperiosteal anterior maxillary incision 2 cm beneath the apex incision is made adjacent

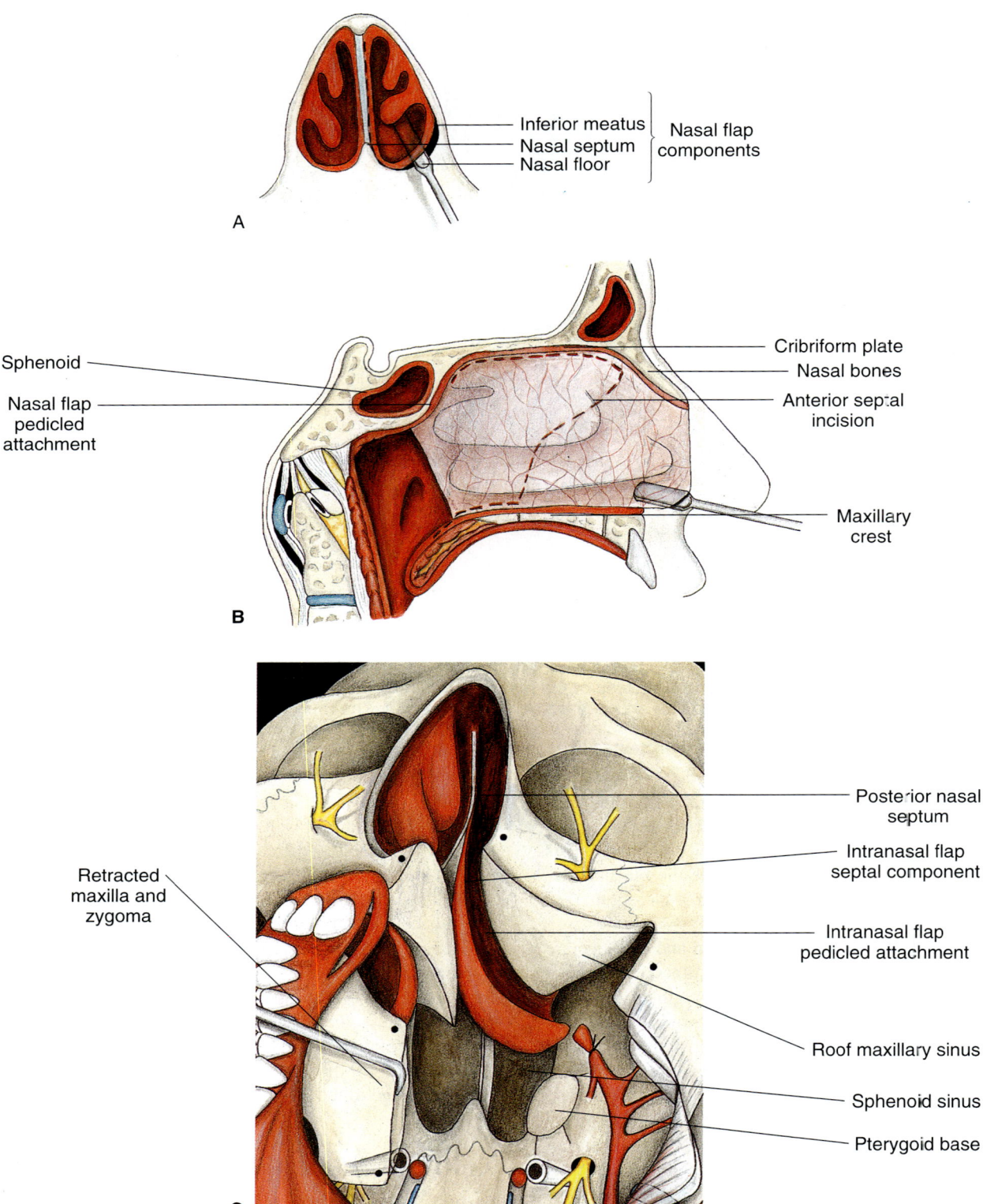

FIG. 3. Transnasal flap construction. **A:** Elevation of mucoperiosteum from lateral wall of nose in the inferior meatus, nasal floor, and septum. **B:** Septal component of the nasal flap detached from the posterior nasal septum beneath the cribriform plate and pedicled lateral to the sphenoid. **C:** Intranasal flap construction continues after the maxillotomy exposure. The flap has been elevated from the lateral inferior meatal wall, floor of the nose, and the posterior nasal septum.

to the central incisor teeth. This 2-cm–wide bipedicled mucoperiosteal flap is elevated from the maxilla and will serve as a hinge for rotation of the maxilla after the maxillary osteotomy. It may be centrally divided if manipulation of the flap or the maxilla is troublesome.

The cheek flap, consisting of skin, subcutaneous tissue, periosteum, and oral mucosa, is elevated from the anterior maxilla to the level of the infraorbital nerve and the inferior rim of the orbit, exposing the zygoma and its masseter attachment, as well as the lateral wall of the maxilla to the pterygoid plate. Medially, these tissues are elevated from the nasal dorsum to the nasofrontal suture and detached from the nasal pyriform aperture so that enough of its adjacent soft tissue will be preserved to permit closure of the defect at the completion of the operation.

Exposure of the Lateral Wall of the Maxilla, Lateral Pterygoid Plate, and Internal Maxillary Artery

The masseter muscle is detached from the body of the zygoma to its arch. Retraction of the masseter muscle exposes the coronoid process of the mandible. For additional exposure, the coronoid is usually removed to the level of the mandibular foramen with a large rongeur after division of its temporalis muscle attachment. Not only is exposure increased by removal of the coronoid, but it facilitates ligation of the internal maxillary artery and creation of a bony soft tissue tract behind the maxilla through which a Gigli saw is passed to divide the maxilla. It does not lead to limitation of jaw mobility any more than if it was not removed (Fig. 4).

With the head extended, buccal fat is removed to expose or palpate the lateral pterygoid plate. The lateral pterygoid muscle is electrocoagulated and detached from its insertion on the lower half of the lateral pterygoid plate and maxilla, with care taken to identify the internal maxillary artery. Exposure with a long Richardson or narrow Deaver retractor is helpful. The numerous veins in the area are exposed and compressed with cottonoid sponges and a large Yankauer suction. They are electrocoagulated as the internal maxillary artery is mobilized; the artery is usually identified in the upper third of the pterygomaxillary fissure deep to the attachment of the lateral pterygoid muscle to the greater wing of the sphenoid, and above the attachment of the lateral pterygoid muscle to the lower half of the lateral pterygoid plate. The artery is below the sometimes palpable infratemporal crest, and travels transversely. It lies above the foramen ovale in the pterygomaxillary fissure and must be differentiated from the mandibular nerve. Its viable posterior segment contributes blood supply to the temporalis muscle and is preserved. The artery is clipped and divided anteriorly. If not immediately identified, it may be ligated after division of the maxilla.

Positioning of Upper Gigli Saw

Each wall of the maxillary sinus below the level of the infraorbital nerve is simultaneously divided with a Gigli saw. To accomplish this, two options are available, related to whether the saw is positioned anterior or posterior to the pterygoid plates. The authors prefer to place the saw anteriorly in the pterygomaxillary fissure. In this position, the saw divides the maxilla through the middle meatus and with less difficulty than if it is positioned posteriorly. In the posterior position, it divides the maxilla through the inferior meatus in a way identical to the LeFort I fracture.

A soft tissue and bony tract is prepared for positioning the Gigli saw. After ligating the internal maxillary artery and identifying the lateral pterygoid plate, the pterygomaxillary fissure is palpated. A no. 22 urethral sound is engaged in the fissure and passed into the pterygopalatine fossa. An index finger in the nasopharynx palpates the eustachian tube. Manipulation of the sound with one hand and confirmation of its anatomic point of entrance above the eustachian tube with the other permits the sound to be passed successfully into the nasopharynx. The same may be accomplished if the sound is passed posterior to the pterygoid plates. This sound or an alternative instrument passes through the pterygomaxillary fissure and the pterygopalatine fossa into the lumen of the nasopharynx with less difficulty if its handles are positioned inferiorly and parallel with the vertical ramus of the mandible. In this position, its tip is less likely to abut the adjacent bony skull base. Should difficulty be encountered in establishing this tract, other alternatives are available. A curved, 1-in. chisel is placed in the pterygomaxillary fissure, the adjacent bone divided, and the fissure enlarged. A small mastoid gouge or chisel may be passed through the pterygomaxillary fissure, into the pterygopalatine fossa, and driven into the nasopharynx. If necessary, the pterygoid plates or the posterior wall of the maxillary sinus may be divided.

Passage of the urethral sound through this defect enlarges the tract and permits passage of the Gigli saw behind the maxilla into the nasopharynx. Creation of the tract inferiorly in the pterygomaxillary fissure reduces the risk of damage to the internal maxillary artery, unless it is clipped before this dissection.

One of several instruments may be used as a ligature carrier for positioning the Gigli saw. An orthopedic wire carrier, a no. 14 Tuohy spinal needle, a thyroid ligature carrier, or a large, curved, long (9 in.) Kelly forceps have been used.

The orthopedic wire carrier is preferred (Fig. 5A). It is a curved, partially tubed instrument that can accommodate and transport a Gigli saw when the eye loop of the saw is compressed. This instrument is introduced into the tract made by the urethral sound and chisels and into the nasopharynx. Again, the position of the point of entrance of the wire carrier into the nasopharynx is confirmed by palpation. It is visualized by elevating the soft palate with a Love or Senturia retractor. Should this maneuver be troublesome, the pterygomaxillary attachment is again divided with a chisel, and the wire carrier repositioned. Care should be taken to prevent the carrier from entering the maxillary sinus, and preferably the carrier should be positioned behind it. The Gigli loop is grasped with forceps and transported into the oropharynx.

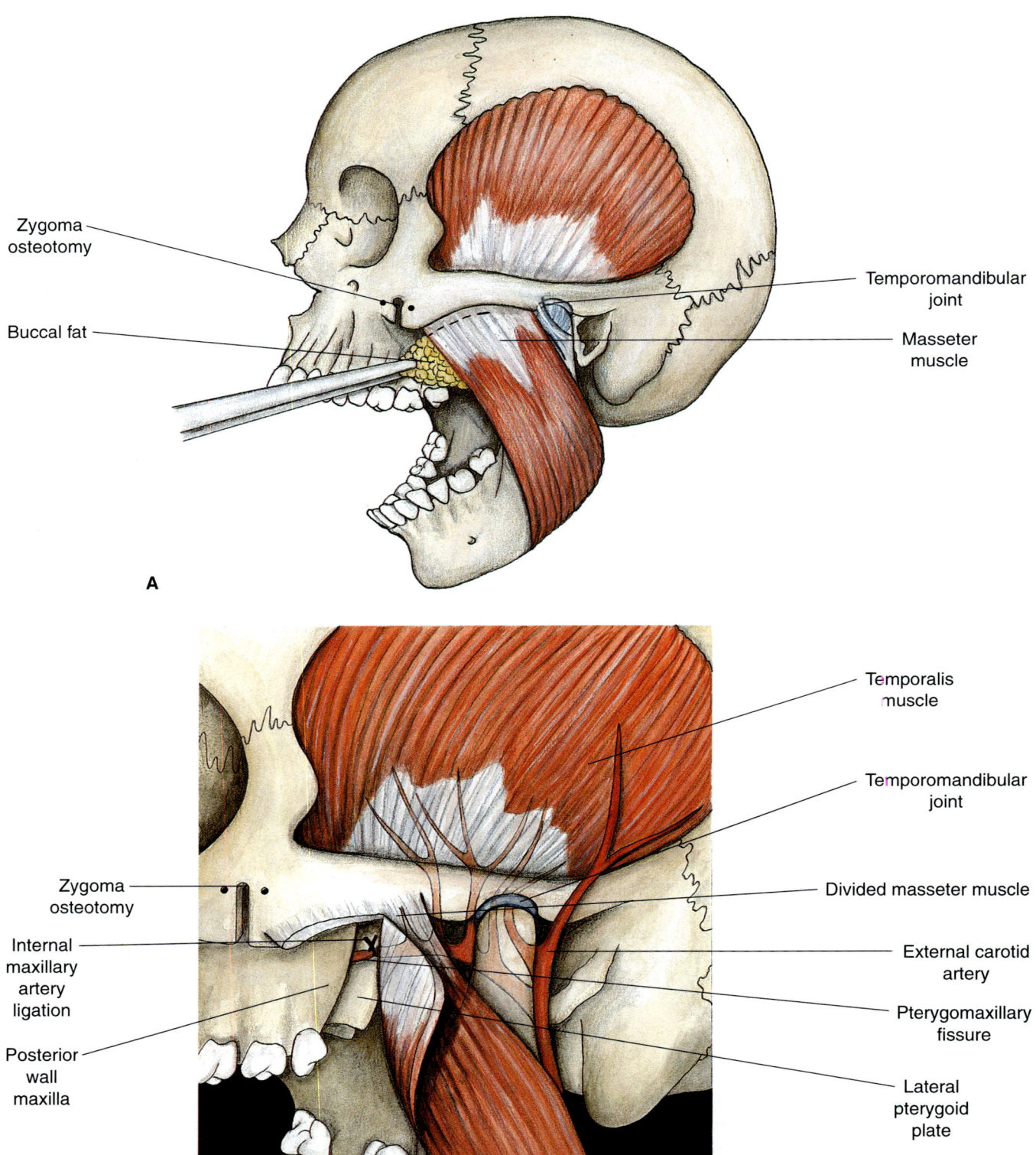

FIG. 4. A: Buccal fat removal to gain exposure in the pterygoid region medial to the masseter muscle. **B:** The infratemporal fossa is exposed medial to the zygomatic arch. The anterior masseter muscle is detached from the zygoma. Retraction of these tissues permits removal of the coronoid process of the mandible and its temporalis attachment. Partial division of the pterygoid muscle reveals the posterior wall of the maxillary sinus, lateral pterygoid plate, and the pterygomaxillary fissure. The anterior internal maxillary artery is clipped.

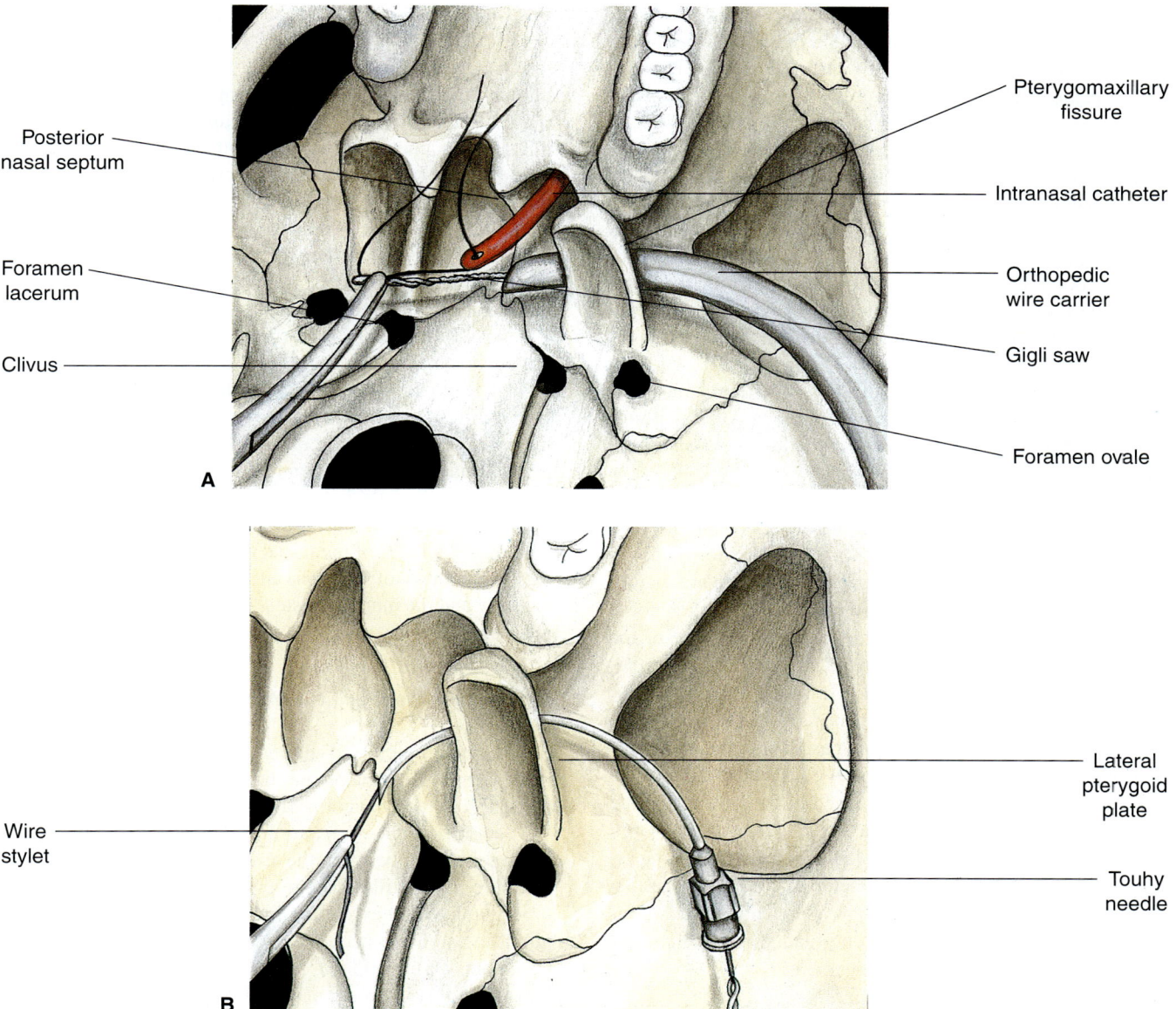

FIG. 5. A: The upper Gigli saw is positioned. An orthopedic wire carrier loaded with the medial arm of the Gigli saw is directed into the nasopharynx through the pterygomaxillary fissure anterior to the pterygoid plates. An intranasal catheter is tied to the Gigli saw loop. Soft palate retraction or manipulation of these instruments into the oropharynx for the silk tie approximation of the Gigli saw and the catheter is usually necessary. **B:** A no. 14 Touhy needle threaded with a no. 20 wire stylet. The Gigli saw is attached to the stylet. Retrograde traction on the wire positions the saw anterior to the pterygoid plate as the needle and stylet are removed.

The carrier is removed. A rubber catheter is passed through the nose into the nasopharynx and oropharynx. The Gigli loop and the catheter are joined with a silk suture. Traction on the catheter elevates and positions the medial arm of the saw in the nose at the level of the ascending process of the maxilla in the middle meatus. A broad ligament clamp may be substituted for the catheter to position the saw. The body of the zygoma is perforated with a drill just below the level of the infraorbital foramen. This perforation is extended to and through the inferior margin of the zygoma. This produces a notch to accommodate the lateral arm of the Gigli saw. The Gigli saw now completely surrounds the maxilla anterior to the pterygoid plates and, if maintained in the initial zygomatic perforation when the bone is divided, ensures division of the lateral nasal wall in the middle meatus. It is important to maintain the Gigli saw in the zygomatic perforation so that the level of division of the lateral nasal wall in the middle meatus is ensured.

Should the orthopedic carrier be unavailable, a specially prepared no. 14 Tuohy spinal needle may be used (see Fig. 5B). Its stylet is removed and a no. 20 or 22 wire is substituted. With the wire in place, the needle and wire are manipulated to produce a gentle curve, with care being taken not to produce a "crack" or break in the needle at the site of the bend. The wire in the needle helps to prevent this, and molding the needle around a medicine glass or a rounded instrument handle is a helpful maneuver. As with the orthopedic carrier, the needle and the wire are passed into the nasopharynx anterior or posterior to the pterygoid plates. The needle is removed. The Gigli saw is attached to the wire extending into the nasopharynx and, by traction on this wire, the Gigli saw is positioned into the perforated zygoma. As with the orthopedic wire carrier, a nasal catheter is attached to the medial arm of the Gigli saw. Traction on the catheter positions the saw in the nose. Again, a long-bladed broad ligament clamp may be substituted for the catheter.

The authors originally used a large, curved, sharp-pointed, right-angled thyroid ligature carrier to maneuver a no. 2 silk suture and the Gigli saw into position. Sometimes the instrument was too short. A large, long, curved Kelly or a broad ligament clamp have also been used without uniform success. It is wise, however, to be aware of these various instruments and have them available should additional techniques be required. Should these instruments not be available, the maxilla may be divided with an oscillating saw after exposure of its lateral wall to the pterygomaxillary fissure and the pyriform aperture at the middle meatus. The saw divides the lateral and anterior maxillary walls and finally the medial wall of the maxilla in the middle meatus to the medial pterygoid plate. The maxilla is then separated from the pterygoid process with a curved osteotome. As previously described, the lower half of the zygoma is divided and allowed to remain attached to the maxilla (Fig. 6).

Positioning of Lower Gigli Saw

A medium-sized, curved Kelly forceps is passed beneath the already elevated nasal floor mucoperiosteum from the pyriform aperture of the nose, through the soft palate perforation at the junction of the hard and soft palate, and into the oral cavity. On occasion, the forceps may be directed through the same perforation from the oral cavity side and the Gigli saw passed through the nose with the aid of a nasal speculum. The saw is engaged between the blades of the clamp. Traction on the clamp positions the saw to divide the hard palate through the initial mucoperiosteal hard palate incision from the posterior margin of the hard palate up to the lingual side of the interdental space between the two central incisor teeth. Beyond this point, the hard palate is divided with a thin-bladed reciprocating or Stryker saw between the incisor teeth, beneath the bipedicled mucoperiosteal flap to the homolateral side of the anterior nasal spine, with care being taken to preserve the roots of the teeth and the nasal spine (Fig. 7). The attachment of the mucoperiosteum of the hard palate on each side of the initial incision remains intact. This reduces the risk of an oronasal fistula. The hard palate osteotomy and the mucoperiosteal incision should not be in apposition.

Preliminary Plating of the Maxilla

Before completely dividing the maxilla, preparation is made for its subsequent stabilization. A vertical incision is made through the zygoma from its perforation downward. This completes the division of the upper maxilla after incision of the bone between the arms of the upper Gigli saw.

Appropriate drill holes are placed on each side of the anterior hard palate, ascending process of the maxilla, and zygoma incisions to accommodate miniplates. The titanium miniplates are positioned, secured in place with screws, and removed for subsequent permanent application at the end of the procedure.

Maxillary and Pterygoid Plate Osteotomies

The angles of the Gigli saws may be varied. The saws adapt better to movement as their cutting angles are increased. Movement is initiated without tension on the saws as they are moved back and forth. Grasping the saw with a hemostat near either side of the pterygoid plates is a helpful initiating maneuver. If division of the bone is unsuccessful, the plates may be divided with chisels as previously described.

Before incision of the upper maxilla, the patient's head is rotated laterally to the contralateral side and firmly held against the operating table. Adequate retraction of the facial soft tissue prevents their injury as a sawing motion is made

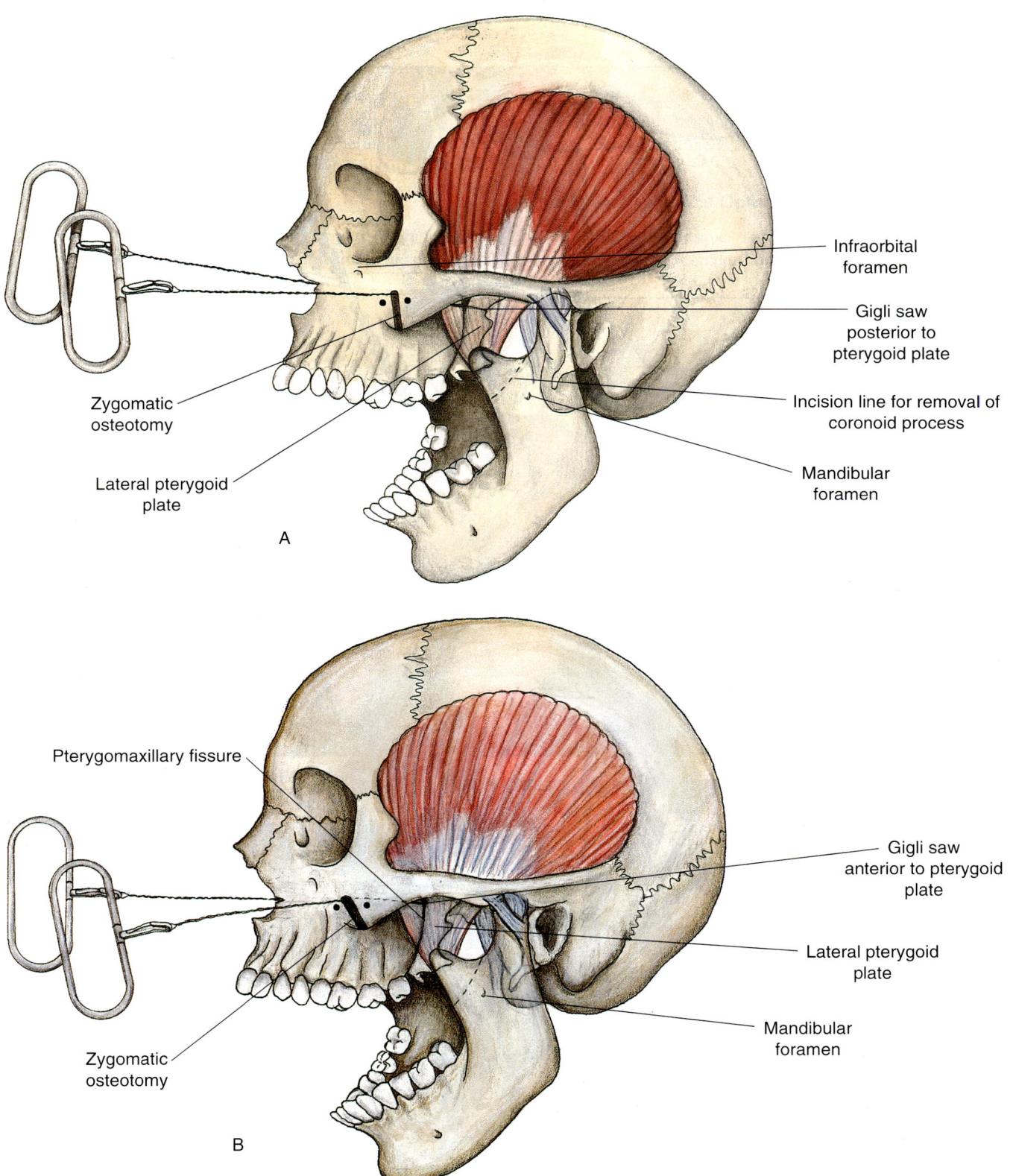

FIG. 6. A: The upper Gigli saw is positioned. Each wall of the maxilla below the level of the infraorbital foramen is simultaneously divided with the Gigli saw positioned behind the pterygoid plates. The saw's medial arm is placed in the inferior meatus of the nose and its lateral arm in the perforated zygoma. The coronoid process of the mandible is removed above the mandibular foramen before insertion of the Gigli saw. **B:** The upper Gigli saw may be positioned anterior to the pterygoid plates. The saw's medial arm is placed in the middle meatus of the nose and its lateral arm in the perforated zygoma. Coronoid excision as above.

These additional maneuvers permit uninterrupted exposure of this area from the roof of the sphenoid to the fourth or fifth cervical vertebra, the infratemporal fossa, the space between the common carotid arteries, the hypoglossal nerves, and the anterior margin of the foramen magnum without interference of exposure by the soft palate or compromise of its contralateral blood supply.

In the face of a positive preoperative diagnosis and confirmation of the extent of disease by maxillotomy exposure, an appropriate surgical technique for removal of the clearly defined tumor must be selected. This subject is discussed only partially in this chapter in the introduction, and in the sections on Indications, Technique, Advantages, Disadvantages, and Comments.

Special instruments designed to maintain continuous retraction and exposure are necessary. These include the multibladed Leylar and Crockard self-retaining retractors, an operating microscope with a 400-mm lens attachment, and a fluoroscope with a C-arm attachment. Special instruments for the removal of bone and tumor should be available and should include those designed for electrocoagulation, the CO_2 laser, a high-speed bone drill, an irrigation suction system, and an ultrasonic aspirator. Microtechnical instruments for dural closure are especially important.

After control of bleeding, several anatomic landmarks should be identified. Confirmation of these landmarks for orientation throughout the procedure is exceptionally helpful. The *midline of the skull base* is in line with the vomer attachment to the anterior face of the sphenoid and its continuation into the nasal septum. The midline continues to the midline of the anterior rim of the foramen magnum. *The base of the pterygoid plates* is attached to the junction of the greater wing and body of the sphenoid. Behind its medial plate is the *foramen lacerum*, which contains the internal carotid artery, and behind or lateral to its lateral plate is the *foramen ovale*, which contains the mandibular nerve. The *middle compartment* of the skull base is bounded laterally by the lateral wall of the sphenoid sinus, medial pterygoid plate, petrooccipital fissure, the anterior margin of the *occipital condyle*, and the anterolateral margin of the foramen magnum. It is primarily composed of the body of the sphenoid and the clivus. The *lateral compartment* is bounded medially by the petrooccipital fissure and laterally by the petrosphenoid fissure. It primarily contains the petrous division of the temporal bone with its adjacent foramen lacerum anteriorly and carotid canal posteriorly. Lateral to the lateral compartment is the infratemporal fossa below the greater wing of the sphenoid and the infratemporal crest. It primarily contains the temporalis and pterygoid muscles, the internal maxillary artery, and the mandibular nerve (Fig. 10).

Complete clivectomy with tumor removal is the procedure of choice when the tumor primarily originates in or secondarily involves the bony clivus, the adjacent clival dura, or extends extracranially or intracranially to compress the brainstem (Fig. 11). Should this require incision or excision of the dura (Fig. 12), a meticulous microsurgical dural repair, as watertight as possible, should be accomplished after tumor removal (Fig. 13). This may be done by primary closure of the defect with or without a fascial graft (Fig. 14). Drilling holes in the adjacent bone to anchor sutures for dural closure is fraught with difficulty and is frequently impossible. If the dural repair is not watertight, the defect may be reinforced with transposition of a fibromuscular temporalis flap or the nasal mucoperiosteal flaps. Free grafts of fat, bone, cartilage, fascia, or muscle may be required to fill remaining surgical defects at the operative site. Postoperative lumbar spinal drainage is required in selected patients.

Extradural and extracranial tumors that are encapsulated or infiltrative, originating from the skull base or extending from the paranasal sinuses, require local excision. Cavitation with the CO_2 laser or the ultrasonic aspirator may be necessary depending on the consistency and vascularity of the neoplastic process.

Wound Closure

Bleeding is carefully controlled with pressure, bipolar and Bovie cautery, Gelfoam and thrombin, Surgicel, and the application of bone wax. The internal maxillary artery may require ligation with a clip. As described in the technique, the wound is packed with abdominal fat. The buccal fat is replaced. If fat is not available, the defect is lined with rayon and filled with a gauze pack saturated with an antibiotic ointment.

Miniplates are applied to the maxilla. A supplementary upper arch bar may occasionally be required for additional maxillary stability.

The gingivobuccal gutter and palate incisions are closed with interrupted chromic suture or Vicryl.

The intranasal circumferential incisions are carefully approximated with interrupted 0000 catgut to prevent stenosis.

An adhesive external nose splint is applied.

POSTOPERATIVE CARE

In the recovery room and the intensive care unit, the head of the bed is elevated. The vital signs are monitored and treated appropriately. Blood replacement may be required. In general, intensive care may be required no longer than 3 days (usually only 1 day), depending on the patient's neurologic status. In some instances, a lumbar drain is necessary if a craniotomy and dural replacement were required.

The cotton in the nares is removed and replaced as frequently as necessary to maintain nasal and facial cleanliness. An icecap to the nose and cheek discourages bleeding and edema of these structures. This is usually discontinued after 48 hours. On the third or fourth postoperative day, enough of the nasal fat is removed to provide an adequate nasal airway. The texture of the fat contributes to its ease of removal without hemorrhage. Nasal saline irrigations are begun the following week and are continued until the washing is clear.

Extended Unilateral Maxillotomy Approach / 225

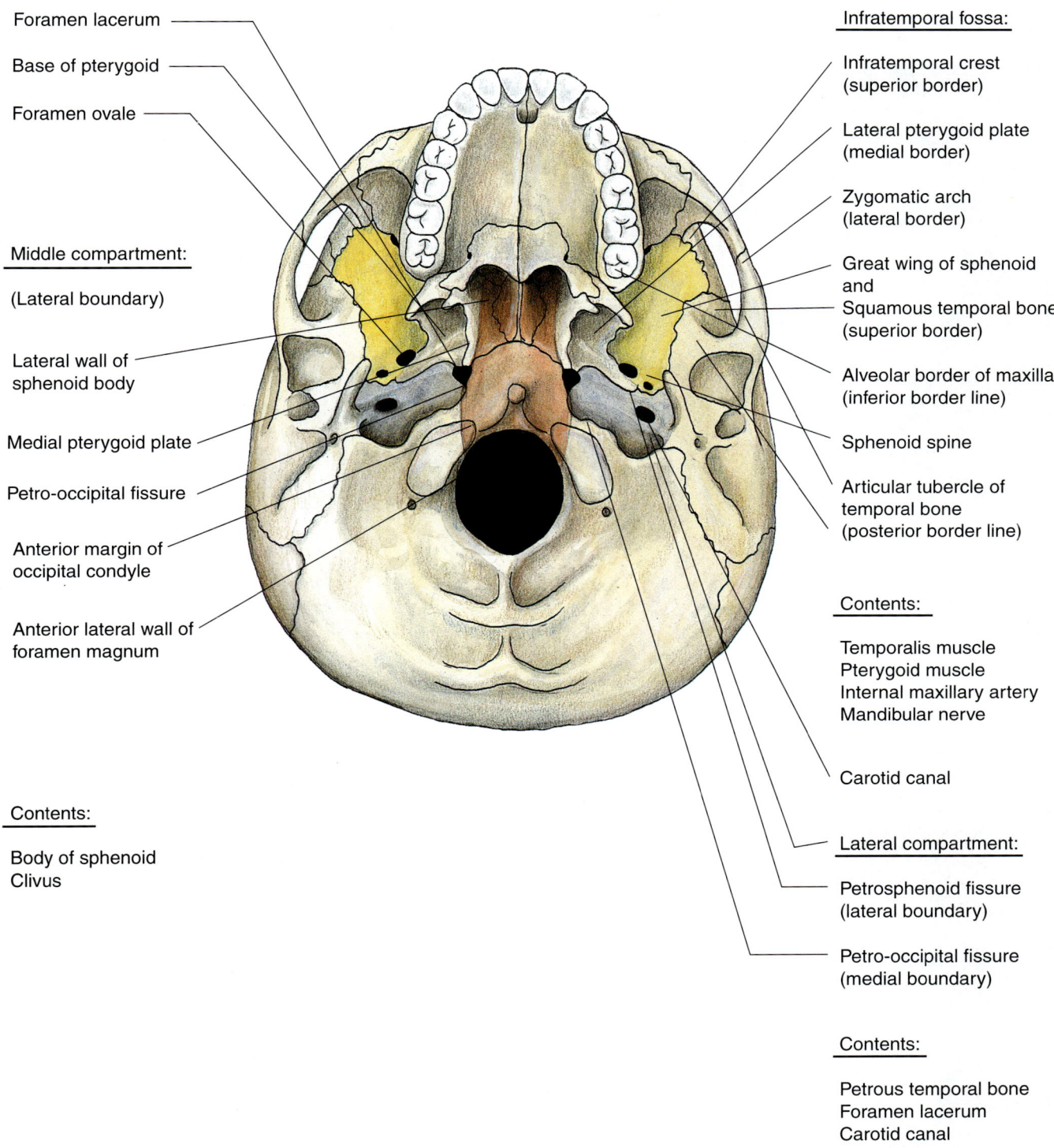

FIG. 10. Important anatomic landmarks that are helpful in preventing serious complications during aggressive surgical procedures for the removal of skull base tumors.

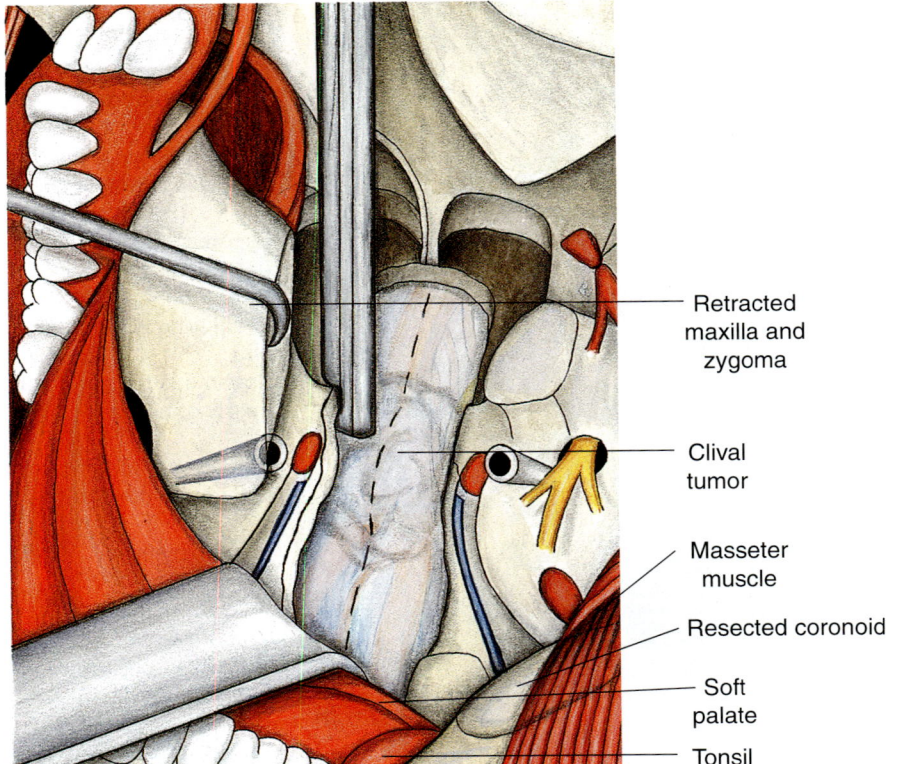

FIG. 11. Surgical exposure of a clival tumor beneath the dura.

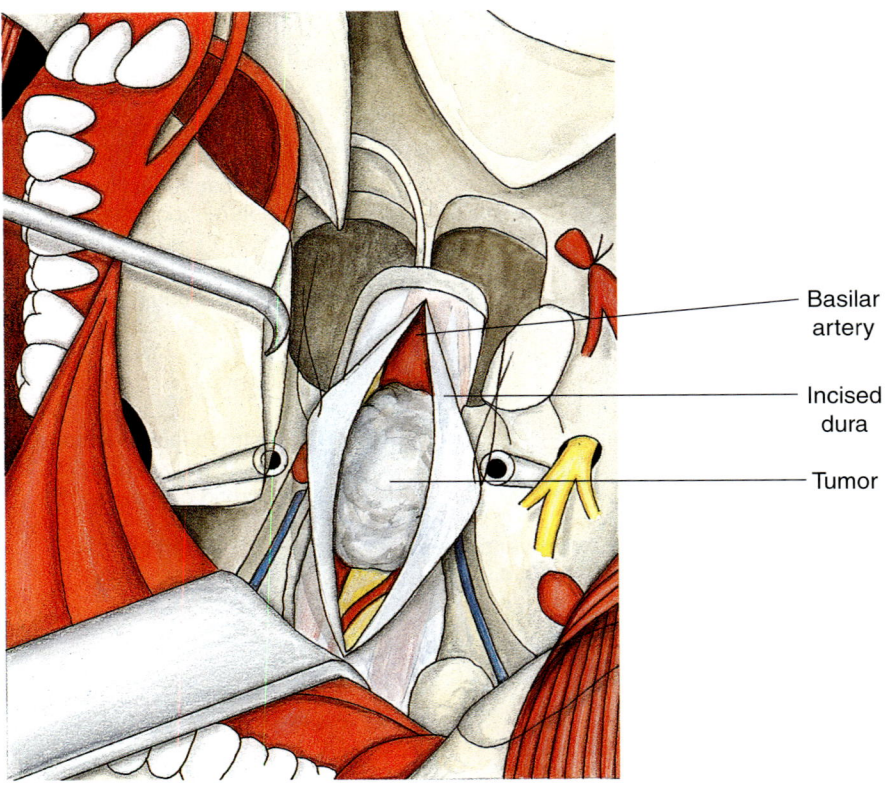

FIG. 12. Dura over the clivus is incised to expose the tumor.

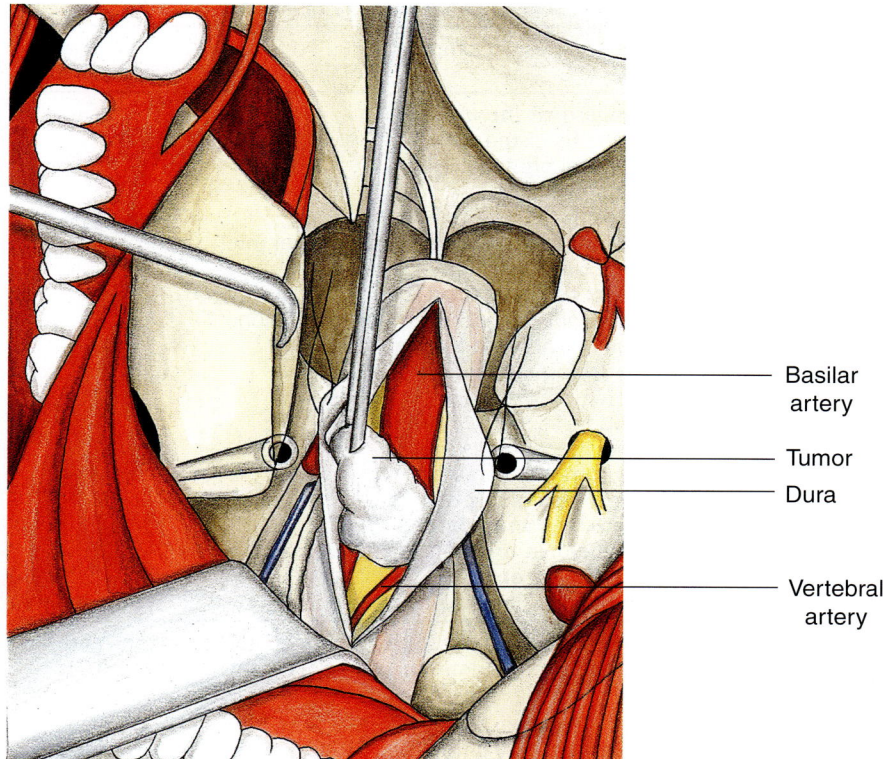

FIG. 13. Tumor removal.

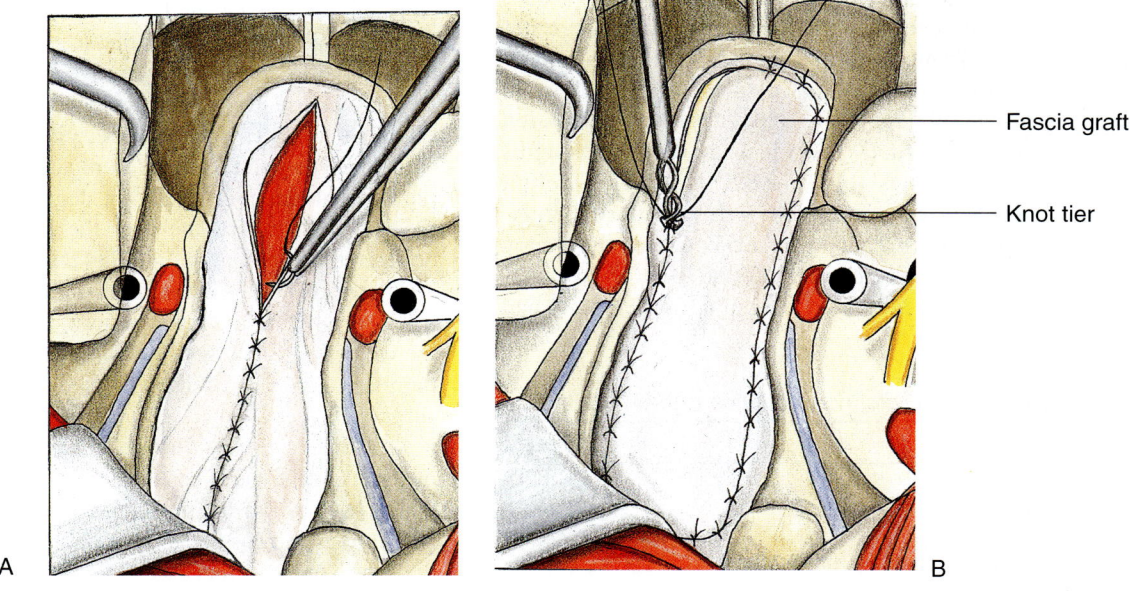

FIG. 14. A: Dural closure. **B:** Fascia graft sutured into dural defect.

Routine nasal and sinus cleansing may be required. The adhesive nasal splint is removed in 1 week.

The oral cavity is cleansed with half-strength peroxide or other appropriate mouthwash. Cleansing of the suture line with a Water-Pik spray is advisable. Jaw motion rehabilitation with the Intraoral Therabite System (Therabite Corporation, Bryn Mawr, PA) to prevent mandibular hypomobility is begun immediately and continued for 2 to 3 months. This discourages restricted jaw motion. Additional dental care is directed by the oral surgeon.

Analgesics, sedatives, antiemetics, and continued antibiotic medications are prescribed as required.

A full liquid diet and clear fluids are begun on the day after surgery if and when bowel sounds return. Soft foods are prescribed after healing of the oral cavity wounds.

Early ambulation is encouraged and is begun the day after surgery.

Magnetic resonance imaging or computed tomography scans are ordered at the discretion of the neurosurgeon.

A lumbar drain is inserted by the neurosurgeon in appropriate patients.

COMPLICATIONS

Since 1988, the authors have used the extended maxillotomy in 30 selected cases (Table 4). Complications observed in these cases occurring immediately after surgery and within a 6-month period of follow-up involved three major areas: (a) healing of the maxilla, (b) sinonasal anatomy, and (c) neurologic function (Table 5).

The incidence of complications occurring in this series of patients included a minor degree of gingival breakdown (one patient), loss of two teeth (one), trismus (one), stiffness of the temporomandibular joint (five), nasal tip depression (two), cerebrospinal fluid (CSF) leakage (two), meningitis (one), pneumocephalus (one), new cranial nerve deficit (two), and other neurologic deficits (two). Medical complications included pneumonia and sepsis (one), pulmonary embolus (one), and myocardial infarction (one). Two deaths occurred in the series attributed to a pulmonary embolus and a myocardial infarction. Blood loss was directly related to the extent and vascularity of the neoplastic processes approached by the maxillotomy exposure, and not to the technique itself.

Side effects that may occur with the procedure are nasal crusting, stiffness of jaw motion, and transient sensory impairment of the palate and cheek. Preservation of the inferior turbinates and reduction of the size of the sinonasal defect with fat will control postoperative crusting as the result of improved nasal air humidification. Immediate rehabilitation of jaw motion after surgery, directed by the oral surgeon and using the Therabite System, eliminates ankylosis of the temporomandibular joint. Varying degrees of sensory impairment of the face ipsilateral to the maxillotomy result predominantly from manipulation of the infraorbital nerve (V2) and occasionally the mandibular division (V3) of the trigeminal nerve within the infratemporal fossa. The anesthesia of the palate is related directly to surgical trauma. Sensory impairment typically resolves over a 3- to 6-month period after surgery.

Problems with maxillary healing and sinonasal anatomy occurred in the early cases of the authors' series and have been resolved with improvement in technique. Gingival breakdown and loss of teeth have not been observed since the gingivobuccal incision was made through the mucoperiosteum at its apex, and the maxilla was divided through the middle meatus 5 mm above the apical roots of the teeth. Anticipated eustachian tube dysfunction leading to otitis with effusion may be prevented by performing a homolateral myringotomy with insertion of a pressure ventilating tube through the tympanic membrane at the beginning of the procedure. Preservation of the septal spine, the maxillary crest,

TABLE 4. *Maxillotomy experience (1988–1995)*

Lesion	No. of cases
Chordoma	10
Meningioma	6
Chondrosarcoma	2
Prolactin-secreting pituitary tumor	2
Juvenile angiofibroma	2
Chondromyxoid fibroma	1
Fibrosarcoma	1
Epidermoid carcinoma	1
Fibrous dysplasia	1
Craniocervical junction abnormality	3
Meningoencephalocele	1
Total	30

TABLE 5. *Complications of extended maxillotomy[a]*

Complication	No. of occurrences
Healing of the maxilla	
Necrosis of the maxilla	0
Gingival breakdown	1
Loss of teeth	1
Trismus	1
Stiffness of the temporomandibular joint	5
Nasosinal anatomy	
Nasal tip depression	2
Transient nasolacrimal duct obstruction	1
Eustachian tube dysfunction	2
Neurologic function	
Cerebrospinal fluid	2
Meningitis	1
Pneumocephalus	1
New cranial nerve deficit	2
Other neurologic deficits	2
Medical complicatons	
Pneumonia and sepsis	1
Pulmonary embolus	1 (death)
Myocardial infarction	1 (death)

[a] *Blood loss* was directly related to the extent and vascularity of the tumor, and not to the technique itself.

and the septal cartilage ensures that no external nasal deformity occurs. The authors have observed no permanent complications with division of the nasolacrimal duct or any velopharyngeal incompetence related to the maxillotomy exposure. Anterior nasal septal perforations are prevented by preserving the anterior half of the septum intact and removing its posterior half. Careful approximation of the nasal vestibular skin suture line has eliminated vestibular stenosis.

The preservation of neurologic function has resulted from the avoidance of unnecessary exposure, manipulation, or sacrifice of neuroanatomic structures. The ventral approach to the midline of the skull base has led to only two patients with new, transient cranial nerve VI palsies that completely resolved within several months after surgery. One patient with an extensive intradural chordoma presented with a progressive quadriparesis and lower cranial nerve deficits. After surgery, there was complete quadriplegia that partially resolved over 6 months. A patient with an intradural chondrosarcoma compressing the ipsilateral brainstem experienced a transient monoparesis of the contralateral upper extremity with tumor removal. This focal deficit resolved completely within 2 weeks after surgery.

Prevention of CSF leakage and the potential for meningitis results from watertight closure of dural defects by repair with interrupted suture or application of a sutured fascia lata graft or rotation of unilateral or bilateral intranasal flaps. In earlier cases of this series, vascularized temporalis muscle and fascia were transposed to cover the dural defects. In all cases the muscle and fascia remained viable and prevented CSF fistula formation. One case in which CSF leakage and meningitis occurred involved a patient with a recurrent chordoma previously operated on with subtotal removal, followed by proton beam radiation therapy and the chronic administration of steroids (Table 6).

In all cases in this series undergoing maxillotomy, no necrosis of the maxilla occurred. Although one greater and lesser palatine artery, posterior superior alveolar artery, and palatine branch of the facial artery have been divided, the maxillary segment continues to survive by blood supply from a palatine branch of the ascending pharyngeal artery and from the contralateral soft palate anastomosis.

ADVANTAGES

The extended maxillotomy is a single-procedure, degloving, sublabial technique that is a unilateral, horizontal, modified LeFort I maxillary osteotomy without a soft palate myotomy. In contrast to the LeFort I operation, the authors prefer division of the maxilla through the middle meatus rather than the standard LeFort I incision through the inferior meatus. This permits the inferior turbinate to remain attached to the retracted maxilla. This technique produces exposure that would be gained only by the incorporation of a combination of other procedures. These include transnasal, transseptal (46–50), transethmoidal (48–51), transsphenoidal (47–53), transmaxillary (49,51,54–56), transoral (57–72), direct nasooropharyngotomy (50,52,69,72), transpharyngeal (73), transpalatal (55,74–81), subtotal maxillectomy (1,82), maxillary swing (83–87), transcranial, infratemporal fossa (42,88,89), lateral rhinotomy (90), and the medial maxillectomy (91). This maxillotomy technique also provides more exposure than the bilateral LeFort I maxillotomy with or without a vertical palate osteomyotomy (4,30–39,41,92). It is designed to permit modifications for skull base exposure. A midline soft palate myotomy with the extended unilateral maxillotomy would seem inadvisable because the soft palate contains significant blood vessels that originate from the contralateral side that primarily supply not only the soft palate but the hard palate. Displacement of the soft palate by its attachment to the retracted hard palate and the lower half of the body of the zygoma provides excellent exposure of the extracranial middle and posterior fossa skull base, especially when the posterior nasal septum, the entire lateral nasal wall, the coronoid process of the mandible, and the homolateral pterygoid plates have been removed. Additional exposure is obtained when the maxilla is retracted with its attached inferior turbinate and nasal floor. Dislocation of the entire nasal septum from the anterior maxillary spine and crest is unnecessary to gain this exposure. Even more exposure of this region is provided by division and retraction of the divided retromolar buccal mucosa, soft palate, and the superior pharyngeal constrictor muscle lateral to the palatine tonsil. This is described in the section on Technique.

The exposure of the skull base produced by the extended horizontal maxillotomy is superior to and far more comprehensive than could be achieved by using any single procedure referenced in the literature. These would include the exposure obtained using only a palatal osteomyotomy (47,59,81,92–94), a mandibulotomy (47,95–106), or a transcervical technique (107–116). The extended maxillotomy should not include an extensive craniotomy procedure. Significant additional exposure is not gained by duplicating the procedure on the contralateral side. In fact, fragmentation of the maxilla into more than one segment on one or both sides

TABLE 6. *Management of intradural tumors in 11 patients*

Diagnosis	Dural suture repair	Graft repair	Temporalis muscle
Chordoma	+		
Chordoma	+		
Chordoma[a]			+
Chordoma		+	
Meningioma			+
Meningioma[b]		+	
Meningioma		+	
Meningioma[b]		+	
Meningioma[b]			+
Chondrosarcoma[a]	+		
Meningoencephalocele	+		

[a] Previous surgery plus radiation therapy.
[b] Previous surgery.

increases the risk of maxillary necrosis (25). In younger patients, if the teeth have erupted, the incision does not interfere with growth center maturation.

Importantly, the morbidity associated with the maxillotomy technique is minimal and may be compared to that associated with a transmaxillary procedure for sinus disease. The major morbidity relates to the neurosurgical procedure required for management of conditions at the skull base and cervical spine.

This procedure was primarily developed to gain adequate extracranial middle and posterior fossa exposure of the middle compartment of the skull base for the removal of clival tumors, and for the excellent view it affords of the brainstem and the anterior skull base. It provides exceptional accessibility to many structures from the roof of the sphenoid sinus to the fifth cervical vertebra, between each eustachian tube, the carotid canals, each petrooccipital fissure, the hypoglossal foramina, the occipital condyles, and the anterior margin of the foramen magnum. Other structures exposed by this technique are listed in Table 7.

The superior exposure of the operative field alone establishes an unexcelled mutual working relationship with surgeons in other fields, primarily the neurosurgeon. It provides an unobstructed, wide-field, direct view into a defect, the depth of field and binocular acuity of which are not restricted by the limitations and confinement of adjacent anatomic structures. This exposure of the skull base permits the manipulation of surgical instruments at a comfortable working distance in the depths of the operative field, whereas such freedom of movement is limited in many of the other techniques. This technique permits the multibladed, self-retaining Leylar neurosurgical and Crockard retractors to retract tissues in more than one direction for exposure without the necessity of using additional retractors. The mobilized maxilla and the lower half of the body of the zygoma remain attached to the soft palate and may be retracted inferiorly, medially, or laterally to gain additional exposure (117) of the medial and lateral compartments of the skull base for removal of primary skull base tumors or secondary tumors that may have extended into this region from adjacent areas. It also permits reconstruction of the defect with temporalis muscle or intranasal mucoperiosteal flaps, as well as with bone, cartilage, and skin grafts.

This access does not limit application of state-of-the-art neurosurgical techniques for the correction of surgical problems that include excision of neoplasms and correction of bony defects. The use of the laser, a high-speed surgical drill, and the operating microscope are not restricted. The carotid artery may be mobilized in its canal and covered with an appropriate graft.

Tumors extending to the medial wall of the jugular foramen may be approached. A vertebral basilar aneurysm (31) may be clipped. A clival dural defect can be sutured watertight or reconstructed with an appropriate graft.

An intradural clival tumor ventral to the brainstem may be removed. In the authors' series, there were 11 such cases. Without this exposure for management of these conditions, life-threatening complications are to be expected.

Through this approach, the entire zygoma may be temporarily excised and replaced, and the coronoid process of the mandible is frequently removed for additional exposure, as well as bone about the infraorbital foramen as it is microfragmented and the nerve mobilized, retracted, and elevated with the degloved soft tissues to a higher level. Bone from the orbital floor may be removed with preservation of its periosteum for more exposure.

Blood loss has not been a major problem and has been controlled by preoperative injection of the soft tissues in the surgical field, the greater palatine canals, the anterior and posterior ethmoid arteries, and the infratemporal fossa with lidocaine containing 1:100,000 epinephrine, and also by ligating the internal maxillary artery in the infratemporal fossa before or after division and retraction of the maxilla. Electrocoagulation of bleeding vessels and the application of topical vasoconstrictors, clotting agents, and bone wax are also helpful to control bleeding. Blood loss associated with the surgical approach has not been a major complication.

The maxilla is accessible for application of titanium plates that provide excellent dental occlusion. Appropriate management of the retracted maxilla as described in the Technique section discourages the development of an oronasal fistula. This operation preserves the apical roots of all the teeth, the nasal spine, and an adequate blood supply to the maxilla.

This exposure permits positioning of the Gigli saw in the middle meatus of the lateral nasal wall, below the infraorbital foramen, and 5 mm above the apex of the roots of the teeth to divide the maxilla. The teeth are preserved. After seating the saws into position, the maxilla may be divided in a few seconds. Other options have been developed for the removal of neoplasms that extend from the nasopharynx into the maxilla. The posterior bony nasal septum may be removed for more contralateral exposure as the bilateral septal mucoperiosteal flaps are preserved, rotated, and positioned into the sphenoclival defect. Additional fragments of the palatine bone, the attached maxillary crest, and maxilla may be removed for further exposure if there is difficulty in visualizing the adjacent lateral pharyngeal wall or positioning the retractor.

Lateral access to the retropharyngeal space with retraction of the tonsillar pillars, palatine tonsil, superior constrictor muscle, soft palate, maxilla, and zygoma is feasible for exposure of the spine to the fourth cervical vertebra. This technique may result in paralysis of the soft palate due to division of the palatal nerve branches from the pharyngeal nerve plexus. This plexus consists of nerves from the bulbar portion of the accessory nerve, and filaments from the branches of the glossopharyngeal, sympathetic, and external branches of the superior laryngeal nerve from the vagus. A sutured fat graft to the nasal surface of the soft palate compensates to some degree for the velopharyngeal incompetence.

Through this exposure, it is advantageous to pack the sur-

TABLE 7. *Anatomic structures that may be encountered in the extended maxillotomy procedure*

I. **Bones**
  A. Sphenoid
    1. Roof
    2. Basisphenoid
    3. Pterygoid processes, medial and lateral
    4. Greater wing
    5. Sinus
    6. Infratemporal crest
    7. Anterior wall
    8. Sphenoid crest
  B. Ethmoid
    1. Sinus—anterior
    2. Sinus—middle
    3. Sinus—posterior
    4. Superior turbinate
    5. Middle turbinate
    6. Lamina papyracea
    7. Perpendicular plate
    8. Cribriform plate
  C. Maxilla (sinus)
    1. Walls
      a. Anterior
      b. Posterior
      c. Medial
      d. Lateral
      e. Superior (orbital floor)
      f. Inferior (hard palate)
    2. Orbital rim
    3. Inferior orbital foramen
    4. Ascending process
    5. Crest
  D. Occipital
    1. Basioccipital
    2. Clivus
    3. Condyles
  E. Temporal
    1. Petrous
  F. Vertebrae
    1. Cervical
      a. 1, 2, 3, 4, and 5
  G. Mandible
    1. Body
    2. Coronoid process
  H. Zygoma
    1. Inferior orbital rim
    2. Frontal process
    3. Arch
  I. Nasal
    1. Right and left
  J. Vomer
  K. Palatine
II. **Muscles**
  A. Buccinator
  B. Facial
  C. Longus capitus
  D. Levator veli palatini
  E. Pterygoid
    1. Internal
    2. External
  F. Superior pharyngeal constrictor
  G. Temporalis
  H. Tensor veli palatini
III. **Fascia**
  A. Prevertebral
  B. Pterygomandibular raphe

IV. **Ligament**
  A. Anterior longitudinal
V. **Nerves**
  A. Trigeminal
    1. Maxillary division
      a. Zygomatic
      b. Sphenopalatine
      c. Posterior superior alveolar
      d. Infraorbital
        1. Anterior superior alveolar
        2. Middle superior alveolar
      e. External nasal
      f. Greater superficial petrosal
      g. Deep petrosal nerve
      h. Nerve of pterygoid canal
      i. Sphenopalatine ganglion
        1. Palatine nerves
        2. Posterior superior nasal branch
        3. Pharyngeal nerve
        4. Nasopalatine
    2. Mandibular nerve
      a. Masseter branch
      b. Deep temporal
      c. Buccinator nerve
      d. Lingual
      e. Inferior alveolar
  B. Abducent
  C. Hypoglossal
VI. **Arteries**
  A. External carotid
    1. Ascending pharyngeal
      a. Palatine branch
    2. Internal maxillary
      a. Deep temporal
      b. Pterygoid branches
      c. Masseteric
      d. Buccinator
      e. Posterior superior alveolar
      f. Infraorbital
      g. Descending (greater) palatine
      h. Pharyngeal
      i. Sphenopalatine
  B. Internal carotid
VII. **Veins**
  A. Inferior petrosal sinus
  B. Internal maxillary
  C. Pterygoid plexus
VIII. **Fossae**
  A. Pterygopalatine
  B. Infratemporal
  C. Extracranial skull base
    1. Anterior
    2. Middle
IX. **Foramina**
  A. Infraorbital
  B. Lacerum
  C. Magnum
  D. Ovale
  E. Sphenopalatine
  F. Spinosum
X. **Fissures**
  A. Infraorbital
  B. Petrooccipital
  C. Pterygomaxillary

(continued)

TABLE 7. *Continued.*

XI. **Space**
    A. Parapharyngeal—above angle of mandible
XII. **Structures**
    A. Paranasal sinuses
        1. Sphenoid
        2. Ethmoid
        3. Maxillary
    B. Oral cavity
        1. Palate
            a. Hard
            b. Soft
        2. Teeth
        3. Gums
        4. Tongue
        5. Lips
        6. Fauces
            a. Glossopalatine arch (anterior pillar)
            b. Pharyngopalatine arch (posterior pillar)
            c. Palatine tonsils
            d. Palatine aponeurosis
                1. Levator velum palatini
                2. Tensor veli palatini
                3. Muscle of uvula
                4. Glossopalatinus
                5. Pharyngopalatine
        7. Pharynx
            a. Nasopharynx
                1. Pharyngeal recess
                2. Torus of auditory tube
                3. Pharyngeal osteum of auditory tube
                4. Adenoid
        8. Oropharynx
            a. Superior pharyngeal constrictor
    C. Nose
        1. External
            a. Right and left nasal bones
            b. Frontonasal suture
            c. Ascending process maxilla
            d. Lower lateral cartilage
                1. Medial feet
                2. Ala cartilage
            e. Upper lateral cartilage
        2. Interior
            a. Nasal spine
            b. Maxillary crest
            c. Septum
                1. Nasal cartilage
                2. Perpendicular plate of ethmoid
                3. Vomer
                4. Sphenoid crest
                5. Anterior nasal spine
                6. Posterior
            d. Lateral nasal wall
                1. Turbinates
                      a. Upper, middle, and lower
                2. Meatus
                      a. Upper, middle, and lower
            e. Cribriform plate
            f. Floor of nose
            g. Inferior conchus

---

gical defect with 2- to 4-cm strips of abdominal fat. The fat is sticky enough to adhere to the walls of the surgical defect. It is soft enough to conform to the defect, solid enough to control bleeding, and, in contrast to rayon, its surface is smooth enough to be removed with minimal discomfort and bleeding. On the fourth or fifth postoperative day, the nonadherent fat in the lumen of the nose and nasopharynx is removed to maintain a nasal airway. The magnification provided by an operating microscope is helpful in selecting the appropriate fatty material to be removed and in leaving behind fat that has already become adherent to the walls of the defect.

Removal of the posterior nasal septum and reducing the size of the sinonasal defect with fat permits an improved moisturizing effect from the remaining turbinates. This also discourages crusting and superficial infection. For this reason, whenever possible, each inferior turbinate should be preserved. Unlike in the extended maxillotomy, the inferior turbinates are routinely removed for better exposure in the LeFort I procedure. Several authors have alluded to the excessive intranasal crusting in their patients. Six of 11 reports (30–36,39,41,54,85) indicate that the inferior turbinates were removed as a routine part of the LeFort I procedure. Although each report does not address the subject as a major complication, it is likely that crusting confronted these patients and possibly could have been controlled or eliminated if the inferior turbinates had not been removed.

Unlike in the infratemporal fossa procedure, the hearing is preserved, as well as all of the cranial nerves; the only neurologic complication related to cranial nerve function is some degree of temporary sensory impairment of the cheek.

Although the access and closure times are not short, the technique is not difficult to master. The degloving technique (26,28,29,39,49,117) eliminates facial scars and may avoid complications associated with keloid formation.

The morbidity is not excessive. The operation is well tolerated by the patient, who may be discharged from the hospital in less than a week. Tracheostomy, percutaneous gastrostomy, and nasogastric feeding tubes have been discontinued. The nasal airway is adequately maintained. Dysphagia and aspiration have not been troublesome. Early ambulation is important and is readily achieved.

The extended maxillotomy exposure is less extensive than the transcervical, mandibulotomy, maxillary swing, extensive craniotomy, and craniofacial disassembly procedures. Traction on vital intracranial structures through a craniotomy for exposure and tumor removal may be life threatening, in contrast to the exposure and tumor removal afforded by this extracranial, transclival, transpharyngeal approach.

DISADVANTAGES

Infiltrative lesions of the skull base that extend into and through many fissures, foramina, and bones are rarely completely removed. *En bloc* excision of many of the malignant and aggressive tumors cannot be accomplished with a good margin of normal tissue without the risk of death from injury to important adjacent life-sustaining structures.

Except in rare instances, it is likely that the extended maxillotomy approach would be considered too extensive to be combined with an extensive intracranial procedure.

Even in the face of the adequate exposure created by the maxillotomy, the neurosurgeon must become adept at manipulating the operating microscope, appropriate instruments, and the laser in a surgical field of this depth.

Temporary restricted jaw motion does occur, but can be managed without excessive morbidity when exercises are initiated in the early postoperative period.

The lengthy duration of the procedure (7–16 hours) and the excessive blood loss (450–4000 ml) are attributed primarily to the nature of the skull base tumor and its adherence to highly vascular structures.

The extended maxillotomy is more extensive than the transnasal, transseptal, transsphenoidal, transsinus, transpalatal, transpharyngeal, and lateral rhinotomy techniques. If only partial exposure of the clivus is required for biopsy or palliative removal of a neoplasm, or for correction of a minor bony abnormality, a more conservative technique should be selected.

COMMENTS

A multiplicity of surgical procedures have been developed by a number of surgeons trained in different specialties that are designed to achieve a multitude of goals in the treatment of patients with craniospinal disease. Many of the conditions are life threatening. Complete eradication of the disease has been the primary goal. Unfortunately, the results have frequently been disappointing, especially in the field of oncology.

The opportunity to remove extracranial skull base neoplasms that may or may not have extended for a short distance intracranially with an exceptionally good margin of normal tissue beyond evidence of disease is limited. Contamination and seeding of neoplastic cells by extirpative techniques, including bone drills and other manipulative maneuvers, cannot be avoided as the surgeon attempts to eliminate all evidence of the neoplasm, especially for those lesions within the bony clivus. Techniques for the removal of low-grade malignant tumors or even histologically benign tumors that mimic malignant lesions by their local aggressiveness remain inadequate and unrewarding. Nevertheless, it is the obligation of the surgeon at the request of the patient to select and use a method of management that offers the best chance for cure and, if not, palliation. Radiation therapy may play an important role should the tumor be sensitive to it and if it has been incompletely removed.

The authors are unable to document in the literature reports that identify an adequate series of patients with a follow-up period sufficient to compare the different treatment modalities with the aim of selecting the one modality or combination of modalities that generates the highest percentage of cures with the least morbidity. Most reports in the skull base literature describe only a case report, or give an account of more than one, and sometimes less than ten patients with a multiplicity of diagnoses. Other reports identify small patient populations with the same diagnosis that have been followed for such short periods of time that the effectiveness of their management is indeterminate.

Gay et al. (118) have reported the largest series of chordomas and chondrosarcomas of the cranial base. A variety of extensive surgical approaches were used to effect the greatest degree of tumor removal. Staged operations with a combination of approaches were used in 52% of the cases. Only 3% of the patients had transfacial procedures. The recurrence-free survival rate for all tumors was 80% at 3 years. Couldwell and Fukushima (119) reported a retrospective study of 109 petroclival meningiomas surgically approached through a number of lateral skull base exposures. Gross total removal of tumor was achieved in only 69% of the cases, with recurrence or progression of disease occurring in 13% of the patients over a 6.1-year follow-up. Perioperative death occurred in 4 patients, and there were 56 significant complications in 35 other patients. The ability to perform a curative operation was limited by involvement of the cavernous sinus, encasement of intracranial vasculature, and pial invasion of the brainstem. Similar observations had previously been made by Sekhar and Narayana (120).

For this chapter, the authors selected only the extended maxillotomy for discussion. It is a procedure designed to give the surgeon adequate exposure for removal of primary extracranial neoplastic disease of the skull base. It continues to have fewer limitations than most of the other beautifully developed and described anterior and lateral skull base approaches. Even with adequate exposure of the region, the surgeon continues to be challenged to remove completely all evidence of neoplastic disease infiltrating the same crevices, fissures, foramina, and fossae, regardless of how extensive or conservative an exposure is selected. The extended maxillotomy provides more exposure than most of the transseptal, maxillary swing, infratemporal fossa, bilateral maxillary osteotomy with or without palatal osteomyotomy, transoral, transnasopharyngotomy, transsinus, lateral rhinotomy, medial maxillectomy, transnasal, transpalatal, transcervical, and mandibulotomy procedures, and with minimal morbidity. In addition, the exposure can be increased by removing the homolateral pterygoid plates, coronoid process of the mandible, the posterior nasal septum, and the entire lateral nasal wall, except for the inferior turbinate and nasal floor, which are temporarily retracted with the maxilla and with the homolateral soft palate. The zygoma may also be tentatively removed and replaced. If necessary, the exposure could be repeated for removal of residual disease. It is not nearly as extensive a procedure as the translocation techniques described by Beals and Joganic (121), Janecka and Sekhar (122), and Arriaga and Janecka (123). The transfacial approach described by Wei et al. (83,84), Brown et al. (85), and Altemir (86) for the removal of extracranial disease and the craniotomy procedures (124–138) described for the removal of intracranial disease have a greater morbidity. Many of these procedures were developed and influenced by the work of Tessier et al. (139). Each of these procedures is well documented and, in selected patients, may be superior to the extended maxillotomy. Technical limitations to the removal of aggressive infiltrative disease at the skull base continue to challenge the surgeon and the patient, regardless of the exposure.

In the authors' experience, a unilateral horizontal maxillotomy (extended maxillotomy) provides more exposure than a bilateral one, especially when the entire posterior nasal septum and the homolateral pterygoid plates are removed and the inferior turbinate is permitted to remain attached to the retracted maxilla. Dislocation of the anterior septum is usually unnecessary. Retraction for exposure of the skull base, sinonasal area, and the infratemporal fossa is best accomplished with the multibladed Leylar and Crockard retractors. The maxilla is divided through the middle meatus, in contrast to the LeFort I incision, which transects the inferior meatus. To preserve the adjacent teeth, the maxilla should be divided 4 to 5 mm above their apical roots, and perhaps this is another reason for division of the maxilla at a higher level. The osteotomy does not pass through a growth center (32).

The authors have come to appreciate the importance of improved humidification of the nasal airway to limit or prevent postoperative nasal crusting associated with superficial infection of the walls of the surgical defect. Preservation of the inferior turbinate and reduction of the size of the surgical defect practically eliminate this handicap for the patient. The size of the surgical defect is reduced not only by preservation of the inferior turbinates but by the application of multiple small fat grafts. These 2- to 4-cm strips of abdominal fat are made to adhere to the wall of the defect and exposed dura. Additional fat is introduced into the lumen of the sinonasal defect. The fat not only adheres to the walls of the defect, but is soft enough to occupy space, solid enough to serve as a substitute for a rayon nasal pack to control bleeding, and its texture is smooth enough to be easily removed. Montgomery's (140) experimental evidence indicates that varying amounts of fat will survive and that the remaining fat is replaced by fibrous tissue, especially in those implants that are severely traumatized. He reports that adipose tissue seems to resist infection. It will completely obliterate a frontal sinus after sinusectomy. The fat survives by revascularization.

The authors are pleased that patient morbidity has lessened since they discontinued the use of a postoperative nasogastric tube, percutaneous esophageal gastrostomy, pharyngotomy, and a tracheostomy. Ambulation and rehabilitative jaw exercises are begun the day after surgery and have eliminated restriction of jaw motion.

In light of the investigative work of Lanigan and West (141), Bell et al. (22), and Nelson et al. (24), the blood supply to the maxilla is better understood. The authors have taken advantage of this new information and their technique has been modified accordingly. As a result, the authors' patients have not been troubled with postoperative hemorrhage, maxillary necrosis, permanent oronasal fistula, loss of teeth, or nasal vestibular stenosis. Pending further investigation, care should be taken not to divide the soft palate in the midline in association with a unilateral extended maxillotomy for fear of interference with the blood supply to the homolateral palate. It seems feasible, however, that there should be abundant anastomoses between the soft palate vessels and the greater palatine artery branches, even if this artery is ligated. Division of the adjacent lateral wall of the oropharynx with its soft palate attachment and retraction of the palate toward the midline carries with it less risk of palate necrosis. On the other hand, Brown et al. (85), Wei et al. (83,84), and Altemir (86) use a similar approach with their maxillary swing procedure. They detach the maxilla from the soft palate and allow it to remain attached to the cheek flap. Its blood supply is from the transverse branch of the external maxillary artery. Necrosis of the maxilla did not complicate healing, and the soft palate remained intact.

Since elimination of the Weber-Fergusson incision, facial scarring has been eliminated. To promote maximum blood supply to the maxilla and in light of the investigative work mentioned previously, the authors make a special effort to permit as much mucoperiosteum of the maxilla as possible to remain in contact with the bone. These tissues are important for the transportation of anastomotic vessels. For this reason, the initial sublabial incision is made at the very apex of the gingivobuccal gutter. A compression dental plate applied to the hard palate would compromise its blood supply and should be avoided.

Surgical exposure and ligation of the internal maxillary artery is preferable before division of the maxilla. This exposure is sometimes difficult. It is made less difficult if the coronoid process of the mandible is removed above the level or entrance of the inferior maxillary nerve and vessels. This maneuver does not increase the limitation of postoperative jaw motion. Although ankylosis of the temporomandibular joint has been eliminated with rehabilitation of jaw motion by the Therabite device, the occasional patient experiences stiffness of jaw motion.

The development of the bilateral septal, floor of the nose, and lateral nasal wall flaps that are based on the soft tissues attached to the lateral wall of the sphenoid has proved exceptionally helpful in assisting in reinforcing the closure of the dural defect in the sphenoclival area.

SUMMARY

Given the numerous modalities of treatment that have been designed for the management of the many craniocervical/skull base conditions affecting the patient, the surgeon must select a method of management that satisfies the goals that have been established by the surgeon and the patient. The surgical procedure selected should provide adequate exposure for correction of the abnormality, a watertight dural closure if possible, and satisfactory reconstruction of the surgical defect, and it should permit postoperative rehabilitative management. To accomplish this, the surgeon must take into account the biologic nature of the condition to be treated, the extent of the disease, his or her experience, as well as the morbidity and mortality rates and the economic resources of the patient and his or her family.

REFERENCES

1. Cocke EW Jr, Robertson JH, Robertson JT, Crook JP. The extended maxillotomy and subtotal maxillectomy for excision of skull base tumors. *Arch Otolaryngol Head Neck Surg* 1990;116:92.
2. von Langenbeck B. Beitrage zur Osteoplastik: Die osteoplastische Resektion des Oberkiefers. In: Goschen A, ed. *Deutsche Klinik*. Berlin: Reimer, 1859.
3. von Langenbeck B. Osteoplastische Resektion des Oberkiefers. *Deutsche Klinik* 1861;29:281.
4. Cheever DW. Nasopharyngeal polypus attached to the basilar process of occipital and body of the sphenoid bone successfully removed by a section, displacement, and subsequent replacement and reunion of the superior maxillary bone. *Boston Medical and Surgical Journal* 1867;8:162.
5. Moloney F, Worthington P. The origin of the LeFort I maxillary osteotomy: Cheever's operation. *Journal of Oral Surgery* 1981;39:731.
6. Lanz O. Osteoplastische Resektion bei der Oberkiefer nach Kocher. In: Lucke R, ed. *Deutsche Zeitschrift für Chirurgie*. Leipzig: Vogel, 1893:423.
7. Partsch C. Eine neue Methode temporarer Gaumen-Resektion. *Archiv für Klinische Chirugie* 1898;57:847.
8. LeFort R. Etude experimentale sur les fractures de la machoire superieure. *Revue de Chirurgie* 1901;23:208.
9. Löwe L. Weitere Mitteilungen über die Ausraumnug der Nase vom Munde her. In: Schech P, Schrotter L, eds. *Monatsschrift für Ohrenheilkunde*. Berlin: Verlag von Oscar Coblentz, 1902:420.
10. Pincus W. Beitrag zur Klinik und Chirurgie des Nasen-Rachenraumes. *Klinische Chirurgie* 1907;82:110.
11. Wassmund J. *Lehrbuch der praktischen Chirurgie des Mundes and der Kiefer*. Leipzig: Meusser, 1935:215.
12. Axhausen G. Zur Behandlung veralteter disloziert veheilter Oberkieferbrueche. *Deutsche Zahn- und Kieferheilkunde* 1934; 1:334.
13. Steinkamm W. *Pseudo-Progenie und ihre Behandlung diss*. Berlin: 1938.
14. Gillies HG, Rowe NL. L'osteotomie du maxillaire superieur envisagee essentiellement dens les cas de bec-de-liere totale. *Revue de Stomatologie* 1954;55:545.
15. Dingman RO, Harding RL. The treatment of malunited fractures of the facial bones. *Plast Reconstr Surg* 1951;7:505.
16. Cupar I. Die chirurgische Behandlung der form- und stellungsueranderungen des Oberkiefers. *Österreichische Zeitschrift für Stomatologie* 1952;10:473.
17. Obwegeser HL. The temporal approach to TMJ, the orbit, and the retromaxillary–infracranial region. *Head and Neck Surgery* 1985;7:185.
18. Hogeman KE, Wilmar K. Die Vorverlagerung des Oberkiefers zur Korrektur von Gebibanomalien. In: Fortsch R, Kiefer U, eds. *Gesichtschir Hrsg*. Stuttgart: Schuchardt, K Thieme, 1967.
19. Pfeifer G. Die chirurgische Spätbehandlung des deformierten Oberkiefers nach früheren Spaltoperationen. *Deutsche Zahn- und Kieferheilkunde* 1969;53:34.
20. Drommer RB. The history of the LeFort I osteotomy. *Journal of Maxillofacial Surgery* 1986;14:119.
21. Bell WH, LeFort I. Osteotomy for correction of maxillary deformities. *Journal of Oral Surgery* 1975;33:412.
22. Bell WH, Fonseca RJ, Kennedy JW III, Levy BM. Bone healing and revascularization after total maxillary osteotomy. *Journal of Oral Surgery* 1975;33:253.
23. Bell WH, Finn RA, Scheideman GD. Wound healing associated with LeFort I osteotomy. *J Dent Res* 1980;59(A):459.
24. Nelson RL, Path MG, Ogle RG, Waite DE, Meyer MW. Quantitation of blood flow after LeFort I osteotomy. *Journal of Oral Surgery* 1977;35:10.
25. Lanigan DT, Hey JH, West RA. Aseptic necrosis following maxillary osteotomies: report of 36 cases. *J Oral Maxillofac Surg* 1990;48:142.
26. Casson PR, Bonnano PC, Converse JM. The mid-face degloving procedure. *Plast Reconstr Surg* 1974;53:102.
27. Conley J, Price JC. Sublabial approach to the nasal and nasopharyngeal cavities. *Am J Surg* 1979;138:615.
28. Maniglia AJ. Indications and techniques of mid-facial degloving. *Arch Otolaryngol Head Neck Surg* 1986;112:750.
29. Price JC, Holliday MJ, Johns ME, Kennedy DW, Richtsmeier WJ, Mattox DE. The versatile mid-face degloving approach. *Laryngoscope* 1988;98:291.
30. Wood GD, Stell PM. The LeFort I osteotomy as an approach to the nasopharynx. *Clin Otolaryngol* 1984;9:59.
31. Archer DJ, Young S, Uttley D. Basilar aneurysms: a new transclival approach via maxillotomy. *J Neurosurg* 1987;67:54.
32. Belmont JR. The LeFort I osteotomy approach for nasopharyngeal and nasal fossa tumors. *Arch Otolaryngol Head Neck Surg* 1988;114:751.
33. Uttley D, Moore A, Archer DJ. Surgical management of midline skull base tumors: a new approach. *J Neurosurg* 1989;71:705.
34. Brown DH. The LeFort I maxillary osteotomy approach to surgery of the skull base. *J Otolaryngol* 1989;18:289.
35. Morril KW, Foster J, Haid RW. The LeFort I osteotomy as an approach to the mid-cranial base for tumor resection: Case report. *J Oral Maxillofac Surg* 1993;51:82.
36. Sasaki CT, Lowlitcht RA, Astrachan DI. LeFort I osteotomy approach to the skull base. *Laryngoscope* 1990;100:1073.
37. Sandor GKB, Charles DA, Lawson VG. Transoral approach to the nasopharynx and clivus using the LeFort I osteotomy with mid-palatal split. *Int J Oral Maxillofac Surg* 1990;19:352.
38. James D, Crockard HA. Surgical access to the base of skull and upper cervical spine by extended maxillotomy. *Neurosurgery* 1991;29:411.
39. Anand VK, Harkey HL, Al-Mefty O. Open-door maxillotomy approach for lesions of the clivus. *Skull Base Surgery* 1991;1:217.
40. O'Reilly GO, Crockard HA, Lightman S, James DR, Phillips RH, Smith M. Excision of a clival and upper cervical pheochromocytoma by an extended maxillotomy approach: a case report. *Skull Base Surgery* 1993;3:87.
41. Catalano PJ, Biller HF, Sachdev V. Access to central skull base via a modified LeFort I maxillotomy: the palatal hinge flap. *Skull Base Surgery* 1993;3:60.
42. Fisch U, Fagen P, Valvanis A. The infratemporal fossa approach for the lateral skull base. *Otolaryngol Clin North Am* 1984;17:513.
43. Schuller DE, Goodman JH, Brown BL, Frank JE, Ervin-Miller KJ. Maxillary removal and reinsertion for improved access to anterior cranial base tumors. *Laryngoscope* 1992;102:203.
44. Mann WJ, Gilsbach J, Seeger W, Floel H. Use of malar bone graft to augment skull base access. *Archives of Otolaryngology* 1985;111:30.
45. Sami LL, Gircis H. Transzygomatic approach for nasopharyngeal fibromata with extrapharyngeal extension. *J Laryngol Otol* 1965;79:782.
46. Joseph M. Pedicled rhinotomy for exposure of the clivus. In: Schmidek HH, Sweet WH, eds. *Operative neurosurgical techniques*. 3rd ed. Philadelphia: WB Saunders, 1995:469.
47. Snow RB, Patterson RR. Surgical treatment of tumors of the clivus and basioccipital region. In: Schmidek HH, Sweet WH, eds. *Operative neurosurgical techniques*. 2nd ed. New York: Grune & Stratton, 1988:635.

48. Lee KJ, Goodrich I, Pensak M. Pituitary surgery: current status including transsphenoidal surgery. *Am J Otolaryngol* 1984;5:138.
49. Papel ID, Kennedy DN, Cohn EC. Sublabial transseptal transsphenoidal approach to the skull base. *Ear Nose Throat J* 1986;65:107.
50. Laws ER Jr. Transsphenoidal surgery for tumors of the clivus. *Otolaryngol Head Neck Surg* 1984;92:100.
51. Kennedy DW, Cohn ES, Papel ID. Transsphenoidal approach to the sella. *Laryngoscope* 1984;94:1066.
52. Lalwani AK, Kaplan MJ, Gutin PH. The transsphenoidal approach to the spheroid sinus and clivus. *Neurosurgery* 1992;31:1009.
53. Hardy J. Transsphenoidal hypophysectomy. *J Neurosurg* 1971;34:582.
54. Crockard HA. The transmaxillary approach to the clivus. In: Sekhar LN, Janecka IP, eds. *Surgery of cranial base tumors*. New York: Raven Press, 1993:235.
55. Crumley RL, Gutin PH. Surgical access for clivus chordoma: the University of California, San Francisco experience. *Arch Otolaryngol Head Neck Surg* 1989;115:295.
56. Sataloff RT, Bowman C, Baker SR, Osterholm J. Transfacial resection of intracranial tumor. *Am J Otol* 1988;9:222.
57. Weissler MC. Transoral approaches to the skull base. *Ear Nose Throat J* 1991;70:587.
58. Miller E, Crockard HA. Transoral transclival removal of anteriorly placed meningiomas at the foramen magnum. *Neurosurgery* 1987;20:966.
59. Pastzor E, Vajda P, Piffko P, Horvath M, Gador I. Transoral surgery for craniocervical space-occupying processes. *J Neurosurg* 1984;60:276.
60. Mullan S, Naunton R, Hekmat-Panah J, Vailati G. The use of an anterior approach to ventrally placed tumors in the foramen magnum and vertebral column. *J Neurosurg* 1966;24:536.
61. Crockard HA. The transoral approach to the base of the brain and upper cervical cord. *Ann R Coll Surg* 1985;167:321.
62. Crockard HA, Bradford R. Transoral transclival removal of a schwannoma anterior to the craniocervical junction: case report. *J Neurosurg* 1985;62:293.
63. Crockard HA, Sen CN. The transoral approach for the management of intradural lesions at the craniovertebral junction: a review of seven cases. *Neurosurgery* 1991;28:88.
64. Crockard HA. Transoral approach to intra- and extradural tumors. In: Sekhar LN, Janecka IP, eds. *Surgery of cranial base tumors*. New York: Raven Press, 1993:225.
65. DeLorenzo N, Fortuna A, Guidetti B. Craniovertebral junction malformations: clinicoradiological findings, long-term results and surgical indications in 63 cases. *J Neurosurg* 1982;57:603.
66. Eisemann ML. Spheno-occipital chordoma presenting as a nasopharyngeal mass: a case report. *Annals of Otology* 1980;89:271.
67. Hadley MN, Spetzler RF, Sonntag VK. The transoral approach to the superior cervical spine: a review of 53 cases of extradural cervicomedullary compression. *J Neurosurg* 1989;71:16.
68. Haselden FG, Brice JG. Transoral clivectomy: a case report. *Journal of Maxillofacial Surgery* 1978;6:32.
69. Handa J, Suzuki F, Nioka H, Koyamy T. Clivus chordoma in childhood. *Surg Neurol* 1987;28:58.
70. Gilsbach J, Eggert HR. Transoral operations for craniospinal malformations. *Neurosurg Rev* 1983;6:199.
71. Delgado TE, Buchheit WA. Surgical management of tumors in and around clivus via transoral approach. *Contemporary Neurosurgery* 1982;4:1.
72. Cook BR, Vries JK, Martinez AJ. Malignant fibrous histiocytoma of clivus: case report. *Neurosurgery* 1987;20:632.
73. Menezes AH, VanGilder JC. Transoral–transpharyngeal approach to the anterior craniocervical junction. *J Neurosurg* 1988;69:895.
74. Guthkelch AN, Williams RG. Anterior approach to recurrent chordomas of the clivus: technical note. *J Neurosurg* 1972;36:670.
75. Precechtel A. Transpalatine operation for choanal atresia. *Annals of Otolaryngology* 1938;87:1014.
76. Ruddy LW. A transpalatine operation for congenital atresia of the choanae in the small child or infant. *Archives of Otolaryngology* 1945;41:432.
77. Tu GY, Hu YH, Xu GZ, Ye M. Salvage surgery for nasopharyngeal carcinoma. *Arch Otolaryngol Head Neck Surg* 1988;114:328.
78. Donald PJ, Bernstein LB. Transpalatal excision of the odontoid process. *Transactions of the American Academy of Ophthalmology and Otolaryngology* 1978;86:729.
79. Loeb HW. *Operative surgery of nose, throat and ear*. St. Louis: CV Mosby, 1917:1.
80. Wilson CP. The approach to the nasopharynx. *Proc R Soc Med* 1951;44:353.
81. Kennedy DW, Papel ID, Holliday M. Transpalatal approach to the skull base. *Ear Nose Throat J* 1986;65:125.
82. Cocke EW Jr, Braund RR. Superior maxillary resection. In: Cooper P, ed. *The craft of surgery*. 2nd ed. Boston: Little, Brown & Company, 1964:82.
83. Wei WI, Lam KH, Sham JST. New approach to the nasopharynx: the maxillary swing approach. *Head Neck* 1991;13:200.
84. Wei WI, Ho CM, Yuen PW, Fung CF, Sham JST, Lam KH. Maxillary swing approach for resection of tumors in and around the nasopharynx. *Arch Otolaryngol Head Neck Surg* 1995;121:638.
85. Brown AMS, Lavery KM, Millar BG. The transfacial approach to the post-nasal space and retromaxillary structures. *Br J Oral Maxillofac Surg* 1991;29:230.
86. Altemir HF. Temporal disarticulation pedicled to cheek of the upper maxilla(s) as transfacial way of approach to the mainly retromaxillary regions and other indications: a new technique. *Estoma* 1982;3:75.
87. Altemir FH. Transfacial access to the retromaxillary area. *Journal of Maxillofacial Surgery* 1986;14:165.
88. Fisch U. The infratemporal fossa approach for nasopharyngeal tumors. *Laryngoscope* 1893;93:36.
89. Donald PJ. Infratemporal fossa and skull base. In: Donald PJ, ed. *Head and neck cancer: management of the difficult case*. Philadelphia: WB Saunders, 1984:277.
90. Maran AGD. Surgical approaches to the nasopharynx. *Clin Otolaryngol* 1983;8:417.
91. Denker A, Kahler O. *Handbuch*.
92. Hayakana T, Kamikawa K, Ohniski T, Yoshimine T. Prevention of post-operative complications after a transoral transclival approach to basilar aneurysms: technical note. *J Neurosurg* 1981;54:699.
93. Alonso WA, Black P, Connor GH. Transoral transpalatal approach for resection of clival chordoma. *Laryngoscope* 1971;81:1626.
94. DiLorenzo N, Palantinsky E, Bardelia L, Malei A. Benign osteoblastoma of the clivus removed by a transoral approach: case report. *Neurosurgery* 1987;20:52.
95. Krespi YP, Har-El G. Surgery of the clivus and anterior cervical spine. *Arch Otolaryngol Head Neck Surg* 1988;14:73.
96. Krespi YP, Har-El G. The transmandibular–transcervical approach to skull base. In: Sekhar LN, Janecka IP, eds. *Surgery of cranial base tumors*. New York: Raven Press, 1993:261.
97. Krespi YP, Levine TM, Oppenheimer R. Skull base chordomas. *Otolargyngol Clin North Am* 1986;19:797.
98. Krespi YP, Sisson GA. Transmandibular exposure of the skull base. *Am J Surg* 1984;148:534.
99. Attia EL, Bentley RC, Head T, Mulder D. A new external approach to the pterygomaxillary fossa and parapharyngeal space. *Head and Neck Surgery* 1984;6:884.
100. Biller HF, Lawson W. Anterior mandibular-splitting approach to the skull base. *Ear Nose Throat J* 1986;65:134.
101. Kremen A. Surgical management of angiofibroma of nasopharynx. *Ann Surg* 1952;138:672.
102. Delgado TE, Garrido E, Harwick RD. Labiomandibular transoral approach to chordomas in the clivus and upper cervical spine. *Neurosurgery* 1981;8:675.
103. Arbit E, Patterson RH Jr. Combined transoral and median labiomandibular glossotomy approach to the upper cervical spine. *Neurosurgery* 1981;8:672.
104. Wood BG, Sadar ES, Levine HL, Dohn DF, Tucker HM. Surgical problems of the base of the skull base. *Archives of Otolaryngology* 1980;106:1.
105. Yumoto E, Okamura H, Yanagihara N. Transmandibular transpterygoid approach to the nasopharynx, nasopharyngeal space and skull base. *Ann Otol Rhinol Laryngol* 1992;101:383.
106. McAfee PC, Bohlman HH, Riley LH Jr. The anterior retropharyngeal approach to the upper part of the cervical spine. *J Bone Joint Surg Am* 1987;69:1371.
107. Southwick WO, Robinson RA. Surgical approaches to the vertebral bodies in the cervical and lumbar regions. *J Bone Joint Surg Am* 1957;39:631.
108. Stevenson GC, Stoney RJ, Perkins RK, Adams JE. A transcervical transclival approach to the ventral surface of the brainstem for removal of a clivus chordoma. *J Neurosurg* 1966;24:544.

109. Lesoin F, Jomin M, Pellerin P. Transclival transcervical approach to the upper cervical spine and clivus. *Acta Neurochir* 1986;80:100.
110. Harwick RD, Miller AS. Craniocervical chordomas. *Am J Surg* 1979;138:512.
111. Wissinger JP, Danoff D, Wisiol ES, French LA. Repair of aneurysm of the basilar artery by a transclival approach. *J Neurosurg* 1967;26:406.
112. Fox JL. Obliteration of midline vertebral artery aneurysm via basilar craniectomy. *J Neurosurg* 1967;26:406.
113. Komisar A, Tabaddor K. Extrapharyngeal (anterolateral) approach to cervical spine. *Head and Neck Surgery* 1983;6:600.
114. Fee WE Jr, Roberson JB Jr, Goffinet DR. Long-term survival after surgical resection for recurrent nasopharyngeal cancer after radiotherapy failure. *Arch Otolargyngol Head Neck Surg* 1991;117:1233.
115. Fee WE Jr, Gilmer PA, Goffinet DR. Surgical management of recurrent nasopharyngeal carcinoma after radiation failure at the primary site. *Laryngoscope* 1988;98:1220.
116. Biller HF, Shugar JMA, Krespi YP. A new technique for wide field exposure of the base of the skull. *Archives of Otolaryngology* 1981;107:698.
117. Paavolainen M, Malmberg H. Sublabial approach to the nasal and paranasal cavities using nasal pyramid osteotomy and septal transection. *Laryngoscope* 1986;96:106.
118. Gay E, Sekhar LN, Rubinstein E, et al. Chordomas and chondrosarcomas of the cranial base: results and follow-up of 60 patients. *Neurosurgery* 1995;36:887.
119. Couldwell WT, Fukushima T. Petroclival meningiomas: surgical experience in 109 cases. *J Neurosurg* 1996;84:20.
120. Sekhar LN, Narayana KS. Surgical excision of meningiomas involving the clivus: pre-operative and intra-operative features as predictors of post-operative functional deterioration. *J Neurosurg* 1994;81:860.
121. Beals SP, Joganic EF. Transfacial exposure of anterior cranial fossa and clival tumors. *BNI Quarterly* 1992;8:2.
122. Janecka IP, Sekhar LN. Anterior and anterolateral craniofacial resection. In: Sekhar LN, Janecka IP, eds. *Surgery of cranial base tumors.* New York: Raven Press, 1993:147.
123. Arriaga MA, Janecka IP. Facial translocation approach to the cranial base: the anatomical basis. *Skull Base Surgery* 1992,1:26.
124. Al-Mefty O, Fox JL, Smith RR. Petrosal approach for petroclival meningiomas. *Neurosurgery* 1988;22:510.
125. Cushing HW, Eisenhart L. *Meningiomas: their classification, regional behavior, life history, and surgical end results.* Springfield, IL: Charles C Thomas Publisher, 1938.
126. Derome PJ, Guiot GL. Surgical approaches to the sphenoidal and clival areas. *Adv Tech Stand Neurosurg* 1979;6:101.
127. Fisch U. Infratemporal fossa approach to tumors of the temporal bone and base of the skull. *J Laryngol Otol* 1978;92:949.
128. Hitselberger WE, House WF. A combined approach to the cerebellopontine angle: a suboccipital/petrosal approach. *Archives of Otolaryngology* 1966;84:267.
129. House WF, De La Cruz A, Hitselberger WE. Surgery of the skull base: transcochlear approach to the petrous apex and clivus. *Archives of Otolaryngology* 1978;86:770.
130. Kawase T, Shiobara R, Toya S. Anterior transpetrosal/transtentorial approach for spheno/petroclival meningiomas: surgical method and results in 10 patients. *Neurosurgery* 1991;28:869.
131. King TT. Combined translabyrinthine/transtentorial approach to acoustic nerve tumors. *Proc R Soc Med* 1970;63:780.
132. Malis LI. Suboccipital subtemporal approach to petroclival tumors. In: Wilson CB, ed. *Neurosurgical procedures: personal approaches to classic operations.* Baltimore: Williams & Wilkins, 1992:41.
133. Sakaki S, Takeda S. Extended middle fossa approach combined with a suboccipital craniectomy to the base of the skull in the posterior fossa. *Surg Neurol* 1987;28:245.
134. Samii M, Ammirati M, Mahran A. Surgery of petroclival meningiomas: a report of 24 cases. *Neurosurgery* 1989;23:12.
135. Rosomoff HL. The subtemporal transtentorial approach to the cerebellopontine angle. *Laryngoscope* 1971;81:1448.
136. Sen CN, Sekhar LN. An extreme lateral approach to intradural lesions of the cervical spine and foramen magnum. *Neurosurgery* 1990;27:197.
137. Spetzler RF, Daspit CP, Pappas CTE. Combined supra- and infratentorial approach for lesions of the petrous and clival regions: experience with 46 cases. *J Neurosurg* 1992;76:588.
138. Yasargil MG, Mortara RW, Curcic M. Meningiomas of basal posterior cranial fossa. *Adv Tech Stand Neurosurg* 1980;7:3.
139. Tessier P, Guiot J, Derome D. Orbital hypertelorism: definite treatment of orbital hypertelorism by craniofacial or by extracranial osteotomies. *Scand J Plast Reconstr Surg* 1973;7:39.
140. Montgomery WW. *Surgery of the upper respiratory system.* Philadelphia: Lea and Febiger, 1971:106.
141. Lanigan DT, West RA. Management of post-operative hemorrhage following the LeFort I maxillary osteotomy. *Journal of Oral and Maxillofacial Surgery* 1984;42:367.

CHAPTER 13

Subcranial Extended Anterior Approach for Skull Base Tumors: Surgical Procedure and Reconstruction

Joram Raveh, Kurt Laedrach, Tateyuki Iizuka, and Franz Leibinger

The extended anterior subcranial approach differs significantly from more traditional approaches to the skull base in that it allows a broad inferior–anterior access to the skull base planes with tumor exposure along all borders, as opposed to the transfrontal superior route. The authors initially used the subcranial approach in 1978 for the treatment of high-velocity skull base trauma and certain craniofacial anomalies. In 1980, the authors expanded the indications to include the subcranial–subfrontal approach for the resection of various skull base tumors. Osteotomy of the frontonasoorbital external skeletal frame provides optimum anterior access to the orbital and sphenoethmoid planes and to the nasal and paranasal cavities, while avoiding frontal lobe retraction and external facial incisions characteristic of transcranial and transfacial approaches. The improved visualization of the anterior skull base and sphenoclival region facilitates *en bloc* tumor removal, exposure of the optic nerve, exposure of the anteromedial aspect of the cavernous sinus, and watertight realignment of the anterior cranial base dura. Because extensive frontal lobe manipulation and external facial incisions are avoided with this approach, intensive care unit and overall hospital stay is reduced, related complications are minimized, and postoperative cosmetic appearance is enhanced. The extended anterior subcranial method is therefore an excellent alternative to traditional transfacial–transcranial skull base approaches for the skull base tumors confined to these locations.

The subcranial approach was first introduced in 1978 by the senior author (J.R.) for treatment of traumatic disruption of the anterior skull base (1–7). It was later used for correction of congenital and acquired craniofacial anomalies (8–12), and in 1980 it was adapted to the combined removal of various malignant and benign skull base tumors (13–16). Along the evolutionary continuum, the subcranial approach differs significantly from more traditional otolaryngologic and neurosurgical approaches (17–25) and from a number of more recently reported modifications of these techniques (26–29). The differences lie not so much in the location of the frontal craniotomy and nasoorbital osteotomies, because most of the bone flap variations that allow transfrontal access are now well known (30–35), but in the surgical exposure and direction of operative approach. The extended subcranial approach allows broad anterior and inferior exposure of all the planes, including the anterior ethmoid roof up to the clivus, as well as across both orbital roofs toward the temporal bone, which permits precise intradural and extradural tumor resection. This is accomplished by dural detachment from this approach with practically no frontal lobe retraction. The subcranial extended anterior approach enables optimal visualization of the tumor borders toward the dura as well as along the nasal and maxillary sinus extensions. The simultaneous exposure of the cranial as well as caudal aspects of the tumor enables radical *en bloc* removal as well as preservation of the optic nerve, chiasm, and carotid arteries, if these structures are not directly involved. The avoidance of facial incisions coupled with adequate drainage of the subcranial compartment, orbital cone, and paranasal spaces reduces the incidence of such complications as visible scars, mucus retention/empyema, and infection, as well as the development of pressure within the orbital cone leading to an apex syndrome.

In this chapter, the indications for this approach, the technique, and various aspects concerning reconstruction are highlighted.

J. Raveh, K. Laedrach, T. Iizuka: Department of Craniomaxillofacial, Facial Plastic and Reconstructive Surgery, Otolaryngology, Head and Neck Surgery, University of Bern, 3010 Bern, Switzerland.

F. Leibinger: Research Institute, Institute Leibinger GmbH, Friburg, Germany.

PREOPERATIVE EVALUATION

All patients are evaluated by a team that includes members from the departments of radiation therapy, otolaryngology, and neurologic surgery. Computed tomography scans with bone algorithms and magnetic resonance imaging are performed. Neuroangiography, preoperative embolization, or carotid occlusion, depending on the cerebral blood flow measurements, are performed when appropriate. After the extent of the lesion and the degree of involvement of adjacent structures are defined, the decision is made regarding surgical procedure. The choice of surgical procedure is a combined otolaryngologic–neurosurgical decision, and the location, size, and extent of intracranial expansion of the lesion dictate the borders of the proposed nasofrontal osteotomy and the necessity of combining other skull base and craniofacial approaches. Both the neurosurgical and otolaryngologic elements of the team are responsible for postoperative and follow-up patient care.

SURGICAL TECHNIQUE—TUMOR RESECTION AND RECONSTRUCTION—GENERAL ASPECTS AND RELATED ANATOMY

The subcranial approach affords anterior access to and exposure of the skull base planes and the subcranial compartment, including the nasal lumen, as shown in Fig. 1A,B. The first step consists of raising a bicoronal flap in the subperiosteal plane, taking care to preserve the pericranium for possible use during reconstruction. The flap is dissected down to the frontozygomatic suture lines bilaterally and to the rhinion and piriform apertures in the midline. The periorbita is dissected from the superior, medial, and lateral walls of the orbit back to the apex on either side, and the anterior ethmoid arteries are ligated. Raising the scalp and face flap induces traction of the orbital contents to a certain degree, but this is harmless. In contrast, a procedure such as lateral permanent retraction of the globes that puts pressure on the orbital contents should be performed carefully and only intermittently. Damage to the optic nerve and orbital contents can be avoided, as is confirmed by the authors' results, as well as their experience with hundreds of cases of skull base trauma and hyperteloric anomalies managed using this same subcranial approach. Depending on the size and extent of both the lesion and frontal sinus, the outline of the nasofrontal segment is planned (see Fig. 1B) and titanium microplates or miniplates (see Fig. 1C) for subsequent bone fixation are adapted and drilled. The osteotomy line of the bone flap may be deliberately extended cranially and laterally, depending on tumor extension. Bur holes are then made, and with a dissector protecting the frontal lobe dura at all times, osteotomies are made across the frontal bone, down to and along the orbital roofs, down the medial orbital wall, and along the nasomaxillary grooves just anterior to the lacrimal duct (see Fig. 1A,D). A vertical osteotomy performed anterior to the crista galli allows detachment of the frontonasal segment, avoiding damage to the sagittal sinus or dural tears. Depending on the tumor location, two types of osteotomies are distinguished as follows:

1. *Type I*: Osteotomy of the frontonasal segment, leaving the posterior frontal sinus wall to be removed in a second step (Fig. 2A,B). This procedure is indicated if the tumor involves the posterior wall. The external skeletal frame is removed after dissection of the posterior wall under direct vision, safely and far enough from the tumor borders.
2. *Type II*: One-stage removal of the frontonasal segment, including the posterior frontal sinus (see Fig. 2A,C,D). This procedure is indicated in tumors not involving the posterior wall or having major intracranial extension, making a broad access necessary. The osteotomy borders can be deliberately extended cranially and laterally. Further, in those cases in which the posterior wall is not involved and the tumor is confined to the sphenoid and clival planes.

Both osteotomy types should be performed meticulously and the dura protected by dissectors inserted along the orbital roofs and the conjunction of the posterior frontal sinus wall and ethmoid roof so as not to sever the dura. Dural tears should be avoided by all means because during the further process this often results in a pealing-off and damaging of the dura along relatively large areas. Using the tumor borders as guides, the dura is divided circumferentially around the olfactory groove and the involved dura, followed by severing of the olfactory filaments. For unilateral tumors, the contralateral olfactory filaments may be preserved. If there is no intracranial extension, the olfactory filaments and dura are separated subcranially from the floor of the anterior cranial fossa, starting at the crista galli and back to the planum sphenoidale, without extensive frontal lobe manipulation. Bone from the orbital and ethmoid roofs is removed to facilitate this dissection. The anterior step-by-step exposure enables not only clear definition of the tumor borders but the exposure of vital structures, such as the optic nerve, lateral sphenoid walls, carotid arteries, and chiasm. The clivus can be optimally assessed as well as the nasal lumen, palate, and maxillary sinuses, enabling *en bloc* removal of tumor. With the dura protected by a slim dissector, osteotomy of the planum sphenoidale is a relatively easy procedure. The medial optic nerve canal wall is also unroofed by this access, and the optic chiasm and nerves can be exposed bilaterally. The anatomic configuration after resection is shown in Fig. 2E-H (coronal plane). A schematic drawing and cadaver dissection of the sagittal planes (see Fig. 2I,J) depict the advantages of the subcranial anterior exposure. To avoid unnecessary pressure to the globe as well as herniation and damage to the periorbital tissue during drilling and further manipulations underneath the skull base, the authors developed special retractors (Fig. 3). Both elastic blades can be shifted apart to fit the orbital cavity, thus avoiding herniation of the periorbital fat tissue.

BASIC ASPECTS OF RECONSTRUCTION

Small dural defects are sutured, whereas larger defects resulting from intradural tumor involvement are patched with fascia lata. A second large fascia lata flap is applied using fibrin glue to seal the entire anterior skull base defect, which reaches from the exposed frontal lobes up to the clival area. The lateral borders of the fascia must be adapted between the dura and the lateral resection borders of the orbital roof and sphenoid plane to avoid herniation and provide a watertight seal to the subcranial compartment. To facilitate fascia application, the authors developed an applicator (Fig. 4A) that is inserted with the fascia layer up to the clivus. The intraoperative view depicting the fascia layer *in situ* is shown in Fig. 4B—the fascia lata borders have not yet been inserted between the dura and the osseous resection borders.

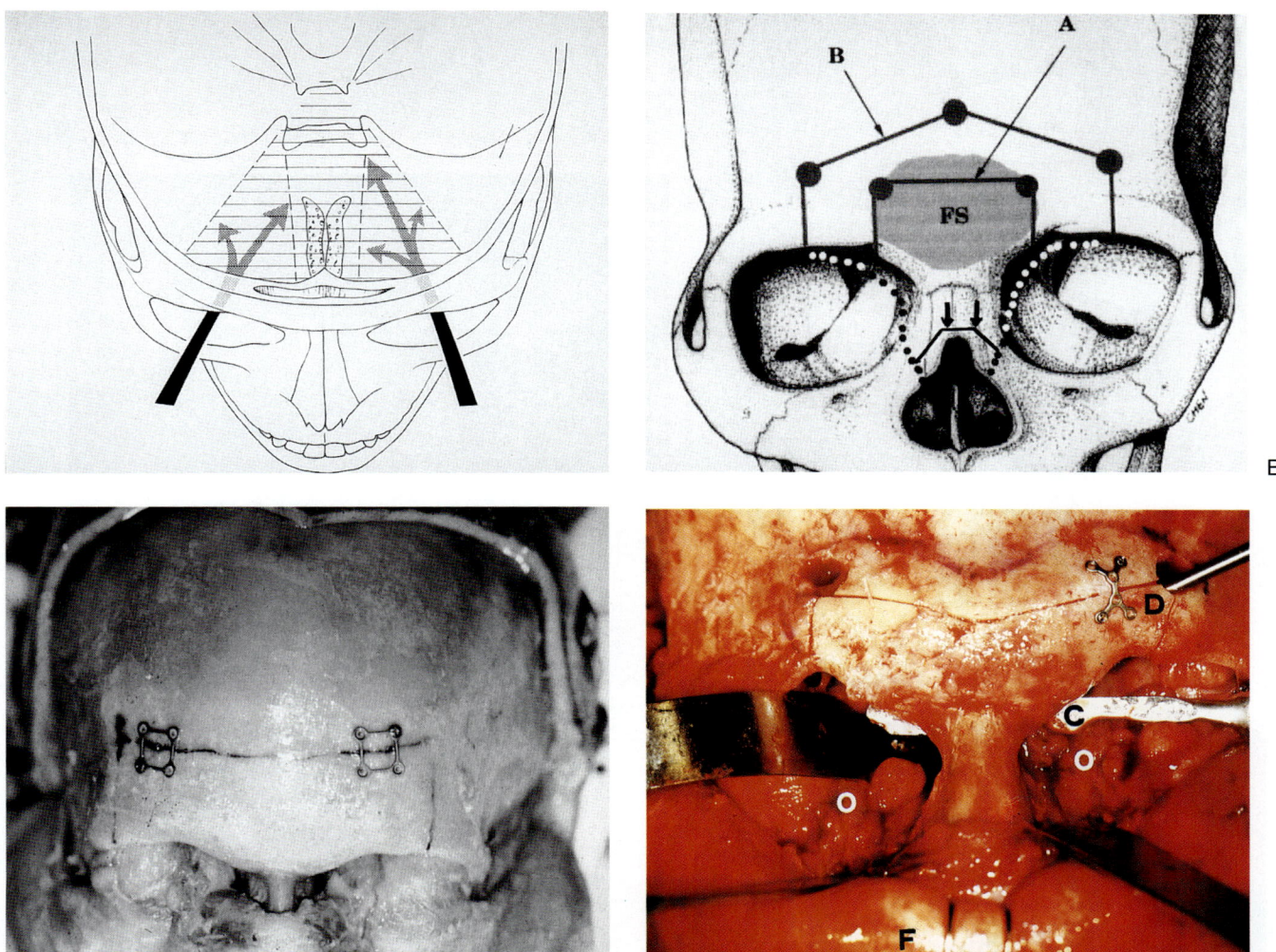

FIG. 1. **A:** Schematic illustration of the subcranial approach and extent of the exposure along the skull base planes. **B:** Schematic illustration of frontonasal segment osteotomies. The frontal bone osteotomy borders (A,B) depend on tumor location and can be extended deliberately. *Dotted lines* indicate orbital roof and lateral nasal wall osteotomies. *Arrows* indicate the osteotomy line, which leaves an anterior part of the nasal bone intact (for indications, see text). **C:** Application of titanium plates (Institute Leibinger GmbH) before osteotomy enables exact repositioning of the segment. **D:** Coronal flap (*F*) and exposure of the orbital cavity and the nasal frame up to the tip of the nose. *O*, retracted orbit; *D*, dissector inserted into the bur hole to protect the dura during the osteotomies; *C*, chisel indicating the osteotomy anterior to the crista galli.

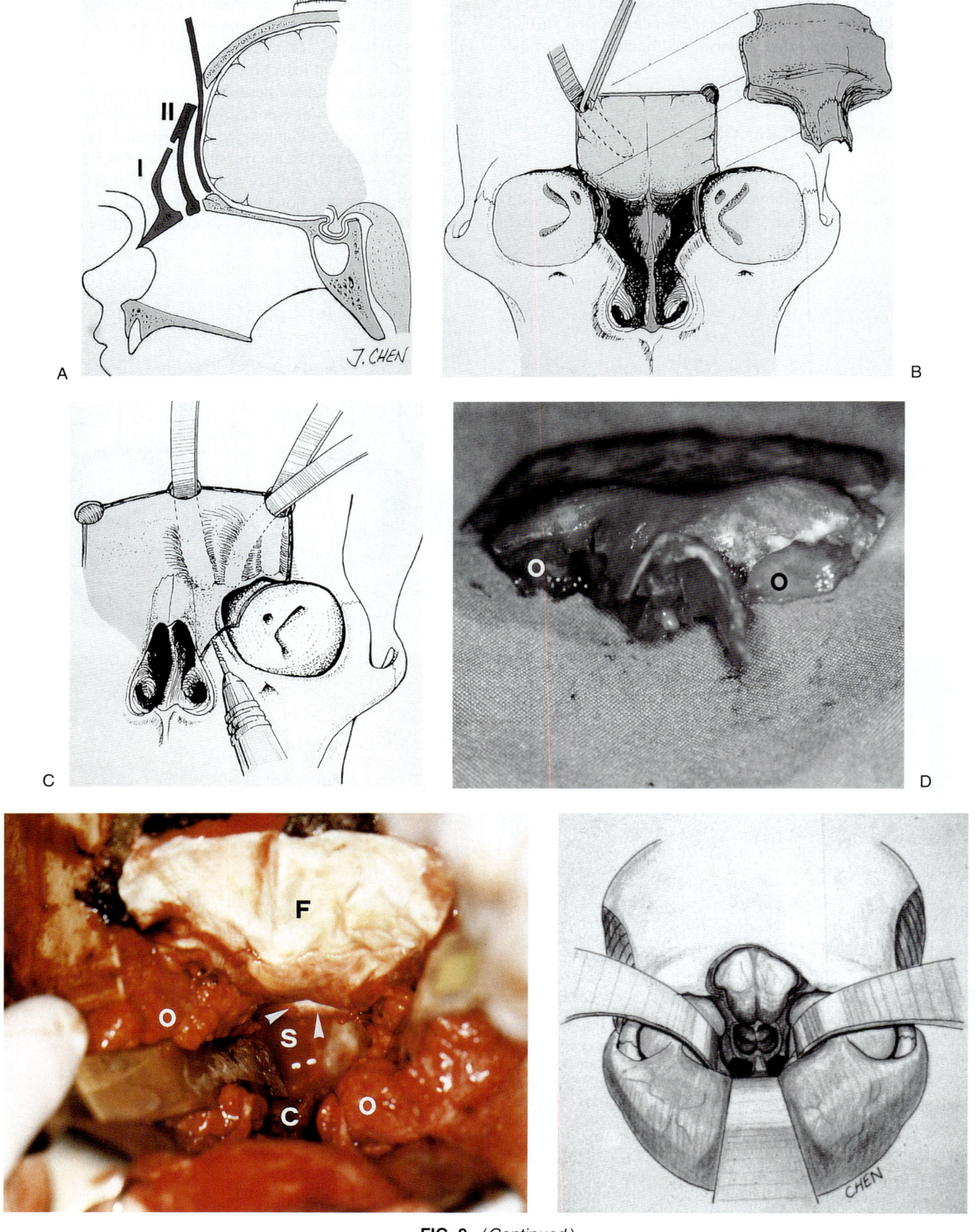

FIG. 2. (*Continued.*)

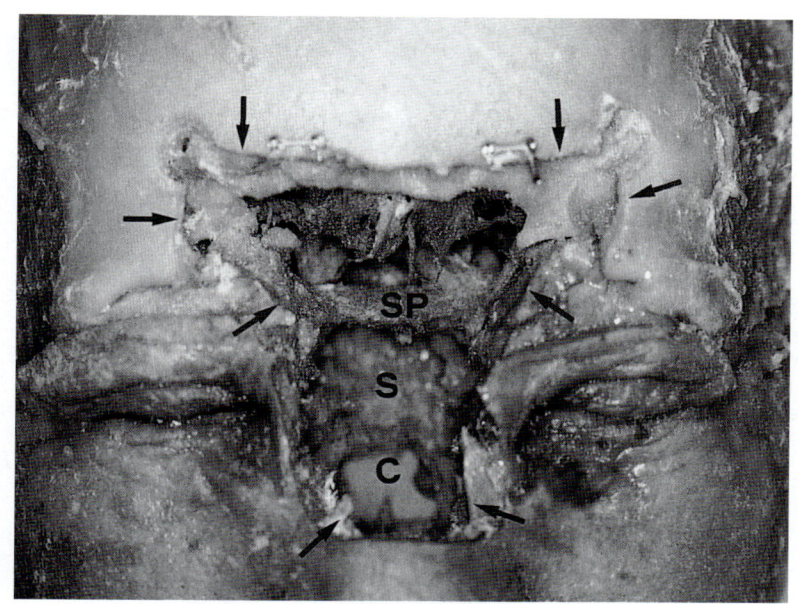
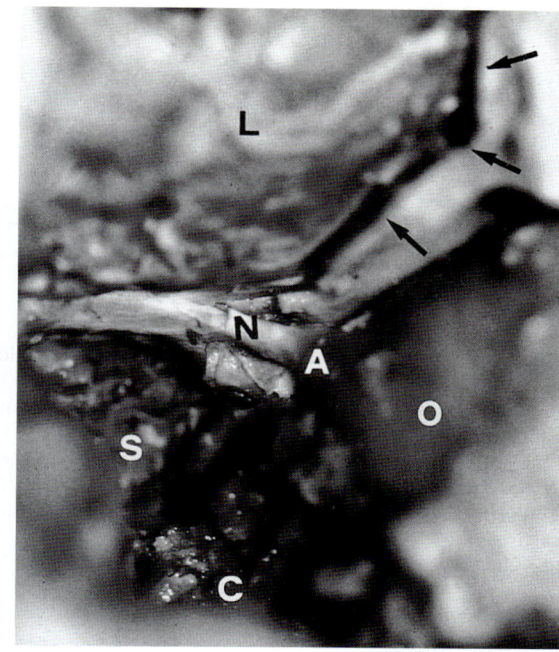
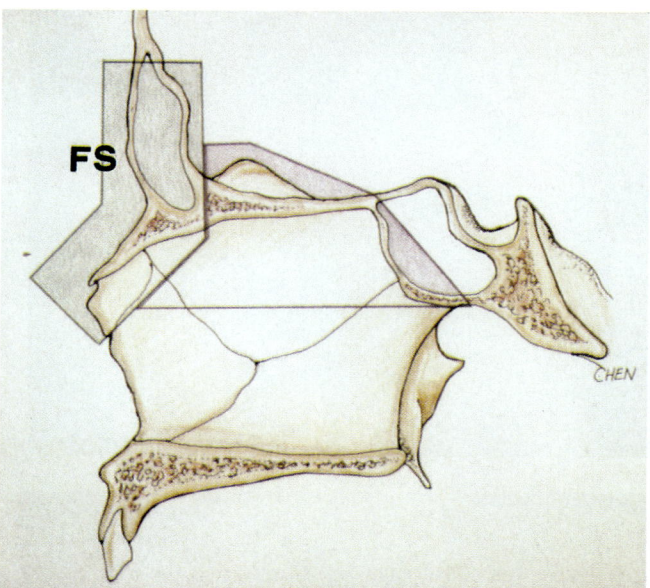
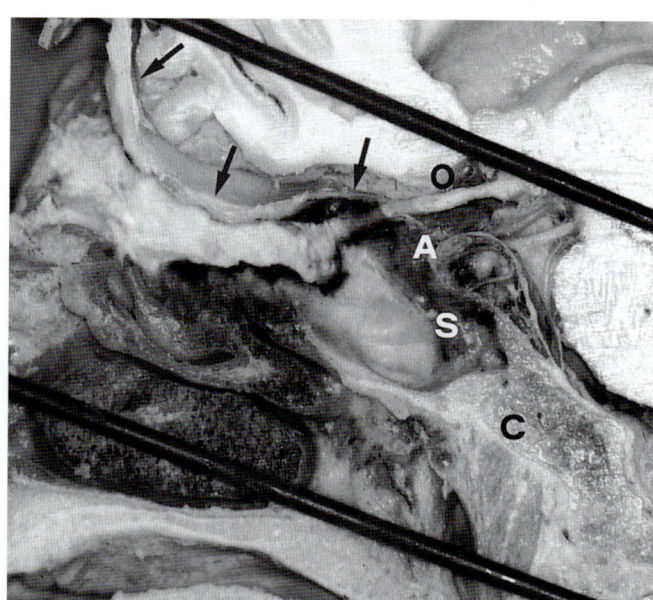

FIG. 2. *Continued.* **A:** Type I and II osteotomies. The type I osteotomy includes removal of the external frontonasal frame and leaves the posterior wall intact. The type II osteotomy includes the posterior wall. For indications, see text. **B:** Type I osteotomy with stepwise removal of the posterior wall. The dura is disattached and always protected by a dissector, including the orbital and ethmoid roof. **C:** Type II segment osteotomy, including the posterior wall. The dissectors protect the dura along the osteotomy lines. **D:** Removed frontonasal segment (in a patient) showing the osteotomy borders along the orbital (*O*) roofs. **E:** Intraoperative view after tumor resection showing a fascia lata layer (*F*) already applied to the frontal lobes. The sella (*arrowheads*), the posterior sphenoid wall (*S*), and superior part of the clivus (*C*) are clearly visible. *O,* retracted orbits. **F:** Schematic drawing indicating the extent of the exposure provided by this approach. **G:** Corresponding anatomic configuration in a cadaver. *Arrows* indicate osteotomy borders after removal of the nasofrontal segment. *Sp,* posterior border of the resected sphenoid plane; *S,* posterior sphenoid walls; *C,* clivus. **H:** Cadaver dissection shows the generous exposure that enables optimal visualization of the optic nerve and chiasm. *Arrows* indicate osteotomy borders along the frontal bone and orbital roof. *O,* orbit; *A,* apex; *N,* optic nerve and conjunction toward the chiasm; *L,* frontal lobe; *S,* posterior sphenoid wall; *C,* clivus. **I:** Schematic drawing of the sagittal plane. Removal of the frontonasal segment (*FS*) provides optimal visualization of the nasal lumen and sphenoclival area. **J:** Cadaver dissection after removal of the frontonasal segment. The posterior frontal sinus wall and the ethmoidosphenoid planes were left intact to preserve the correct anatomic configuration (*arrows*). This area is always removed to provide optimal exposure of the sphenoclival region. Exposure and visualization of the optic nerve (*O*), carotid artery (*A*), sphenoid (*S*), clivus (*C*), and nasal lumen by this access are optimal.

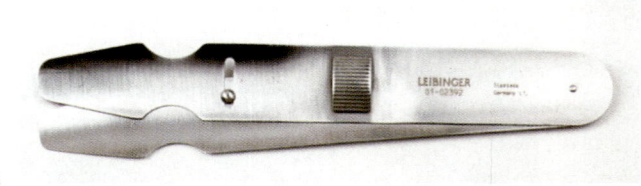
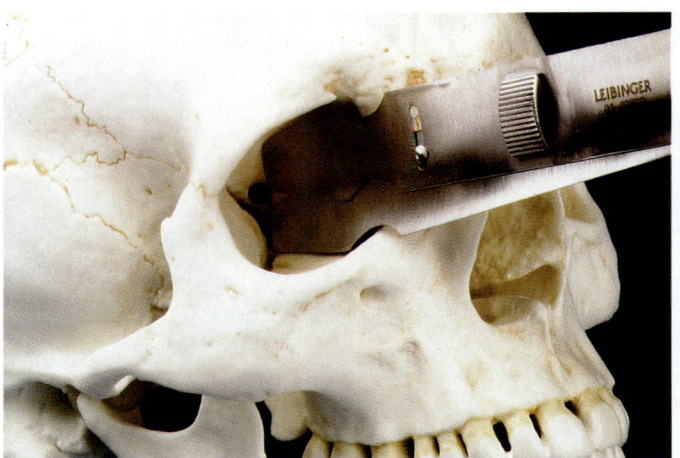

FIG. 3. A: Orbital retractor developed in cooperation with Institute Leibinger. The blades can be spread and the different elastic features of each enable optimal adjustment toward the orbital cone. **B:** The retractor *in situ*. The major advantage is that herniation of periorbital fat tissue toward the subcranial compartment can be avoided, as well as damage to the tissue during the drilling process.

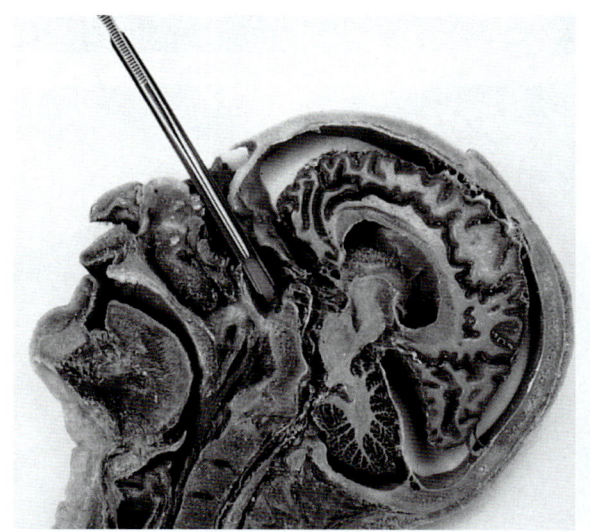
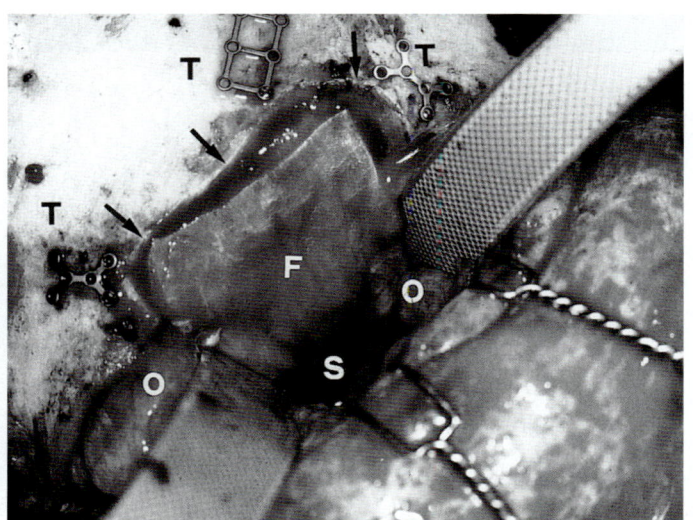
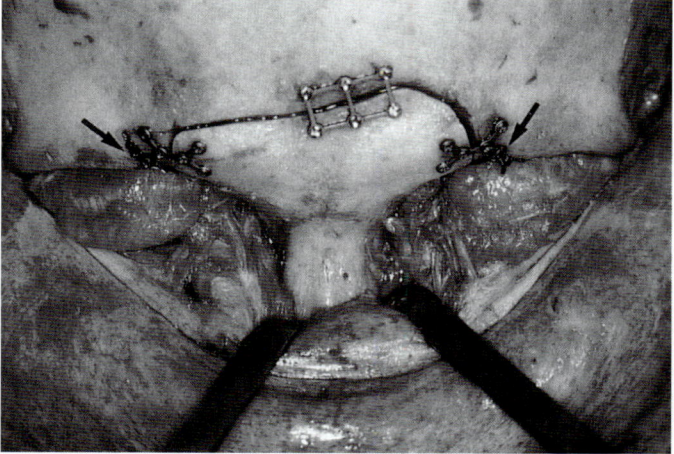

FIG. 4. A: Fascia lata applicator developed in cooperation with Institute Leibinger. It is a pick-up with a slim branch and a broad branch that facilitates the application of fascia layers to the sphenoclival and frontal lobes. **B:** Intraoperative view of the anterior part of the first fascia layer (*F*) already adapted to the frontal lobes. *S*, sphenoid; *O*, retracted orbits. *Arrows* indicate osteotomy borders of the frontal segment. *T*, preadapted titanium plates. **C:** Drawing depicting canthal ligament fixation. After replacement of the nasofrontal segment, the canthal ligament (*C*) is fixed by a thread guided underneath the skull base to the contralateral frontal sinus wall/supraorbital rim. **D:** Same patient as in Fig. 4B with repositioned frontonasal segment. *Arrows* indicate each canthal ligament thread fixed to the contralateral supraorbital rim.

Only in very extensive resections of the skeletal skull base frame or frontal lobe defects free or pedicled osseomyocutaneous flaps are necessary. Polyethylene tubes are inserted bilaterally into the subcranial compartment and externalized through the nasal lumen. These tubes are left in place for 8 months, allowing frontal drainage to avoid development of an apex syndrome or later mucus retention.

The medial orbital walls are reconstructed with lyophilized cartilage grafts only in those cases in which total removal of the wall was necessary or if the periosteum had to be resected. This procedure is unambiguous in such cases to avoid enophthalmos or strabismus. After removing all of the mucosa from the undersurface, the nasofrontal segment is exactly repositioned, reproducing the original configuration. This position is ensured by the previously adapted titanium microplates or miniplates (see Fig. 4B). Canthal ligament fixation is accomplished by placing a nonabsorbable suture through the ligament and then guiding the suture under the nasofrontal segment to the contralateral anterior frontal sinus wall (see Fig. 4C). Bilateral tightening of the suture results in medial, downward, and inward pull, thus achieving correct positioning of the canthal ligaments along the vertical, horizontal, and sagittal planes. The intraoperative view after correct osteosynthesis and contralateral canthal ligament fixation with sutures is shown in Fig. 4D.

ISSUES RELATED TO TUMOR LOCATION, CONSEQUENT OSTEOTOMY, AND RECONSTRUCTION

Tumors Located Posterior to the Ethmoid, Sphenoid, and Clivus

The giant cell tumor case illustrated in Fig. 5 is representative for this type of location. As depicted in axial, coronal, and sagittal magnetic resonance imaging (MRI) and computed tomography (CT) scans, the tumor extends intracranially, with partial resorption of the sphenoid plane, lateral sphenoid walls, and clivus and direct adjacency to the optic nerves, carotid arteries, and cavernous sinus. In such cases, extension of the frontonasal segment osteotomy as shown in Fig. 5B is sufficient for optimal exposure of the tumor. Furthermore, if no anterior or nasal lumen involvement is manifested, an anterior bridge of the nasal bone can be left intact. The intraoperative view after removal of the tumor (see Fig. 5C) reflects the advantage of a generous exposure. Resection of the ethmoid roof and the involved sphenoid plane enables optimal visualization of the optic nerve and chiasm conjunction, as well as the posterior sphenoid walls and clivus. Exposure and resection of the tumor from the anterior to the distal direction as well as downward enables direct visualization of the tumor borders from various angles and, as in this case, enables meticulous removal of the tumor along the medial optic nerve canal, the sphenoid wall, and the carotid prominence, despite the fact that the bone has grossly been resorbed. Histologic examination confirmed that all borders were tumor free. Comparison of preoperative and postoperative MRI and CT scans (see Fig. 5D-N) shows absence of tumor and the presence of fascia lata and Gelfoam layers. The reconstruction in such cases is relatively simple because the frontonasal segment can be exactly replaced and fixed with the titanium plates that were adapted before the osteotomy (see Fig. 5O). The further aspects of skull base management and canthal ligament fixation are the same as described previously (see Fig. 4). The patient's appearance is shown in Fig. 5P,Q. Three years after surgery, the patient is tumor free with good aesthetic and functional results.

Tumors Involving All Anterior Skull Base Planes with Intracranial as Well as Nasal Lumen and Maxillary Sinus Extension

In this category, multiple issues with regard to tumor resection as well as reconstruction need to be considered, including:

- Fragmentation due to tumor involvement of the frontal and nasal bones makes replacement by bone grafts necessary.
- Tumor extension toward the nasal lumen and maxillary sinuses often makes simultaneous resection of the orbital floor, anterior maxillary sinus wall, and the palate necessary.
- Lateral infratemporal fossa and pterygopalatine extension makes a combined LeFort I osteotomy or lateral approach necessary.
- Reconstruction makes the application of free, pedicled, or revascularized grafts/flaps necessary.

The exposure afforded by the subcranial approach enables radical tumor resection and reconstruction, obviating further transfacial procedures such as lateral rhinotomy or midface splitting, thus avoiding visible skin incisions and damage to intact structures.

Each of the following cases illustrates the various factors alluded to previously, demonstrating the best choice of methods to fulfill the surgical requirements.

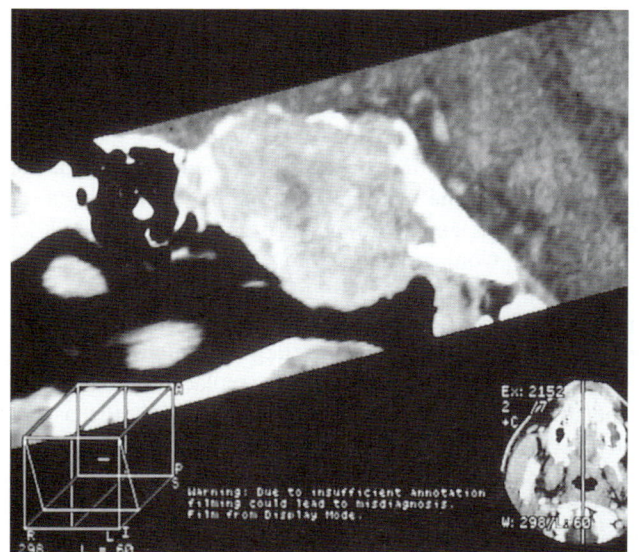

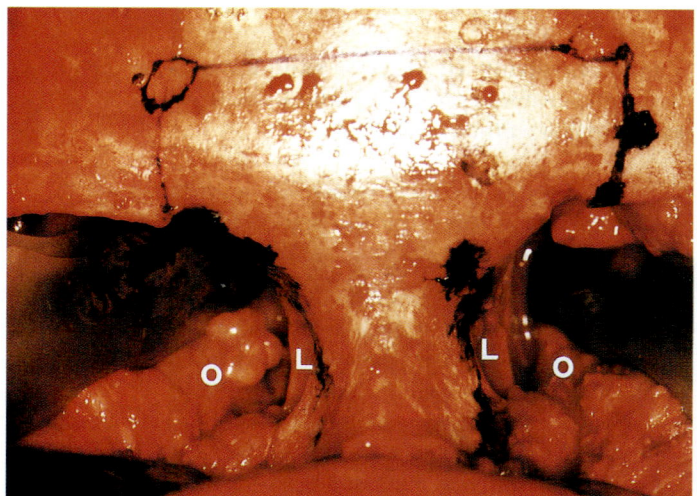

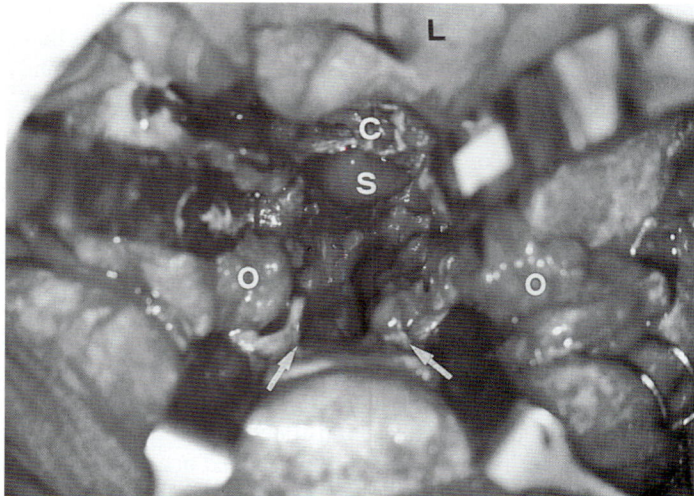

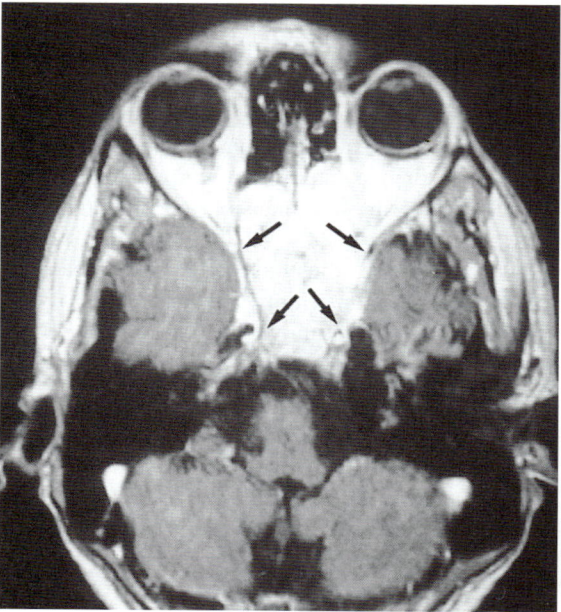

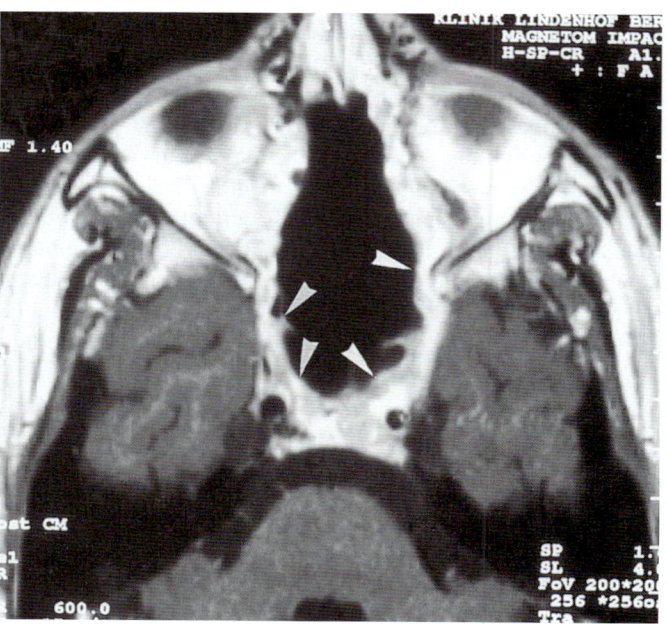

FIG. 5. Representative case for the surgical management of tumors located in the posterior ethmoid and sphenoclival region. **A:** Parasagittal computed tomography (CT) scan showing a giant cell tumor located in the sphenoid plane, posterior sphenoid wall, and clivus. Bone erosion is manifested. **B:** Osteotomy borders of the frontonasal segment. *O*, retracted orbit after exposure of the cone; *L*, lacrimal duct canal. **C:** Intraoperative appearance after tumor removal. *L*, anterior lobes covered by a pad; *O*, retracted orbits revealing the defect borders after resection of the ethmoid compartment and roof and the sphenoid plane, along with intracranial tumor extension (no intradural involvement) and the sella floor; *S*, the posterior sphenoid wall; *C*, partially removed anterior clivus bone. *Arrows* indicate anterior resection borders of the apertura piriformis. **D:** Preoperative axial magnetic resonance image (MRI) indicating the adjacency of the tumor with the carotid arteries, particularly on the left, and with the optic nerves (*arrows*). **E:** Postoperative MRI indicating absence of tumor and showing fascia lata layers (*arrowheads*). The medial optic nerve canal walls and the bone along the carotid arteries prominence—lateral sphenoid walls was removed and aligned with an additional fascia layer.

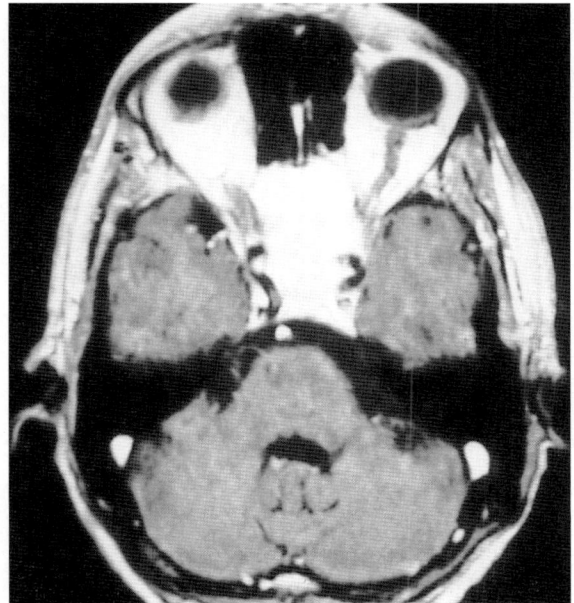
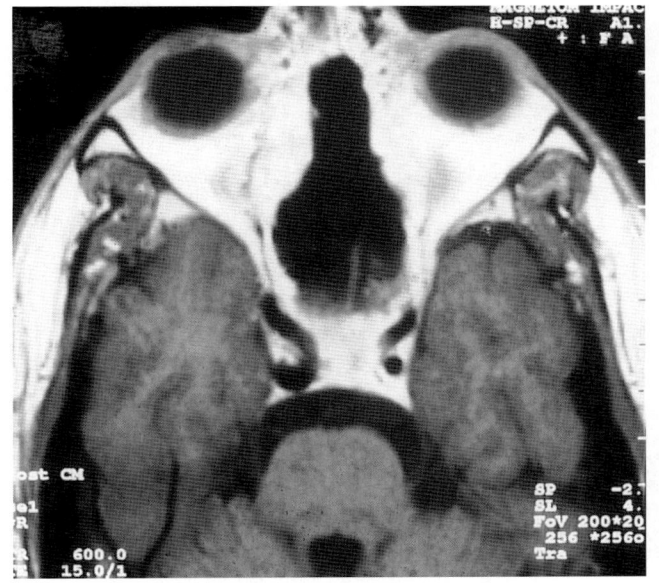
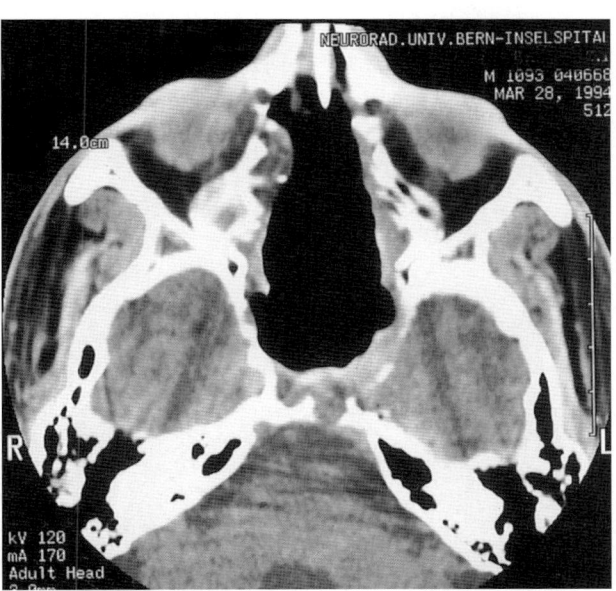

FIG. 5. *Continued.* **F–H:** Additional preoperative **(F)** and postoperative **(G)** MRIs and CT scan **(H)** confirming radical tumor removal.

(figure continues)

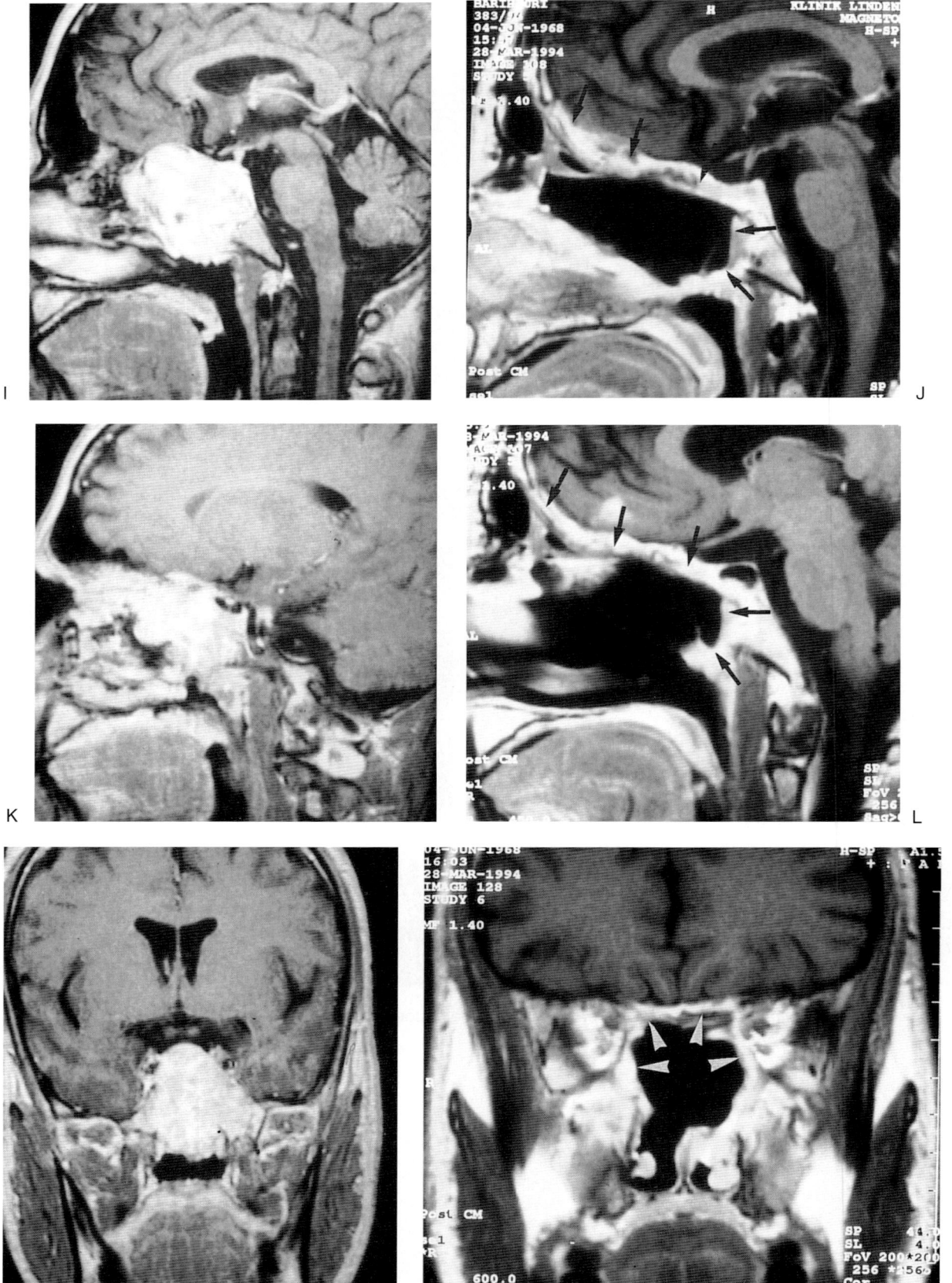

FIG. 5. *Continued.* **I–L:** Preoperative and postoperative sagittal MRIs. Note absence of tumor. Fascia lata layers applied to the frontal lobes and sphenoclival area can be seen (*arrows*). **M,N:** Preoperative and postoperative coronal MRIs indicating the extent of tumor, and the fascia layers (*arrowheads*) after tumor removal.

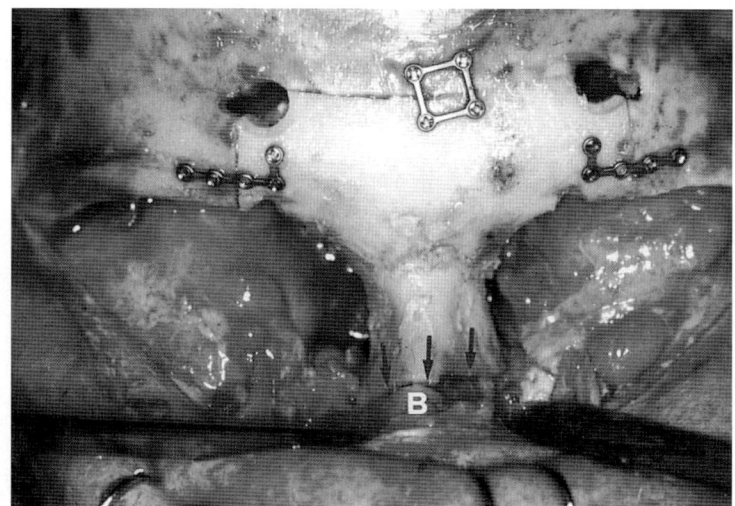
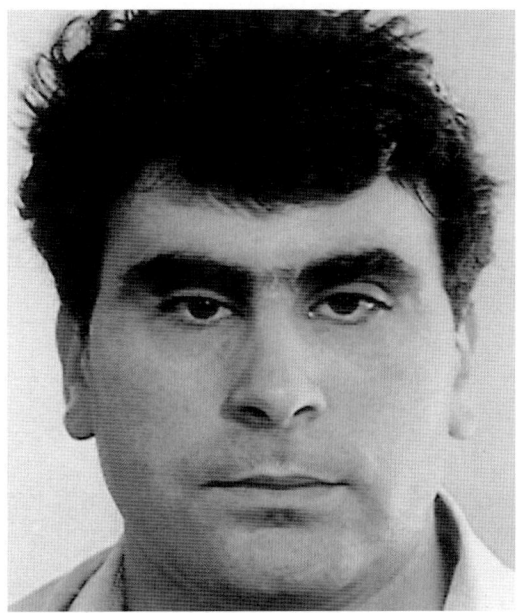
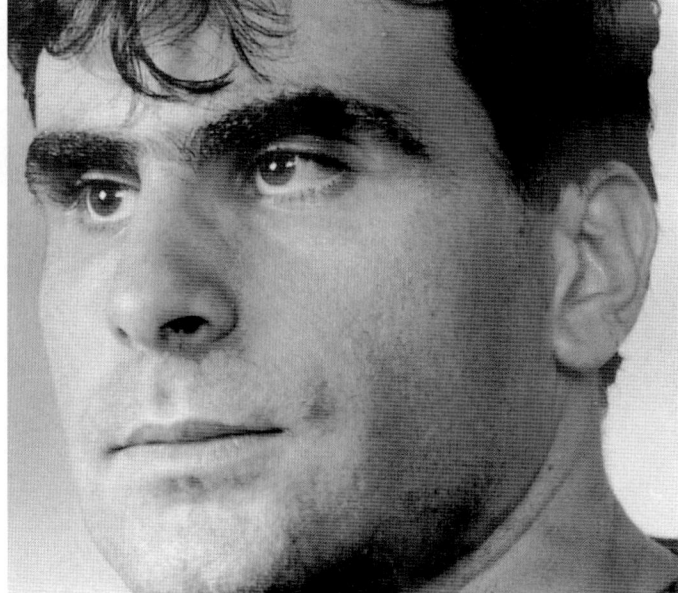

FIG. 5. *Continued.* **O:** Appearance after replacement and fixation of the frontonasal segment. In this case, the osteotomy (*arrows*) was performed leaving an anterior bridge (*B*) intact. For indications, see text. **P,Q:** The patient's postoperative appearance. Note correct configuration of the frontonasal area and canthal ligaments. The frontal photograph was intentionally performed at an angle to depict the slight enophthalmos. There is no double vision.

CASE 1

This case, illustrated in Fig. 6, demonstrates the surgical management of an extensive esthesioneuroblastoma. Intracranial as well as intranasal extension along with partial resorption of the nasal buttress are shown in Fig. 6A. Further involvement of the medial orbital walls and maxillary sinus extension including the orbital floor were evident. The intraoperative view after the removal of the tumor by the subcranial approach is shown in Fig. 6B. The extent of the resection along the skull base and radical tumor removal are documented in Figs. 6C-F. Because tumor extension toward the nasal lumen was well defined and encapsulated, only the nasal–maxillary sinus floor mucosa in direct contact had to be removed. Because the mucosa turned out to be tumor free, the hard palate was not resected. Alignment of the bone toward the lumen was done using a pedicled buccal fat pad layer (36) (see Fig. 6F). Reconstruction of the medial orbital wall as well as the orbital floor on the right was performed with lyophilized cartilage layers. Substitution of the tumor-involved frontonasal segment was accomplished with external table bone grafts. The Y-shaped titanium miniplate developed in cooperation with the Leibinger Institute is most suitable for the fixation of the grafts up to the tip of the nose.

CASE 1 (Continued)

Because the plate has been adapted before the osteotomy, reshaping of the grafts and their fixation enable the exact reproduction of the preoperative configuration (see Fig. 6G,H). The external table provides sufficient bone graft material even in more extensive frontal bone defects, as shown in a different case (see Fig. 6I). Meticulous reconstruction is crucial for correct reproduction of an aesthetic appearance, as shown in Fig. 6J-M.

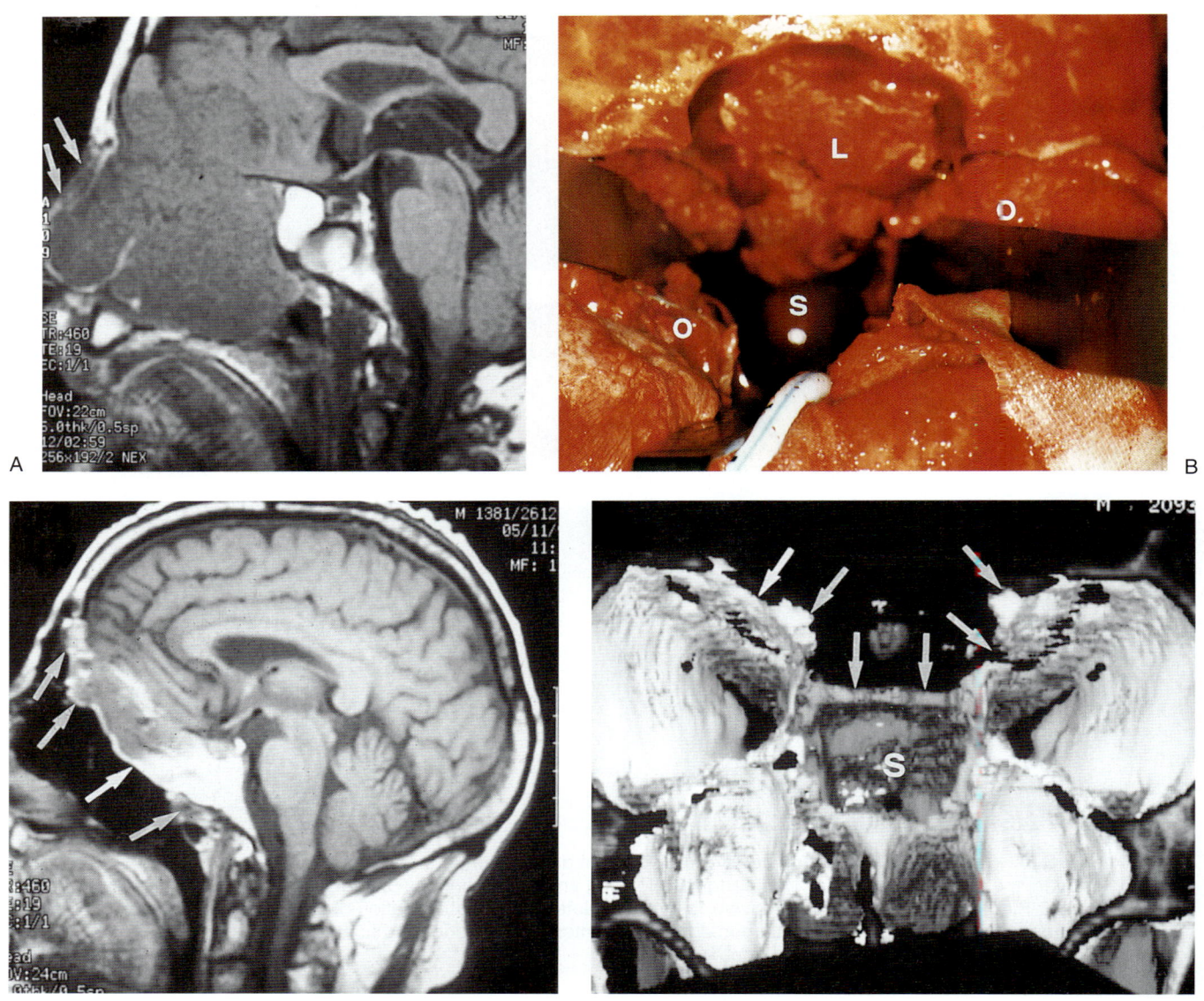

FIG. 6. Case 1. **A:** Preoperative sagittal magnetic resonance image (MRI) showing intracranial and nasal lumen extensions of an esthesioneuroblastoma and involvement and resorption of the nasal bone (*arrows*). **B:** Intraoperative appearance after tumor removal. *O*, retracted orbits; *L*, frontal lobes and first fascia lata layer; *S*, posterior sphenoid wall. **C:** Postoperative sagittal MRI. Note absence of tumor. Fascia lata layers and the nasal external table bone grafts (*arrows*) are seen. **D:** Three dimensional computed tomography scan showing the borders of the resected skull base (*arrows*). *S*, posterior sphenoid wall.

CASE 1 (Continued)

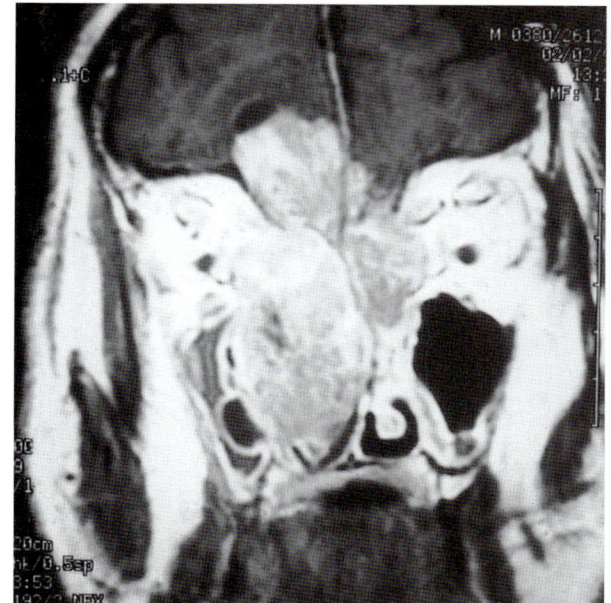
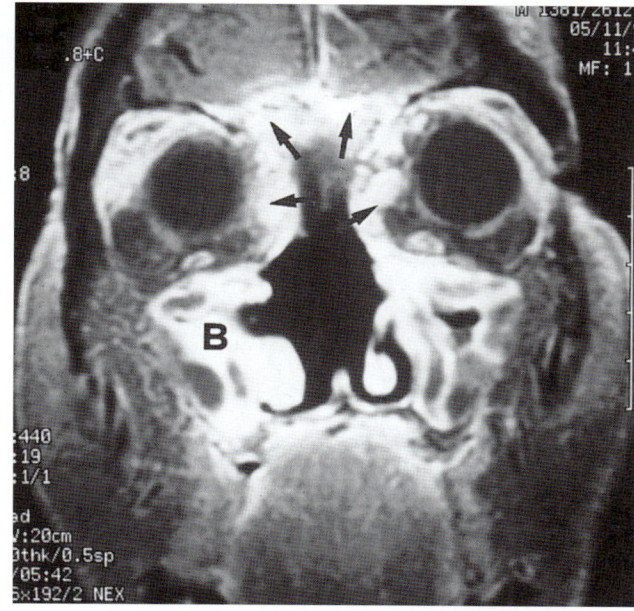
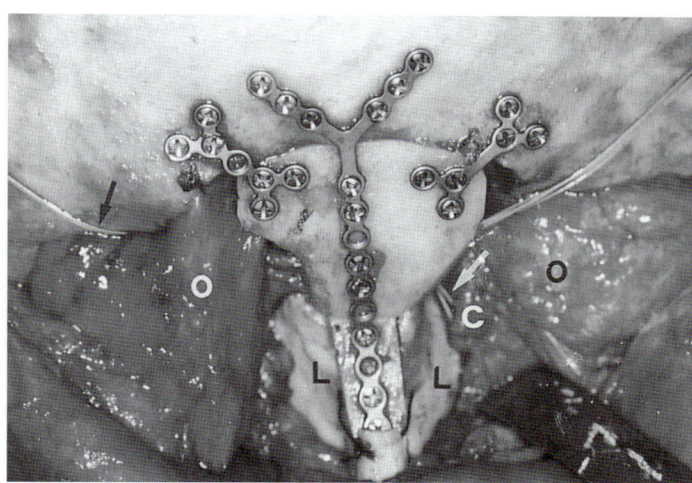
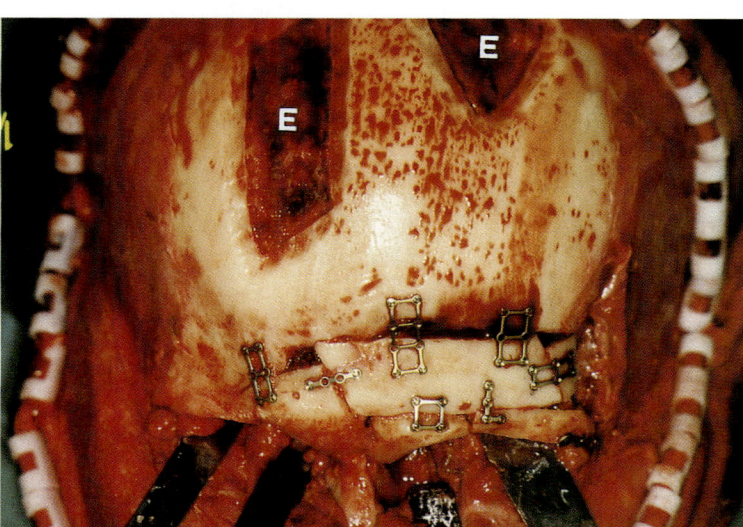

FIG. 6. Case 1. *Continued.* **E:** Preoperative coronal MRI showing nasal and maxillary sinus involvement. **F:** Postoperative coronal MRI showing fascia lata layers and lyophilized cartilage grafts along the medial orbital wall and floor (*arrows*). *B*, pedicled buccal fat pad for lining of the palate/maxillary sinus floor. **G,H:** Tumor involvement of the frontonasal frame necessitated reconstruction with external table bone grafts. The preadapted Y-shaped titanium plate (Institute Leibinger GmbH) for fixation of the grafts and reconstruction of the lateral nasal walls (*L*) is crucial for a satisfactory aesthetic result. *O*, orbit. *Arrows* indicate the thread applied to the left canthal ligament (*C*) guided underneath the skull base to be fixed to the contralateral supraorbital rim (see Fig. 4c). **I:** Intraoperative view showing the frontonasal reconstruction in larger defects. *E*, external table donor site (in a different patient).

(figure continues)

CASE 1 (Continued)

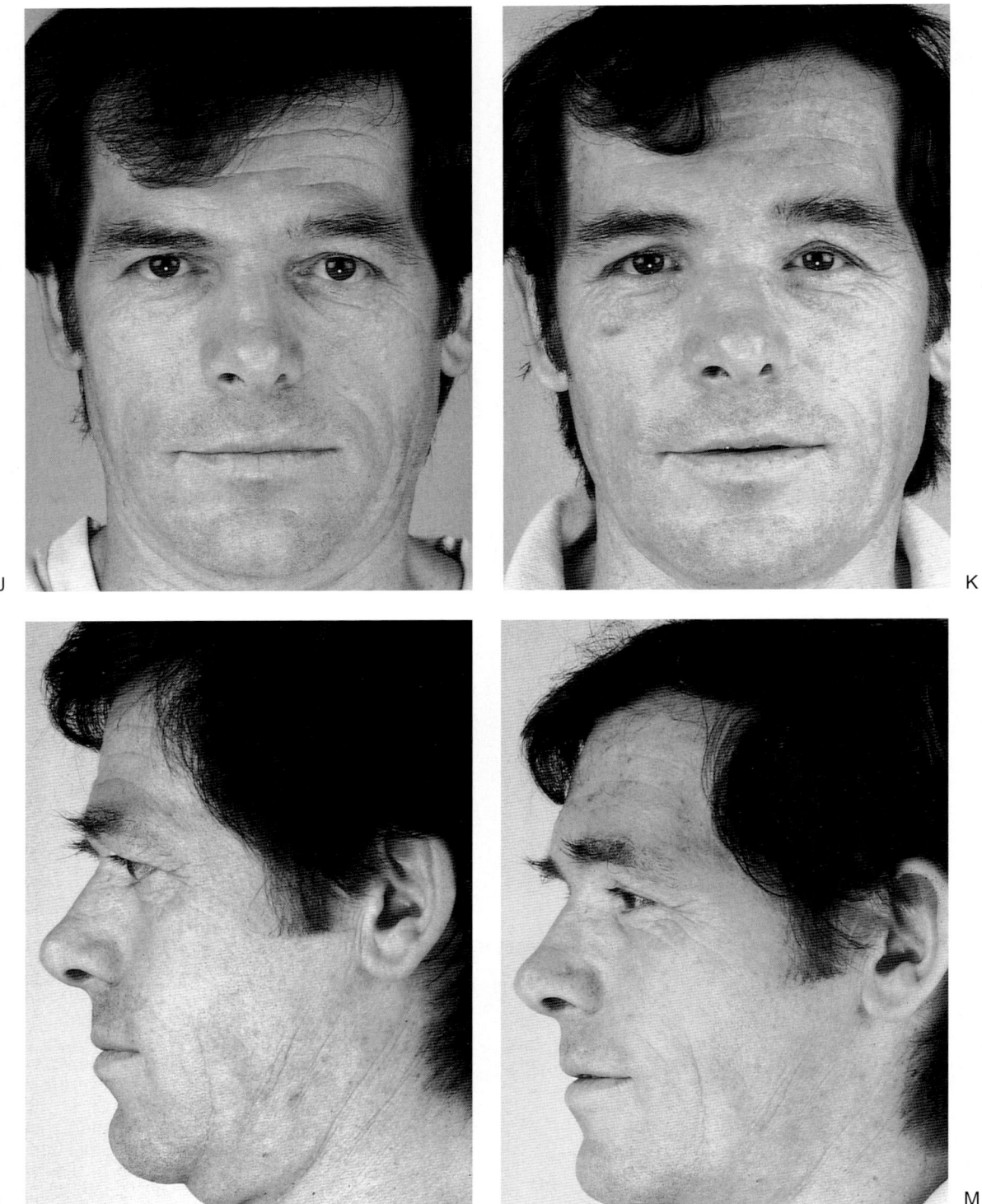

FIG. 6. Case 1. *Continued.* **J,K:** Frontal views before surgery and 3 weeks after surgery **(J)** with correct frontonasal configuration. Slight edema of the upper and lower eyelids is still seen **(K)**. **L,M:** Lateral views before **(L)** and after surgery **(M)**.

CASE 2

In this case (Fig. 7), the tumor—squamous cell carcinoma previously operated on elsewhere—involved the skull base as well as the palate and the nasal frame (see Fig. 7A). The intraoperative appearance after tumor removal (see Fig. 7B), including resection of the ethmoidosphenoid plane, shows the fascia lata already applied along the skull base up to the posterior sphenoid wall and clivus, as well as to the orbital roofs. By this approach, *en bloc* removal of the hard palate along with the tumor was, because of the broad exposure, relatively easy to perform. In Fig. 7C, the tongue is pulled through the palatine defect up to the skull base and is clearly visible. Reconstruction of the palatine defect in such cases is best performed using a temporalis vessel-pedicled external table graft, as shown in Fig. 7D (a different case). The flap is inserted underneath the zygomatic arch. Depending on the size of the bone

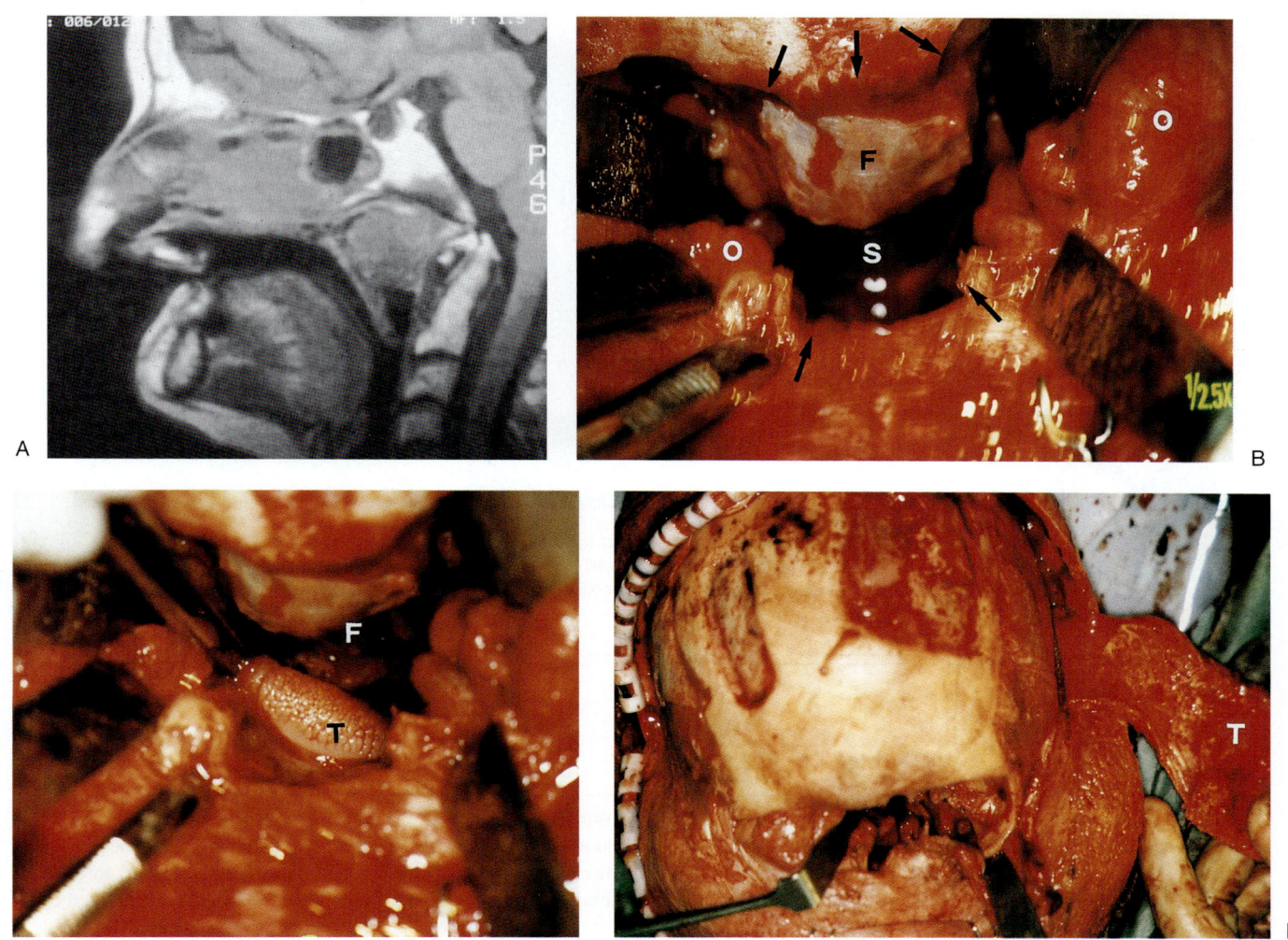

FIG. 7. Case 2. **A:** Sagittal magnetic resonance image (MRI) showing a squamous cell carcinoma involving the anterior skull base, nasal lumen, and palate. This patient was previously operated on elsewhere. **B:** Intraoperative view after tumor removal. *F,* fascia lata applied to the frontal lobes and skull base planes; *O,* retracted orbits; *S,* posterior sphenoid wall. *Arrows* indicate superior frontal and inferior frontonasal segment osteotomy borders. **C:** Appearance after tumor removal along the nasal cavity along with resection of the palate through same subcranial access. *T,* the tongue pulled through the defect up to the fascia (*F*) aligning the frontal lobe. **D:** Reconstruction of such defects: free external table grafts for substitution of the frontonasal segment, and external table flap (*T*) pedicled by temporal vessels and guided underneath the zygomatic bone, for reconstruction of the palatine defect (different patient).

(figure continues)

CASE 2 (Continued)

graft, the zygoma, including the arch, has to be osteotomized to permit this procedure, and is then refixed with plates and free external table grafts for the back of the nose. The postoperative CT scan in Fig. 7E (same patient as in Fig. 7A-C) shows the cavity after tumor resection as well as part of the plates used for the fixation of nasal bone grafts, which substituted for the tumor-involved frontonasal segment. Another postoperative CT scan of the same patient (see Fig. 7F) demonstrates the palatine bone grafts *in situ* with the dental implants that have simultaneously been inserted in the same primary surgical session. Thus, secondary surgery can be avoided and the osseointegration of the implants is optimal. Furthermore, because the dental suprastructure and dental reconstruction are applied 3 months after surgery, function and physiologic loads minimize resorption of the bone grafts. Replacement of the palatine mucosa has to be done using a cutaneous revascularized free skin flap—in this case, a radialis forearm flap was preferred.

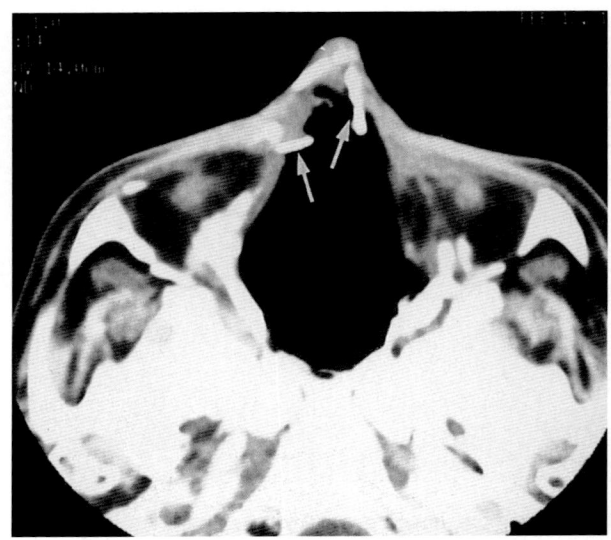 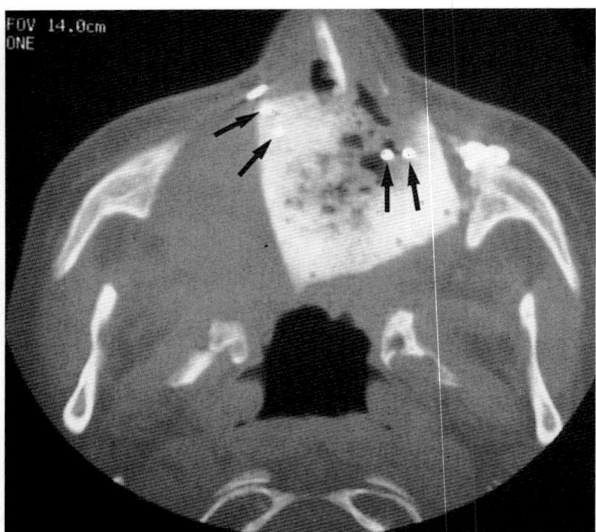

FIG. 7. Case 2. *Continued.* **E:** Postoperative computed tomography (CT) scan showing absence of the tumor. *Arrows* indicate the anterior part of the plates used for fixation of the frontonasal free bone grafts. **F:** Postoperative CT (lower level) showing the pedicled external table graft *in situ* with the simultaneously applied dental implants (*arrows*).

CASE 3

The patient in case 3 presents a skull base tumor with intracranial as well as nasal and maxillary sinus extension, necessitating bone grafting for reconstruction of the orbital cone.

In this case, esthesioneuroblastoma involving the skull base, nasal lumen, and maxillary sinus (Fig. 8A) made resection of the orbital floor and anterior maxillary sinus wall, as well as hemiresection of the palate, necessary. The extent of the radical resection is manifested in Fig. 8B, which also shows absence of tumor. In this level of the MRI, the bone transplants applied in the same session are not clearly represented. The external table bone grafts for the reconstruction of the supraorbital rim, orbital floor, anterior maxillary sinus wall, and lateral palatine defect were applied by the transconjunctival and intraorbital approach (Fig. 8C). The grafts are clearly depicted in the same patient's CT scans (Fig. 8D,E).

CASE 3 (Continued)

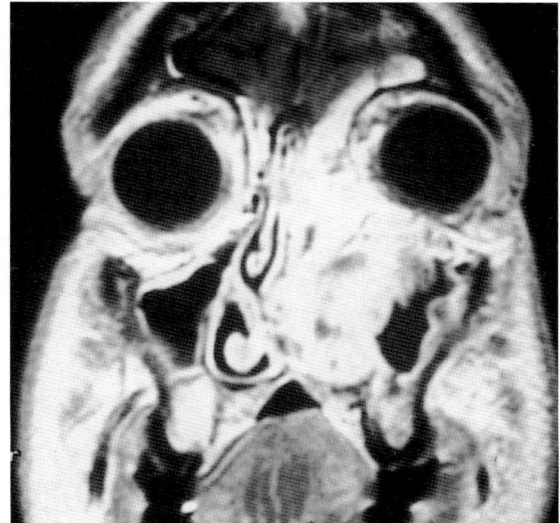
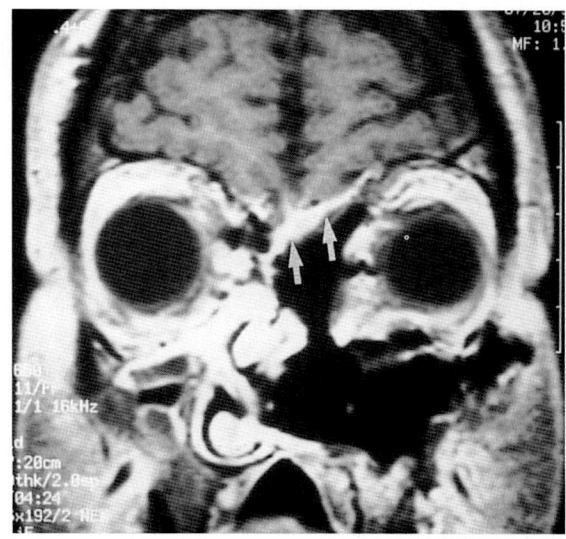
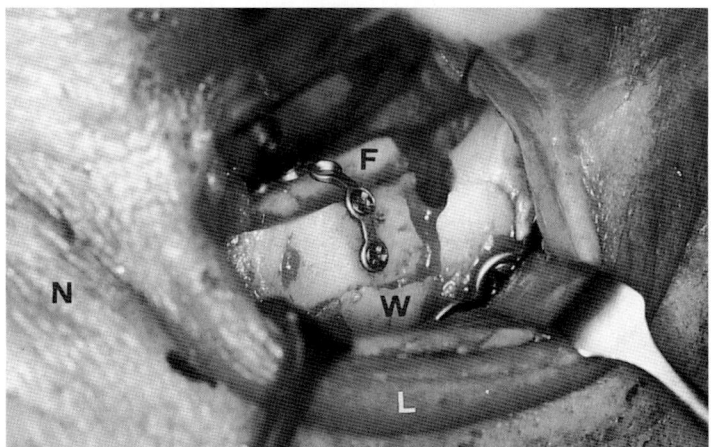

FIG. 8. Case 3. **A:** Preoperative coronal magnetic resonance image (MRI) showing extension of an esthesioneuroblastoma toward the nasal and maxillary sinus cavity, involving the medial orbital wall and floor as well as the palate. **B:** Postoperative MRI showing the extent of the resection; note absence of tumor and presence of fascia lata layers (*arrows*). The bone grafts are only partially seen on this level. **C:** Intraoperative view showing the transconjunctival approach. *L*, lower lid; *N*, lateral nasal wall. The infraorbital rim, floor of orbit (*F*), and anterior maxillary sinus wall (*W*) are fixed by titanium plates. **D,E:** Postoperative coronal and axial computed tomography scans showing the applied pedicled palatine (*P*) and free orbital floor and anterior maxillary sinus wall external table grafts (*arrows*). The advantages of the subcranial approach in avoiding additional transfacial approaches are convincing.

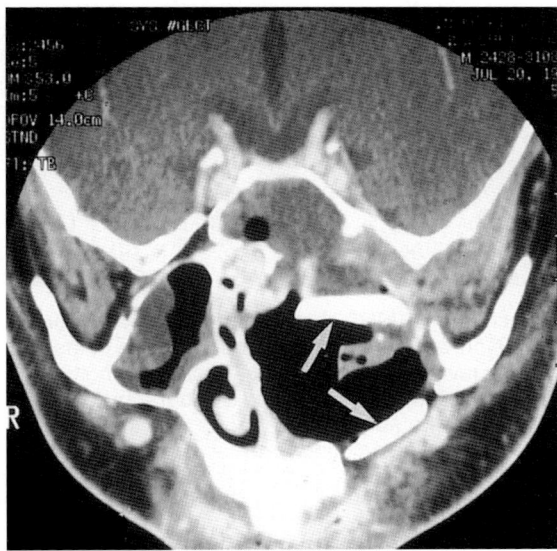
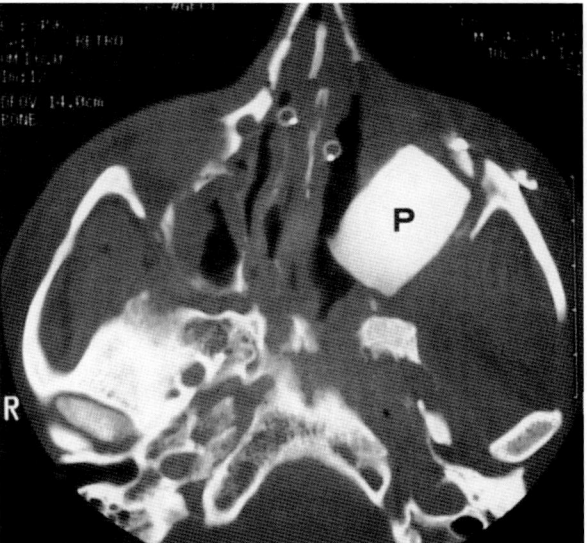

CASE 4

In this case (Fig. 9), a juvenile angiofibroma tumor was located in the nasal-maxillary sinus lumen as well as the skull base up to the sphenoclival area. Preoperative and postoperative MRI and CT scans depict the extent of the resection. To achieve a radical resection, the medial wall and orbital floor on both sides as well as the palate–maxillary sinus floor on the right side had to be removed. An external table graft was applied to the palate defect on the right side and aligned with the maxillary sinus lumen by a pedicled fat pad layer (see Fig. 9D). For the reconstruction of the medial and orbital floor on both sides, a combination of lyophilized cartilage layers and external bone grafts was preferred (see Fig. 9E). The patient's preoperative and postoperative appearance is shown in Fig. 9F-I.

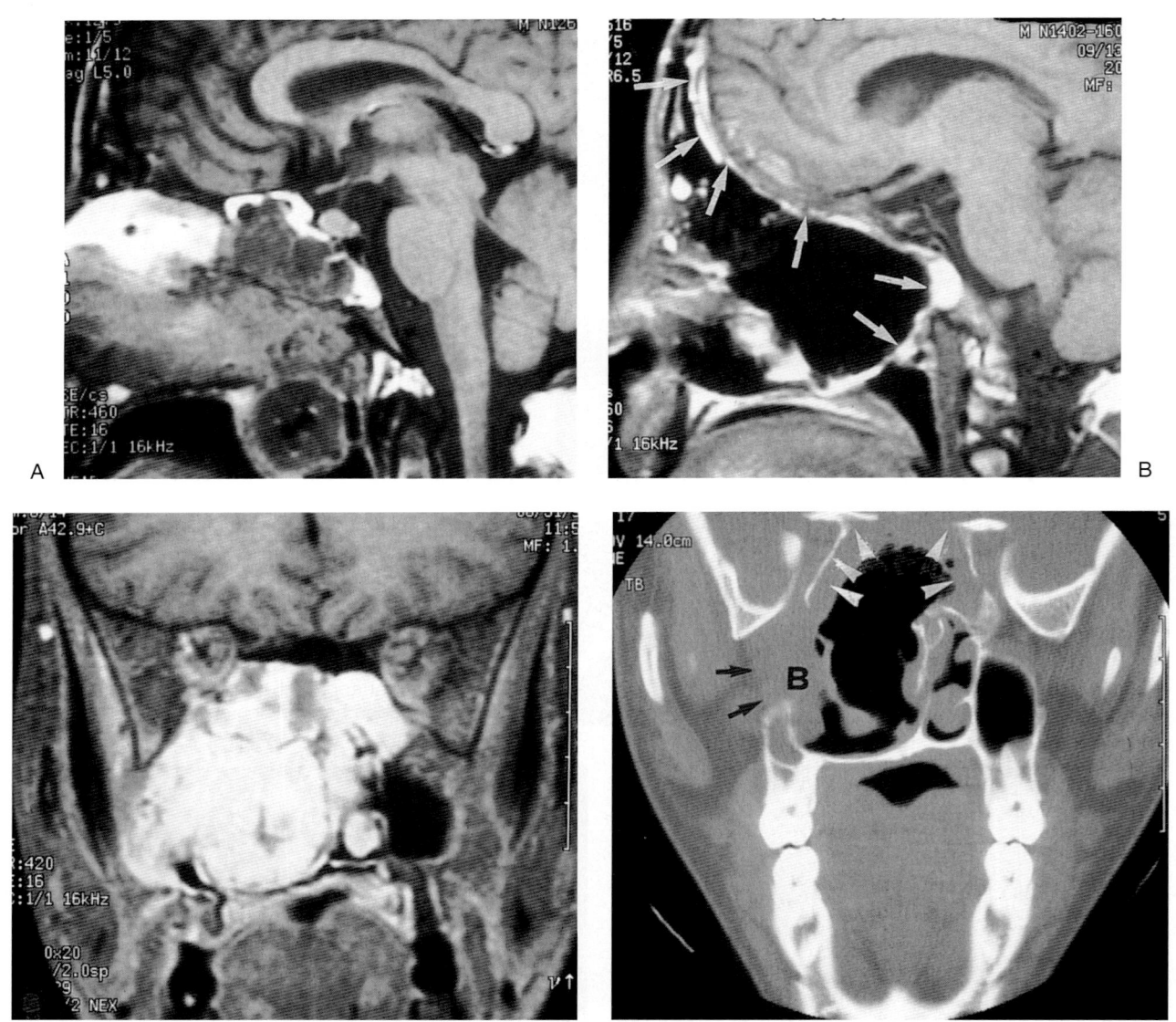

FIG. 9. Case 4. **A:** Preoperative sagittal magnetic resonance image (MRI) showing tumor with anterior and sphenoclival extensions. **B:** Postoperative sagittal MRI. Note absence of tumor and presence of fascia lata layers (*arrows*). **C:** Preoperative coronal MRI showing juvenile angiofibroma tumor involving the skull base, nasal lumen, and maxillary sinus. **D:** Postoperative coronal computed tomography scan showing absence of tumor and the extent of the resection along the sphenoid plane, as well as fascia lata layers (*arrowheads*). Through the resected retromaxillary pterygopalatine area (*arrowheads*), the pedicled buccal fat pad (*B*) is seen lining the palatine bone graft.

CASE 4 (Continued)

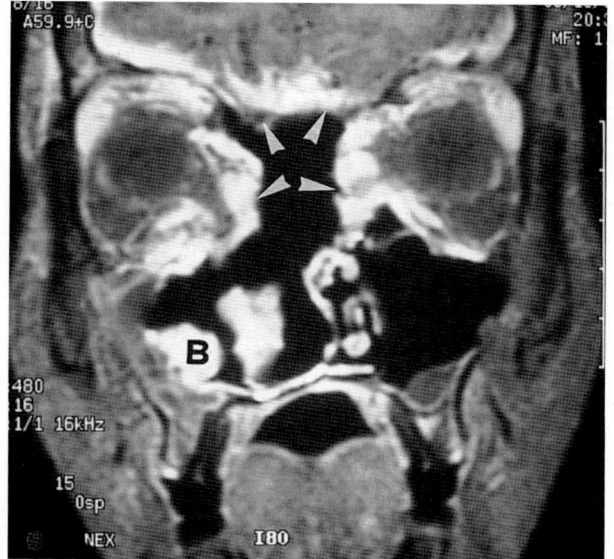

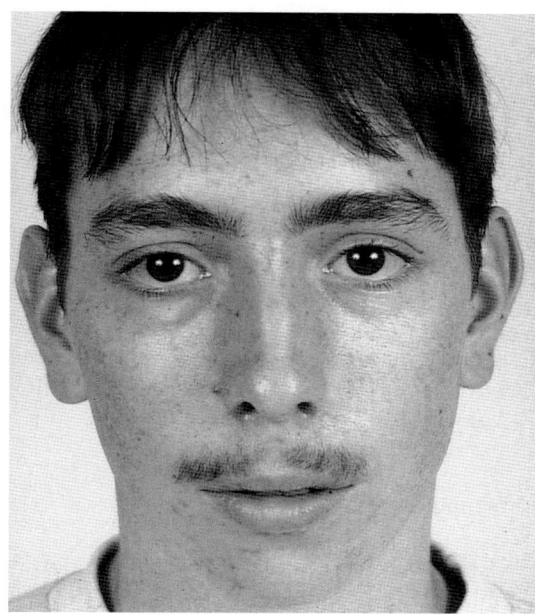
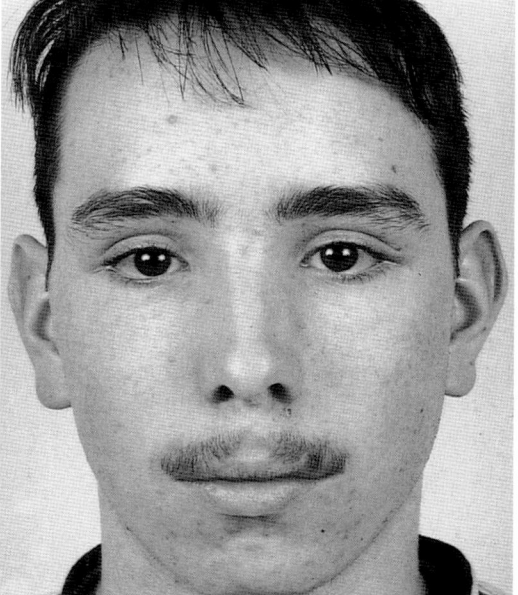

FIG. 9. Case 4. *Continued.* **E:** Deeper MRI level showing absence of tumor. Note fascia lata layers applied to the dura (*arrowhead*), as well as the buccal fat pad (*B; arrows*). **F–I:** Patient's preoperative and postoperative appearance, indicating adequate reproduction of the preoperative appearance.

(figure continues)

CASE 4 (Continued)

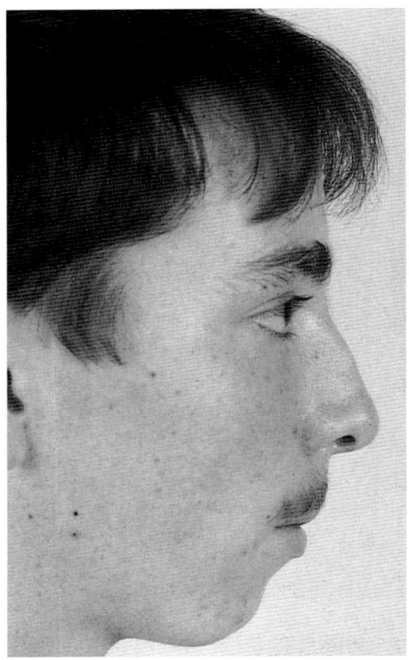
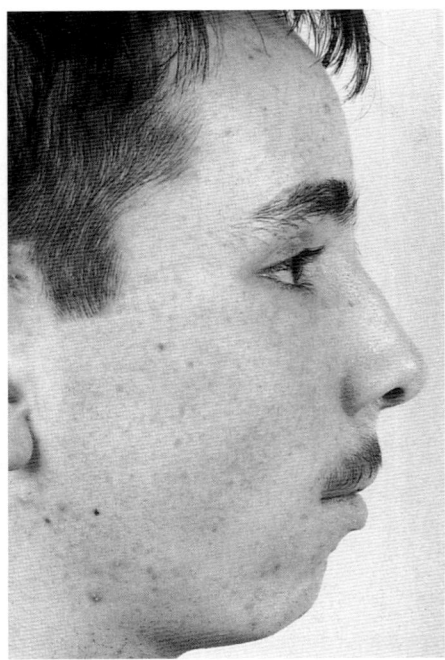

FIG. 9. Case 4. *Continued.*

RESULTS

In this study, only the 104 cases surgically treated by the extended anterior approach up to 1993 are included. A further 45 cases treated between 1993 and 1995 are still in the process of evaluation. Not included are the cases operated on by the lateral approach. The follow-up corresponds to a previous publication (15).

Patient Population

The patients ranged in age from 4 to 83 years, with a mean age of 61.8 years. There were 59 male and 45 female patients. Fig. 10 shows the histologic composition of the lesion, of which 57 were benign and 47 malignant tumors. Figure 10 also shows the location of the tumors with respect to the skull base. Thirty patients received radiation therapy (11 before surgery, 19 after surgery), 3 patients underwent chemotherapy, and 9 patients had had previous operations for tumor ablation.

Patient Follow-up

The state of disease at follow-up is indicated in Table 1. Fifty-one (89%) of 57 patients with benign and 31 (68%) of 47 patients with malignant lesions were alive with no evidence of disease. Mean follow-up time in months is indicated in parentheses in the table. Because frontal lobe retraction was avoided, immediate postoperative recovery was accelerated. Even in the case of large tumors with extensive resection, the stay in the intensive care unit was reduced to an average of 2 days, and hospital stay was limited to 11 to 12 days.

Postoperative Complications

Early and late postoperative complications are listed in Table 2. Recurrent cerebrospinal fluid (CSF) leakage occurred in three patients; in one patient accidental removal of nasal packing on postoperative day 1 resulted in an immediate CSF leak. This patient was treated by lumbar CSF drainage, and the leak was successfully controlled. In the second and third cases, inadequate primary dural repair and fascia lata alignment resulted in early CSF leakage. In two other cases a pneumocranium was manifested, and revisions were necessary.

Frontal lobe contusion with edema was observed in one patient who underwent combined transfrontal–subcranial resection. Temporary postoperative seizures occurred in one patient. In two patients, epidural infections occurred and were successfully treated with antibiotic drugs. There were no brain abscesses. Cranial nerve dysfunction (other than ol-

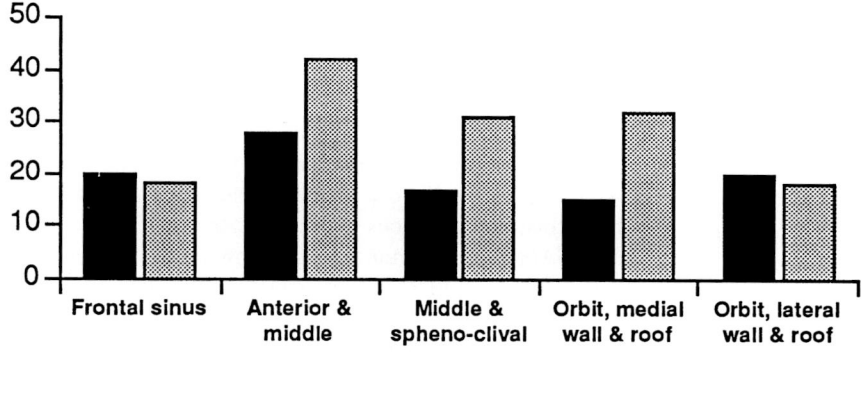

FIG. 10. Histologic types and localization of anterior skull base tumors.

factory) was observed in eight patients and included three optic, one trochlear, two abducens, and two oculomotor nerves affected. The three cases of early optic nerve dysfunction were related to tumor removal at the optic canal or chiasm, and all resolved with time. In the other five patients, compensation occurred and no secondary corrections were necessary. The optimum inferior exposure afforded by the subcranial approach allowed preservation of contralateral olfactory filaments during unilateral tumor resection. In two patients with benign and five patients with malignant tumors, anosmia was not observed as a sequela of skull base tumor removal. None of the patients required facial incisions, and the authors have not observed nasofrontal segment bone resorption in any of their patients to date.

DISCUSSION

The subcranial extended approach and osteotomy of the frontonasoorbital external skeletal frame provides an optimum anterior access to the anterior skull base and sphenoclival region, as well as to the nasal and paranasal cavities.

TABLE 1. Tumor diagnosis and survival[a]

Histology	A&W	AWD	DOD	DOC	No. of cases
Benign					
Adenoma	4 (19)				4
Angioma	6 (13)				6
Angiofibroma	7 (12)			1 (10)	7
Fibrous dysplasia	4 (21)				4
Giant cell tumor	1 (3)				1
Inverted papilloma	11 (22)	3 (20)		1 (18)	14
Meningioma	7 (24)	1 (36)			8
Neurofibroma	1 (5)				1
Osteoma	12 (10)				12
Total	51	4		2	57
Percent	89	7		4	100
Malignant					
Adenocarcinoma	6 (37)	2 (30)	3 (6)		11
Adenoid cystic carcinoma	2 (30)	2 (15)			4
Basal cell carcinoma	2 (15)				2
Clear cell carcinoma	1 (13)				1
Esthesioneuroblastoma	7 (13)			1 (63)	8
Melanoma	2 (30)	1 (14)		1 (36)	4
Non-Hodgkin's lymphoma	2 (34)				2
Sarcoma	4 (10)	1 (8)			5
Squamous cell carcinoma	6 (24)	2 (11)	2 (8)		10
Total	32	8	5	2	47
Percent	68	17	11	4	100
Total cases	**83**	**12**	**5**	**4**	**104**

A&W, alive without disease; AWD, alive with disease; DOD, died of disease; DOC, died of other causes.
[a] Numbers in parentheses indicate mean follow-up period in months.

Table 2. Postoperative complications (N = 104)

Complications	No. of cases
Early	
Cerebrospinal fluid leaks	3
Frontal lobe contusion/edema	1
Epidural infection	2
Pneumocranium	2
Pulmonary embolism	1
Partial local flap necrosis	2
Cutaneous fistula	2
Temporary siezures	2
Optic nerve dysfunction	3
Late	
Frontal sinus dysfunction	1
Epiphora	1
Cranial nerve dysfunction	
Olfactory	73
Oculomotor	2
Abducens	2
Trochlear	1
Optic	0

Accurate delineation of tumor margins and dural excision are facilitated by this approach. Because the tumor borders are exposed from the anterior to posterior as well as from the cranial to distal (and vice versa) directions, accurate visualization of the optic nerves along the canal and chiasm and the carotid arteries, and the prevention of unnecessary damage, comprise major advantages. In cases of unilateral lesions, the contralateral olfactory filaments can often be preserved. Optic nerve exposure and decompression by removal of the medial optic nerve canal walls is readily performed. The subcranial approach can be combined with an intraoral access or a LeFort I osteotomy for lateral retromaxillary–sphenopalatine extensions. Thus, *en bloc* removal of virtually all tumor extensions, including those into the epipharyngeal and clival area, while sparing the optic chiasm, is facilitated.

Because of the broad exposure obtained, further transfacial approaches are unnecessary. Skull base tumors have been surgically approached in various ways since the early 1970s. The transbasal–transethmoidal approach to the skull base, initially described by Escher (19,37) and Naumann (22), has been well known to otolaryngologists since the late 1940s. In 1972, Derome et al. (18) described the transbasal removal of sphenoethmoid tumors using a similar technique. Jane et al. (38), Jackson (33), and others (30–32,34,35) have described various orbital osteotomies for access to intracranial and extracranial skull base lesions. Combinations of transcranial and transfacial approaches were initially reported by Smith et al. (39), Ketcham et al. (40), and Van Buren et al. (41), and later by Donald (42). Modifications of these techniques by Sekhar et al. (29) and Rinehart et al. (28) have appeared in the literature. All of these techniques differ slightly in the planning and positioning of the facial and cranial osteotomies, and all except the subcranial method advocate a transfrontal approach with unavoidable retraction of the frontal lobes, even when an attempt is made to minimize such manipulation. In addition, the accepted methods of transfacial approach, such as the lateral, superior, and midline rhinotomies, require significant external facial incisions that are completely avoided by the subcranial extended exposure.

Transfrontal access also implies that the tumor is exposed in a superior to inferior direction. On the one hand, particularly for tumors located underneath the sphenoid plane and clivus, this direction does not provide the necessary visualization. Apart from tumor extension toward the nasal lumen, the epipharynx and maxillary sinuses cannot be assessed. This also makes further combined transfacial procedures necessary. On the other hand, in transfacial approaches, the exposure is performed in the anterior to posterior direction, providing insufficient exposure of tumor borders, particularly for sphenoclival and intracranial tumor extensions. This factor, as well as the exposure of the optic nerves, optic chiasm, and carotid arteries, often implies a piecemeal removal of the tumor. In contrast, the subcranial extended approach provides tumor exposure from all directions, thus enabling optimal visualization of the tumor and the adjacent vital structures, and avoiding frontal lobe retraction. Delfini et al. (26) and Pinsolle et al. (27) have described and confirmed the advantages of the same subcranial exposure in small series, although they did not refer to any of the current authors' previous publications.

The subcranial exposure also allows for watertight alignment of the dura and anterior skull base after ablative surgery, with an infrequent incidence of postoperative CSF leakage and epidural infection. The frontal subcranial polyethylene drainage tube has proved effective in limiting late infectious sequelae such as chronic sinusitis, mucocele, or brain abscess. Centripetal medial canthal ligament fixation as well as the avoidance of all external facial scars has improved postoperative cosmetics tremendously, and is a distinct advantage over more traditional transfacial methods such as lateral rhinotomy and midline–midface osteotomy. Because the authors' procedure requires little or no frontal lobe retraction, postoperative brain edema and intensive care unit and total hospital stay are reduced, and postoperative recovery is accelerated.

ACKNOWLEDGMENTS

The authors thank the Department of Neuroradiology (Prof. G. Schroth) for outstanding support and cooperation, and Dr. J. Chen (Department of Otolaryngology, Sunnybrooke Health Center, Toronto, Ontario, Canada) for the superb quality of the drawings.

REFERENCES

1. Raveh J. Das einzeitige Vorgehen bei der Wiederherstellung van Frontobasal-Mittelgesichtsfrakturen. Modifikationen und Behandlungsmodalitäten. *Chirurgie* 1983;117:779.
2. Raveh J, Laedrach K, Vuillemin T, et al. Management of combined frontonaso-orbital/skull base fractures and telecanthus in 355 cases. *Arch Otolaryngol Head Neck Surg* 1992;118:605.

3. Raveh J, Neiger M. Die Wiederherstellung bei schweren Gesichtsschädelverletzungen. *Schweizer Monatsschrift fur Zahnheilkunde* 1981;91:206.
4. Raveh J, Reidli M, Markwalder TM. Operative management of 194 cases of combined maxillofacial-frontobasal fractures: principles and modification. *J Oral Maxillofac Surg* 1984;42:555.
5. Raveh J, Vuillemin T. Subcranial management of 395 combined frontobasal-midface fractures. *Arch Otolaryngol Head Neck Surg* 1988; 114:1114.
6. Raveh J, Vuillemin T. The surgical one-stage management of combined cranio-maxillo-facial and frontobasal fractures: advantages of the subcranial approach in 374 cases. *J Craniomaxillofac Surg* 1988;16:160.
7. Laedrach K, Annino D, Raveh J, Zingg M, Vuillemin T, Leibinger K. Advanced approaches to cranio-orbital injuries. *Facial Plastic Surgery Clinics of North America* 1995;3:107.
8. Raveh J. Neue Aspekte der kraniofazialen Chirurgie. *Schweiz Monatsschr Zahnmed* 1986;96:406.
9. Raveh J, Vuillemin T. Advantages of an additional subcranial approach in the correction of craniofacial deformities. *J Craniomaxillofac Surg* 1988;16:350.
10. Vuillemin T, Raveh J. The subcranial approach for the correction of hypertelorism. *Journal of Craniofacial Surgery* 1990;1:91.
11. Raveh J. Specific procedures: craniofacial congenital anomalies—subcranial osteotomy approach. In: *Principles and practice of ophthalmic plastic and reconstructive surgery*. Philadelphia: WB Saunders, 1993;16D:8;3.
12. Raveh J, Imola M, Laedrach K, Zingg M, Vuillemin T. Update on corrections of craniofacial anomalies. *Facial Plastic Surgery Clinics of North America* 1995;3:17–38.
13. Raveh J, Laedrach K, Speiser M, et al. The subcranial approach for fronto-orbital and anteroposterior skull base tumors. *Arch Otolaryngol Head Neck Surg* 1993;119:382.
14. Raveh J, Vuillemin T. The subcranial–supraorbital temporal approach for tumor resection. *Journal of Craniofacial Surgery* 1990;1:53
15. Raveh J, Turk JB, Laedrach K, et al. Extended anterior approach for skull base tumors: long-term results. *J Neurosurg* 1995;82:1002.
16. Laedrach K, Raveh J. Advantages of the combined subcranial/transfrontal approach for frontal skull base tumor resection. In: *Acta volume of the IV International Congress of the International Society of Cranio-Maxillofacial Surgery*. Bologna: Mondozzu Editore, 1992;4:293.
17. Blackblock JB, Weber RS, Lee YY, et al. Transcranial resection of tumors of the paranasal sinuses and nasal cavity. *J Neurosurg* 1989; 71:10.
18. Derome P, Akerman M, Anquez L, et al. Les tumeurs spénoethmoidales: possibilités d'exérèse et de réparation chirurgicales. *Neurochirurgie* 1972;18[Suppl 1]:1.
19. Escher F. Ein Beitrag zur Versorgung frontobasaler Hirnverletzungen. *Pract Otorhinolaryngol* 1944;6:326.
20. Jackson IT, Marsh WR, Hide TAH. Treatment of tumors involving the anterior cranial fossa. *Head and Neck Surgery* 1984;6:901.
21. Lyons BM, Donald PJ. Radical surgery for nasal cavity and paranasal sinus tumors. *Otoiaryngol Clin North Am* 1991;24:1499.
22. Naumann HH. Chirurgie der Nasennebenhöhle. In: Naumann HH, ed. *Kopf und Halschirurgie*. Stuttgart: Thieme, 1974;2:409.
23. Schramm VL Jr, Myers EN, Maroon JC. Anterior skull base surgery for benign and malignant disease. *Laryngoscope* 1979;89:1077.
24. Sekhar LN, Janecka IP, Jones NF. Subtemporal–infratemporal and basal subfrontal approach to extensive cranial base tumours. *Acta Neurochir* 1988;92:83.
25. Irish JC, Gullane PJ, Gentili F, et al. Tumors of the skull base: outcome and survival analysis of 77 cases. *Head and Neck Surgery* 1994;16:3.
26. Delfini R, Ianetti G, Belli E, et al. Cranio-facial approaches for tumors involving the anterior half of the skull base. *Acta Neurochir* 1993;124:53.
27. Pinsolle J, San-Galli F, Siberchicot F, et al. Modified approach for ethmoid and anterior skull base surgery. *Arch Otolaryngol Head Neck Surg* 1991;117:779.
28. Rinehart GC, Jackson IT, Potparic Z, et al. Management of locally aggressive sinus disease using craniofacial exposure and the galeal frontalis fascia-muscle flap. *Plast Reconstr Surg* 1993;92:1219.
29. Sekhar LN, Nanda A, Sen CN, et al. The extended frontal approach to tumors of the anterior, middle, and posterior skull base. *J Neurosurg* 1992;76:198.
30. Alaywan M, Sindou M. Fronto-temporal approach with orbito-zygomatic removal: surgical anatomy. *Acta Neurochir* 1990;104:79.
31. Al-Mefty O. The supraorbital-pterional approach to skull base lesions. *Neurosurgery* 1987;21:474.
32. Hakuba A, Lui SS, Nishimura S. The orbitozygomatic infra-temporal approach: a new surgical technique. *Surg Neurol* 1986;26:271.
33. Jackson IT. Craniofacial osteotomies to facilitate resection of tumors of the skull base. In: Wilkins RH, Rengachary SS, eds *Neurosurgery update I*. New York: McGraw-Hill, 1990;277.
34. Johns ME, Kaplan MJ, Park TS, et al. Supraorbital rim approach to the anterior skull base. *Laryngoscope* 1984;94:1137.
35. Tessier P, Guiot G, Rougerie J. Ostéotomies cranio-naso-orbito-faciales: hypertélorisme. *Ann Chir Plast* 1967;12:103.
36. Vuillemin T, Raveh J, Ramon Y. Reconstruction of the maxilla with bone grafts supported by the buccal fat pad after tumour resection. *J Oral Maxillofac Surg* 1988;46:100.
37. Escher F. Clinical classification and treatment of the frontobasal fractures. In: *Disorders of the skull base region*. Stockholm: Almqvist & Wiksell, 1969:33.
38. Jane JA, Park TS, Pobereskin LH, et al. The supraorbital approach: technical note. *Neurosurgery* 1982;11:537.
39. Smith RR, Klopp CT, Williams JM. Surgical treatment of cancer of the frontal sinus and adjacent areas. *Cancer* 1954;7:991.
40. Ketcham AS, Hoye RC, Van Buren JM, et al. Complications of intracranial facial resection for tumors of the paranasal sinuses. *Am J Surg* 1966;112:591.
41. Van Buren JM, Ommaya AK, Ketcham AS. Ten years' experience with radical combined craniofacial resection of malignant tumors of the paranasal sinuses. *J Neurosurg* 1968;28:341.
42. Donald PJ. Craniofacial surgery for head and neck cancer. In: Johnson JT, Blitzer A, Ossoff RH, et al, eds. *American Academy of Otolaryngology–Head and Neck Surgery: instruction courses*. St. Louis: CV Mosby, 1989;2:225.

CHAPTER 14

Cranioorbital Approach

Alfred P. Bowles, Jr. and Vinod K. Anand

The cranial base is an anatomically complex region encompassing arteries and nerves that intertwine with an irregular bony topography. To improve exposure to lesions in the cranial base, a number of frontolateral approaches have been used based on techniques that incorporate the orbital roof. Several of the techniques used have been reintroduced, modified, and revised to provide surgeons with accessible avenues to lesions in the anterior and middle fossa. With the frontolateral approaches, as with other skull base approaches, the basic premise is that the bone is expendable, not the brain, and with this philosophy, bone flaps incorporating the orbital bone can be created for improved exposure, followed by unroofing of the sphenoid wing and optic canal, with skeletonization of the anterior clinoid as needed. The advantage in removing bone extensively and gaining access under the frontal and temporal lobes is the resultant shortening of the distance to the targeted lesion with minimization of brain retraction.

Different techniques have been described for the initial bone flap to provide anterior and lateral exposure, and these techniques include frontal or frontotemporal bone with the orbital roof, with or without a zygomatic osteotomy, and with the orbital roof removed as a separate bone flap or in continuity with the frontal or frontotemporal bone flap. The frontolateral exposures have been designated by several different names (i.e., cranial–orbital, orbitocranial, supraorbital, cranioorbital–zygomatic, and others); however, the purpose of all the flaps and the subtle differences between techniques is to provide increased exposure beneath the frontal and temporal lobes.

A. P. Bowles, Jr.: Department of Neurosurgery, University of Mississippi Medical Center, Jackson, Mississippi 39216.
V. K. Anand: Department of Surgery, Division of Otolaryngology, University of Mississippi Medical Center, Jackson, Mississippi 39216.

CRANIOORBITAL ZYGOMATIC APPROACH

The cranioorbital–zygomatic (COZ) approach was introduced and popularized at the authors' institution by Dr. Ossama Al-Mefty, and the authors continue to use the COZ approach and modifications derived exclusively for lesions involving the anterior and middle fossa. The COZ approach is a composite of at least four different approaches that can be tailored to meet the specific requirements of a given lesion. The approach is ideally suited for lesions in the sellar, suprasellar, parasellar, and retrosellar regions, and for lesions extending into the cavernous sinus. Access to the floor of the middle fossa is also provided and, with extradural dissection, the petrous canal and petrous apex can be identified. The posterior aspect of the cavernous sinus is accessible, and intradural exposure of the petrous bone is available as far back as the internal acoustic meatus. Intradurally, the third and fourth cranial nerves can be exposed extending from the cerebral peduncle and entering into the cavernous sinus; drilling through the petrous tip medial to the carotid artery and anterior to the internal auditory meatus (Kawase's triangle) can provide access to the upper pons (1).

The COZ approach, which represents a modification of the supraorbital approach revised by Jane et al. (2), has been outlined and detailed in several other reports (3–10). Specific details of the techniques used at the authors' institution follow.

Patient Position

The patient is placed supine with the head at the foot end of the table and with the table rotated 180 degrees away from the anesthesiologist: rotating the operating field away from the anesthetic equipment increases the degree of operative maneuverability. With the head at the foot end of the table, the surgeon has more comfortable leg and knee space while seated at the microscope. A lumbar drain is placed that is connected to a drainage collection bag. The authors usually drain off 10 to 15 ml of cerebrospinal fluid (CSF) just before dissection of the dura away from the inner table of the bone

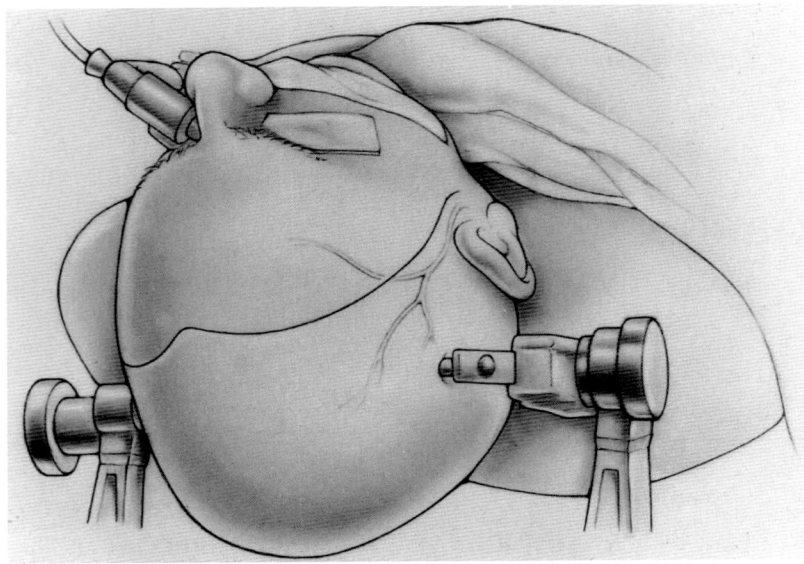

FIG. 1. Illustration of the bicoronal skin incision with the ipsilateral incision placed in front of the trunk of the superficial temporal artery at the level of the zygoma. The bicoronal skin incision, which starts at the level of the zygoma and is carried contralaterally behind the hairline to the supratemporal line, preserves the trunk and posterior branch of the superficial temporal artery. The incision that starts at the level of the zygoma ipsilaterally is placed so that the frontal branches of the facial nerve are also preserved.

flap. An additional 15 to 20 ml of CSF may be drained after the dura is opened for greater brain relaxation. With the lumbar drain in place, furosemide (Lasix) or mannitol usually is not given. However, the P_{CO_2} is maintained from 27 to 28 mm Hg. The skin over the abdomen and leg ipsilaterally is prepared and draped for a potential harvest of free fat graft, fascia lata, saphenous vein, sural nerve, or free rectus abdominis, which may be needed for subsequent reconstruction. The table is adjusted so that the patient's trunk and head are elevated 20 degrees. Once immobilized with three-point pin fixation, the head is carefully hyperextended 5 to 10 degrees and rotated anywhere from 10 to 60 degrees contralaterally, depending on the targeted lesion. The head may only need to be rotated 0 to 10 degrees for access to the floor of the anterior fossa. The head should be rotated 20 to 30 degrees to maximize access to the optic chiasm and sellar regions. The head may be rotated even further for exposure to the cavernous sinus. With the head and neck extended and rotated, the supraorbital margin and pterional region are placed at the highest point, and after opening the dura and wide sylvian fissure dissection, the frontal and temporal poles open up under the weight of gravity, exposing the sylvian cistern.

Skin Incision and Pericranial Flap

After the head and neck have been prepared and draped, a bicoronal skin incision is made, beginning 1 cm anterior to the tragus at the level of the zygomatic arch ipsilaterally, with the incision carried behind the hairline to just below the superior temporal line contralaterally (Fig. 1). The position of the ipsilateral incision is such that only the anterior branch of the superficial temporal artery is cut, with preservation of the trunk and posterior branches, which would be located behind the incision. The superficial temporal vessels are preserved in the event that an extracranial–intracranial microvascular bypass is necessary. With the incision placed 1 cm anterior to the tragus, the trunk of the superficial temporal artery lies posterior to the incision, and the superior branches of the facial nerve are anterior to the incision. The incision is carried through the skin and galea but not the pericranium. The areolar tissue is dissected away from the galea remaining adherent to the pericranium for a thicker pericranial graft. The skin flap is reflected anteriorly along with the frontal branch of the facial nerve, which has been dissected subfascially (Fig. 2). Both superficial and deep layers of the temporalis fascia are incised approximately 1.5 cm distal and parallel to the zygomatic arch and lateral rim over the orbit. The frontal branch lies within the fat pad between the superficial and deep fascial layers. Both superficial and deep layers of the temporalis fascia are incised above the zygomatic arch and posterior to the lateral orbital rim. The frontal branch lies within the fat pad between the superficial and deep fascial layers. While transitioning from the superficial to the deep layers of the temporalis fascia, the frontal branch is at considerable risk anteriorly. Therefore, this zone transitioning occurs posterior to the midpoint between lateral orbital rim and preauricular crease, and all the superficial tissue is reflected anteriorly. Incisions are then made through the pericranium, with the pericranium dissected free from the occipital bone and reflected anteriorly over the scalp flap and preserved for later reconstruction (Fig. 3A). The intact base of the pericranial flap is dissected free from the roof and lateral orbit, and the deep fascial layer with the frontal branch of the facial nerve superior to this layer is dissected subperiosteally across the frontal and malar process and body of the zygoma (see Fig. 2). With a high-speed drill (C_1 attachment, Midas Rex), a cuff of bone is drilled around the supraorbital foramen, freeing the supraorbital nerve, which is reflected anteriorly (see Fig. 3B). The temporalis muscle fasciae are dissected away from the superior surface of the body of the zygoma, leaving the masseter attached to the inferior surface of the zygoma. Oblique osteotomies are then

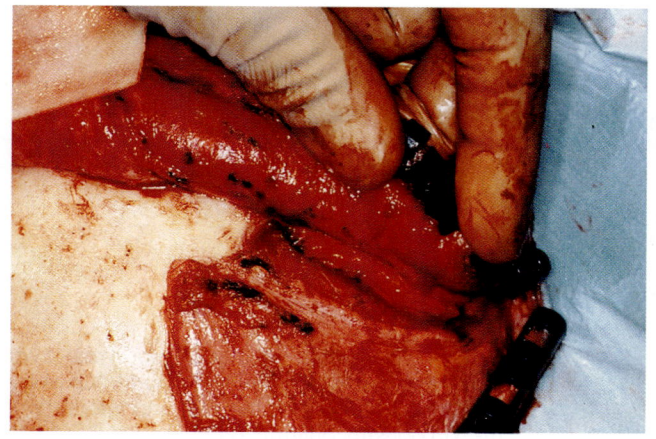
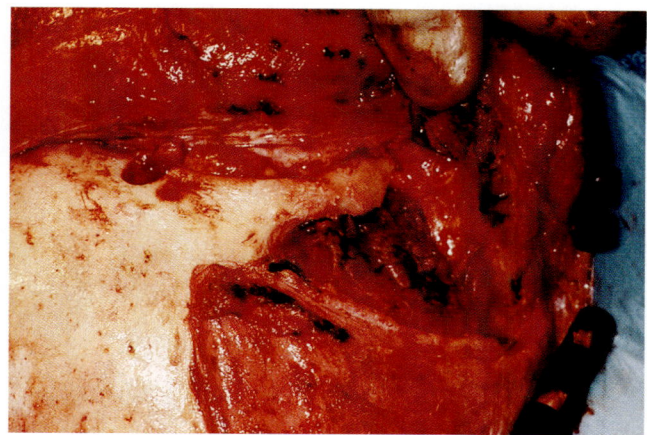
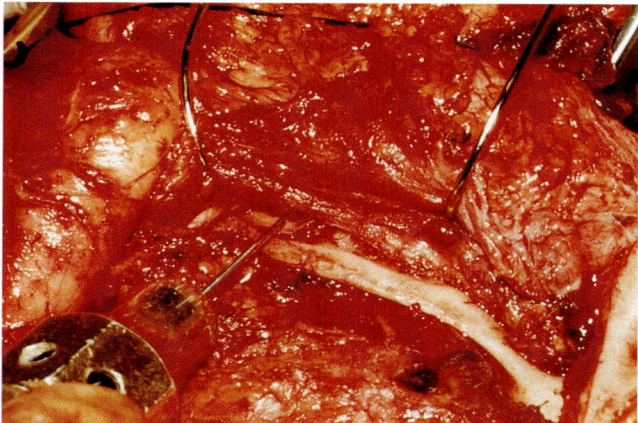

FIG. 2. Intraoperative photomicrographs of the subfascial dissection along the lateral rim of the orbit and body of the zygoma. In **(A)**, an incision through both the superficial and deep fasciae of the temporalis muscle is cut parallel to the lateral rim of the orbit and zygomatic arch and dissected subperiosteally across the lateral rim of the orbit **(B)** and the body of the zygoma **(C)**. The upper branches of the facial nerve continue in the superficial and deep fasciae of the temporalis muscle within the fat pad between the two fascial layers; when these layers are dissected anteriorly and subperiosteally across the bone, the upper frontal branches are preserved. With the body of the zygoma exposed **(C)**, oblique osteotomies can be placed because the upper zygoma can be retracted inferiorly.

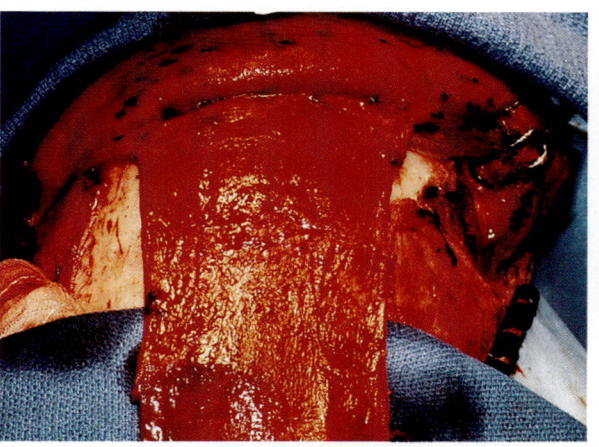
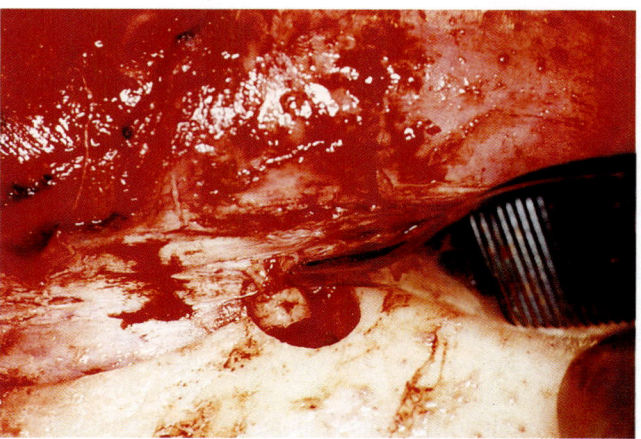

FIG. 3. A: Intraoperative photograph of the pedicle of pericranium that has been dissected subperiosteally away from the skull along each superior temporal line. **B:** To protect the supraorbital nerve, a cuff of bone is drilled around the supraorbital foramen, which is reflected anteriorly with the pericranial graft.

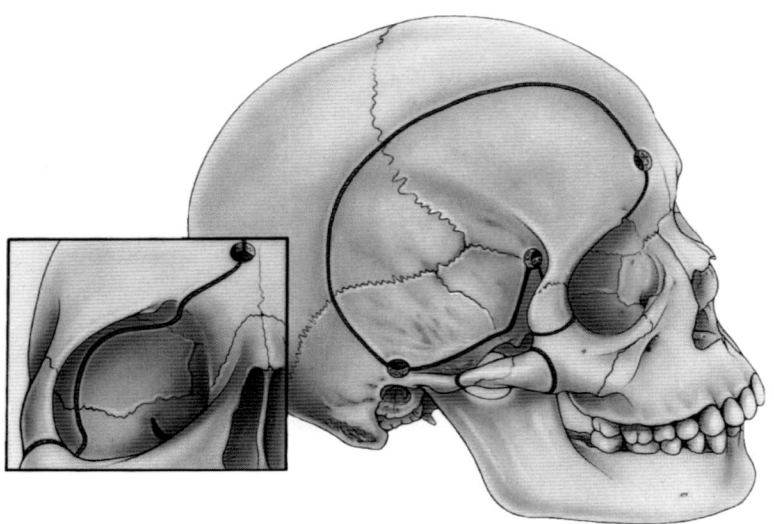

FIG. 4. Illustration of the cranioorbital–zygomatic approach. The frontotemporal flap is outlined in continuity with the roof and lateral rim of the orbit, with oblique osteotomies along the body of the zygoma. Osteotomy through the roof of the orbit is demonstrated (*inset*). (Reproduced from ref. 9, with permission.)

placed at either end of the zygoma (see Fig. 2C), and with retraction of the zygoma, improved basal exposure of the middle fossa is provided. The temporalis muscle is then dissected from the calvarium, exposing the junction of the zygomatic, sphenoid, and frontal bone.

Bone Flap

A supraorbital–pterional bone flap is generated that consists of frontotemporal bone in continuity with the anterior, superior, and lateral rims of the orbit (Fig. 4). Four bur holes are made, with the first placed in the location of MacCarty's keyhole. The first bur hole is made in the temporal fossa, medial to the frontozygomatic suture (keyhole), and should expose the dura of the frontal fossa, and the anterior orbital area with the periorbita separated from the dura by the root of the orbit. The second bur hole is placed in the inferoposterior portion of the squamous temporal bone just above the roof of the zygoma. The third bur hole is then placed superior to the second bur hole along the superior temporal line. The last bur hole is made in the midline just above the nasion with perforation of the anterior and posterior walls of the frontal sinus. For cosmetic reasons, the authors usually attempt to make this hole as small as possible with a small drill bit. The second, third, and fourth bur holes are connected with a craniotome using the footplate, and then an osteotomy is made with a high-speed drill extending along the base of the temporal fossa to the sphenoid ridge, connecting bur holes one and two.

With a high-speed drill, an osteotomy is made through the lateral wall of the orbit just superior to the malar prominence and extended to the keyhole at the level of the inferior orbital fissure. An osteotomy is then extended from the fourth bur hole above the nasion through both walls of the frontal sinus, extending inferiorly and medially to the orbital roof. The oblique osteotomy from the fourth bur hole to the orbit is directed to the supraorbital foramen, lateral to the trochlear groove on the undersurface of the orbit. Finally, the anterior roof of the orbit is cut across with an osteotome, starting from the lateral margin of the roof at the keyhole and cutting transversely across the roof to the medial border of the orbit. The supraorbital temporal bone flap is then removed.

With removal of the frontal bone, the frontal sinus is exposed. The mucosa of the sinus is exenterated with a cutting bur and the posterior wall removed (cranialization) and then plugged with muscle, fat, or antibiotic-soaked Gelfoam. All instruments exposed to the frontal sinus are removed and resterilized, and surgical attire replaced. The remainder of the orbital roof is then removed as a posterior orbitotomy with a high-speed drill (Fig. 5). A medial cut is made in the

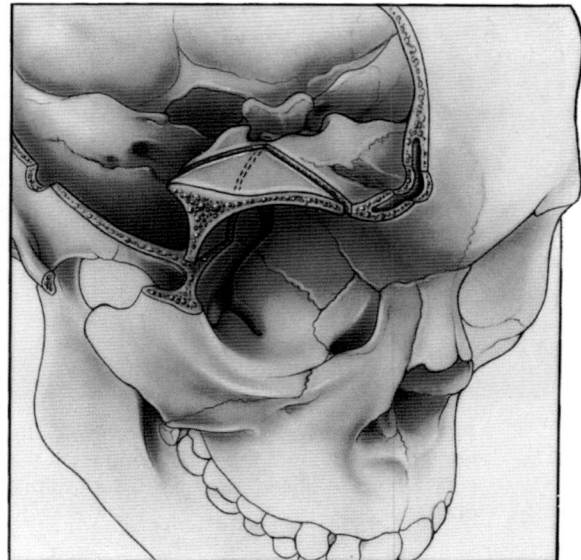

FIG. 5. After removal of the supraorbitopterional bone flap, the remaining portion of the roof and lateral orbital wall is removed as a posterior orbitotomy and reattached to the cranial flap at the end of the procedure. (Reproduced from ref. 9, with permission.)

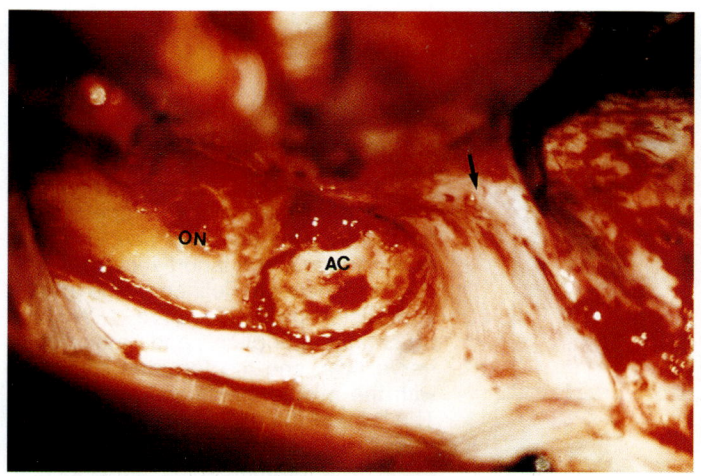 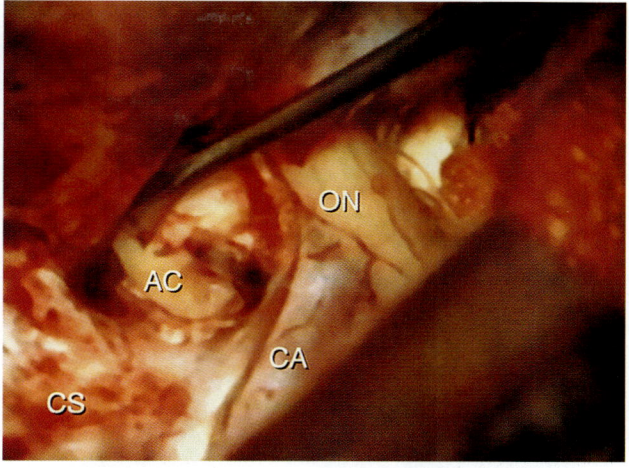

FIG. 6. Intraoperative photograph (A) of the superior orbital fissure (arrow), which has been unroofed. The optic canal has been unroofed as well, exposing the optic nerve (ON), and the anterior clinoid (AC) has been drilled down to its base. Another operative photograph (B) shows the intradural removal of the remaining base of the anterior clinoid in relation to anatomic landmarks—the optic nerve (ON), the carotid artery (CA), and the cavernous sinus.

roof of the orbit and extended posteriorly. The second cut is made at the base of the lateral orbital wall along the inferior orbital fissure. The cuts are then connected across the sphenoid ridge above the superior orbital fissure. A posterior orbitotomy is then reattached to the bone flap (see also Fig. 13B) for orbital reconstruction.

Drilling of the Sphenoid Bone

To provide greater access to the cavernous sinus optic canals and interpeduncular cisterns, the authors usually completely remove the sphenoid ridge, which is drilled away with a high-speed air drill under the microscope (Fig. 6A). Drilling is continued with unroofing of the superior orbital fissure and skeletonization of the anterior clinoid. The anterior clinoid may be removed extradurally or intradurally, or both, with exposure of the subclinoid segment of the carotid artery below (see Fig. 6B). After the superior orbital fissure is opened, the optic canal can also be unroofed extradurally, with exposure of the optic nerve. To unroof the optic canal safely, the authors usually use a small diamond drill bit with continuous irrigation.

Exposure of the Intrapetrous Carotid Artery

When operating on lesions involving the cavernous sinus, proximal control of the internal carotid artery (ICA) can be achieved with exposure of the intrapetrous ICA. Exposure of the ICA within the intrapetrous canal may also provide the site for potential venous bypass grafting of the cavernous ICA. With the bone flap removed and the body of the zygoma retracted inferiorly, the anterior roof of the middle fossa can be visualized after the dura is dissected away from the bone. Within Glasscock's triangle, the petrous can be carefully drilled, exposing the ICA below (Fig. 7).

With microscopic magnification, the dura is elevated from the floor of the temporal fossa in a mediobasal direction. The middle meningeal artery should be identified and followed back to the foramen spinosum. The artery is coagulated and cut, and the foramen packed with bone wax. The temporal dura is then elevated further medially, with dissection limited anteriorly by the trigeminal ganglion and cranial nerve V3. The foramen ovale is then identified with cranial nerve V3 exiting through it. Just medial and posterior to the foramen spinosum, the greater and lesser superficial petrosal nerves should be identified exiting from the facial hiatus (Fig. 8), and these nerves are sharply cut to avoid traction on the greater superficial petrosal nerve to the geniculate ganglion, which could result in facial paralysis (see Fig. 8B). The dura is then elevated posteriorly and medially to expose the arcuate eminence of the petrous bone, and with the greater superficial petrosal nerve, the posterior aspect of the trigeminal ganglion and mandibular nerve, a line drawn between the foramen spinosum and arcuate eminence forms the border of the posterolateral (or Glasscock's) triangle (11). In this triangle and just medial and parallel to the greater superficial petrosal nerve, the bone of the petrous canal is unroofed with a diamond drill bit under constant irrigation. The horizontal portion of the petrous ICA is then exposed (see Fig. 6A). In a significant number of cases, the bone is absent, and the periosteum covering the ICA is exposed when the dura is elevated. Once the petrous canal is unroofed, a 60-cm, 2-Fr Fogarty arterial embolectomy catheter (Baxter Health Care Corporation, McGraw Park, IL) can be inserted (11). In general, 1.0 to 1.5 cm of bone is unroofed to expose the ICA properly. The catheter is inserted extraarterially between the outer wall of the vessel and the wall of the carotid

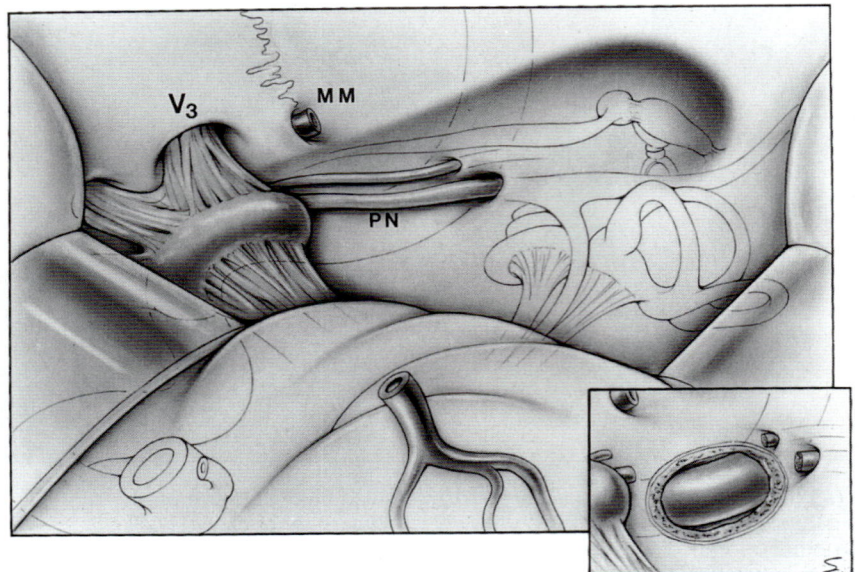

FIG. 7. Illustration of the intrapetrous internal carotid artery exposed in Glasscock's triangle; the landmarks for Glasscock's triangle are defined by the greater superficial petrosal nerve (*PN*), the trigeminal ganglion and mandibular nerve (*V₃*), and the foramen spinosum with the middle meningeal artery (*MM*). The dura of the middle fossa is elevated from the floor, exposing Glasscock's triangle. The foramen spinosum is located and the middle meningeal artery cut and coagulated. The petrosal nerves are sharply incised and then the carotid artery unroofed (*inset*).

canal, 5 to 10 mm proximal to the carotid canal (Fig. 9A). The distal end of the catheter is connected to a three-way stopcock and attached to a syringe with saline. The balloon can be inflated with 0.2 ml of saline and the stopcock closed to provide temporary occlusion of the ICA (see Fig. 9B).

Intradural Dissection

Before opening the dura, an additional 10 to 20 ml of CSF is drained through the lumbar catheter for further brain relaxation as needed. A curvilinear incision is then made extending from the basal frontal region across the sylvian fissure to the basal temporal region. A large piece of Surgicel is placed over the periorbita and then the dura is reflected anteriorly over the periorbita and tacked into place, with further retraction of the orbital contents. Using sharp dissection, the sylvian fissure is opened, and the frontal and temporal poles separated. The authors usually place a self-retaining retractor lightly on the temporal lobe and begin dissection on the frontal side of the sylvian vein. The dissection is then directed in a deeper orientation, allowing identification of a cortical arterial branch, which is then followed down to the middle cerebral artery. With the middle cerebral artery identified, dissection is continued anteriorly along the middle cerebral artery with the sylvian cistern opened from a deep to superficial orientation, and with dissection progressing anteriorly.

With the superior and lateral rims of the orbit removed, the sphenoid wing and superior orbital fissure unroofed, the transsylvian dissection can be extended far superiorly. With the head and neck in 10 to 15 degrees of extension and with the bony removal and wide superior sylvian fissure dissec-

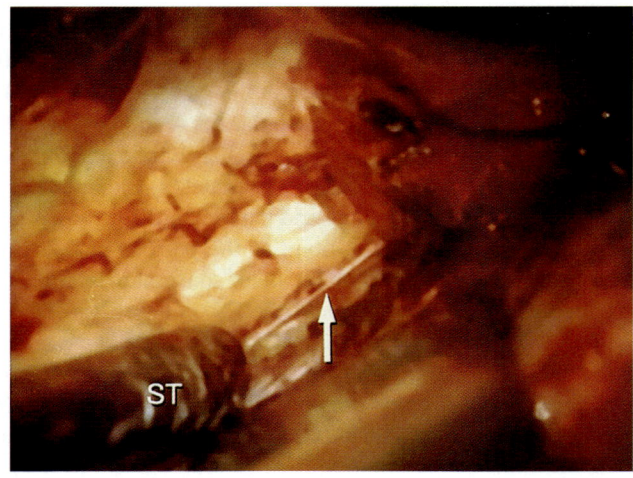
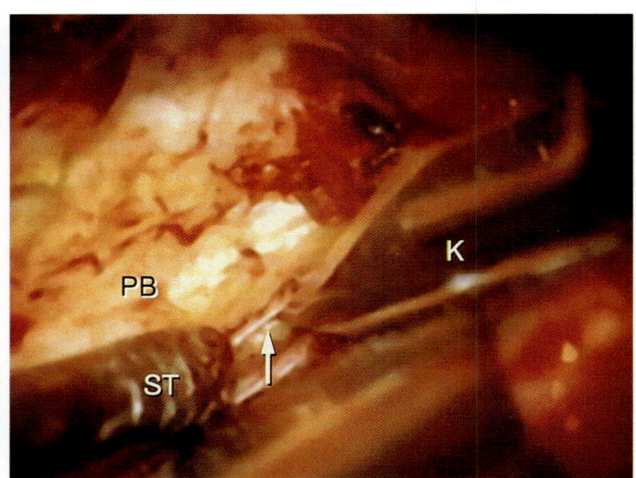

FIG. 8. Intraoperative photograph of the greater superficial petrosal nerve (*arrow*) **(A)**, and with a subsequent incision by knife (*K*) **(B)**. At the base of the greater superficial petrosal nerve is the suction tip (*ST*) with the nerve along the petrosal base (*PB*).

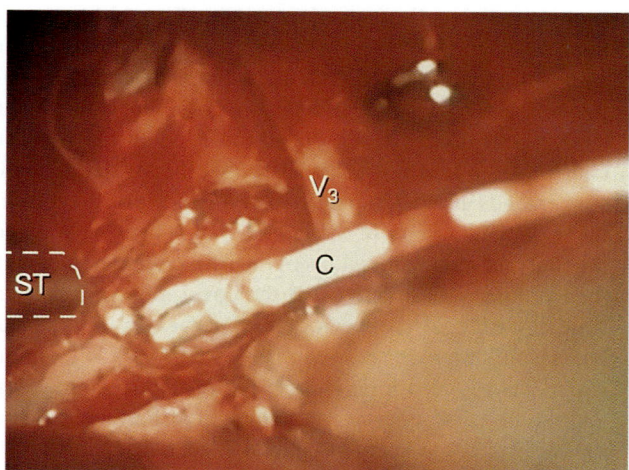 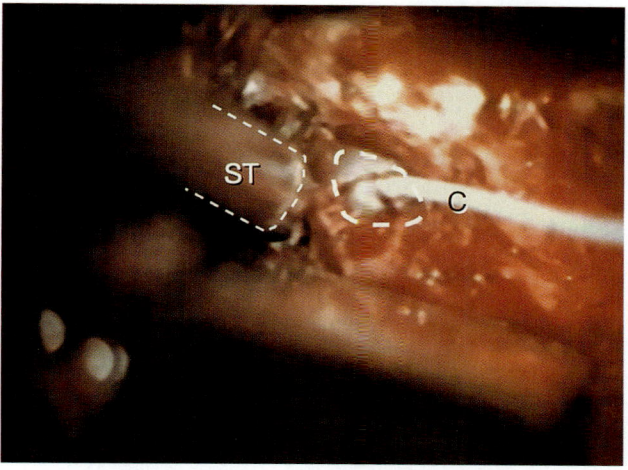

FIG. 9. A: After the landmarks for Glasscock's triangle have been visualized and the petrous canal identified, the bone over the carotid artery is unroofed and a Fogarty embolectomy catheter (*C*) is placed extraarterially within the canal. In Glasscock's triangle, the mandibular nerve (V_3) is seen in relation to the catheter. **B:** Enhanced operative photograph shows expansion of the extraarterial catheter balloon within the canal. The suction tip (*ST*) is also shown at the base.

tion, the frontal and temporal poles readily separate under the influence of gravity. The frontal lobe may be gently supported with a self-retaining retractor; however, the elevation requirements are minimal, with an added distance of 1.5 cm or less required for exposure. Multidirectional viewing (Fig. 10) is then provided with surgical dissection possible by multiple routes, including subfrontal, subtemporal, and transsylvian avenues, in front of the chiasm, behind the chiasm, and into the lamina terminales.

Entering the Cavernous Sinus

The COZ approach is well suited for lesions, especially tumors, involving the cavernous sinus, providing superior and lateral entry into the cavernous sinus. In cavernous sinus surgery, proximal distal control of the carotid artery is crucial for "safe surgery"; control of the carotid artery is achieved by exposing the horizontal segment of the petrous ICA through Glasscock's triangle, and the subclinoid segment of the ICA. After the posterior roof of the orbit is removed, a thin rim of bone remains over the optic canal and superior orbital fissure. A diamond drill bit is used to unroof completely the optic canal and superior orbital fissure extradurally, and then the anterior clinoid is drilled away to expose the subclinoid segment of the ICA. The anterior clinoid is initially skeletonized to allow the diamond drill extradurally to core out the middle and leave a thin shell. Drilling is continued on the inferior strut of the lesser wing beneath the

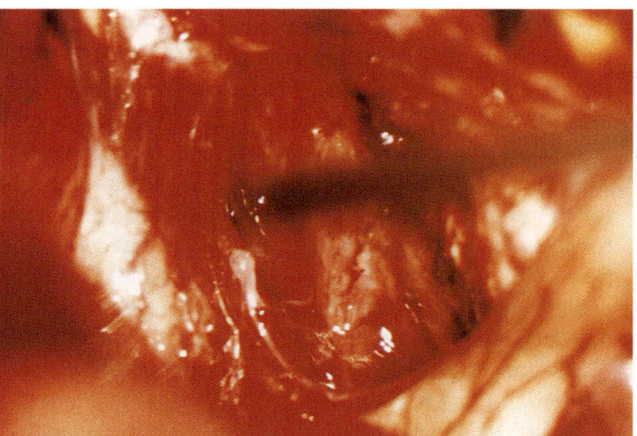 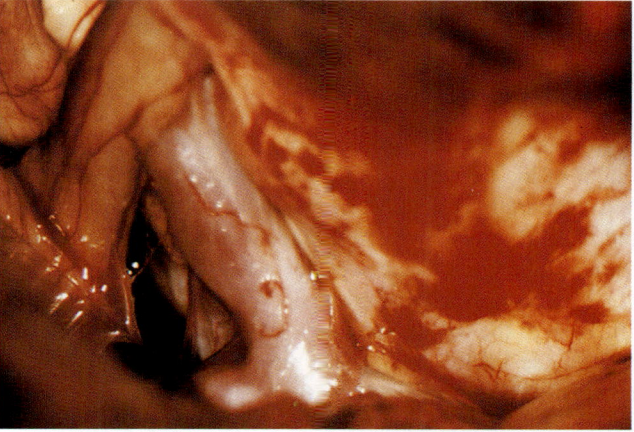

FIG. 10. Intraoperative photographs showing the multidirectional views that may be provided from the cranioorbital–zygomatic approach, with exposure of the optic nerves, chiasm, and infundibulum (**A**), and carotid artery and cavernous sinus (**B**).

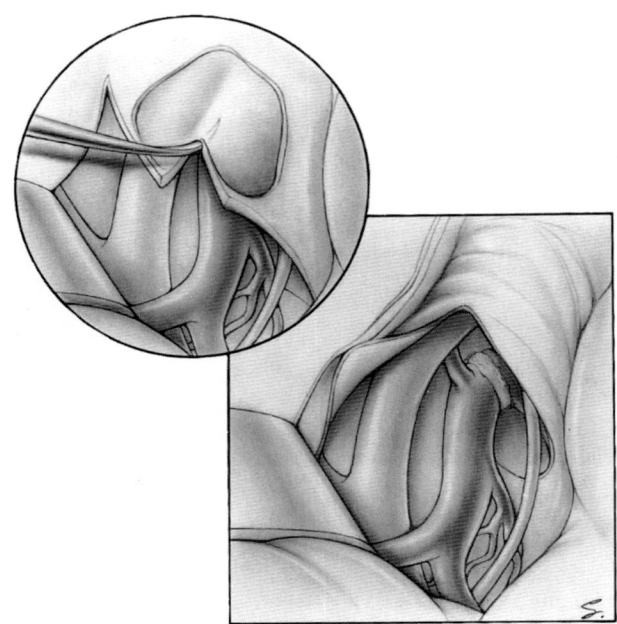

FIG. 11. After the anterior clinoid has been completely removed, the subclinoid segment of the carotid artery is exposed. With incision of the falciform fold (*inset*), the optic nerve can be mobilized medially, further exposing the ophthalmic artery and carotid artery as it enters the cavernous sinus. The carotid artery can then be followed in the cavernous sinus through the superior route in a retrograde fashion.

optic nerve and disconnects the anterior clinoid, which then can be removed by subperiosteal dissection.

Marked by proximal and distal rings, the subclinoid section of the ICA is exposed extradurally. The anterior clinoid can be removed extradurally or intradurally. For surgery involving tumors, the authors usually remove the entire anterior clinoid extradurally; for aneurysms that extend underneath the clinoid, two thirds of the anterior clinoid is removed extradurally and the remainder is drilled away intradurally.

Entry into the cavernous sinus depends on the lesion and its origin; however, in most cases, the authors enter the cavernous sinus through a superior or lateral entry, or both. With the subclinoid segment of the ICA exposed and the optic canal unroofed, the dural sheath of the optic nerve is then incised, starting at the falciform fold and extending along the length of the nerve (Fig. 11). The distal ring anchoring the ICA subdurally is untethered and, with both the optic nerve and carotid artery mobilized, excellent entry into the cavernous sinus through the superior wall is provided (see Fig. 11). Medial mobilization of the optic nerve also allows identification of the origin and course of the ophthalmic artery.

With the lateral entry, after the optic nerve and carotid artery have been mobilized by incising the dura propria, the lateral wall of the oculomotor foramen of the third cranial nerve is unroofed with a sickle knife, and the outer layer of the lateral wall of the cavernous sinus is pulled away laterally from the first and second divisions of the fifth cranial nerve, exposing Parkinson's triangle (Fig. 12A). Alternatively, with the free edge of the tentorium visualized and the course of the third and fourth cranial nerves identified entering the cavernous sinus, an incision can be made through the lateral wall of the cavernous sinus beneath the projected course of the fourth cranial nerve (see Fig. 12B). The incision extends about 7 mm anteriorly and posteriorly and, similarly, the outer layer of the lateral wall is peeled away from the first and second divisions of the fifth cranial nerve, which then provides good access to the cavernous sinus through Mullan's triangle (between cranial nerves V1 and V2) and Parkinson's triangle (between nerves IV and V1). A natural gap exists between the first division of the trigeminal nerve and the fourth cranial nerve, and deep in Parkinson's triangle, the cavernous segment of the ICA can be identified with the sixth cranial nerve on the lateral wall of the ICA. The gap is usually enlarged to expose the ICA and the sixth cranial nerve; however, sometimes the ICA is located between Mullan's triangle or the gap between the first and second divisions of the trigeminal nerve.

The lateral exposure can also be increased by further peeling back the outer layer of the lateral wall. Drilling of the posterior clinoid provides an avenue to the cavernous sinus lateral to the carotid artery and third cranial nerve, and drilling of the petrous tip anterior to the internal auditory canal (Kawase's triangle) exposes the posterior aspect of the cavernous sinus and the posterior fossa.

Reconstruction and Closure

If the frontal ethmoid or sphenoid sinuses are opened during the approach or removed because of involvement with disease, communication between the paranasal sinuses and intradural space is prevented with the reconstruction using a free fat graft and fascia lata. Sinus mucosa is exenterated and packed with fat and fibrin glue. A fascial graft is then laid intradurally and secured with sutures to the basal dura, and the graft is spread to cover the frontal and temporal fossa and sutured to the frontal and temporal dura. The preserved pericranial flap in the frontal region is then turned over the frontal sinus, periorbita, and extended over any defect in the floor of the anterior fossa. The authors have also reconstructed large defects in the anterior fossa with a split-thickness bone graft sandwiched between the pericranium and galea that was dissected away from skin. Defects in the floor of the middle fossa to the infratemporal and sphenopalatine fossae are reconstructed by enveloping the defects along the floor with a pedicle of the temporalis muscle. Similarly, a pedicle graft of temporalis muscle may be sutured to close a defect through Kawase's triangle.

Several calvarial and central dural tack-ups are placed after the dura has been closed in a watertight fashion. Basal temporal dural tack-ups are also secured to the undersurface of the temporalis muscle. The bone flap with posterior orbitotomy attached is reattached to the cranial vault with plates and screws, and the temporalis muscle (if not used for re-

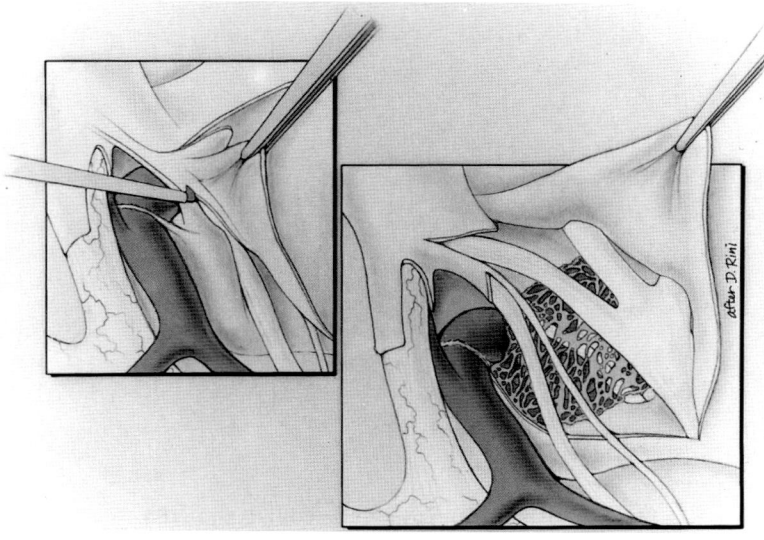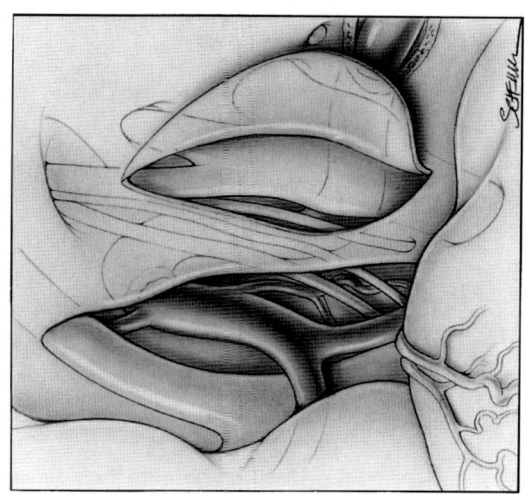

FIG. 12. The cavernous sinus can be entered laterally through Parkinson's triangle by mobilizing the dura and unroofing the third cranial nerve, with the outer layer of the lateral wall of the cavernous sinus peeled laterally to provide full exposure of cranial nerves III and IV and the first and second divisions of cranial nerve V (A). Alternatively, an incision can be made through the lateral wall of the cavernous sinus beneath the projected course of cranial nerve IV, with the dura peeled away over Parkinson's triangle between cranial nerves III and IV superiorly and the first division of the trigeminal nerve inferiorly (B).

construction of the floor of the middle fossa) is returned to its anatomic position and secured at the bone along the superior temporal line. The zygomatic arch is then repositioned and secured with miniplates and screws, and galea and skin are closed.

CRANIOORBITAL APPROACHES FOR TUMORS

The craniooorbital approaches have been successfully used for several different tumors involving anterior and middle cranial fossae. Most tumors in this location are benign (i.e., meningiomas, neurilemomas) or malignant but locally confined (i.e., chordomas, esthesioneuroblastomas); however, carcinomas and metastatic lesions are also encountered. Frontolateral approaches incorporate the orbital roof and provide greater access to tumors underneath the frontal and temporal lobes. With modifications of the craniooorbital bone flap (i.e., changing the position and size of the flap), incorporation of the posterior orbitotomy or zygomatic osteotomy, and variations in the degree of sphenoid unroofing, the craniooorbital approaches can be specifically tailored to optimize the exposure of a given tumor.

The technical aspects of the COZ approach incorporate most of the techniques required for all craniooorbital approaches and, by including all or part of the steps required with or without modifications, the COZ approach can define a tailored approach specific for a tumor and can be dictated by location and disease. Several of the modifications derived from the COZ theme are grouped accordingly for tumor type and location, and are described in the following sections.

Supraorbital Approach

The supraorbital approach is well suited for small to moderately sized tumors involving the sellar and suprasellar regions and the lamina terminales. Typical tumors encountered that could be suitably exposed include tuberculum sellae meningiomas, craniopharyngiomas, and pituitary and hypothalamic tumors. Exposure is also provided for large orbital neoplasms, tumors of the orbital apex, and optic canal lesions.

With the supraorbital approach (Fig. 13), the authors typically create two separate bone flaps:

1. A craniooorbital flap that includes the superior and lateral orbital rim
2. A smaller, more posterior flap that includes the remainder of the roof and lateral wall of the orbit (posterior orbitotomy)

The technical aspects of the supraorbital approach used at the authors' institution are similar to the techniques described for the COZ, except that the bone flap is smaller and fewer steps are required.

For tumors involving the sellar and suprasellar regions and the planum sphenoidale, the patient is placed supine, brow up, with the head extended to allow the frontal lobes to fall backward. The incision, harvest of the pericranial pedicle flap, and subfascial dissection are as described for the COZ. However, only the lateral rim of the orbit is exposed to the level of the malar process of the zygoma, and the craniooorbital bone developed is smaller, omitting the incorpora-

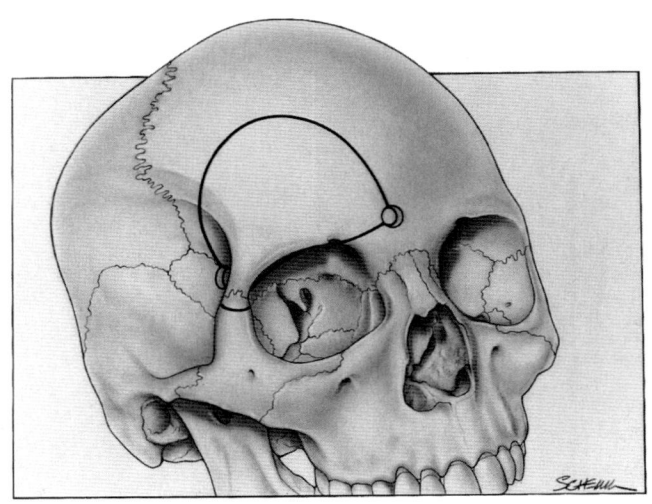 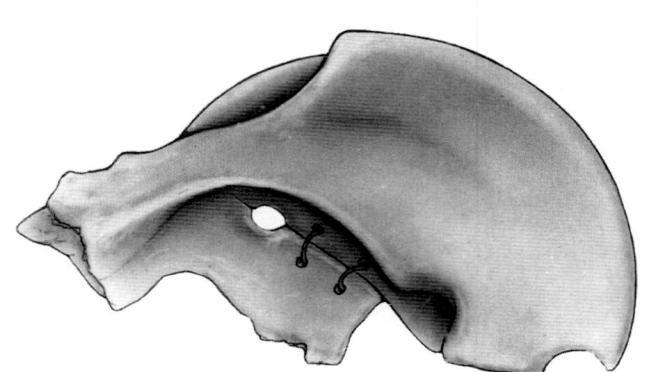

FIG. 13. Illustration of the supraorbital bone flap (A), and with posterior orbitotomy reattached (B).

tion of temporal bone. Two bur holes are made: the first is made at the site of MacCarty's keyhole, and the second is made in the frontal bone above the nasion. With the craniotome, the cranial holes are interconnected through the frontal bone about 4 cm above the supraorbital rim with osteotomies made through the anterosuperior aspect of the roof and lateral rim of the orbits. Entry into the frontal sinus is managed as described previously. The osteotomy through the outer rim of the orbit is made at the base, just above the malar process of the zygoma (see description of COZ approach). The posterior orbitotomy, described in the COZ approach, facilitates an even lower basal approach. The superior orbital fissure can be unroofed and the anterior clinoid skeletonized and removed, if needed. Because of midline exposure, both optic nerves are easily seen, and the optic canals can be unroofed extradurally with optic nerve decompression.

In the original description of the supraorbital approach by Jane et al. (2), only a single bone flap comprising the superior and lateral orbital rim is removed. Additional removal of the posterior of the orbit, as discussed previously, has been termed the "superolateral cranioorbital approach" by Al-Mefty and colleagues (8,12). The cranioorbital flap, which includes the superior and lateral orbital rims, provides low basal exposure with minimal frontal lobe retraction. With removal of the posterior aspect of the orbital roof, basal exposure is increased, especially to the planum sphenoidale, tuberculum sellae, and optic canal. Removal of the orbital roof is required for exposure to the orbit with the supraorbital approach, anatomic landmarks are better oriented with the brow up (i.e., visualization of the optic chiasm and lamina terminales), and whether the entire roof of the orbit should be removed is determined based on the tumor at hand.

As an example, the authors have used the supraorbital approach with posterior orbitotomy for a patient with a tuberculum sellae meningioma (Fig. 14). The patient presented with headaches and declining vision. Low basal exposure was achieved so that the tumor could be easily devascularized at the base across the ethmoid plate, planum sphenoidale, and tuberculum sellae, and then removed. Both optic canals were carefully unroofed with a diamond drill bit under constant irrigation. The tumor was completely removed without leaving any residual lesion (see Fig. 14C).

Bifrontal Cranioorbital Approach

For large and giant tumors involving the anterior fossa, the supraorbital approach can be incorporated into a bifrontal flap with or without a unilateral posterior orbitotomy. Tumors extending across the floor of the anterior fossa, such as olfactory groove meningiomas, are more easily exposed by bifrontal flap. Malignant tumors that extend into the anterior fossa from the face or into the orbit can also be exposed with a bifrontal flap with craniofacial resection.

With the bifrontal cranioorbital approach, the supraorbital bone is incorporated as a bifrontal flap (Fig. 15). Five bur holes are made, the first at the location of MacCarty's keyhole, and the second through the frontal bone just above the orbital ridge. Bur holes are made through bone adjacent to the location of the superior sagittal sinus from 5 to 8 cm above the nasion. The last bur hole is placed just above the nasion. The authors use a Midas Rex drill with an M_3 attachment for the bur holes; however, for cosmetic reasons, smaller holes are made into the frontal sinus just above the nasion and in the frontal bone just above the orbital ridge. An osteotomy is made across the lateral rim of the orbit and extending into the keyhole. Although the bur holes are interconnected with a craniotome, the authors usually drill directly over the sinus, connecting adjacent bur holes with a B_1 attachment of the Midas Rex drill without the foot plate. As described previously, an osteotomy is made across the ante-

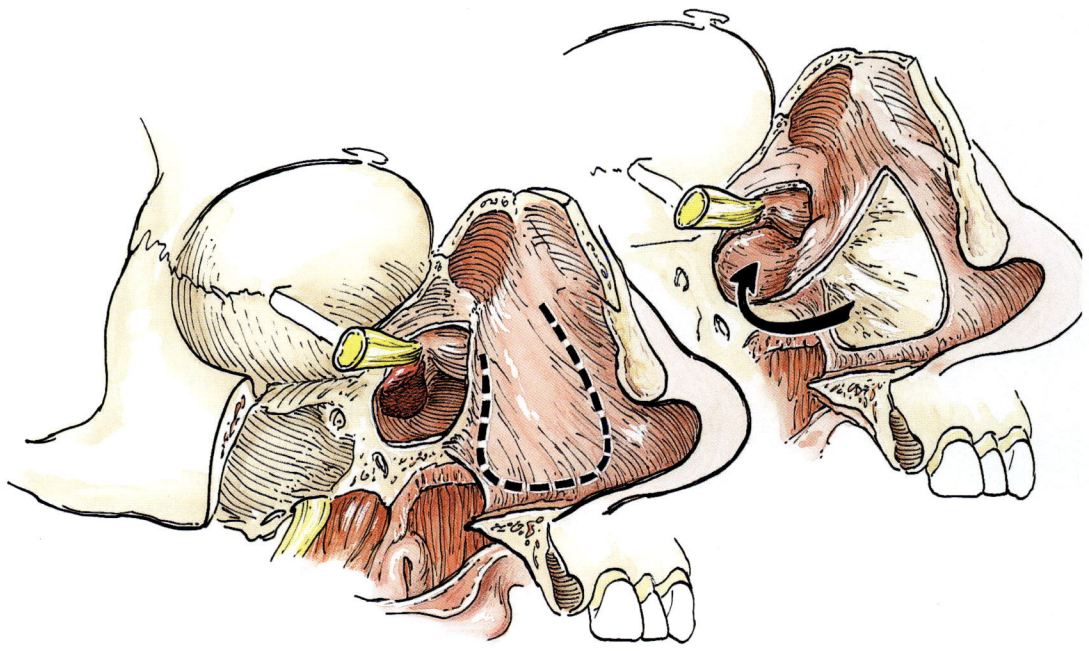

FIG. 32. Septal flap pedicled posterosuperiorly and rotated into nasopharyngeal defect.

Dural closure is performed in the fashion previously outlined. The orbit and denuded cheek area are skin grafted. Exposed dura, especially when grafted, and carotid must be covered by viable tissue. The sphenoid sinus is packed with a free abdominal fat graft and the anterior opening plugged with a bone or cartilage graft from the nasal septum or maxillary bone uninvolved by tumor and removed previously for exposure. A septal flap of mucoperiosteum pedicled on the vomer, or even preserved rostral sphenoid mucosa, the nasopharyngeal vault, or the nasal side of the soft palate can be rotated 180 degrees into the defect (Fig. 32).

A preformed palatal obturator is fixed to the remaining teeth or residual palate.

Type III

The most extensive type of subcranial approach includes resection of both the maxilla and the mandible. The exposure

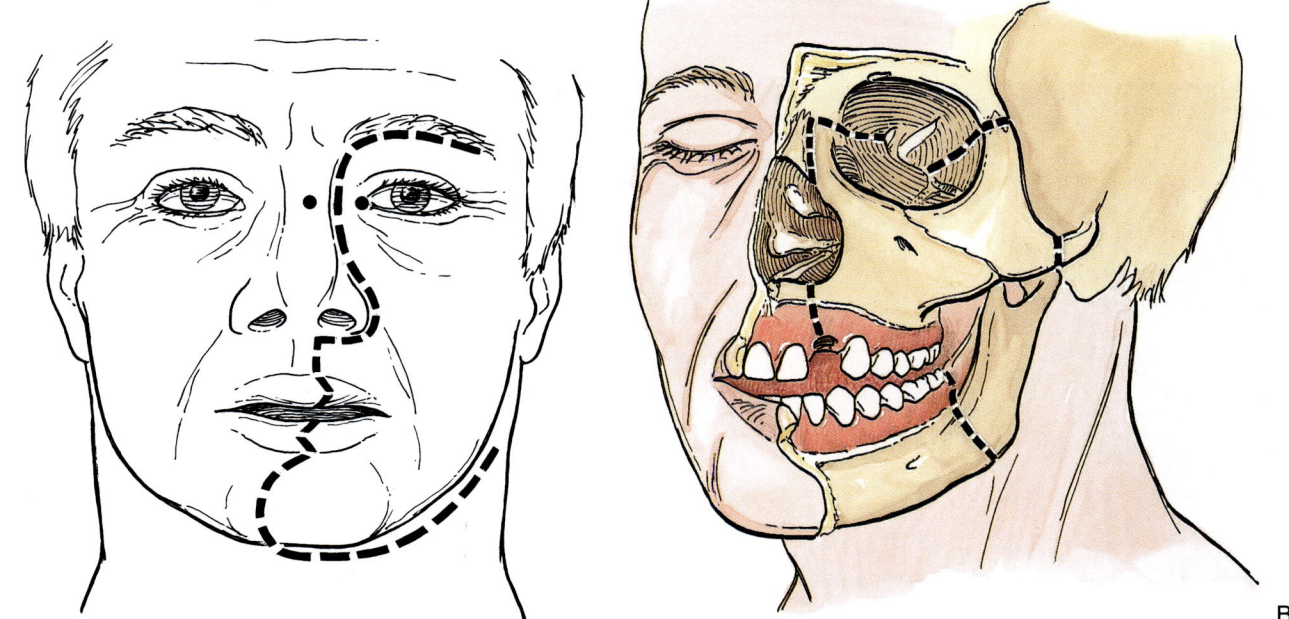

FIG. 33. Type III incision. **A:** Facial incision. **B:** Intraoral incision.

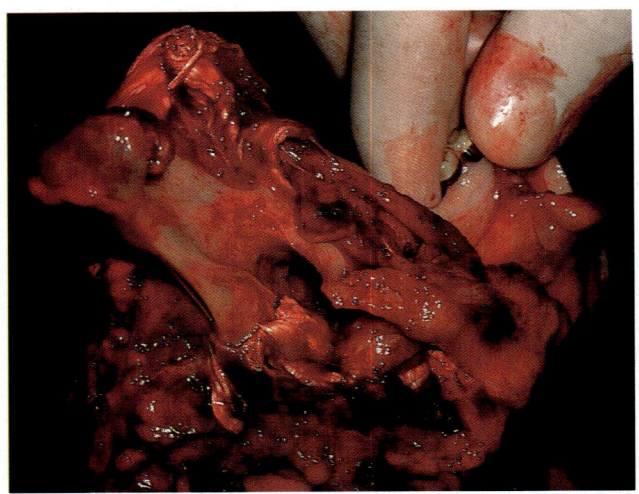

FIG. 34. Extensive perineural spread of cancer of lip along mental and inferior alveolar nerve, requiring hemimandibulectomy as part of type III excision.

of the subcranial floor of both the anterior and middle fossa afforded by this approach is extensive. This resection is done for very large, invasive upper aerodigestive tract malignancies whose intracranial involvement is usually small compared with the subcranial component. A radical neck dissection is done in continuity with the subcranial block if metastasis is present or if a high frequency of occult nodal spread is anticipated.

A Weber-Fergusson incision is extended intraorally and into the pharynx to encompass whatever oral or pharyngeal tumor exists. It is carried along the gingivobuccal sulcus through the oral buccal mucosa from the pharynx to the midline of the lip (Fig. 33). The lower lip is split, creating a dart in the vermilion border, and the incision is carried around the natural crease of the chin button, extending in a curvilinear manner into the upper neck.

The maxillectomy is performed, often with an orbital exenteration (done in 50% of the author's cases) as previously described. The extent of partial mandibulectomy varies with local extent of tumor. Because most neoplasms originate in the lateral oropharynx, nasopharynx, palate, or deep in the infratemporal fossa, most mandibular resections include the condyle, ramus, and angle. Occasionally, a recurrent tongue cancer or alveolar ridge tumor with extensive perineural spread may require mandibular body resection as well (Fig. 34).

On some occasions, only the posterior maxilla is involved, and a Weber-Fergusson incision is not required. The distal alveolus and posterior wall with pterygoid plates attached are removed intraorally, similar to the procedure described by Day and Donald (4). The exposure of the skull base is then similar to that described by Gluckman et al. in Chapter 17 of this text.

In the standard type III approach, a much wider extent of the skull base is exposed. The internal carotid artery and internal jugular vein are isolated in the upper neck and are individually loosely encircled by soft catheters. Pharyngeal, lingual, palatal, and buccal soft tissues are resected in continuity with the mandible and maxilla. The immediate subcranial and intracranial portion of the tumor is amputated from the main specimen in the "modified *en bloc*" resection method described previously (Fig. 35). Bearing in mind the amount of bony destruction and soft tissue tumor extension portrayed in the preoperative CT and MRI scans and that visualized with the main tumor specimen removed, subcranial and intracranial resection proceeds.

Bony limits of tumor invasion are defined, keeping in mind that although direct bone erosion occurs with aggressive neoplasms, the most common avenues of spread are

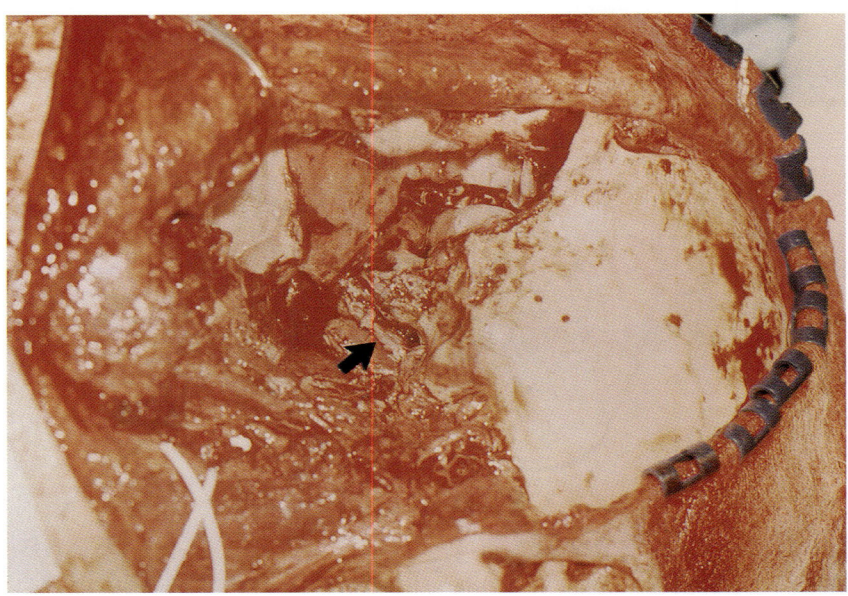

FIG. 35. Example of tumor extension visualized after main mass of neoplasm resected. *Solid arrow* shows petrous carotid artery with tumor on it.

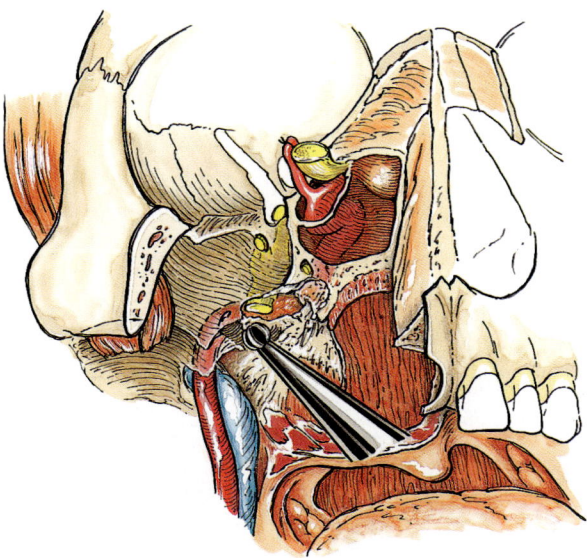

FIG. 36. Drilling away of the bone of the carotid canal.

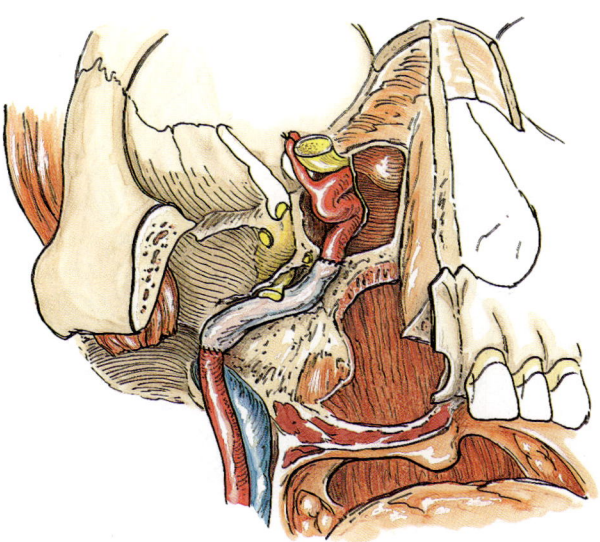

FIG. 38. Diagram showing vein graft.

through vascular and neural foramina. Therefore, careful exploration of the carotid canal, jugular foramen, foramen spinosum, and especially the foramen ovale is important. A clear view of the foramen ovale may now be obtained because of the removal of the hemimandible and pterygoid muscles. The foramen rotundum and optic canal may also be involved. Extension of tumor along the trigeminal nerve branches is commonly seen. Gross Meckel's cave and cavernous sinus involvement are often revealed in the preoperative MRI scans, but microscopic invasion is rarely portrayed (5). The internal carotid artery may be followed from the carotid canal to the foramen lacerum and thence to the cavernous sinus by drilling away the carotid canal bone from below (Fig. 36). Starting at the fibrous ring in the upper extremity of the neck, the artery is followed superiorly through the foramen until it starts to make its bend into its horizontal course. Bone is further removed up to the foramen lacerum, where the vessel again becomes vertical as it enters the intracranial cavity in the cavernous sinus (Fig. 37). If the carotid is invaded by tumor, it is removed and replaced with a saphenous vein graft (Fig. 38). If the cavernous sinus is invaded, it is removed in its entirety with frozen-section control of margins.

Jugular vein invasion is followed into the jugular foramen, with care taken to plug the inferior petrosal sinus with hemostatic gauze as dissection proceeds subtemporally into the sigmoid sinus. Once in the sigmoid, hemostasis in the sinus is ensured by a plug of hemostatic gauze (Fig. 39). Figure 40 illustrates a patient with malignant schwannoma who underwent a type III resection. Compromise of the lower cranial nerves emanating from the jugular foramen is inevitable when resecting malignancy in this area. Thyroplasty and cricopharyngeal myotomy may be done at a later time to improve speech, prevent aspiration, and aid in swallowing.

Meckel's cave dissection may need to be followed by trigeminal trunk dissection over the petrous ridge. Such extensive dissection may need to be aided by a temporal or temporal–occipital craniotomy. The latter might best be done as a second stage. Eustachian tube involvement can be resected from the nasopharyngeal to the tympanic end using this approach.

Temporal lobe dura and a portion of the lobe itself can be removed with this exposure. The amount of temporal lobe resection is limited to the silent areas, and extent of tumor is usually predictable by MRI.

Wound closure requires a watertight seal between the in-

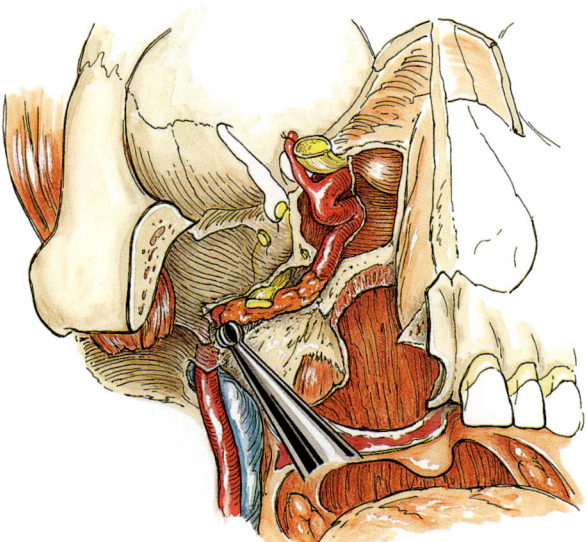

FIG. 37. Internal carotid artery is exposed from the cavernous sinus to the fibrous ring in the neck.

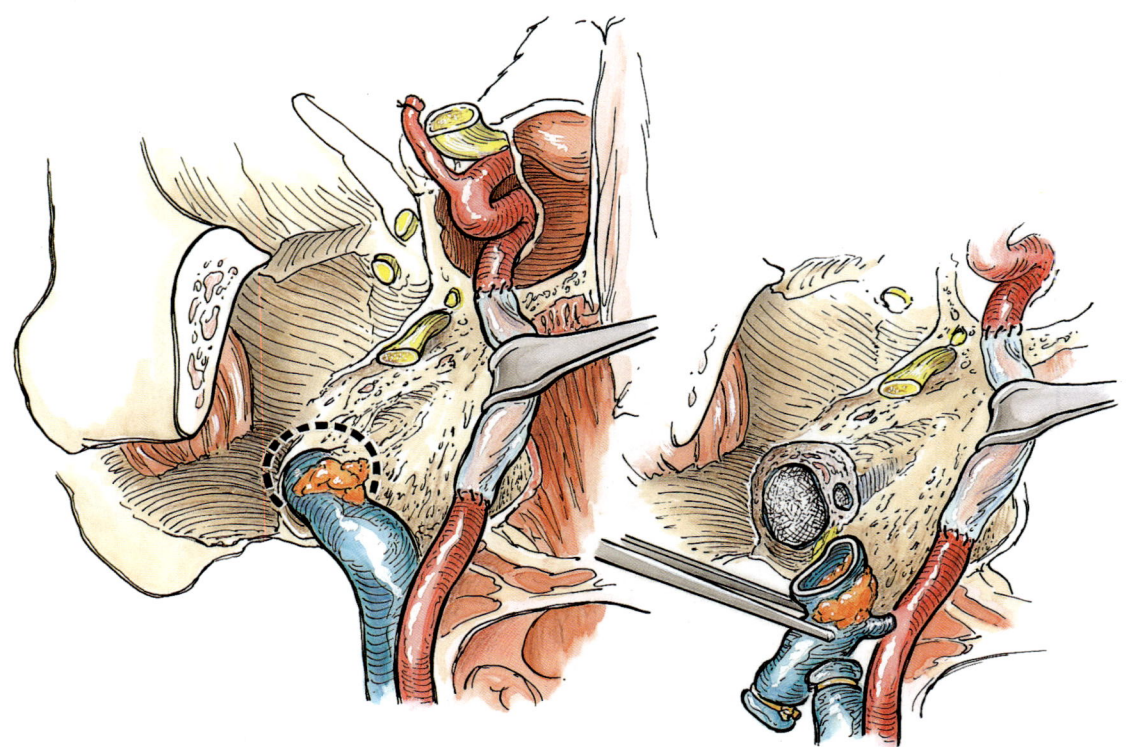

FIG. 39. Jugular vein resection with a hemostatic gauze plug in the inferior petrosal sinus. **A:** Carotid retracted with graft and tumor being resected from jugular fossa. **B:** Jugular bulb occluded, internal jugular vein tied off, and inferior petrosal sinus sealed with hemostatic plug.

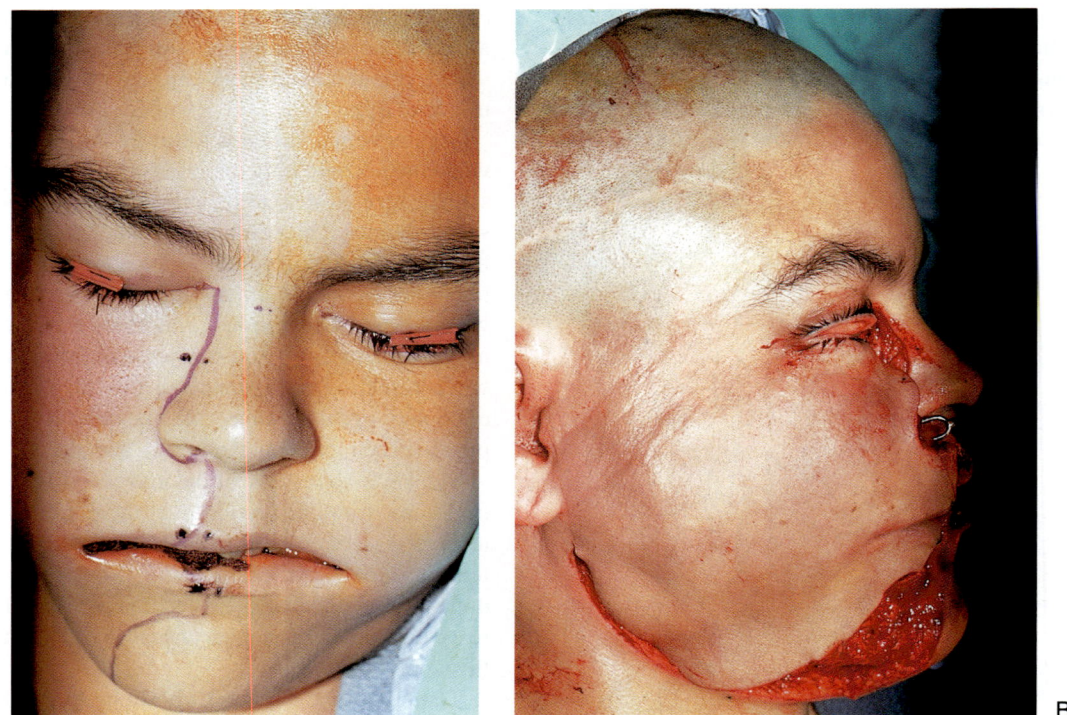

FIG. 40. Tumor involvement of middle fossa floor and internal carotid artery in patient with a malignant schwannoma of the infratemporal fossa. **A:** Initial incision marked out. **B:** Incision made.

(figure continues)

FIG. 40. *Continued.* **C:** Tumor exposed. **D:** Tumor removed. **E:** Skull base exposure with internal carotid artery involvement. Suction pointing to the tumor on the carotid artery in the foramen lacerum. **F:** Saphenous vein graft in place.

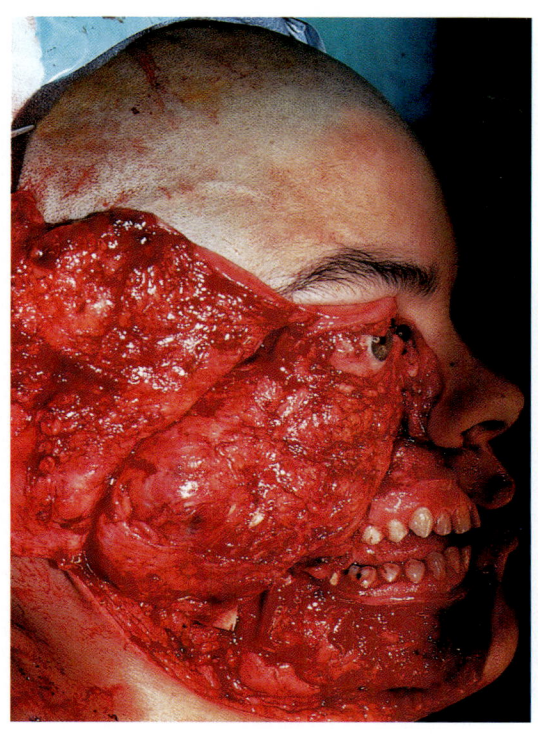
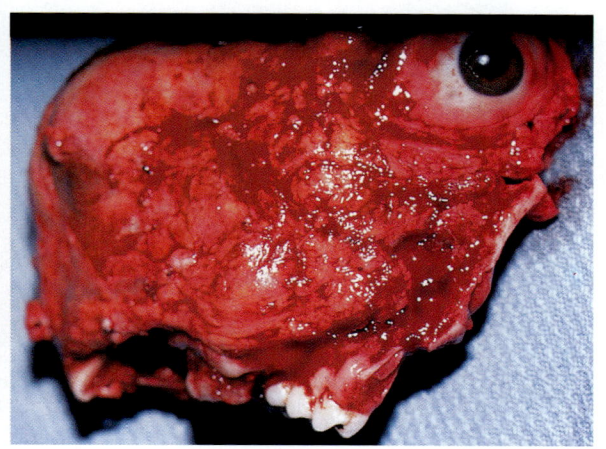
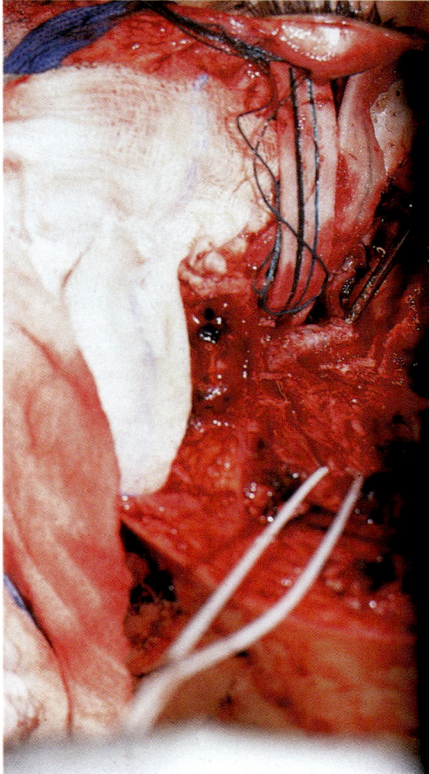
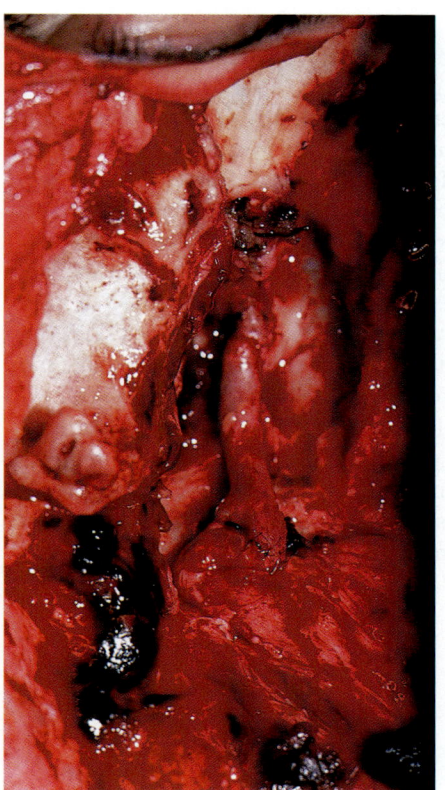

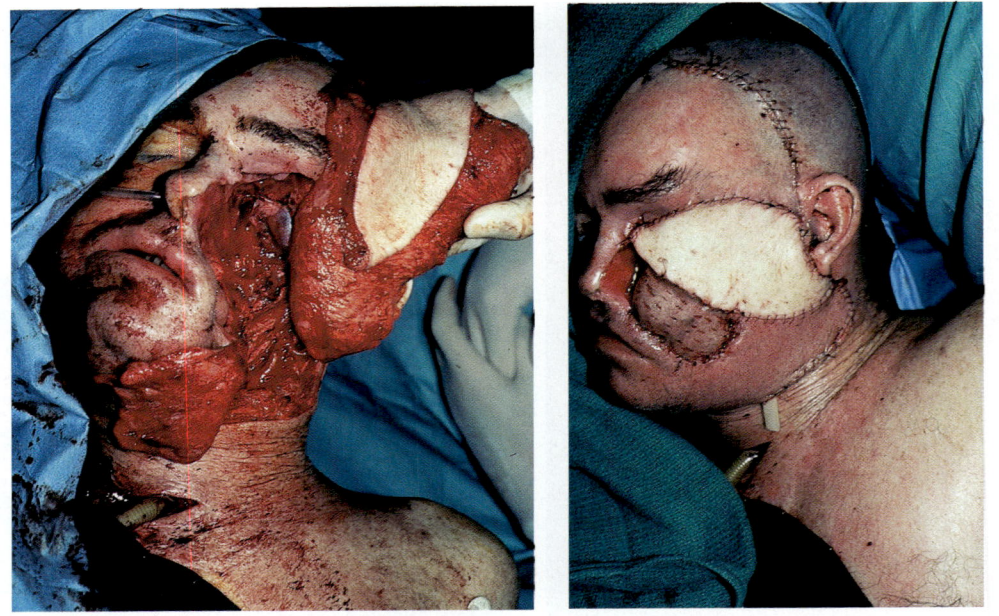

FIG. 41. Latissimus dorsi free flap used to repair massive subcranial defect after type III resection. **A:** Flap elevated and about to be placed in defect. **B:** Flap sutured into defect.

tracranial cavity and the widely exposed, extensively exenterated upper aerodigestive tract. These patients are usually failures of past surgery and radiation therapy, so wound healing may be a problem. Vascularized free tissue transfer is the answer to this problem in most cases. Resected dura is replaced with fascia or preserved cadaveric dura. Large soft tissue replacement is often required for the subcranial repair. The latissimus dorsi free flap (Fig. 41) provides excellent bulk with an epithelial lining. The rectus abdominis flap with an overlying skin graft or intact abdominal skin is useful as well. The muscle is turned to the side of the dural repair and the skin is sutured to any cutaneous defect or used as a cavity liner. A deepithelialized bridge interposed at the level of the skin repair can provide both facial cutaneous replacement and cavity lining.

The results of this approach vary according to the extent of tumor involvement, with the most favorable lesions being the small ones that have minimal subcranial extent, and the large ones requiring type III excision carrying the worst prognosis.

REFERENCES

1. Krespi YP, Sisson GA. Transmandibular exposure of the skull base. *Am J Surg* 1984;148:534–538.
2. Schramm VL Jr. Anterior craniofacial resection. In: Jackson CG, ed. *Surgery of skull base tumors.* New York: Churchill Livingstone, 1991:67–83.
3. Raveh J, Turk JB, Lädrach K, et al. Extended anterior subcranial approach for skull base tumors: long term results. *J Neurosurg* 1995;82:1002–1010.
4. Day T, Donald PJ. Posterior bimaxillary composite resection for squamous cell carcinoma of the retromolar trigone. *Head Neck* (*submitted for publication*).
5. Nemzek W, Hecht S, Grandour-Edwards R, Donald PJ. Perineural spread of head and neck tumors: how accurate is MR imaging? *Am J Neuroradiol* (*in press*).

CHAPTER 16

Infratemporal Fossa—Middle Cranial Fossa Approach

Paul J. Donald

Probably the most difficult and complex of all the approaches in skull base surgery is the infratemporal fossa–middle cranial fossa approach. It is also the most versatile, giving access not only to all of the subcranial tissues that underlie the middle fossa floor from the zygoma to the nasopharynx, but to the contents of the middle cranial fossa from the lesser sphenoid wing to the tentorium, including the petrous ridge and cavernous sinus. The clivus is widely exposed, and cutting the tentorium can expose the upper brainstem.

Considerable credit must be given to the originators of this operation. Ugo Fisch of Zurich designed the infratemporal fossa approach and first presented it in 1977 (1). It forms the basis for all the approaches to the lateral and inferolateral skull base that have been developed since. The first well coordinated intracranial and extracranial approach to this region was designed by Victor Schramm (2) and Laligam Sekhar when they were both at the University of Pittsburgh. They modified Fisch's approach, creating an excellent simultaneous exposure of the intracranial and extracranial aspects of the middle fossa through a small but strategically placed craniotomy. The removal of this bony barrier improved maneuverability in both the intracranial and extracranial compartments. The procedure described in this chapter is markedly similar to Schramm and Sekhar's operation, with some modifications.

Patients who require this operation for malignant disease usually have a more extensive lesion than those who need anterior fossa skull base surgery. They often require longer periods of time in the intensive care unit and a more prolonged hospital stay. The keystone structures that are responsible for many of the problems arising from this surgery are the cavernous sinus and the internal carotid artery (ICA).

Resection of either or both of these structures may leave the patient with substantial deficits. In malignancy, the entire sinus often needs to be removed, creating an immobile and sometimes insensate eye with ptosis of the upper lid. The cornea, therefore, is extremely prone to injury, not only from unappreciated trauma but also from sympathetic dystrophy secondary to autonomic denervation. If the original tumor is an extension from a lesion in the paranasal sinuses, then the orbit is usually exenterated and these sequelae are not an issue. Management of the carotid is still unsettled, but arterial invasion usually mandates resection in cases of malignancy and grafting rather than sacrifice, even in the presence of a negative balloon test occlusion (BTO) and favorable single-photon emission computed tomography (SPECT) scan (see Chapter 7).

It is only fair to interject at this juncture that the resection of the cavernous ICA and cavernous sinus in the face of malignancy, especially squamous cell carcinoma, remains highly controversial.

CLINICAL PRESENTATION

Patients who require this approach present with a wide variety of disease processes. The primary consideration in this chapter is tumor. The tumors may be benign or malignant, and may originate intracranially from dura or calvarial bone or extracranially from the manifold soft tissues that occupy the subcranial area. Chapter 3 describes the types and behavioral characteristics of these various tumors. Most common among the intracranial neoplasms that extend extracranially are meningioma, chordoma, chondroma, and chondrosarcoma. Among the extracranial tumors that extend intracranially are schwannoma, often of the trigeminal nerve; parotid tumors, both benign and malignant, especially from the deep lobe; and squamous cell carcinomas from the paranasal sinuses, nasopharynx, and temporal bone. Meta-

---

P. J. Donald: Department of Otolaryngology–Head and Neck Surgery, and Center for Skull Base Surgery, University of California, Davis Medical Center, Sacramento, California 95817.

static deposits in high lymph nodes from any head and neck site, but more often from the nasopharynx or paranasal sinuses, may erode through the middle fossa skull base. Rarely, metastases from distant sites such as breast, prostate, or kidney may present as a pathologic node at the skull base. A rather curious inflammatory lesion may present itself as a skull base neoplasm both in symptomatology and in radiographic appearance. This is a variant of the so-called Tolosa-Hunt syndrome (Fig. 1). The author's team has had four such patients in their experience, all of whom resolved on steroid therapy.

Unfortunately, the presenting symptoms of lesions in this area are often subtle. Many patients complain of pain only in the region of the infratemporal fossa, ear, or behind the eye. This symptom is often passed off as myofascial dysfunction or "temporomandibular joint" (TMJ) syndrome. Trismus secondary to pterygoid muscle invasion or direct involvement of the mandibular branch of the trigeminal nerve may still be mistaken for these syndromes. Any patient with a past history of carcinoma of the nasopharynx or oropharynx must be viewed with a high index of suspicion when presenting with pain in the infratemporal fossa.

Special attention should be focused on the patient with oropharyngeal carcinoma who, after the standard therapy of composite resection and postoperative radiation therapy, presents with pain deep in the infratemporal fossa. The clinician should especially be alerted if the pain is new. There is often little to find on physical examination other than an occasional increase in trismus. Because the inferior alveolar nerve has been sacrificed in the initial resection, the only remaining sensory nerve from V3 is the auriculotemporal, which may also have been injured at surgery. Such patients should have magnetic resonance imaging (MRI). Because of

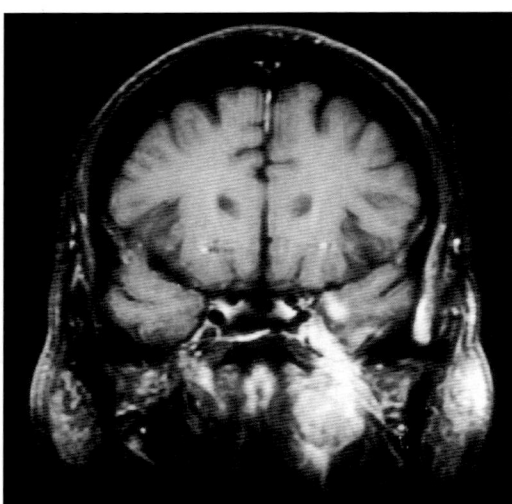

FIG. 1. Magnetic resonance image in coronal plane showing what appears to be a tumor of the infratemporal fossa involving the mandibular branch of the trigeminal nerve and the cavernous sinus. Surgical exploration revealed only inflammation.

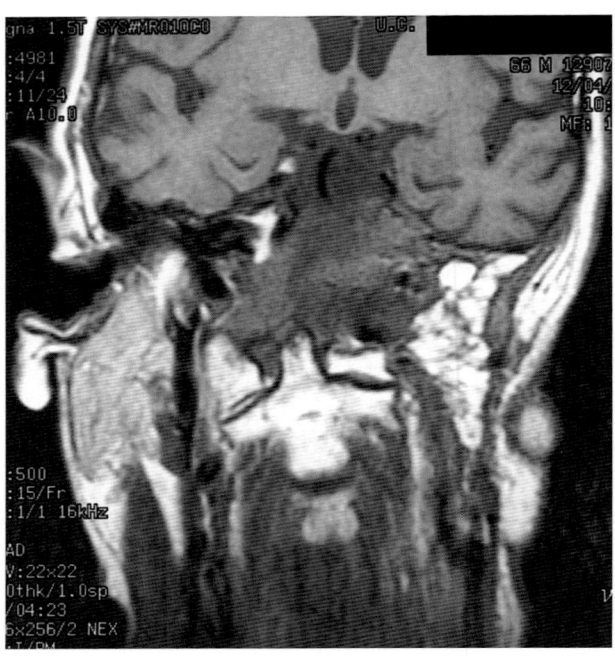

FIG. 2. Magnetic resonance image showing extensive, recurrent tumor in deep lobe of parotid gland that resulted in facial nerve paralysis and extension to the odontoid of C2.

the obscuring distortions of the past surgery and radiation, it is often difficult to distinguish fibrosis and edema from tumor, even with gadolinium contrast (see Fig. 8, Chapter 5). Often, serial MRIs at 6-week to 3-month intervals are the only means by which to make a diagnosis. Unfortunately, valuable time may be lost as the tumor continues to grow and is constantly at risk of metastasis. Analysis by positron emission tomography (PET) scanning may be of great assistance here (3).

Carcinoma of the temporal bone may be subtle or patently obvious (see Figs. 3 and 30, Chapter 5). The symptom of painful otorrhea unresponsive to vigorous local therapy is highly suspect. Temporal bone carcinoma is covered in Chapter 20, but it is important to mention that anterior extension can involve the infratemporal fossa.

As in temporal bone carcinoma, malignancies in the infratemporal fossa may present with a facial nerve paralysis. This is especially true of parotid gland carcinomas. Recurrent carcinoma or tumors of the deep lobe often involve the facial nerve. Paresis or complete paralysis of the entire nerve, indicating main trunk invasion, is usually the rule (Fig. 2).

Extension of tumor through the foramen ovale along the third division of the trigeminal nerve can produce numbness over its sensory distribution and, by spread through the gasserian ganglion, hypesthesia of both the second and first divisions of the trigeminal nerve. This manifests itself initially as numbness over the chin and lower face and then advances to numbness over the midface, especially the area subserved by the infraorbital nerve with V2 involvement and the forehead and cornea if V1 is affected. Once the tumor has reached the gasserian ganglion in Meckel's cave, extension

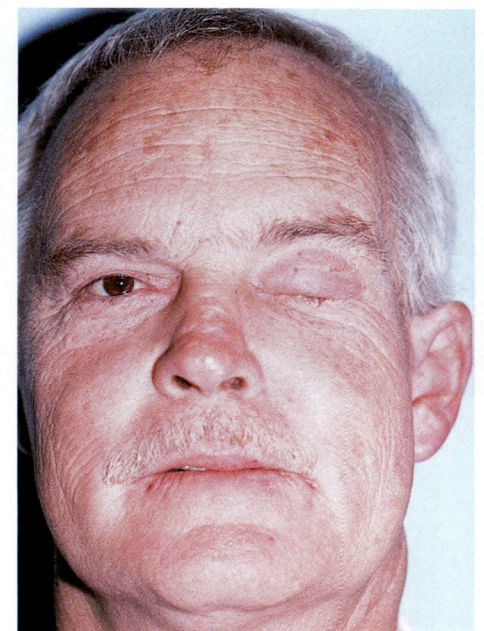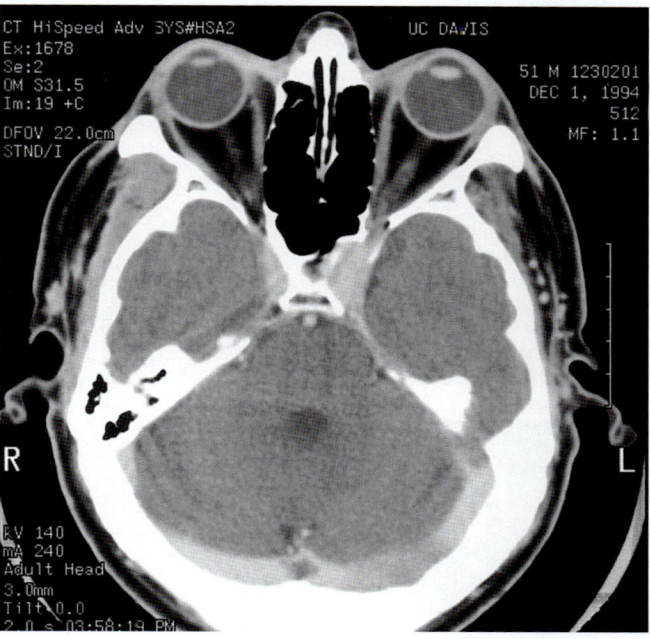

FIG. 3. Patient with extension of squamous cell carcinoma along the infraorbital nerve to produce numbness of all three divisions of the trigeminal nerve, as well as complete ophthalmoplegia and ptosis of the upper eyelid. **A:** Frontal view of patient. **B:** Computed tomography scan showing cavernous sinus invasion.

into the cavernous sinus is imminent. Once this occurs, paralysis of the oculomotor, trochlear, and abducens nerves often follows. Ptosis and ophthalmoplegia are the result (Fig. 3).

Tumor extension directly from the nasopharynx usually follows the foramen lacerum. The subsequent invasion of the cavernous sinus commonly produces abducens nerve paralysis with a lateral rectus palsy (Fig. 4). Invasion of the lateral wall of the sinus results in affliction of cranial nerves III and IV, and eventually involvement of V2, V3, and the optic nerve with extension superiorly.

Invasion of the carotid artery is usually asymptomatic. Rarely is the tumor so advanced as completely to occlude the vessel. Were that to occur, a stroke may ensue. This is possible even with reduced flow in a patient with already compromised cerebral circulation.

Involvement of temporal dura commonly produces unremitting, intense headache (Fig. 5). Because much of the temporal lobe is "silent," brain invasion gives little in the way of differentiating signs and symptoms.

With metastatic tumor to high internal jugular, parapharyngeal, or retropharyngeal lymph nodes, lower cranial nerves may be affected. Extracapsular tumor spread from these nodes may erode skull base bone and invade the jugular foramen, producing symptoms secondary to affliction of cranial nerves IX, X, XI, and, with spread to the adjacent hypoglossal canal, XII. The cervical sympathetic may be involved, producing Horner's syndrome. Clinical investigation of these patients, after a thorough head and neck and neurologic examination, includes a thorough general medical assessment. If a tumor is deemed operable, two other medical circumstances preclude an attempt at infratemporal fossa–middle cranial fossa excision. The first is the presence of distant metastasis and the second is general lack of medical fitness. General debility from extensive physiologic aging, severe cardiovascular disease, poorly controlled diabetes, or incipient renal or hepatic failure is a contraindication to surgery. A final contraindication to surgery is lack of patient commitment. Some natural reluctance to undergo such an extensive procedure is anticipated, but a lackluster attitude on the part of the patient, coupled with perhaps overzealous enthusiasm of family or friends, should be carefully assessed before consideration of surgery.

Magnetic resonance imaging with gadolinium contrast and, if indicated, fat suppression should be complemented by fine-cut computed tomography scanning through the skull base. The coronal plane is most helpful in clearly outlining carotid involvement and cavernous sinus invasion. Bony detail is best delineated with computed tomography, and soft tissue invasion by MRI. Gadolinium contrast is extremely helpful in differentiating tumor from adjacent soft tissue, especially in recurrent or persistent disease. A word of warning is necessary, however, regarding these studies; there are false-negative and false-positive scans. Moreover, the studies do not always accurately delineate the extent of tumor.

Chapter 19 of this text is already devoted to the management of the ICA. There are many methods of evaluating the patency of the circle of Willis but, more important, the surgeon must assess the amount of blood flow from collateral circulation if the ICA on the tumor side is removed. The gold standard has been BTO of the ICA using radioactive xenon

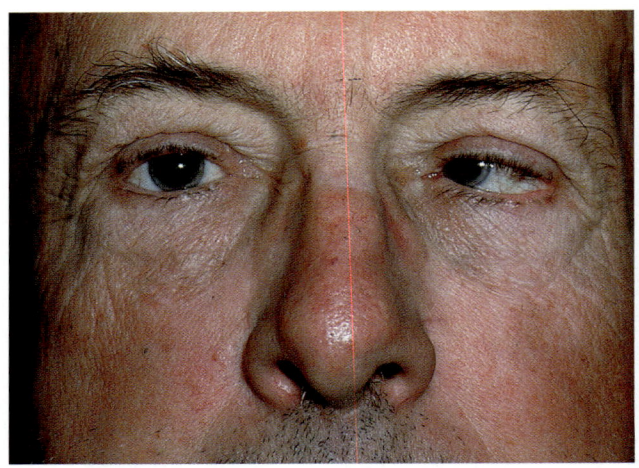
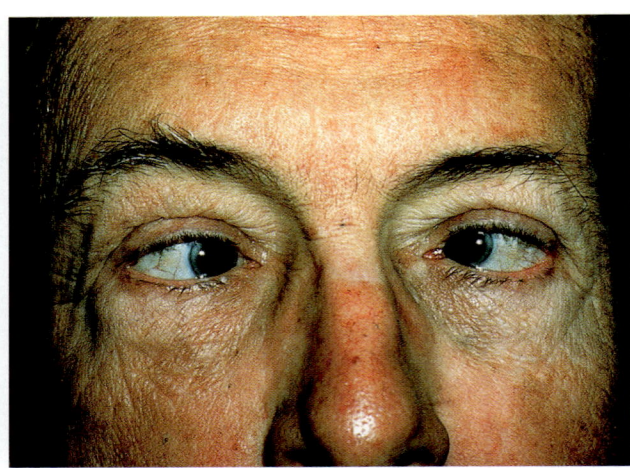
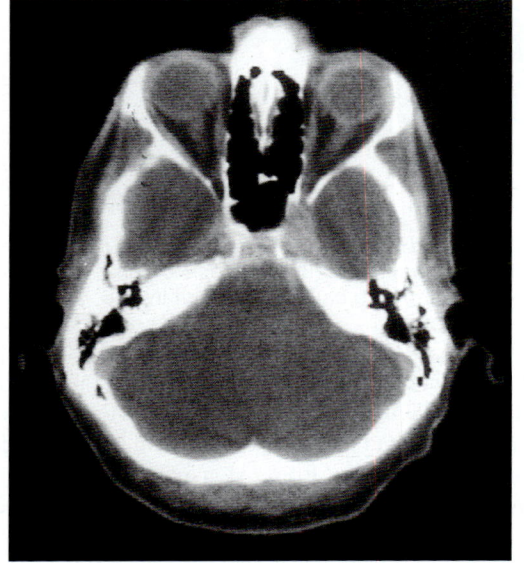

FIG. 4. Patient with a lateral rectus muscle palsy of the eye secondary to direct invasion of the cavernous sinus through the foramen lacerum by a nasopharyngeal carcinoma. **A:** Straight-ahead gaze. **B:** Lateral gaze, revealing lateral rectus palsy of left eye. **C:** Computed tomography scan demonstrating carcinoma of nasopharynx invading cavernous sinus.

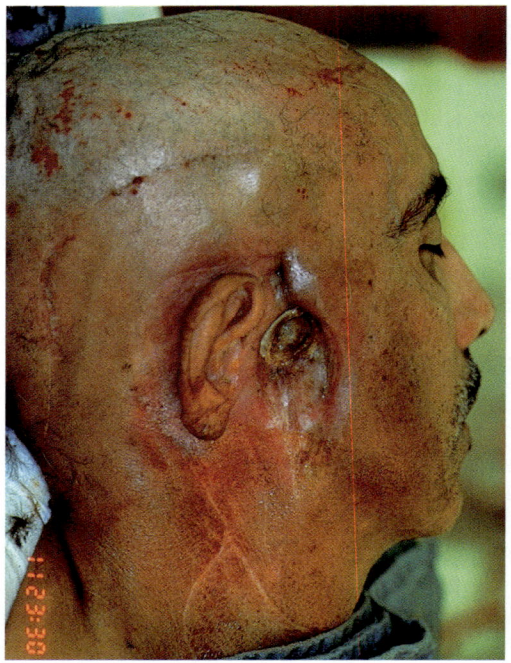
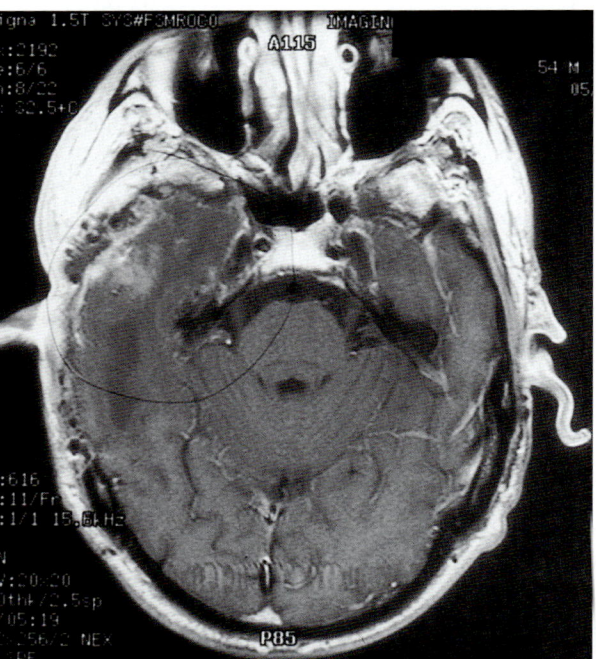

FIG. 5. A: Middle-aged man with recurrent temporal bone carcinoma presenting with excruciating cranial pain. **B:** Magnetic resonance image showing extensive dural involvement and brain invasion.

TABLE 1. *Sensitivity of positron emission tomography scanning in head and neck and skull base cancer*

Type of disease	False-positive results	False-negative results	Error rate
Primary	1/8	2/8	38%
Recurrent	2/22	1/29	14%
Regional metastases	3/12	2/18	17%
Distant metastases	2/11	1/18	10%

to provide a calculation of cerebral blood flow before and after temporary occlusion. Xenon studies are notoriously difficult to perform because of frequent fluctuations in gas concentrations and problems with the measuring equipment. Much more practical has been the use of SPECT with technetium-99m hexamethylpropyleneamine oxime (HMPAO) contrast (see Chapter 7). This has produced predictable results for the author's team, and is their investigative method of choice. For a more complete analysis of investigation of the ICA, see Chapters 7 and 19.

The investigative tool most recently incorporated into the team's armamentarium is the PET scan. Because of the avidity of tumor cells for glucose, a nonmetabolizing, radioactive, fluoridated analogue is given and subsequent PET scans are done. In the author's experience, the accuracy for the detection of previously untreated primary disease is 87%, and for recurrent or persistent disease, 86%. The false-positive and false-negative rates and sensitivity are given in Table 1.

As with all skull base tumor patients, extensive discussion between the patient and the head and neck surgeon, the neurosurgeon, and the plastic surgeon ensues. It is important for the patient to understand the arduousness of the procedure, what functions will be lost, what cosmetic deformities will result, and what other treatment options exist. For malignant tumors, skull base surgery often remains the only chance for cure. The surgeon must be realistic—not overenthusiastic, but encouraging—when discussing options with these often desperate patients.

SURGICAL PROCEDURE

Preparation

As in most of the author's skull base patients, there is a routine preoperative set of procedures that includes tracheostomy, the placement of a lumbar subarachnoid drain, and instillation of Frost temporary tarsorrhaphy sutures in the eyelids (see Fig. 2, Chapter 29). Unless fixation pins are insisted on by the neurosurgeon, a Mayfield horseshoe head rest is used for ease of surgical access. Central venous pressure and arterial lines are usually placed, and any cranial nerve monitoring devices inserted. Electroencephalography electrodes are sutured or stapled to the scalp to monitor cerebral electrical activity in cases of possible ICA sacrifice.

An extensive surgical preparation is usually necessary, including a head shave with a scrub of the entire face, head, neck, and anterior chest. The abdomen is also prepared if a rectus abdominis flap is to be used as a vascularized free tissue transfer for reconstruction. Often, both legs are scrubbed in anticipation of the possible harvest of split-thickness skin, fascia lata, or saphenous vein grafts (Fig. 6).

Incision

The standard skin incision can be of two types, depending on the location of the lesion. For more anteriorly located lesions such as deep-lobe parotid tumors, lesions invading the foramen ovale, or nasopharyngeal carcinoma, the incision extends in a curvilinear fashion from the vertex of the skull, in front of the ear in a preauricular crease, and under the lobule of the ear, then curves forward in the upper neck, resembling a modified Blair incision for parotidectomy (Fig. 7A,B). The posterior incision goes behind the ear 2 to 4 cm, similar to the incision described by Fisch and extending into the neck toward the hyoid. Lesions such as temporal bone carcinomas, extensive glomus jugulare tumors, and clival chordomas are examples of when to use the posterior incision (see Fig. 7C,D). A lazy-S is subtended into the neck if a radical neck dissection is to accompany the procedure.

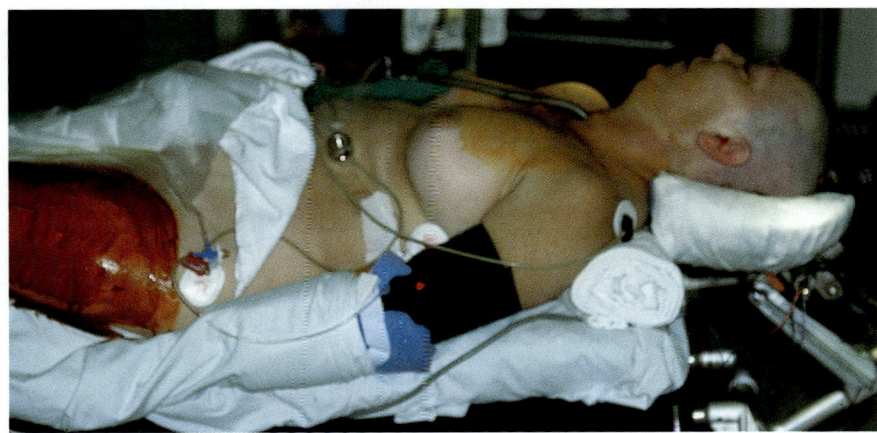

FIG. 6. Patient with multiple sites surgically prepared, including the site of craniofacial cervical incision and graft or flap donor sites.

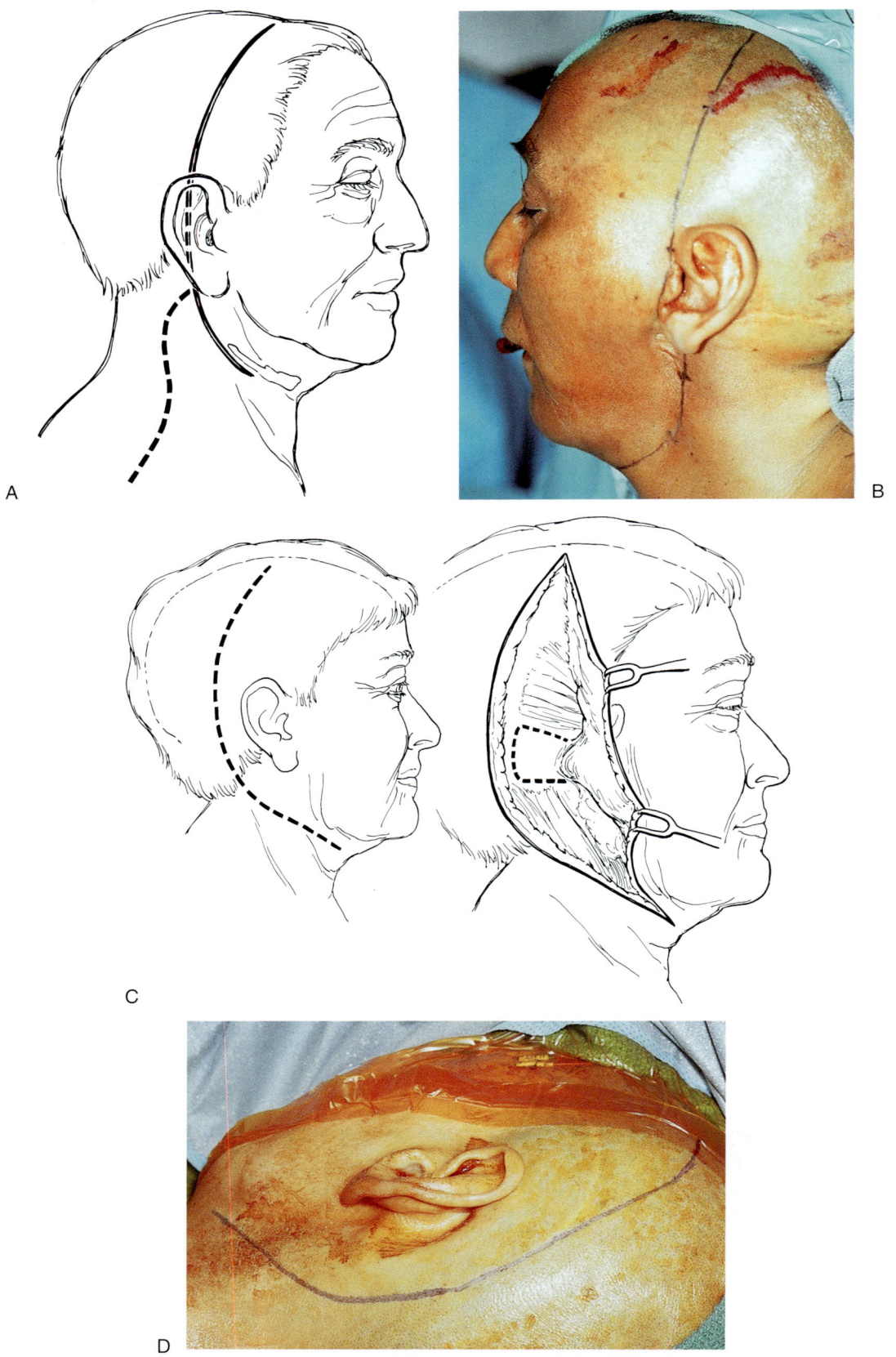

FIG. 7. Incision for middle temporal fossa–infratemporal fossa approach. **A:** Line drawing of anterior incision. Lazy "S" incision added if neck dissection is required. (From Donald PJ. Craniofacial surgery for head and neck cancer. In: Johnson JT, Blitzer A, Ossoff RH, Thomas JR, eds. *AAO-HNS instructional courses.* Vol. 2. St. Louis: CV Mosby, 1989:244, with permission.) **B:** Anterior incision in patient with recurrent deep lobe parotid carcinoma extending into the middle cranial fossa. **C:** Line drawing of posterior incision. **D:** Posterior incision in patient with glomus jugulare tumor with marked intracranial extension. Dotted line outlines mastoid periosteal flap for closure of the external auditory canal.

The scalp incision goes to the level of the pericranium. As the flap is developed, the temporalis muscle is identified (Fig. 8). The superficial and deep temporalis fascia are incised in a semilunar manner to include the frontal branch of the facial nerve, which emerges approximately 1.5 cm in front of the auricle and arches into the frontalis muscle approximately 2 to 2.5 cm above the brow (Fig. 9). This protects the nerve from injury.

The cervicofacial portion of the incision proceeds superficially to the platysma and superficial muscular aponeurotic system (SMAS) fascia in a plane similar to that in a superficial plane face lift. This is carried forward anteriorly to a point from the angle of the mandible to the lateral orbital rim (Fig. 10). When using this anterior incision, a decision whether to cut across the external auditory canal (EAC) is made, usually predicated on the necessity of exposing the ICA. The posterior incision always cuts across the canal because carotid exposure is usually necessary (Fig. 11).

External Auditory Canal Obliteration

In most instances of both the anterior and posterior incision, exposure of the petrous portion of the ICA is required. This is best facilitated by exposing and later obliterating the eustachian tube. A decision regarding elimination of the middle ear cleft and the EAC or preservation of a nonventilated middle ear cleft and the permanent instillation of a ventilating tube is often difficult. For ease of management and decreased frequency of complications, there is little question that obliteration is the treatment of choice. In those patients desiring hearing preservation and in young patients, maintenance of the integrity of the middle ear and EAC and the use of a ventilating tube is preferable.

If the EAC is to be obliterated, it is best done at this juncture. The obliteration technique described by Fisch is easy to perform with predictable results, and is illustrated in Fig. 12. This is certainly the preferable technique in nasopharyngeal carcinoma or in patients who are failures of prior radiation therapy.

Internal Carotid Artery and Internal Jugular Vein Exposure

Attention is now turned to the neck where the internal jugular vein (IJV) and ICA are identified and dissected superiorly as close as possible to the skull base foramina through which they pass. Care is taken to avoid damage to cranial nerves IX through XII during the dissection. Soft rubber catheters are placed around these vessels for later control of bleeding, if necessary (see Fig. 3, Chapter 29). The upper end of this dissection may need to be postponed until the mandibular condylectomy is done. Eventually the ICA needs to be exposed to visualize the fibrous ring and the entrance of the artery into the skull at the carotid foramen (Fig. 13). Similarly, the IJV is dissected to the jugular foramen.

Temporalis Elevation

The temporalis muscle body is exposed in its entirety. In over half the cases, it serves as the major reconstructive flap that separates the middle cranial fossa from the upper aerodigestive tract. Maintaining its viability is essential, and inte-

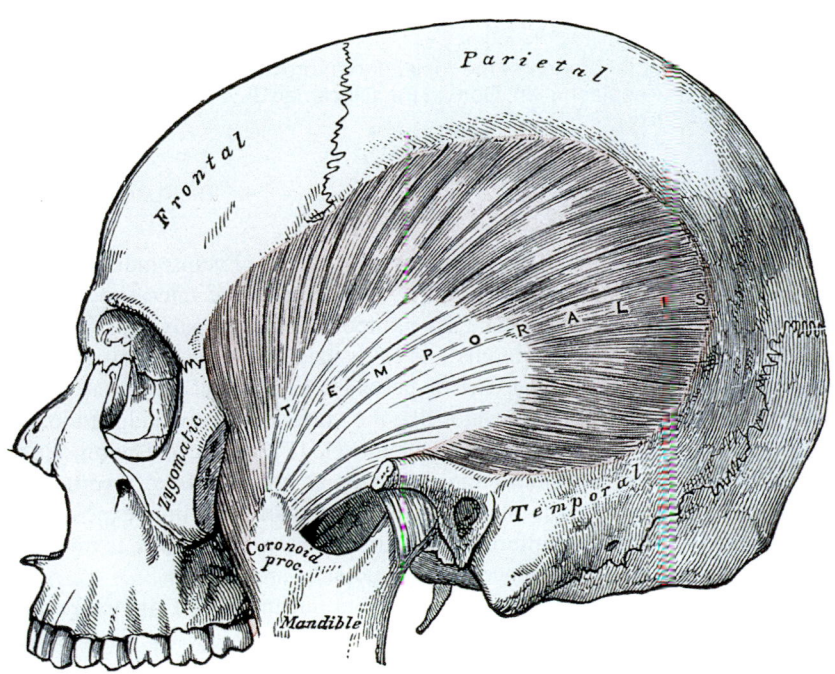

FIG. 8. Temporalis muscle. Note the large, fan-shaped configuration of the muscle, with the bulk of its insertion being on the coronoid process. (From Goss CM. *Gray's anatomy.* 29th American ed. Malvern, PA: Lea & Febiger, 1973, Figure 6.5, with permission.)

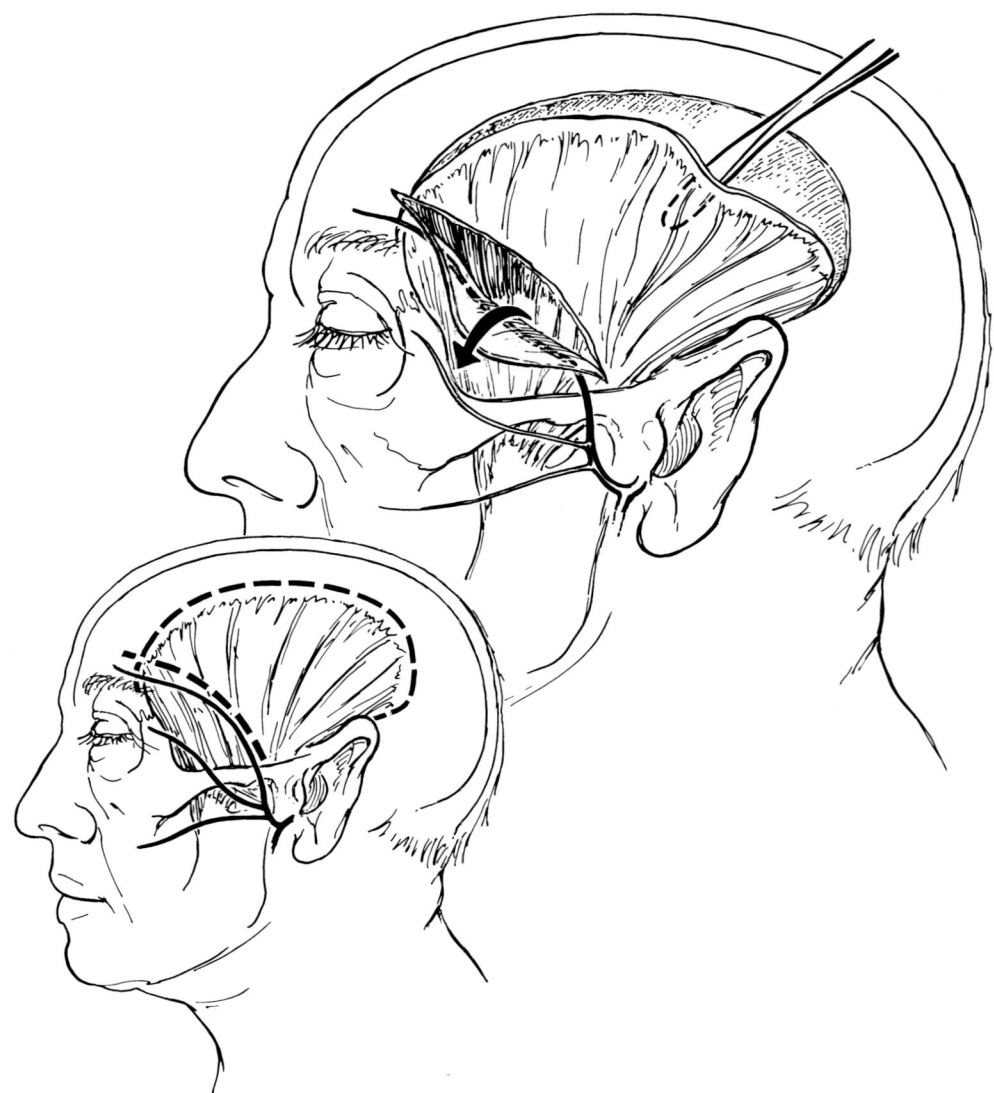

FIG. 9. Incision of temporalis fascia to include the frontal branch of the facial nerve, precluding it from injury. (From Donald PJ. Skull base surgery for sinus neoplasms. In: Donald PJ, Gluckman JL, Rice DH, eds. *The sinuses*. New York: Raven Press, 1995:479.)

gral to that is an understanding of its blood supply. The superior supply from the superficial temporal artery and branches of the postauricular artery is unavoidably eliminated during the muscle elevation. The integrity of the inferior supply through the deep temporal branches is assiduously maintained. These deep branches emerge from the internal maxillary artery both directly posteriorly and anteriorly to the foramen ovale (Fig. 14). The posterior artery exits the internal maxillary just anterior to this artery's emergence from under the neck of the mandible. The anterior deep temporal leaves the internal maxillary just before its disappearance into the pterygomaxillary fissure. In an attempt to achieve hemostasis of the prolific bleeding often encountered from the pterygoid plexus of veins, indiscriminate cautery in this area may compromise the anterior deep temporal artery. The use of bipolar cautery is advised.

The temporalis muscle is elevated in its entirety, usually with a 2-cm cuff of pericranium. Careful elevation with a broad, flat elevator like the von Langenbeck helps to maintain the integrity of the muscle (Figs. 9, 15). The muscle is elevated along the calvarium as it curves from a vertical to an oblique plane. Further dissection, and thus exposure of the deep inferior part of the infratemporal fossa, is impeded by the presence of the zygomatic arch.

In highly invasive tumors, infiltration of the temporalis muscle may be observed at this point (Fig. 16). The muscle

INFRATEMPORAL FOSSA–MIDDLE CRANIAL FOSSA APPROACH / 317

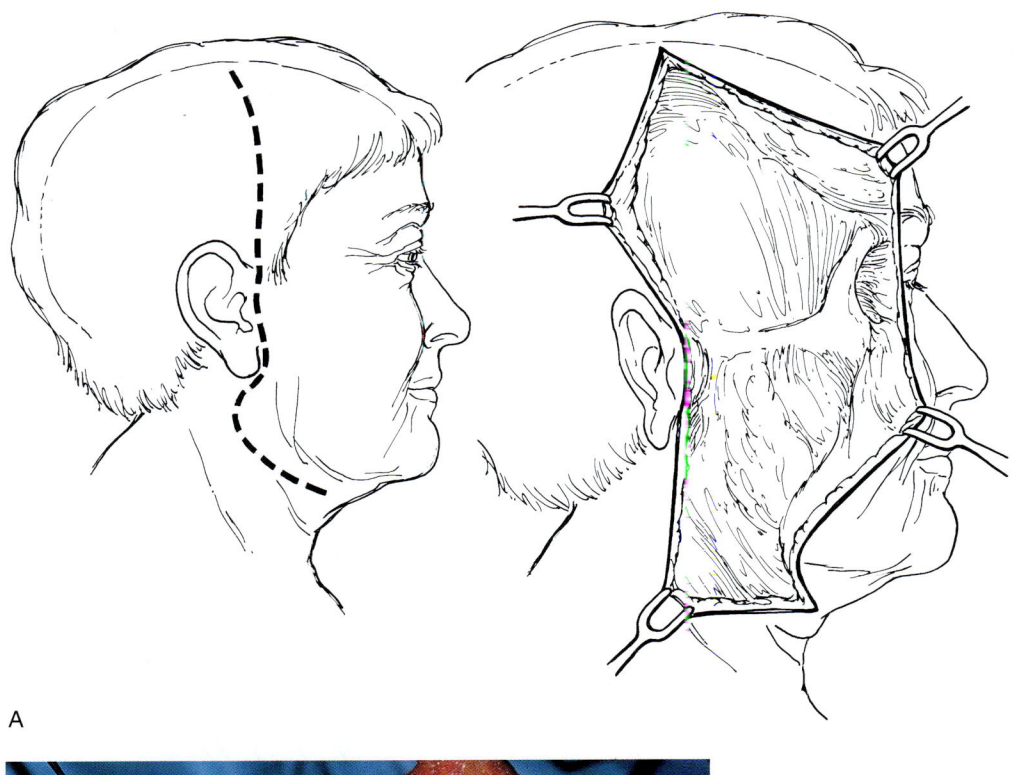

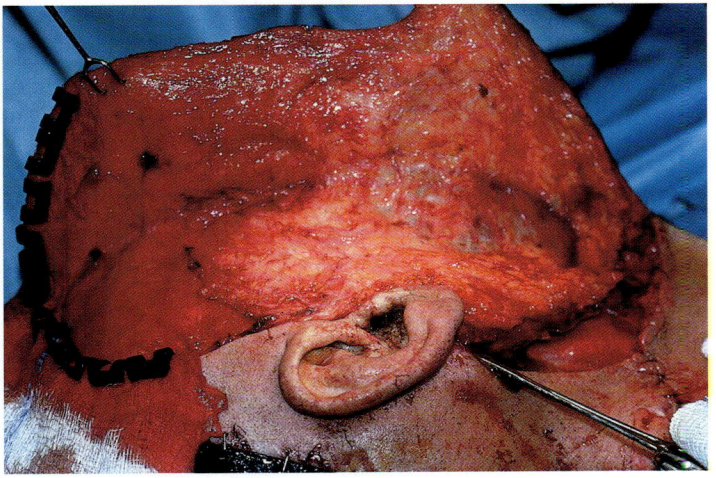

FIG. 10. Anterior elevation of cervicofacial skin flap from the angle of the mandible to the lateral orbital rim. **A:** Line drawing. **B:** Patient with elevation complete.

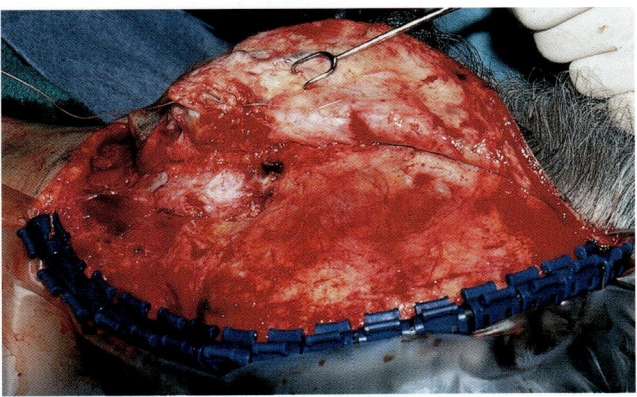

FIG. 11. Posterior incision with external auditory canal amputation and closure (see also Fig. 12). Internal carotid artery exposure is anticipated.

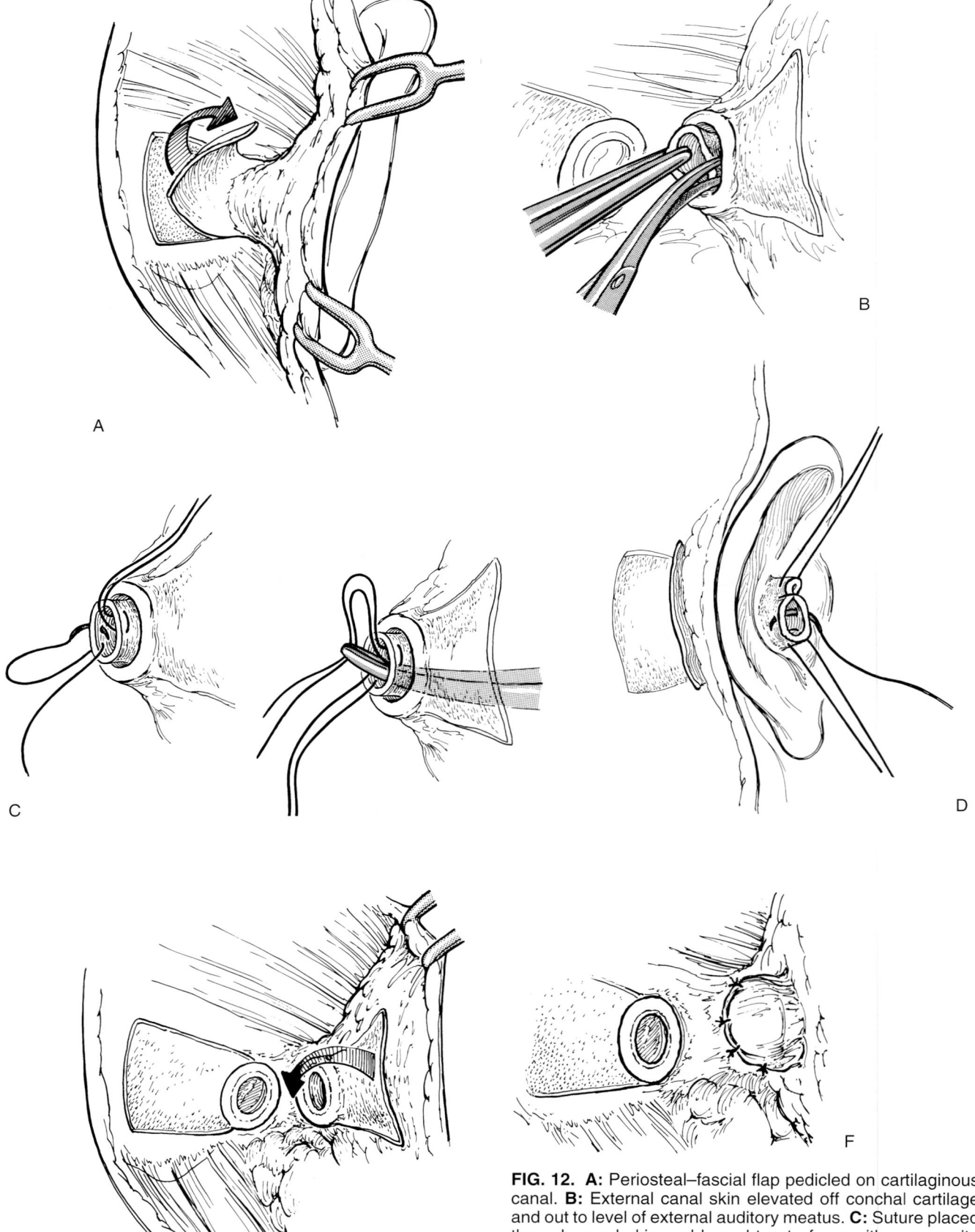

FIG. 12. A: Periosteal–fascial flap pedicled on cartilaginous canal. **B:** External canal skin elevated off conchal cartilage and out to level of external auditory meatus. **C:** Suture placed through canal skin and brought out of ear with a mosquito clamp. **D:** External auditory canal (EAC) skin closed. **E:** Periosteal–fascial closure over EAC. **F:** Closure complete.

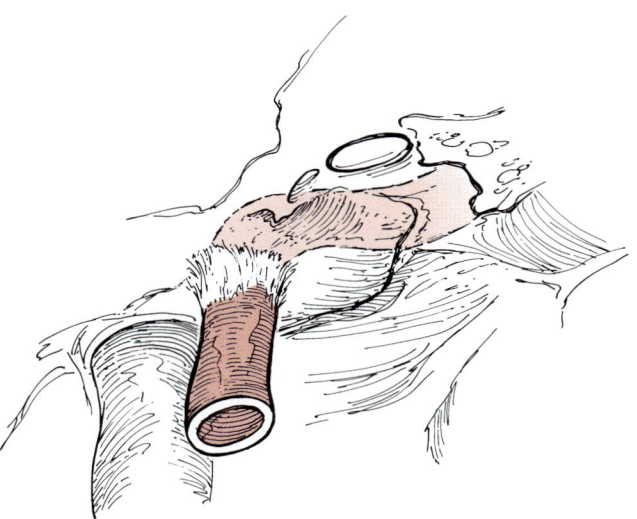

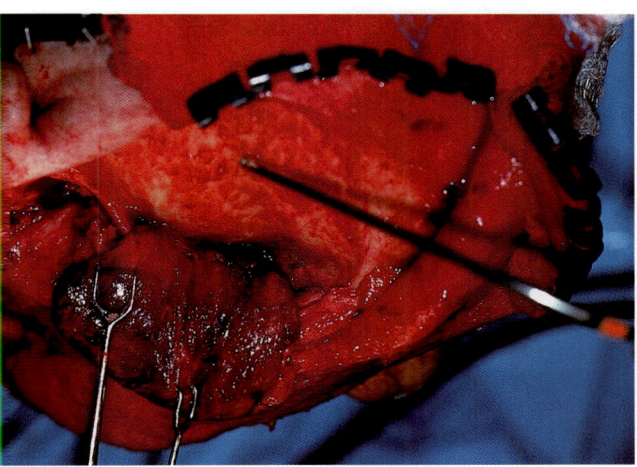

FIG. 13. Internal carotid artery with fibrous ring as it enters the carotid foramen. Internal jugular vein enters the jugular foramen posterolaterally.

FIG. 15. Temporalis elevated, but further dissection impeded by the presence of the zygomatic arch.

then must become part of the resection. If tumor involvement is suspected by preoperative studies, then, if oncologically sound, pericranium adjacent to the muscle is preserved.

Zygomatic Ostectomy

To open the depths of the infratemporal fossa, the zygomatic arch, including a part of the body and the orbital process, is removed in a piece (Fig. 17). Incision of periosteum is followed by a subperiosteal elevation from just in front of the articular process to the posterior part of the malar eminence, superiorly around the lateral orbital rim and immediately adjacent lateral orbital wall. Care is taken to preserve the periorbita without perforation and to protect it gently with a malleable retractor during subsequent drilling. Drill holes are placed in the arch and the orbital rim in anticipation of placing miniplates for later reconstruction (Fig. 18).

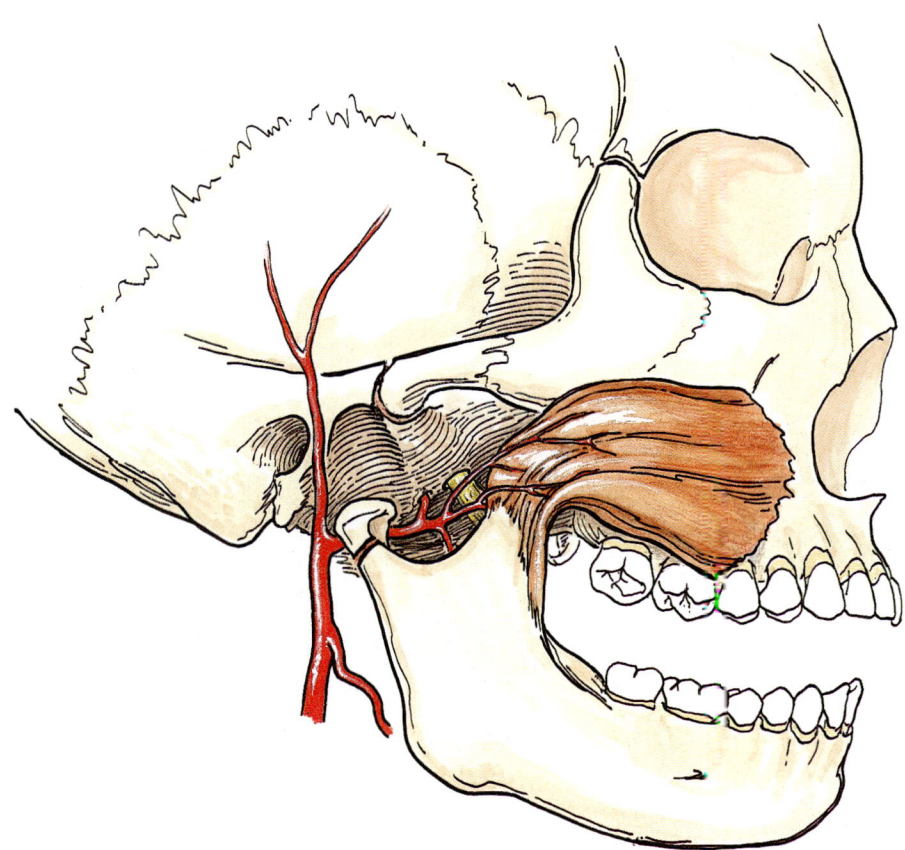

FIG. 14. Blood supply to the temporalis muscle.

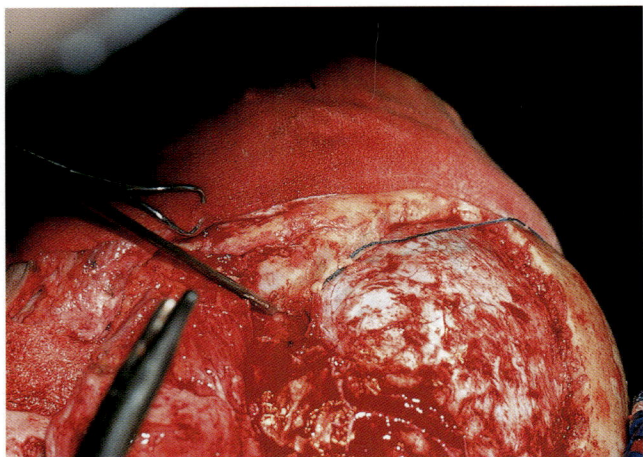

FIG. 16. Highly infiltrative adenoid cystic carcinoma of the ethmoid sinuses invading the orbital apex, middle cranial fossa, and temporalis muscle.

A fine-blade power saw or the B_5 attachment to the Midas Rex is used to cut across the posterior arch just anterior to the articular eminence (Fig. 19). The sagittal saw or the Midas Rex cutting tool then cuts across the lateral orbital rim above the zygomaticofrontal suture. This is carried approximately 2 to 4 mm deep until the thin lateral orbital wall is encountered (Fig. 20). This cut is extended down the lateral orbital wall just inside the rim until the inferior orbital fissure is reached (Fig. 21). The final cut is through the posterior portion of the zygomatic body, carried from the beginning of the malar eminence to the inferior orbital fissure, usually switching from the B_5 to the B_1 attachment (Fig. 22). The last vestiges of soft tissue are removed from their attachments to the zygoma, and the bone is removed (Fig. 23) and stored in a saline-soaked sponge until the reconstructive phase.

Mandibular Condylectomy

The last step in removing impediments to the deep infratemporal fossa is the mandibular condylectomy. Some controversy surrounds the management of the condylar process and the TMJ. In the opinion of some surgeons, incision of the TMJ and inferior retraction of the meniscus and condylar head provides adequate exposure and preserves joint integrity. There have, however, been some reports of stiffness, pain, and TMJ dysfunction resulting from this technique. Removal of the condyle and disk has, in this author's experience, resulted only in some lateral sway on full opening of the jaw, and no pain or malfunction (Fig. 24).

The key point in removing the condyle is to avoid cutting the internal maxillary artery that runs just deep to the condylar neck. Because destroying this vessel devascularizes the temporalis muscle, its protection is vital. The secret to the vessel's preservation is a subperiosteal dissection.

Some of the insertion of the lateral pterygoid muscle that penetrates the anterior surface of the TMJ capsule is dissected away with the cautery. The periosteum is incised along the anterior and lateral aspects of the condylar head by going through the temporomandibular ligament and the joint capsule. Sharp dissection with an elevator such as the Obwegeser allows dissection around the mandibular neck (Fig.

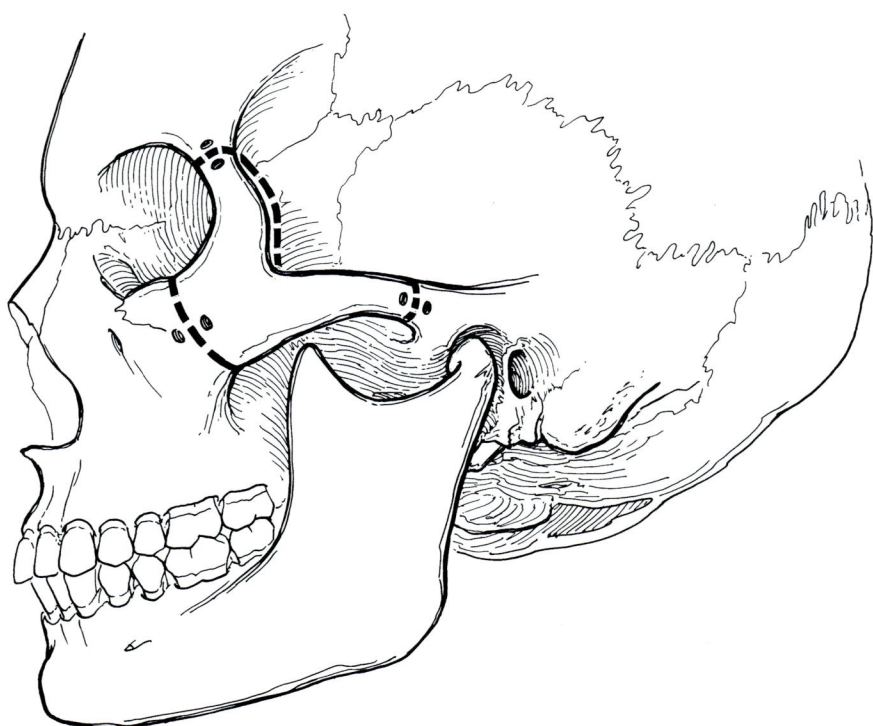

FIG. 17. Diagram illustrating the cuts in zygomatic ostectomy. Bone is preserved for later reconstruction. Note holes drilled for wire ligation. At least two holes are required if plate osteosynthesis is used. (From Donald PJ. Skull base surgery for sinus neoplasms. In: Donald PJ, Gluckman JL, Rice DH, eds. *The sinuses*. New York: Raven Press, 1995: 481.)

INFRATEMPORAL FOSSA–MIDDLE CRANIAL FOSSA APPROACH / 321

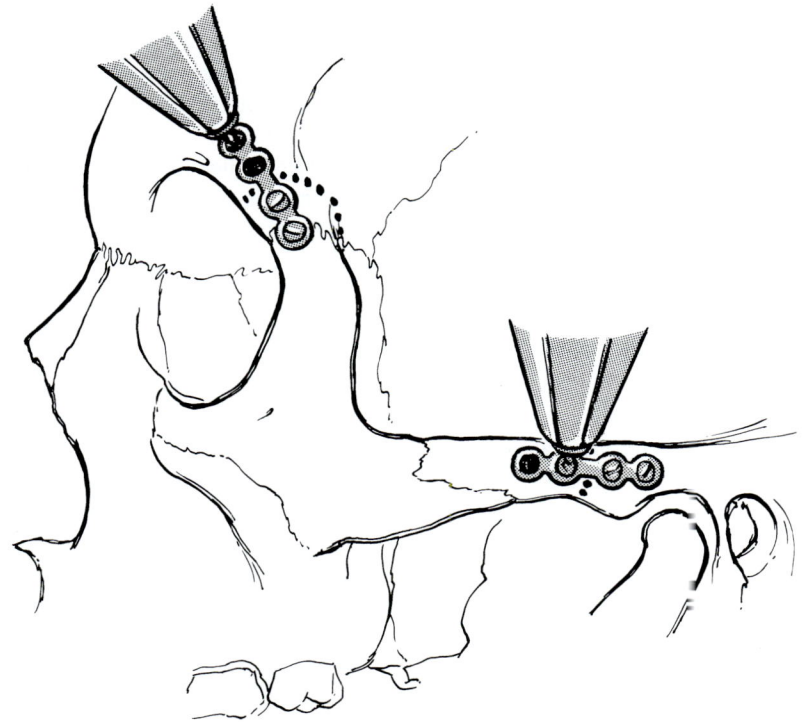

FIG. 18. Holes being drilled and plates applied, then removed for later osteosynthesis with the completion of the operation.

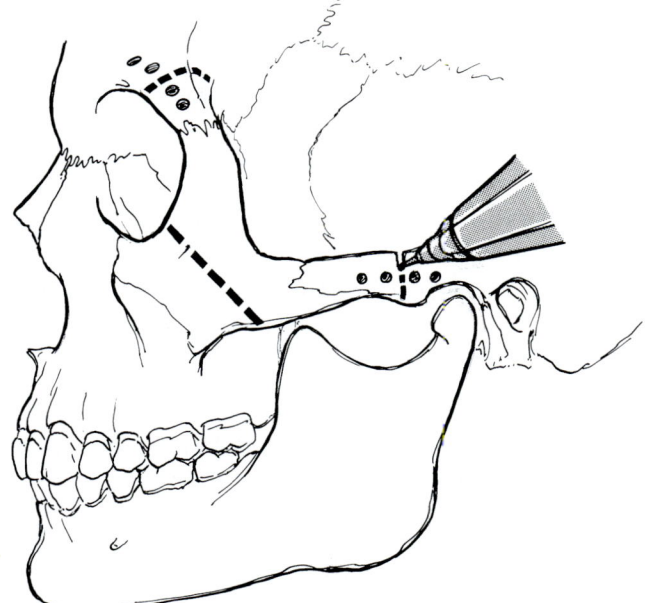

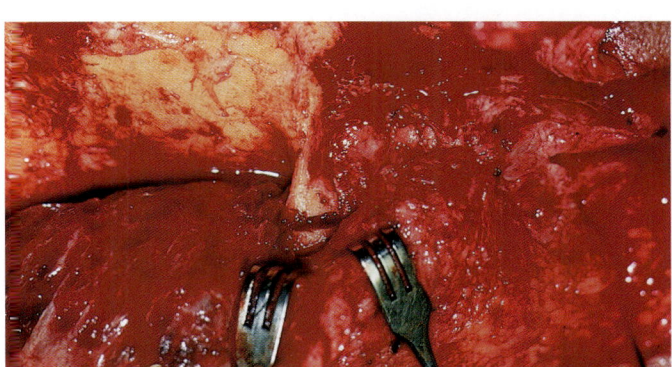

FIG. 19. Cut in front of articular eminence. **A:** Diagram. **B:** Completion of cut in patient.

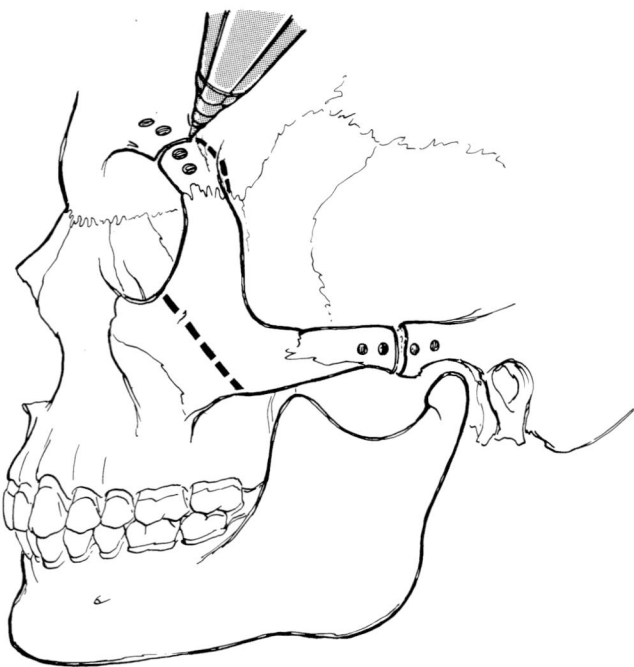

FIG. 20. Cutting tool cuts across the orbital rim to a depth of 2 to 4 mm until the thin lateral wall bone is encountered.

25). A malleable retractor is placed deep to the neck and the cutting tool used to transect it just below the condyle. Removal of the condyle is completed by dissecting the remaining soft tissue attachments on the deep and posterior surface of the joint. Both condyle and meniscus are removed. This exposes the glenoid fossa and opens the dissection of the subcranial part of the middle cranial fossa floor (Fig. 26).

Exposure of Subtemporal Trapezoid

With the zygomatic arch and the condyle removed, the temporalis muscle can be dissected down to its insertion on the coronoid process and anterior surface of the mandibular ramus. As this dissection continues and the muscle is carefully retracted inferiorly, an exposure of the undersurface of the sphenoid and temporal bones is gradually achieved (Fig. 27). The glenoid fossa is cleared of residual soft tissue, especially to expose the anteromedial aspect of the fossa, which leads to the sphenoid spine. Deep and anterior to the spine is the middle meningeal artery—the posteromedial target of the dissection at this point. A few millimeters anterior to it is the foramen ovale and the emergence of cranial nerve V3, the second medial target structure. Soft tissue dissection from the lateral orbital wall inferiorly leads to the origin of the pterygoid plates, the superior surfaces of the pterygoid muscles, and the pterygoid venous plexus.

Before describing the craniotomy, it is probably prudent to review those anatomic structures of the undersurface of the skull that form the floor of the middle cranial fossa. Head and neck surgeons, especially those with otolaryngologic backgrounds, have extensive training in the anatomy of the temporal bone. However, in traditional training, the undersurface of the bone and especially that of the sphenoid adjacent to it usually receive little attention.

If a line connects the articular eminence to the hamulus of the medial pterygoid plate, from this point to the occipital condyle and from thence to the mastoid process and back to the eminence, a trapezoid is inscribed (Fig. 28). All the important neurovascular structures relevant to the middle fossa skull base are contained within the confines of this figure. The two target structures for the inferomedial extent of the craniotomy, namely the foramen spinosum and foramen ovale, are seen as a direct line is made anteriorly from the anteromedial extremity of the glenoid fossa.

At this point, if doubt exists concerning intracranial spread of tumor up the mandibular branch of the trigeminal nerve, then this branch should be sampled for biopsy. If subcranial tumor is present, then the bone around the foramen ovale is drilled away and the nerve is exposed at the level of the middle fossa dura on the floor of Meckel's cave. The nerve is amputated at this point and sent for frozen-section histologic analysis (Fig. 29). If positive, the the craniotomy proceeds, with the first step being the otologic exposure.

Otologic Exposure

With the EAC transected at the bony–cartilagenous junction, the auricle is retracted posteriorly. There is often a few millimeters of thick canal skin, often with some remnants of conchal cartilage that need to be excised into the bony EAC. If the ear is to be obliterated, less care needs to be exercised in excising this skin because the entire remaining medial canal skin, in addition to the tympanic membrane, is to be removed. The operating microscope is brought in for the next phase.

When the middle ear is to be preserved, an anterior tympanomeatal flap is constructed (Fig. 30). The flap is cut through two incisions in the canal skin at approximately 6 and 12 o'clock, and connected laterally. The inferior incision is carried to the annulus and the superior incision approximately 2 mm short of the notch of Rivinus. The skin sleeve is dissected down the anterior canal wall to the tympanic annulus from the hypotympanic level up to the anterior mallear fold. The skin is elevated over the bone of the scutum and posteriorly to promote flap mobilization. The annulus is prized from its sulcus and the anterior hypotympanum and the entire protympanum exposed. The tympanomeatal flap is reflected posteriorly to provide full exposure of the tympanic portion of the eustachian tube and the hemicanal of the tensor tympani above it.

Two bony incisions in the EAC are constructed. The superior one starts at the squamosal part of the temporal bone directly above the EAC at 12 o'clock. The cut progresses through the bone until the temporal lobe dura is exposed for

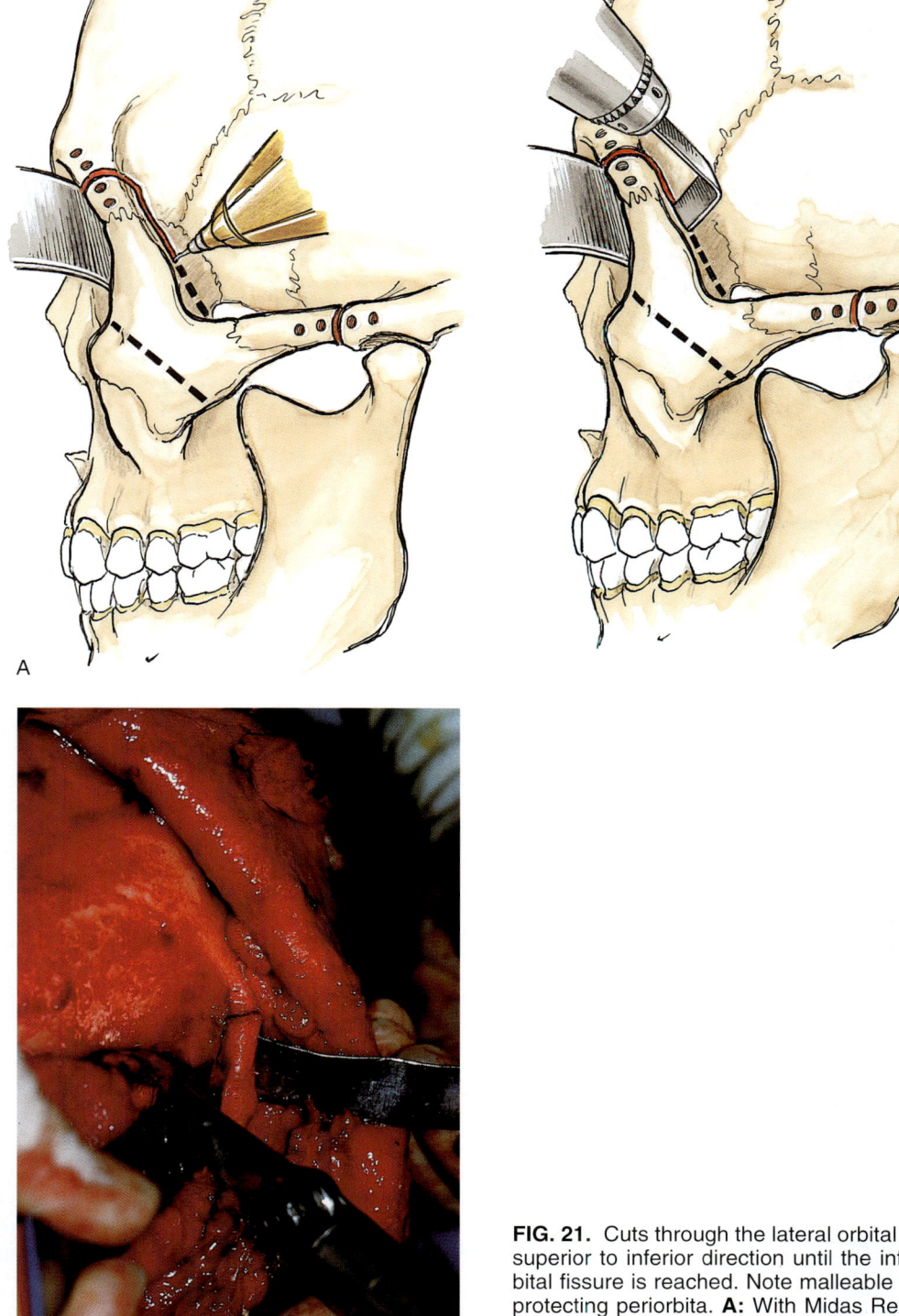

FIG. 21. Cuts through the lateral orbital wall in a superior to inferior direction until the inferior orbital fissure is reached. Note malleable retractor protecting periorbita. **A:** With Midas Rex cutting tool. **B:** With sagittal saw. **C:** Sagittal saw cut in patient.

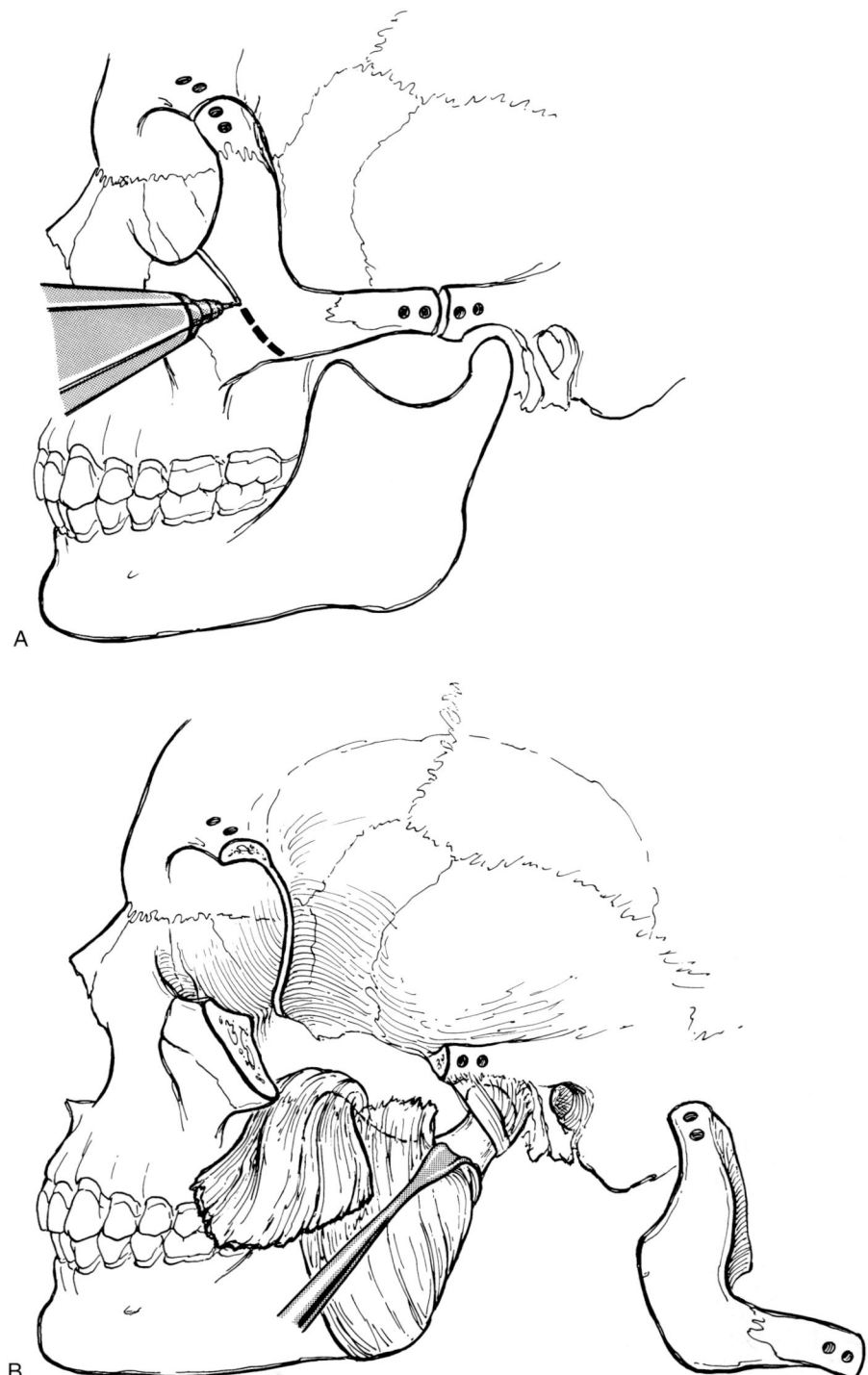

FIG. 22. Final cut through the posterior malar eminence extending to the inferior orbital fissure. **A:** Diagram illustrating cut. **B:** Bony excision complete.

INFRATEMPORAL FOSSA–MIDDLE CRANIAL FOSSA APPROACH / 325

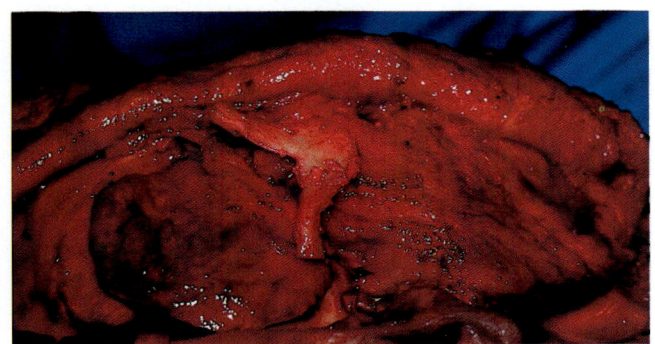

FIG. 23. Zygomatic excision complete in patient.

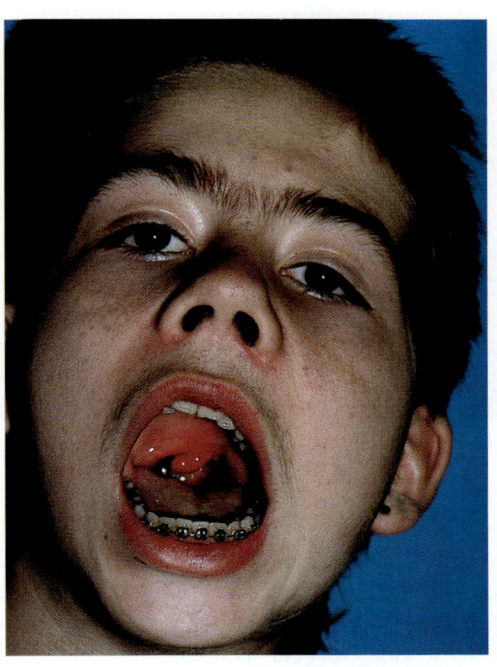

FIG. 24. Typical example of patient after condylectomy in infratemporal fossa–middle cranial fossa approach. Note no trismus but slight lateral sway on full opening.

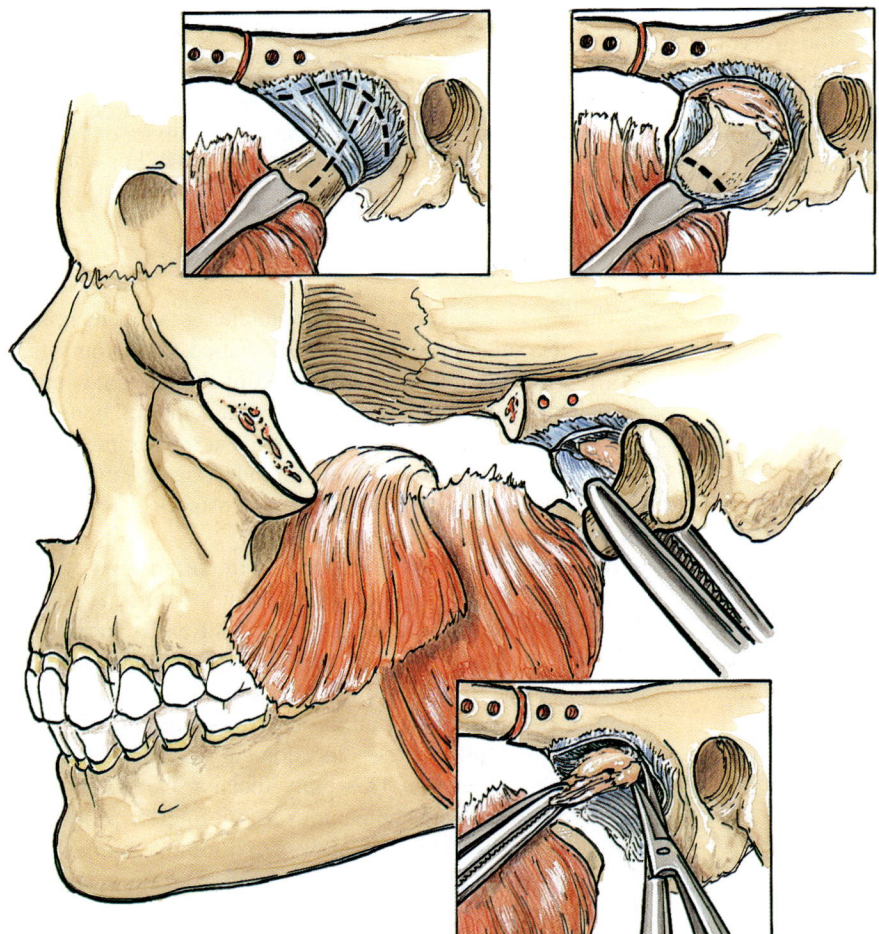

FIG. 25. Condylectomy: Lateral aspect of the temporomandibular joint capsule is opened and connected to a vertical incision in the periosteum of the mandibular neck. The condylar neck is transected and the condyle removed. The meniscus and attached soft tissue are removed.

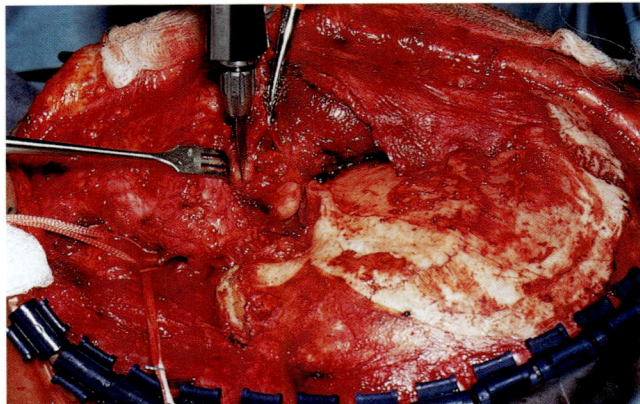

FIG. 26. Condyle removed.

a few millimeters and the floor of the middle fossa is reached. A drill cut is directed from this point to the anterior part of the epitympanum anterior to the mallear head. It is even better to angle this cut such that it goes through posterior zygomatic root cells, missing any view of the malleus at all. The anterior mallear ligaments are cut when exposed and the bur carried over the hemicanal of the tensor tympani, taking great care to stay anterior to the cochleaform process and thus missing the facial nerve. The hemicanal is transected and a deep groove made in the superior wall of the protympanum.

Inferiorly, a bur cut is made in the EAC bone at about 7:30 that goes through the tympanic bone into the glenoid fossa. The cut proceeds medially down the canal and into the inferior aspect of the protympanum at about 7 o'clock. The tympanic annulus is transected at this point and a fissure is again made in the protympanum, but less deep than the superior one in order to miss damaging the ICA. The subsequent craniotomy cuts will join up with these incisions in the temporal bone.

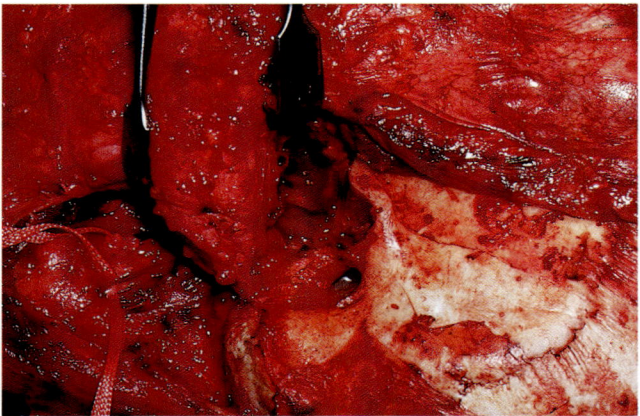

FIG. 27. View of infratemporal fossa with temporalis dissected down to coronoid process. Zygoma and condyle have been removed.

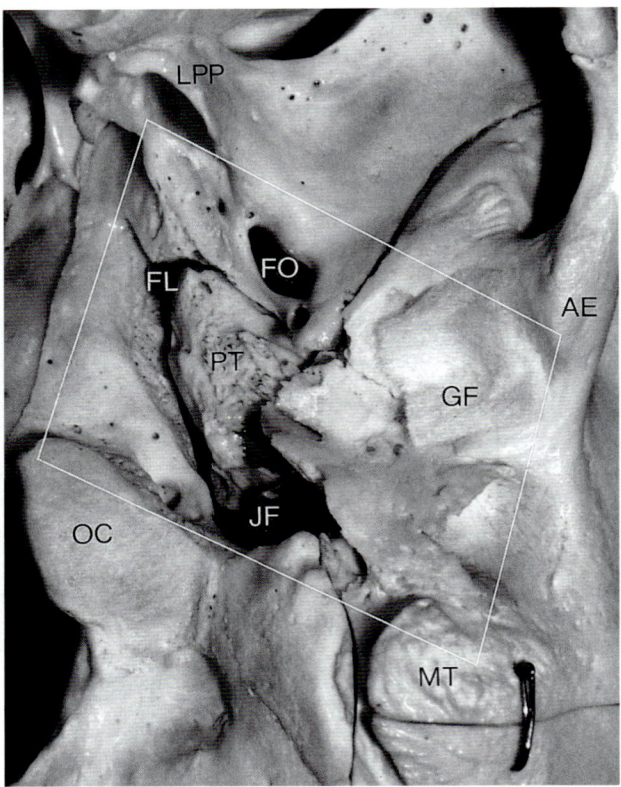

FIG. 28. The subtemporal trapezoid. *LPP,* lateral pterygoid plate; *AE,* articular eminence; *MT,* mastoid tip; *OC,* occipital condyle; *FL,* foramen lacerum; *FO,* foramen ovale; *GF,* glenoid fossa; *JF,* jugular foramen; *PT,* petrous tip. (From Donald PJ. *Head and neck cancer: management of the difficult case.* Philadelphia: WB Saunders, 1984:286, with permission.)

Craniotomy

The key to the exposure of the middle fossa and its immediate subcranial structures is an L-shaped craniotomy that has a vertical component comprised of the greater wing of the sphenoid and squamosal aspect of the temporal bone, and a short horizontal component that ends at the foramen ovale and foramen spinosum. Often a modest-sized craniotomy provides adequate exposure. The size usually is predicated on intracranial tumor extent.

Initially, it is advisable to perform the inferior part of the craniotomy, only a part of which exposes dura. A switch from the otologic round bur to the Midas Rex B_5 attachment enhances the speed at which these inferior bony cuts can be made. A through-and-through incision is made through the anterior EAC bone into and through the glenoid fossa plate. The complete full-thickness incision cut stops at the level of the tympanic annulus. This bony incision carries into the mesotympanum from the annulus to the inferior protympanum at a depth of approximately 2 to 3 mm. A similar incision of the same depth is made in the glenoid fossa and carried from the annulus to the foramen spinosum. Too deep a cut endangers the ICA. The middle meningeal artery is

INFRATEMPORAL FOSSA–MIDDLE CRANIAL FOSSA APPROACH / 327

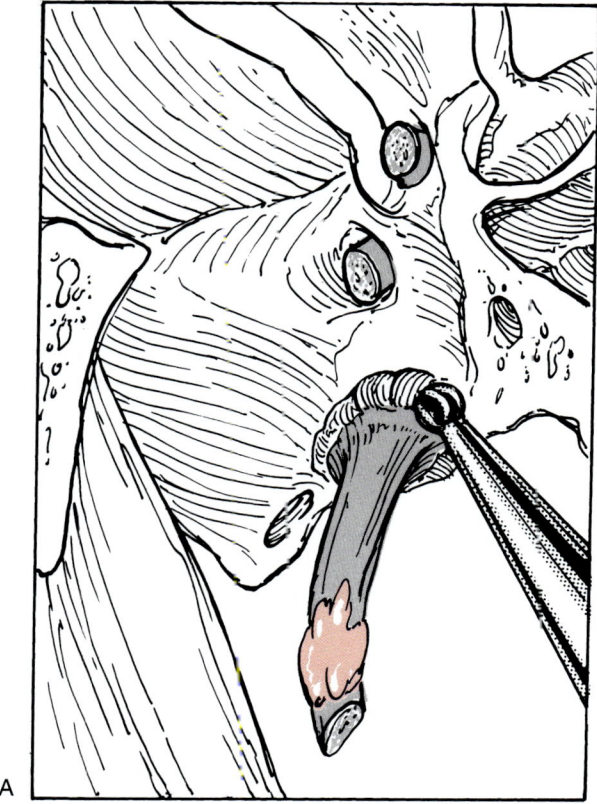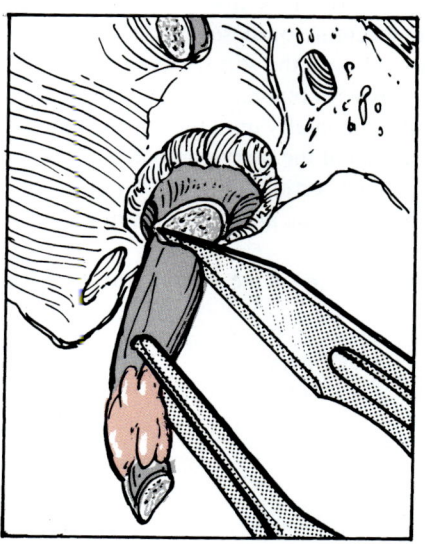

FIG. 29. A: The bone from the edges of foramen ovale is drilled away to expose the mandibular branch of the trigeminal nerve's emergence from the dural sleeve from Meckel's cave on the middle fossa floor. **B:** The nerve is amputated flush with the dura and sent for frozen-section histologic analysis.

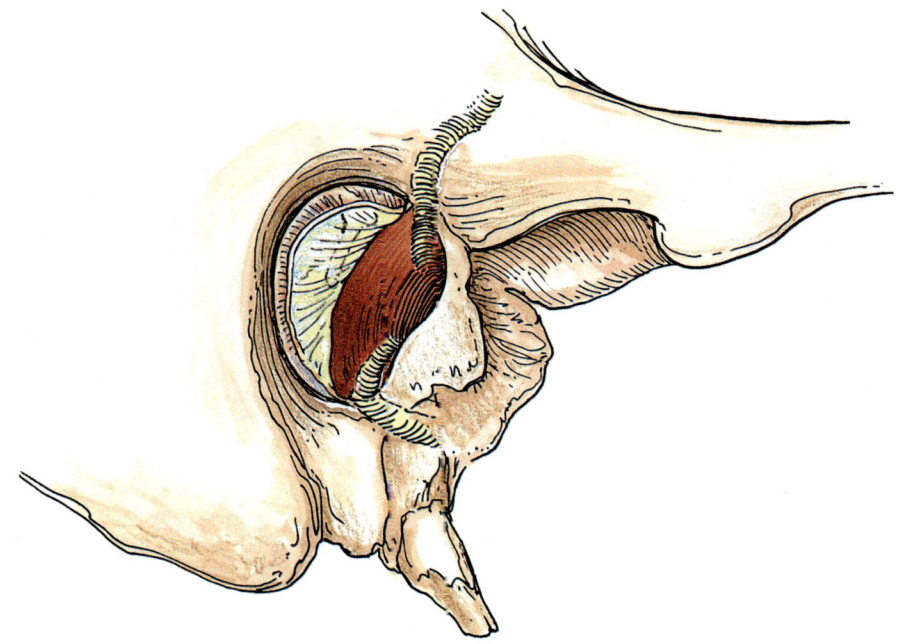

FIG. 30. Anterior tympanomeatal flap retracted, exposing the tympanic opening of the eustachian tube. The superior and inferior cuts into the protympanum are outlined.

clipped or coagulated with the bipolar cautery. The foramen spinosum is connected to the posterior lip of the foramen ovale (Fig. 31). The dura is exposed in this incision from the foramen spinosum anteriorly. Sometimes venous extensions of the cavernous sinus may invest the foraminal portion of V3. Inadvertent rupture of these vessels often occurs during the bony cuts and even the soft tissue extension. The bleeding usually stops with bipolar cautery. Anteriorly, this incision is carried horizontally until the cutting tool reaches just above the insertion of the pterygoid plates. This point marks the beginning of the vertical course of the craniotomy. It will proceed superiorly in the anterior reach of the infratemporal fossa.

The inferior portion of the craniotomy has been mostly done, and now the superior part over the greater sphenoid wing and squamosal temporal bone proceeds (Fig. 32). How high the craniotomy extends is mainly predicated on the degree of invasion of temporal lobe dura. Often, only the dura of the floor of the middle fossa is involved, and only a more limited craniotomy is required.

A bur hole is made at or inferior to the pterion with the M_5 bur of the Midas Rex or a standard craniotome. Dural elevation permits the introduction of the footed handpiece and the craniotomy proceeds in a posterior superior loop until it ends at the dural exposure at the top of the otologic incision superior to the EAC. The handpiece is removed and reinserted into the bur hole and directed inferiorly to the previously made cut above the pterygoid plates.

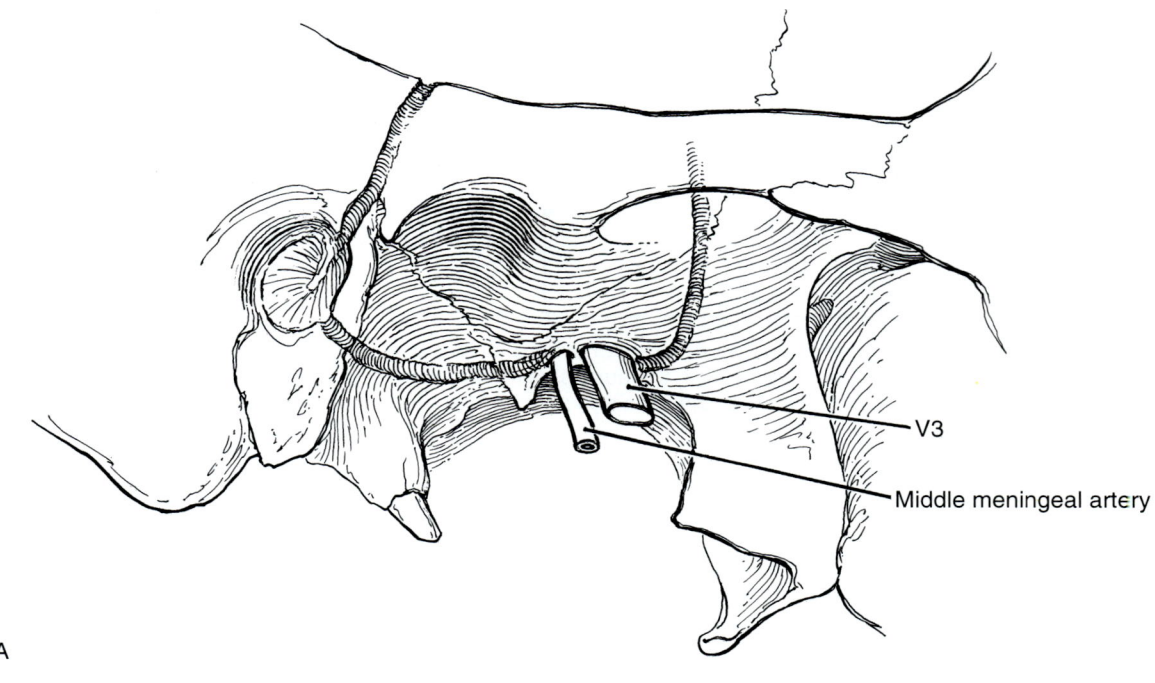

A

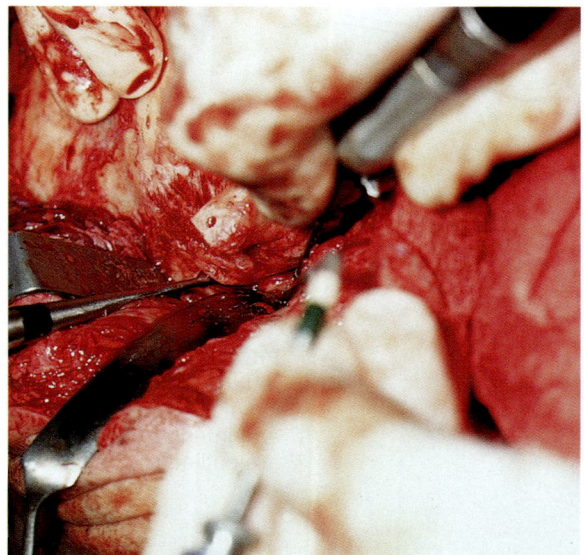

B

FIG. 31. Inferior cut connecting foramen spinosum to foramen ovale. **A:** Close-up view of inferior aspect of cut through the external auditory canal and glenoid fossa, and connecting the foramen spinosum to the foramen ovale. (From Donald PJ. Skull base surgery for sinus neoplasms. In: Donald PJ, Gluckman JL, Rice DH, eds. *The sinuses.* New York: Raven Press, 1995:483.) **B:** In patient.

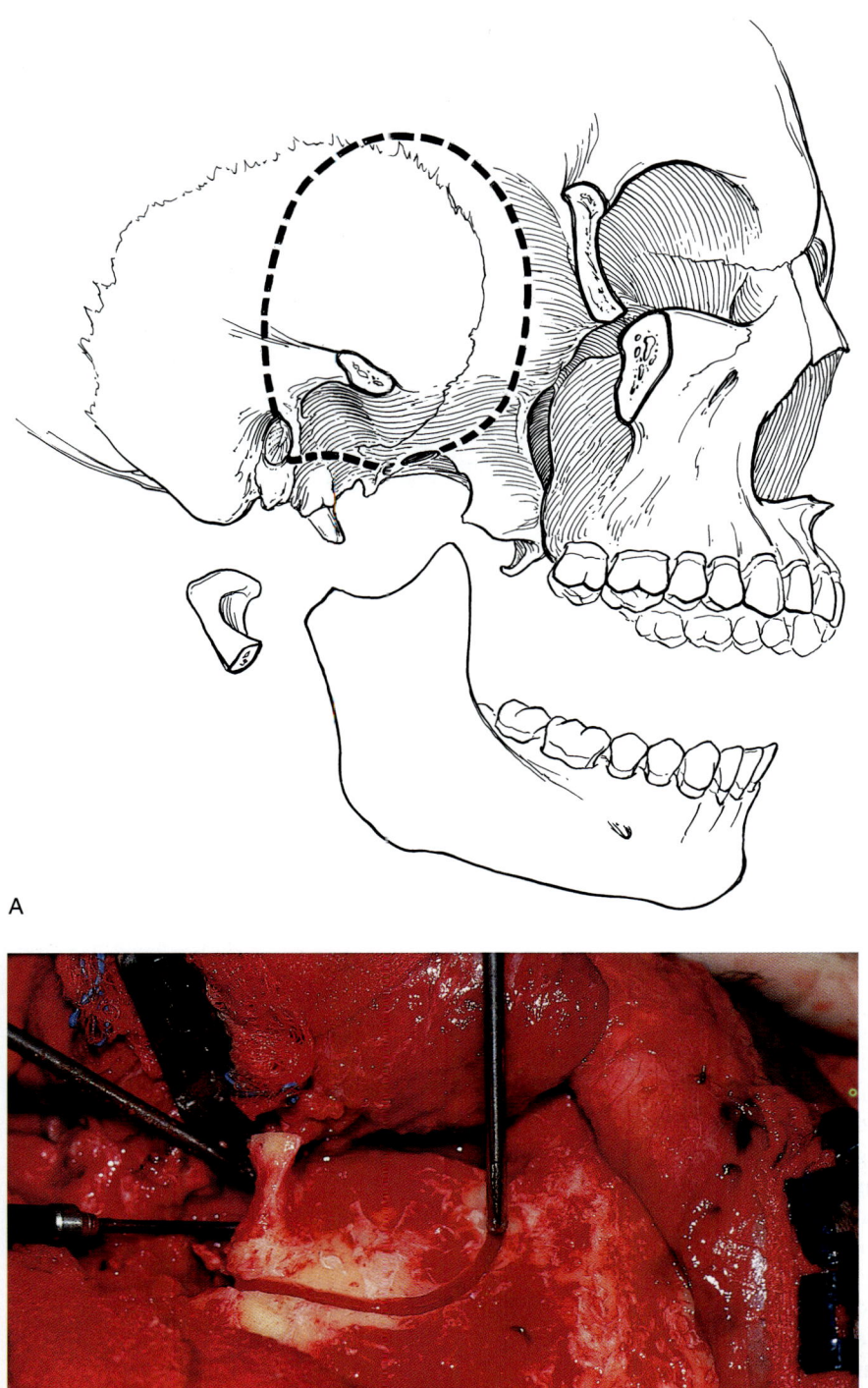

FIG. 32. L-shaped craniotomy. A: Diagram outlining cuts. B: Craniotomy outlined in patient.

Careful dural elevation is done at the periphery of the bone cuts, with special attention given to its brittleness in the elderly. A broad elevator is used to dissect the dura from the superior craniotomy incision to the middle fossa floor. A gentle prying motion fractures the craniotomy bone flap through the previously drilled faults in the temporal bone (Fig. 33). The fracture will be through the lateral wall of the bony eustachian tube. This is a crucial maneuver. The open eustachian tube reveals the bulge of the ICA canal in its medial wall. Sometimes the bony wall is dehiscent and carotid pulsations can be visualized through the tubal mucosa. This relationship is the vital key to the safe dissection of the carotid. At this point, the vertical portion of the artery is bending into the horizontal part.

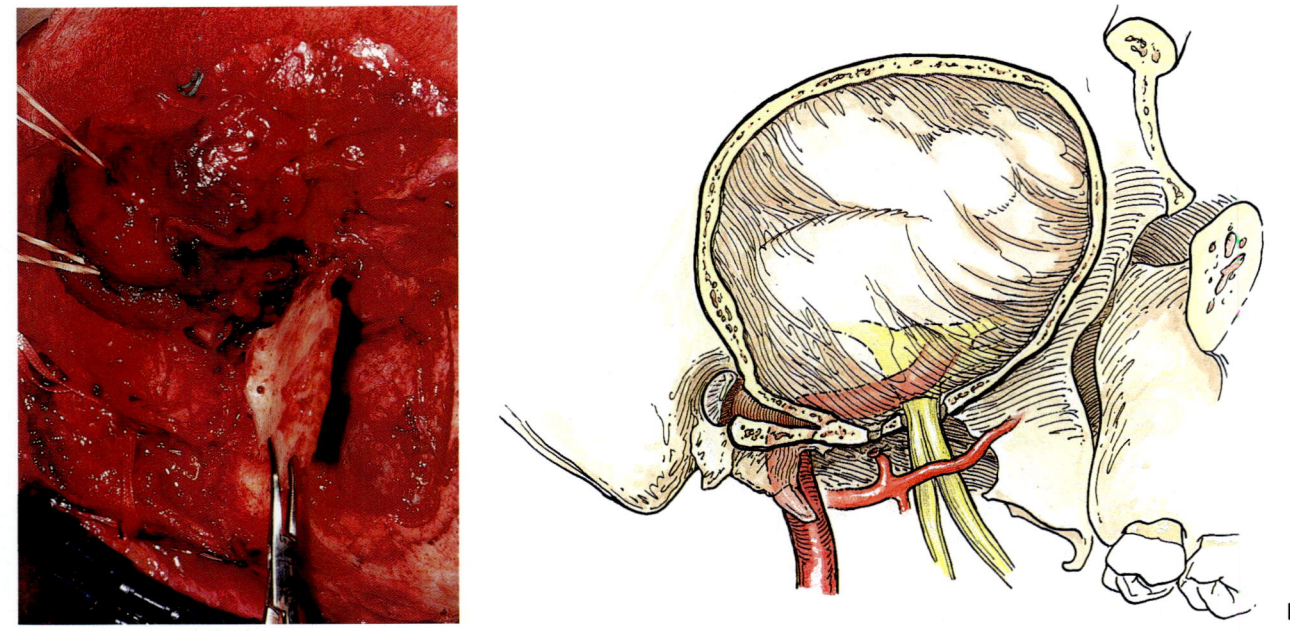

FIG. 33. Craniotomy performed. **A:** Elevator prying craniotomy flap in patient. **B:** Flap removed. Note the bone flap has been fractured across the eustachian tube. V3 is exposed as it emanates from its dural sleeve.

The cut through the foramen ovale shows the mandibular branch of the trigeminal nerve as it approximates the dura that invests it.

Carotid Dissection and Eustachian Tube

Two principal structures make middle fossa surgery difficult: the ICA and the cavernous sinus. The ICA is exposed as much as is necessary to resect all tumor. Once identified in the medial wall of the bony eustachian tube, the vertical portion of the artery is uncovered by beginning at the fibrous ring at the carotid foramen and working superiorly to the tube. The carotid canal is progressively exposed by removing bone first laterally, then anteriorly, posteriorly, and even medially when required.

The bony eustachian tube is now removed with the drill, gradually exposing the ICA. The artery often parallels the tube for a short distance, but then the tube angles inferiorly and away from the vessels. The bony tube quickly gives way to cartilage because the latter comprises two thirds of its length. The cartilage is a little more difficult to drill, but is excised as far as is necessary to expose the artery. In nasopharyngeal carcinoma and other tumors with tubal involvement, usually all of the cartilaginous tube is excised and the bone in which it nestles is removed wide of all tumor invasion. This approach is especially suited to nasopharyngeal carcinoma resection because the entire eustachian tube, the origins of the palatal muscles, and all adjacent bone can be widely resected. In all other approaches to nasopharyngeal malignancy, this is not possible. This is the most direct and by far the safest method to encompass this disease. The artery lies under a very thin layer of bone on the middle fossa floor. The bone here is often dehiscent in spots. In its more medial course, it underlies the gasserian ganglion, which may need to be sacrificed if carotid involvement by tumor extends this far (Fig. 34).

The bony removal continues under microscopic control up to the foramen lacerum. The artery then resumes a vertical course through the middle fossa floor into the cavernous sinus. The artery is now fully mobilized (when required by tumor involvement) from the fibrous ring to the foramen lacerum (Fig. 35A). Any middle fossa floor invaded by tumor is resected.

The tough periosteal lining of the carotid canal provides a firm barrier to the penetration of even the most malignant tumors. As described in Chapter 4, the connective tissue and adventitia of the artery all provide barriers to tumor extension. The treatment algorithm in Table 2 describes the decision-making approach to patients with ICA invasion by tumors of various degrees of malignancy. Most patients can have the carotid spared if tumor invasion is only into the periosteum. Low-grade malignancies, even with penetration of arterial adventitia, permit arterial sparing. Carotid penetration or even adventitial involvement by high-grade malignancies such as squamous cell carcinoma require carotid artery resection.

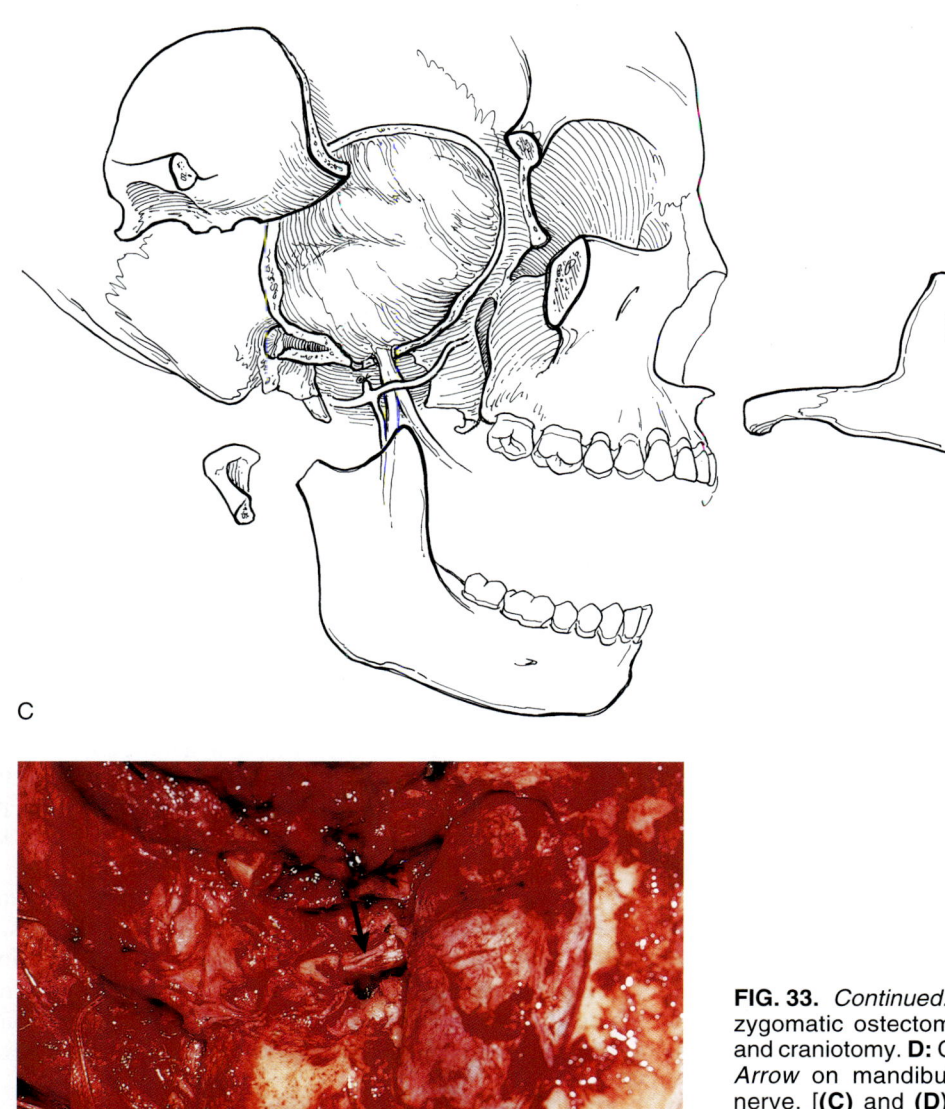

FIG. 33. *Continued.* **C:** Summary of steps thus far: zygomatic ostectomy, mandibular condylectomy, and craniotomy. **D:** Craniotomy complete in patient. *Arrow* on mandibular branch of the trigeminal nerve. [**(C)** and **(D)** from Donald PJ. Skull base surgery for sinus neoplasms. In: Donald PJ, Gluckman JL, Rice DH, eds. *The sinuses.* New York: Raven Press, 1995:485 **(C)**, 486 **(D)**.]

The management of carotid invasion has undergone some evolution since the early to mid-1980s. For a long time, invasion of the carotid by malignancy was thought to carry the stigma of a hopeless prognosis. Some studies following patients with carotid involvement in the neck have revealed a prognosis of about 20% to 25% 2-year and longer tumor-free survival (3,4). No good follow-up study of the prognosis of patients with intracranial carotid involvement and resection has been done. Using the cervical carotid paradigm in such tumors, a similar outcome might be expected if all tumor is excised with adequate margins. Unfortunately, intracranial carotid resection has met with limited success in the author's series. A redesign of the operation, increasing the radicality of resection of the cavernous sinus in which the ICA resides, may improve results.

Decisions regarding carotid artery management center around two main features. The first is the biology of the tumor in question, and the second involves the anatomic site of invasion. For the most part, benign tumors and low-grade malignancies tend to have pushing rather than infiltrating borders. The acinic cell and adenoid cystic carcinomas tend to be quite infiltrative extracranially, but are a pushing, less aggressive type of tumor intracranially. Squamous cell carcinomas and malignant melanoma, on the other hand, are more locally aggressive. The anatomic location along the course of the carotid also determines the extent of resection. The fibrous ring at the entrance to the skull base is very dense and thick, providing a protective barrier to the penetration of even squamous cell carcinoma. Sometimes the ring can be dissected to the arterial media and the tumor encom-

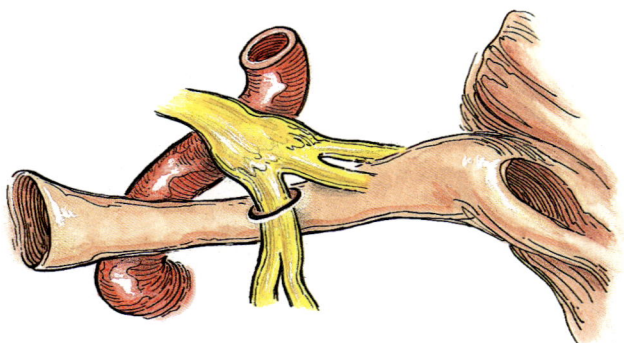

FIG. 34. Diagram summarizing the course and relationships of the petrous internal carotid artery to key structures. It is crossed anterolaterally by the eustachian tube and mediosuperiorly by the gasserian ganglion.

TABLE 2. *Treatment algorithm based on tumor histologic type and depth of carotid canal invasion*

1. Periosteum of canal	→ Artery preservation
2. Adventitia	
Benign	⎱ Artery preservation
"Low-grade malignancy"	⎰
High-grade malignancy	→ Artery resection Resection + graft
3. Media	→ Artery resection Resection + graft

passed. The petrous course of the carotid also has a configuration that resists tumor penetration. Janecka and Prassad did an excellent study elucidating the anatomy of the petrous canal (see Fig. 14, Chapter 4). The inner surface of the canal is lined with periosteum. A loose connective tissue containing a few small nutrient blood vessels connects the periosteum to the denser collagenous tissue comprising the arterial adventitia. Next comes the arterial media and intima. The vessel is suspended within the canal and possesses three barriers for tumor to breach before actual arterial invasion takes place. Table 2 depicts a treatment algorithm based on tumor histologic type and depth of invasion of the carotid canal.

The cavernous carotid has very thin connective tissue on most of its wall. The medial wall is plastered to the cavernous sinus dura and is intimately related to the intracranial side of the lateral wall of the sphenoid sinus. Spread of tumor to the main body of the cavernous sinus usually leads to carotid invasion. The arterial wall is thin and easily penetrated by tumor.

The safety of ICA excision in its cranial course without the placement of a graft is very much open to question. Even a negative BTO coupled with a satisfactory SPECT scan or xenon flow scan indicating adequate flow does not guarantee the avoidance of stroke. This is especially true during periods of unplanned postoperative hypotension (see Fig. 35B). If the artery must be excised, the current wisdom is to use an interposition graft. The saphenous vein is probably the best graft material, although synthetics may be used.

Once removed, the graft is placed quickly while the patient is under barbiturate coma (Fig. 36). The patient is heparinized during graft placement, then reversed with protamine once all leaks have been sealed. Clamp time is kept to a minimum.

The carotid resection and graft are done with microscopic control. All preliminary steps such as vascular sutures, instruments, and alternative graft materials must be readily at hand before clamping of the vessel. Adequate exposure at the distal and proximal ends of the artery, leaving room to clamp, then excise the vessel with an adequate cuff to sew, is

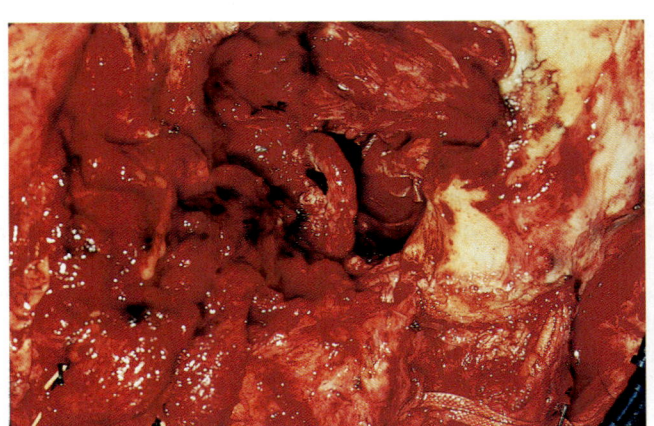
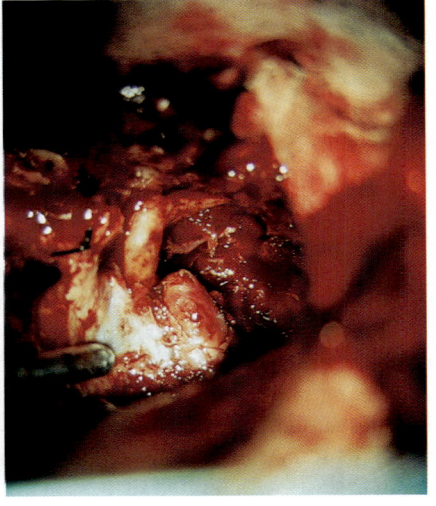

FIG. 35. **A:** Petrous internal carotid artery (ICA) dissected to the foramen lacerum. **B:** View of cavernous sinus under microscope just before resection of the ICA. The patient died of a stroke 48 hours after surgery after an episode of hypotension.

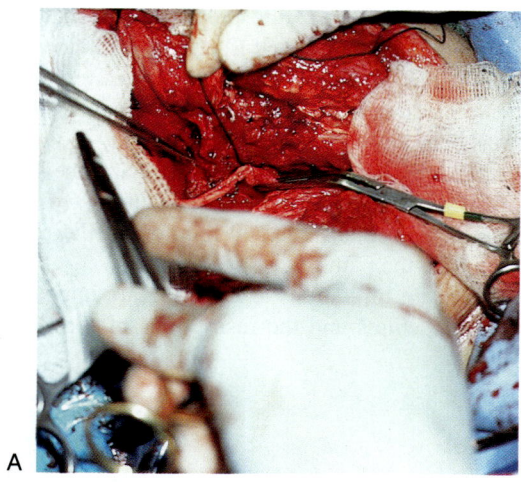
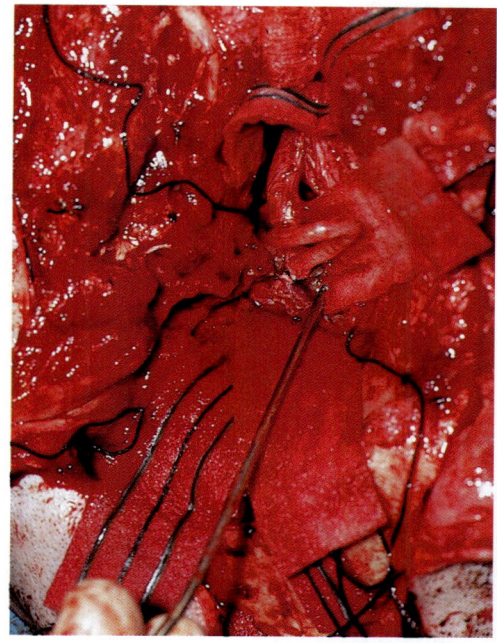

FIG. 36. Internal carotid artery (ICA) replaced with saphenous vein. **A:** Vein graft being sewn in place. **B:** Flow in graft restores continuity of ICA flow.

ensured. Total mobilization of the artery from the cervical part to the cavernous portion facilitates this. Once both anastomoses are completed, the clamps are removed, the leaks oversewn, and Gelfoam patches soaked in thrombin are placed around the suture lines.

Cavernous Sinus

The cavernous sinus resection often precedes the management of the carotid. The artery is freed from its canal, and if tumor persists beyond the petrous part, the cavernous sinus is resected. Small outpouchings of the sinus (see Figs. 10 and 24, Chapter 4) project along the three branches of the trigeminal nerve as they enter their foramina. In addition, there are a myriad of connections to other veins and dural sinuses. Minimal invasion at these sites can limit the amount of the sinus removed. Frozen-section examination of these margins is critical.

Major invasion of the sinus (Fig. 37) tends to compress the venous structures within, and dissection proceeds rather easily until the invasive edge is reached. The profuse hemorrhage characteristic of this structure is then encountered. Not only must the soft tissue component of the sinus be removed, but the adjacent bone as well.

Cavernous dissection is done under the operating microscope in a slow and methodical manner. Because of its propensity for brisk hemorrhage, it must be removed piecemeal. Once the relatively avascular areas of frank tumor involvement are passed, the sinus that still possesses microscopic residua is systematically removed. Bleeding is often profuse and troublesome. A small area of sinus is cleared, thrombin-soaked Gelfoam pledgets are placed and held over that area with a cottonoid, and the adjacent area of the sinus then removed. Liberal use of the bipolar cautery and hemostatic gauze aids in hemorrhage control. Each grossly normal piece of tissue removed is submitted for frozen-section analysis. In this way, little by little, the entire cavernous sinus is removed. With major involvement of the sinus, the carotid will need removal in most cases. The lateral wall of the sphenoid sinus, a portion of the middle fossa floor, a portion of

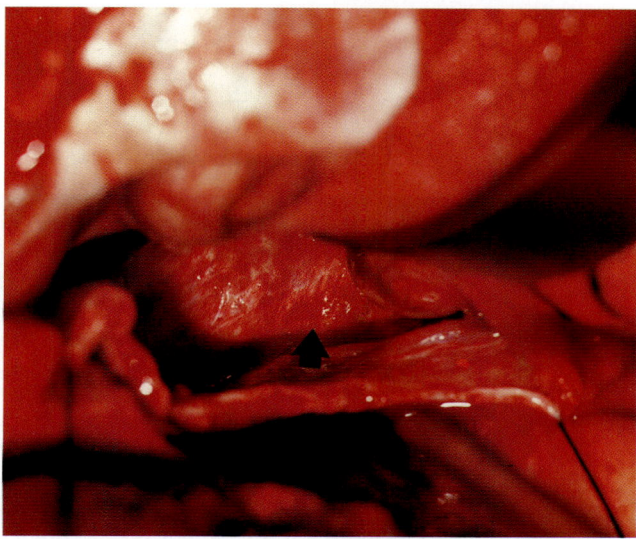

FIG. 37. Cavernous sinus (*arrow*) full of nasopharyngeal carcinoma.

the petrous tip, and, at times, the bone surrounding the superior orbital fissure are removed. Hemostasis is required at the basilar plexus, the superior petrosal sinus, the circular sinus, ophthalmic veins, and the vein of Vesalius. In addition, two or more cerebral veins enter the sinus as well and may require control.

Dura and Brain Resection

Dural invasion varies from minimal involvement at the neural and vascular foramina at the sites of entry into the intracranial space, to widespread involvement characteristic of recurrent tumors after full-course radiation therapy. Sometimes the dura is replaced almost entirely by tumor tissue. The pushing nature of the upper aerodigestive tract tumors has been fully discussed in Chapter 4. A cuff of 5 to 10 mm of grossly healthy dura is excised and the periphery examined by frozen-section analysis. Often grossly normal dura has tumor extensions and requires further resection as dictated by the pathologist's report.

Certain limitations to resection are imposed by vital central structures and the restrictions of certain reconstructive

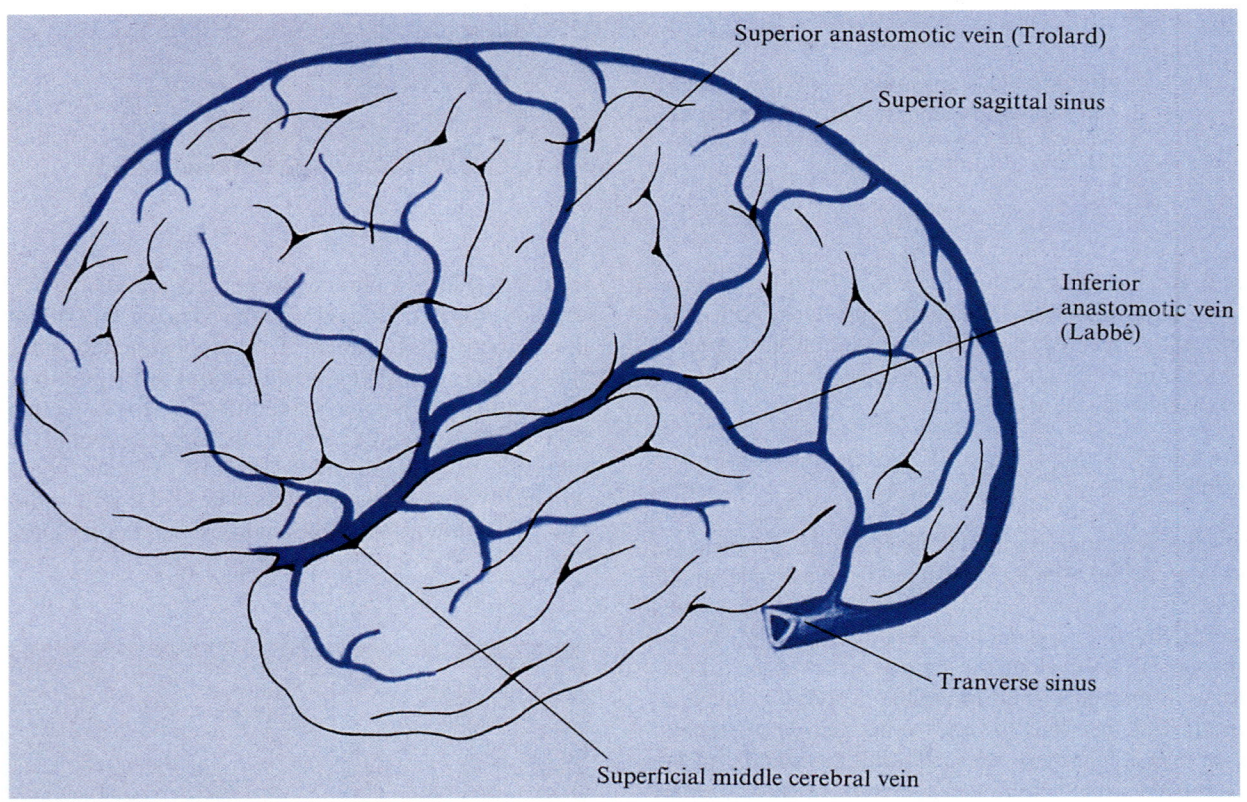

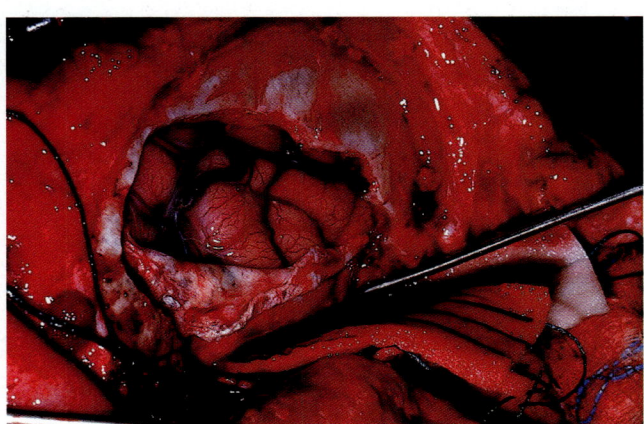

FIG. 38. A: The inferior anastomotic vein of Labbé draining into the sigmoid sinus. **B:** The vein of Labbé, seen in a patient with a dural tear.

options. In the middle fossa, the two major structures that impede further dural excision are the vein of Labbé and the superior sagittal sinus. The vein of Labbé, or inferior anastomotic cerebral vein, drains into the lateral sinus at a variable distance from the sigmoid sinus (Fig. 38). If the superior anastomotic vein of Trolard is not patent or is of small caliber, the vein of Labbé will be the only vein draining the entire ipsilateral cerebral hemisphere. To sacrifice it would then result in a massive infarction and often death. Cerebral venography may establish the venous drainage pattern in those patients in whom the vein of Labbé is in jeopardy.

The superior sagittal sinus can usually be safely obliterated in the anterior fossa from the anterior fossa floor up to the coronal suture. The middle fossa component cannot be ligated because in most instances it will lead to quadriplegia and often death. Fortunately, few skull base tumors extend that far (Fig. 39).

The second dural restriction concerns the potential for dural reconstruction and the provision of a watertight seal. As dural resection along the clivus and under the brainstem increases in extent, there is a progressive increase in difficulty in obtaining a sound dural closure. A cerebrospinal fluid (CSF) leak at this site is an open avenue to the nasopharynx, which possesses one of the highest concentrations of pathogenic bacteria in the entire upper aerodigestive tract (5,6). Tissue glue helps, but a suture line is superior in strength. For most fibrin glues, the adhesive strength is lost in about 1 week.

Brain resection is controversial. Much of the reluctance is a reflection of the neurosurgical experience with primary brain tumors. Most of these lesions are multifocal in character, with a large primary site and multiple satellite lesions in discontinuity. A sufficient margin of healthy, uninvolved tissue that skirts all areas of tumor involvement is often not feasible without engendering serious neurologic side effects. As detailed in Chapter 4, upper aerodigestive tract carcinomas have a more pushing type of edge and can be encompassed by a narrower resection margin.

Silent areas of the brain such as the frontal lobes and the anterior part of the temporal lobes can be sacrificed with impunity. As the more posterior aspect of the temporal lobe is reached, especially on the dominant side, speech disturbance may be encountered. As seen in Chapter 4, local control can be achieved with brain resection in a high percentage of patients. Meningeal carcinomatosis in the author's experience is a distinctly rare event, having been seen in only two cases.

Reconstruction

The key procedure in the reconstruction is to separate the intracranial cavity from the upper aerodigestive tract with a watertight seal whenever possible. Infection will not only produce meningitis or, worse, an abscess, but may cause spontaneous rupture of the ICA. An arterial graft is particularly vulnerable to such exposure. Fascia lata, temporalis fascia, or allograft is used to patch resected dura (Fig. 40). Careful suturing, especially on the inferior aspects above the clivus, is essential. The closure may be augmented with tissue glue.

The next layer comprises muscle. The temporalis muscle, if preserved, is placed under and across the craniotomy site. The pericranial cuff is sutured to the basipharyngeal fascia of the nasopharynx (Fig. 41). In this way, the potential dead space left by resected soft tissues under the sphenoid bone

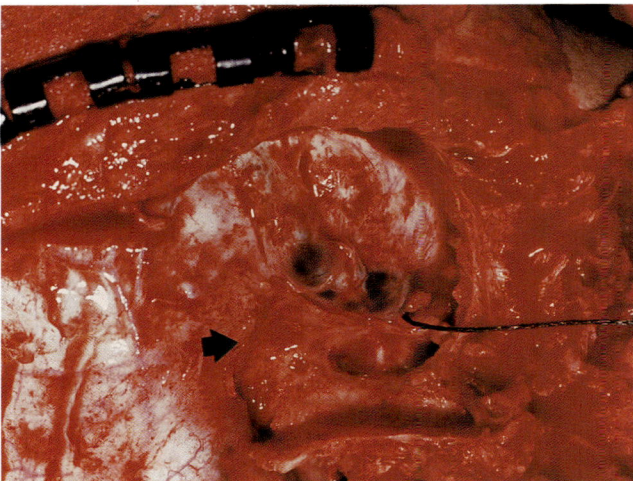

FIG. 39. Adenoid cystic carcinoma with extensive spread in dura close to the superior sagittal sinus (*arrow*).

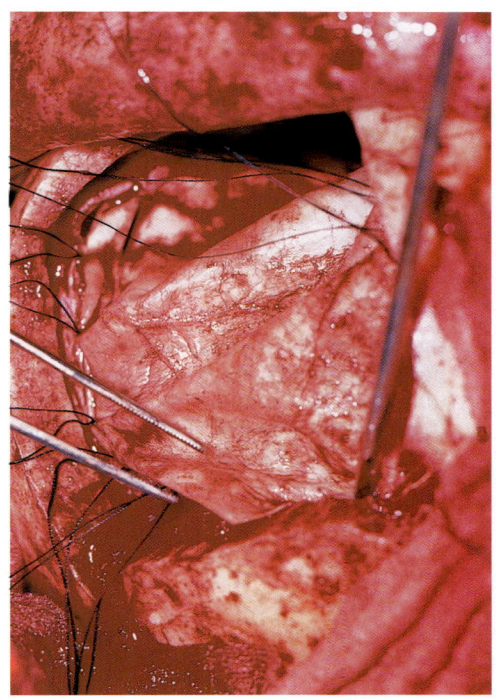

FIG. 40. Dura of temporal lobe patched with lyophilized dura.

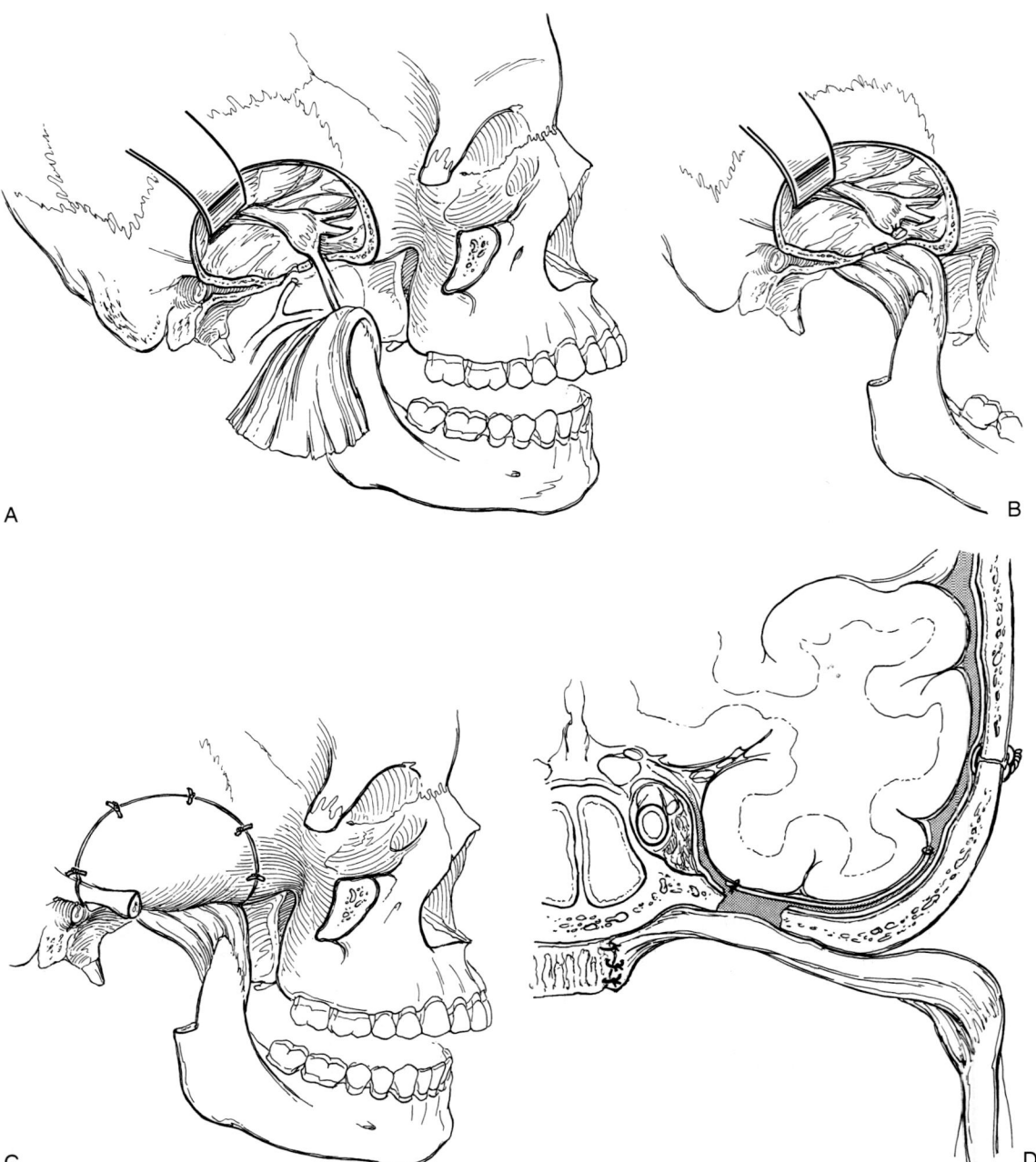

FIG. 41. A: Temporalis muscle flap. **B:** The temporalis muscle is placed across the craniotomy defect below the middle fossa floor and into the nasopharynx. **C:** Craniotomy flap restored and muscle flap turned in. **D:** Coronal view showing suture of pericranial attachment of the temporal muscle to the basipharyngeal fascia. (From Donald PJ. Skull base surgery for sinus neoplasms. In: Donald PJ, Gluckman JL, Rice DH, eds. *The sinuses.* New York: Raven Press, 1995:487.)

can be obliterated. The integrity of the muscle is carefully ensured before this step.

Other myogenous or musculocutaneous flaps can be alternatively used if the temporalis flap has questionable viability. The sternocleidomastoid muscle has been used when the resection has not progressed too far medially from the foramen ovale. It is too short to reach the nasopharynx. Its blood supply from the occipital artery should be preserved. A cuff of clavicular periosteum helps hold the sutures.

The posterior trapezius flap has been well described by Netterville and Jackson (see Chapter 32) and provides excellent muscle bulk and cutaneous cover when skin involvement requires wide excision. The drawback lies in the repositioning of the patient that is needed during this phase of the operation. The pectoralis major musculocutaneous flap produces satisfactory reconstruction, especially if there is extensive pharyngeal resection or cutaneous loss (Fig. 42). The patient's upper torso and neck length must, however, be compatible so that there is sufficient flap length to allow a tension-free closure. The muscle bulk of both this and the trapezius flap amply efface the subcranial deficit. Unfortunately, flap length has often been a problem.

The most utilitarian flap is the rectus abdominis myogenous free flap, which can bring skin if required (Fig. 43). Bringing fresh vascularized tissue into the wound greatly enhances healing. Although there is often a resulting facial asymmetry created by the muscle bulk and the skin paddle that is commonly brought up as an indicator of flap viability, this can be revised at a later date, producing a fine cosmetic result (Fig. 44). The flap is usually pedicled on the deep inferior epigastric artery and vein and is sewn into the external carotid artery and IJV. The donor site is reinforced with Marlex mesh when below the arcuate line. The anterior rectus sheath remnants are approximated when possible, and the skin usually closed primarily. The flap is inset so that the

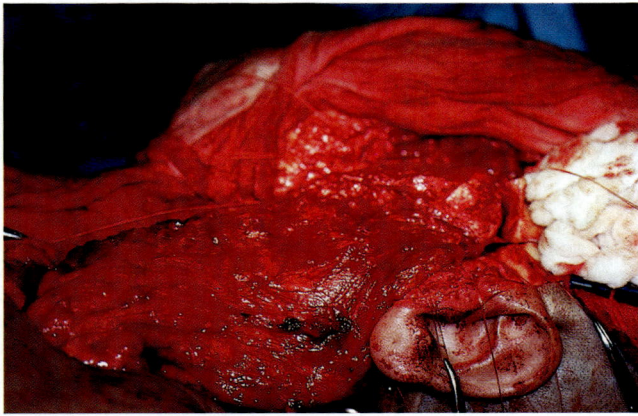

FIG. 42. Pectoralis major musculocutaneous flap used to reconstruct infratemporal fossa and undersurface of the middle fossa. A large skin paddle was required to reconstruct the pharynx from the nasopharynx to the vallecula.

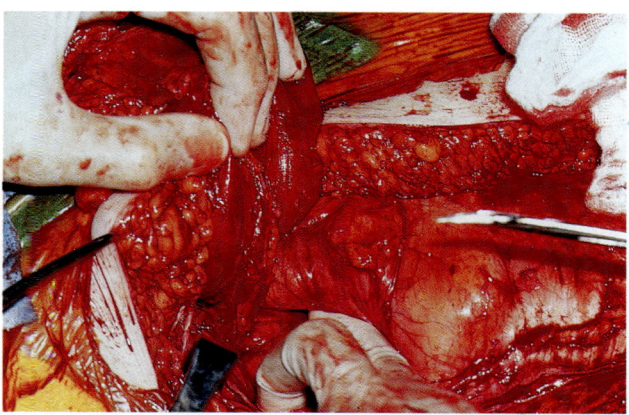

FIG. 43. Rectus abdominis flap being elevated.

muscle extends into the resected nasopharynx, and secured as well as possible to the pharyngobasilar fascia. The vital point is to ensure that an adequate paddle of soft tissue is interposed between the dural repair, the exposed ICA, and the upper aerodigestive tract. Sometimes, the skin paddle is required to line the pharynx when it is extensively resected. Whenever possible, muscle is carried superiorly into the infratemporal fossa to aid in ablating the cosmetic defect caused by the absence or atrophy of the temporalis muscle.

The skin paddle is checked frequently in the first 36 hours for viability and the pedicle monitored with Doppler ultrasonography. This is a vigorous flap that usually has excellent vessels of large caliber; flap failure is rare.

The zygoma and the craniotomy bone flaps are returned and secured with miniplates (Fig. 45). The inferior aspect of the L-shaped craniotomy flap is often partially missing because of bone erosion by tumor and subsequent osseous resection to ensure tumor-free margins. The muscle flap fills in the dead space and adds support.

Skin closure is then done and the wound drained with a closed system of suction drainage. Careful attention is paid to removing all eustachian tube remnants before wound closure. If the middle ear space is to be maintained, a ventilating tube is placed. If the ear is to be ablated, all middle ear mucosa and ossicles are removed as well as the tympanic membrane and residual canal skin. A mastoidectomy is done if not already performed, with the usual precautions taken to protect the facial nerve.

The lumbar drain is usually discontinued at about 72 hours unless a CSF leak occurs. If a leak does not stop in 3 days, the patient is returned to the operating room for repair. Antibiotic prophylaxis is continued for 24 hours after surgery, then discontinued. Suction drains are removed once the output is below 20 ml daily. Wounds are dressed with antibiotic ointment daily. The tracheostomy and nasogastric tube are discontinued as soon as airway jeopardy has passed and oral alimentation can ensue.

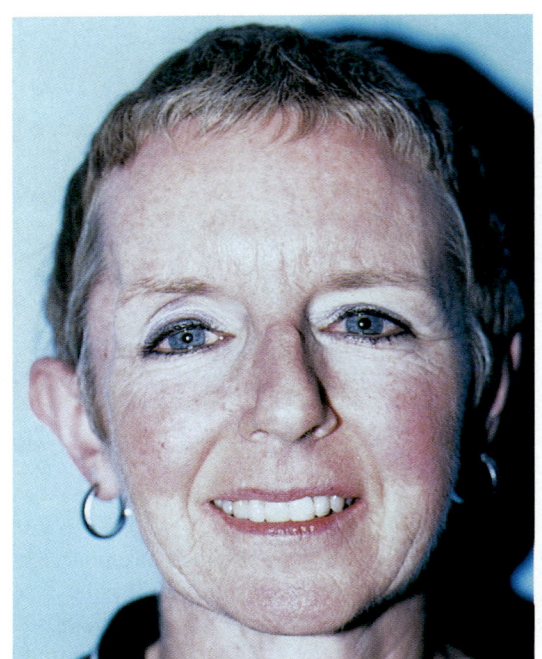
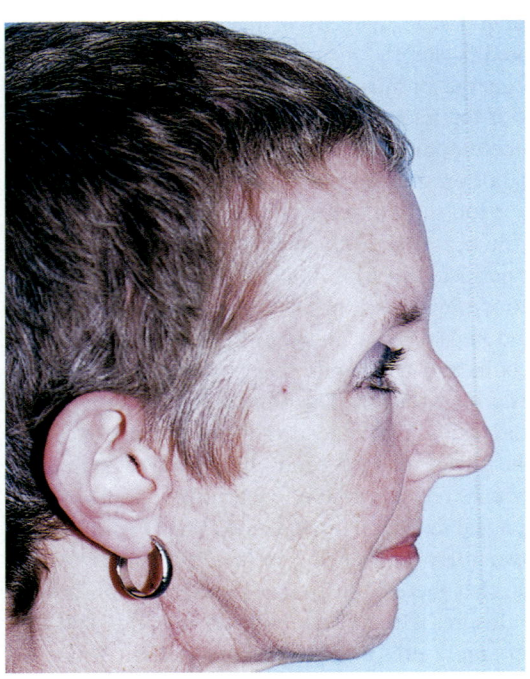

FIG. 44. A,B: Patient, 1 year after infratemporal fossa–middle cranial fossa resection and reconstruction with a rectus abdominis flap. The skin monitor has been removed and the scar revised in a manner similar to rhytidectomy.

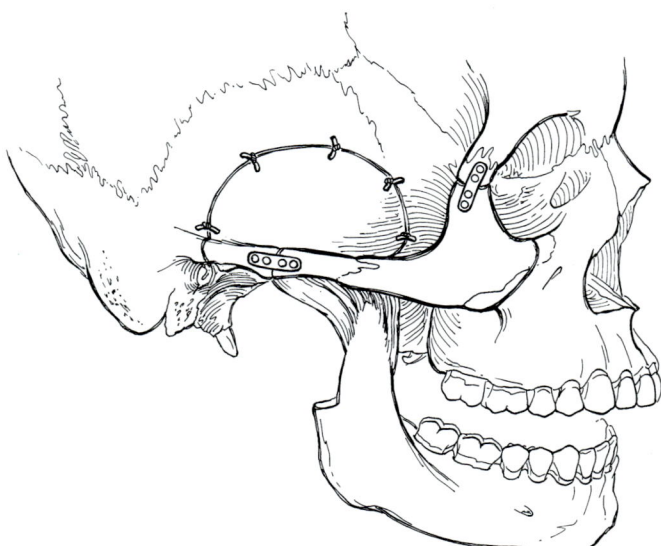

FIG. 45. Zygoma and craniotomy flaps restored and fixed in place with miniplates. (From Donald PJ, Gluckman JL, Rice DH, eds. *The sinuses*. New York: Raven Press, 1995:487.)

CONCLUSIONS

The middle cranial fossa–infratemporal fossa procedure is a somewhat complex and elaborate operation. In the author's opinion, it provides the best exposure to the middle fossa floor and contents. Carotid and cavernous exposure is optimized and subcranial resection can extend from the posterior ethmoids to C2 and include all the subcranial soft tissues, including those adjacent to the posterior maxillary wall and the posterior aspect of the maxillary sinus itself.

Two-year tumor-free survival rates are approximately 40%. The complications regarding carotid artery resection and the cavernous sinus have been described. CSF leaks are uncommon; meningitis and epidural and brain abscesses are rarer still. (See Chapter 29 for a complete discussion.)

REFERENCES

1. Fisch U. Infratemporal fossa approach for extensive tumors of the temporal bone and base of the skull. In: Silverstein H, Horell H, eds. *Neurological surgery of the ear.* Birmingham: Aesculapius, 1997:34–53.
2. Schramm VL. Infratemporal fossa surgery. In: Sekhar LN, Schramm VL, eds. *Tumors of the cranial base: diagnosis and treatment.* Mount Kisco, NY: Futura Publishing Co., 1987:421–437.
3. Nyak UK, Donald PJ, Stevens D. Internal carotid artery resection for invasion of malignant tumors. *Archives of Otolaryngology* 1995;121:1029–1063.
4. Biller HF, Urken M, Lawson W, Halimov M. Carotid artery resection and bypass for neck carcinoma. *Laryngoscope* 1988;98:181–183.
5. Rice DH. Microbiology. In: Donald PJ, Gluckman JL, Rice DH, eds. *The sinuses.* New York: Raven Press, 1995:57–64.
6. Tierno PM. Microbiology of the nose and paranasal sinuses. In: Goldman JL, ed. *Rhinology.* New York: John Wiley & Sons, 1987:79–97.

CHAPTER 17

Transmandibular Approach

Jack L. Gluckman, Lyon L. Gleich, and Keith M. Wilson

Access to large tumors involving the middle compartment of the extracranial skull base, particularly if there is lateral extension into the infratemporal fossa and parapharyngeal space, can be difficult. The transmandibular–transcervical approach permits not only wide exposure of this area but control of the great vessels that traverse this region.

The key to this technique is the mandibular osteotomy and lateral swing of the mandibular segments, which has been used by head and neck cancer surgeons for many years. It was first described in 1936 by Roux and then modified and refined over the years (1,2) to the point that it is now a standard component of the surgical armamentarium for cancers of the oral cavity and pharynx. This evolution has been facilitated by newer techniques of mandible stabilization, particularly the use of plates, which have minimized the morbidity and particularly the nonhealing originally associated with this technique.

In 1981, Biller et al. (3) first described this approach for wide-field exposure of the anterior skull base and infratemporal fossa. This technique, which included a median labiomandibulotomy with "mandibular swing" and detachment of the pharynx from the skull base by dividing the eustachian tube, resulted in excellent exposure and great safety, and since that time has been embraced by many skull base surgeons. In the authors' institution, it remains a commonly performed approach for large anterior skull base tumors with lateral infratemporal fossa extension.

RATIONALE

The extracranial skull base can best be regarded as consisting of a midline compartment and two lateral compartments separated by the internal carotid arteries (4) (Fig. 1). The lateral compartments consist of the greater wing of the sphenoid and the petrous portion of the temporal bone. The middle compartment consists of the body of the sphenoid, clivus, and occipital condyles. Although many approaches are available to the middle compartment, they are limited in their ability to attain lateral exposure and safe control of the great vessels. Likewise, the lateral approaches to the lateral compartments are limited in their inferior and medial exposure.

The transmandibular approach provides an excellent wide-field exposure to this area with easy identification and control of the great vessels and cranial nerves. Its major indication is in large tumors involving both the middle and lateral compartments.

The exposure that is achieved with the transmandibular approach extends from the ipsilateral infratemporal fossa to the contralateral medial pterygoid plate, and from the anterior cranial fossa to the lower clivus and anterior cervical spine down to C7.

INDICATIONS

Tumors arising in the midline from the sphenoid, clivus, anterior foramen magnum, and upper cervical vertebra with extension into the lateral compartment; tumors arising in the lateral compartment (i.e., lesions of the infratemporal fossa, inferior surface of the temporal bone, and pterygomaxillary fossa), as well as parapharyngeal space tumors can all be easily accessed using the transmandibular approach (3,5–7).

Which tumors are amenable to wide-field craniofacial resection is the subject of some debate; suffice to say that the high-grade carcinomas and sarcomas with extensive skull base invasion probably should not be subjected to this type of surgery except under certain circumstances, but many low-grade malignant and benign tumors can be completely resected by this technique. In addition, other conditions, such as invagination of the odontoid process, internal carotid artery aneurysm, and foreign bodies, can be approached this way.

J. L. Gluckman, L. L. Gleich, K. M. Wilson: Department of Otolaryngology–Head and Neck Surgery, University of Cincinnati, Cincinnati, Ohio 45267.

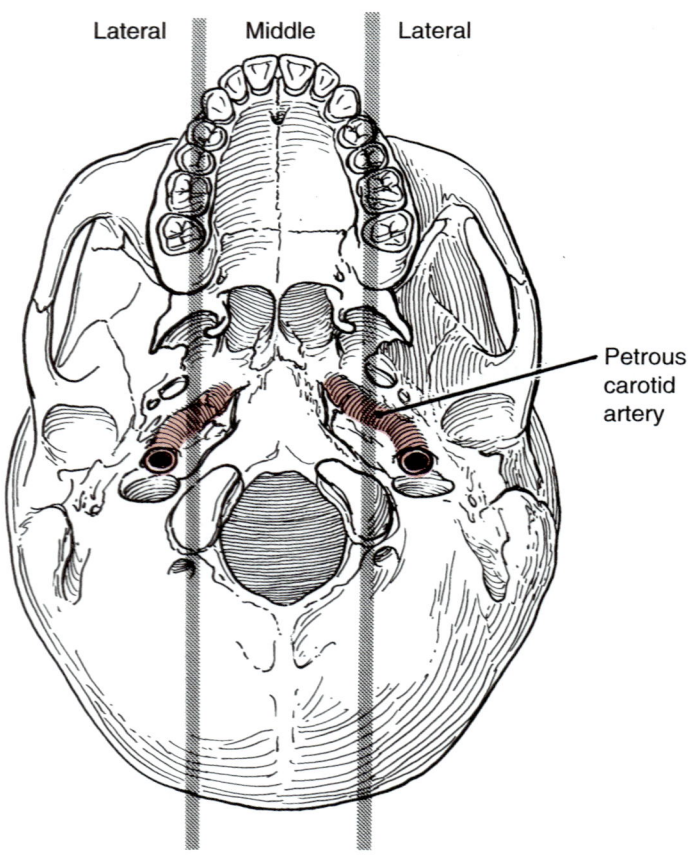

FIG. 1. The compartments of the extracranial surface of the skull base separated by the internal carotid arteries.

PREOPERATIVE EVALUATION

Evaluation of the Tumor

The preoperative evaluation depends on the individual patient and usually includes full clinical examination, computed tomography scan, magnetic resonance imaging, and biopsy. If the possibility exists for carotid artery resection or resection of the cavernous sinus, the cerebral blood flow should be assessed by arteriography, and balloon occlusion performed if deemed necessary.

Evaluation of the Mandible

The status of the patient's dentition should be carefully assessed because this may determine the site and type of the osteotomy (i.e., which tooth to extract, and whether the teeth can be used for fixation). In older patients, the degree of atrophy of the mandible may also dictate the type of osteotomy and the plating configuration to be used for fixation.

Evaluation of the Patient

As in all surgery, the patient's general physical and mental health must be evaluated before undertaking any procedure. Informed consent should be obtained, including all risks and realistic expectations of success. This should include the risks of bleeding, injury to cranial nerves, and impaired healing at the osteotomy site.

TECHNIQUE

Depending on the type and extent of the tumor, the craniotomy is usually performed first to ensure resectability. Once it is deemed appropriate to proceed with the transmandibular–transcervical approach, a tracheostomy is performed.

Labiomandibulotomy

A curvilinear incision is made from the mastoid tip to the submental region, passing two fingerbreadths below the mandible. The incision should extend through the platysma and fascia overlying the submandibular gland and the superior flap elevated in this plane to protect the marginal mandibular nerve. The lip-splitting incision can be made vertically through the midline or curved around the ipsilateral mental crease, which is the authors' technique of choice (Fig. 2).

The sternocleidomastoid muscle is then retracted laterally and the carotid sheath and its contents identified. Vascular loops are loosely placed around the common and internal

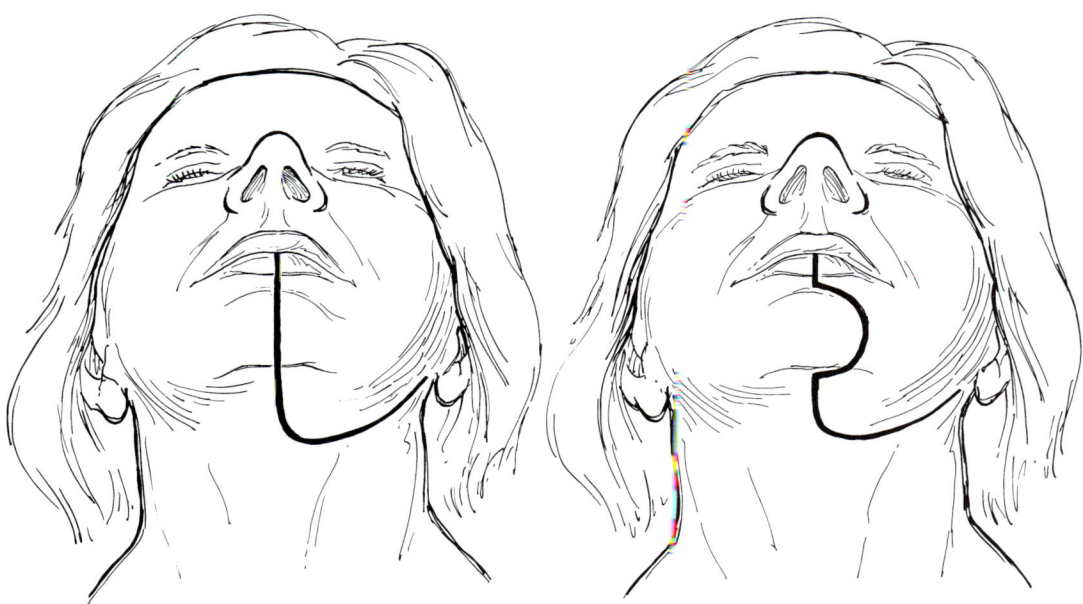

FIG. 2. Cervical and lip-splitting skin incision options.

carotid arteries as well as the jugular vein to facilitate control of these vessels if this should become necessary. Care is taken to expose and protect the vagus, spinal accessory, and hypoglossal nerves.

The lip-splitting incision is completed and the mandibular periosteum is incised anterior to the mental foramen. The periosteum is elevated anteriorly and posteriorly, ensuring that the mental nerve is not compromised (Fig. 3). A decision now has to be made as to the optimal site and configuration of the osteotomy. The state of dentition and the amount of mandibular atrophy govern this decision.

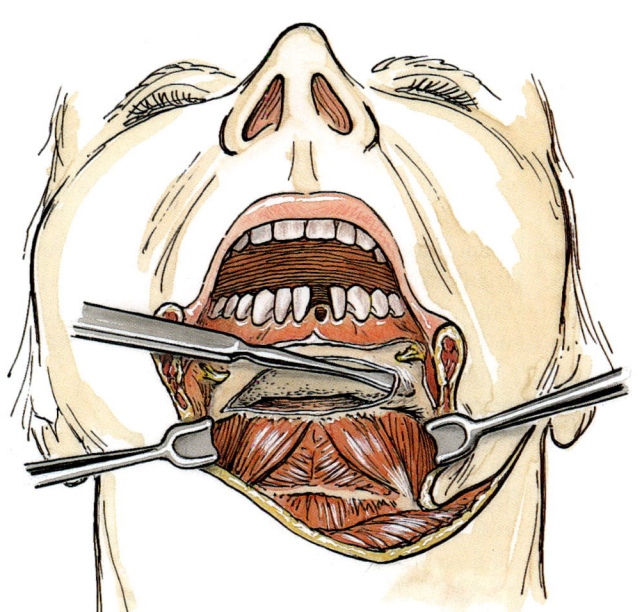

FIG. 3. Exposure of the potential osteotomy site with preservation of the mental nerve.

The mandibulotomy may be performed in a stair-step or notched fashion to increase postoperative stability; however, with newer plating techniques, a straight vertical midline osteotomy probably yields comparable stability (8) (Fig. 4). The optimal site for the osteotomy is anterior to the mental foramen up to and including the midline. If the patient has dentition, it is possible to create the osteotomy directly between two teeth; however, it is the authors' opinion that it is best to remove a tooth (usually the lateral incisor or canine) at the osteotomy site, rather than risking losing both teeth on either side of the osteotomy. If possible, the osteotomy should be made at the site of a previous extraction. Once the configuration and site of the osteotomy have been decided, the plates are chosen and placed, and holes drilled. The bone cut is made with an oscillating saw and fine chisel.

At this stage, a mucosal incision is made in the lateral floor of the mouth extending posteriorly toward the anterior tonsillar pillar. It is important to preserve a cuff of mucosa on the alveolar ridge to permit a watertight closure when the incision is closed (Fig. 5). The mandible is now swung laterally by dividing the mylohyoid and digastric muscles. The mucosal incision is then progressively extended along the anterior pillar until adequate exposure is obtained. The pterygoid muscles may need to be divided to obtain adequate visualization of the infratemporal fossa. Note that the floor of mouth mucosal incision is lateral to the submandibular duct and gland, which are kept intact.

Skull Base Exposure

As the mandible is retracted, the parapharyngeal space comes into view. The styloid process is fractured at its base and removed. The internal carotid artery, internal jugular

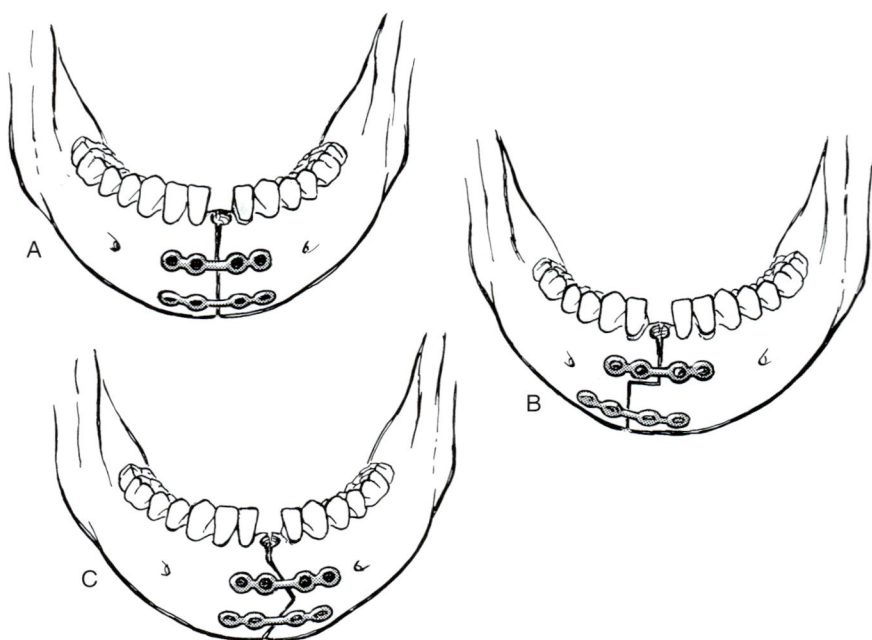

FIG. 4. Types of osteotomies. **A:** Vertical. **B:** Stair-step. **C:** Notched.

vein, and vagus, spinal accessory, hypoglossal, and glossopharyngeal nerves are then traced superiorly to the skull base.

As the dissection continues superiorly, the pharynx is noted to be tethered by the cartilaginous eustachian tube and levator veli palatini and tensor veli palatini muscles. These structures can then be divided if necessary, with care taken to protect the internal carotid artery. The pharynx can then be rotated medially, exposing the midline compartment of the skull base (Fig. 6).

The approach can be extended to expose the posterior nasal cavity by removing the pterygoid plates and posterior hard palate and incising into the posterior nasal mucosa. Removal of the maxillary tuberosity facilitates exposure of the pterygopalatine fossa. The sphenoid and maxillary sinuses can also be exposed by this approach, and of course various maxillotomy and maxillectomy procedures can be combined with this approach.

The craniofacial resection of the tumor is then accomplished. The intrapetrous internal carotid artery may be completely exposed in its vertical and horizontal segments. Although portions of the skull base can be removed piecemeal from below, usually the entire thickness of bone is removed with a combined craniofacial resection.

Closure

The age-old axiom that the key to successful craniofacial surgery is successful closure, certainly holds true in this technique.

If a significant skull base defect has been created, then this has to be meticulously reconstructed. Dura should be reconstructed and then various muscle flaps, either pericranial or temporalis, used to reinforce this. If the defect is large, a free rectus abdominis flap may be necessary. The authors rarely replace the resected bone.

If a significant pharyngeal wall defect results, it is reconstructed using a pectoralis major myocutaneous flap or cutaneous free flap, depending on the size and site of the defect.

The superior constrictor muscle is then reattached to the base of the skull and the pharynx sutured to the prevertebral fascia. When closing the floor of mouth incision, it is important to suture the floor of mouth mucosa not only to the cuff of the alveolar ridge mucosa, but to the alveolar ridge periosteum to prevent dehiscence. The mandible is then reap-

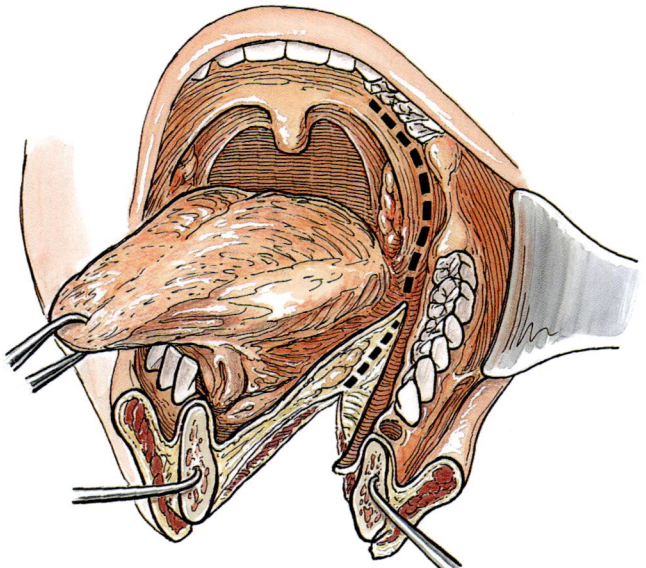

FIG. 5. Release incision through the mucosa of the floor of mouth.

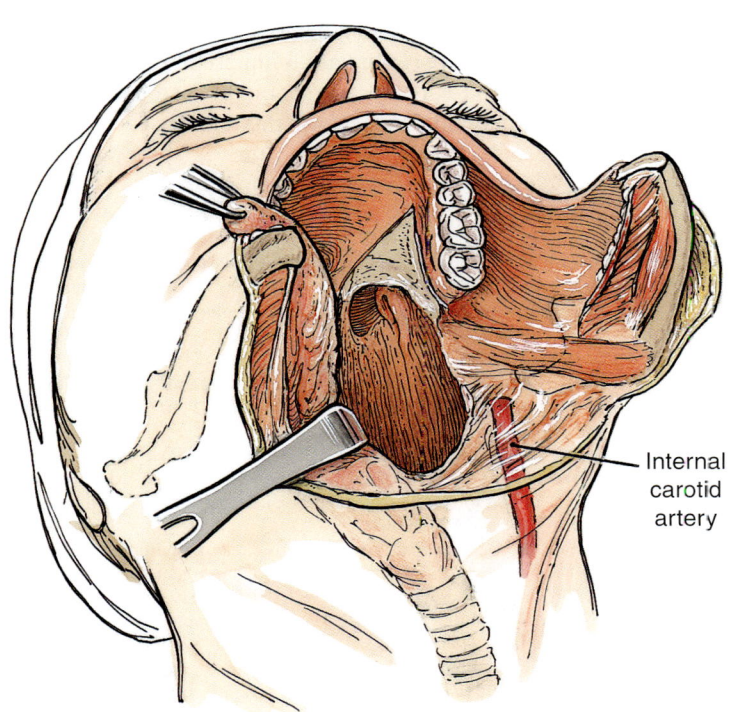

FIG. 6. Exposure of the infratemporal fossa and parapharyngeal space, together with midline compartment after retraction of the pharynx.

proximated using the previously fitted plates. In general, the authors do not put the patient into intermaxillary fixation.

A dermal graft may be placed for carotid protection and the neck incisions closed in layers. The lip is reapproximated by first reattaching the orbicularis oris by means of a permanent suture (e.g., 3.0 nylon) and then realigning the vermilion border accurately. The tracheostomy tube is maintained until the patient clearly has a safe airway. A nasogastric tube is maintained until the patient can tolerate an oral diet; if multiple cranial nerve palsies have occurred, placement of a gastrostomy should be considered.

COMPLICATIONS

Serous Otitis

This results if the eustachian tube has been transected; a long-term tympanostomy tube is needed for relief of this problem.

Cerebrospinal Fluid Leak, Intracranial Infection, and Pneumocephalus

As in all craniofacial resections, inadequate reconstruction can result in intracranial infection, cerebrospinal fluid leak, and even the development of pneumocephalus. This procedure is no exception. Prevention is very important and consists of a meticulous, watertight closure. Most leaks settle spontaneously, but, if not already present, a lumbar drain will need to be inserted, and occasionally open exploration and direct closure are indicated.

Cranial Nerve Injury

Cranial nerves may be intentionally sacrificed or inadvertently injured during the tumor resection. Of these, vagal injury with secondary dysphonia and dysphagia with aspiration is the most devastating. Although some suggest that prophylactic vocal medialization should routinely be performed (9), the authors usually do not perform this but rather give the patient a trial of swallowing. Older patients with multiple cranial nerve palsies usually require surgical intervention including gastrostomy, but the younger patients do quite well without surgery.

Temporomandibular Joint Dysfunction

Temporomandibular joint dysfunction can result from excessive lateral traction during the mandibular swing. This is due to disruption of the joint ligaments and compression of the articular capsule. In addition, division of the muscles of mastication for exposure can result in functional asymmetry and further malocclusion, aggravating the temporomandibular joint dysfunction. Early initiation of range-of-motion exercises of the jaw may reduce joint fibrosis. Splints, dentures, bite blocks, and antiinflammatory agents may be used to reduce these symptoms (10–12). The prophylactic injection of intraarticular steroids seems to reduce this complication.

Mandibulotomy Complications

Healing of the mandible after osteotomy requires appropriate repair and fixation. Although most osteotomies heal well without any sequelae, malunion or nonunion can have devastating consequences. For this reason, the following steps should be taken:

1. Avoid excessive elevation of the mandibular periosteum at the osteotomy site, which may devascularize the osteotomy site.
2. Design the osteotomy with care. Stair-step and notched osteotomies result in improved contact surface and good alignment and stabilization. Vertical osteotomies result in less bone removal, but are associated with greater rotational forces from distractional influences (8,13,14). If a vertical osteotomy is used, intermaxillary fixation should perhaps be used. Although it is technically possible to perform the osteotomy between two teeth, it is probably safer to remove a tooth to avoid the potential for infection at the site (15).
3. Ensure adequate stabilization. Although both wires and plates have their proponents for optimal stabilization (16,17), most favor plating as the technique of choice (14). Tension bands can be placed in dentate patients for added fixation.

Improper stabilization can result in malpositioned segments and nonunion. If movement of the mandibular segments is detected early in the postoperative period, exploration and refixation should be performed (15). Although malpositioned segments may not result in major problems in the edentulous patient because a denture can be fashioned to accommodate the malunion, in the dentulous patient the resulting malocclusion may cause pain at the osteotomy site and at the temporomandibular joint (10).

Rarely, osteomyelitis may develop at the osteotomy site, in which case necrotic tissue and nonviable bone should be debrided, antibiotics commenced, and external fixation applied. After the infection is controlled, bone grafting is indicated. Hyperbaric oxygen may aid healing in these patients.

In conclusion, the authors believe that the transmandibular–transcervical approach has an important role in contemporary skull base surgery, and should be included in the armamentarium of all who perform this surgery.

REFERENCES

1. Trotter W. Operations for malignant diseases of the pharynx. *Br J Surg* 1929;16:485–495.
2. Spiro RH, Gerold FP, Strong EW. Mandibular "swing" approach for oral and oropharyngeal tumors. *Head and Neck Surgery* 1981;3:371–378.
3. Biller HF, Shugar JMA, Krespi YP. A new technique for wide-field exposure of the base of the skull. *Archives of Otolaryngology* 1981;107:698–702.
4. Som PM, Shugar JMA, Parisier SC. A clinical radiographic classification of skull base lesions. *Laryngoscope* 1979;89:1066–1076.
5. Krespi YP, Sisson GA. Transmandibular exposure of the skull base. *Am J Surg* 1984;148:534–538.
6. Yumoto E, Okamura H, Yanagihara N. Transmandibular transpterygoid approach to the nasopharynx, parapharyngeal space, and skull base. *Ann Otol Rhinol Laryngol* 1992;101:383–389.
7. Franklin DJ, Moore GF, Fisch U. Jugular foramen peripheral nerve sheath tumors. *Laryngoscope* 1989;99:1081–1087.
8. McGregor IA, MacDonald DG. Mandibular osteotomy in the surgical approach to the oral cavity. *Head and Neck Surgery* 1983;5:457–462.
9. Netterville JL, Stone RE, Luken ES, Civantos FJ, Ossoff RH. Silastic medialization and arytenoid adduction: the Vanderbilt experience. *Ann Otol Rhinol Laryngol* 1993;102:413–424.
10. Sataloff RT, Myers DL, Roberts BR. Pain following surgery of the skull base. *Otolaryngol Clin North Am* 1984;17:613–625.
11. Niparko JK, Mattox DE. Complications of lateral skull base surgery. In: Eisele DW, ed. *Complications in head and neck surgery*. St. Louis: Mosby–Year Book, 1993:619–620.
12. Bell WE. *Temporomandibular disorders: classification, diagnosis, management*. 3rd ed. St. Louis: Mosby–Year Book, 1990.
13. Komisar A, Shapiro BM. Complications of midline mandibulotomy. *Ear Nose Throat J* 1988;67:521–523.
14. Sullivan PK, Rabian R, Driscoll D. Mandibular osteotomies for tumor extirpation: the advantages of rigid fixation. *Laryngoscope* 1992;102:73–80.
15. Sessions RB, Hudkins C. Complications of surgery of the oral cavity. In: Eisele DW, ed. *Complications in head and neck surgery*. St. Louis: Mosby–Year Book, 1993:218–222.
16. Shah JP, Kumaraswamy SV, Kulkarni V. Comparative evaluation of fixation methods after mandibulotomy for oropharyngeal tumors. *Am J Surg* 1993;166:431–34.
17. McCann KJ, Irish JC, Gullane PJ. Complications associated with rigid fixation of mandibulotomies. *J Otolaryngol* 1994;23:210–215.

CHAPTER 18

Anterior Subcranial (Transbasal—Derome) Approach

Ricardo Ramina, João J. Maniglia, Ari A. Pedrozo, and Murilo S. Meneses

Editor's Note: *The editor's treatment philosophy regarding the management of aggressive malignant tumors invading the intracranial space is at variance with the authors of this chapter. Combined chemotherapy and radiation therapy is usually met with failure when the cancer is this advanced. Aggressive resection of the cavernous sinus and excision of the petrous and cavernous carotid artery is done when these structures are invaded. The artery is replaced with a graft of Gore-tex or saphenous vein (see Chapter 16). En bloc resections of many skull base malignancies with significant central spread are usually impossible. A modified en bloc resection with frozen-section monitoring is a highly successful method of control (see Chapter 4) and is the editor's method of choice. The insurance of tumor-free margins is the goal—however achieved.*

Tumors of the anterior skull base frequently may involve the paranasal sinuses, orbit, and clivus. Surgical treatment of these lesions is often difficult and requires a multidisciplinary approach to achieve radical tumor removal and adequate reconstruction of the skull base. These tumors are located in a "frontier region," involving extracranial and intracranial structures. When they are treated independently by ear–nose–throat, head and neck surgeons, neurosurgeons, and ophthalmologists, only incomplete tumor removal or a biopsy is most frequently achieved. Multidisciplinary treatment by a skull base team, however, gives the best chance for total removal of the lesion, preservation of important neurovascular structures, and reconstruction of the skull base. Choosing the correct surgical approach is one of the most important ways of achieving the best result.

The transbasal approach was initially developed by Tessier et al. (1) in 1960 for treatment of craniofacial abnormalities. In 1963, Ketchman et al. (2) described a combined intracranial and extracranial approach to the anterior skull base for the treatment of malignant tumors. Derome (3,4) modified and used it for surgical removal of tumors of the anterior and middle skull base. Several modifications have been introduced, and many denominations, such as frontobasal, subcranial, transbasal, craniofacial, and others have been used (5–9). Since these early reports, several authors have extended the indications and modified this surgical approach (8–13). This procedure has become the approach of choice for tumors involving the craniofacial region, and can be extradural, intradural, or combined (14).

The major advantages of this procedure are wide exposure of the anterior cranial base with minimal retraction of the brain, and the possibility of reconstructing the whole anterior skull base with a galea–periosteum flap and bone, which provides an excellent cosmetic result with no visible skin scar. The main disadvantage of this approach can be loss of olfaction (15), which is seen with large lesions that require bilateral olfactory denervation. In small and more laterally situated lesions, it may be possible to preserve at least one olfactory nerve. The possibility of creating a communication between the intradural space and the paranasal sinuses is the most dangerous complication. Meningoceles or encephaloceles with brain herniation may develop if the skull base is not adequately reconstructed.

INDICATIONS AND CONTRAINDICATIONS

The indications for this surgery are very broad and include congenital abnormalities, traumatic lesions, CSF fistulas, infection, some vascular lesions, and tumors (9,11,16–18). Lesions of the midline that involve the paranasal sinuses, orbit, anterior portion of the clivus, anterior cranial fossa, and sellar and suprasellar regions can be surgically treated using this procedure. This approach permits wide exposure from

---

R. Ramina, A. A. Pedrozo, M. S. Meneses: Skull Base Surgery Foundation, Curitiba 80240, Brazil.
J.J. Maniglia: Department of Otolaryngology, Universidade Federal do Paraná, Curitiba, Paraná 80440-080, Brazil.

the frontal sinus down to the foramen magnum/C1 region (4,14). Lesions extending lateral to the internal carotid artery, cavernous sinus, petroclival region, and the posterior inferior portion of the clivus can be removed by a combined approach in the same or a second operative procedure (9,11,14).

The tumors can be benign or malignant. Another group comprises the very large (usually recurrent) benign lesions and the slow-growing malignancies. For benign tumors, radical piecemeal or *en bloc* resection with maximal preservation of nerves and vessels is the goal of surgery. With malignant processes, the lesion has to be removed *en bloc*, with a safety margin of healthy tissue. A major surgical procedure is justified in these cases only if total removal of the lesion can be anticipated with acceptable morbidity.

Invasion of the cavernous sinus or the internal carotid artery by high-grade malignant tumors usually is a contraindication to surgery. Palliative surgery may be indicated in cases of large, recurrent, benign tumors and slow-growing malignant lesions. Sacrifice of one infiltrated, but functioning, optic nerve or internal carotid artery is justified only if radical removal of the lesion can be achieved.

SURGICAL CONSIDERATIONS AND OPERATIVE TECHNIQUE

Surgical Considerations

The *extradural* subcranial approach is used for extradural tumors such as osteomas, fibrous dysplasia, chordomas, and chondrosarcomas, malignant tumors of the paranasal sinuses, traumatic lesions, CSF fistula, infections, and congenital abnormalities. Small dural lacerations (traumatic lesions) are repaired through this procedure.

The *intradural* subcranial approach is indicated when the lesion remains solely intradural. The indications include craniopharyngiomas, large pituitary adenomas, olfactory groove and tuberculum sellae meningiomas, and others.

The *combined* subcranial approach is used when the tumor invades the skull base dura and bone and its removal establishes a communication between the intradural space and the paranasal sinuses. Esthesioneuroblastomas, invasive meningiomas, and malignant processes are examples of tumors that may require this approach.

Operative Technique

The Approach

General anesthesia with oral endotracheal intubation is used in all patients. Tracheostomy is rarely used. The oral cavity is packed with gauze. Both the face and the head are prepared with povidone–iodine solution. Antibiotic therapy, beginning the night before, is routinely used and continued for 3 days after the surgery. The patient is placed in the dorsal decubitus position with the neck extended, and the head secured in a head holder above heart level. A bicoronal incision is made beginning anterior to the tragus at the level of the zygoma. The skin flap is dissected in the subperiosteal plane and turned down anteriorly at level of the orbital rims and glabella. The galea and periosteum are incised at a level higher than the skin incision to obtain a very long flap. The supraorbital foramen is identified, and the supraorbital nerve and artery are preserved (Fig. 1). This foramen is frequently incomplete, and the nerve and artery are dissected free with the pericranium. Sometimes the foramen is opened using a small osteotome and the neurovascular pedicle released with the bicoronal flap.

A large galea–periosteum flap that includes a small portion of the anterior temporalis fascia is dissected, remaining attached to the supraorbital region. It is used to cover the floor of the anterior fossa, the paranasal sinuses, and orbits to reconstruct the dura at the end of the operation. This flap is a modification of the traditional galea–periosteum flap because it includes the temporalis fascia. This large, vascularized flap is very useful for covering the whole anterior cranial fossa and supports the bone fragments used for reconstruction of the surgical defect in the anterior fossa (Fig. 2).

A bicoronal craniotomy is carried out; the frontal bone includes both orbital rims and a large portion of the orbital roof on both sides. Three bur holes are drilled: two holes are placed in the "key point" (after coagulating and dissecting a small portion of the temporalis muscle), 1 cm below the superior temporal line, in the temporal fossa, behind the lateral orbital rim. The third bur hole is placed over the sagittal sinus approximately 6 cm from the nasion. A bur hole over the frontal sinus is avoided by cutting the bone in the region of the glabella with a small cutting bur or an oscillating saw (Fig. 3). The bur holes are connected using the Gigli saw or craniotome. The periorbita is bilaterally dissected from the orbital roof. The anterior two thirds of the orbital roof is cut using a small curved osteotome and high-speed drill. Both

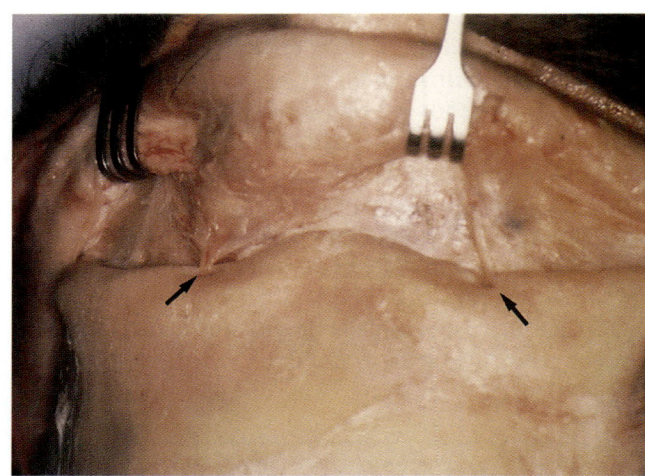

FIG. 1. Cadaver specimen showing both supraorbital nerves (*arrows*).

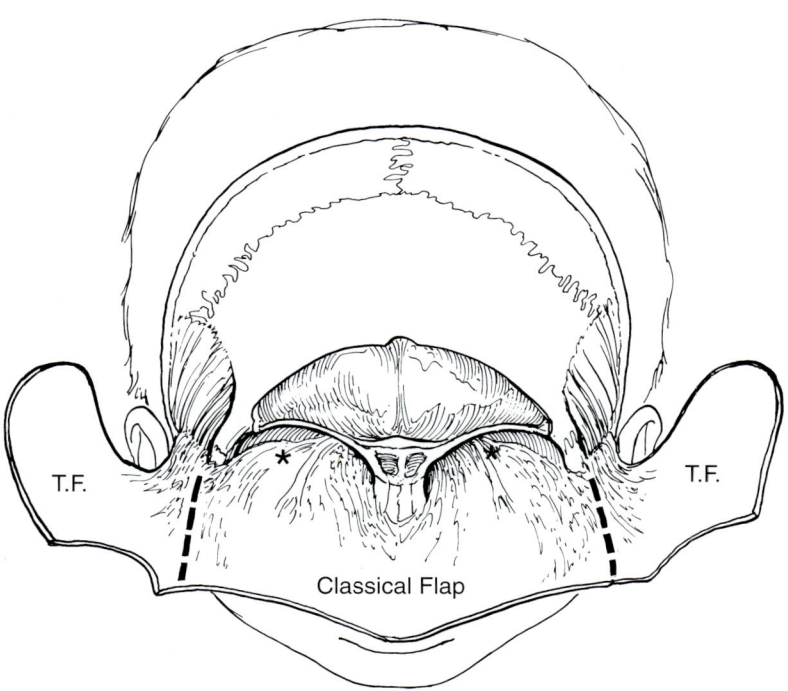

FIG. 2. Modified galea–periosteum flap. The temporal fascia (*T.F.*) remains attached to the "classic flap" (*asterisks*) periorbita.

orbital roofs are connected with the opening in the nasion region using a high-speed drill. The bicoronal craniotomy bone is removed (Fig. 4). The frontal sinus mucosa is totally removed with a bur from its inner table. The frontal sinus is completely cranialized by removing the posterior wall of the sinus with rongeur and cutting burs. In cases in which the frontal sinus is infiltrated by the tumor, this portion of the lesion can be easily resected at this point. At this stage of the operation, surgical variations are performed according to the histologic type and extension of the lesion.

Extradural Approach

The basal dura mater is detached from the anterior cranial fossa floor and crista galli. One or two olfactory nerves are sectioned, depending on the lesion's extension. The dura over the lamina cribrosa, ethmoid roof, and orbit is elevated up to the planum sphenoidale and the anterior clinoid processes, exposing both optic nerves extradurally. The crista galli and the lamina cribrosa are removed using the high-speed drill and a fine leksell. If the lesion infiltrates the olfactory bulbs, they are resected intradurally. Possible dural lacerations during this dissection are sutured or grafted using temporalis fascia. Self-retaining retractors are positioned. This extradural approach completely exposes the anterior cranial base from orbit to orbit. It allows exposure of nasal septum, both nasal fossae, and the nasopharynx. Removal of the facial portion of the lesion is often possible without any

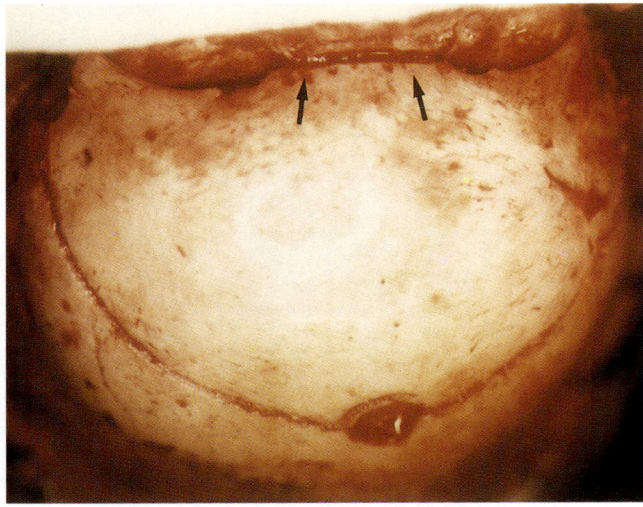

FIG. 3. Bicoronal craniotomy. The bone in the region of the glabella is cut with an oscillating saw (*arrows*).

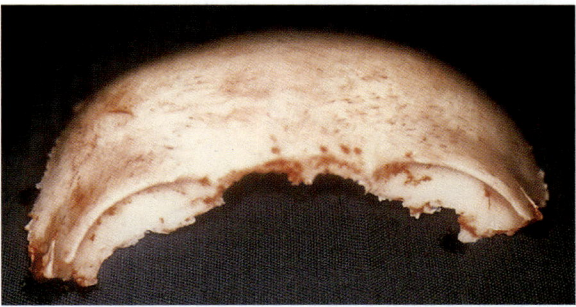

FIG. 4. Craniotomy bone including both orbital rims and a portion of the orbital roof.

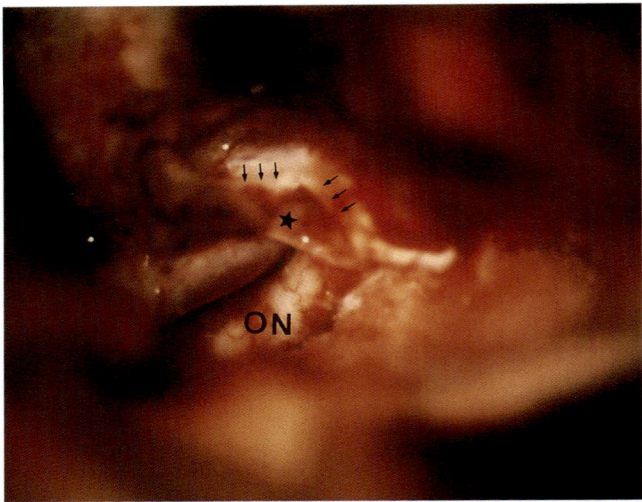

FIG. 5. Exposure of the clinoid portion of the internal carotid artery and dural ring around the vessel (*asterisk*). The anterior clinoid process was removed intradurally (*arrows*). ON, optic nerve.

Both ethmoid sinuses can be totally removed, and the sphenoid sinus is exposed by resection of the planum sphenoidale. Tumors in the sphenoid sinus region and in the clivus (midline) are removed using this procedure.

Some lesions (e.g., adenoid cystic carcinoma) may extend into the middle fossa, following the second branch of the trigeminal nerve (V2) into the gasserian ganglion. Extradural dissection of the floor of the middle fossa is carried out and the second division of the trigeminal nerve (V2) identified. In some cases, a small temporal craniectomy may be necessary to expose the third division of the trigeminal nerve (V3) after coagulation and cutting of the middle meningeal artery. The superior orbital fissure and the clinoid portion of the internal carotid artery are identified by extradural dissection with removal of the lateral aspect of the greater sphenoid wing and intradural drilling of the anterior clinoid process (Fig. 5). This gives access to the cavernous sinus and infratemporal fossa.

The sphenoid sinus can be entered in two ways: through a midline approach after removal of planum sphenoidale, or laterally through the floor of the middle fossa between V2 and V3. The intersphenoid septum is resected with a rongeur, and tumor in the sphenoid sinus and lower clivus can be removed with microsurgical techniques. Some lesions, such as chondrosarcomas and chordomas, may extend down to the jugular foramen. The extradural portion of these tumors can be removed using this approach.

additional facial approach. The medial aspect of the orbit can be approached after removal of the lamina papyracea and ligature of the anterior and posterior ethmoid vessels. The optic nerve canal is identified and decompressed under the microscope using diamond burs and irrigation. The superior orbital fissure may be opened.

Case Reports

CASE 1

A 9-year-old girl complained of visual loss in the right eye. Neurologic examination showed amaurosis on the right eye and visual decrease on the left. Atrophy of the right optic papilla was noted. Magnetic resonance imaging (MRI) demonstrated a very large cystic lesion in the sphenoid sinus and pituitary region (Fig. 6).

On July 10, 1994, an extradural subcranial approach was performed. A huge cystic mass was completely removed and the cranial base reconstructed. The postoperative visual acuity improved in the left eye. The right amaurosis remained unchanged.

Histologic examination of the specimen was diagnostic for aneurysmatic bone cyst. Follow-up examination 18 months after the surgery with computed tomography (CT) scan confirmed total removal of the lesion (Fig. 7). The visual acuity remained unchanged in the right eye.

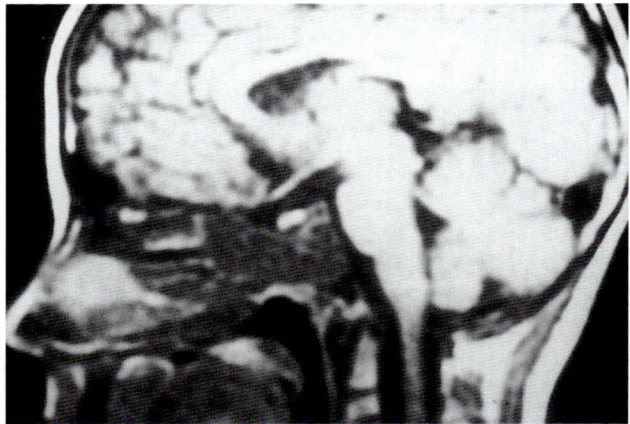

FIG. 6. Case 1. Preoperative T1-weighted magnetic resonance image with gadolinium administration shows a large cystic lesion in the sphenoid region with extension and destruction of the clivus. No contrast enhancement was observed. The histologic diagnosis was aneurysmatic bone cyst.

CASE 1 (Continued)

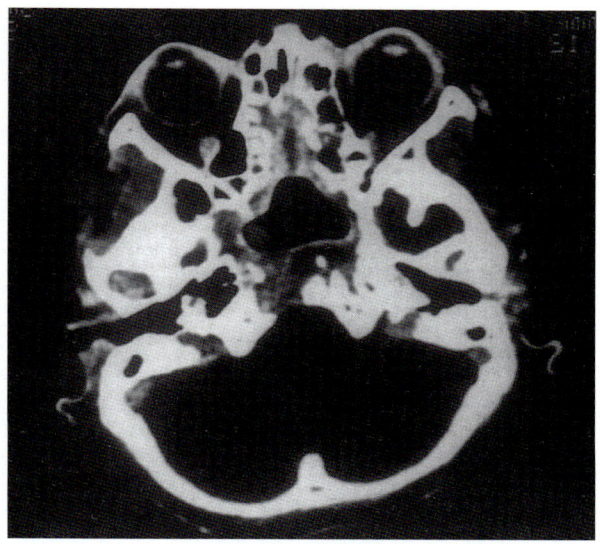

FIG. 7. Case 1. Postoperative computed tomography scan showing total removal of the aneurysmatic bone cyst in the sphenoid sinus/clivus region.

CASE 2

This 17-year-old boy presented with a progressive visual loss in the left eye over a period of 4 months. Visual acuity in the right eye started to decrease, and 2 months before admission to the authors' clinic, he complained of loss of olfaction. CT scanning revealed a very large tumor occupying the sphenoid and ethmoid sinuses, anterior portion of the clivus, and both orbits (Fig. 8). No dural invasion could be demonstrated by CT.

In December, 1989, the lesion was completely removed through an extradural subcranial approach. The medial orbital walls and orbital roofs were infiltrated by the lesion and were removed. The orbital fissure and optic canals were opened on both sides. After total resection of the lesion, the anterior cranial base was reconstructed with a galea–periosteum flap (Figs. 9, 10). The histologic diagnosis was chondrosarcoma.

The patient underwent radiation therapy after the surgery, and a local frontal abscess developed secondary to a bony sequestrum. Fragments of bone used for reconstruction of the frontal sinus had to be removed and the infection was successfully treated with antibiotics. The bone used for reconstruction of the anterior fossa floor was covered by temporalis fascia, was not infected, and could be left in place. On follow-up examination and CT scan (Fig. 11) 6 years after surgery, there was no evidence of tumor recurrence and the patient had no additional neurologic deficit.

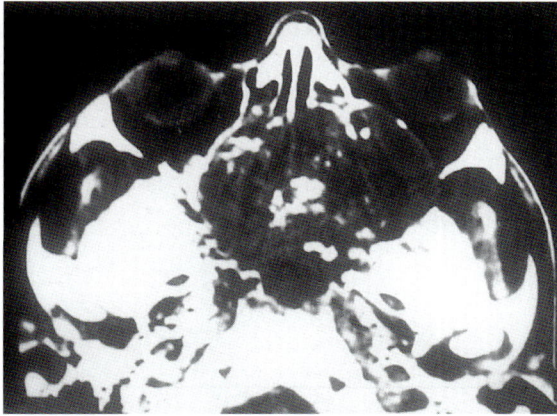

FIG. 8. Case 2. Preoperative computed tomography scan showing a large tumor in the ethmoid/sphenoid sinus region with extension to both orbits. Calcifications can be observed. The histologic diagnosis was chondrosarcoma.

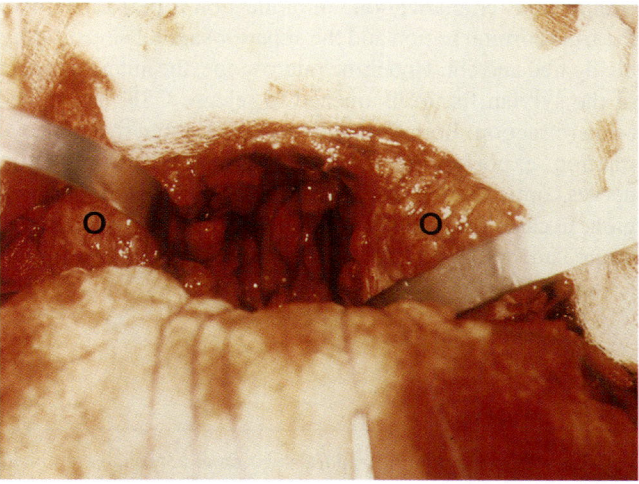

FIG. 9. Case 2. Intraoperative photograph after total removal of a large chondrosarcoma showing the large defect in the anterior cranial base and both orbits (O).

CASE 2 (Continued)

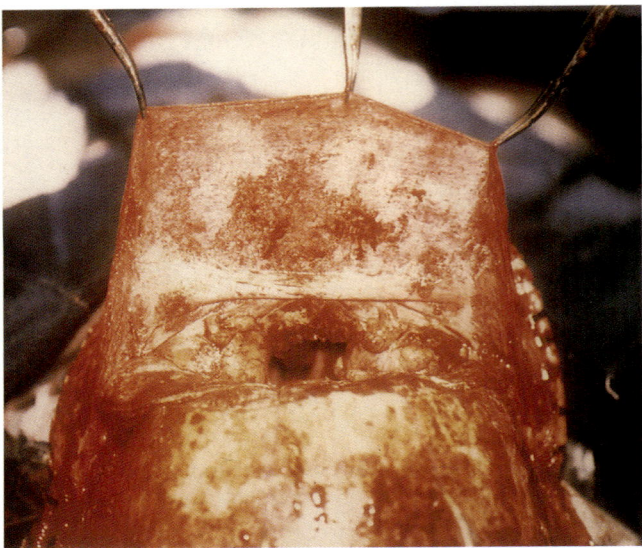

FIG. 10. Case 2. Reconstruction of the anterior cranial base with vascularized galea–periosteum flap.

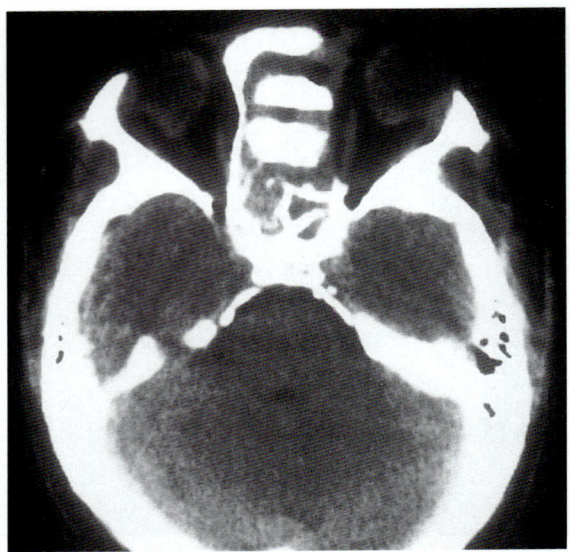

FIG. 11. Case 2. Postoperative computed tomography scan after total removal of chondrosarcoma showing the bone fragments used for reconstruction of the anterior cranial base.

Intradural Approach

The subcranial approach is also used for intradural tumors like pituitary adenomas, craniopharyngiomas, meningiomas, chordomas, chondrosarcomas, and others. In cases of severe craniofacial trauma with contusion or laceration of the frontal lobes, this procedure allows wide exposure for inspection of the intradural compartment and dural reconstruction.

After bilateral craniotomy involving both orbital rims and frontal sinus cranialization, dural incision is performed over the frontoorbital region and the superior sagittal sinus is double ligated and cut. Under the microscope, the anterior aspect of the sylvian fissure is opened to release CSF and reduce brain retraction. Both frontal lobes are elevated by gentle retraction, exposing the whole anterior fossa, the olfactory nerves, optic nerves, carotid arteries, and the pituitary region. In cases of sellar lesions (e.g., craniopharyngiomas, pituitary adenoma, and tuberculum sellae meningiomas), at least one olfactory nerve can be preserved.

Removal of the lesion in the sellar and parasellar region is possible after identification of the optic nerves and internal carotid arteries. An ultrasonic aspirator is used for the intracranial portion of the tumor. In some cases, such as in malignant lesions, the anterior portion of the cavernous sinus is invaded through the superior orbital fissure. This intracavernous portion of the tumor can be exposed and removed through this approach. The internal carotid artery is identified in the clinoid region by intradural removal of the anterior clinoid process after opening the superior orbital fissure. Resection of invaded internal carotid artery and nerves of the superior orbital fissure may be carried out in cases of malignancy. A preoperative balloon occlusion test is performed and, if necessary, a bypass between the petrous portion or cervical portion of the internal carotid artery and the middle cerebral artery (M1 and M2 segments) can be performed using a saphenous graft. In the authors' opinion, however, this procedure should be carried out only in cases of benign tumors or low-grade malignancies.

Case Reports

CASE 3

This is an example of an extradural subcranial approach combined with an intradural presigmoid access. A 42-year-old man presented with numbness around the mouth and cervical pain. CT scanning and MRI showed a very large tumor in the clivus region, reaching the jugular foramen and extending into the sphenoid sinus. The tumor caused compression of the brainstem (Fig. 12).

On October 22, 1992, an extradural subcranial approach was carried out (Figs. 13–15). Total removal of the extradural portion of the lesion was possible. The dura was infiltrated in the posterior clivus region, and no attempt was made to remove this part of the lesion because of danger of CSF fistula. Reconstruction was performed using galea–periosteum flap, bone, and abdominal fat. The

CASE 3 (Continued)

remaining intradural portion was removed in a second stage using a presigmoid approach (Fig. 16).

The histologic diagnosis was chordoma. In spite of radical removal and postoperative radiation therapy, the lesion recurred and the patient died 2.5 years after the operation.

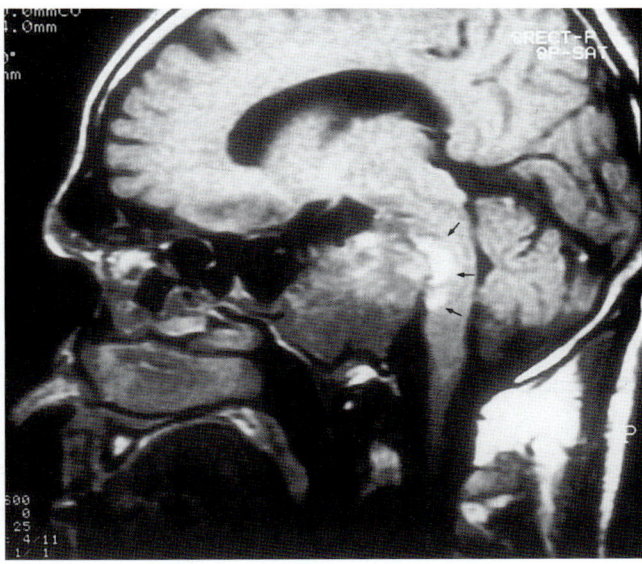

FIG. 12. Case 3. Preoperative T1-weighted magnetic resonance image with gadolinium administration showing a large chordoma of the clivus compressing the brainstem (*arrows*). Minimal gadolinium enhancement is observed.

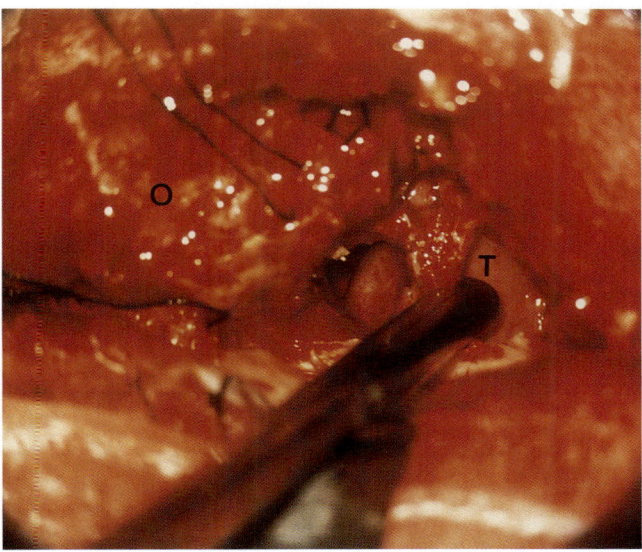

FIG. 13. Case 3. Intraoperative photograph showing extradural approach to the sphenoid sinus filled by the tumor (*T*). The intersphenoid septum is being removed with a Kerrison rongeur. The planum sphenoidale was drilled out. *O*, orbit.

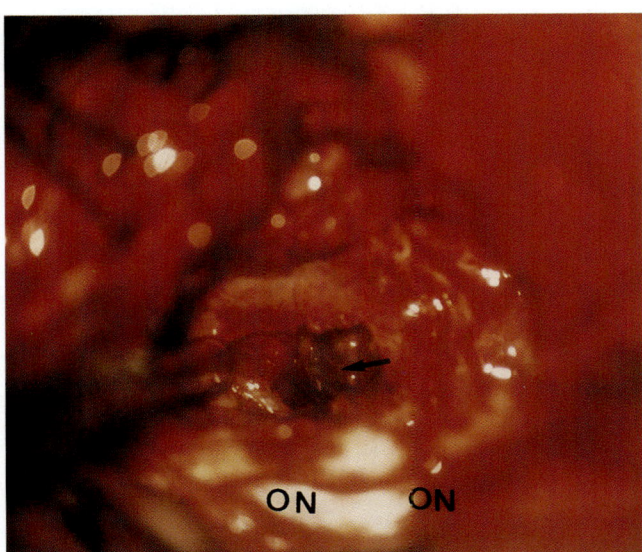

FIG. 14. Case 3. Intraoperative photograph after removal of the extradural portion of a clival chordoma that extended into the jugular foramen (*arrow*). *ON*, extradural exposure of both optic nerves.

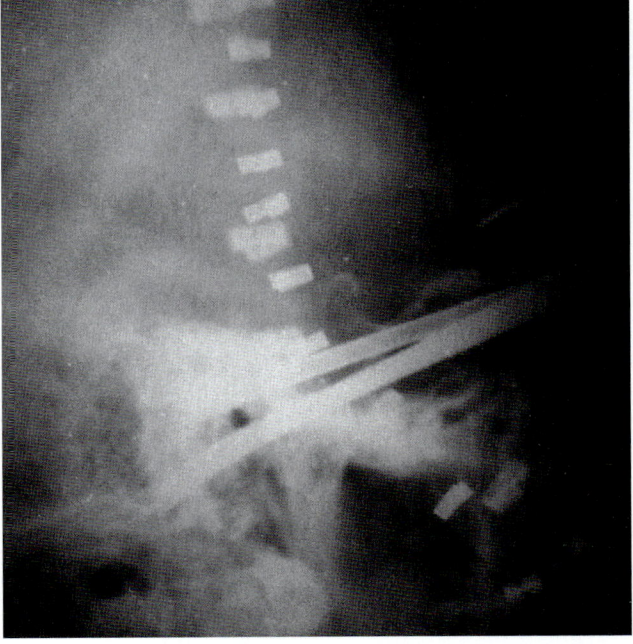

FIG. 15. Case 3. Intraoperative radiograph showing the extradural subcranial approach from the frontal sinus, through the sphenoid sinus and reaching the jugular foramen.

CASE 3 (Continued)

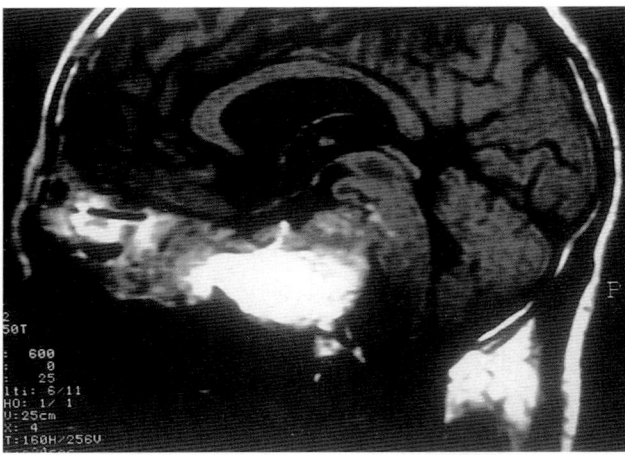

FIG. 16. Case 3. Postoperative T1-weighted magnetic resonance image with gadolinium administration demonstrating total removal of the extradural portion of the lesion. The ethmoid and sphenoid sinuses are filled with abdominal fat. The intradural (retrosellar) portion of the lesion was removed in a second surgical procedure using a presigmoid approach.

CASE 4

This 6-year-old girl showed signs of hypopanpituitarism and progressive visual loss in both eyes. Neuroradiologic and endocrinologic evaluation revealed the presence of a very large tumor in the sellar region with compression of the brainstem (Fig. 17). The diagnosis of a craniopharyngioma was suspected.

On August 20, 1992, an intradural subcranial approach was performed (Figs. 18, 19). Radical removal of the lesion was possible with preservation of the pituitary stalk (Fig. 20).

After surgery, the patient's vision improved markedly, and hormonal reposition with cortiron, tirotin, and growth hormone was initiated.

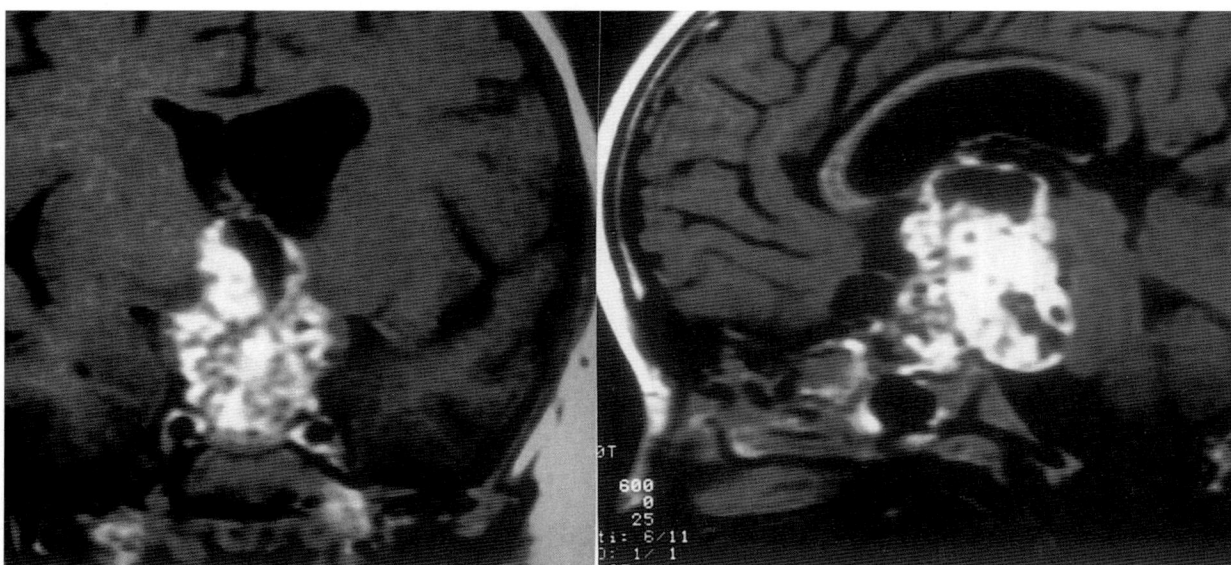

FIG. 17. Case 4. Preoperative T1-weighted magnetic resonance image with gadolinium administration showing a huge tumor in the sellar, suprasellar, and prepontine regions. The lesion had solid portions that enhanced with gadolinium, and cysts. The tumor extended from the sella up to the lateral ventricles. The histologic diagnosis was craniopharyngioma.

CASE 4 (Continued)

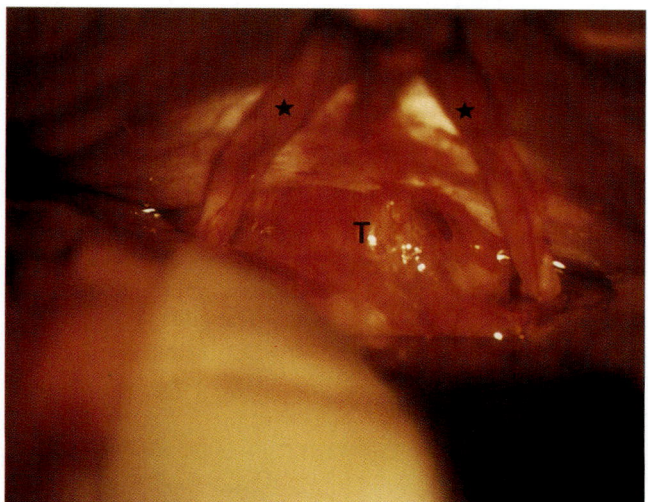

FIG. 18. Case 4. Subcranial intradural exposure of a large craniopharyngioma (*T*) with preservation of both olfactory nerves (*stars*).

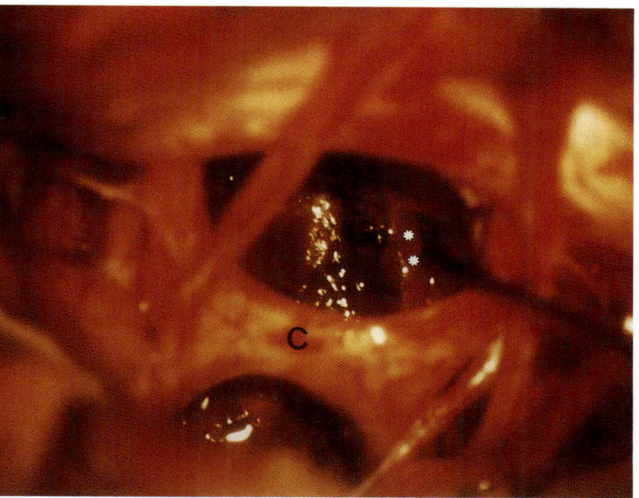

FIG. 19. Case 4. Intraoperative photograph. The craniopharyngioma was totally removed using a subcranial intradural approach. The optic chiasm (*C*) and the pituitary stalk (*asterisks*) were preserved.

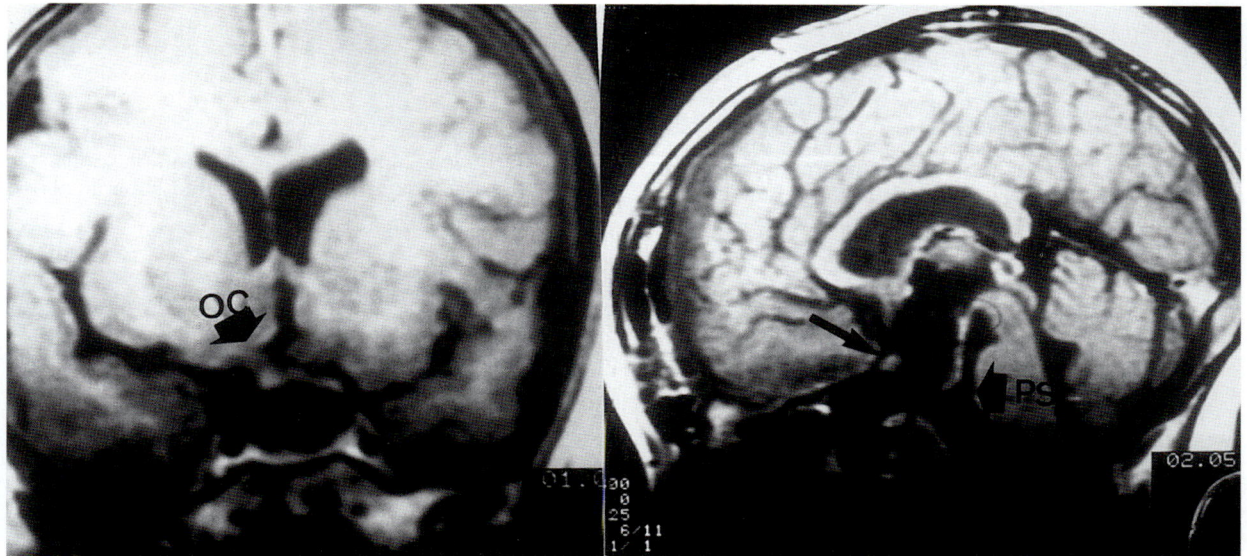

FIG. 20. Case 4. Postoperative T1-weighted magnetic resonance image with gadolinium administration after total removal of a large craniopharyngioma. The optic chiasm (*arrow; OC*) and the pituitary stalk (*arrow; PS*) can be observed.

Combined Approach

If necessary, the authors use transfacial approaches in combination with the subcranial exposure to extend the operation to include access to the maxillary sinus, pterygopalatine fossa, infratemporal fossa, and middle cranial fossa. The authors prefer to use degloving techniques and transmaxillary access for benign tumors and slow-growing and low-grade malignant tumors. The Weber-Fergusson incision is used for more malignant lesions in which a radical operation is necessary (e.g., for total maxillectomy including orbital exenteration and reconstruction). In cases of esthesioneuroblastomas, the dura is opened for resection of the olfactory bulbs, with intraoperative frozen-section histologic studies obtained to ensure safe margins and removal of intradural tumor (19). Some aggressive meningiomas invade the floor of the anterior cranial base, the paranasal sinuses, and the intradural compartment. Removal of the lower part (maxillary sinuses) of these lesions requires transfacial approaches. Aggressive pituitary adenomas may infiltrate the ethmoid and the sphenoid sinuses. In these cases, a combined subcranial–transfacial approach is also used. Reconstruction of dura and cranial base is one of the most important steps of this approach. Communication of the intradural compartment with the paranasal sinuses may cause CSF fistula and meningitis.

Case Report

CASE 5

This 42-year-old man presented with bleeding from the nose. Rhinoscopy and CT scan (Fig. 21) revealed a large tumor occupying the nasal fossa with infiltration of the right orbit and anterior cranial base. A biopsy was taken and an esthesioneuroblastoma was diagnosed.

In November, 1988, a combined frontobasal/degloving approach was performed and the lesion completely removed (Figs. 22, 23). Radiation therapy was administered after the operation. The patient had no additional neurologic deficit or signs of recurrence in the control MRI examination 7 years after surgery (Fig. 24).

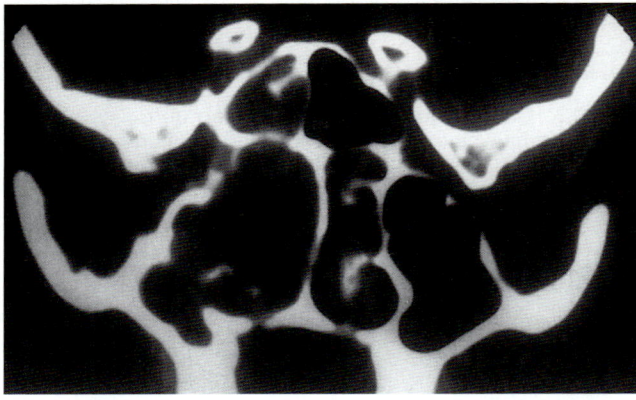

FIG. 21. Case 5. Coronal computed tomography scan with contrast enhancement showing a tumor in the nasal fossa, sphenoid sinus, and right orbit. The histologic diagnosis was esthesioneuroblastoma.

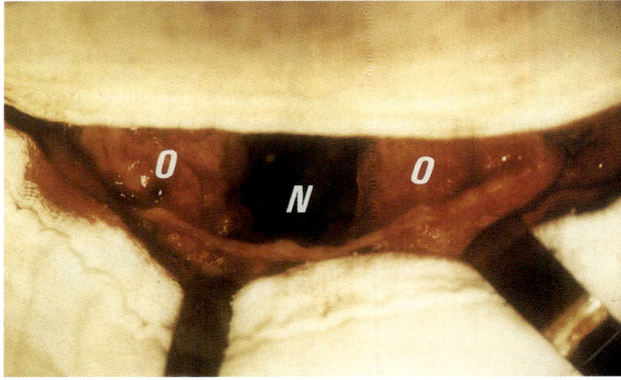

FIG. 22. Case 5. Intraoperative photograph showing total removal of the lesion using a combined subcranial/degloving approach. *O*, orbit; *N*, nasopharynx.

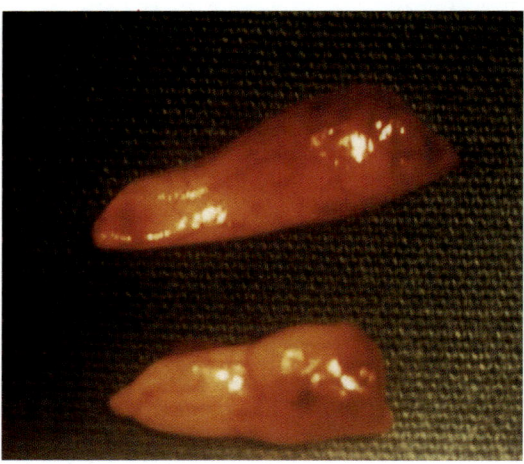

FIG. 23. Case 5. Surgical specimen of both resected olfactory nerves and bulbs. Both nerves were infiltrated by the tumor.

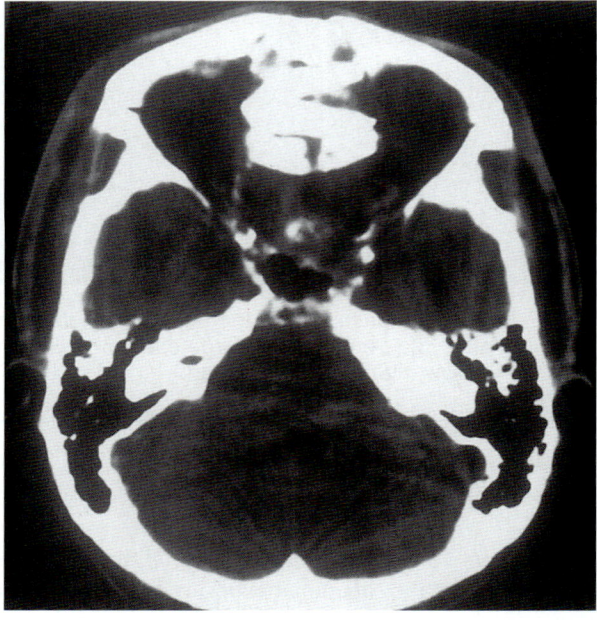

FIG. 24. Case 5. Postoperative computed tomography scan after radical removal of esthesioneuroblastoma. The anterior cranial base was reconstructed with bone fragments.

Reconstruction

Reconstruction of the large defect in the frontobasal approach is of paramount importance. The dura is sutured primarily whenever possible, or a temporalis fascia graft is used. The modified pedicled galea–pericranium flap is then rotated to cover the whole anterior fossa. Reconstruction of large bone defects of the anterior fossa is necessary in the authors' experience because of the resulting dead space and to avoid delayed meningoceles, encephaloceles, and meningitis. Bone for this purpose is taken from the inner table of the frontal craniotomy bone. It is removed with an oscillating saw or small high-speed drill. In some cases, such as in children, it can be obtained from the iliac bone; this has the advantage of providing both cancellous and cortical bone. Over this flap, bone grafts from the inner table of the frontal bone are placed and covered with the temporalis fascia attached to the galea–pericranium flap (Fig. 25).

Reconstruction of the supraorbital margins and orbital roofs is not necessary because they remain in the craniotomy in one piece. If they are infiltrated by the lesion and have to be removed, they can be reconstructed with iliac graft or with split rib graft. The nasal cavities and the oropharynx are packed with tetracycline-soaked gauze. This packing is left in place for 7 days.

For patients with a large defect of the anterior skull base, a spinal lumbar catheter for continuous CSF drainage is inserted. This system is usually removed 3 days after surgery. The bifrontal craniotomy is closed in routine fashion.

TABLE 1. *Cases operated on using subcranial approach*

Lesion	No. of cases
Menigiomas	12
Pituitary adenomas	8
Craniopharyngiomas	7
Chordomas/chondrosarcomas	5
Malignant tumors	8
Fibrous dyplasia	4
Osteoma/ossifying fibroma	2
Esthesioneuroblastoma	2
Aneurysmatic bone cyst	1
Cerebrospinal fluid fistula	4
Trauma	4
Total	57

CASE MATERIAL

From 1987 to 1995, 57 patients were operated on using a subcranial approach in the authors' institution (Table 1).

COMPLICATIONS

Complications related to this approach include CSF fistula and meningitis, infection, postoperative enophthalmos, hypertensive extradural pneumocephalus, cosmetic defects, and loss of olfaction.

In the authors' series, there were two cases of postoperative extradural infection. These patients had delayed extradural infection in the frontal sinus region. One of these patients with a malignant tumor underwent radiation therapy after the operation; the other patient was successfully treated with antibiotics. Meningitis, CSF fistula, postoperative enophthalmos, and pulsatility of the eyeball were not observed in the authors' patients. The cosmetic results are very satisfactory because the orbital rim and the bifrontal craniotomy are removed in one piece. Avoiding the bur hole over the frontal region gives a better aesthetic result. There was no mortality in this series.

CONCLUSION

The subcranial approach is the procedure of choice for most patients with anterior skull base lesions. The presence of intracranial and extracranial invasion with involvement of the clivus, pterygoid plates, anterior cavernous sinus, and sellar region is not a contraindication to this approach. Such an extensive surgical procedure, however, is not indicated when a highly malignant tumor is present or when it invades the cavernous sinus bilaterally. The use of this procedure or its combination with different approaches depends on the exact location of the lesion as well as its histologic nature (5,16,20–22).

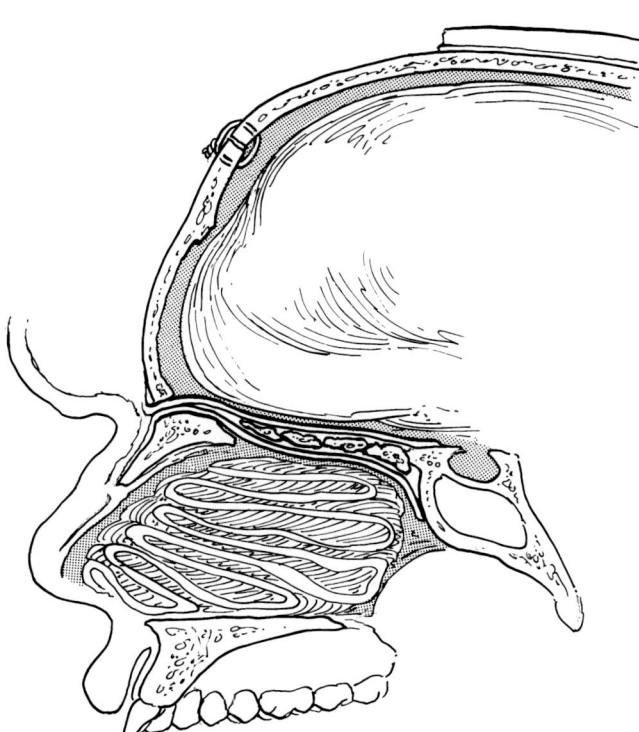

FIG. 25. Reconstruction of the anterior skull base with galea–periosteum flap (from below) and temporalis fascia (from above). In between are bone fragments from the inner table of the frontal bone.

In malignant lesions and giant benign tumors, the decision between complete tumor removal or subtotal resection for decompression of intracranial structures, with radiation therapy and chemotherapy, is based on careful preoperative evaluation. CT and MRI are performed for precise determination of tumor extension and involvement of neurovascular structures at the skull base. Digital subtraction angiography with balloon occlusion test is indicated when sacrifice of the internal carotid artery may be necessary. Intranasal biopsy should be considered when a malignant lesion is suspected. In cases of highly malignant tumors, the authors do not recommend a very large surgical procedure. Alternative therapy with radiation therapy and chemotherapy is carried out after biopsy. In cases of large benign lesions, radical removal is always attempted. Radical removal is not possible in some patients because of invasion of vital structures. In these cases, decompression of the involved structures and postoperative radiosurgery or radiation therapy may be the best treatment option.

The main advantages of this surgical approach are exposure of the whole anterior cranial base and paranasal sinuses with minimal retraction of the frontal lobes; the possibility of combining other surgical procedures for removal of tumors that invade the paranasal sinuses, clivus, middle fossa, and anterior portion of the cavernous sinus and nasopharynx; and very good reconstruction of the anterior cranial base with excellent cosmetic results.

The "one-piece" frontoorbital bone craniotomy permits reconstruction of the orbital roof, avoiding pulsatile exophthalmos. An excellent cosmetic result is obtained because the orbital rims remain attached to the frontal bone. Reconstruction of the large bony defect of the anterior cranial base should always be done to prevent meningoceles and encephaloceles that may cause delayed CSF fistula and meningitis.

For pure intradural lesions, such as aggressive pituitary adenomas, meningiomas, and craniopharyngiomas, this approach is also useful because dissection of both olfactory nerves is performed and wide bilateral exposure is obtained with minimal brain retraction. Both internal carotid arteries and optic nerves are identified and can be preserved. Removal of tumor infiltration into the sphenoid sinus is possible after drilling of the planum sphenoidale.

Tumor infiltration of the petrous bone, posterior fossa, intradural clivus region, and cavernous sinus with involvement of the internal carotid arteries are the main limitations for this procedure. In these cases, the authors effected the subcranial exposure with different surgical approaches. Anterior facial and lateral approaches are performed, usually during the same operative procedure. Posterior fossa approaches are carried out in a second operation some days later.

Loss of olfaction is produced in most patients when there is infiltration of the lamina cribrosa. It is, however, well tolerated in most cases. It can be avoided if there is no tumor infiltration in at least one olfactory nerve. In cases of large pituitary adenomas, craniopharyngiomas, and tuberculum sellae meningiomas, careful dissection of the olfactory nerves with preservation of function may be possible and should always be attempted. The mortality and morbidity associated with this surgical procedure are very low and usually related to postoperative CSF fistula and infection. The multidisciplinary teamwork of neurosurgeons, ear–nose–throat, head and neck surgeons, ophthalmologists, and plastic surgeons permits a more radical and safer approach to avoid these complications.

REFERENCES

1. Tessier P, Guiot G, Derome P. Orbital hypertelorism: definite treatment of orbital hypertelorism by craniofacial or by extracranial osteotomies. *Scandinavian Journal of Plastic and Reconstructive Surgery* 1973;7:39–58.
2. Ketchman AS, Wilkins RH, Van Buren JM, Johnson RH, Smith RR. A combined intracranial facial approach to the paranasal sinuses. *Am J Surg* 1963;106:698–703.
3. Derome P. Les tumeurs spheno-ethmoidales. *Neurochirurgie* 1972;18[Suppl 1]:1–164.
4. Derome PJ. Transbasal approach to tumors invading the skull base. In: Schmidek HH, Sweet WH, eds. *Operative neurosurgical techniques*. 3rd ed. Philadelphia: WB Saunders, 1995:427–441.
5. Benzil DL, Robotti E, Forcht DT, Sullivan P, Bevivino JR, Knuckey NW. Early single-stage repair of complex craniofacial trauma: experimental and clinical study. *Neurosurgery* 1992;30:166–173.
6. Cheesman AD, Lund VJ, Howard DJ. Craniofacial resection for tumors of the nasal cavity and paranasal sinuses. *Head and Neck Surgery* 1986;8:429–435.
7. Jackson IT, Marsh WR, Hide TA. Treatment of tumors involving the anterior cranial fossa. *Head and Neck Surgery* 1984;6:901–913.
8. Raveh J, Vuillemin T. The subcranial-supraorbital and temporal approach for tumors resection. *Journal of Craniofacial Surgery* 1990;1:53–59.
9. Sekhar LN, Sen C, Snyderman CH, Janecka IP. Anterior, anterolateral, and lateral approaches to extradural petroclival tumors. In: Sekhar LN, Janecka IP, eds. *Surgery of cranial base tumors*. New York: Raven Press, 1993:157–223.
10. Persing JA, Jane JA, Levine PA, Cantrell RW. The versatile frontal sinus approach to the floor of the anterior cranial fossa. *J Neurosurg* 1990;72:513–516.
11. Raveh J, Vuillemin T, Sutter F. The subcranial management of combined fronto-basal-midface fractures. *Arch Otolaryngol Head Neck Surg* 1988;114:1114–1122.
12. Samii M. Neurosurgical aspects of tumors of the base of the skull. In: Youmas JR, ed. *Neurosurgical surgery*. Philadelphia: WB Saunders, 1990:3639–3653.
13. Sundaresan N, Sachdev V, Krol G. Craniofacial resection for anterior skull base tumors. In: Schmidek HH, Sweet WH, eds. *Operative neurosurgical techniques*. 3rd ed. Philadelphia: WB Saunders, 1995:415–425.
14. Ramina R. The transfrontal basal approach to skull base surgery. Presented at the Sacramento Skull Base Surgery Symposium, Sacramento, California, June 25–30, 1995.
15. Spetzler RF, Herman JM, Beals S, Joganic E, Milligan J. Preservation of olfaction in anterior craniofacial approaches. *J Neurosurg* 1993;79:48–52.
16. Delfini R, Missori P, Iannetti G, Ciapetta P, Cantore G. Mucoceles of the paranasal sinuses with intracranial and orbital extension: report of 28 cases. *Neurosurgery* 1993;32:901–904.
17. Jan M, Dweik A, Destrieux C, Djebbari Y. Fronto-orbital sphenoidal fibrous dysplasia: case report. *Neurosurgery* 1994;34:544–543.
18. Morita A, Ebersold MJ, Olsen KD, Foote RL, Lewis JE, Quast LM. Esthesioneuroblastoma: prognosis and management. *Neurosurgery* 1993;32:706–711.
19. Meneses MS, Thurel C, Mikol J, et al. Esthesioneuroblastomas with intracranial extension. *Neurosurgery* 1990;27:813–820.
20. Delashaw JB Jr, Tedeschi H, Rhoton AL. Modified supraorbital craniotomy: technical note. *Neurosurgery* 1992;30:954–956.
21. Lalwani AK, Kaplan MJ, Gutin PH. The transsphenoethmoid approach to the sphenoid sinus and clivus. *Neurosurgery* 1992;31:1008–1012.
22. Price JC. The midfacial degloving approach to the central skull-base. *Ear Nose Throat J* 1986;65:174–180.

CHAPTER 19

Work-up and Management of the Internal Carotid Artery in Neoplastic and Vascular Lesions

Laligam N. Sekhar and Sorin D. Bucur

When the internal carotid artery (ICA) is extensively involved by neoplasms or vascular lesions of the cranial base area, a careful preoperative work-up, a plan of intraoperative management, and well developed microsurgical techniques are essential to avoid complications. The most dreaded complications of such management are carotid blowout resulting in severe hemorrhage and death, or, more commonly, stroke secondary to the ischemia produced by occlusive or embolic problems.

PHYSIOLOGY OF CEREBRAL CIRCULATION

The brain receives a blood flow averaging 50 to 55 ml/100 g of brain tissue/minute. The blood flow is much higher to the gray matter, in the range of approximately 70 to 75 ml/100 g/minute, and much lower in the white matter, in the range of 15 to 20 ml/100 g/minute. The blood flow to the brain is closely coupled to its metabolic state; the requirements of blood flow to the brain decrease with decreasing cerebral metabolic rate. Situations of decreased metabolic rate are anesthesia, barbiturate coma, hypothermia, and coma due to severe brain injuries. When the brain tissue does not receive adequate blood flow, permanent injury and cell death can occur, producing neurologic deficits. This is called a "stroke."

The brain can tolerate a range of lowered blood flows for varying periods of time. In experimental models, the electrical activity of brain cells ceases when the blood flow drops to between 15 to 20 ml/100 g/minute. When such reduction is prolonged, permanent damage can occur. In the human brain, a reduction of the blood flow below 15 to 20 ml/100 g/minute results in a burst suppression pattern on the electroencephalogram (EEG) and a prolongation of somatosensory evoked potential (SSEP) responses to the hemispheres. Reduction of brain blood flow below a threshold of 10 ml/100 g/minute, even for a short period of time, can result in permanent brain damage. Such brain injury is due to excessive activation of the calcium ion system in the brain cells and eventually results in loss of cellular membrane integrity, with the intravascular transudation of sodium ions and permanent disabling of the electrical conducting mechanism. This leads to a cascade of events that include lipid peroxidation, the generation of free radicals, and other deleterious events that are mostly irreversible. The goal of ICA management before and during surgery is to prevent the reduction of cerebral blood flow below a critical flow threshold.

At a vascular level, strokes from carotid occlusion can occur because of the severe reduction of blood flow, or because of the occurrence of a thromboembolic phenomenon. The latter is a more common mechanism of stroke. In this situation, a clot forms inside the carotid artery and propagates up into the middle cerebral artery (MCA) and its branches, or small pieces of clot break off and migrate into the peripheral vessels, blocking the blood flow to the various vessels.

When a carotid artery is temporarily occluded, collateral circulation in the brain can frequently provide blood flow for varying periods of time. Such collateral circulation is derived from the external carotid artery, the contralateral ICA, or the basilar artery, through the arteries of the circle of Willis and the ophthalmic artery. Unfortunately, such collateral circulation is inadequate in 10% to 30% of patients. The collateral circulation can be improved for periods of time by artificially inducing hypertension, about 30 to 40 mm Hg above the baseline. In addition, during anesthesia, the re-

L. N. Sekhar, S. D. Bucur: Department of Neurological Surgery, The George Washington University Medical Center, Washington, D.C. 20037.

quirements for blood flow can be diminished by reducing the metabolic demand using barbiturate- or etomidate-induced coma, or by means of mild or even severe hypothermia with cardiac circulatory arrest.

If the carotid artery is permanently occluded, however, thromboembolic mechanisms can operate conjointly with ischemic mechanisms to cause a stroke.

GENERAL PRINCIPLES

The goal of the management of a carotid artery involved by a neoplasm or giant aneurysm is, first, to preserve the artery, and second, if the artery cannot be preserved, to replace it with an alternative source of blood flow. Another method that has been used by others and also by the current authors in the past is to occlude the artery permanently, based on the presumed adequacy of the collateral circulation.

Whether the carotid artery can be dissected free of tumor depends on several factors: the arterial segment involved, whether the artery is completely encased or encased and narrowed, whether an arachnoid plane is present around the artery to enable its dissection, the histologic nature of the tumor, and previous treatment.

Encasement of the upper cervical and petrous segments of the ICA allows the artery to be dissected in some cases because of the presence of a periadventitial plane in the upper cervical segment and periosteum of the petrous internal artery canal. Encasement of the intracavernous carotid artery can be more problematic. Even though there is an adventitial plane present, there is no periadventitial tissue to protect the artery from invasion. Tumors that encase this segment of the artery may invade the adventitia, which also carries the vasa vasorum (blood supply to the wall) of the artery. The supraclinoid ICA lies in the subarachnoid space, and a delicate arachnoid plane is present between the artery and tumor, in a previously unoperated or nonirradiated patient. In such previously untreated cases, the artery can be dissected free of tumor.

The nature of the tumor encasing the artery is important. Meningiomas encasing the carotid artery frequently invade the adventitia, but the artery is protected by the arachnoid membrane in the subarachnoid space. Previous surgery or radiation therapy destroys the arachnoid plane, making the dissection impossible. Chordomas and chondrosarcomas, if they have not been previously operated, can frequently be dissected away from the ICA even when they completely encase it. However, when previous radiation therapy has been used, dissection is frequently impossible. Schwannomas encase the ICA rarely, but when such encasement occurs, they can always be dissected from the artery. Cavernous angiomas are rare lesions, but can be dissected free from the artery when they encase it. Malignant tumors, such as adenoid cystic carcinomas and squamous cell carcinomas, may be dissectable from the artery, but for oncologic reasons the artery frequently has to be excised when it is encased by the tumor.

PREOPERATIVE EVALUATION

The magnetic resonance imaging scan is the most important noninvasive test in evaluating carotid artery and other vascular encasement. T2-weighted images are particularly useful. Magnetic resonance imaging can also provide information about the water content of the tumor; in the case of benign tumors, this can be a useful indicator of whether the tumor can be dissected from the artery. Magnetic resonance angiography can also reveal the course of the artery through the tumor.

Cervical and cerebral angiography are important elements of the preoperative work-up. During angiography, the radiologist evaluates the blood supply to the tumor and the collateral pathways. If the artery is encased by tumor, an occlusion test of the artery with clinical evaluation is frequently performed. The value of the carotid occlusion test is controversial, but in the hands of experienced neuroradiologists, the test seems to be quite safe. Intravenous heparin is administered before the test (one tablet of aspirin also may be administered orally) to prevent any endothelial injury form the test. The test is carried out by temporary occlusion of the carotid artery for 15 to 20 minutes. Simultaneously, the other sources of collateral supply—namely, the external carotid artery, the contralateral ICA, and the vertebral artery—are injected with contrast to see which vessels are supplying the hemisphere during the period of test occlusion. The patient is examined clinically to determine if there are any neurologic deficits. If any develop, the test is terminated immediately. Some investigators perform balloon occlusion tests with induced hypotension to simulate dire perioperative conditions; however, because this process increases the risk of the test, the authors do not favor it.

The balloon occlusion test may be combined with other measurements of the adequacy of collateral flow. The gold standard here is xenon blood flow examination, which is not available in most institutions. Single-photon emission computed tomography (SPECT) scanning, which is available in most institutions, provides a qualitative indication of the adequacy of blood flow. Only a qualitative comparison of the information from the ipsilateral hemisphere with that of the contralateral hemisphere is possible, and no quantitative information is available from SPECT scanning. However, SPECT scans can be performed quite easily and are widely available. Transcranial Doppler ultrasound studies of MCA flow velocity have also been obtained as an indicator of collateral flow, but no correlation studies between transcranial Doppler and xenon-determined blood flow have been performed. It appears that transcranial Doppler is probably too sensitive to reductions in flow. No studies correlating transcranial Doppler or SPECT with the risk of carotid occlusion have been reported. The authors' protocol is simply to perform a clinical balloon occlusion test with simultaneous demonstration of the angiographic source of collateral circulation.

MANAGEMENT OF THE INTERNAL CAROTID ARTERY

Before and during an operation, the surgeon has to make a decision about whether the artery can be preserved. In the case of malignant tumors encasing the carotid artery, this decision is made before the surgery. In such patients (e.g., those with squamous cell carcinoma or adenoid cystic carcinoma encasing the carotid artery), the authors place a saphenous vein bypass graft from the cervical ICA, bypassing the region of the tumor, to the M3 segment of the MCA. The tumor-involved segment of the ICA is simultaneously occluded (Figs. 1–5). Approximately 1 or 2 weeks later, the operation to remove the tumor is performed without any complications.

With other tumors, such as meningiomas, chordomas, and chondrosarcomas, the authors usually make an attempt to peel the tumor from the artery during the operation. Nor-

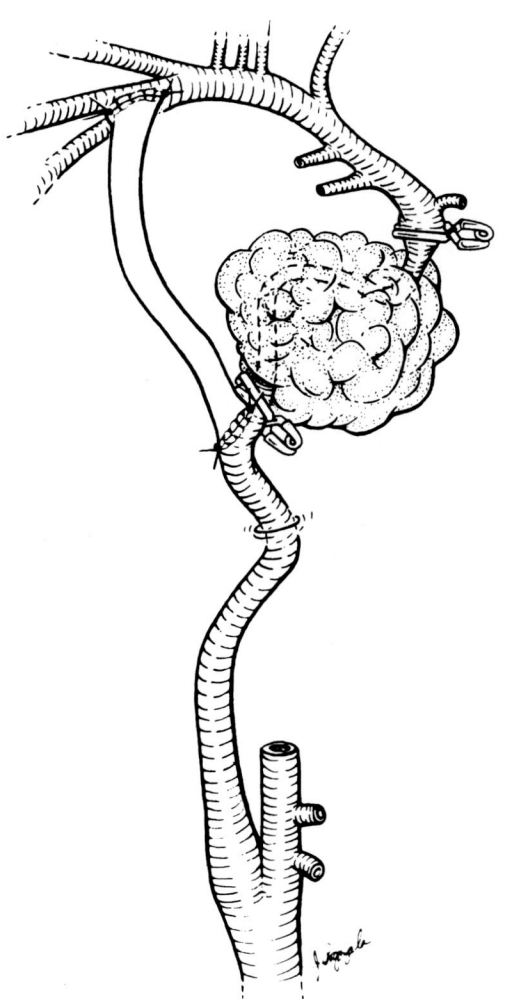

FIG. 2. Schematic drawing showing the strategy of saphenous vein graft bypass from the petrous internal carotid artery (ICA) to the M2 segment of the middle cerebral artery in case of complete encasement of the petrous and cavernous ICA by a tumor. (Copyright 1995 Laligam N. Sekhar, MD.)

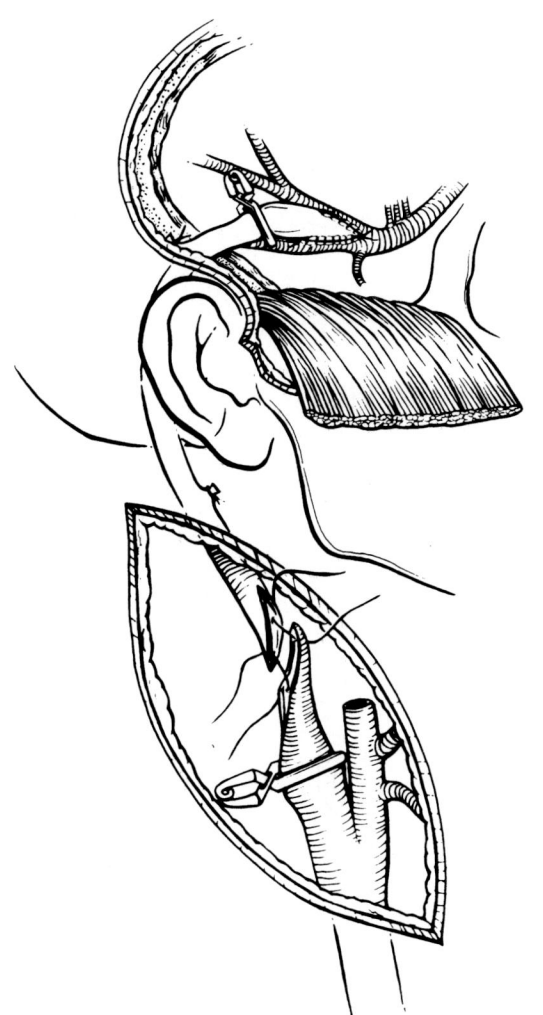

FIG. 1. Schematic drawing showing the trajectory of the graft through a tunnel shaped in the retroauricular area. (Copyright 1995 Laligam N. Sekhar, MD.)

mally, such dissection is carried out from the normal to the abnormal area, with preparation made for proximal and distal control to trap the artery temporarily in the event of vascular injury. The anesthesiologist must also prepare for the induction of barbiturate or etomidate coma, induced hypertension, and mild hypothermia to protect the brain during temporary vascular occlusion. If the artery is not dissectable, it is replaced with a saphenous vein graft. Such a graft may be a direct interposition graft (Figs. 6, 7), or a bypass graft as previously described.

The authors no longer perform elective carotid artery occlusion based on preoperative assessment of collateral circulation; their experience in this area has been reported previously. The authors found that despite the best measures of collateral circulation, the incidence of stroke was still unacceptably high.

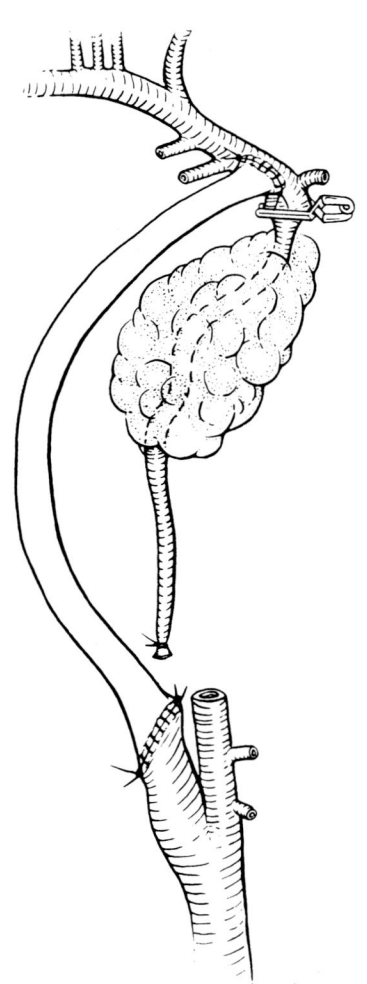

FIG. 3. Schematic drawing showing cervical internal carotid artery (ICA) to supraophthalmic ICA vein graft bypass, with the ICA sacrificed. (Copyright 1995 Laligam N. Sekhar, MD.)

FIG. 4. Schematic drawing showing arteriotomy at the level of the M2 middle cerebral artery bifurcation, and the position of the graft to ensure additional retrograde flow. (Copyright 1995 Laligam N. Sekhar, MD.)

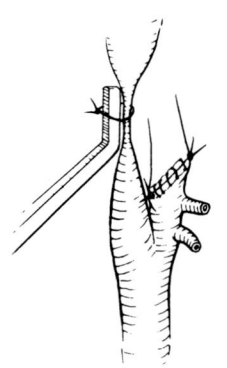
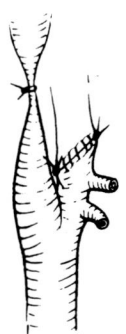
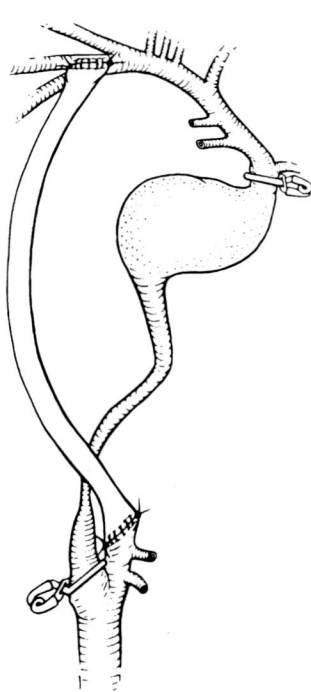

FIG. 5. Schematic drawing showing the saphenous vein bypass strategy between the external carotid artery and the M2 segment of the middle cerebral artery, with different modalities of internal carotid artery (ICA) ligation, in a case of giant cavernous ICA aneurysm. (Copyright 1995 Laligam N. Sekhar, MD.)

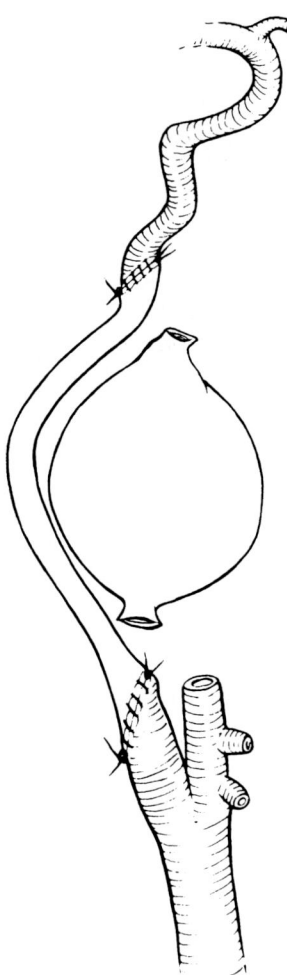

FIG. 6. Schematic drawing showing cervical internal carotid artery (ICA) to cervical ICA interposition graft bypass for a giant cervical ICA aneurysm or pseudoaneurysm. (Copyright 1995 Laligam N. Sekhar, MD.)

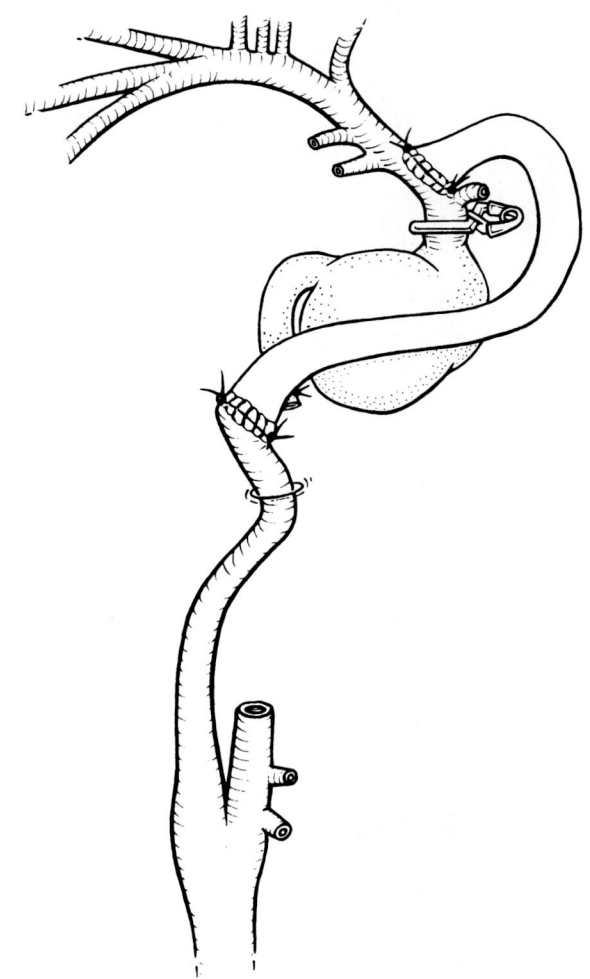

FIG. 7. Schematic drawing showing petrous internal carotid artery (ICA) to supraophthalmic ICA interposition graft bypass in a case of giant cavernous ICA aneurysm. (Copyright 1995 Laligam N. Sekhar, MD.)

CASE REPORTS

CASE 1

This 30-year-old woman presented with a cavernous sinus syndrome secondary to a recurrent chondrosarcoma involving the sphenocavernous area (Fig. 8). The intracavernous ICA was encased and narrowed by the tumor (Fig. 9). An initial operation was performed to replace the ICA with a saphenous vein bypass graft from the cervical ICA to the M2 segment of the MCA (Figs. 10, 11). At a subsequent operation 5 days later, the tumor was resected completely. The patient recovered well, but with a worsening of her cranial nerve IV function. No recurrence has been observed over the last 3 years (Figs. 12–14).

CASE 1 (Continued)

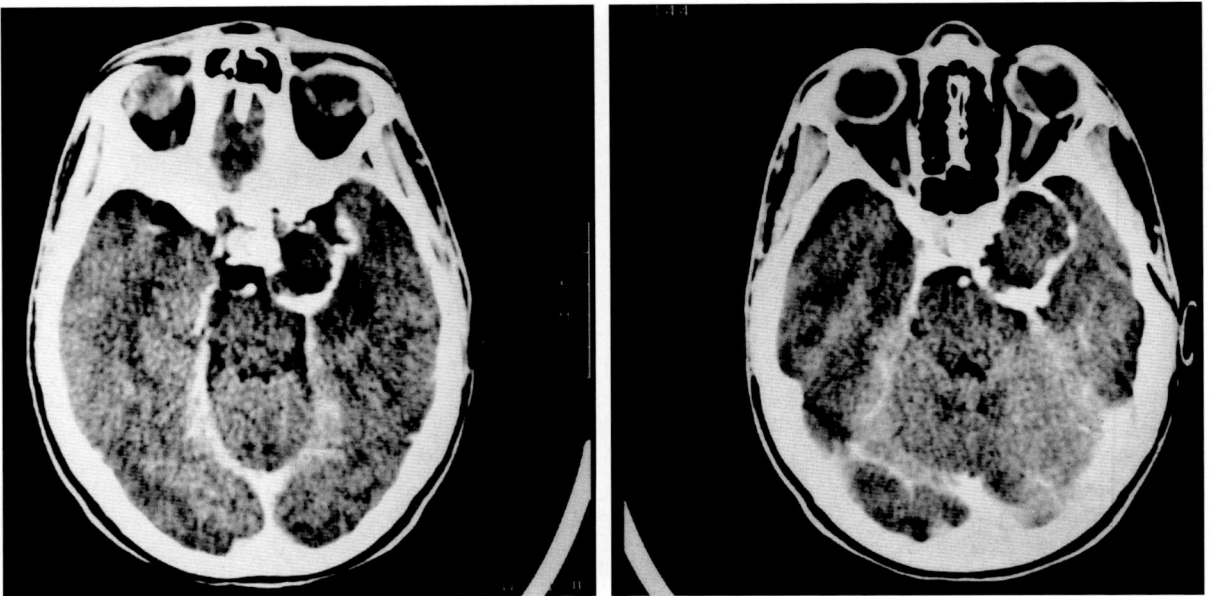

FIG. 8. Case 1. **A,B:** Preoperative enhanced computed tomography scans showing tumor in the left sphenocavernous area.

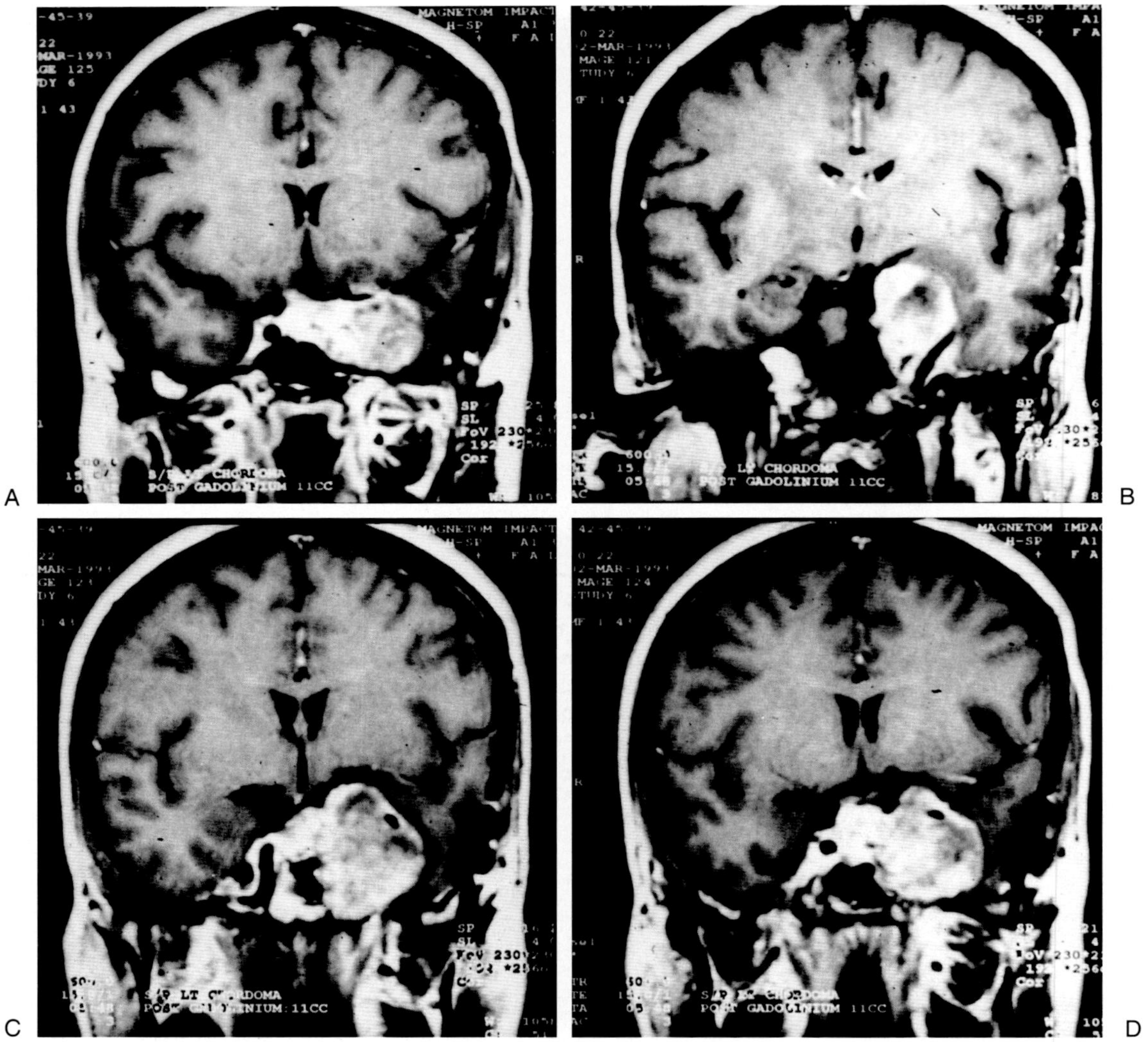

FIG. 9. Case 1. **A–D:** Preoperative coronal magnetic resonance images showing extension of the tumor with encasement and narrowing of the cavernous internal carotid artery.

CASE 1 (Continued)

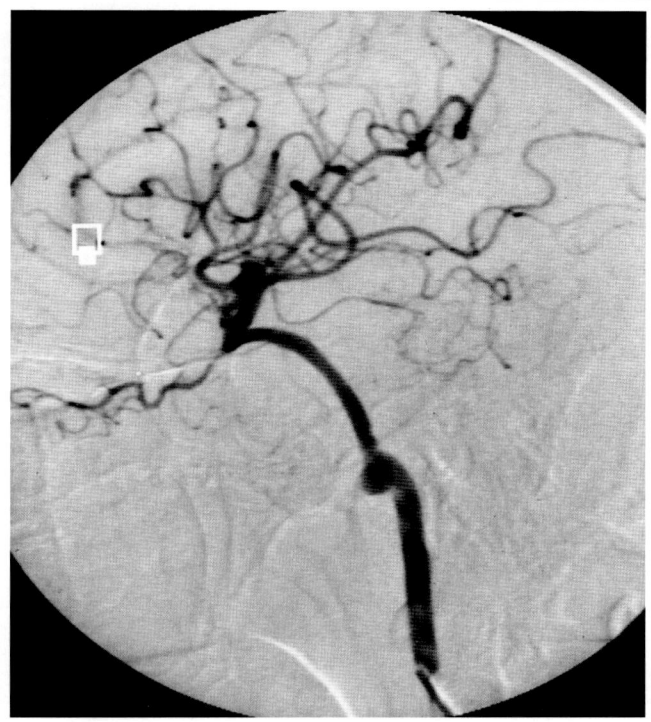

FIG. 10. Case 1. Intraoperative angiogram demonstrates good flow through the graft.

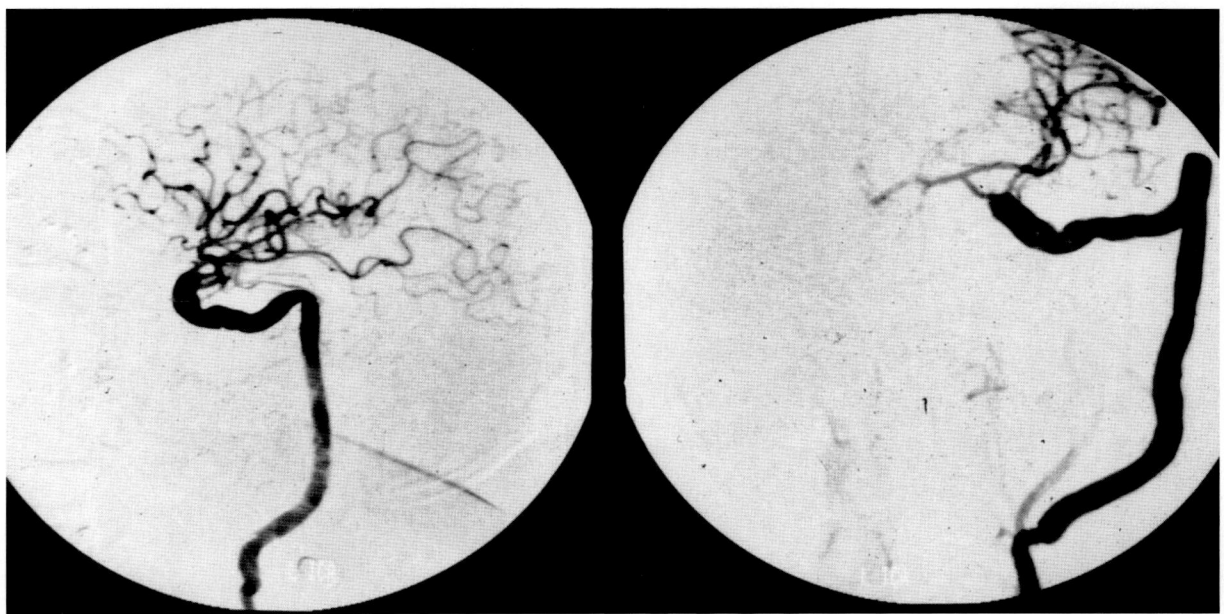

FIG. 11. Case 1. **A,B:** Postoperative angiogram.

CASE 1 (Continued)

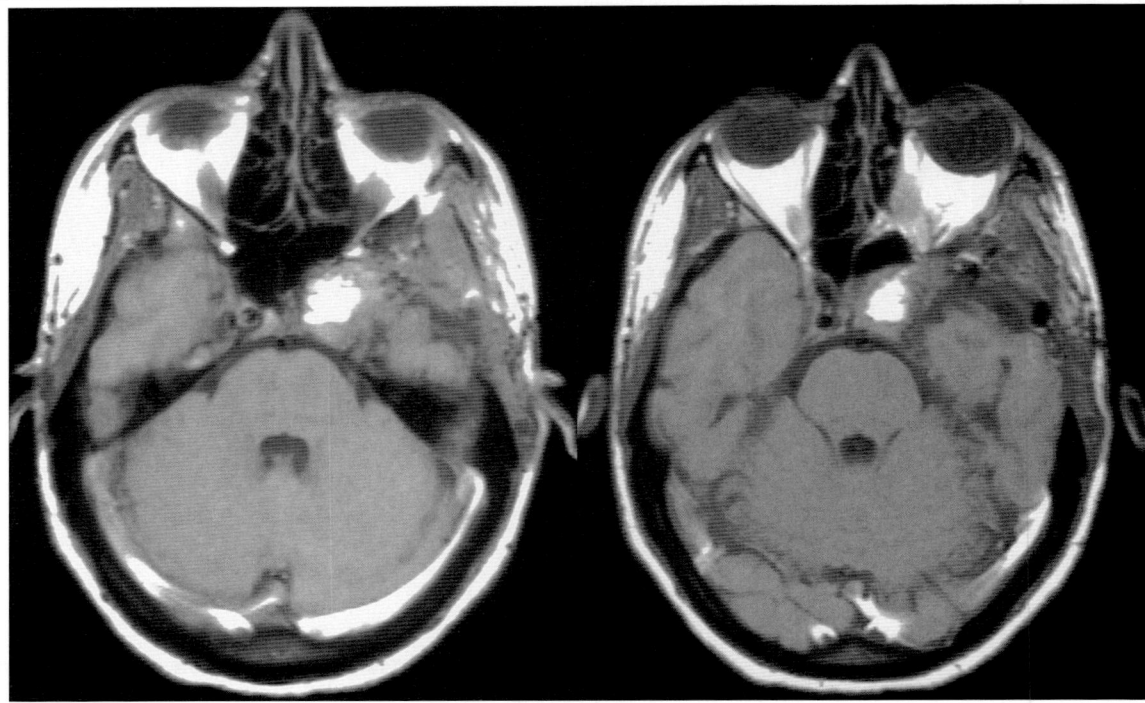

FIG. 12. Case 1. **A:** Postoperative axial magnetic resonance image (MRI) showing complete resection of the tumor. **B:** Postoperative axial MRI showing the position of the vein graft.

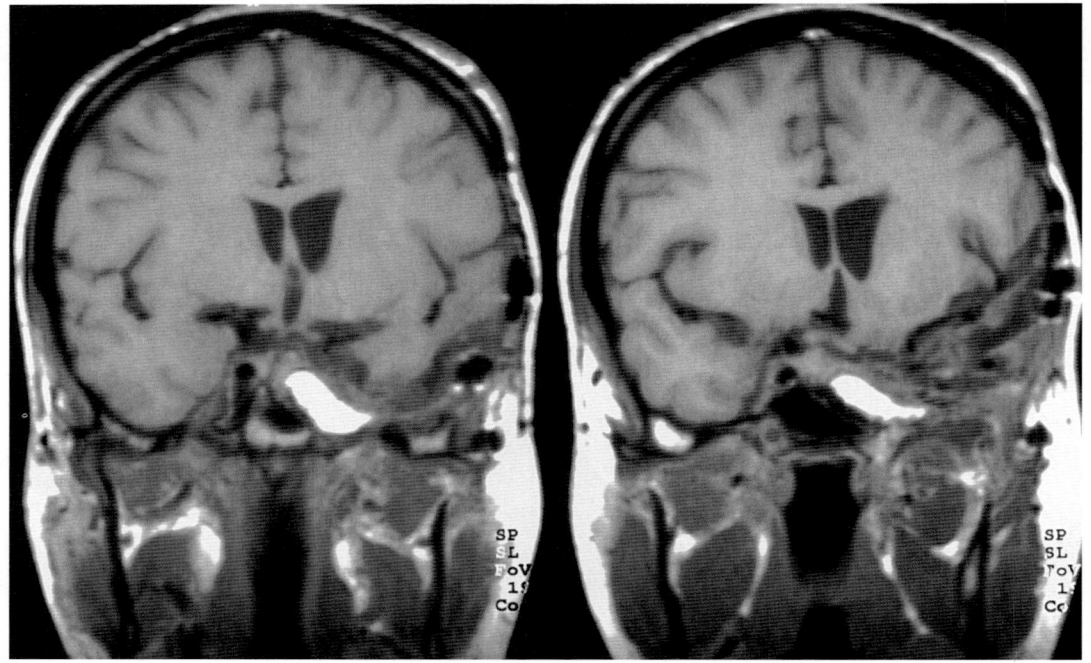

FIG. 13. Case 1. **A,B:** Postoperative coronal magnetic resonance images showing complete resection of the tumor. The enhanced region represents the fat graft used for reconstruction.

CASE 1 (Continued)

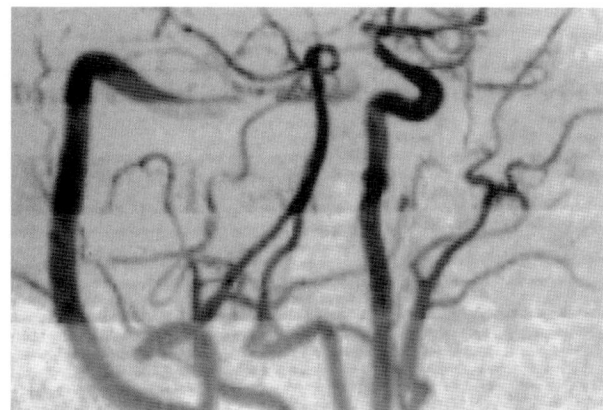

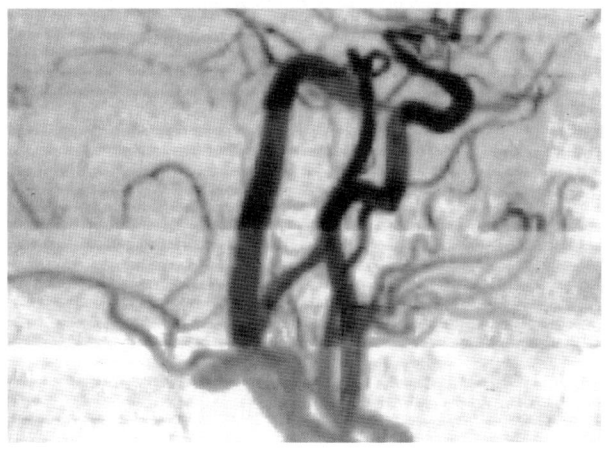

FIG. 14. Case 1. **A,B:** Follow-up magnetic resonance angiograms demonstrating patency of the vein graft.

CASE 2

This 40-year-old patient had been treated with biopsy and radiation therapy 8 years previously for an extensive adenoid cystic carcinoma. He presented with an extensive regrowth involving the cavernous sinus, petroclival area, and the infratemporal fossa (Figs. 15–17). The petrous and cavernous ICA segments were involved by the tumor. He tolerated balloon test occlusion of the left ICA clinically with good collateral flow demonstrated from the other side (Figs. 18, 19). Because of the risk of stroke and ICA

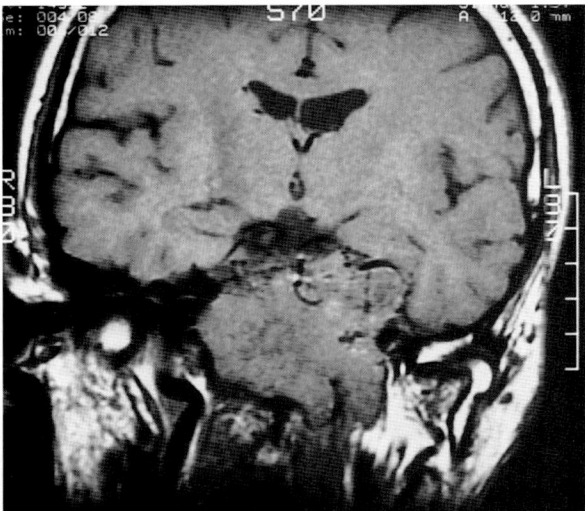 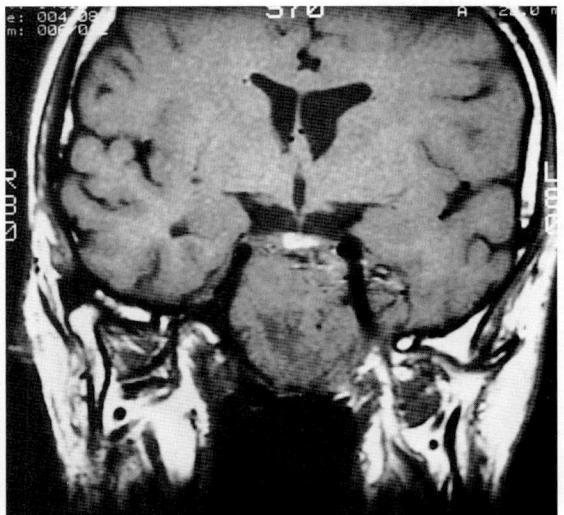

FIG. 15. Case 2. **A,B:** Preoperative coronal magnetic resonance images show extension of the tumor into the cavernous sinus and infratemporal fossa.

CASE 2 (Continued)

rupture, a saphenous vein graft bypass running behind the ear was performed initially (Fig. 20), and this was followed by gross total tumor resection through a preauricular infratemporal approach, and reconstruction with a rectus abdominis free flap (Fig. 21). The patient recovered well without additional neurologic deficit. Follow-up intravenous chemotherapy was performed. However, 2 years later, he had extensive local and systemic tumor recurrence and died, despite further chemotherapy.

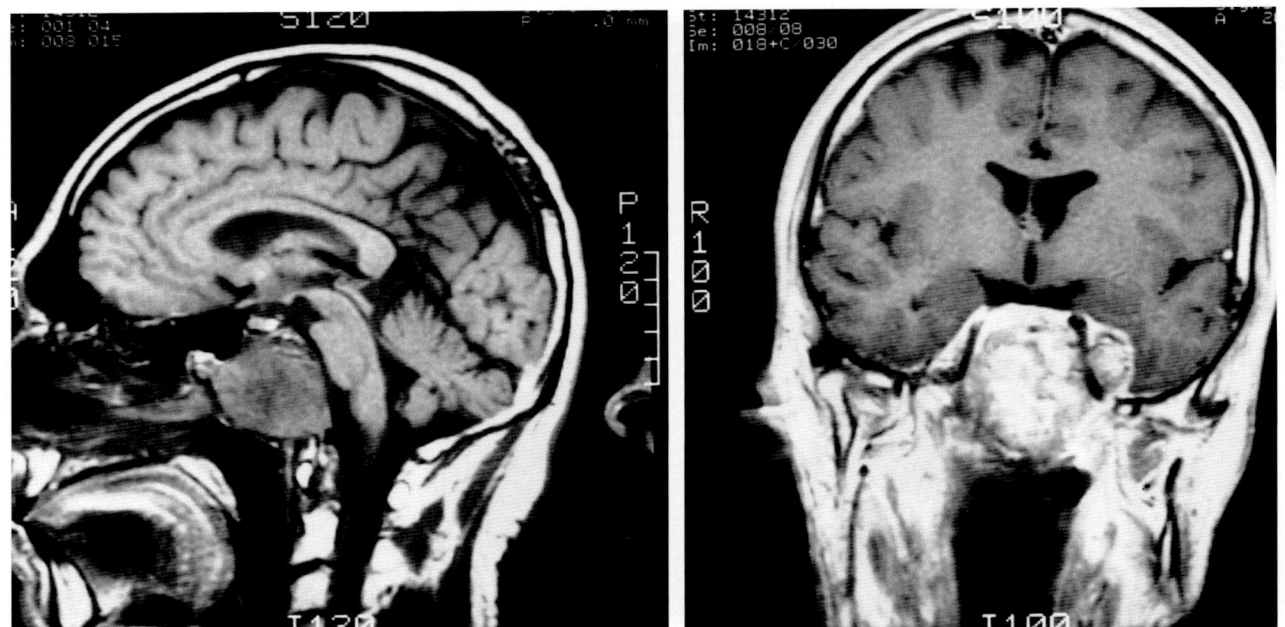

FIG. 16. Case 2. Preoperative sagittal magnetic resonance image (MRI) **(A)** shows extension of tumor in the petroclival area, and coronal MRI **(B)** demonstrates encasement of the internal carotid artery by the tumor.

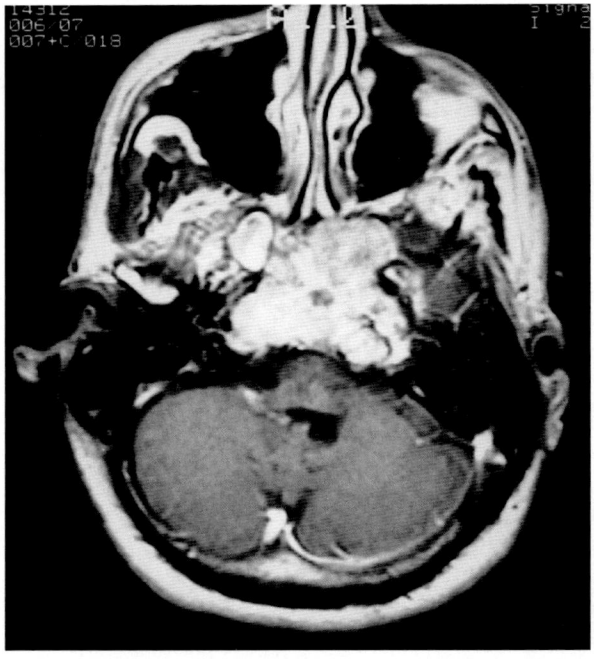

FIG. 17. Case 2. Preoperative axial magnetic resonance image.

CASE 2 (Continued)

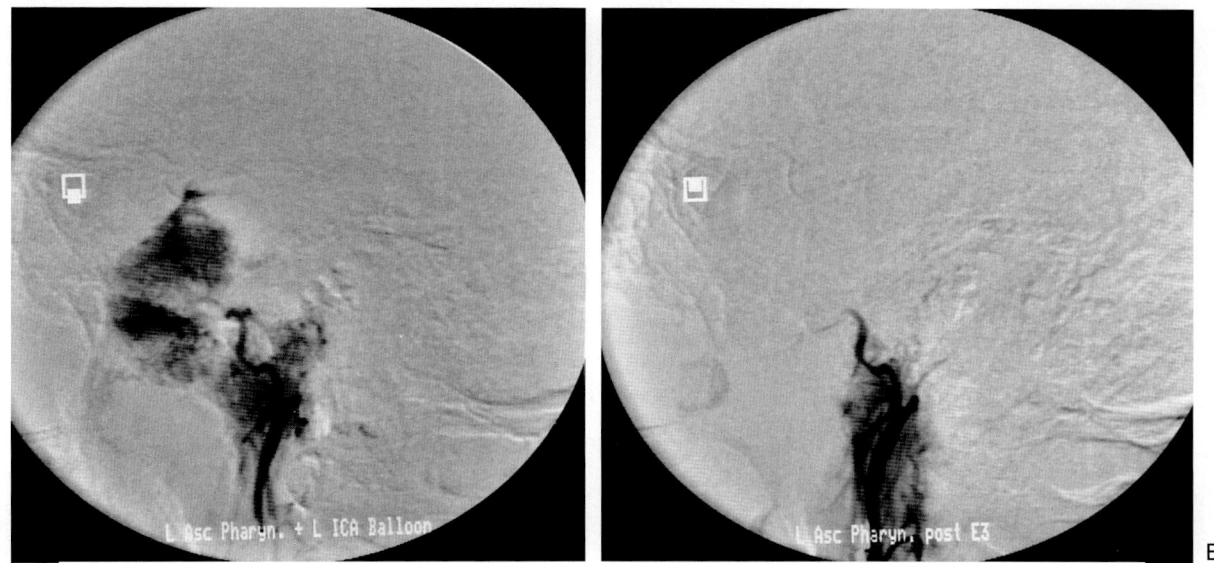

FIG. 18. Case 2. Preoperative supraselective angiograms showing vascularization of the tumor from the left ascending pharyngeal artery **(A)**, and injection after embolization **(B)**.

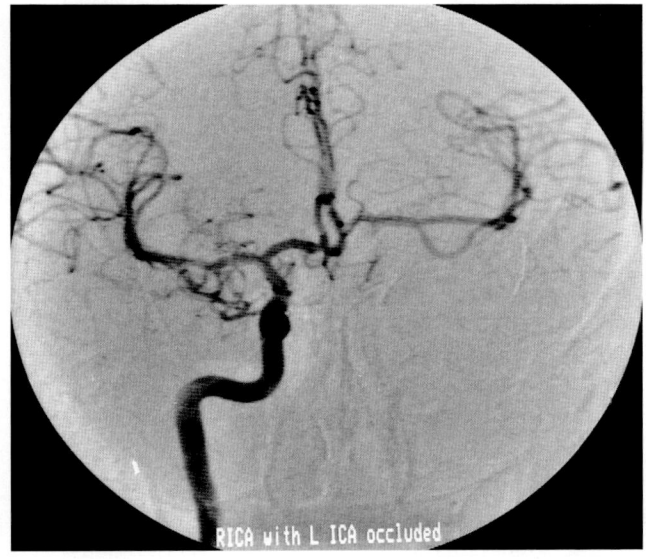

FIG. 19. Case 2. Anteroposterior view of right internal carotid artery (ICA) injection during balloon test occlusion of the left ICA, showing excellent collateralization through anterior communicating artery.

CASE 2 (Continued)

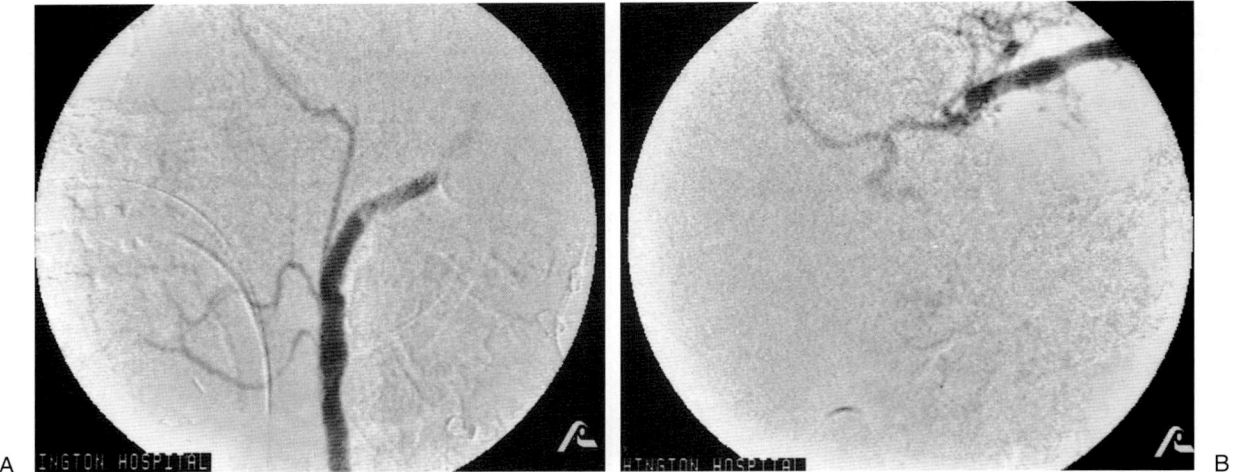

FIG. 20. Case 2. **A,B:** Intraoperative angiograms demonstrating the patency of the graft.

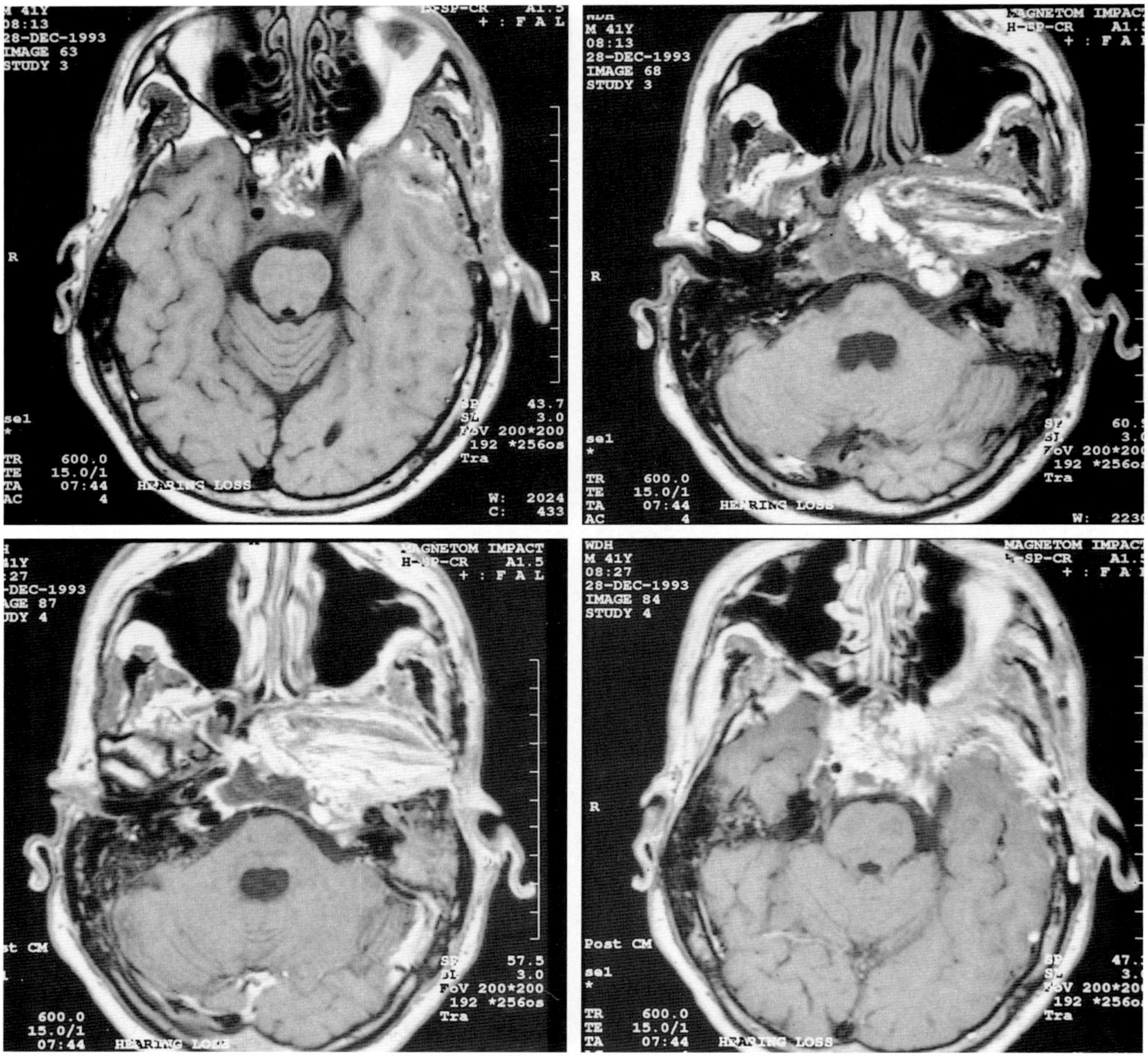

FIG. 21. Case 2. **A–D:** Postoperative axial magnetic resonance images showing gross resection of the tumor, and the muscle flap in the middle fossa used for reconstruction.

CASE 3

This 31-year-old woman had an extensive meningioma of the jugular foramen and the upper cervical area. A biopsy had been performed at another institution, after which she sustained a spinal accessory nerve palsy. The tumor was growing progressively in size (Figs. 22, 23). The upper cervical ICA was encased and narrowed by the tumor, and she failed a carotid occlusion test, manifesting a neurologic deficit during the occlusion. An ICA to MCA bypass was performed in preparation for the tumor resection, after dissection of the ICA from the tumor proved impossible. However, this graft exhibited poor flow (Fig. 24), and eventually occluded 2 weeks after surgery. The tumor was subsequently resected by a combined transjugular, infratemporal, and upper cervical approach. The abnormal segment of ICA was resected and reconstructed by means of a vein graft from the cervical to the petrous ICA (Figs. 25, 26). During temporary ICA occlusion, induced hypertension, mild hypothermia, and barbiturate-induced coma were used for brain protection. Her postoperative course was complicated by cranial nerves IX and X palsy, but she made an excellent recovery without having a stroke. The brain protection techniques used during the operation were effective in preventing a stroke during the period of temporary ICA occlusion.

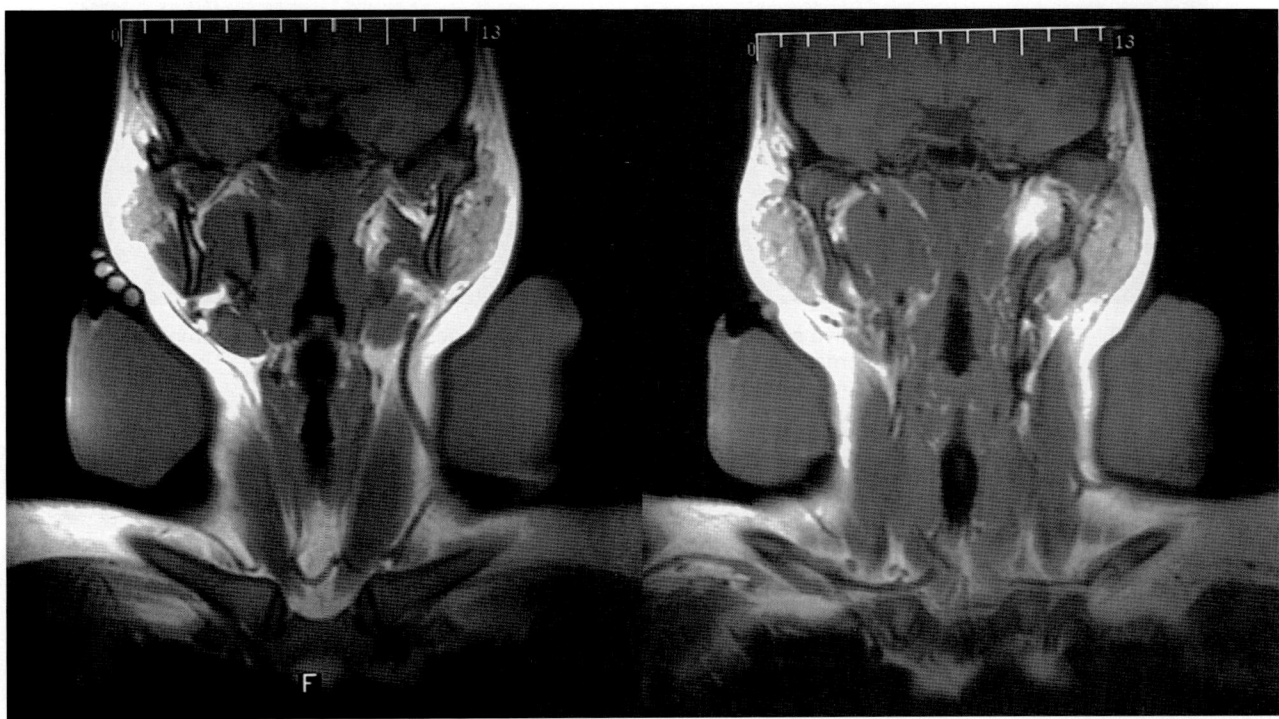

FIG. 22. Case 3. **A,B:** Preoperative coronal magnetic resonance images showing extension of the tumor in the infratemporal fossa.

CASE 3 (Continued)

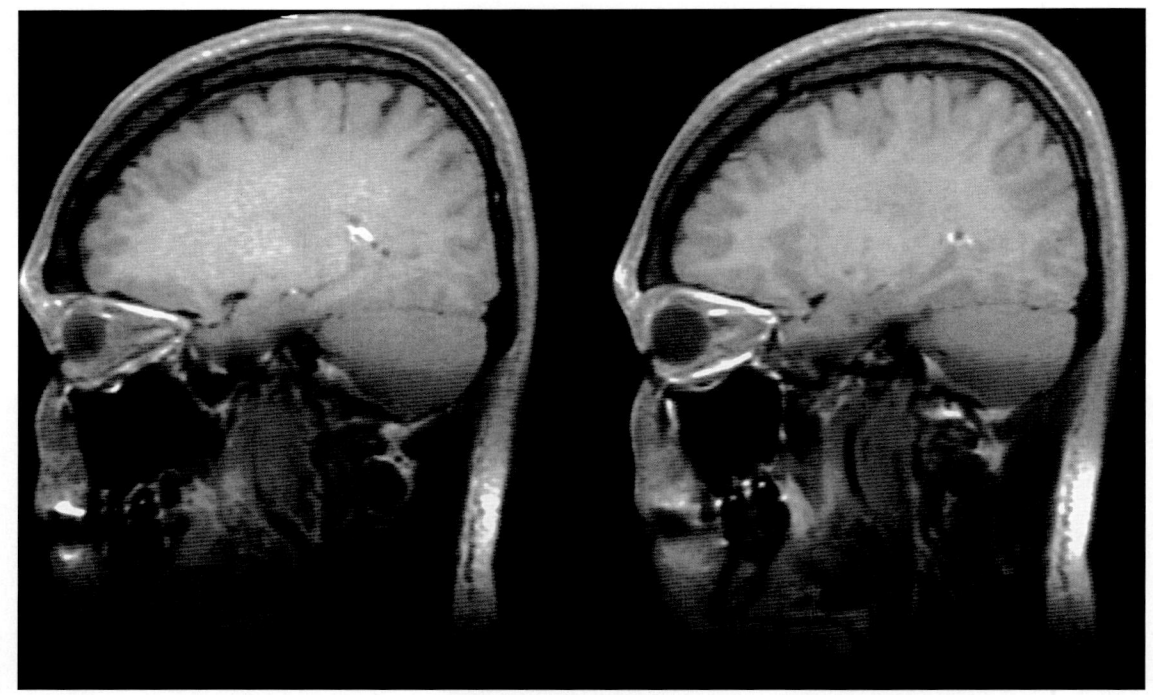

FIG. 23. Case 3. **A,B:** Preoperative sagittal magnetic resonance images demonstrate encasement and displacement of the cervical internal carotid artery by the tumor.

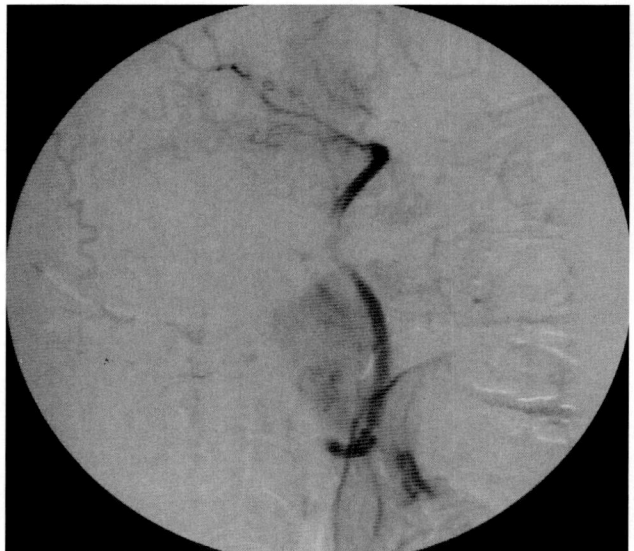

FIG. 24. Case 3. Postoperative angiogram of the first stage, demonstrating poor flow through the graft.

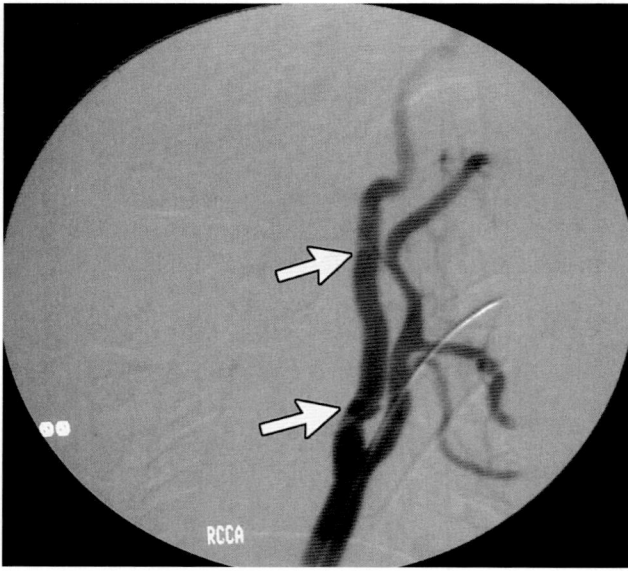

FIG. 25. Case 3. Postoperative angiogram after complete removal of the tumor and reconstruction of the cervical internal carotid artery. *Arrows* indicate locations of the proximal and distal anastomoses.

CASE 3 (Continued)

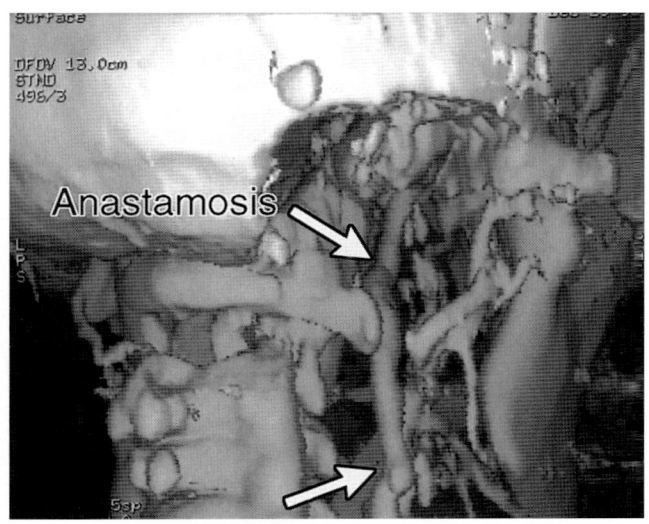

FIG. 26. Case 3. Postoperative three-dimensional computed tomography scan showing the graft.

OPERATIVE TECHNIQUE

Patients who require a significant ICA dissection during tumor removal undergo neurophysiologic monitoring using EEG and SSEP. The patient's head is placed in a radiolucent-pin head holder and a femoral artery sheath is placed by the neuroradiologist, in preparation for intraoperative angiography. The cervical internal and external carotid arteries are exposed. The greater saphenous vein is either exposed in the thigh for a distance of 20 cm, or the thigh area is at least prepared for possible extraction of the vein graft. If saphenous vein is not available, the radial artery can be used.

During the operation, dissection of the tumor is attempted if it is a benign tumor or of the cartilaginous variety (chordoma or chondrosarcoma). With malignant tumors, a bypass is performed electively if ICA resection will be required during the tumor resection.

If a saphenous vein bypass of the ICA is performed, the authors prefer a vein graft from the cervical ICA to the M2 segment of the MCA because the temporary occlusion time of the ICA is minimized. Occlusion of the M2 segment of the MCA for less than 50 minutes under brain protection techniques is well tolerated. If the patient has absolutely no collateral circulation, the external carotid artery or the vertebral artery may be used for the proximal anastomosis. If the M2 segment of the MCA is less than 3 mm in diameter, the supraclinoid ICA is used for the distal anastomosis, or a radial artery graft may be used.

During vascular occlusion, the patient's blood pressure is raised 20%, 2,000 U of heparin and 1 g of methylprednisolone are given intravenously, and metabolic suppression of the brain is induced with barbiturate, etomidate, or propofol, to achieve burst suppression on the EEG. If changes occur in the SSEP during the operation, ischemia of the deep brain regions is indicated, and the temporary clips may need to be repositioned, or the blood pressure raised further.

The distal anastomosis is performed first, with the graft preferably placed into a bifurcation of the MCA. After completing the anastomosis, a temporary clip is placed on the vein graft close to the MCA, and flow is resumed through the MCA. The vein graft is then brought to the neck through a retroauricular tunnel, and the proximal anastomosis is performed.

After the anastomosis is completed, the temporary clips are removed, and graft flow is checked by means of intraoperative Doppler probe and angiography. If adequate flow is not demonstrated, the problem must be corrected during surgery.

After surgery, the patient is maintained on subcutaneous heparin for a week, and then perpetually on 325 mg of aspirin daily.

RESULTS OF VEIN AND RADIAL ARTERY GRAFTING

One hundred twenty-two vein and artery grafts were performed by the senior author from 1985 through 1997 for the management of skull base tumors and aneurysms of the anterior or posterior circulation. The results of the grafting procedures cannot be compared with those of vascular occlusion procedures because many patients with poor collateral circulation were treated by grafting. Intraoperative angiography, and the lessons learned from the correction of intraoperative vein grafts, improved the patency rate of the grafts from 90% to 98% and reduced the stroke rate from 13% to 9%, even though more and more complex lesions have been treated in more recent years. Strokes with major deficits (Glasgow outcome score of 3) have occurred in only 5% of the group.

CONCLUSION

Management of the ICA in skull base and vascular surgery has been greatly improved by vein and artery bypass techniques. Further improvements in brain protection techniques and in our understanding of vascular physiology will result in further benefits for patients with difficult lesions.

BIBLIOGRAPHY

DeVries EJ, Sekhar LN, Janecka IP, Schramm VL, Horton JA, Eibling DE. Elective resection of the internal carotid artery without reconstruction. *Laryngoscope* 1988;989:960–966.

Erba SM, Horton JA, Latchaw RE, et al. Balloon test occlusion of the internal carotid artery with stable xenon/CT cerebral blood flow imaging. *AJNR Am J Neuroradiol* 1988;9:533–538.

Gormley WB, Sekhar LN. Augmentation of cerebral vascular reserve with bypass grafting in the treatment of tumors, aneurysms, and occlusive disease. *Critical Reviews in Neurosurgery* 1995;5:333–341.

Iwai Y, Sekhar LN, Goel A, Cass S. Vein graft replacement of the distal vertebral artery. *Acta Neurochir (Wien)* 1993;120:81–87.

Kotapka MJ, Kalia KK, Martinez AJ, Sekhar LN. Infiltration of the carotid artery by cavernous sinus meningioma. *J Neurosurg* 1994;81:252–255.

Sekhar LN, Iwai Y, Wright D, Bloom M. Vein graft replacement of the middle cerebral artery after unsuccessful embolectomy: case report. *Neurosurgery* 1993;33:723–727.

Sekhar LN, Patel SJ. Permanent occlusion of the internal carotid artery during skull-base and vascular surgery: is it really safe? [Editorial]. *Am J Otol* 1993;14:421–422.

Sekhar LN, Sen CN, Jho HD. Saphenous vein graft bypass of the cavernous internal carotid artery. *J Neurosurg* 1990;72:35–41.

Sen C, Sekhar LN. Direct vein graft reconstruction of the cavernous, petrous, and upper cervical internal carotid artery: lessons learned from 30 cases. *Neurosurgery* 1992;30:732–743.

Steed DL, Webster MW, DeVries EJ, et al. Clinical observations on the effect of carotid artery occlusion on cerebral blood flow mapped by xenon computed tomography and its correlation with carotid artery back pressure. *J Vasc Surg* 1990;1:38–44.

SECTION III
Posterior Fossa Approaches

CHAPTER 20

Temporal Bone Resection

Aongus J. Curran, Patrick J. Gullane, Manohar L. Bance, and Paul J. Donald

Malignant tumors affecting the temporal bone are rare and account for only 0.05% of head and neck carcinomas (1). Owing to this rarity, a complete understanding of the pathophysiology of the disease is lacking. Diagnosis is usually at a late stage because the signs and symptoms of malignancy are often initially similar to those associated with chronic suppurative otitis media or otitis externa. The lack of a coherent staging system when comparing different reports makes an accurate comparison of the various treatment options difficult. Politzer gave the first detailed account of the disease in 1883, and is also credited with recognizing the importance of chronic suppurative otitis media as a common etiologic factor in its development (2). In this century, Parsons and Lewis contributed significantly to the surgical principle of *en bloc* resection of the lateral skull base, and Lederman introduced the important role radiation therapy has to play in the management of this aggressive group of tumors (3,4).

Since the late 1970s, there have been significant technical refinements and advances in cranial base surgery (5,6). The improved exposure and safety of approaches coupled with better anesthesia and an ability to reconstruct large defects with free and pedicled myocutaneous flaps has resulted in a reduction in functional and aesthetic morbidity. Modern imaging involving both computed tomography (CT) and magnetic resonance imaging (MRI) allows more precise localization and treatment planning for these tumors, which are now frequently managed by a multidisciplinary team that usually involves a combination of head and neck surgeons, neurosurgeons, and plastic surgeons. The most widely accepted operative concept is to free the involved temporal bone from its surrounding venous sinuses, protect the internal carotid artery (ICA) and brainstem, and avoid injury to cranial nerves. Typically, the patient also receives preoperative or postoperative radiation therapy. Although this has resulted in an improved quality of life for patients, the impact of these advances on survival is unknown. A recurring theme in previous reports is that diagnosis is often late in the natural history of the disease, and this is reflected in the frequently encountered poor prognosis.

The aim of this chapter is to present the clinical features of temporal bone malignancy that necessitate temporal bone resection, the options in management, and the controversies that surround this area. Particular emphasis is placed on tumors arising in the external auditory meatus, middle ear, and mastoid, and no attempt is made to detail the clinical features and management of malignancies involving the pinna. Although these lesions are much more common, the principles of management and complications associated with these tumors are somewhat different. Benign tumors are mentioned for completeness, whereas the management of glomus tumors is described elsewhere (see Chapter 24).

ANATOMY

Temporal Bone

The temporal bone occupies the center of the lateral skull base, with vital neurovascular structures passing to and from the brain through its substance (Fig. 1). It is a single bone that possesses tympanic, mastoid, zygomatic, and petrous portions. Each temporal bone articulates with its neighboring sphenoid, parietal, occipital, and zygomatic bones. It articulates with the condyle of the mandible by the glenoid fossa on the undersurface of the squamous portion of the bone as the temporomandibular joint (TMJ).

The temporal bone has many important relationships to neighboring structures, including:

1. *Medially*, the cerebellopontine angle and the brainstem are found.

A. J. Curran, P. J. Gullane, M. L. Bance: Department of Otolaryngology, The Toronto Hospital, and the University of Toronto, Toronto, Ontario, M5G 2C4 Canada.

P. J. Donald: Department of Otolaryngology—Head and Neck Surgery, and Center for Skull Base Surgery, University of California, Davis Medical Center, Sacramento, California 95817.

2. *Inferiorly* are the great vessels and the contents of the neck.
3. *Laterally* are the external auditory meatus and auricle.
4. *Anteroinferiorly* lies the infratemporal fossa, which contains the pterygoid muscles, the mandibular division of the trigeminal nerve, the internal maxillary artery, and the pterygoid venous plexus.
5. *Posteriorly*, the cerebellum is housed in the posterior cranial fossa, with the lower cranial nerves (VII–XII) surrounded by venous sinuses.
6. *Superiorly*, the temporal lobe is housed in the middle cranial fossa with cranial nerves II to VI.

The ICA enters the skull base at the carotid foramen (Figs. 1, 2). Here it passes through the petrous part of the temporal bone anteromedial to the jugular foramen and medial to the styloid process. The vessel then turns through 90 degrees, becoming horizontal medial to the eustachian tube within the temporal bone. It then turns again to emerge at the foramen lacerum as it enters the cavernous sinus. During its intratemporal course, it gives off the caroticotympanic artery, and within the cavernous sinus it gives off cavernous arteries. Vascularized tumors such as glomus tumors and nasopharyngeal angiofibroma are often supplied by these vessels, which can subsequently become significantly enlarged.

The temporal bone is closely related to the jugular bulb and the sigmoid sinus. At its superior end, the sigmoid sinus receives venous blood from the transverse (lateral) and superior petrosal sinuses (see Fig. 2). Mastoid emissary veins often communicate across the calvarium between the sigmoid sinus and posterior auricular veins. The jugular bulb becomes the internal jugular vein after the union of the sigmoid and inferior petrosal sinuses, and only a thin plate of bone separates it from the ICA.

The facial nerve has the longest bony course of any peripheral nerve in the body. Meatal, labyrinthine, middle ear, and mastoid components make up its intratemporal course. With the eighth cranial nerve (cochleovestibular), it leaves the pons and enters the porus of the internal auditory canal accompanied by the nervus intermedius and the internal labyrinthine artery and vein (see Fig. 2). It lies in the anterosuperior quadrant at the fundus above the cochlear branch of the eight nerve superior to the crista transversalis. The nerve then courses anteriorly to the geniculate ganglion and is ensheathed by an extension of the subarachnoid space with cerebrospinal fluid (CSF) to this point. The geniculate ridge, a sharp, bony prominence, separates the labyrinthine from the tympanic segments. The latter begins at the geniculate ganglion, where the nerve makes its first extraaxial turn (internal genu) and begins a posterior course. The cochleariform process marks its most anterior limit and is a valuable landmark to locate the nerve in the middle ear. In as many as

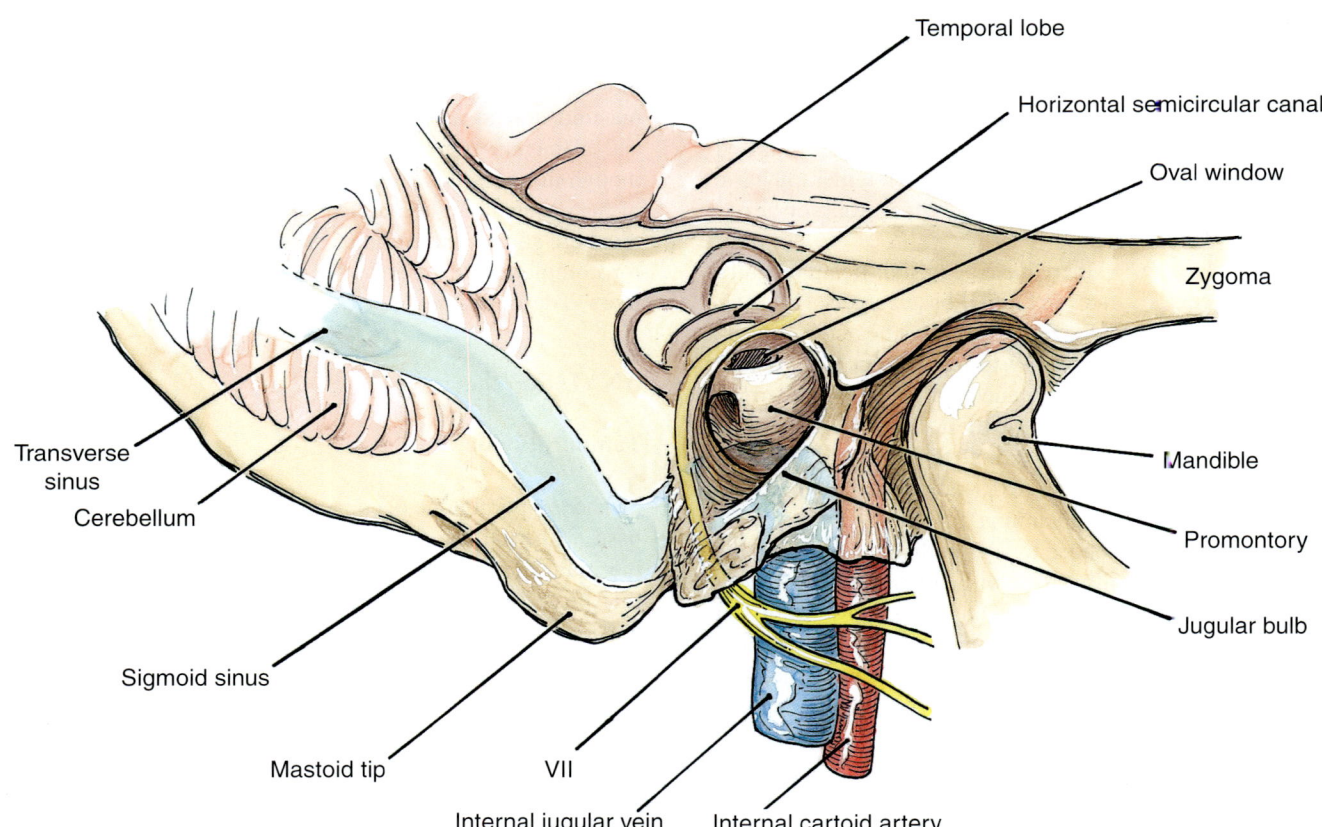

FIG. 1. Coronal section through temporal bone showing relationships of major vessels, brain, mandible, and middle ear.

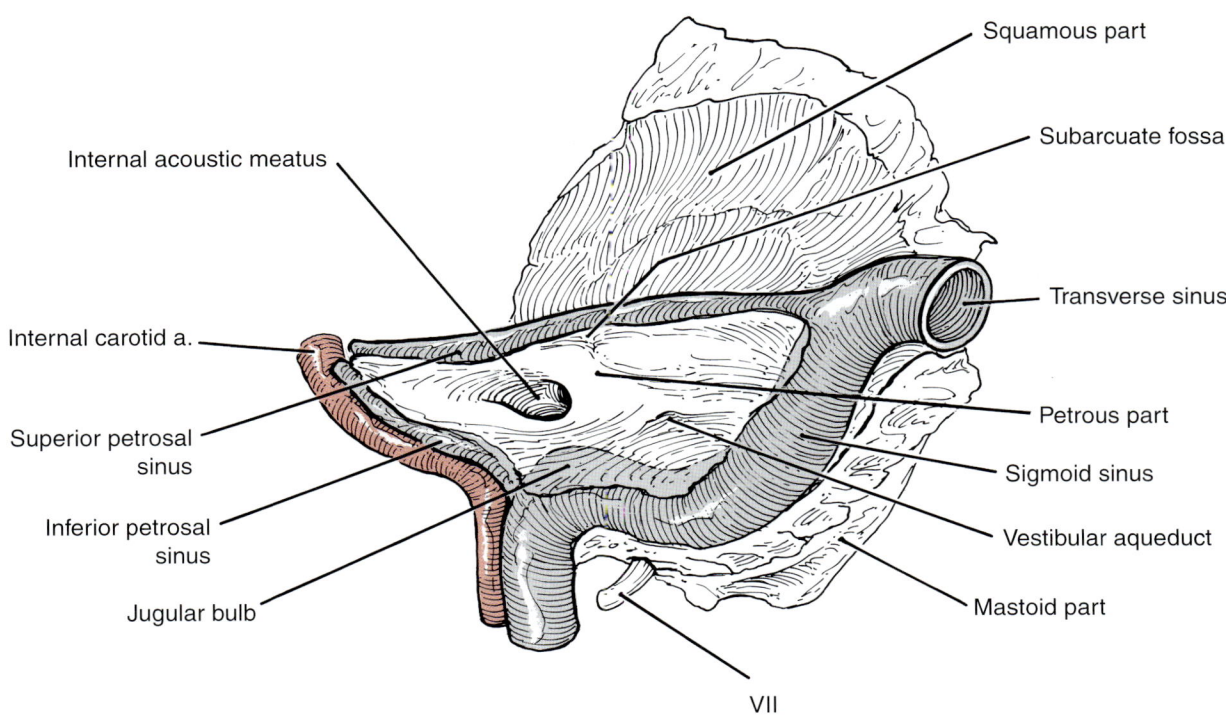

FIG. 2. Temporal bone viewed posteriorly, demonstrating the internal auditory canal and major venous sinuses.

50% of cases, the bone is dehiscent over the nerve during its course through the middle ear. At the pyramidal eminence, the nerve makes its second turn (second genu) to begin its vertical mastoid course to the stylomastoid foramen. As the facial nerve passes through the temporal bone, it supplies the stapedius muscle. Later, it supplies the posterior belly of the digastric muscle and, extratemporally, the muscles of facial expression. In its vertical course, the facial recess lies lateral to the nerve. This is the space bounded between the facial nerve and the chorda tympani nerve, and is an important surgical concept in lateral temporal bone resection. Figure 3 shows the surgical anatomy of this area as seen during mastoidectomy. Entry into the middle ear through this space allows visualization of the middle ear and removal of the middle ear and lateral ear with preservation of the facial nerve. Preganglionic parasympathetic secretomotor and special sensory afferent fibers are carried in the nervus intermedius, which travels with the facial nerve, and are then distributed by the greater superficial petrosal nerve and the chorda tympani. The pterygopalatine ganglion acts as a relay station, carrying secretomotor function from the greater superficial petrosal nerve to the nasal and lacrimal glands. The chorda tympani carries secretomotor fibers to the submandibular ganglion before these fibers reach the sublingual and submandibular glands, and also taste fibers from the anterior two thirds of the ipsilateral tongue.

On the anteromedial surface of the petrous temporal bone lies a shallow depression called Meckel's cave, in which sits the ganglion of the trigeminal nerve (V). Spread of disease to the petrous apex may result in some patients experiencing changes in facial sensation or facial pain. At the jugular foramen, the glossopharyngeal (IX), vagus (X), and accessory (XI) nerves leave together at the base of the temporal bone. A plexus (Jacobson's) is formed on the middle ear promontory by sensory afferent fibers from cranial nerve IX before they exit anteriorly as the lesser petrosal nerve. This innervation of the middle ear by the glossopharyngeal nerve accounts for the phenomenon of referred pain experienced in some pharyngeal disorders.

External Auditory Canal

The external auditory canal (EAC) measures approximately 2.5 cm in an adult and extends from the concha to the tympanic membrane. Cylindrically shaped, the outer one third is cartilaginous and the inner two thirds is bony. The latter is formed by the squamous portion of the temporal bone in its posterosuperior portion, and the remainder by the tympanic plate. The cartilaginous portion extends medially from the concha. Both parts are lined by closely applied skin. Pilosebaceous and ceruminous glands are found only in the outer third, in the cartilaginous portion.

Middle Ear

The middle ear is an air-filled space within the temporal bone containing the malleus, incus, and stapes ossicles with

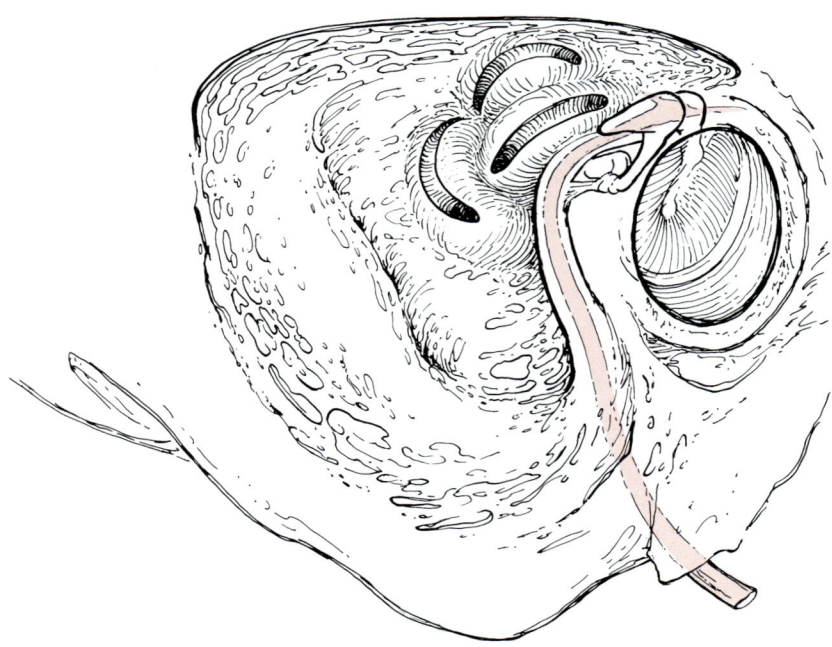

FIG. 3. Surgical anatomy of the mastoid, showing labyrinth (opened), fossa incudis, facial nerve, and facial recess.

their supporting ligamentous attachments. Shaped like a biconcave disc approximately 15 mm in diameter, it is lined by ciliated, columnar, mucus-secreting epithelium. It also contains two muscles, the stapedius and the tensor tympani. Laterally, it is bounded by the tympanic and squamous portions of the temporal bone with the tympanic membrane and medially by the petrous portion and inner ear structures. The medial wall has a number of important landmarks, such as the promontory, the round and oval windows, the ridge of the facial canal, and the processus cochleariformis. Superiorly lies the tegmen tympani, and often only a thin layer of bone separates this space from the middle cranial fossa. The floor of the middle ear is usually made of a layer of bone overlying the jugular bulb. Posteriorly, the middle ear opens into the aditus ad antrum, which passes into the mastoid air cell system. A number of bony canals leave the middle and inner ears and act as potential routes of spread of disease through the skull base. The eustachian tube joins the anterior wall of the middle ear to the nasopharynx, opening posterior to the medial pterygoid plates. From the anterior wall, the caroticotympanic plexus also leaves the middle ear. The eustachian tube lies superolateral to the carotid canal and is separated from the ICA by a thin lamina of bone. Two bony canals, the vestibular and cochlear aqueducts, leave from the inner ear. The former transmits the endolymphatic duct, which leads to the endolymphatic sac on the posterior surface of the temporal bone. The latter connects the perilymph of the scala tympani with the CSF of the posterior fossa.

Lymphatic Drainage of the External Auditory Canal and Middle Ear

The anterior half of the external auditory meatus drains to the lymphatics of the preauricular, superficial, and deep parotid lymph nodes. Drainage then proceeds to the upper echelon of deep cervical nodes. The posterior portions of the canal drain typically to the retroauricular nodes overlying the sternocleidomastoid muscle, and then to upper deep cervical nodes from this site.

The middle ear mucosa with the tympanic portion of the eustachian tube drains primarily to the parotid nodes and then to the upper deep cervical chain. The remainder of the eustachian tube at the nasopharyngeal end drains to the retropharyngeal lymph nodes (including the node of Rouvier), and to the upper deep cervical nodes.

INCIDENCE

The reported incidence of temporal bone malignancy, including tumors involving the EAC, is 0.01% of all reported neoplasms. Ninety percent represent primary tumors and 10% are metastases. Because of the increased numbers of head and neck surgeons, few relatively recent reports contain large numbers of patients compared with early descriptions.

For malignant tumors affecting the EAC, the male:female preponderance varies from 1:1 to 1:15 (7–11), with age ranges between 40 and 75 years (median, 62–68 years) (9,10). Most are squamous cell carcinomas, with approximately 20% being adenoid cystic or adenocarcinomas. Primary basal cell carcinoma arising in the external auditory meatus is unusual, and malignant melanoma is rare (7). There are no reliable data regarding racial preponderance.

A number of reports state that malignant disease in the middle ear and mastoid is twice as common in men than women (7,12,13). Up to 20% of cases are in the pediatric age group, and thus the average age of involvement is altered by this statistic. Most tumors in the pediatric age group are rhabdomyosarcomas, whereas most in the adult group are squamous cell carcinomas. This results in a bimodal distribution of tumor incidence, with one peak for childhood non-squamous malignancies and another in the fifth to sixth decades for squamous cell carcinomas.

ETIOLOGY

External auditory canal malignancy is associated with chronic inflammatory conditions such as otitis externa. It is possible that carcinogens such as aflatoxin produced by the *Aspergillus* fungus may have a role to play in some cases (14). Chronic chromate burns from repeated matchstick abuse and accidental exposure to radium paint used during World War II for illuminating watch dials are other known potential causes of such malignancies (15).

Politzer in 1883 first noted that malignancy of the middle ear and mastoid had a definite association with chronic suppurative otitis media (2). In 38% to 57% of patients, a chronic discharge is present before the development of malignancy (10,13). It is hypothesized that chronic inflammation alters the immunologic behavior of the middle ear cleft, resulting in a propensity for malignant change. Rarely is carcinoma identified in the presence of a normal intact tympanic membrane or without a prior history of otorrhea. Conventional external-beam radiation therapy for unrelated head and neck disease and therapeutic radium implants can also lead to the development of middle ear malignancy (15,16). In the past, radium seed implants were used to treat adenoid hyperplasia, predisposing the mastoid and middle ear to malignant change by the slow emission of radioactive alpha particles (15).

CLINICAL FEATURES

Cancer of the external auditory meatus and temporal bone is rarely diagnosed at an early stage. Tumors involving the temporal bone usually originate from the external canal and invade inward. Often, prolonged medical therapy for non-specific symptoms such as otorrhea and pruritus occurs. When more advanced symptoms such as intractable pain, facial paralysis, sensorineural hearing loss, severe vertigo, or tinnitus with bloody discharge occur, the clinician is usually alerted to the diagnosis. Unrelenting and deep temporal bone pain is characteristic and signifies bony or dural invasion. The duration of symptoms until diagnosis varies from 4 months to 4 years (10). A history of previous mastoid surgery is not uncommon, and often the diagnosis is made after several biopsy attempts because secondary infection, hemorrhage, and tissue necrosis distort the histopathologic assessment.

Clinical examination usually reveals an ulcer or polypoid tissue in the external auditory meatus associated with a tympanic membrane perforation. In up to 50% of cases the tumor is not visible otoscopically. Hearing loss may be conductive, sensorineural, or mixed, depending on tumor location (1). Trismus is usually indicative of disease extending into the TMJ or the infratemporal fossa, affecting the medial or lateral pterygoid muscles. The fissures of Santorini within the canal enable disease to transgress this area without difficulty, and parotid extension may present with a slight fullness in the gland substance. Tumors of the mastoid tend to advance rapidly through the cellular system to the posterior cranial fossa, and palsies of cranial nerves VII, IX, X, and XI represent advanced disease and poor prognosis (17,18). On occasion, tumor can spread down the eustachian tube and mimic a nasopharyngeal primary. The inner ear, being composed of compact bone, is resistant to invasion until late in the disease process.

PATIENT EVALUATION

Once histologic confirmation has been achieved by biopsy, the extent of disease is determined clinically and radiologically. A complete head and neck examination is necessary and includes examination of both ears and an evaluation of hearing with tuning forks and audiometry. The nose, oral cavity, pharynx, and larynx are examined. Facial nerve function is evaluated and the neck palpated for nodal involvement. Although assessing the local extent of the disease is often the first priority, it is important to exclude secondary lung, liver, and bone involvement. In general, if radical excision is contemplated, distant metastases are usually considered a contraindication to surgical cure. Radiography of the chest (posteroanterior and lateral) is necessary to assess for metastases, a second primary tumor, and acute or chronic pulmonary disease. Radiologic assessment with plain films of the mastoid and skull base has no role to play with the advent of CT and MRI, and is mentioned only in a historical context. Hypocycloidal tomography, once the gold standard for providing detailed views of temporal bone anatomy, has largely been superseded by high-resolution CT. Combining thin-slice (1.5 mm), high-resolution CT and MRI has revolutionized imaging of the temporal bone.

A CT scan and MRI assess the extent of the primary: its relationship to the dura, brain, facial nerve, carotid artery, and sometimes the presence of cervical metastases (Fig. 4). CT findings vary from demonstrating localized areas of bony erosion in the walls of the external auditory meatus, to involvement of the middle ear and mastoid. It is important to determine by CT if the bony septum between the eustachian tube or the floor of the middle ear and the ICA is eroded. Extension through the tegmen to the middle cranial fossa and posteriorly to the lateral sinus, as well as petrous apex, carotid canal, and jugular fossa involvement also can be assessed. An accuracy rate of 98% was reported when preoperative assessment of tumor extent was checked against operative and histologic findings (8). CT is also a valuable tool in delineating spread to the infratemporal fossa, parotid gland, and the retropharyngeal or cervical nodal chain. Similar to other head and neck sites, a limitation arises in the ability of CT to differentiate soft tissue inflammation from tumor in the absence of bony erosion.

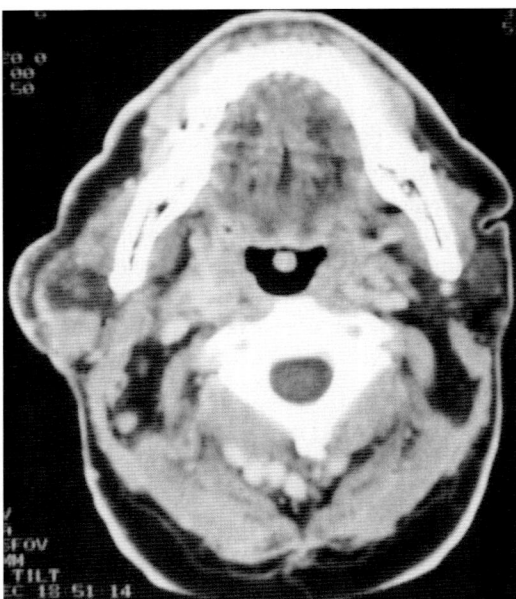

FIG. 4. Recurrent carcinoma of right temporal bone in a 52-year-old man. Computed tomography scan demonstrates erosion of temporal bone from carcinoma and previous mastoidectomy.

The superior soft tissue differentiation afforded by MRI is a major advantage of this imaging modality over CT, especially with the tumor-enhancing effects of paramagnetic contrast agents such as gadolinium-DPTA. The use of this agent helps to define tumor from brain and from the inflammatory and reactive changes frequently seen before and after surgery. In addition, MRI provides valuable information concerning ICA or sigmoid sinus patency by the presence or absence of flow void signals, which is also helpful when combined with contrast enhancement for determination of cavernous sinus involvement. MR angiography, with its absence of ionizing radiation and detailed information, is beginning to replace conventional angiographic techniques. As CT and MRI continue to complement each other and technological advances such as three-dimensional reconstructions, it is conceivable that further refinements will improve surgical and radiation therapy planning, as well as postoperative assessment.

STAGING

No coherent staging system for temporal bone malignancy has been accepted by either the American Joint Committee on Cancer or the Union Internationale Contre le Cancer. This makes any rational comparison of previous reports difficult and any meaningful statistical analysis impossible. Previous attempts at staging systems have been criticized principally because reported series included small numbers, an assortment of differing histologic types, metastatic lesions, and differing anatomic sites (18,19). Both Goodwin and Jesse (18) and Stell and McCormick (19) proposed staging systems based on their series of cases. The latter found no difference in survival between patients with tumors of the external ear and those with middle ear tumors when corrected for stage. Despite the pitfalls of previous staging systems, advances in diagnostic imaging have greatly aided preoperative assessment and staging of patients with temporal bone malignancy. Arriaga et al. (8) found high-resolution CT was an accurate indicator of histopathologically proven tumor invasion. Twelve anatomic sites of the temporal bone were studied. When radiologic findings were compared with operative and histopathologic findings, there was a 98% correlation. The 12 sites for EAC malignancy and the proposed staging system are documented in Table 1.

No staging system for temporal bone malignancy proper exists at present, although a number of conclusions can be made from previous reports. The extent of local disease, the patient's general medical condition, the histologic type, lymphatic involvement, and the presence of distant metastases are all important prognostic factors (19). Five-year survival rates vary from 28.3% with disease of the EAC to 36.8% with primary middle ear involvement (7,8,20). At the time of diagnosis, temporal bone malignancy must be considered aggressive and at an advanced stage.

TABLE 1. *Proposed anatomic/radiologic staging system for external auditory canal malignancy*

Anatomic regions
External auditory canal
  Anterior canal
  Superior canal
  Posterior canal
  Inferior canal
Infratemporal extension
  Middle ear
  Otic capsule
  Mastoid
  Jugular fossa
  Carotid canal
  Tegmen ± middle fossa
  Posterior fossa

Propsed staging system

T1	Limited to the EAC without bony erosion or soft tissue extension.
T2	Tumor with limited EAC erosion or CT evidence of less than 0.5 cm soft tissue involvement.
T3	Tumor eroding the full thickness of the EAC with greater than 0.5 cm soft tissue involvement or with tumor involvement of the middle ear, mastoid, or facial nerve.
T4	Tumor eroding the cochlea, petrous apex, medial wall of the middle ear, carotid canal, jugular foramen or dura, or extensive involvement of soft tissue > 0.5 cm.
N	Any nodal involvement is a poor prognostic factor. Despite an early T staging, the presence of positive nodes implies advanced disease.
M	When distant metastases are present.

EAC, external auditory canal.

HISTOLOGIC TYPES

Squamous Cell Carcinoma

Squamous cell carcinoma is the most common malignancy affecting the EAC and middle ear (Fig. 5). When arising in the external auditory meatus, it predominantly affects its bony portion. Typically, a highly infiltrative pattern is seen histologically with poorly demarcated margins. Most (62.5%) are moderately differentiated, 25% are well differentiated, and 12.5% are poorly differentiated. The degree of tumor differentiation has not been shown to affect prognosis (9). The tumors that originate in the middle ear are highly infiltrative and aggressive and usually cause widespread bony destruction. The compact bone of the otic capsule and the petrous apex appears relatively resistant to tumor destruction until late in the disease process. The dura of the middle cranial fossa also appears to resist invasion, although the tegmen not infrequently is breached. Often tumor surrounds the carotid artery and spreads along the petrosal nerves to the parotid and TMJ.

Table 2 provides a list of the most frequently reported tumors involving the temporal bone from a number of reported series.

Basal Cell Carcinoma

Basal cell carcinomas typically arise in the concha, pinna, or postauricular region of the ear and it is uncommon for these lesions to originate in the canal or middle ear. Although often regarded as innocuous lesions by many, basal cell carcinomas have a propensity to spread along tissue plains, invade bone, and behave in an aggressive manner. Any basal cell carcinoma arising in the external auditory meatus or middle ear cleft must be considered an aggressive type and treated in this fashion.

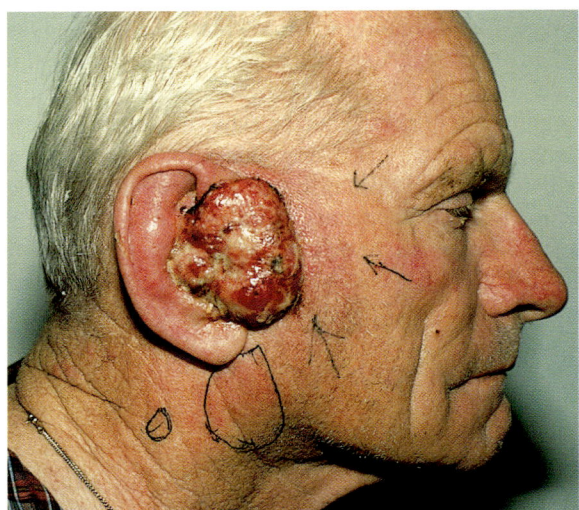

FIG. 5. Squamous cell carcinoma of the external ear invading temporal bone.

TABLE 2. *Common malignancies of the external auditory canal and temporal bone*

Squamous cell carcinoma
Basal cell carcinoma
Malignant tumors of glandular origin
    Adenoid cystic
    Ceruminous adenocarcinoma
Sarcomas
    Rhabdomyosarcomas
    Chondrosarcomas
    Osteosarcomas
Rare tumors
    Malignant melanoma
    Lymphomas
    Langerhans' cell histiocytosis
    Carcinoid tumors
    Verrucous carcinoma
    Giant cell tumors
    Chordoma

Tumors of Glandular Origin

For many years, "ceruminoma" has been used to denote both benign and malignant tumors arising in the ceruminous glands. This has led to confusion regarding the prognosis of neoplasms arising in the ceruminous glands. Benign lesions, ceruminous adenomas, and pleomorphic adenomas (mixed tumors) tend to arise in the sixth decade of life and are less common than malignant glandular tumors of the canal and middle ear (21). The latter types, adenoid cystic carcinomas and ceruminous adenocarcinomas, arise earlier in life and are believed to develop from eccrine sweat glands or ceruminous glands.

Adenoid Cystic Carcinoma

This tumor is the most common malignant lesion of glandular origin to arise in the EAC. Historically, the lesion was often misdiagnosed, resulting in inadequate treatment and numerous recurrences. Commonly, the lesion involves cranial nerves and intracranial contents by the time it is diagnosed because of the affinity of adenoid cystic carcinoma for invading perineural tissue. Adenoid cystic carcinoma occurs in middle-aged people, with equal distribution between men and women. In over 90% of cases, severe pain is a presenting feature. Despite wide resection, local recurrences and pulmonary metastases are typical features.

When found in the middle ear cleft, these tumors have usually arisen as a result of perineural spread from another site. It is possible that tumors can arise *de novo* in the middle ear cleft because ectopic glandular tissue, known as choristoma, has been described. In theory, ectopic glandular tissue can become trapped within the developing temporal bone, and may proliferate in later life. This salivary tissue is associated with anomalies of the seventh nerve pathway and congenital ossicular abnormalities (22). Another suggestion has been that the tissue represents an aberrant bud of parotid gland (23).

Similar to other sites in the head and neck region, there are three histologic patterns of adenoid cystic carcinoma that correlate with prognosis. The well differentiated, unencapsulated variety is the most common, with a propensity for infiltrating neural structures and perivascular spaces and invading tissue plains. This type gives a "Swiss cheese" histologic appearance to the affected tissue. A better prognosis is often associated with a cribriform pattern when a mantle of cells surrounds a central core of hyalinized tissue. Those tumors with a solid cellular pattern and an anaplastic appearance have the worst prognosis clinically (24).

The timing of metastatic spread varies considerably, and reports of systemic metastases appearing 30 years after the diagnosis exist. The lungs are the most common site of spread, although kidney, brain, cervical nodes, and bone are also affected. Surprisingly, patients may live for considerable periods with pulmonary metastases without significant symptoms, in contrast to other tumor types that have spread to this site.

Ceruminous Adenocarcinomas

These rare tumors affect men and women with equal frequency and usually around the fifth decade of life. The presentation is similar to other tumors of the EAC. Histologically, the finding of invasion of surrounding structures distinguishes them from benign ceruminous adenomas, which they resemble. Microscopic glandular, cystic, or papillary patterns are found.

Adenocarcinoma

This tumor is rarely found arising from the middle ear and occurs more commonly in women than men. The average age at presentation is approximately 40 years, and it is important to consider a metastatic origin (14). When arising behind an intact tympanic membrane, this lesion may initially have the appearance of a facial neuroma, a cholesterol granuloma, or a glomus tumor (25). Glomus tumors typically have a "moth-eaten" appearance on CT and may exhibit a smooth, scalloped enlargement of the jugular fossa. Malignant invasion by adenocarcinoma tends to show a more aggressive pattern of bony invasion.

Sarcomas

Sarcomas are rare tumors that arise primarily from poorly differentiated connective tissue, fat, muscle, synovium, vascular endothelium, or the supporting tissue of peripheral nerves. Those involving the EAC and temporal bone are extremely rare. The introduction of immunohistochemical staining in conjunction with conventional histologic methods has helped pathologists to reach accurate diagnoses in cases that in the past had been diagnostic dilemmas. Children (male more than female) are most often affected, with the usual presentation being a polyp in the external auditory meatus. Rhabdomyosarcoma is the most common tumor in this group, and the prognosis is generally poor. Other sarcomas affecting the temporal bone include neurofibrosarcomas, malignant fibrohistiosarcomas, leiomyosarcomas, and malignant schwannomas.

Rhabdomyosarcoma

This highly aggressive malignant tumor occurs primarily in children and accounts for 5% to 15% of childhood neoplasia. These tumors are locally destructive and invasive. In contrast to adults, in whom rhabdomyosarcomas involve the limbs, most children are affected in the head and neck region. The orbit, paranasal sinuses, and oral cavity are the most frequently affected sites, with temporal bone involvement accounting for 7% (26). In the middle ear, the stapedius and tensor tympani muscle are thought to be the sites of origin of this tumor. Twenty-five percent of cases originate near the eustachian tube and may not cause aural symptoms until late in the disease (27).

The median age for tumor occurrence is around 4 years, with a slight male over female preponderance. A typical presentation is with a purulent aural discharge, a mass in the EAC, and hearing loss. Failure of an attack of acute otitis media to subside with the presence of a mass should alert the clinician to this diagnosis. Because of the similarities with common middle ear disease, the diagnosis is often missed. Often a general anesthetic is necessary in young children to make an accurate tissue diagnosis. Multiple cranial nerve palsies are indicative of skull base involvement, and unfortunately 20% of patients have systemic metastases at the time of diagnosis. Meningeal involvement is associated with a poor prognosis because brain parenchymal spread has often occurred at this stage (28). Four tumor types are found histologically: pleomorphic, embryonal, alveolar, and botryoid. The embryonal subtype is the most common, and usually a mixture of each type is present in any individual lesion. A combination of chemotherapy (vincristine, dactinomycin, cyclophosphamide, and doxorubicin) and high-dose radiation therapy (4,000 cGy) is the treatment of choice. Limited resection may also be necessary in selected cases. A 47% 5-year survival rate can be achieved with this modality of treatment. Intrathecal chemotherapy and intracranial radiation therapy are being evaluated in an attempt to reduce tumor recurrence (28).

Chondrosarcoma

These tumors of cartilaginous origin usually arise during the sixth decade of life, primarily from the external auditory meatus. They are believed to originate from persistence of fetal cartilaginous chondrocranium, which develops during the fifth week of fetal life (29). Benign chordomas have a similar histologic appearance with chondroid matrices, and can cause confusion in the initial pathologic diagnosis. A pattern of aggressive clinical behavior distinguishes chondrosarcomas from the benign lesion. A radical surgical resection to prevent recurrence is usually necessary. Radiation therapy is not a reliable treatment option as a primary modality, although it can be used for residual disease; there are reports of remissions in some low-grade lesions.

Osteosarcoma

Osteogenic sarcoma represents the most common malignant tumor to involve bone, although the head and neck region is rarely affected. Typically the mandible is the site of involvement when the head and neck area is involved. Rare cases of temporal bone involvement have been described in the literature, and require a radical resection with combined radiation therapy when identified.

Rare Tumors

A number of rare tumors involving the EAC and temporal bone have been described in the world literature as case reports. Some benign tumors that have a locally aggressive nature are also described for completeness.

Malignant Melanoma

Primary malignant melanoma arising in the EAC is a rare entity compared with its incidence in other body sites (30). The lack of exposure to ultraviolet radiation in this region presumably has a protective influence against malignant transformation. Melanoma involving the middle ear reflects metastatic spread, and facial nerve palsy as a result of neural invasion has been reported.

Chordoma

Chordomas are rare tumors thought to develop from the embryonic remnants of the notochord. Some cases of these lesions arising in the temporal bone have been described, although they usually arise in the axial skeleton. More commonly seen is direct spread of chordoma to the petrous bone from the clivus. A high local recurrence rate after resection is reported, although they tend to grow slowly, if aggressively. The chondroid chordoma is a well differentiated variety that has a better prognosis than a true chordoma (31).

Fibrous Dysplasia

Monostotic or, less commonly, polyostotic fibrous dysplasia may involve the temporal bone in 20% of patients with head and neck involvement by this condition. The hearing loss is primarily conductive as a result of narrowing of the EAC and usually presents in the first two decades of life. Radiologic expansion of the temporal bone is characteristic, with cortical narrowing. Progressive canal narrowing may lead to cholesteatoma formation and necessitate surgical intervention.

Carcinoid Tumors of the Middle Ear Cleft

Eleven case reports in the literature describe primary carcinoid tumors of the middle ear, with a slight male preponderance. Presentation is with a sensation of aural fullness and hearing loss. Usually the tympanic membrane is not perforated but laterally displaced. Systemic features of carcinoid, such as flushing, wheezing, or diarrhea, are not described. The tumor is slow growing and behaves in a benign manner, with a 96% 5-year survival rate after resection (32). Radiation therapy is not recommended unless the disease has spread beyond the temporal bone or resection margins were incomplete. Reresection is preferable to radiation therapy.

Verrucous Carcinoma of the Middle Ear

This clinically aggressive and locally invasive tumor is histologically classified as benign. No basement membrane invasion or cytologic evidence of atypia are present microscopically. Verrucous carcinoma exhibits a papillomatosis, keratinizing squamous epithelium with acanthosis, hyperkeratosis, and parakeratosis (33). Grossly, the lesion is indistinguishable from well differentiated squamous cell carcinoma, with a soft, friable appearance and papillary frond formation.

A wide surgical resection is recommended to prevent local recurrence. Radiation therapy is not recommended. A progression to invasive squamous cell carcinoma has been described after radiation therapy for these lesions in other head and neck sites.[1]

Langerhans' Cell Histiocytosis

Eosinophilic granuloma, Hand-Schüller-Christian disease, and Letterer-Siwe disease make up a group of disorders called Langerhans' histiocytosis (histiocytosis X). A localized pattern of histiocytic proliferation is seen in eosinophilic granuloma, with a diffuse pattern in Hand-Schüller-Christian disease and Letterer-Siwe disease. Over 70% of eosinophilic granulomas are diagnosed before the age of 20 years, and most before 5 years of age (29). Letterer-Siwe disease presents before the age of 3 years, and Hand-Schüller-Christian disease before the age of 5 years. A

---

[1] **Editor's note:** *The editor does not recommend radiation therapy in the case of recurrent disease. Reresection is the treatment of choice.*

history of chronic otorrhea with a friable EAC mass are the typical features. CT scanning demonstrates lytic, circumscribed bone lesions. Localized eosinophilic granuloma can be treated with surgical curettage and low-dose radiation therapy. Systemic disease requires chemotherapy with prednisolone, vinblastine, methotrexate, or cyclophosphamide. A poor prognosis is associated with presentation at a younger age group and systemic disease, but the prognosis is excellent in localized eosinophilic granuloma (34).

Secondary Carcinoma of the Temporal Bone

Occasionally the temporal bone is the site of secondary tumor involvement by direct invasion, hematogenous dissemination, or lymphatic or CSF spread. The temporal bone contains marrow, and sites such as the petrous apex with a constant sluggish blood flow may serve as prime areas for metastatic growth. Carcinoma of the breast, thyroid, lung, stomach, larynx, prostate, uterus, nasopharynx, and kidney are known to spread to the temporal bone.

Tumors in adjacent anatomic sites may invade the temporal bone directly. Carcinoma of the parotid may spread to bony channels or potential anatomic spaces such as the fissures of Santorini and Huschke's foramen. Lymphomas may invade from the nasopharynx and produce symptoms from perineural invasion or eustachian tube dysfunction. Meningeal carcinomatosis or intracranial primary tumors may spread to involve the temporal bone. The former is usually associated with multiple cranial nerve palsies due to diffuse infiltration of the subarachnoid space.

The presentation is not dissimilar to that of primary malignancy of the temporal bone. Often, severe pain, facial paralysis, and otorrhea are the the initial symptoms. Gradenigo's syndrome (affecting cranial nerves V and VI) or variations of Collet-Sicard syndrome (involving cranial nerves IX, X, XI, and XII) may be seen. Inner ear extension is associated with sensorineural hearing loss, tinnitus, and vertigo. Trismus is present when the TMJ is invaded.

MANAGEMENT

The Carotid Artery

Central to the successful management of the patient with temporal bone malignancy is correct management of the carotid artery. Before any attempted surgical resection, a detailed knowledge of the carotid artery and its possible involvement must be obtained. Whether the carotid artery can be preserved or should be resected, reconstructed, or both, are key questions in the oncologic decision-making process. Despite the advances in diagnostic imaging since the late 1970s, it is still difficult to predict which patients are likely to have permanent neurologic damage (i.e., stroke) as a consequence of ICA occlusion, and also which patients are likely to benefit from a revascularization procedure.

Clearly, a patient with a history of amaurosis fugax, a previous cerebrovascular accident, or transient ischemic attacks is more likely to suffer a permanent neurologic deficit should ICA occlusion be necessary. Conventional angiography, dynamic brain scans, and balloon occlusion techniques with somatosensory cortical evoked potentials (SCEP), transcranial Doppler ultrasonography, SPECT scanning, or stable xenon/CT cerebral blood flow imaging are valuable investigations to assess the risks of ICA occlusion (35–37).

Conventional Angiography

During this procedure, the patency of the circle of Willis and the collateral circulation of the cerebral hemispheres are assessed by studying the ipsilateral and contralateral ICAs in addition to the vertebral arteries. An indication of the collateral circulation may be gained by compressing the ipsilateral ICA and simultaneously injecting dye into the contralateral artery. Tumor invasion may be seen as a stenosis or an irregularity of the vessel wall. The presence of an atherosclerotic plaque in the contralateral artery is usually considered to be an indication for a carotid endarterectomy. Unfortunately, angiography reveals the anatomic details of the circle of Willis as well as vessel diameters, but gives no information on blood flow, and is thus a poor predictor of the vigor of cerebral circulation when one carotid is occluded.

Dynamic Brain Scans

Intravenous injection of technetium-99 glucoheptonate is performed while the ipsilateral ICA is occluded digitally. The collateral blood flow through the circle of Willis to the hemisphere with its blood supply occluded is compared with that of the opposite, unoccluded side.

Carotid Occlusion Studies

Studies determining the effect of ICA occlusion on intracranial circulation and the indications for vascular reconstruction were initially performed in the operating room during a major ablation. Changes in the SCEPs and the arterial pressure recorded in the distal stump of the ICA were used as parameters to decide if reconstruction was necessary. Cortical potentials were recorded 2 minutes before ICA occlusion and then every 90 seconds after occlusion of the vessel for 10 minutes. Maintenance of stump pressure above 50 mm Hg and unchanged SCEPs were indicative of adequate collateral circulation, and reconstruction of the artery was not undertaken. A drop in stump pressure below 50 mm Hg and a greater than 50% attenuation in SCEPs were indications for reconstruction of the ICA. It is now known that SCEPs do not predict which patients will tolerate a permanent occlusion of the ICA, and merely indicate the ability to tolerate a transient occlusion of blood flow (35).

At present, preoperative evaluation of clinical responses and SCEPs is performed using balloon occlusion angiography. A nondetachable balloon is introduced on a double-lumen Swan-Ganz catheter and the patient responses to occlusion are recorded. In the presence of neurologic symptoms or alterations in SCEPs, complete ICA resection without prior bypass surgery would be contraindicated. Attempts to improve the predictive ability of balloon occlusion testing have centered on inducing controlled hypotension, which reflects perioperative cerebral perfusion. In addition, Erba et al. have described xenon/CT cerebral blood flow imaging (37). This investigation is believed to give reliable information on cerebral blood flow reserve after occlusion. A number of patient groups were defined on the basis of this test:

- Group I: No change in cerebral blood flow after occlusion of the ICA
- Group II: A mild to moderate symmetric reduction in cerebral blood flow in all parts of the brain
- Group III: A significant reduction in blood flow that was greater in the cerebral hemisphere on the side of the occlusion
- Group IV: Occurrence of neurologic abnormalities when the balloon was initially inflated, requiring termination of the investigation

Despite negative findings in these investigations, approximately 10% of patients experience permanent neurologic deficit after resection of the ICA. Some of these episodes are related to reduced cerebral blood flow during periods of hypotension. Brain retraction, vascular spasm, emboli, and intraoperative hypotension may account for this damage. The risk of emboli can in theory be reduced by keeping the distal stump of the ICA as short as possible.

Surgical Considerations

In the absence of a widely accepted staging system, clinical experience dictates the management decisions in these rare and diverse malignant tumors. In general, surgery or radiation therapy, alone or in combination, are the treatment options. Tumors confined to the EAC are considered localized in the absence of middle ear cleft invasion or facial nerve involvement. The steps in the decision-making process involve the following:

1. Histopathologic confirmation of malignancy
2. Radiologic determination of disease extent and metastatic spread
3. A realistic appraisal of whether surgery is aimed at palliation or cure
4. The need to include the parotid, TMJ, infratemporal fossa, neck exploration, carotid artery, and dural or cerebral resection or reconstruction as part of the planned resection
5. The necessity or type of reconstruction options
6. A radiation oncology consultation in anticipation for postoperative radiation
7. A neurosurgery consultation if skull base surgical resection needed
8. An internal medicine, cardiology, or anesthesiology consultation

A number of surgical approaches are feasible that largely depend on the extent of the tumor. Complete surgical resection with a clear microscopic margin is the preferred initial primary treatment goal in a patient with a resectable cancer. For small tumors, radiation therapy is an alternative. When resection is contemplated, a team comprising a head and neck surgeon, neurosurgeon, neurootologist, and plastic surgeon may be required. In general, four types of resection are performed. These are excisional biopsy (including sleeve resection), lateral temporal bone resection, subtotal temporal bone resection, and total temporal bone resection. Figures 6 and 7 schematically depict lateral temporal bone resection and subtotal temporal bone resection, the two most commonly performed procedures.[2]

Excisional Biopsy

Rarely, when a tumor is small and does not invade bone or cartilage, it can be excised with an adequate margin of normal skin. This is usually basal cell in type. A so-called sleeve excision can be done (Fig. 8).

Lateral Temporal Bone Resection

The aim of this procedure is to resect a tumor confined to the EAC or tympanic membrane while conserving both labyrinthine and facial nerve function without compromising tumor margins. Ideally, this procedure is of value when a tumor arises in the postauricular sulcus, the concha, and the EAC, or when disease has just invaded the mastoid cortex or tympanic plate, but has not invaded the middle ear and mastoid air cells. When tumor is confined to the EAC, a more extensive resection does not improve survival (38). The following steps are necessary successfully to complete this resection, which involves a progressive dissection to verify the extent of the tumor and resecting only the temporal bone that is adjacent to tumor.

The first step of the procedure is to outline the lesion emanating from the EAC with an adequate margin of skin and conchal cartilage (Fig. 9). Incisions are extended superiorly and inferiorly to permit adequate exposure for mastoidectomy, condylar resection, and parotidectomy, when these latter two adjunctive procedures are required. The superior extension into the scalp is required if the zygomatic root is invaded or limited middle fossa exposure is necessary. The remnant of the pinna is left attached to the skin flap (Fig. 10).

---

[2]**Editor's note:** *Radiation therapy for small lesions is selected only if patients refuse surgery. Surgery for small lesions results in better than a 90% local control rate.*

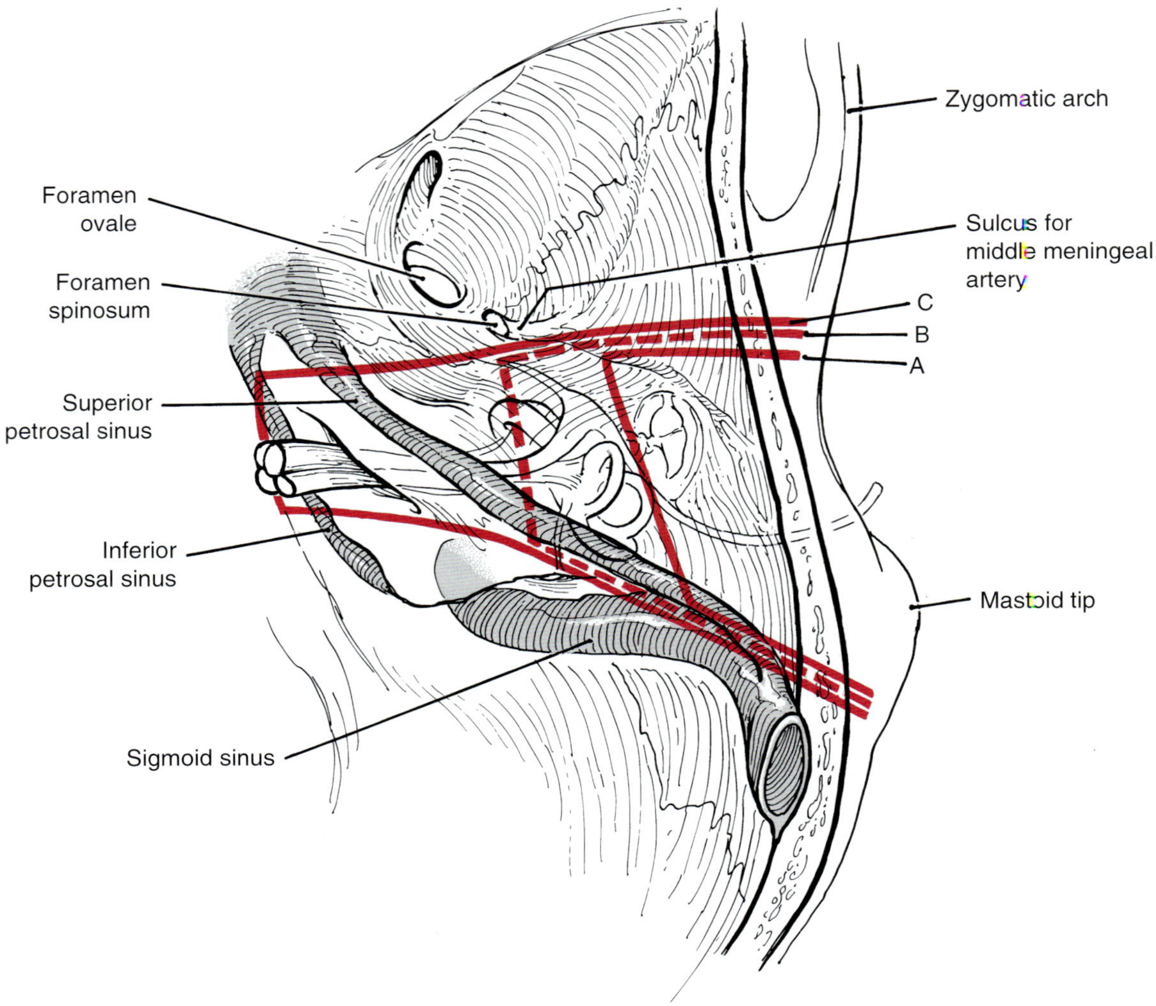

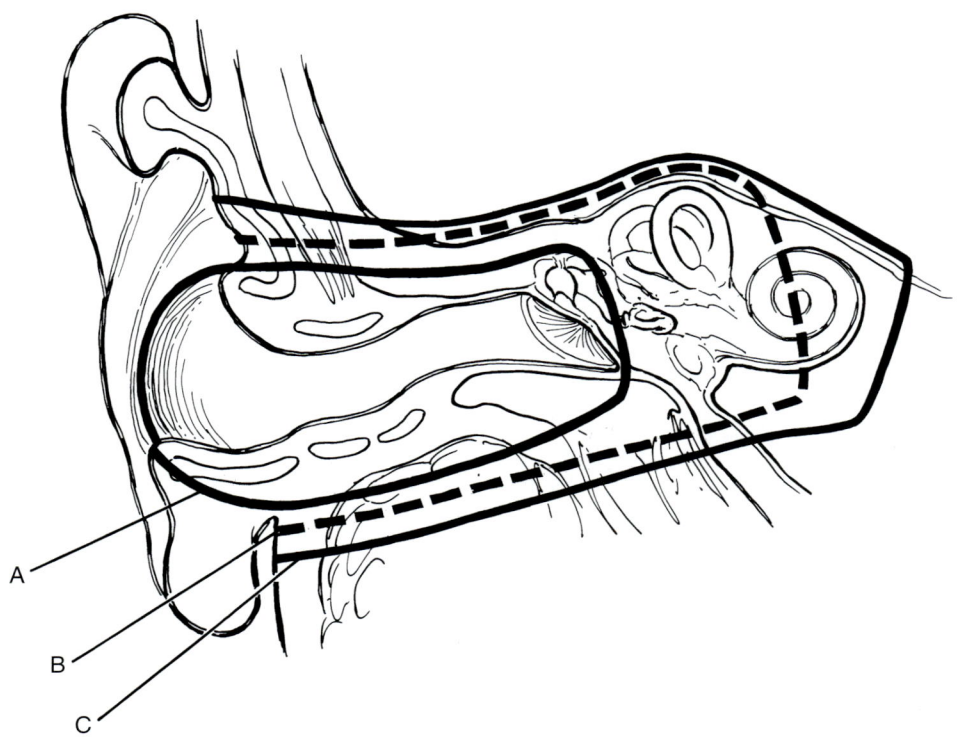

FIG. 6. Axial schematic representation of extent of resection for lateral (*A*), subtotal (*B*), and total (*C*) temporal bone resections.

FIG. 7. Coronal schematic representation of extent of resection for lateral (*A*), subtotal (*B*), and total (*C*) temporal bone resections.

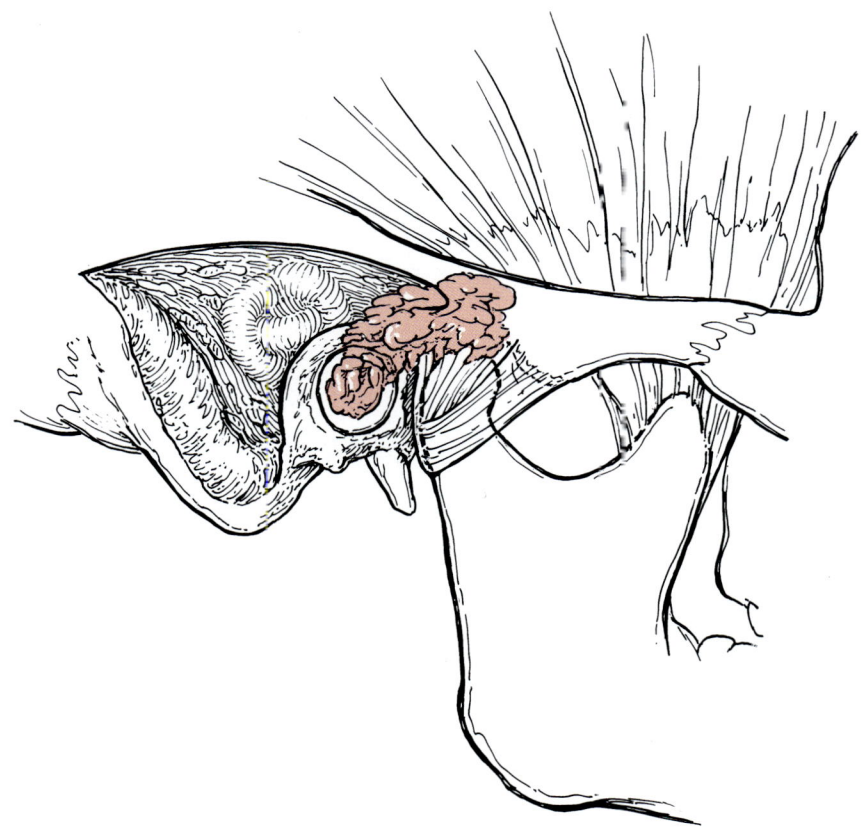

FIG. 14. Mastoidectomy completed, but zygomatic root shows evidence of invasion.

mentioned, a mandibular condylectomy is done that includes the condyle, meniscus, glenoid fossa, capsular ligaments, and insertion of the lateral pterygoid muscles (see Fig. 12). Although controversial, it is probably wise to do a parotidectomy with facial nerve sparing in most cases of carcinoma of the EAC. The easy passage of tumor through the fissures of Santorini in the cartilaginous external canal to the parotid make the gland particularly vulnerable to tumor spread, and thus parotid resection is an important aspect of safe tumor clearance.

The final stage of tumor resection is at hand. In the usual type of tumor without zygomatic extension, a fissure is cut with the bur from the anterior attic into the glenoid fossa. A similar fissure is made from the inferior extremity of the facial recess toward the hypotympanum, taking care to stay lateral to the facial nerve (Fig. 15). In most cases, the tympanic membrane requires excision. In those few cases in which the membrane is spared, the fissure cut is made lateral to the tympanic ring. A series of osteotome cuts superiorly, inferiorly, and posteriorly is made (Fig. 16A). The final osteotome is placed in the posterior fissure and driven into the glenoid fossa (see Fig. 16B). The specimen fractures away from the main body of the temporal bone and is removed from the last soft tissue attachments at the TMJ (see Fig. 16C).

With zygomatic extension, mandibular condylectomy is usually necessary and a more extensive resection is required. The resection is outlined in (Fig. 17). Great care must be taken to stay lateral to the eustachian tube and to come across the mesotympanum close to the tympanic annulus to avoid injury to the internal jugular vein and ICA. Fissures are cut through the glenoid fossa and tympanic bone, connecting the posterior fissure made inferior to the facial recess and the fissure at the zygomatic root. A fascia graft is placed over the stapes in an attempt to reconstruct the tympanic membrane. Split-thickness skin is applied to the mastoid cavity, and the scalp advanced into the defect as well (Fig. 18).

Complete Temporal Bone Resection

The next most common operation done after the lateral temporal bone resection is the subtotal operation. This procedure is done when tumor invades the middle ear and mastoid. This operation is based on the principles established by Lewis in the original operation (3). The importance of his contribution of this procedure—heroic in proportion at the time—cannot be overemphasized. One of the basic modifications to Lewis' original procedure is the use of the high-speed air drill.

A complete mastoidectomy is done despite the fact that the origin of the tumor may have been the auricle or the periauricular skin. The first resection block before the mastoidectomy will then be the margin of healthy skin and soft tissue surrounding the tumor, and the tumor is amputated at

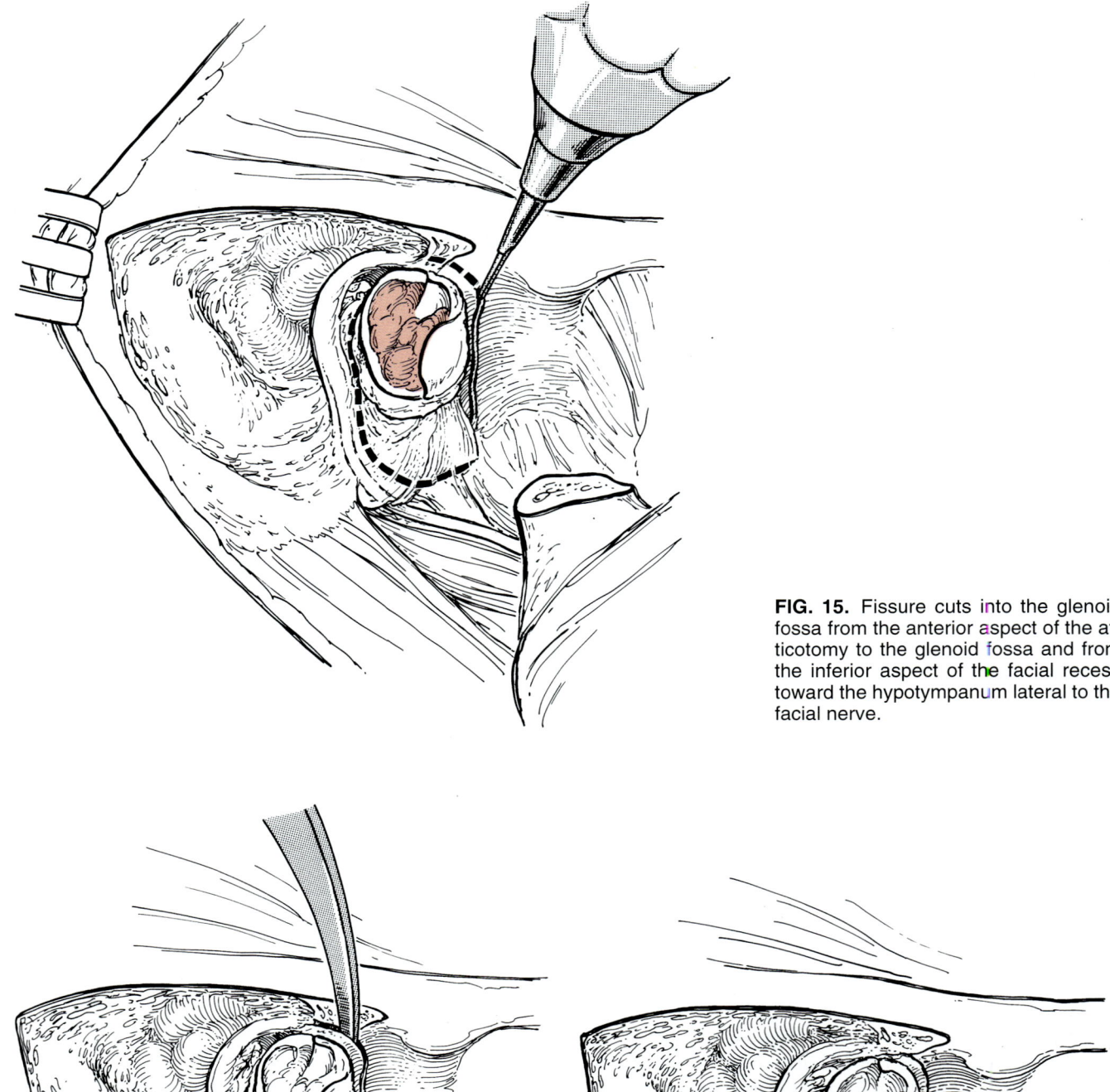

FIG. 15. Fissure cuts into the glenoid fossa from the anterior aspect of the atticotomy to the glenoid fossa and from the inferior aspect of the facial recess toward the hypotympanum lateral to the facial nerve.

FIG. 16. Lateral temporal bone resection with zygomatic root, condyle, and glenoid fossa removed. **A:** Fissures cut and osteotomes placed. Note successive osteotome cuts superiorly, inferiorly, and finally anteriorly. **B:** An osteotome is placed in the fissure inferior to the facial recess and driven anteriorly into and through the anterior bony canal into the glenoid fossa.

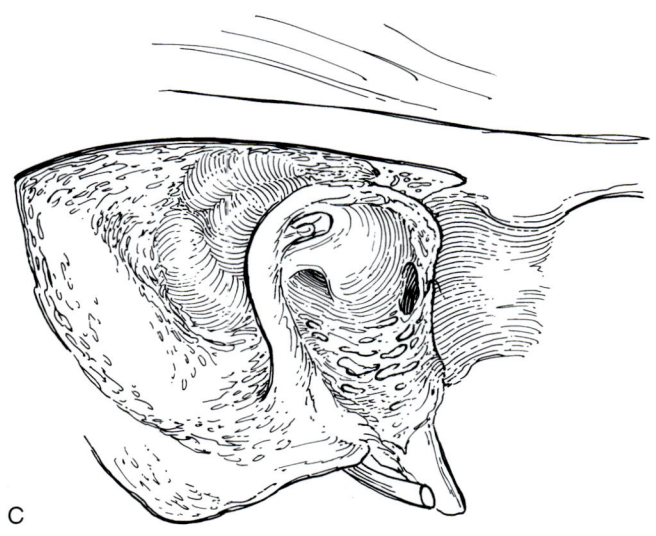

FIG. 16. *Continued.* **C:** Resection completed.

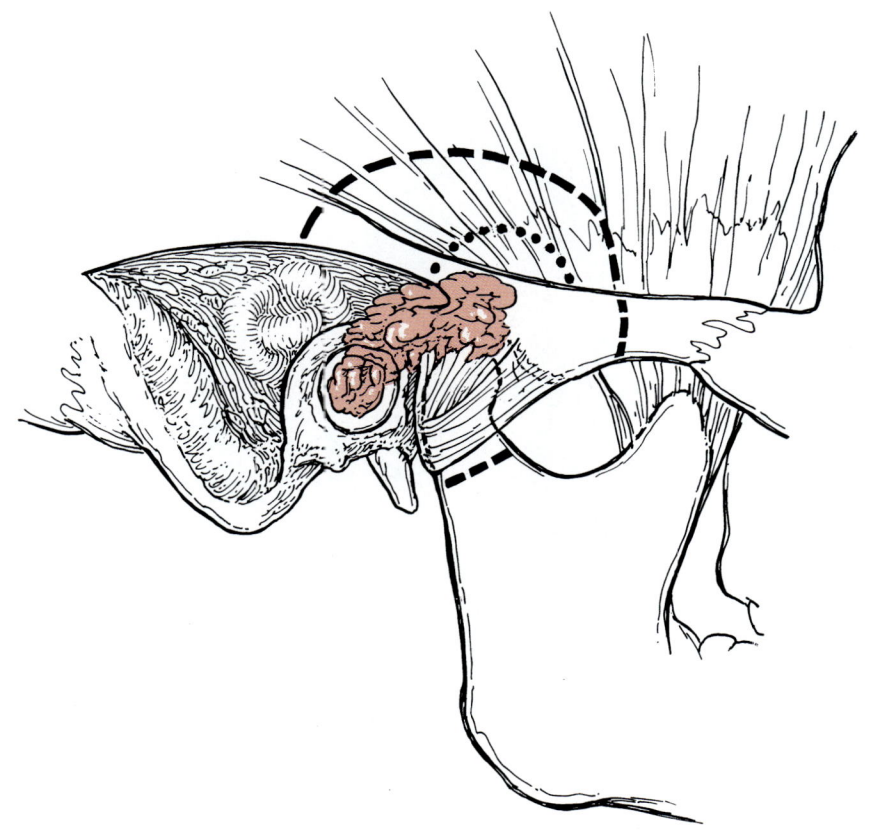

FIG. 17. More extensive involvement of tissues adjacent to external auditory canal is diagrammed and cuts in the calvarium, zygomatic arch, and condyle are outlined. Dashes over the temporal squama indicate the craniotomy, and the dots outline the proposed ostectomy.

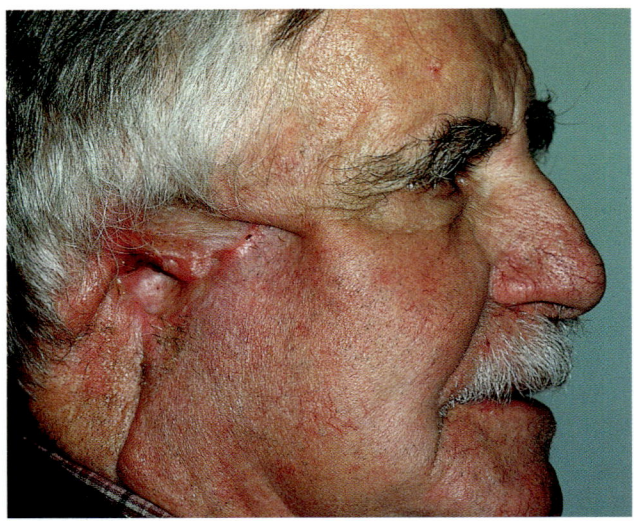

FIG. 18. Patient 6 months after extended lateral temporal bone resection with partial resection of zygoma, as outlined in Fig. 17. Wound was closed with scalp advancement and healed split-thickness skin graft.

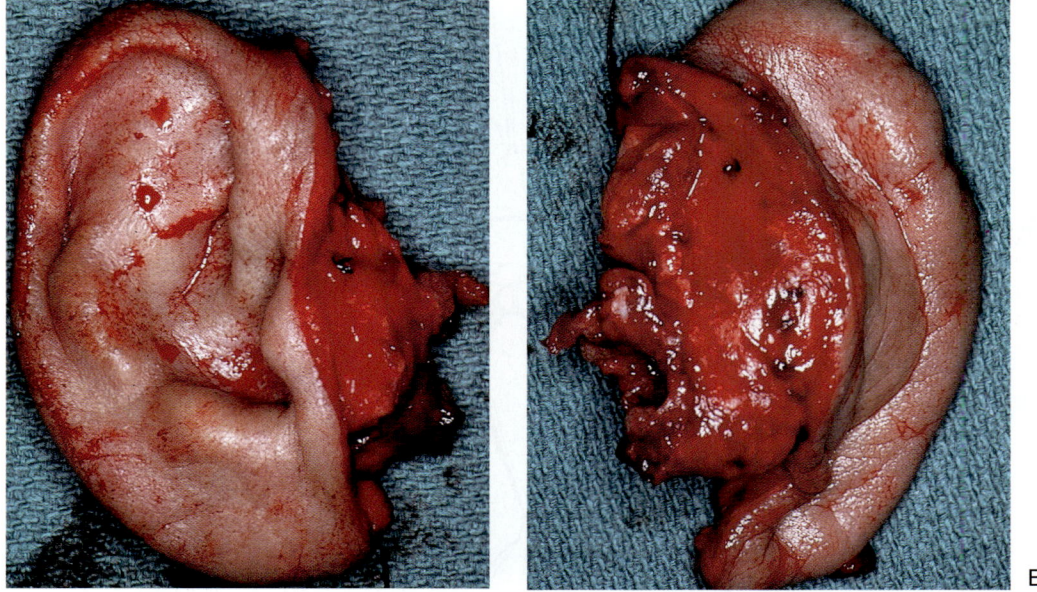

FIG. 19. First block resection of lateral tissues, including involved auricle, periauricular skin, and soft tissues, to facilitate more precise temporal bone resection. **A:** Soft tissue block. **B:** Mastoidectomy done. Residual cancer left in temporal bone before subsequent complete removal.

the level of the cartilaginous canal and tumor-breached mastoid cortex (Fig. 19). As is mentioned throughout this text, total clearance of tumor by negative frozen-section and eventually negative permanent-section margins ensures total tumor removal and a low incidence of local tumor recurrence. To struggle with a large tumor mass that interferes with adequate visualization, especially when that necessitates unnecessary sacrifice of normal uninvolved tissue for the sake of the *en bloc* principle, is unwarranted. A series of "*en bloc* resections" with tumor only at the deep margin continues until all malignancy is cleared.

Complete encompassment of all disease in the mastoid is effected. Invasion through the tegmen mastoideum and tympani is not uncommon because this route presents a path of least resistance to tumor spread (6) (Fig. 20). Tumor may invade the sigmoid sinus or the lateral sinus through the sigmoid plate (Fig. 21). The resection of the lateral sinus must proceed with great care because the vein of Labbé enters the sinus at a variable distance from the top of the sigmoid sinus. Removal of the vein may result in severe motor deficits or even death, depending on the integrity of the superior cerebral vein of Trollard.

Below the tentorium, extension of tumor may penetrate the cerebellar dura, and a more extensive removal of the occipital bone will be necessary to provide exposure for resection (Fig. 22). The exposure may require a dissection following the sigmoid sinus to the jugular bulb and even into the neck. Penetration from the jugular fossa into the carotid canal often means the addition of the infratemporal fossa approach for optimal exposure.

Exposure of the zygomatic root, mandibular condylectomy, and parotidectomy are done in a similar fashion to the lateral resection.

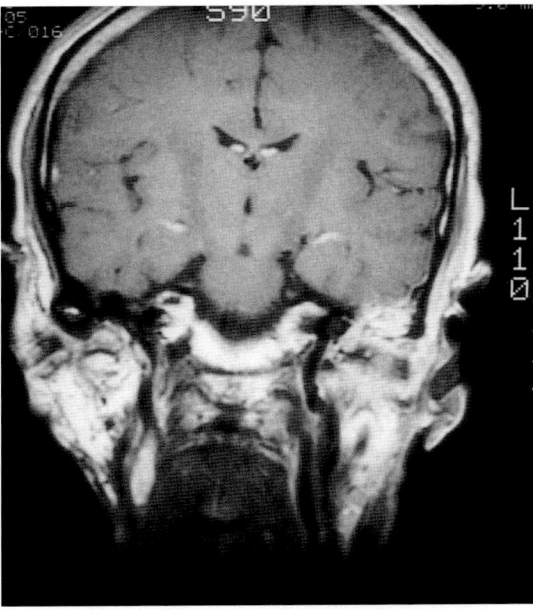

FIG. 20. Coronal magnetic resonance image showing penetration of tumor through tegmen mastoideum and overlying dura and into brain.

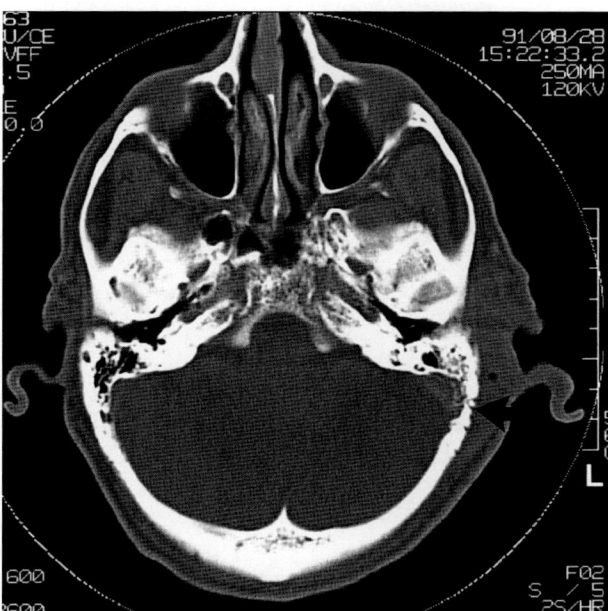

FIG. 21. Axial computed tomography scan showing temporal bone and scalp tumor penetrating the skull in region of lateral venous sinus on the left.

Control of the medial aspect of resection is accomplished by a small, limited middle fossa craniotomy whose size is dictated by the extent of dural invasion (Fig. 23).

Temporal Craniotomy

The temporal craniotomy is most expeditiously outlined according to the method described by Montgomery (39). A cutting bur is used to outline a small bony incision in the temporal squama. The incision should extend in a smooth arc from the sinodural angle to a point 4 cm above the EAC, and then arch forward to the cut in the zygomatic arch (see Fig. 23). Before extending the cut to the dura, the intracranial fluid volume is diminished by extracting CSF through a previously placed lumbar drain, through a lumbar puncture, or by use of an osmotic diuretic such as mannitol.

Next, the inner table of skull is carefully cut through and the bone flap carefully dissected from the underlying dura. This is usually fairly easy to do, except in the elderly, in whom the dura is brittle and adherent to the skull. This part of the procedure may be done either by the neurosurgeon or the head and neck surgeon. The author prefers to cut the bone flap himself and leave the rest to the neurosurgeons, because they seem to think that a bigger craniotomy is desirable. The purpose of this operative step is to control the superior petrosal sinus and the middle meningeal artery, detect and resect any dural invasion or temporal lobe extension if possible, and establish the medial margin of resection. As the temporal lobe dura is elevated from the floor of the middle fossa and retracted with a Teflon-coated retractor, the superior petrosal sinus is prized from its fissure in the posterosu-

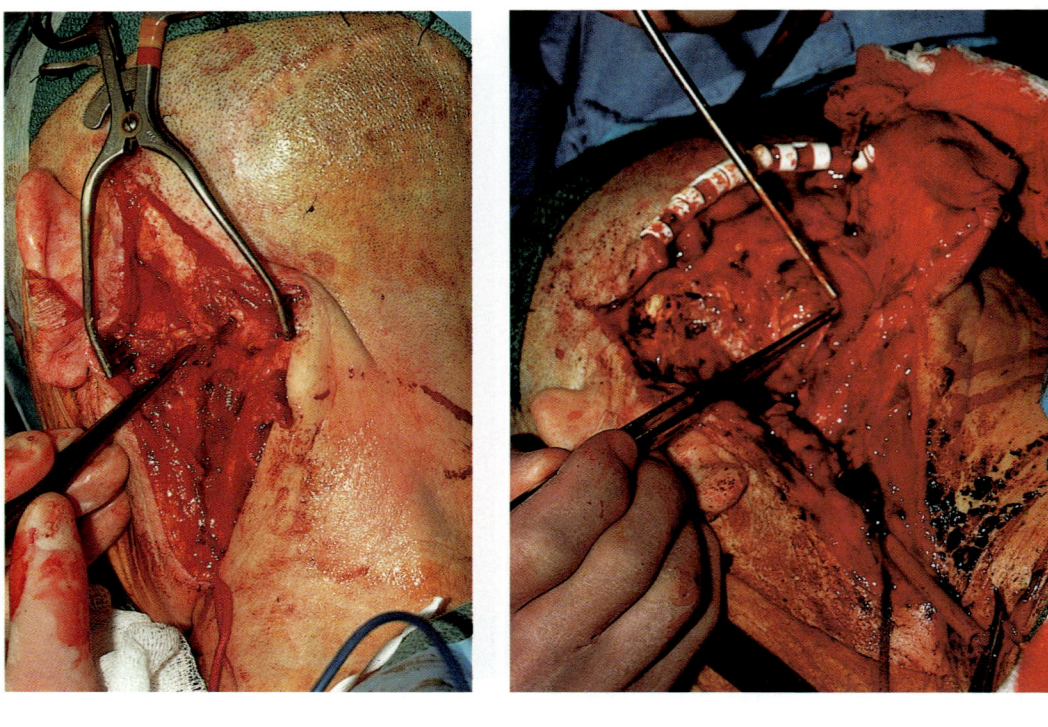
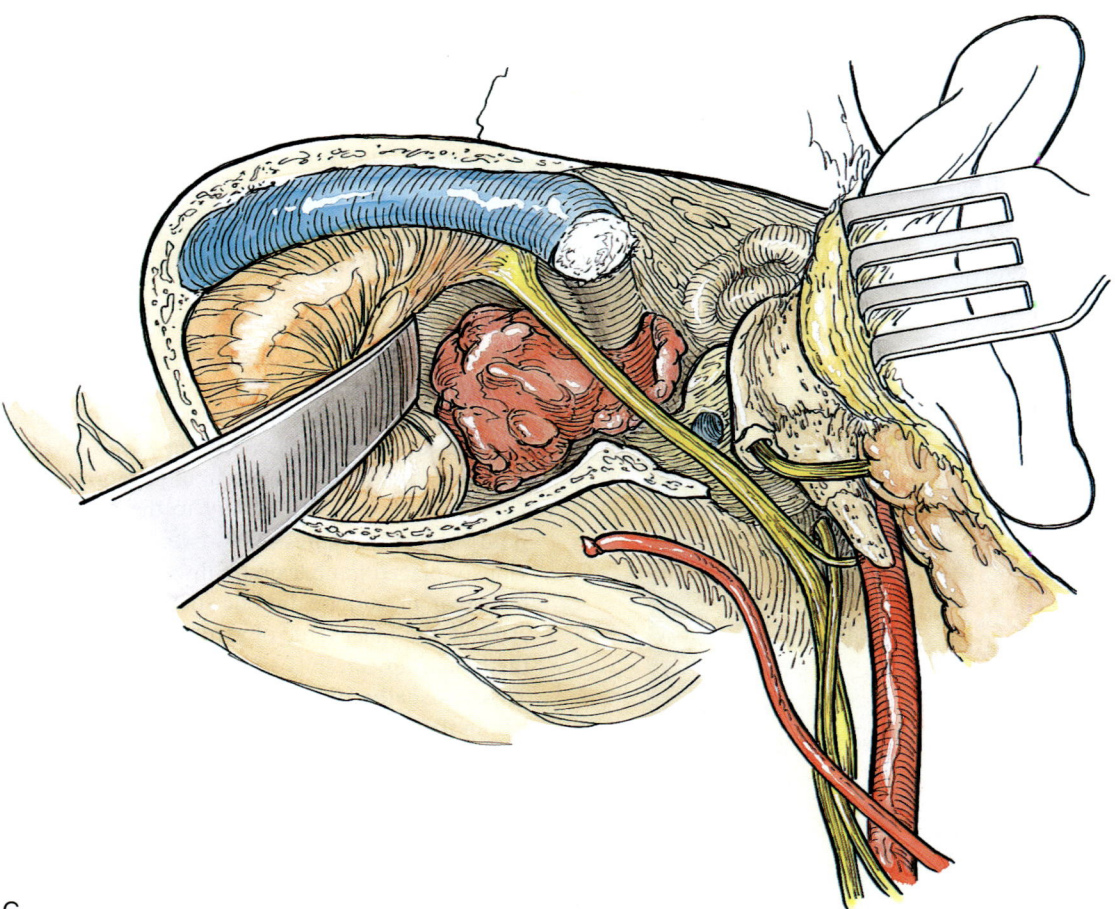

FIG. 22. More extensive posterior craniotomy must be carried into the occiput to resect effectively cerebellar dura invaded by tumor. **A:** Modified postauricular incision. Extended mastoidectomy; pointer on tumor. **B:** Occipital craniotomy as an extension of the presigmoid exposure achieved by complete mastoidectomy. (From Donald PJ. *Head and neck cancer: management of the difficult case.* Philadelphia: WB Saunders, 1984:248.) **C:** Drawing illustrating exposure and cerebellar retraction.

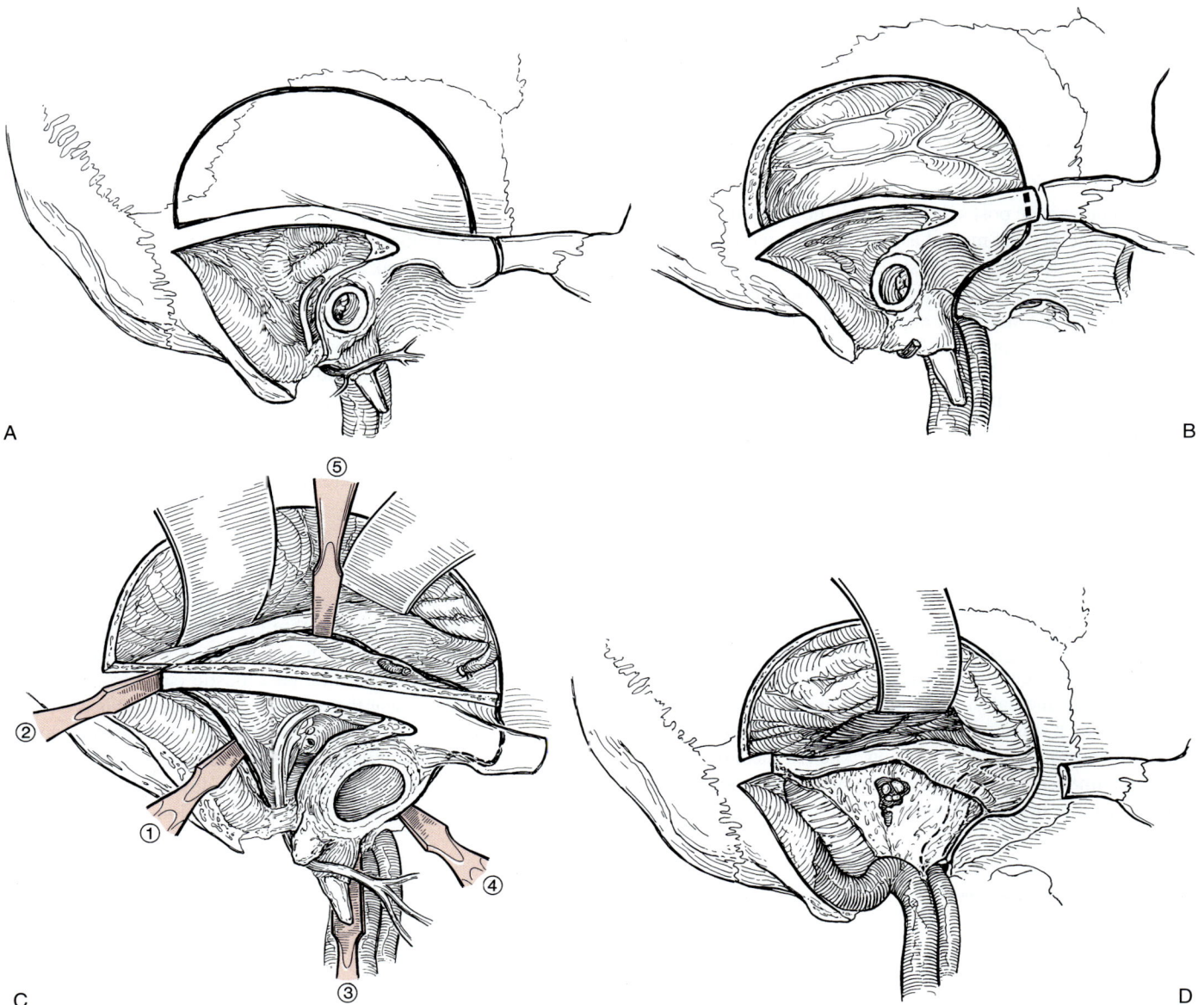

FIG. 23. A: The temporal craniotomy is outlined with the cutting bur. **B:** Craniotomy flap removed. The glenoid fossa is cut across medially, and the incision often transects the eustachian tube and proceeds into the middle cranial fossa. The inferior aspect of the fissure is carried down to the level of the medial aspect of the styloid process. **C:** The five osteotome cuts necessary to excise the bone are outlined. **D:** Defect after excision. (From Donald PJ. *Head and neck cancer: management of the difficult case.* Philadelphia: WB Saunders, 1984:241–243.)

perior extremity of the temporal bone (see Figs. 7–23). This elevation proceeds toward the cavernous sinus and Meckel's cave, judiciously avoiding both.

Exposure of the middle fossa floor to the portion of temporal bone medial to the arcuate eminence is done with the dural elevator.

All aspects of the circumference of the temporal bone are now outlined, and final bony cuts may now be made.

Final Bony Cuts

This critical part of the resection is where most surgical disasters occur. The problem is that the internal cuts that sever the temporal bone from the skull run adjacent to the course of the ICA and the jugular bulb. Injury to the latter structure is no great problem because bleeding can be controlled from below by the umbilical tape and from above through tamponade of the sigmoid or lateral sinuses. However, hemorrhage from a rent in the ICA can be life threatening because bleeding can be only partially controlled in the neck. Moreover, occlusion of the vessel may result in stroke and even death.

Osteotome cuts are initiated at the following sites (see Fig. 23C):

1. A cut is made posteriorly through the back surface of the bone at its most medial aspect, through the most medial limit of cerebellar plate skeletonization.
2. From cut no. 1, a superiorly directed bony incision is made to the sinodural angle. A cut through the tegmen mastoideum connects this to the craniotomy and is carried medially.
3. A cut is then made inferiorly just lateral to the styloid process and directly lateral to the jugular bulb. This cut is directed superiorly and slightly medially.
4. A cut is made anteroinferiorly through the fissure in the glenoid fossa.
5. For the "coup de grace," a cut is made superiorly through the floor of the middle fossa, just medial to the arcuate eminence.

These bony incisions are best made with an osteotome. The instrument is guided toward the theoretical center of the temporal bone near the internal acoustic meatus by being angled slightly medially. A gentle tapping with the mallet is followed by a slight twisting of the osteotome. This results in a more controlled type of incision. The cut medial to the arcuate eminence has to penetrate the otic capsule and thus requires a more brisk blow with the hammer.

Anteroinferiorly, the cutting and twisting motion of the osteotome usually results in the bone splitting along the plane of the initial ascending portion of the ICA. The bone is most commonly transected through either the cochlea or the internal auditory canal.

Cavity Ablation

If the bone transection is too medial in the internal auditory canal, a CSF leak may result. A fat graft taken from the subcutaneous area of the abdomen and placed at the site of the leak is usually an effective plug.

Temporalis muscle flaps may be used to ablate the cavity. However, the cavity should not be so effaced that possible tumor recurrences might be obscured in their early stages.

The most important aspect of closure is the careful replacement of any resected dura with fascia, together with the securing of a watertight closure of any rents.

Hypoglossal-to-Facial Nerve Anastomosis

Full temporal bone resection always necessitates transection of the facial nerve. Although some thought may be given to cable grafting the nerve, this connection must extend from the proximal internal acoustic canal to the transected main trunk near the resected parotid bed. This is a difficult maneuver, and the author elects in most cases to do a hypoglossal-to-facial nerve crossover anastomosis.

The hypoglossal nerve is cut as far down in the neck as possible so the anastomosis will be tension free. The ap-

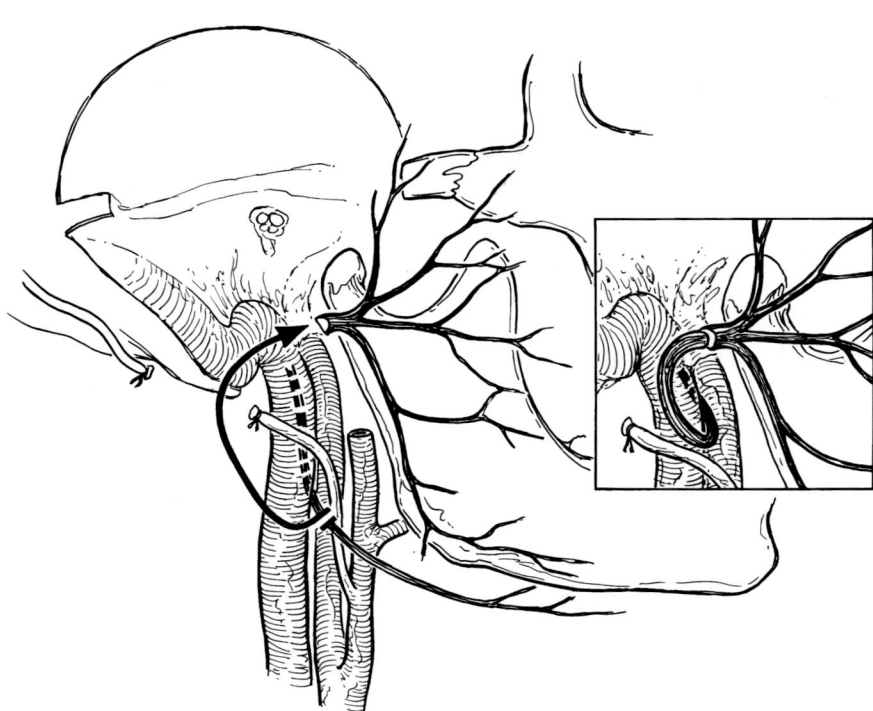

FIG. 24. Total temporal bone resection with hypoglossal-to-facial nerve crossover anastomosis. (From Donald PJ. *Head and neck cancer: management of the difficult case.* Philadelphia: WB Saunders, 1984:244.)

proximation is made under microscopic control using 10-0 nylon sutures. Approximately 10 sutures are placed through the epineurium of these nerves (Fig. 24).

Closure

When a portion of the auricle remains, the flap is returned and the gap created by the conchal and external canal skin excision is bridged with a split-thickness skin graft. The graft is inverted into the cavity and packed with iodoform- or antibiotic-impregnated gauze packing. The graft is sutured to the auricular cut edges, and the remaining wound in the neck and scalp is closed with interrupted sutures.

The neck is drained and a large pressure dressing applied, or suction drains are used. Excision of the entire auricle occasionally presents a problem in closure. Because most patients with temporal bone carcinoma are elderly, an elevation of the facial skin similar to that of a face lift enhances flap advancement. When this is not enough, a relaxation incision can be done and a bipedicled scalp flap advanced into the wound. The donor site on the skull is skin grafted, and the wound closed and drained.

Total Petrosectomy

The most extensive temporal bone cancers are fortunately rarely seen. These tumors involve all or some of the internal acoustic canal, the ICA, the superior or inferior petrosal sinuses, the cavernous sinus, and any of the surrounding dura, the falx, or the temporal lobe of the brain. Controversy continues concerning the advisability of brain, ICA, and cavernous sinus resection. In the authors' experience, the prognosis is adversely affected by involvement of these areas, but resection is still considered warranted even if only as a palliative effort. Details of carotid resection and the management of cavernous sinus involvement are found in Chapter 16, and these issues are not discussed in detail here.

The preparation for the resection is similar to that for the subtotal temporal bone resection (Fig. 25). Posteriorly, cerebellar plate removal continues to a point just lateral to the porus acusticus. Superiorly, the superior petrosal sinus is elevated to its point of entrance into the cavernous sinus. In the process, Meckel's cave is exposed and the proximity of Dorello's canal is reached. If uninvolved, cranial nerves V and VI are carefully protected. Involvement of the cranial nerve V is not uncommonly seen, and the gasserian ganglion may need to be removed.

Careful elevation of the lateral aspect of the cavernous sinus is necessary so that the final osteotome cut does not lacerate the sinus. The various extensions of the sinus to the foramina of the third and sometimes second divisions of the trigeminal nerve may need to be coagulated with the bipolar cautery and packed off with thrombin-soaked Gelfoam pledgets or hemostatic gauze.

Anteriorly, exposure of the middle fossa floor provides

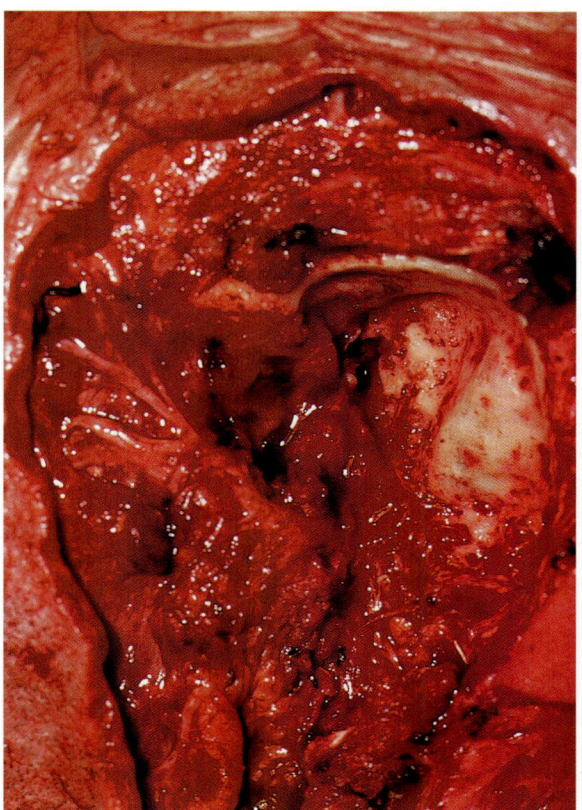

FIG. 25. Patient after complete mastoidectomy and parotidectomy with cranial nerve VII exposure and middle fossa craniotomy, now ready for complete petrosectomy.

exposure of the foramen spinosum. The middle meningeal artery can be clipped, tied, or coagulated. Exposure of the foramen ovale requires zygomatic ostectomy to provide infratemporal fossa exposure.

Inferiorly, careful attention is given to clear delineation of the ICA and internal jugular vein, and rubber catheters are used to circle these vessels in the neck. If either vessel is invaded at this point, the "modified *en bloc*" resection principle is invoked, and in the initial phase of total petrosectomy, any tumor involvement of either the vein or artery is left to be addressed at the next phase of resection.

Osteotome cuts are made lateral to or just through the most lateral aspect of the internal auditory canal. These are done both posteriorly and superiorly (Fig. 26) near the petrous apex. The fracture along the carotid canal is even easier in those cases with ICA invasion by tumor. The bone tends to fracture along this line of weakness. With removal of the bone, CSF begins to leak from the internal auditory canal.

With removal of bone, only a rudiment of the petrous apex remains (Fig. 27). The remaining bone, and that of its articulation with the sphenoid, is removed with a drill. The carotid canal is drilled away if involved and the carotid removed and grafted. The cavernous sinus is removed by the neurosurgeon. Clival erosion is removed by the drill. Per-

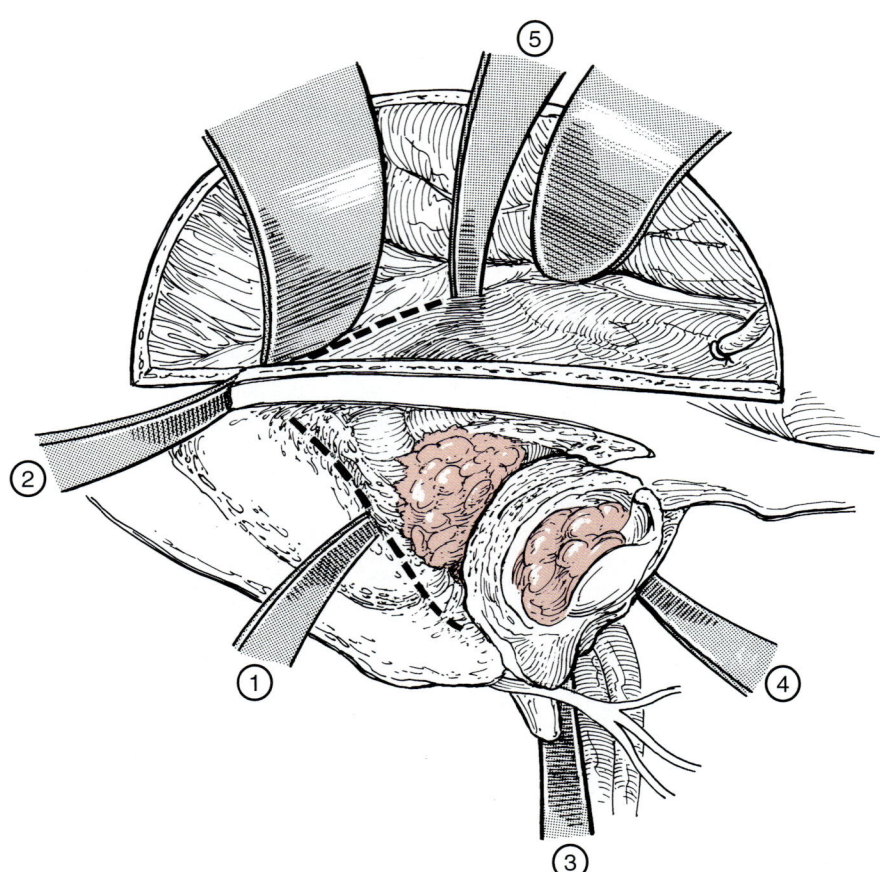

FIG. 26. Osteotome cuts (1) through cerebellar plate, (2) along tegmen mastoideum, (3) through tympanic bone just lateral to the internal carotid artery and internal jugular vein, (4) through the glenoid fossa, and (5) medial to superior semicircular canal adjacent to cavernous sinus.

ineural invasion is traced in a central direction until tumor-free margins are obtained.

Reconstruction involves dural grafting, but a watertight seal between the often incomplete dural closure and the nasopharynx is not uncommon. Complete eustachian tube removal is usually necessary. Closure from the nasopharynx and augmentation of dural closure may occasionally be achieved with fat grafts. Usually a temporalis muscle flap or a rectus abdominis free flap effects closure and seals any CSF leakage. Meticulous postoperative eye care is essential, especially when the facial nerve and trigeminal ganglia have been resected.

The Neck

Management of the neck is an important issue in the management of these tumors. Unfortunately, it is often not addressed in publications in this area. Although many publications quote cervical lymphatic metastases in the range of 10% to 20%, the authors' belief is that this incidence is higher. The American Society for Head and Neck Surgery and The Society of Head and Neck Surgeons have published guidelines for management of the neck (40). For N0 neck disease, an ipsilateral upper neck dissection (level 2 and 3 nodes) is recommended. For N1 disease, an ipsilateral modified radical dissection with preservation of cranial nerve XI,

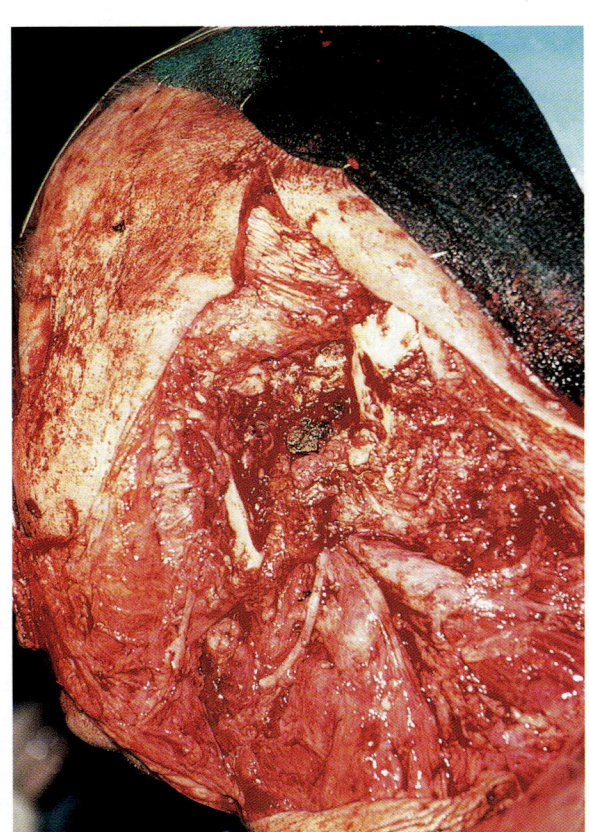

FIG. 27. Bony remnant after total petrosectomy.

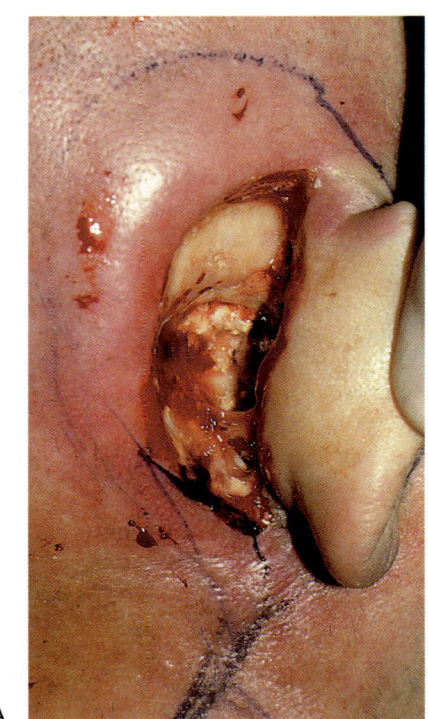
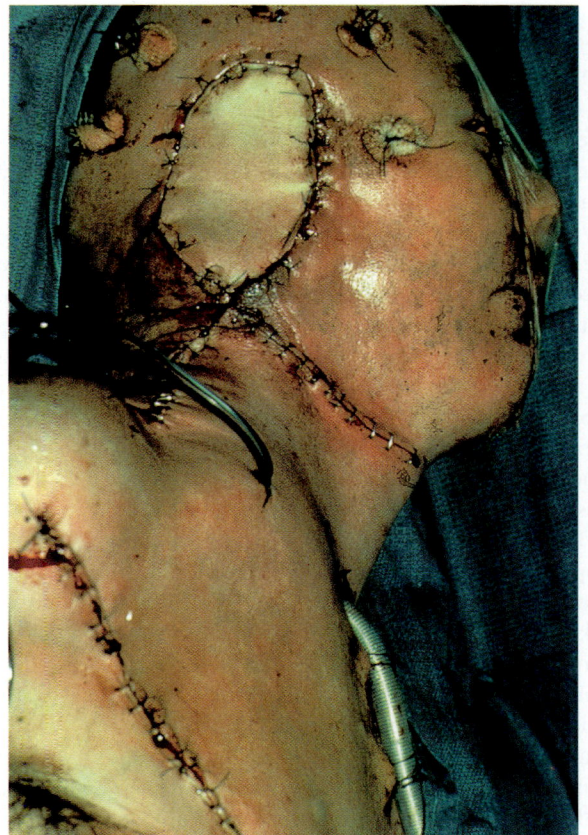
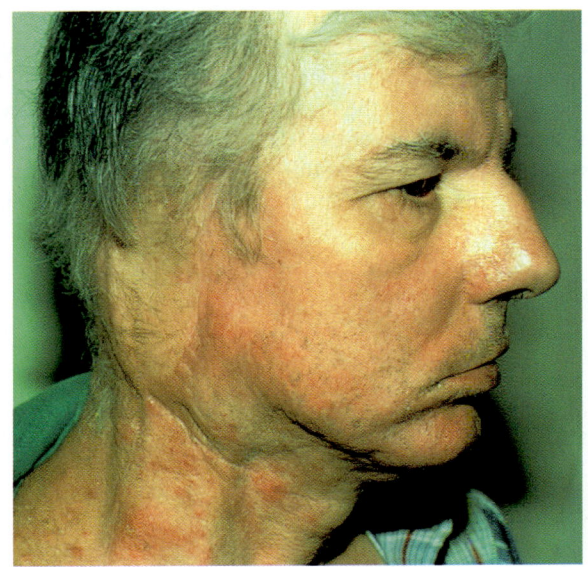

FIG. 28. Pectoralis major myocutaneous flap reconstruction of temporal bone defect. **A:** Before resection. **B:** After insetting of flap. **C:** Postoperative appearance at 3 years.

the sternocleidomastoid muscle, and internal jugular vein is preferred. For N2,3 disease, preservation of these structures is also recommended whenever possible, although a radical neck dissection may be necessary.[3]

---

[3]**Editor's note:** *The editor's philosophy is more radical than that of the other authors of this chapter. The N1 disease is treated by a radical neck dissection modified by preservation of the spinal accessory nerve when possible. For N2 and N3 disease, not only is a radical neck dissection done, but the occipital nodes are removed.*

Reconstruction

The head and neck surgeon of the 1990s has a vast array of reconstructive techniques available after ablative resections, and these may involve regional, primary, and free flap reconstruction. Reconstruction aims at covering exposed dura, preventing CSF leakage, and replacing surgical dead space with healthy, vascularized tissue. This reduces the morbidity associated with these procedures by reducing complications, and thus improves quality of life. Myocutaneous axial flaps such as the pectoralis major flap (Fig. 28) largely replaced local temporalis and deltopectoral flaps during the 1980s (41). To reach the lateral skull base, this flap (based on the pectoral branch of the acromiothoracic artery) must be stretched to an extreme, and this may result in partial necrosis at a critical anatomic site. As free tissue transfer became more widely available, this flap became less widely used. The trapezius myocutaneous flap (Fig. 29) based on the transverse cervical vessels and the latissimus dorsi flap provide excellent bulk and soft tissue cover. They remain alternatives less commonly used to reconstruct the lateral skull base. The need to alter the position of the patient during the procedure, coupled with a technically difficult elevation, has not led to widespread adoption of these reconstructive options. Free tissue transfer is the preferred reconstructive option for lateral skull base defects. Free rectus abdominis or myocutaneous flaps provide reliable one-stage reconstruction of complex temporal bone defects. Vessels suitable for anastomosis can be easily obtained from the cervical vessels, and good tissue bulk is provided by these flaps. Larger and more extensive tumors previously deemed inoperable are now being resected. Complications such as CSF leakage are reduced, and the provision of healthy tissue to the ablation site allows postoperative radiation therapy to be safely instituted (42). Patients requiring complete resection of the auricle may be candidates for the osseointegrated, bone-anchored implants developed by Branemark et al. (43). These implants are placed once good tissue cover has been achieved, and cosmesis is excellent once a bone-anchored prosthesis is placed.

Despite the advances in technical aspects of surgery for these tumors, it is not known whether long-term survival is improved. No single institution has sufficient data to allow a meaningful analysis of results. Resection in cases of petrous apex involvement appears to be of reasonable value. In a series of 14 total temporal bone resections reported by Malata et al. (44), 9 (64%) had a tumor free survival when followed for an average of 70 months.

COMPLICATIONS

By paying careful attention to preoperative evaluation and adhering to sound oncologic principles, many of the complications and emergencies associated with the treatment of temporal bone malignancies can be avoided. Intraoperative hemorrhage, cerebrovascular accidents, and CSF leakage are the primary complications associated with temporal bone surgery. Hemorrhage during surgery usually occurs from the jugular bulb or sigmoid sinus. The immediate importance of this bleeding stems from the fact that air embolism may occur with consequent life-threatening arrhythmias or hemodynamic changes. Simple pressure, a muscle plug, or bone wax packed into the area is often enough to tamponade these low-pressure bleeds. Occasionally, the sigmoid sinus needs to be ligated below the entry of the superior petrosal sinus for adequate venous control.

Cerebrospinal fluid leakage may result whenever the subarachnoid space is opened, and carries a risk of meningitis. Complete obliteration of the middle ear space, repairing torn dura, sealing dead space with vascularized tissue, and observing meticulous wound closure help to minimize this complication. If CSF rhinorrhea occurs, a compression dressing and trial of a lumbar drain for a number of days may be warranted to reduce the CSF pressure and allow spontaneous closure. Rarely, a second surgical exploration with attention to the region of the eustachian tube may be needed.

Whenever the ICA is ligated, resected, or both, despite reconstruction, a full-blown cerebrovascular accident (stroke) may develop and have devastating consequences for the pa-

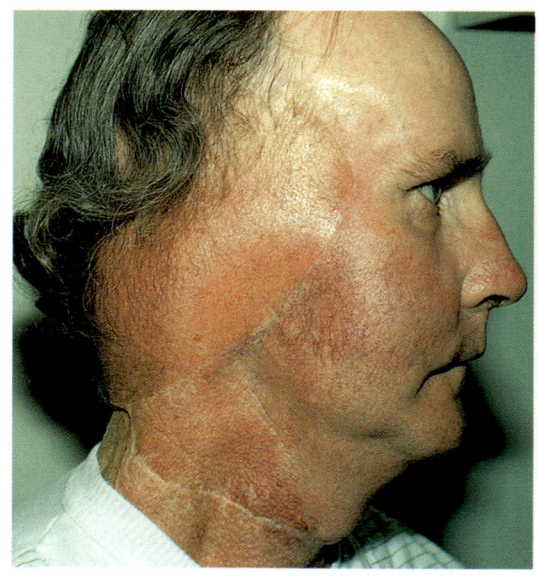 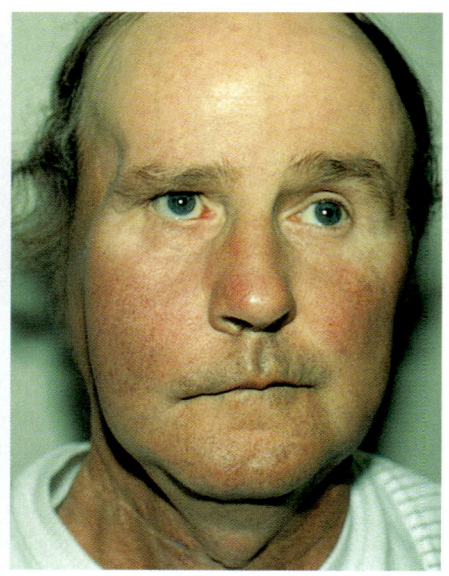

FIG. 29. A,B: Trapezius myocutaneous flap reconstruction of temporal bone defect.

tient. Thromboembolic phenomena from atheroma, air embolism, or blood clot are potential causes. Cerebral hypoperfusion caused by perioperative hypotension and vascular spasm may have detrimental sequelae in a patient with a marginal collateral circulation. Bypass grafts need to be kept as short as possible when used, and anastomosed in an end-to-end fashion to reduce turbulent blood flow.

After major resections, patients often lose any residual cochleovestibular function. Vertigo in the immediate postoperative period is not uncommon, and ataxia from the abrupt vestibular loss may persist for several months until compensation from the functioning opposite labyrinth occurs. Elderly patients are particularly prone to this persistent disequilibrium.

Single or multiple cranial nerve deficits may be present before surgery as a result of tumor invasion of the skull base or after surgery because of surgical trauma. Early recognition of swallowing dysfunction and potential aspiration is important because appropriate preventive means can minimize aspiration pneumonia.

Facial Nerve Injury and Rehabilitation

Loss of facial nerve function with its associated psychological sequelae, alterations in speech, and mastication problems is expected after major resections. Primary intraoperative reconstructive options include interposition sural or greater auricular nerve cable grafts between the proximal and distal ends of the facial nerve. Other reconstructive options include facial-to-hypoglossal (VII–XII), facial-to-accessory (VII–IX), or a cross-facial sural nerve interposition graft. Depending on the individual case, these procedures are usually performed at a later stage and usually within 6 months of the initial surgery (45).

Myths and misconceptions surround the role of these reconstructive methods in the delayed case. Usually when a useful facial nerve is absent or long-term facial paralysis has resulted in mimetic atrophy and fibrosis, alternatives to reinnervation are required. In these cases, the rehabilitation techniques include static and dynamic procedures (46).

Dynamic procedures involve regional muscle transfer (masseter or temporalis) when available. Gold-weight lid-loading and eyelid-spring implantation help to prevent corneal abrasion and are useful as early rehabilitation methods for the paralyzed eye. Although tarsorrhaphy is a time-honored method of corneal protection, it has an unpleasant cosmetic result and may restrict lateral visual fields. Tarsorrhaphy has to a large degree been replaced by the preformed upper-eyelid gold-weight implants (0.75–1.2 g) which provide adequate corneal protection in patients with minimal lid retraction. A major advantage of this method is the ease with which the implant can be removed should facial nerve function recover spontaneously. Failure rates (including extrusion) are usually less than 10% (46,47). Eyelid springs are indicated for a more complete or permanent facial paralysis when there is marked lid retraction and a poor Bell's phenomenon. They are technically difficult to insert and remove, if required. Failure rates (including extrusion) are estimated at 15% (46,48).

Static procedures involve the use of fascial or alloplastic (i.e., Gortex) slings and cosmetic procedures such as face lift, brow lift, and lid tightening. An advantage of the alloplastic slings is that they can be temporarily inserted to improve oral competence and minimize drooling in a patient with a facial paralysis. At a later stage, removal is possible should facial function improve.

When facial function is not expected to recover, a combination of static and dynamic procedures is usually required. Every patient requires an individualized approach to rehabilitation, and multiple procedures are usually the norm to achieve a satisfactory cosmetic and functional result.

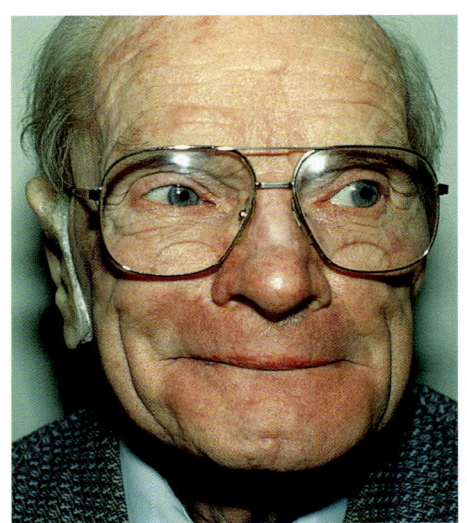
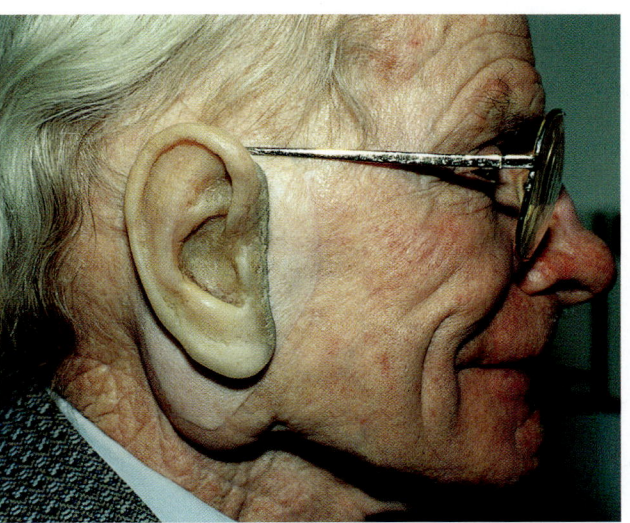

FIG. 30. A,B: Prosthetic reconstruction of the pinna 3 years after a lateral temporal bone resection.

Other Rehabilitation Problems

Hearing rehabilitation may become an issue if the neoplasm is in an only hearing ear. Younger patients may object to cosmetic appearance of a skin graft that may influence the choice of free flap. Osseointegrated prostheses are also an option for long-term cosmesis (Fig. 30). Dental consultation is very useful in managing some of the long-term problems with TMJ dysfunction and masticatory pain. Swallowing therapy and vocal therapy may be useful in the presence of postoperative swallowing dysfunction and aspiration.

RADIATION THERAPY

The precise role of preoperative or postoperative radiation therapy for malignancy involving the temporal bone is unclear. A review (38) has indicated that the addition of radiation therapy to patients with disease confined to the EAC and treated with a lateral temporal bone resection confers no survival advantage. The role of radiation therapy in patients treated with subtotal temporal bone resection was unclear. Radiation therapy is seldom advocated as the sole treatment modality for malignancy of the EAC or temporal bone. Its overall effectiveness is diminished if the bone is invaded by tumor (49). Postoperative radiation therapy may help in improving local control rates in resectable disease, but does not appear to affect recurrence and survival rates if the surgical margins are involved with residual tumor. Lederman (50) and others have recommended that radiation therapy should be used after variants of lateral temporal bone resections have been performed.

Guidelines from The American Society for Head and Neck Surgery and The Society of Head and Neck Surgeons (40) for postoperative radiation therapy include when resection margins are close (less than 5 mm), when proximity of tumor to important structures such as ICA or facial nerve preclude "wide margins," when margins of resection are microscopically positive, and, finally, when there is perineural invasion. In general, these conditions apply to most resections for temporal bone carcinoma.

Radiation therapy is also indicated if there are multiple histologically positive nodes, or evidence of extracapsular spread. In addition, radiation therapy is indicated for most adenoid cystic carcinomas.

Five-year survival rates from radiation therapy alone of 11% contrast to 34% when combined radiation therapy and surgery is used. In theory, suspected micrometastatic disease in the lateral skull base, parotid, or neck may be sterilized by a course of radiation treatment. Once the extent of the tumor has been defined, the optimal target volume can be decided. A typical plan is shown in Fig. 31. Typically, two wedged cobalt-60 fields are applied at right angles, producing a circumscribed high-dose volume. The dose beyond the 130 line reduces rapidly (51).

Complications of radiation treatment include osteoradionecrosis of the surrounding bone, EAC stenosis, and sensorineural hearing loss. Necrotizing otitis externa progressing to skull base osteomyelitis has been described with fatal outcome if untreated. Inadvertent injury to the eyes, brainstem, and central cortex (Fig. 32) may occur because of the radiation fields required for extensive disease control. This type of injury typically occurs in a delayed manner (i.e., ra-

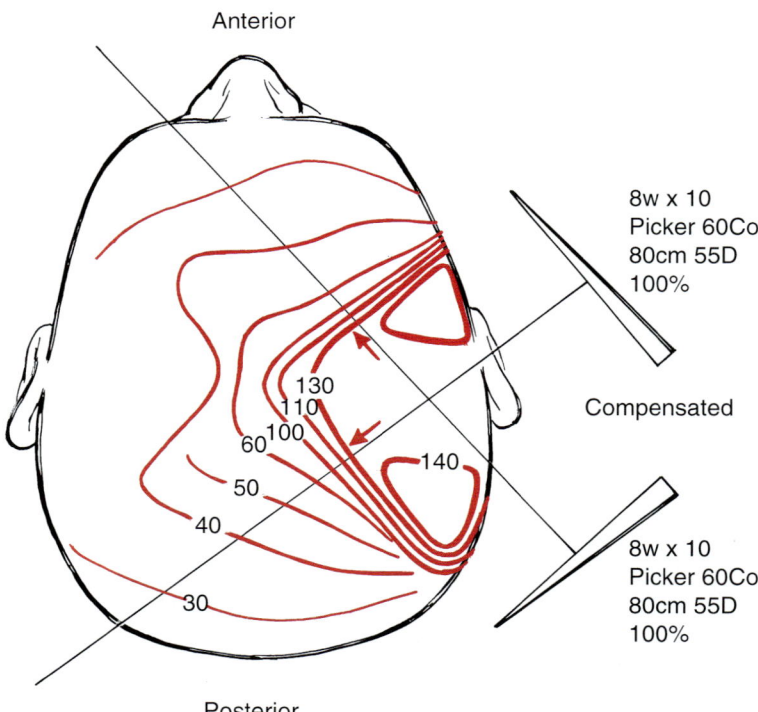

FIG. 31. Typical radiation field plan for treatment of external ear canal and middle ear. High-dose volume is delivered to line 130. Dose beyond this reduces rapidly, minimizing radiation effect to brainstem and cranial nerves.

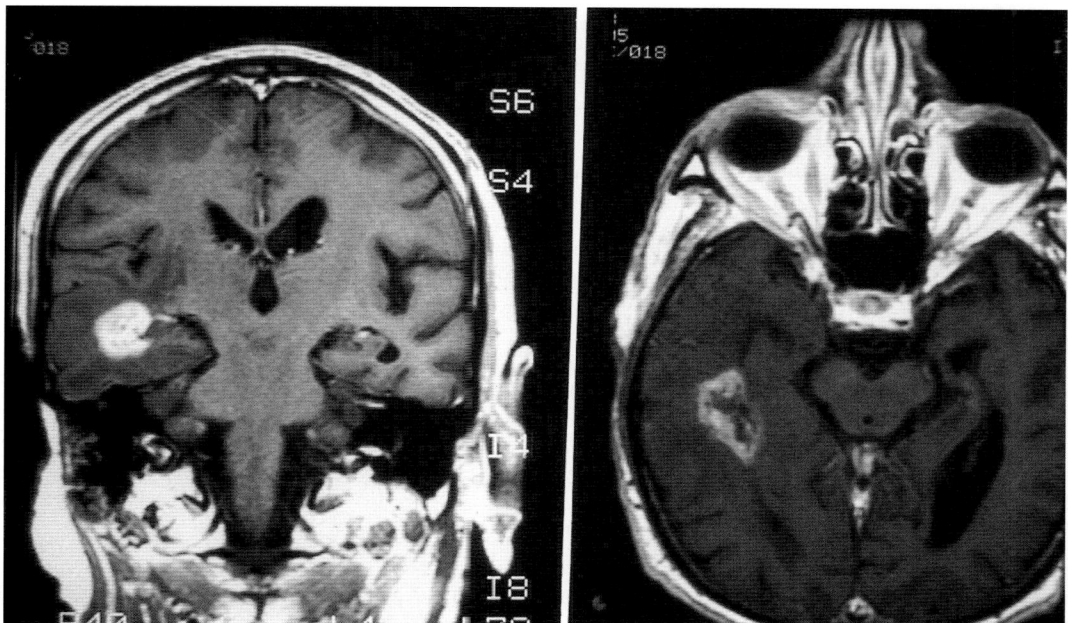

FIG. 32. Coronal and axial computed tomography scans demonstrate radiation necrosis affecting right temporal lobe.

diation-induced cataracts, progressive brain and brainstem necrosis). The facial nerve is usually not affected, although progressive cochleolabyrinthitis may involve the inner ear. Temporal bone malignancy tends to have an unpleasant natural history if left untreated. With time, the tumor becomes gradually larger, more painful, ulcerated, and necrotic. Often a malodorous discharge is socially unacceptable. Once the dura is invaded, intolerable pain makes adequate analgesia an imperative part of the management of these patients A well planned resection may not provide cure, but will result in good palliation of pain secondary to recurrent or residual disease.

CONCLUSIONS

Temporal bone carcinoma is a relatively rare disease. It is a difficult disease to treat and should be managed at major centers with experienced staff, for several reasons. It is difficult for anyone outside these centers to acquire enough experience to manage the complexities of the problem. Concentration of experience also allows patterns to be observed that may be pertinent to staging and trials of different treatment modalities.

The main problems in the treatment of this disease are

1. Early diagnosis: General otolaryngologists and other physicians treating ear disease need continuing education about the often subtle presentation of these neoplasms, and need to maintain a high index of suspicion.
2. Inadequate staging system: It is difficult to compare outcomes of different treatment modalities without a common language in which to describe the extent of the disease. Also, lack of a staging system makes prognostication less scientific.
3. Frequently, dilemmas arise with the management of the carotid artery and facial nerve. These have been addressed in the text, but are another reason these lesions should be treated by experienced surgeons.

Free and myocutaneous flaps have reduced complications such as CSF leaks and wound infections, and improved cosmesis. This has probably been the most significant advance in the surgical treatment of these lesions in the recent past.

Combined radiation therapy and surgery should be considered the treatment of choice for all but early lesions.

REFERENCES

1. Arena S, Keen M. Carcinoma of the middle ear and temporal bone. *Am J Otolaryngol* 1988;9:351–356.
2. Politzer A. *Textbook of diseases of the ear*. London: Balliere Tindall & Cox, 1883. Cassells JP, translator.
3. Lewis JS. Cancer of the ear. *Laryngoscope* 1960;70:551–560.
4. Lederman M. Malignant tumors of the ear. *J Laryngol Otol* 1965;79:85–119.
5. Nuss D, Janecka I, Sekkar L, et al. Craniofacial disassembly in the management of skull base tumors. *Otolaryngol Clin North Am* 1991;24:1465–1497.
6. Shah J. Indications, complications, sequelae and results of cranial base surgery. In: *Proceedings of the 4th international conference on head and neck cancer*. Arlington, VA: The Society of Head and Neck Surgeons, 1996:74–78.
7. Conley J, Schuller D. Malignancies of the ear. *Laryngoscope* 1976;86:1147–1163.
8. Arriaga M, Curtin H, Takahashi H, et al. Staging proposal for external auditory meatus carcinoma based on the preoperative clinical examination and computed tomography findings. *Ann Otol Rhinol Laryngol* 1990;99:714–721.
9. Chen KTK, Dephner LP. Primary tumors of the external and middle ear. *Archives of Otolaryngology* 1978;104:247–252.

10. Boland J, Paterson R. Cancer of the middle ear and the external auditory meatus. *J Laryngol Otol* 1955;69:468–478.
11. Shih L, Crabtree J. Carcinoma of the external auditory canal; an update. *Laryngoscope* 1990;100:1215–1218.
12. Conley J. Cancer of the middle ear. *Annals of Otolaryngology* 1965;74:555–572.
13. Tucker W. Cancer of the middle ear. *Cancer* 1965;18:642–650.
14. Stell P. Epithelial tumors of the external auditory meatus and the middle ear. In: Booth J, ed. *Scott Brown's otolaryngology.* 4th ed. London: Butterworth, 1987:534–545.
15. Ruben R, Thaler S, Holzer J. Radiation induced carcinoma of the temporal bone. *Laryngoscope* 1977;87:1613–1621.
16. Applebaum E. Radiation-induced carcinoma of the temporal bone. *Otolaryngol Head Neck Surg* 1979;87:604–609.
17. Parsons H, Lewis L. Subtotal resection of the temporal bone for cancer of the ear. *Cancer* 1954;7:995–1000.
18. Goodwin W, Jesse R. Malignant neoplasms of the external auditory canal and temporal bone. *Archives of Otolaryngology* 1980;106:675–679.
19. Stell P, McCormick M. Carcinoma of the external auditory meatus and middle ear: prognostic factors and a suggested staging system. *J Laryngol Otol* 1985;99:847–850.
20. Paaske P, Witten J, Schwer S, et al. Results in treatment of carcinoma of the external auditory canal and middle ear. *Cancer* 1987;59:156–160.
21. GW. Tumors arising from glandular structures of the external auditory canal. *Laryngoscope* 1983;93:326–340.
22. Cannon CR, McLean WC. Salivary gland choristoma of the middle ear. *Am J Otol* 1980;1:250–252.
23. Hociota D, Atamar T. A case of salivary gland choristoma of the middle ear. *J Laryngol Otol* 1975;89:1065–1068.
24. Perzin K, Gullane P, Conley J. Adenoid cystic carcinoma involving the external auditory canal. *Cancer* 1982;50:2873–2883.
25. Goebel JA, Smith PG, Kemick JL. Primary adenocarcinoma of the temporal bone mimicking paragangliomas: radiographic and clinical recognition. *Laryngoscope* 1987;96:231–238.
26. Wiatrak BJ, Pensak ML. Rhabdomyosarcoma of the temporal bone. *Laryngoscope* 1989;99:1188–1192.
27. Canalis R, Gussen R. Temporal bone findings in rhabdomyosarcoma with predominantly petrous involvement. *Archives of Otolaryngology* 1980;106:290–293.
28. Raney RB, Lawrence W, Maurer H, et al. Rhabdomyosarcoma of the ear in childhood. *Cancer* 1983;51:2356–2361.
29. May J, Fisch U. Neoplasms of the ear and lateral skull base. In: Bailey BJ, ed. *Head and neck surgery–otolaryngology.* Philadelphia: JB Lippincott, 1993:1564–1577.
30. Freidmann I, Radcliffe A. Otosclerosis associated with malignant melanoma of the ear. *J Laryngol Otol* 1954;68:114–119.
31. Hasegawa M, Nishijima W, Watanabe I, et al. Primary chondroid chordoma arising from the base of the temporal bone. *J Laryngol Otol* 1985;99:485–489.
32. Krouse J, Nadol J, Goodman M. Carcinoid tumors of the middle ear. *Ann Otol Rhinol Laryngol* 1990;99:548–552.
33. Woodman G, Jurco S, Alford B, et al. Verrucous carcinoma of the middle ear. *Archives of Otolaryngology* 1981;107:63–65.
34. Cunningham M, Curtin H, Jaffe R, Stool S. Otologic manifestations of Langerhan's histiocytosis. *Archives of Otolaryngology* 1989;115:807.
35. Atkinson D, Jacobs L, Weaver A. Elective carotid resection for squamous cell carcinoma of the head and neck. *Am J Surg* 1984;148:483–488.
36. Sekhar L, Sen C, Jho H. Saphenous vein graft bypass of the cavernous internal carotid artery. *J Neurosurg* 1990;72:35–41.
37. Erba S, Horton J, Latchaw R, et al. Balloon test occlusion of the internal carotid artery with stable xenon/CT cerebral flow imaging. *AJNR Am J Neuroradiol* 1989;9:533–538.
38. Prasad S, Janecka I. Efficacy of surgical treatments for squamous cell carcinoma of the temporal bone: a literature review. *Head Neck* 1994;110:270–280.
39. Montgomery WW. *Surgery of the upper respiratory tract.* Vol. 1. Philadelphia: Lea & Febiger, 1971:471.
40. The American Society for Head and Neck Surgery and The Society of Head and Neck Surgeons. *Clinical practice guidelines for the diagnosis and management of cancer of the head and neck.* The American Society for Head and Neck Surgery and The Society of Head and Neck Surgeons, 1996.
41. Ariyan S, Sasaki C, Spencer D. Radical en-bloc resection of the temporal bone. *Am J Surg* 1982;142:443–447.
42. Irish J, Gullane P, Gentille F, et al. Tumors of the skull base: outcome and survival analysis of 77 cases. *Head Neck* 1994;16:3–10.
43. Alberktsson T, Branemark P, Jacobson M, et al. Present clinical applications of osseointegrated percutaneous implants. *Plast Reconstr Surg* 1987;9:721–731.
44. Malata CM, Cooter RD, Towns GM, Batchelor AGG. Petrosectomy for invasive tumors: surgery and reconstruction. *Br J Plast Surg* 1996;49:370–378.
45. Fisch U, Mattox D. Petrosectomy and facial nerve rehabilitation in malignant tumors of the retromandibular fossa. In: Bull TR, Myers E, eds. *Plastic reconstruction of the head and neck.* London: Butterworth, 1986:79–97.
46. May M, Sobol S. Reanimation of the paralysed face without the facial nerve. In: Sekhar LN, Janecka IP, eds. *Surgery of cranial base tumors.* New York: Raven Press, 1993; 449-460.
47. May M. Gold weight and wire spring implants as alternatives to tarsorrhaphy. *Archives of Otolaryngology* 1987;13:656–660.
48. May M. Paralysed eyelid reanimation with a close eyelid spring. *Laryngoscope* 1988;98:382–385.
49. Arthur K. Radiotherapy in carcinoma of the middle ear and external auditory canal. *J Laryngol Otol* 1976;90:753–762.
50. Lederman M, et al. Cancer of the middle ear; technique of radiation treatment. *Br J Radiol* 1965;38(456):895–905.
51. Harwood A, Keane T. Malignant tumors of the temporal bone and external ear: medical and radiation therapy. In: Alberti PW, Ruben RJ, eds. *Otologic medicine and surgery.* Vol. 2. New York: Churchill Livingstone, 1988:1389–1408.

CHAPTER 21

Transcervicomastoid Approach

Gale L. Gardner, Edwin W. Cocke, Jr., and Jon H. Robertson

Historically, the surgical management of tumors involving the jugular foramen has constituted a difficult surgical problem. Beginning in the early 1970s, the authors began a multidisciplinary effort to overcome the problem. Using the methods of head and neck surgery, otologic surgery, and neurosurgery, a procedure has evolved that is described in this chapter; it is termed the transcervicomastoid (TCM) approach to the jugular foramen. The authors discuss this evolution of the procedure and the surgical efforts made by others on which the procedure is based. Diagnosis, preoperative evaluation and treatment, surgical anatomy and technique, and outcome and complications are presented.

INDICATIONS AND ALTERNATIVE FORMS OF TREATMENT

The TCM approach is indicated for the removal of any tumor or lesion involving the jugular bulb and adjacent skull base that is thought to be suitable for surgery. The authors have used the procedure for the following conditions:

Types of Tumors	Number
Carcinoma	2
Chondrosarcoma	1
Glomus jugulare tumor	32
Glomus jugulare and vagale tumors	3
Glomus jugulare, vagale, and carotid body tumors	1
Glomus jugulare and carotid body tumors	2
Meningioma	3
Neurofibroma	2
Neuroma of cranial nerve X	1
Total	47

G. Gardner, E. W. Cocke, Jr.: Department of Otolaryngology, Head and Neck Surgery, The University of Tennessee, Memphis, The Health Science Center, Memphis, Tennessee 38103.

J. H. Robertson: Department of Neurosurgery, The University of Tennessee, Memphis, The Health Science Center, and Semmes-Murphey Clinic, Memphis, Tennessee 38103.

The authors believe surgery to be contraindicated when the patient's general health or age precludes a major surgical procedure, when intracranial extension is deemed to be nonresectable, when the tumor involves the vagus nerve and the opposite vagus is nonfunctional, and when internal carotid artery involvement is present and there is inadequate collateral circulation as demonstrated by balloon occlusion test.

Alternative treatments for glomus tumors include radiation therapy and embolization. Although the authors now use preoperative embolization in nearly every instance in which they perform TCM, it may also be considered for palliative purposes under unusual circumstances. In their early experience with TCM for large glomus tumors, the authors used preoperative radiation therapy to reduce vascularity. They continue to use radiation therapy alone for glomus tumor management in patients unable to undergo surgery because of age or poor general health.

EVOLUTION OF THE TRANSCERVICOMASTOID PROCEDURE

This procedure is designed to accomplish tumor removal by (a) resection of overlying soft tissue, (b) removal of bone from over the jugular bulb, and (c) resection of the jugular bulb with *en bloc* removal of tumors involving the bulb or located adjacent to it.

Efforts to develop a systematic surgical approach to the jugular foramen and adjacent skull base began shortly after Guild (1) and Rosenwasser (2) identified glomus tumors as occurring in the temporal bone in the early 1940s. In 1949, Lundgren (3) suggested resection of the jugular bulb. He made reference to Seiffert, who in 1934 reported a case in which he had explored the bulb in a patient having a jugular foramen syndrome, and found tumor filling the bulb.

In 1951 Weille and Lane (4) correctly recognized that glomus tumors may arise from the dome of the jugular bulb. They recommended removal of bone from around the tumor so as to avoid trauma to the tumor itself, but did not recommend removal of the bulb because of the risk of significant hemorrhage.

Capps (5) in 1952 reported a case in which he had approached the skull base for removal of a glomus tumor. He described mobilizing the facial nerve, packing the lateral sinus, ligating the upper end of the internal jugular vein, and attempting unsuccessfully to remove the jugular bulb.

In 1961, Gastpar (6) reported resection of the jugular bulb. Shapiro and Neus (7) in 1963 described operating on a patient with recurrent glomus tumor of the jugular bulb in which they had used an extended incision, rerouted the facial nerve, exposed the hypotympanum and bulb, and accomplished total tumor removal without significant complications and with minimal blood loss.

Gejrot (8) in 1965 described a similar procedure in four cases. He described packing of the upper sigmoid sinus and removal of the lateral wall of the sinus inferiorly, with preservation of the medial (dural) wall to avoid entry into the posterior fossa. He ligated the internal jugular vein in the neck and isolated and removed the tumor, working both from above and below.

In 1968, House (9) reported extensive experience removing glomus tumors through the mastoid and extended facial recess with preservation of the posterior bony canal wall, but without rerouting of the facial nerve.

Portmann (10) in 1968 described removal of a large glomus tumor of the skull base with extension both into the temporal bone and posterior fossa, and pointed out the advantages of combined otologic and neurosurgical participation.

In 1974, Glasscock et al. (11) reported on their experience in which they had combined the methods of House and Shapiro, and had carried out tumor removal with transposition of the facial nerve and preservation of the posterior bony ear canal with exposure through an extended facial recess exposure.

The current authors (12) reported their experience treating 10 patients with glomus tumors of the skull base in 1976 to The Triological Society, and published this in 1977. The authors emphasized removal of soft tissue from the lateral base of the skull adjacent to the jugular foramen, wide removal of bone from over the mastoid and lateral skull base with exposure of the jugular bulb, transposition of the facial nerve, ligation of the upper sigmoid with resection of the lateral wall of the sigmoid inferiorly, ligation of the internal jugular vein in the neck, and resection of the tumor with attempted preservation of cranial nerves IX through XII.

Simultaneously in 1977, Fisch (13) described a similar procedure, but emphasized infratemporal fossa exposure to facilitate exposure of the internal carotid artery and to allow extension of the exposure anteriorly for more extensive and anteriorly placed tumors.

Since that time, the authors and others have continued to use these techniques with various modifications for the surgical management of various lesions occurring in and adjacent to the jugular foramen. It has been the authors' experience that wide exposure of the tumor using the methods

TABLE 1. *Most common presenting symptoms for tumors of the jugular foramen*

Symptom	No. of cases	Mean duration (mo)
Tinnitus	38	48
Hearing loss	35	66
Dizziness	26	41
Ear pressure	22	76
Ear pain	21	28

developed as early as the 1940s, and the use of preoperative embolization combined with careful identification of the lower cranial nerves at the jugular foramen, allow total removal of a high percentage of tumors occurring in this area, with acceptable morbidity in properly selected patients.

DIAGNOSIS AND IMAGING

The clinical presentation of tumors originating in or proximate to the jugular bulb is related not only to the adjacent neurovascular structures present in this area, but to the nature of the tumor mass that is involved. In the authors' series, glomus tumors predominate and produced symptoms reflecting their tendency toward local invasiveness.

This series constitutes 46 patients who underwent surgery for tumors of the jugular foramen, with 1 patient undergoing bilateral surgery for bilateral tumors. All underwent a workup that included a medical history, head and neck examination, audiometric evaluation, and radiographic evaluation. Sampling of the tumor for biopsy through the ear canal was performed before treatment early in this study when preoperative x-ray therapy was being used, for confirmation of type of tumor. All but a few patients in this series underwent preoperative evaluation and postoperative follow-up by a single internist.

The most common presenting symptoms in this series have been tinnitus, hearing loss, dizziness or imbalance, ear blockage, and otalgia, with a mean duration of 53 months (Table 1). The incidence of preoperative cranial nerve dysfunction is indicated in Table 2.

Early in this series, radiographic examination included plain films of the skull base and occasional arteriography and venography. Computed tomography became available in

TABLE 2. *Preoperative cranial nerve dysfunction*

Cranial nerves	No. of cases
VI	1
VII	6
VIII	23
IX	6
X	12
XI	11
XII	12

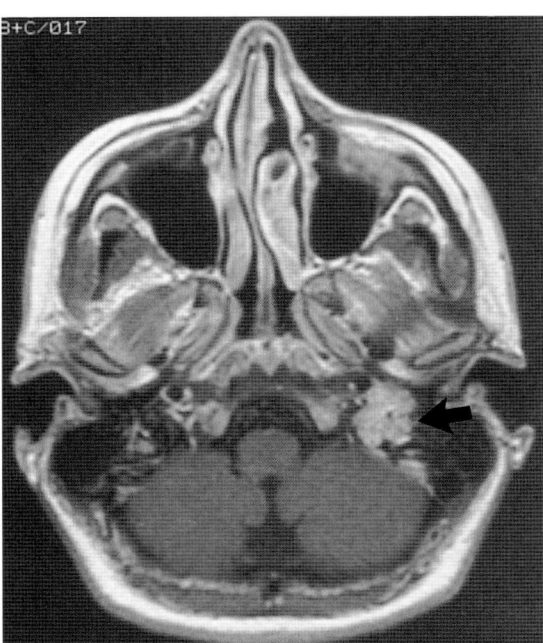

FIG. 1. Magnetic resonance image. *Arrow* indicates soft tissue mass in left jugular foramen area.

the late 1970s and was used with occasional angiography. The authors now depend on magnetic resonance imaging for diagnosis and operative planning (Fig. 1), with occasional computed tomography for bone definition (Fig. 2). Angiography is used if embolization is planned, or if the internal carotid artery is significantly involved (Fig. 3).

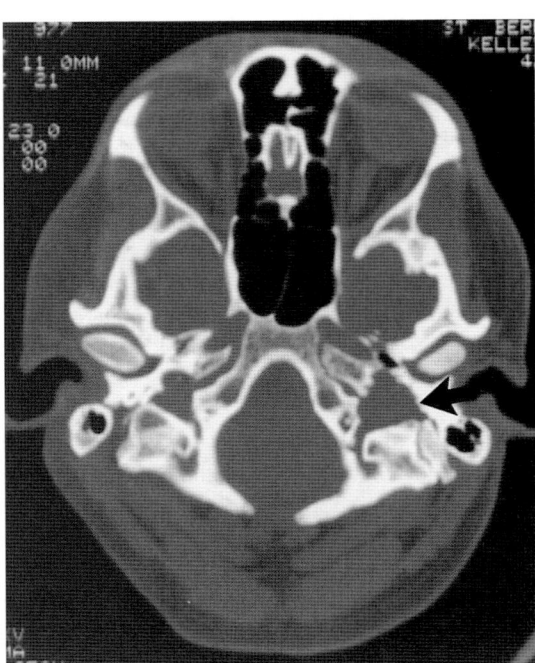

FIG. 2. Computed tomography scan. *Arrow* indicates bone defect in left jugular foramen area.

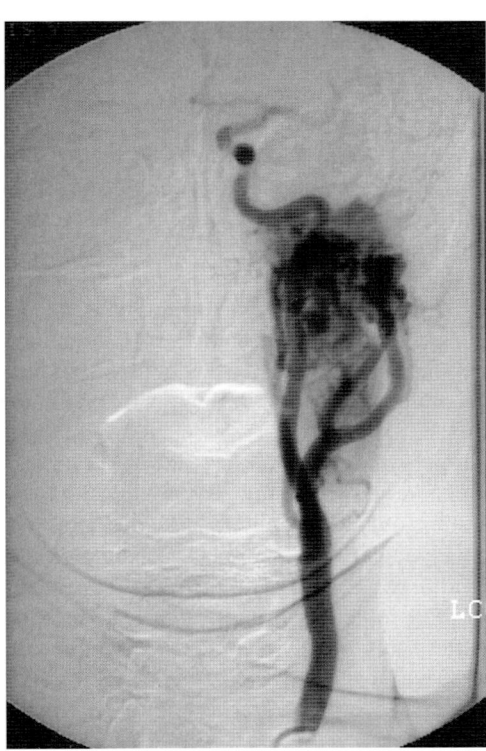

FIG. 3. External carotid arteriogram. Note vascular mass typical of glomus jugulare tumor.

PREOPERATIVE MEDICAL EVALUATION

Preoperative medical evaluation in patients with jugular foramen tumors is predicated on the high incidence of lower cranial nerve deficit before and after surgery in these patients. Emphasis is placed on preoperative evaluation of the upper gastrointestinal tract and lungs because of the high risk of postoperative aspiration secondary to injury to the vagus nerve, particularly in patients with preexisting disease, including hiatal hernia, gastroesophageal reflux, and chronic pulmonary disease. Early in this series, tracheostomy was performed prophylactically in such situations, but much less frequently now.

In older patients with large tumors, in whom blood pressure fluctuation would constitute a problem, a preoperative 24-hour urinary study for norepinephrine and serotonin secretion is performed to rule out a catecholamine-secreting tumor. The authors believe this study should be carried out regardless of whether the patient has a clinical history suggesting pheochromocytoma or carcinoid apudoma. Because medications and physical stress may invalidate test results, time must be allowed for performance of this test under suitable conditions to produce valid results. The alternative is to run the risk of tachycardia and hypertension due to release of norepinephrine by a pheochromocytoma, or hypotension due to the vasodilatory effects of a carcinoid apudoma, as a result of tumor manipulation.

Because of the possibility of significant blood loss, the authors have patients bank two or more units of autologous blood. Hemorrhagic disorders are screened for simultaneously, and treated before surgery. Aspirin is not allowed within 1 week of surgery.

Patients with essential hypertension, in the absence of renal contraindication, are given angiotensin-converting enzyme inhibitors before surgery, thus allowing perioperative and postoperative continuity of intravenous therapy with enalapril. When norepinephrine secretion is identified, α-adrenergic antagonist treatment for 7 to 10 days may control blood pressure elevation. Short–half-life β-adrenergic antagonist is added before and through surgery for control of arrhythmia.

After surgery, the authors emphasize elevation of the head of the patient's bed to prevent cerebrospinal fluid leakage and aspiration. When aspiration is so great a problem as to interfere with deglutition, and nutrition is impaired, a percutaneous endoscopic gastrostomy is placed, either before surgery if this problem is strongly anticipated, or, more frequently, after surgery when the problem occurs.

Preoperative antibiotic treatment is with cefazolin (a cephalosporin), 1 g given intravenously the night before surgery, the morning of surgery, and every 8 hours after surgery.

EMBOLIZATION AND RADIATION THERAPY

Early in this series, the authors treated patients with preoperative x-ray therapy in an effort to reduce vascularity at surgery. Currently, irradiation is used only as a primary mode of therapy for patients who are not surgical candidates because of advanced age or severity of health problems. Sixteen patients in this series have received preoperative radiation therapy.

The authors have used preoperative embolization since the 1970s. It has been particularly helpful with the advent of newer embolization techniques using microcoils and polyvinyl alcohol as the embolizing agents. The authors have noted a striking reduction in bleeding during surgery, and now use embolization on a virtually routine basis. Twelve of the patients in this series received preoperative embolization (Fig. 4).

The authors prefer to embolize those patients with glomus jugulare tumors before surgery. The procedure is performed 1 to 2 days before surgery, and is carried out using subselective arterial catheterization and angiography with a 3-Fr microcatheter to embolize the external carotid branches feeding the tumor. The embolizing material most commonly used is polyvinyl alcohol with or without platinum microcoils.

The most frequent problems associated with this procedure have been nausea with vomiting and facial pain, which have typically resolved within 12 to 18 hours after the procedure. There have been no instances of cerebral injury or cranial nerve dysfunction in this series.

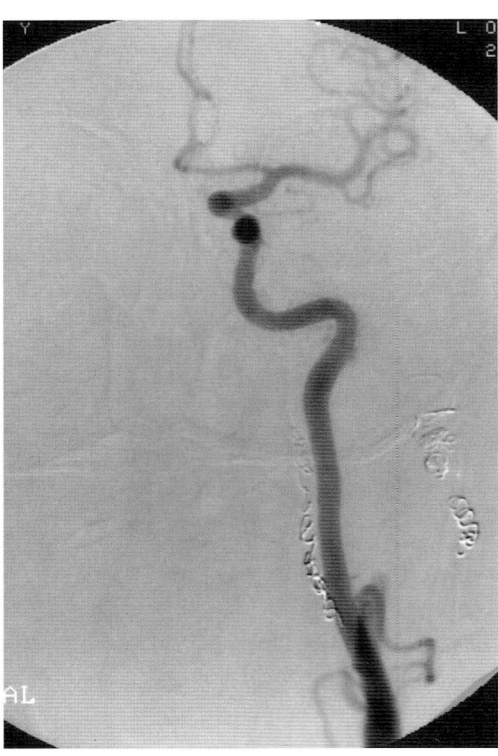

FIG. 4. External carotid arteriogram after embolization. Compare with Fig. 3 (same patient); note marked reduction in vascularity.

ANESTHESIA CONSIDERATIONS

Anesthesia should be carried out in anticipation of a prolonged surgical procedure with the possibility of sudden, dramatic blood loss or air aspiration in a patient subject to probable lower cranial nerve stimulation as well as epinephrine or serotonin secretion. In addition to basic anesthetic monitoring, an arterial line, Foley catheter, peripheral nerve stimulator, and central venous pressure line are placed. Because the jugular vein on one side, if not occluded by tumor, will be surgically divided, the authors use a peripheral vein for central venous pressure monitoring, with placement of a femoral introducer and passage of a Bungedin-Albin air aspiration catheter into the right atrium. A Zoll external pacemaker is also placed to address lower cranial nerve stimulation.

The patient is placed on an egg-crate–padded operating table, with thigh-length thromboembolic stockings and sequential compression boots placed on the lower extremities. Unless the patient is advanced in age or cachectic, an external warming device has not been used.

Anesthesia is induced and maintained by a combination of large doses of narcotic at the beginning of the procedure coupled with reduced inhalation agent and the inclusion of a continuous nonpolarizing muscle relaxant infusion. An ar-

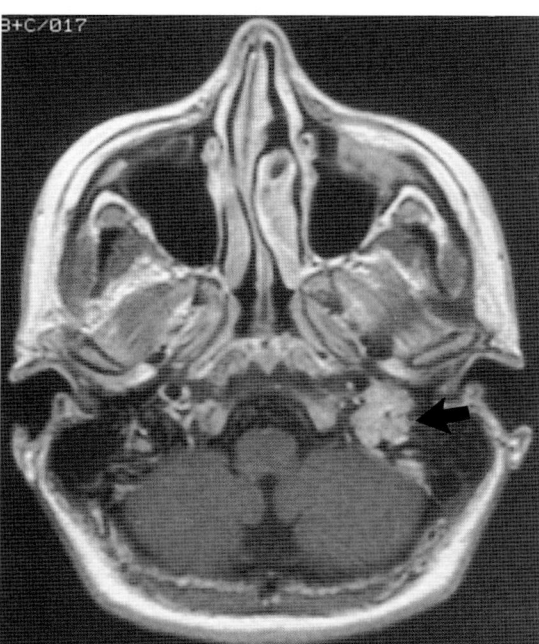

FIG. 1. Magnetic resonance image. *Arrow* indicates soft tissue mass in left jugular foramen area.

the late 1970s and was used with occasional angiography. The authors now depend on magnetic resonance imaging for diagnosis and operative planning (Fig. 1), with occasional computed tomography for bone definition (Fig. 2). Angiography is used if embolization is planned, or if the internal carotid artery is significantly involved (Fig. 3).

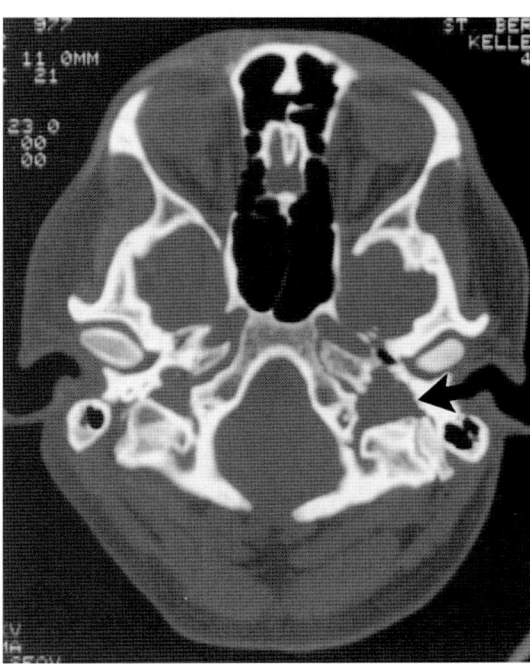

FIG. 2. Computed tomography scan. *Arrow* indicates bone defect in left jugular foramen area.

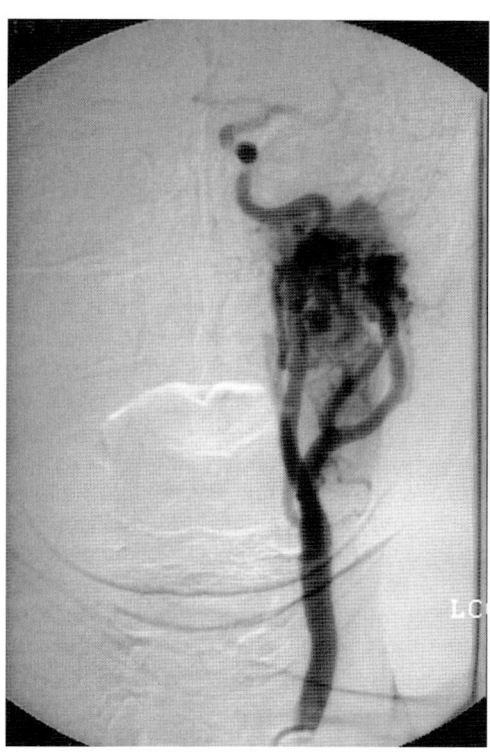

FIG. 3. External carotid arteriogram. Note vascular mass typical of glomus jugulare tumor.

PREOPERATIVE MEDICAL EVALUATION

Preoperative medical evaluation in patients with jugular foramen tumors is predicated on the high incidence of lower cranial nerve deficit before and after surgery in these patients. Emphasis is placed on preoperative evaluation of the upper gastrointestinal tract and lungs because of the high risk of postoperative aspiration secondary to injury to the vagus nerve, particularly in patients with preexisting disease, including hiatal hernia, gastroesophageal reflux, and chronic pulmonary disease. Early in this series, tracheostomy was performed prophylactically in such situations, but much less frequently now.

In older patients with large tumors, in whom blood pressure fluctuation would constitute a problem, a preoperative 24-hour urinary study for norepinephrine and serotonin secretion is performed to rule out a catecholamine-secreting tumor. The authors believe this study should be carried out regardless of whether the patient has a clinical history suggesting pheochromocytoma or carcinoid apudoma. Because medications and physical stress may invalidate test results, time must be allowed for performance of this test under suitable conditions to produce valid results. The alternative is to run the risk of tachycardia and hypertension due to release of norepinephrine by a pheochromocytoma, or hypotension due to the vasodilatory effects of a carcinoid apudoma, as a result of tumor manipulation.

Because of the possibility of significant blood loss, the authors have patients bank two or more units of autologous blood. Hemorrhagic disorders are screened for simultaneously, and treated before surgery. Aspirin is not allowed within 1 week of surgery.

Patients with essential hypertension, in the absence of renal contraindication, are given angiotensin-converting enzyme inhibitors before surgery, thus allowing perioperative and postoperative continuity of intravenous therapy with enalapril. When norepinephrine secretion is identified, α-adrenergic antagonist treatment for 7 to 10 days may control blood pressure elevation. Short–half-life β-adrenergic antagonist is added before and through surgery for control of arrhythmia.

After surgery, the authors emphasize elevation of the head of the patient's bed to prevent cerebrospinal fluid leakage and aspiration. When aspiration is so great a problem as to interfere with deglutition, and nutrition is impaired, a percutaneous endoscopic gastrostomy is placed, either before surgery if this problem is strongly anticipated, or, more frequently, after surgery when the problem occurs.

Preoperative antibiotic treatment is with cefazolin (a cephalosporin), 1 g given intravenously the night before surgery, the morning of surgery, and every 8 hours after surgery.

EMBOLIZATION AND RADIATION THERAPY

Early in this series, the authors treated patients with preoperative x-ray therapy in an effort to reduce vascularity at surgery. Currently, irradiation is used only as a primary mode of therapy for patients who are not surgical candidates because of advanced age or severity of health problems. Sixteen patients in this series have received preoperative radiation therapy.

The authors have used preoperative embolization since the 1970s. It has been particularly helpful with the advent of newer embolization techniques using microcoils and polyvinyl alcohol as the embolizing agents. The authors have noted a striking reduction in bleeding during surgery, and now use embolization on a virtually routine basis. Twelve of the patients in this series received preoperative embolization (Fig. 4).

The authors prefer to embolize those patients with glomus jugulare tumors before surgery. The procedure is performed 1 to 2 days before surgery, and is carried out using subselective arterial catheterization and angiography with a 3-Fr microcatheter to embolize the external carotid branches feeding the tumor. The embolizing material most commonly used is polyvinyl alcohol with or without platinum microcoils.

The most frequent problems associated with this procedure have been nausea with vomiting and facial pain, which have typically resolved within 12 to 18 hours after the procedure. There have been no instances of cerebral injury or cranial nerve dysfunction in this series.

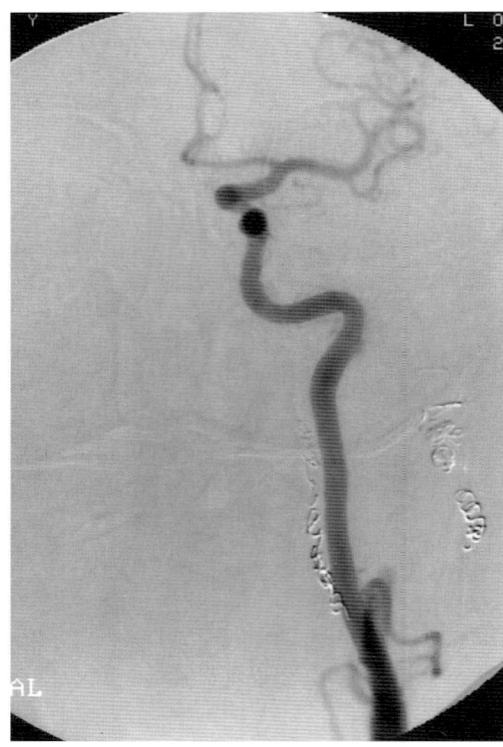

FIG. 4. External carotid arteriogram after embolization. Compare with Fig. 3 (same patient); note marked reduction in vascularity.

ANESTHESIA CONSIDERATIONS

Anesthesia should be carried out in anticipation of a prolonged surgical procedure with the possibility of sudden, dramatic blood loss or air aspiration in a patient subject to probable lower cranial nerve stimulation as well as epinephrine or serotonin secretion. In addition to basic anesthetic monitoring, an arterial line, Foley catheter, peripheral nerve stimulator, and central venous pressure line are placed. Because the jugular vein on one side, if not occluded by tumor, will be surgically divided, the authors use a peripheral vein for central venous pressure monitoring, with placement of a femoral introducer and passage of a Bungedin-Albin air aspiration catheter into the right atrium. A Zoll external pacemaker is also placed to address lower cranial nerve stimulation.

The patient is placed on an egg-crate–padded operating table, with thigh-length thromboembolic stockings and sequential compression boots placed on the lower extremities. Unless the patient is advanced in age or cachectic, an external warming device has not been used.

Anesthesia is induced and maintained by a combination of large doses of narcotic at the beginning of the procedure coupled with reduced inhalation agent and the inclusion of a continuous nonpolarizing muscle relaxant infusion. An armored endotracheal tube is placed in anticipation of frequent need for manipulation of the head.

The vasomotor effects of secreting tumors have been managed with β blockade and antihypertensive agents. Esmolol is the authors' agent of choice for the former, and intravenous nicardipine for the latter.

The goal is to have the patient as alert as possible at the end of the procedure to assess neurologic status promptly. β Blockade and antihypertensive treatment are continued into the postoperative period as indicated.

SURGICAL ANATOMY

An understanding of the neurovascular structures of the neck is important to the exposure of the jugular bulb. Inferior to the bulb, the lower cranial nerves are close to the facial and hypoglossal nerves, the internal jugular vein, and internal carotid artery. Successful dissection in this region is enhanced by recognition of several relatively constant anatomic relationships. The stylomastoid foramen through which the facial nerve exits the skull base is located posterolateral to the base of the styloid process. Cranial nerve IX occupies the medial aspect of the jugular foramen, extends into the neck, and passes lateral to the internal carotid artery. Cranial nerve XI exits the jugular foramen, first lying medial to the jugular vein, and then passing over the anterior surface of that structure before continuing inferiorly under the medial surface of the sternocleidomastoid muscle. Cranial nerve XII exits the hypoglossal canal, passes behind the vagus nerve, and then courses anteriorly toward the tongue. In summary, the nerves exiting the jugular foramen all travel medial to the jugular bulb. In the neck, cranial nerves VII, IX, and XII pass lateral to the internal carotid artery. Cranial nerve X courses in the groove between the jugular vein and the internal carotid artery. Cranial nerve XI crosses anterior to the jugular vein (occasionally posterior) on its way through the sternomastoid muscle, to the posterior triangle of the neck and the trapezius.

The jugular foramen, located in the posterolateral skull base, is bounded anterolaterally by the petrous portion of the temporal bone and posteromedially by the occipital bone. The two jugular foramina are not symmetric, the right side being larger in over two thirds of cases (14,15). This is believed to result from the asymmetry in the size of the transverse and sigmoid sinuses. The jugular foramen is divided into two segments by a fibrous septum, which is infrequently ossified, connecting the jugular process of the occipital bone with the jugular spine of the petrous bone. Di Chiro and colleagues (14) studied 129 dry skulls and noted a bony septum unilaterally in 13.2% of these, and bilaterally in 4.7%. The posterolateral segment, designated the pars venosa, is the larger of the two and contains the jugular bulb, cranial nerves X and XI, as well as the posterior meningeal artery. The anteromedial segment of the jugular foramen is smaller, is designated the pars nervosa, and contains cranial nerve IX and the several venous channels of the inferior petrosal sinus.

Although the exact anatomic location of cranial nerves IX, X, and XI as they traverse the jugular foramen may be variable, in essentially every case they pass medial to the jugular bulb. Cranial nerve IX travels alone, and is located medially and anteriorly to the cranial nerves X and XI, which are closely adherent. Cranial nerve IX exits the skull through a separate bony canal in 6% of cases (15).

The venous structure of the jugular foramen comprises the medial extension of the horizontal limb of the sigmoid sinus into the venous jugular bulb, which extends superiorly, and then inferiorly to pass into the neck as the internal jugular vein. The jugular bulb is housed in the bony jugular fossa, the superior portion of which separates the dome of the jugular bulb from the hypotympanum of the middle ear. The superior extent of the jugular bulb above the level of the horizontal segment of the sigmoid sinus varied between 0.25 and 0.75 in. in a study by Graham (16). The thickness of the bony covering over the dome of the jugular bulb depends on the size of the bulb, a small bulb having a relatively thick bony roof, whereas with a large bulb, the bone may be thin or even dehiscent, so that the venous wall of the bulb may occasionally reach the round window (16). The fallopian canal and contained facial nerve lie just lateral to the jugular bulb, and may be as close as 1 mm to the bulb.

The largest vessel to empty into the jugular bulb, with the exception of the sigmoid sinus, is the inferior petrosal sinus, which opens into the anterior aspect of the jugular bulb usually by multiple channels that pass through the fibrous septum between the pars nervosa and venosa. Occasionally, the vein of the cochlear aqueduct or a branch from the occipital sinus empties into the jugular bulb as well (16). These multiple channels constitute an expected source of bleeding during removal of the tumor and attached jugular bulb from the surrounding jugular fossa and enclosed cranial nerves. Controlled dissection of the tumor from the cranial nerves depends on management of these vascular channels.

SURGICAL TECHNIQUE

Skull Base Exposure

The patient is placed in supine position on the operating table with the head raised 30 degrees to reduce bleeding. The patient's head is placed at the "foot" end of the table in preparation for the otologic phase of the procedure to follow. The shoulders are slightly elevated with padding to improve visibility of the skull base. Hair is shaved from about the ear, neck, and chest to the nipple line. The surgical area is thoroughly cleansed and prepared with agents of the surgeon's choice.

Lidocaine 1% with epinephrine 1:100,000 is injected into the skin and subcutaneous tissues of the upper neck, mastoid, parotid gland, and facial nerve regions, to reduce bleeding during the skin incision and soft tissue phase of the procedure.

The surgical area is again prepared and covered with transparent and cloth drapes that are sutured in place. The abdomen is also prepared and draped in anticipation of harvesting adipose tissue for later wound closure.

Two suctions, a Malis cautery unit, and a Shaw cautery knife should be available during the initial phase of the procedure. The latter has been found to be useful in dissecting the structures of the neck, and particularly in dissecting the adjacent soft tissues from bone as well as from vital structures.

An oblique incision is made through the skin, subcutaneous tissues, and platysma of the upper neck. This incision is placed in an obvious skin crease and extends from the postauricular region almost to the hyoid bone below the level of the tail of the parotid gland. The superior skin flap is elevated, with the skin and subcutaneous tissues being elevated to the mastoid bone and from the parotid fascia to the region of the mandibular angle. A periosteal flap is elevated inferiorly and kept in continuity with the sternocleidomastoid muscle and later used in wound closure. The greater auricular nerve is identified for possible later use as a nerve graft.

The main trunk of the facial nerve is exposed by elevating the tail of the parotid gland from the lateral surface of the sternocleidomastoid muscle and detaching the gland from

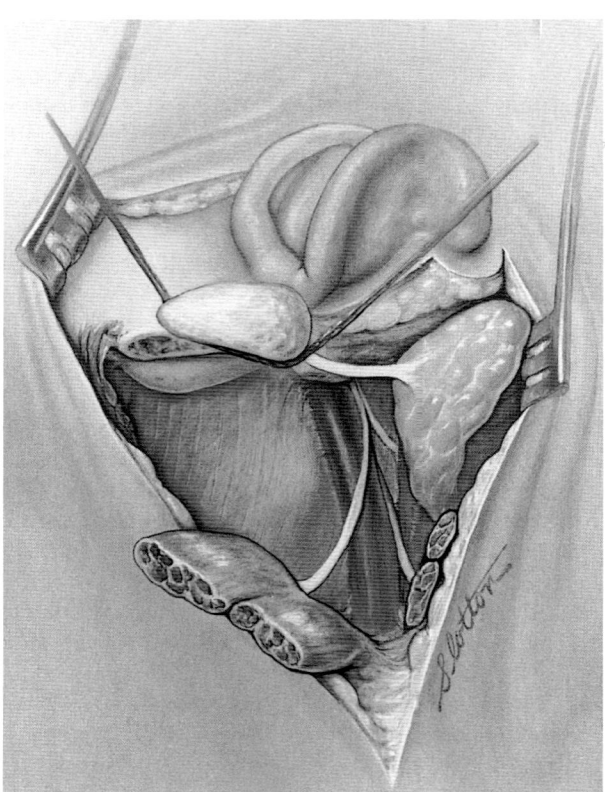

FIG. 6. Exposure of internal jugular vein. Note mastoid tip being resected with Gigli saw.

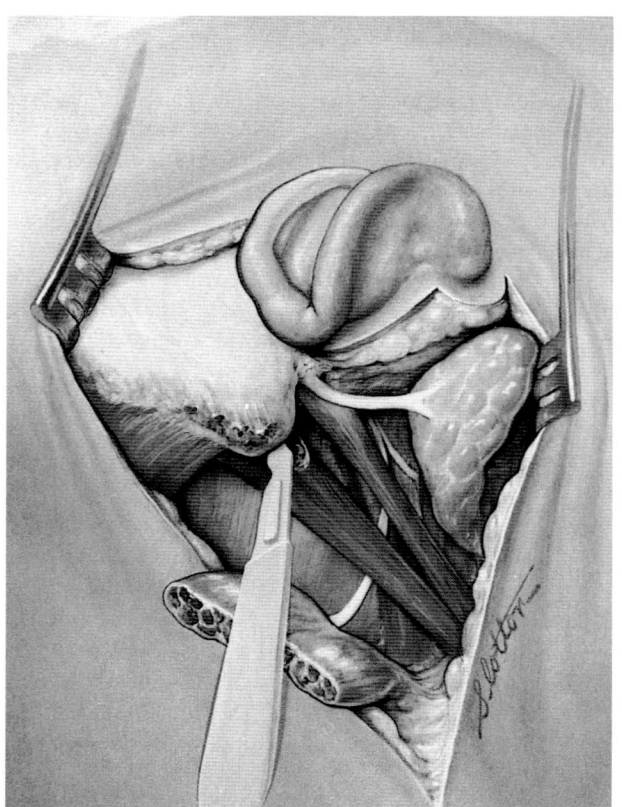

FIG. 5. Superficial dissection of skull base area. Note extensive dissection of facial nerve to its first genu. The authors no longer do this, but rather leave the nerve attached to adjacent soft tissue.

the cartilaginous canal of the external ear to the tympanomastoid fissure. The sternocleidomastoid muscle is partially detached from the mastoid bone as the parotid tail is retracted forward and the mastoid attachment of the posterior belly of the digastric muscle is exposed (Fig. 5).

The main trunk of the facial nerve is identified above and medial to the anterior superior attachment of this muscle to the mastoid bone, and deep to the tympanomastoid fissure. The facial nerve is no longer dissected to its first major division, but rather is left attached to the adjacent soft tissue, as advocated by Brackmann (17). The mastoid tip is removed with a Gigli saw after complete detachment of the sternocleidomastoid muscle and the posterior belly of the digastric muscle from it. Ligation of the occipital artery may be required (Fig. 6).

The styloid process is identified and its attached tendons resected. With the facial nerve and the internal jugular vein in clear view, the styloid process is resected from the skull base with a rongeur. This resection is carried out medial to the stylomastoid foramen and as close to the jugular foramen as possible. The tympanic bone may be removed at this point, or may be removed during the otologic phase to follow.

The neurovascular structures of the upper neck are mobilized as a unit and dissected superiorly to the carotid canal and jugular foreman. The tributaries of the internal jugular vein are mobilized and ligated. Ligation of the internal jugular vein in the neck is deferred until immediately before tumor removal.

The soft tissues of the base of the skull are resected to permit bony exposure of the posterior three fourths of the circumference of the jugular foreman (Fig. 7). The rectus capitis lateralis muscle and the atlantooccipital ligaments are detached from the jugular process of the occipital bone.

An elevator is used to separate the jugular vein from the posterior margin of the jugular foramen and partially from the neurovascular bundle anteriorly. This separation is completed at a later stage when the vein is excised. If the neck is short, the authors prefer to amputate the lateral process of the first cervical vertebra. Before this, the soft tissue on the lateral surface of the transverse process is divided, with care taken to avoid injury to the vertebral artery.

Temporal Bone Exposure

The otologic phase of this procedure is begun by first repositioning the patient and bringing in the microscope and other otologic equipment. For tumors that are 2 cm in diameter or smaller, the membranous ear canal is preserved. The neck incision is continued superiorly as a wide, C-shaped postauricular incision. The soft tissues are elevated and the

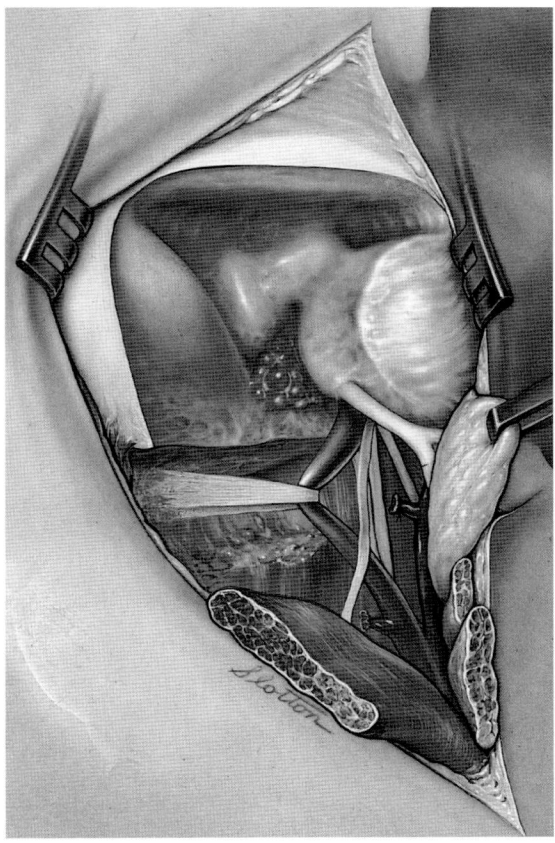

FIG. 8. Initial simple mastoid exposure. Note that membranous and bony ear canal are retained. The sigmoid sinus and mastoid segment of the facial nerve have been skeletonized. Horizontal and posterior semicircular canals are visible.

auricle turned forward. A high-speed electric drill is used to perform a simple mastoidectomy. The sigmoid sinus and mastoid segment of the facial nerve are skeletonized (Fig. 8).

For a tumor larger than 2 cm, the original neck incision would have been continued as a wide, C-shaped postauricular incision initially, with transection of the membranous ear canal at the bony cartilaginous junction, as shown in Fig. 9. Cartilage is excised from the membranous meatus and the meatus closed primarily in two layers.

A diamond bur is used to remove the remaining bone from over the upper two thirds of the sigmoid sinus and from over the mastoid and tympanic segments of the facial nerve (see Fig. 9). If the surgery is being performed for a glomus tumor, and if the tumor has extended posteriorly into the mastoid air cells, either superficial or deep to the facial nerve, great care may be required to differentiate the nerve from the glomus tissue, and to preserve the nerve. The authors are reluctant to sacrifice the facial nerve in this situation when dealing with a benign tumor.

For tumors larger than 2 cm in diameter, the posterior bony canal wall is now removed. The facial nerve is elevated from the fallopian canal, extending from the geniculate ganglion to the stylomastoid foramen, and then turned forward

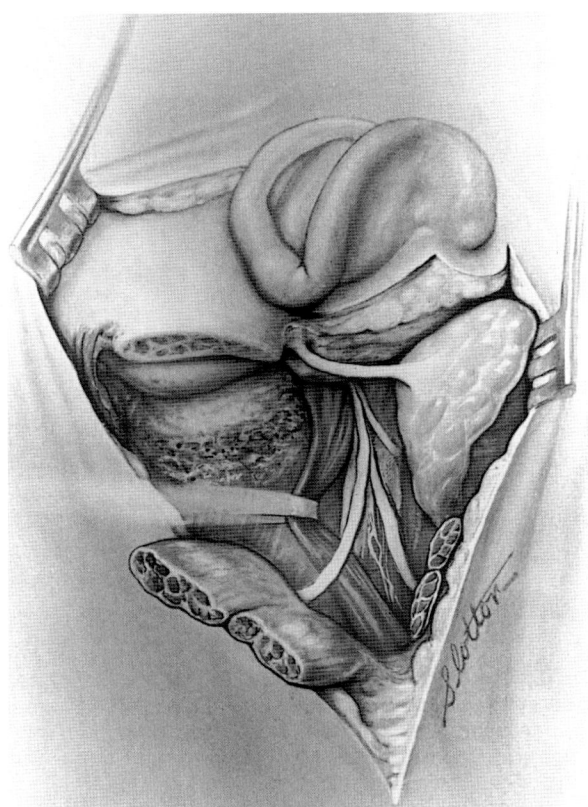

FIG. 7. Soft tissue exposure of skull base. Note that dissection extends to the margin of the jugular foramen.

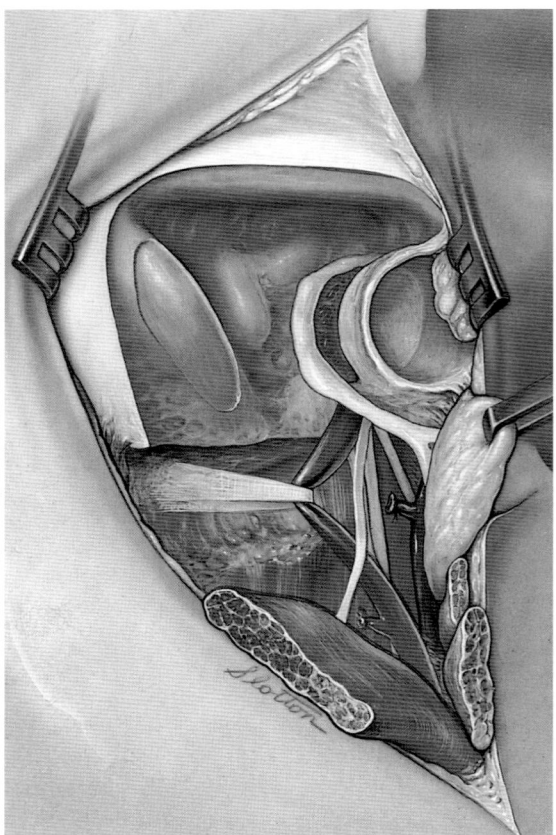

FIG. 9. Dissection for large tumor. Membranous ear canal is being transected and auricle turned forward. Bone has been removed from over the upper sigmoid sinus and from over the mastoid and tympanic segments of the facial nerve.

(Fig. 10). The skin of the external auditory canal is elevated to the level of the tympanic membrane, the middle ear entered, and the incudostapedial joint and tensor tympani tendon sectioned. The ear canal skin, tympanic membrane, malleus, and incus are removed.

For small tumors, the canal wall is preserved, as shown in Fig. 9. As Brackmann has recommended (17), large scissors are used to dissect the nerve and its adjacent soft tissue from the underlying bone. Only the mastoid segment of the facial nerve is mobilized, as Farrior has described (18).

Bone is now removed from the posterolateral skull base, including the base of the lateral aspect of the temporal bone and the jugular process of the occipital bone. Specific landmarks that are removed include the tympanic bone, digastric groove, stylomastoid foramen, posterolateral lip of the jugular foramen, and the lateral wall of the jugular fossa and hypotympanum. This bone removal exposes the soft tissue of the lower one third of the sigmoid sinus, jugular bulb, and tumor within the hypotympanum (see Fig. 10).

The orifice of the eustachian tube is identified, and its mucosal surface carefully denuded. Bone wax and small pieces of temporalis muscle tissue are used to occlude the eustachian tube. This completes the otologic phase of the tumor exposure, with the sigmoid sinus, jugular bulb, internal jugular vein, and associated tumor fully exposed through the base of the skull.

Tumor Removal and Reconstruction

The internal jugular vein is now ligated beyond any intraluminal tumor extension in the neck, passed beneath the spinal accessory nerve, and dissected to the jugular foramen as the neurovascular structures are retracted anteriorly (see Fig. 10). Two small incisions are made in the dura immediately anterior and posterior to the sigmoid sinus, well above any intraluminal tumor mass. Two silk sutures are carefully passed through one of these incisions, into the subarachnoid space medial to the sinus, and brought out through the second dural incision, and the sinus ligated (Fig. 11). The lateral wall of the sigmoid sinus is then resected inferiorly from the point of sinus ligation down to the tumor (Fig. 12).

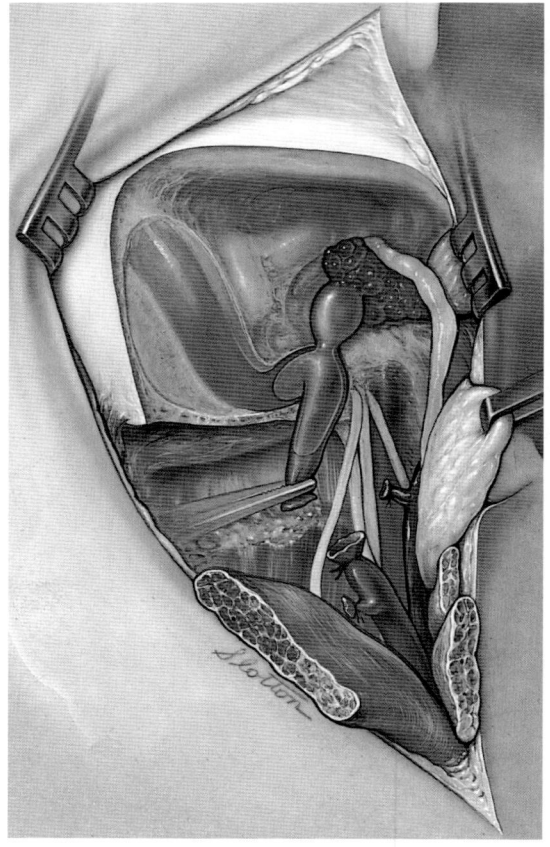

FIG. 10. Continued dissection for large tumor. Facial nerve has been elevated from fallopian canal and turned forward. Bone has been removed from the posterolateral skull base, exposing the lower sigmoid, jugular bulb, and tumor within the hypotympanum. Note that the internal jugular vein has been divided in the neck and dissected to the jugular foramen.

Typically, there is a preserved plane of dissection between the medial surface of the tumor and the lower cranial nerves. Working circumferentially in this plane, using sharp tissue dissection, the surgeon gently dissects the tumor mass free (Fig. 13). Care should be taken to avoid damage to the lower cranial nerves from excessive bipolar coagulation and overpacking with Surgicel. Often there is brisk venous bleeding at this point from the several entrances of the inferior petrosal sinus into the jugular bulb. This should be controlled by packing Surgicel into the venous openings of the sinus (Fig. 14). The tumor cavity is inspected, and any remaining tumor remnants are removed (Fig. 15). If tumor has extended into the posterior fossa, it is removed in continuity with the primary tumor mass in the skull base. If it is necessary to resect dura, a dural graft of pericranium or temporalis fascia is sutured in place.

As Fisch has described (13), a small diamond drill is used to create a groove in the anterior attic wall, and the proximal tympanic segment of the facial nerve is permanently placed within this groove (see Fig. 14) The authors perform this step of the procedure at the time of displacement of the nerve from the fallopian canal, thus protecting it from injury throughout the remainder of the procedure.

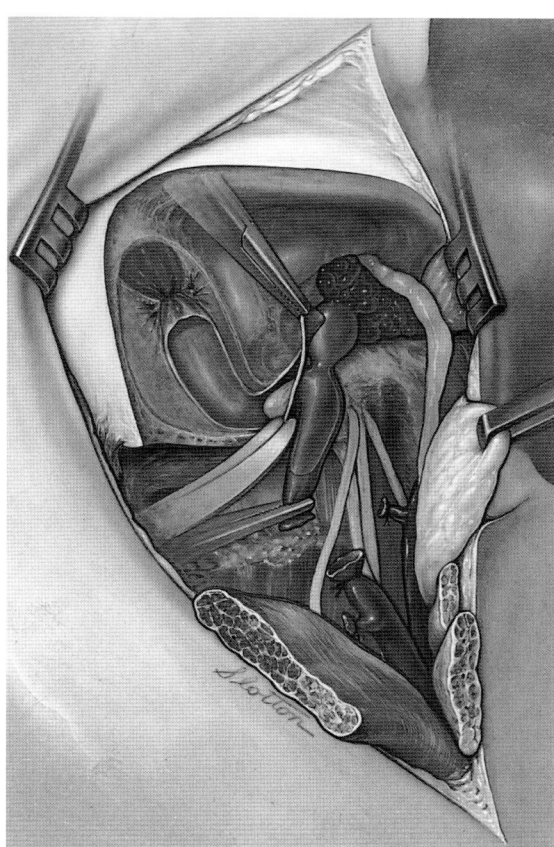

FIG. 12. Lateral wall of the sigmoid sinus is resected inferiorly to the level of the tumor.

If the tumor involves the carotid canal, bone over the lower aspect of the anterior wall of the mesotympanum adjacent to the eustachian tube orifice may be removed to allow exposure of this portion of tumor (see Fig. 15). This step may be performed after primary tumor removal, or may be carried out earlier in the procedure as bone is removed from the surface of the tumor.

The middle ear and mastoid are carefully inspected for residual tumor, which is removed separately, along with any remaining remnants of mucosa. When the posterior canal wall has been removed for a larger tumor, the mastoid and middle ear space is packed with fat and covered by downward rotation of the posterior temporalis muscle and upward mobilization of the previously prepared sternocleidomastoid musculoperiosteal flap. For smaller tumors with preservation of the canal wall, adipose tissue is placed only in the tumor bed, and the middle ear either left undisturbed or the ossicular chain and tympanic membrane reconstructed, depending on the extent of the tumor into the middle ear.

The skin edges are closed in layers, and a Hemovac drain placed into the subcutaneous plane. A spinal drain is placed at the end of the procedure if a dural graft was required, to avoid postoperative cerebrospinal fluid leakage.

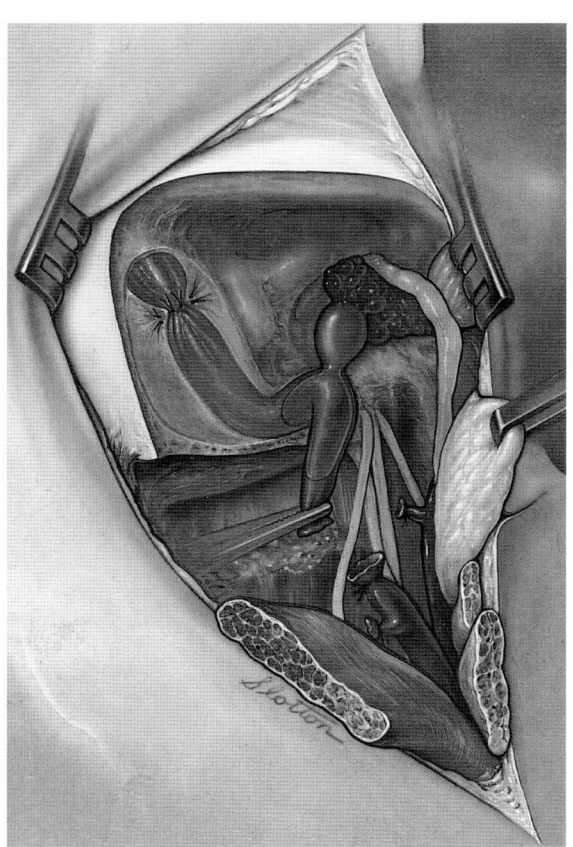

FIG. 11. Sigmoid sinus has been ligated. Note that dural openings anterior and posterior to the sinus are individually closed with sutures.

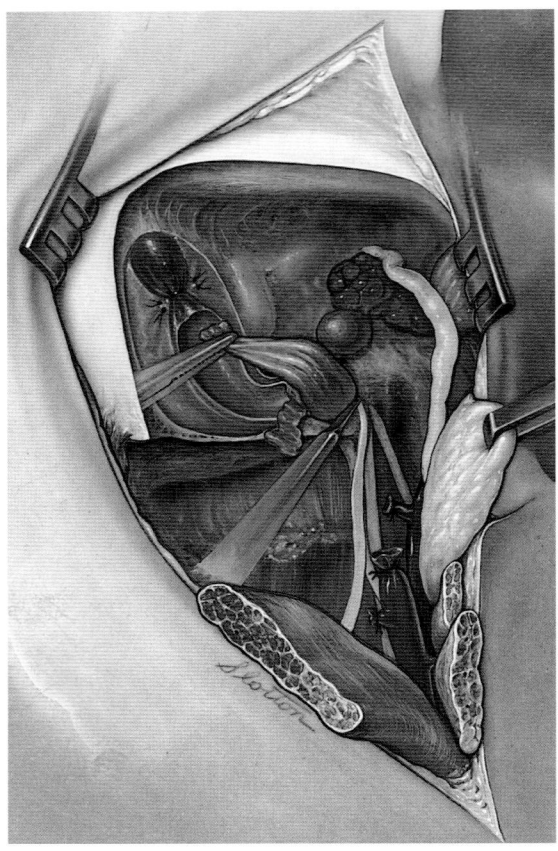

FIG. 13. Tumor dissection. Note use of sharp dissection of the jugular bulb and tumor, with lower cranial nerves in clear view.

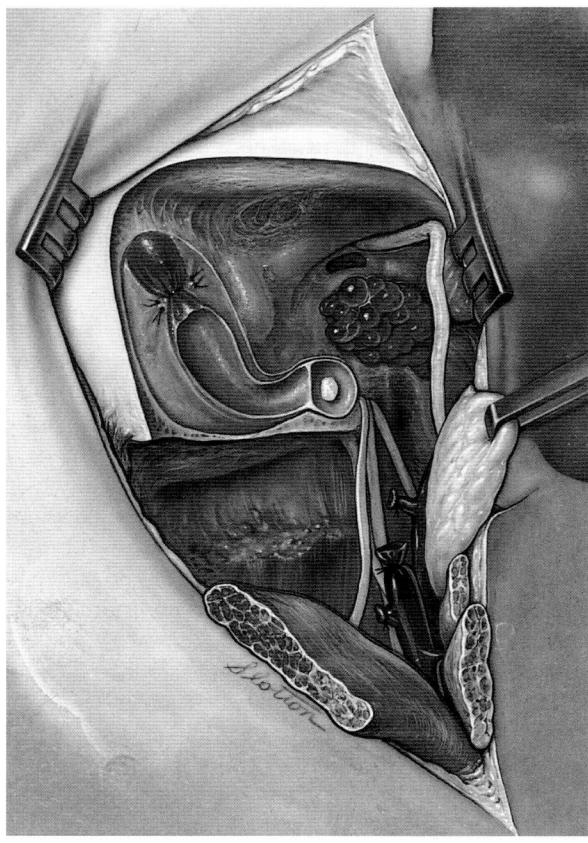

FIG. 14. Primary tumor mass has been removed. Surgicel has been packed into lumen of inferior petrosal sinus. Note groove in anterior attic wall for placement of facial nerve.

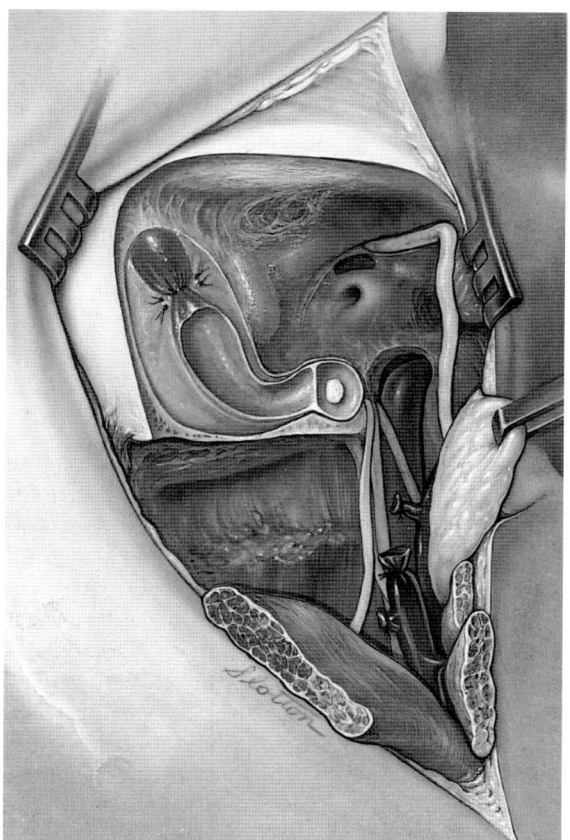

FIG. 15. Completed tumor removal. Facial nerve is permanently displaced anteriorly. Note removal of bone over vertical segment of internal carotid artery, inferior to eustachian tube orifice, when carotid canal is involved by tumor.

RESULTS AND COMPLICATIONS

The conditions requiring this surgery have been listed previously. Between September, 1972, and July, 1994, 46 patients underwent 47 primary skull base surgical procedures using variations of the approach described in this chapter. One of these patients had bilateral tumors and underwent bilateral surgery. Three additional patients also had bilateral skull base tumors, but underwent only unilateral surgery. Eight patients had multicentric tumors (Table 3). Forty-two

TABLE 4. Postoperative complications

Complication	No. of patients
Surgical death	1
Cerebrospinal fluid leak	8
Meningitis	3
Penumonitis	4
Wound problems	8
Eye problems	9
Sensorineural hearing loss	3
Abdominal wall hematoma	1
Seizure	1
Hemiparesis	2
Radiation chrondritis of auricle	1
Pulmonary embolus	3
Tumor recurrence	9
Aspiration problem	10
Ear canal stenosis	2
Septicemia	1
Cranial nerve dysfunction	
VI	4
VII	43
IX	16
X	29
XI	20
XII	20

Note: These complications occurred in 43 patients.

of the 46 patients are alive. Of the four deaths, three were for reasons unrelated to the skull base tumor or to the surgery, one because of pneumonitis and two of cardiovascular causes. The fourth patient died 2 weeks after surgery of a pulmonary embolus secondary to surgery.

Nine patients in this series experienced a total of 13 complications recognized during surgery, including damage to cranial nerves VII (six), IX (one), X (one), and XI (one); injury to the internal carotid artery (two); and displacement of the stapes (two). All postoperative complications are indicated in Table 4.

Of the 47 cases in the series, the facial nerve was anatomically intact after surgery in 38 (81%). In the remaining nine patients (19%), continuity of the facial nerve was lost, and was restored by either end-to-end reanastomosis or by use of a nerve graft. Facial nerve function at the time of the most recent postoperative examination is indicated in Table 5.

Eleven patients have undergone revision surgery (Table

TABLE 3. *Number of multicentric tumors*

Patient	Glomus jugulare	Glomus vagale	Carotid body	Neurofibroma	Meningioma
1	1	1	1		
2	2				
3	1		1		
4				4	1
5	1	1			
6	2	2	2		
7	1	1	1		
8	2	1	2		

TABLE 5. *Postoperative facial nerve function—house classification*

House class	No. of tumors
I	4
II	2
III	28
IV	3
V	0
VI	5
No follow-up	4
Postoperative death	1
Total	47

6). Four patients have received postoperative radiation therapy, and two received postoperative embolization therapy.

Of the 42 living patients in this series, 20 (48%) have been seen in follow-up within the past year; 14 (33%) have been seen within the last 2 to 5 years; 6 (14%) within the last 6 to 10 years; 1 (2%) 12 years ago; and 1 (2%) was never seen after surgery and has been lost to follow-up. Thus, 81% of the patients in this series have been seen in follow-up within the past 5 years (Table 7).

Twenty-six patients (having 27 tumors) were thought to have had total tumor removal at the time of initial surgery, and 20 patients (having 20 tumors) were considered to have had subtotal removals. Tumor recurrence has been diagnosed in 7 of the 26 patients (27%) thought to have undergone total tumor removal initially, with 4 undergoing secondary surgery for this reason. Of the 20 patients undergoing what was considered to be subtotal surgery initially, only 5 have had residual tumor on postoperative imaging studies, and 3 have undergone secondary surgery. Of the total series of 42 living patients, 32 are considered free of disease based on postoperative imaging studies, and 10 are being followed for residual disease.

Further analysis of the 20 patients undergoing what was thought to be subtotal surgery showed 18 to be living at the time of this study. Of these, 7 either had no follow-up imaging studies available or the studies were equivocal, leaving 11 living patients with definitive imaging results. Definite residual disease was shown in 5, but 6 of the original 20 were apparently free of disease. Two of these had received preoperative irradiation, and four had not.

TABLE 6. *Revision surgeries*

Reason for revision surgery	No. of patients	Surgical procedures
Recurrent disease	4	6
Cerebrospinal fluid leakage	3	3
Wound problem	2	5
Hearing problem	3	3
Total	11[a]	17

[a] One patient had two procedures.

DISCUSSION

In the early 1970s, the authors became interested in developing a better method of dealing with jugular foramen tumors in general, and glomus jugulare tumors in particular. The authors proceeded to develop the method described in this chapter, not realizing that many of the features incorporated in this method had been developed a number of years earlier, principally in Scandinavia and the United Kingdom. The authors have attempted to give credit to these efforts in an earlier section of this chapter.

Surgical Approach

It has seemed best to the authors to approach a jugular fossa tumor with surgery directed toward the primary tumor mass in the jugular fossa and foramen, rather than primarily from above through the mastoid. The authors believed that the latter approach would not allow as wide exposure of the primary tumor mass as was preferred. The concept rather was first to remove soft tissue widely over the bone of the skull base that covered the tumor; next, to remove this overlying bone to expose the tumor itself as widely as possible; and finally to remove the tumor. For non-glomus tumors of the jugular foramen that are less vascular, correspondingly less exposure may be required.

The authors have referred to this approach in several ways in the past, originally calling it a combined approach, and later a skull base approach, which they now think is now too generic a term. It is referred to here as a transcervicomastoid approach so as better to identify it as a direct approach through the neck, temporal bone, and skull base. Unless there is extensive involvement of the internal carotid artery, which is usually not the case, there is no necessity to remove the ramus of the mandible and enter the actual infratemporal fossa. The authors therefore do not believe that referring to this and similar approaches as infratemporal fossa approaches is appropriate.

Ancillary Forms of Treatment

Initially, the authors found bleeding to be a major problem in performing this operation for glomus jugulare tumors. For this reason, preoperative radiation therapy was initially used. When embolization became available in the late 1970s, and particularly when its improved methods became available in the 1980s, the authors abandoned preoperative radiation therapy.

In the process, however, x-ray therapy was used as a single mode of therapy for glomus jugulare tumors in older patients and in patients with significant health problems, and the authors have been greatly impressed with how well these patients have done. In fact, several younger, healthy patients were given radiation therapy, with planned surgery to fol-

TABLE 7. *Follow-up results*

Years operated	No. of patients	No. of patients/% seen within: 0–1 year	2–5 years	6–10 years	10–12 years	No follow-up
1972–1974	3	1	1	1	0	0
1975–1979	7	2	2	2	1	0
1980–1984	7	3	3	1	0	0
1985–1989	11	5	3	2	0	1
1990–1994	14	9	5	0	0	0
Total	42	20	14	6	1	1
Percent		48%	33%	14%	2%	2%

low. Radiation, however, became the only form of treatment when the patients refused the planned follow-up surgery. Although the authors do not advocate such treatment for younger patients, it is impressive how well these patients have done over time.

Conservation of Function

The authors have been aware of Glasscock and colleagues' (11) and Farrior's (18) advocacy of preservation of the posterior canal wall with limited mobilization of the facial nerve, to preserve the conductive mechanism and hearing in suitable cases. Until relatively recently, the authors have chosen to remove the posterior canal wall in all cases, to fully mobilize the facial nerve, and to close the ear canal at the meatus. More recently, the authors have pursued Glasscock's and Farrior's concept in treating several patients with smaller tumors, and have been gratified with the results. The authors recommend this approach for smaller tumors, and plan to continue its use.

The authors have referred earlier to Brackmann's method of preserving the soft tissue attachments to the facial nerve to preserve blood supply and facial nerve function. Since adopting this method, the authors have been gratified with the improved postoperative facial nerve function that has resulted, and plan to continue its use as well.

Complications

Early in the authors' series, several instances of postoperative cerebrospinal fluid leakage were encountered that were major problems to manage. Since beginning the use of temporalis muscle and periosteal flaps for closure of the tumor area, this has been a much less frequent and significant problem.

As the results demonstrate, postoperative facial nerve dysfunction has also been a major problem in this series, particularly immediately after surgery. The authors are hopeful that reduced dissection of the facial nerve distal to the stylomastoid foramen, as just discussed, will improve future results.

Recurrence of Tumor

The data indicate a 27% recurrence rate in those patients in whom what the authors believed to be gross total tumor removals were carried out. In the case of glomus tumors, the authors do not believe it is possible, except in rare circumstances, and with very small tumors, to accomplish total histologic tumor removal, even with the sacrifice of adjacent important neurovascular structures; nor do they believe it is justified to sacrifice these structures in glomus tumor surgery, in light of the natural history of these predominantly slow-growing tumors. For example, it would be preferable to treat recurrent disease later, rather than risk life-threatening complications initially by sacrificing the internal carotid artery. The authors suspect that as patients are followed for long periods of time after skull base surgery, particularly for glomus tumors, recurrence rates similar to the one reported here will not be unusual. For this reason, the authors believe that patients who have undergone skull base removal for glomus jugulare tumors should be followed indefinitely. For other tumor types, such as neuromas, long-term follow-up may not be such a critical factor.

Surgical Technique

Early in this series of cases, the surgery was staged because of the duration of the procedure. As the surgical team's experience increased, this became unnecessary, and it is no longer done.

When this procedure was first developed, the authors used a Fogarty catheter to occlude the superior end of the sigmoid sinus while the sinus was divided and then closed. The authors no longer manage the sigmoid sinus in this way, but rather pass two suture ligatures medial to the sinus, and divide the sinus between the ligatures, as Fisch described in his first report (13).

Occasionally in dealing with glomus jugulare tumors, the tumor extends intravascularly either inferiorly down the internal jugular vein or superiorly up the sigmoid and perhaps even into the lateral sinus. Obviously, this must be taken into account and the dissection extended sufficiently to allow complete resection of the intravascular component of the tumor. The authors have not seen this feature with other types of skull base tumors.

Intracranial extension of skull base tumors has not been a significant problem in this series. The authors believe that the wide exposure achieved with this approach, and the participation of a neurosurgeon on the operative team, have allowed intracranial extension to be dealt with in a relatively routine manner.

These data demonstrate a relatively high incidence of immediate postoperative dysfunction of cranial nerves IX through XII, reflecting the fact that tumors of the jugular foramen, particularly glomus tumors, are densely adherent to these nerves. During the authors' early experience, long-term lower cranial nerve dysfunction was a major problem. Because of this, since the early 1980s the authors have made an effort to apply microdissection techniques to separate the tumor from the cranial nerves in the jugular foramen area. The authors believe that this, along with the markedly reduced bleeding seen with more recent embolization techniques, has improved the long-term results in this regard.

If a patient has lost vagus nerve function as a result of preoperative tumor growth, compensation will have usually occurred before surgery, and these cases are less critical in terms of the necessity to preserve nerve structure. The availability of the percutaneous endoscopic gastrostomy technique during the latter part of this study has been a major benefit in dealing with those situations in which it is necessary to sacrifice a functional vagus nerve, and has virtually eliminated the need for tracheostomy.

The authors have no enthusiasm for sacrificing the internal carotid artery for what are generally benign tumors of the skull base, and have rarely done so. Instances in which this artery has been significantly involved by tumor have been quite infrequent in this series. When such is the case, however, an infratemporal fossa approach for exposure has been used, with an attempt to preserve the artery. When preoperative studies indicate significant involvement of the artery by tumor, the authors perform preoperative balloon occlusion studies, and ligate and resect the artery only if feasible and absolutely necessary. The authors have had no experience in repair of the internal carotid artery by grafting.

CONCLUSIONS

During the 25 years that the authors have been engaged in the management of skull base tumors using this approach, they have been gratified by the technical advances that have become available. There is no doubt that further advances will be made. The authors suspect that these will include intravascular interventional methods, which could conceivably make surgery as we know it unnecessary. In the meantime, conventional methods of tumor removal will continue to be used, and will be benefited by adequate surgical exposure. The authors believe that the TCM approach fulfills the requirements for dealing with tumors in this relatively inaccessible area, and recommend its use in appropriate cases.

ACKNOWLEDGMENT

The surgical illustrations were prepared by Daniel Slotton (Los Angeles, CA) at the time of the authors' original report on this work in 1977 (12). Several of the illustrations have been revised by Mr. Slotton for this publication to reflect modifications that have been made in the procedure since its original description.

REFERENCES

1. Guild SR. A hitherto unrecognized structure, the glomus jugularis, in man. *Anat Rec* 1941;79[Suppl 2]:28.
2. Rosenwasser H. Carotid body tumor of the middle ear and mastoid. *Archives of Otolaryngology* 1945;41:64–67.
3. Lundgren N. Tympanic body tumors in the middle ear: tumors of carotid body type. *Acta Otolaryngol (Stockh)* 1949;37:366–379.
4. Weille FL, Lane CS Jr. Surgical problems involved in the removal of glomus-jugulare tumors. *Laryngoscope* 1951;61:448–459.
5. Capps FCW. Glomus jugulare tumors of the middle ear. *J Laryngol Otol* 1952;66:302–314.
6. Gastpar H. Die Tumoren des Glomus Caroticum, Glomus Jugulare-Tympanicum und Glomus Vagale. *Acta Otolaryngol* 1961;[Suppl 167].
7. Shapiro MJ, Neus DK. Technique for removal of glomus jugulare tumors. *Archives of Otolaryngology* 1964;79:219–224.
8. Gejrot T. Surgical treatment of glomus jugulare tumors: with special reference to the diagnostic value of retrograde jugularography. *Acta Otolaryngol* 1965;60:150–168.
9. House W. Panel discussion (McCabe BF, moderator): Rosenwasser H, House W, Witten RM, Hamberger C-A. Management of glomus tumors. *Archives of Otolaryngology* 1969;89:170–178.
10. Portmann M. In: Hamberger C-A, Wersall J, eds. *Disorders of the skull base region.* New York: John Wiley & Sons, 1969:297–298.
11. Glasscock ME, Harris PF, Newsome G. Glomus tumors: diagnosis and treatment. *Laryngoscope* 1974;84:2006–2032.
12. Gardner G, Cocke EW, Robertson JT, Trumbull ML, Palmer RE. Combined approach surgery for removal of glomus jugulare tumors. *Laryngoscope* 1977;87:665–688.
13. Fisch U. Infratemporal fossa approach for extensive tumors of the temporal bone and base of the skull. In: Silverstein H, Norrell H, eds. *Neurological surgery of the ear.* Birmingham, AL: Aesculapius Publishing Co., 1977:34–53.
14. Di Chiro G, Fisher RL, Nelson KB. The jugular foramen. *J Neurosurg* 1964;21:447.
15. Rhoton AL, Buza R. Microsurgical anatomy of the jugular foramen. *J Neurosurg* 1975;42:541–550.
16. Graham MD. The jugular bulb: its anatomic and clinical considerations in contemporary otology. *Archives of Otolaryngology* 1975;101:560–564.
17. Brackmann DE. The facial nerve in the infratemporal fossa. *Otolaryngol Head Neck Surg* 1987;97:15–17.
18. Farrior JB. Infratemporal approach to skull base for glomus tumors: anatomic considerations. *Ann Otol Rhinol Laryngol* 1984;93:616–622.

CHAPTER 22

Petroclival Approach

Madjid Samii and Marcos Tatagiba

The petroclival region is a complex area situated at the junction of the adjacent parts of the sphenoid, temporal, and occipital bones. There has been much discussion about the best way to approach this region, which reflects the difficult challenge this region represents. Different ways have been described in the past, and new approaches have arisen in concert with the modern skull base philosophy.

A number of lesions may originate in the petroclival region, including meningiomas, schwannomas, chordomas, chondrosarcomas, carcinomas, aneurysms, and others (1–4). Before the microsurgical era, tumors involving the petroclival region were considered inoperable (5,6). High surgical mortality and morbidity characterized these lesions, mainly related to large tumor size and involvement of important neurovascular structures (7).

Developments in neuroradiology, skull base approaches, and intensive care have led to a breakthrough in the management of the petroclival lesions. Increasing experience with these lesions has resulted in much information about patient selection for surgery, surgical strategies, and postoperative management.

Different approaches exist to access the petroclival region (8–19). The most important include the transpetrosal retrolabyrinthine (presigmoid), translabyrinthine, and transcochlear approaches, the suboccipital retrosigmoid approach, the subtemporal approach, the combined subtemporal–retrosigmoid approach, the combined subtemporal–presigmoid approach, the middle fossa (anterior transpetrosal) approach, and the preauricular infratemporal approach.

Most of these approaches have been described in other chapters of this text. In this chapter, the authors present a detailed description of the combined subtemporal–presigmoid approach and brief descriptions of the retrosigmoid and the middle fossa approaches to the petroclival region.

M. Samii, M. Tatagiba: Department of Neurosurgery, Hannover Medical School, 30625 Hannover, Germany.

PATIENT SELECTION AND SURGICAL CONCEPT

Petroclival tumors may become very large and extend into the middle cranial fossa, cavernous sinus, tentorial incisura, cerebellopontine angle, internal auditory canal, jugular foramen, foramen magnum, and extracranial spaces (Fig. 1). Using appropriate skull base approaches, a number of these lesions can be totally resected. These lesions still represent a surgical challenge, however. Increasing experience has demonstrated that the indications for surgery may be limited in some patients who do not tolerate an extensive tumor resection.

The most important factors with an impact on surgical resection are the nature and extension of the lesion, involvement of the cavernous sinus and vertebrobasilar system, and the patient's age and condition. Accurate clinical and radiologic investigations are essential to select the patients who can profit from the surgery.

On the basis of the preoperative clinical and radiologic data, the surgical plan is drawn. The strategy, however, may vary according to intraoperative findings. During the surgical procedure, tumor resection largely depends on tumor biology and the interface between tumor and normal tissue.

Despite all advances in neuroradiology, no preoperative tests can depict the tumor consistency exactly, the closeness of the tumor–nerve relation, or involvement of the arachnoid and pial sheaths. Therefore, in deciding whether to perform a radical or partial tumor resection, the surgeon must rely on his or her previous experience with similar cases, and consider both the tumor-intrinsic factors and the patient's expectations.

It is the authors' belief that all attempts should be made at radical resection of these lesions. However, if the tumor shows an infiltrative growth pattern and major neurovascular structures are involved without clinical deficits, the authors prefer a subtotal resection, and not to risk major functions or even the patient's life.

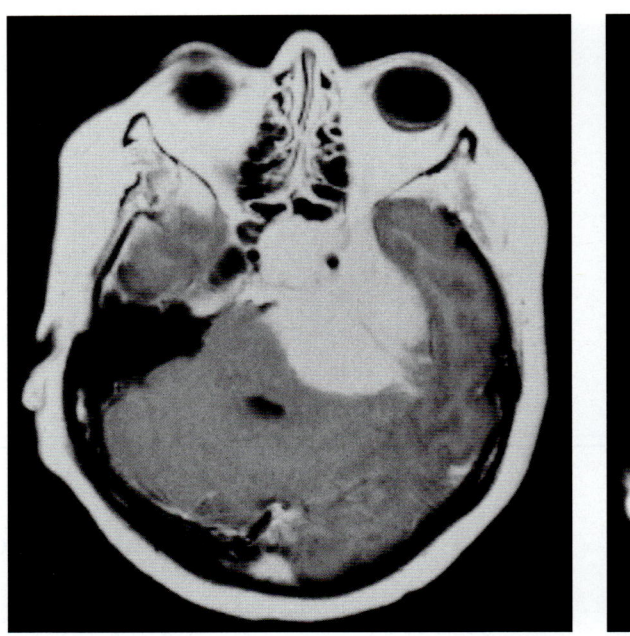
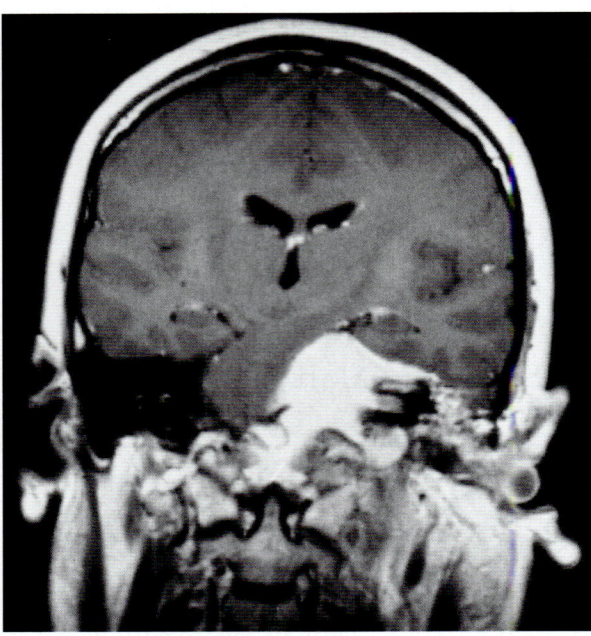

FIG. 1. A: Axial gadolinium-enhanced magnetic resonance image (MRI) of a petroclival meningioma showing extension into the posterior and middle fossae, the cavernous sinus, and extracranial spaces. **B:** Coronal MRI showing craniocaudal tumor extension and extension into the internal auditory canal and the jugular foramen.

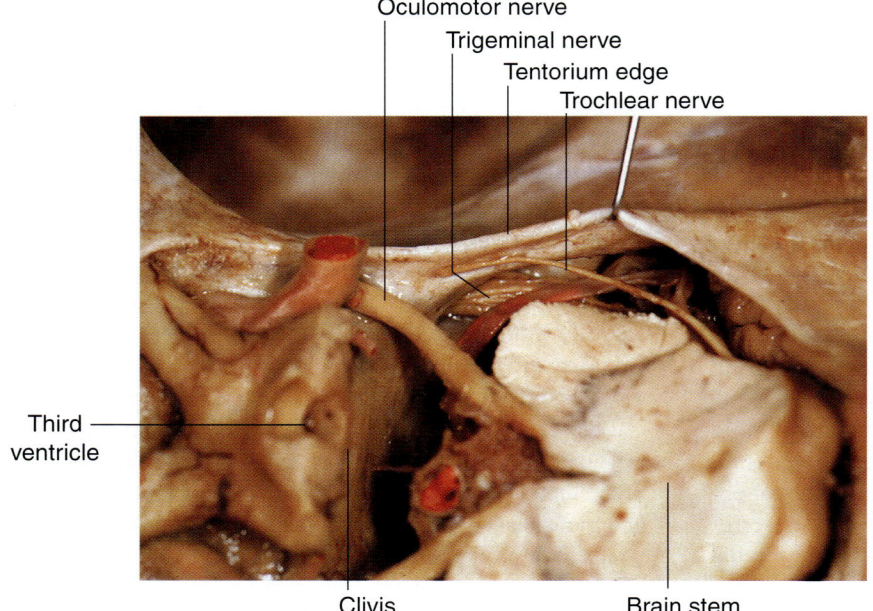

FIG. 2. Cadaver dissection showing the petroclival region from a medial view. The petroclival region is a complex area containing important neurovascular structures, situated at the junction of the clival and petrous bones.

SURGICAL ANATOMY OF THE PETROCLIVAL REGION

The petroclival region is the area situated between the middle and posterior skull base at the junction of the adjacent parts of the sphenoid, temporal, and occipital bones (Fig. 2).

The *extradural* structures related to the petroclival region that affect the surgical approaches are basically the temporal bone and its petrosal structures. The *intradural* structures related to the petroclival region can be divided into three spaces (17): the inferior petroclival space, consisting of the lower clivus and foramen magnum; the middle petroclival space, which comprises the cerebellopontine angle and prepontine area; and the superior petroclival space, which corresponds to the anterior part of tentorial incisura, the sella and parasellar regions, and the floor of the third ventricle.

The petrous bone is the key extradural structure of the petroclival region. Differing from classic descriptive anatomy, the surgical anatomic scheme divides the petrous bone into anterior and posterior portions, according to the major available transpetrosal approaches (20,21).

Anterior Portion of the Petrous Bone

Major anatomic structures of the anterior portion of the petrous bone include the foramen spinosum with the middle meningeal artery anteriorly; the arcuate eminence posteriorly; the petrous carotid artery, which is mostly only partially covered by a thin bone layer; and the superior petrosal sinus, which runs along the medial border of the upper surface of the petrous bone.

The greater petrosal nerve passes below the lateral margin of the trigeminal ganglion. Drilling along the course of the greater petrosal nerve in a dorsal direction exposes the geniculate ganglion, which can be followed in a medial direction to expose the labyrinthine portion of the facial nerve through its course into the internal auditory canal (Fig. 3).

Opening the internal auditory canal and the dura surrounding the contents of the internal auditory canal exposes the intracanalicular portions of the facial and superior vestibular nerves superiorly, and the cochlear and inferior vestibular nerves inferiorly. The superior vestibular and the facial nerves are separated at the fundus of the internal auditory canal by the vertical crest (the so-called "Bill's bar"). The facial and cochlear nerves are in the anterior half, and the superior and inferior vestibular nerves are in the posterior half of the canal. The cochlea lies between the internal auditory canal and the petrous carotid artery, beneath the geniculate ganglion. The labyrinth with the vestibule and the superior semicircular canal lie close posterior to the fundus of the internal auditory canal. The length of the internal auditory canal varies from 8 to 12 mm (average, 10 mm). The average distance between the posterior semicircular canal and the edge of the canal is 7 mm (17).

The bony area between the greater petrosal nerve anteriorly, the carotid artery and the cochlea laterally, and the internal auditory canal and the semicircular canals posteriorly,

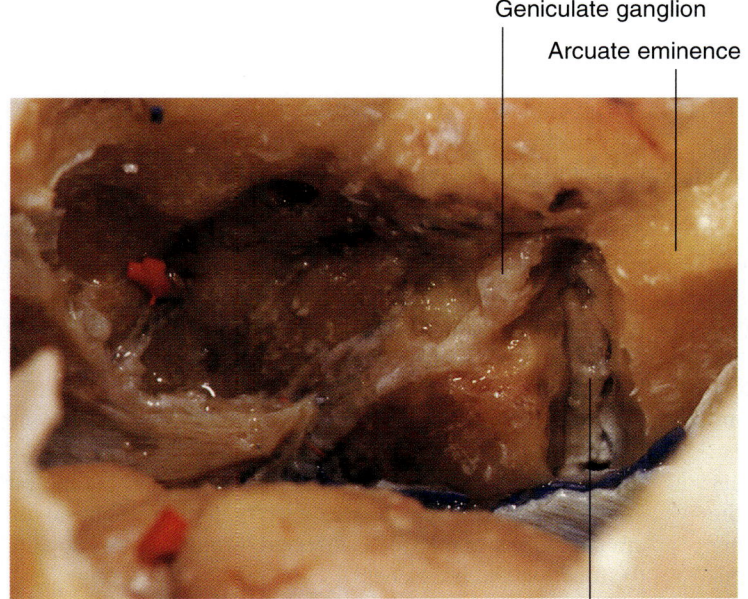

FIG. 3. Cadaver dissection showing the surgical anatomy of the anterior petrous bone. The bone covering the greater superficial petrosal nerve was drilled away, and the nerve followed to the fundus of the internal auditory canal.

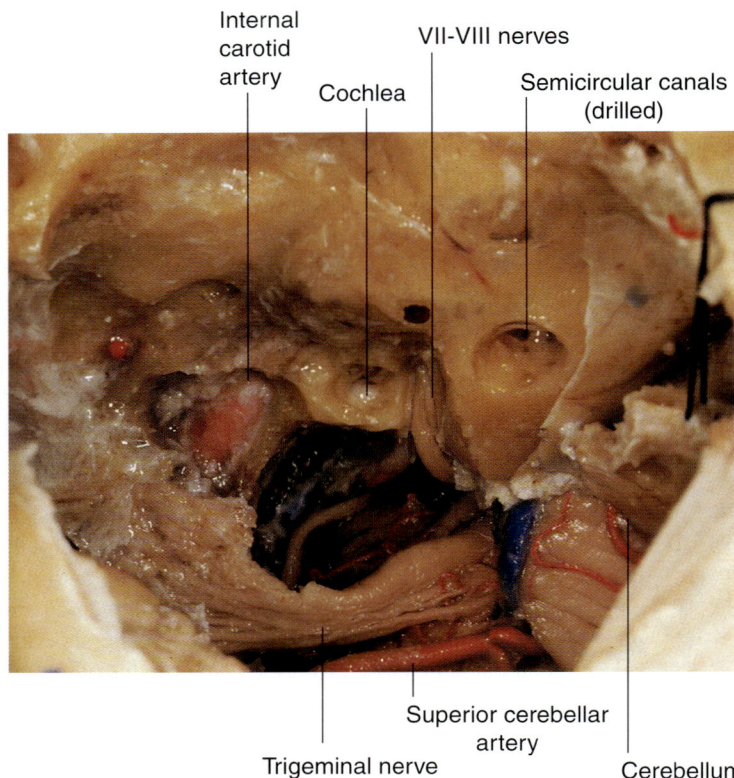

FIG. 4. Cadaver dissection of the anterior petrous bone after drilling the bone between the internal carotid artery and the internal auditory canal, which exposes the cerebellopontine angle structures.

has been called Kawase's triangle. Bone removal at that area exposes the posterior fossa and cerebellopontine angle from above (Fig. 4).

Posterior Portion of the Petrous Bone

The posterior approaches to the petrous bone involve bone removal behind the sigmoid sinus in the retrosigmoid approach, and between the wall of the external auditory canal and the sigmoid sinus in the presigmoid approach.

Decortication of the mastoid and removal of most mastoid air cells exposes the middle fossa plate and the superior petrosal sinus superiorly, the anterior portion of the sigmoid sinus posteriorly, and the plate covering the labyrinth block and facial nerve anteriorly (Fig. 5).

The otic capsule consists of the vestibule, the semicircular canals, and the cochlea. The lateral semicircular canal runs perpendicular to the facial nerve, and the posterior semicircular canal runs parallel to the sigmoid sinus. Lateral to the otic capsule lies the antrum, and inferior to it, the digastric ridge.

The vestibule is separated from the apex of the jugular bulb by an approximately 6-mm bone. The height of the jugular bulb may vary considerably, sometimes reaching the internal auditory canal. Penetration of a high-lying jugular bulb may be the source of severe bleeding or air embolism during surgery. Preoperative identification and careful intraoperative dissection are essential to control this problem (22).

The vertical segment of the carotid artery runs upward in the carotid canal, then curves anteromedially to form the horizontal segment.

CLINICAL ASPECTS

The clinical picture in petroclival lesions is primarily related to the origin and major extension of the lesion (23). Chordomas and chondrosarcomas usually cause diplopia because of cranial nerve VI involvement, whereas meningiomas, trigeminal schwannomas, and epidermoid cysts more frequently produce trigeminal symptoms and hearing problems (2,24,25).

From a topographic point of view, petroclival lesions can be divided into three main types in relation to the middle and posterior fossae.

The first group presents with a major extension into the posterior fossa and cerebellopontine angle. These tumors are more likely to produce hearing loss, tinnitus, cerebellar signs, and facial weakness as early symptoms. The lower cranial nerves may also be affected, producing swallowing dysfunction and hoarseness.

The second group of petroclival tumors presents with major extension into the middle fossa and usually involves the cav-

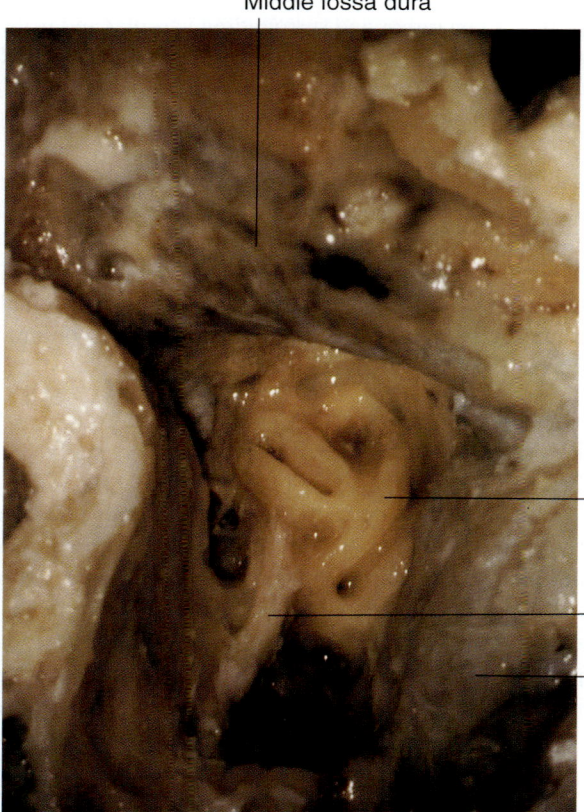

FIG. 5. Cadaver dissection of the posterior petrous bone after drilling away the mastoid to expose the sigmoid sinus, the middle fossa dura, the semicircular canals, and the facial nerve in the fallopian canal.

ernous sinus. These tumors frequently cause trigeminal symptoms (pain or hypesthesia) and diplopia at first presentation.

Finally, large tumors extending both into the middle and the posterior fossae constitute the third group of petroclival lesions. They may affect cranial nerves II through XII, but the most common symptoms are hearing loss and trigeminal problems. In a series of 36 patients with large petroclival meningiomas, 75% of the patients presented with hearing loss, and half of them had trigeminal symptoms (1).

Headache is common to them all.

RADIOLOGY

Computed tomography (CT) and magnetic resonance imaging (MRI) are complementary diagnostic tools in skull base surgery. High-resolution CT with soft tissue and bone algorithms provides indispensable demonstration of bony landmarks of the petrous bone and clivus (Fig. 6). Spiral CT technology allows for three-dimensional representation of the tumor, the intracerebral vessels, and bone structures. When planning the surgical approach, the three-dimensional imaging of spiral CT adds significant spatial information to that obtained by MRI and conventional CT (Fig. 7).

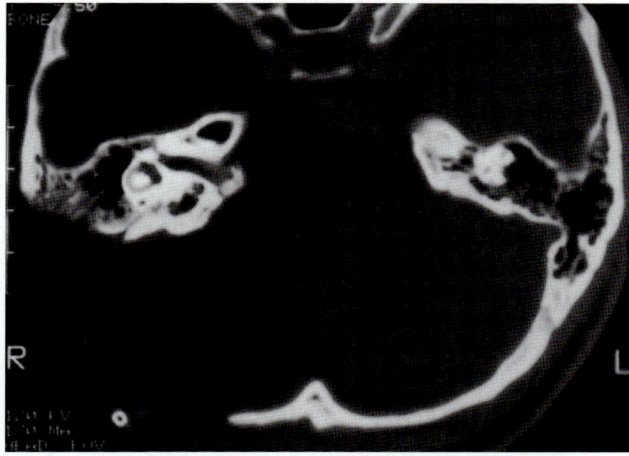

FIG. 6. Axial postoperative computed tomography scan with bone algorithms through the petrous bone. This technique well demonstrates the amount of bone removal and the preserved inner ear structures.

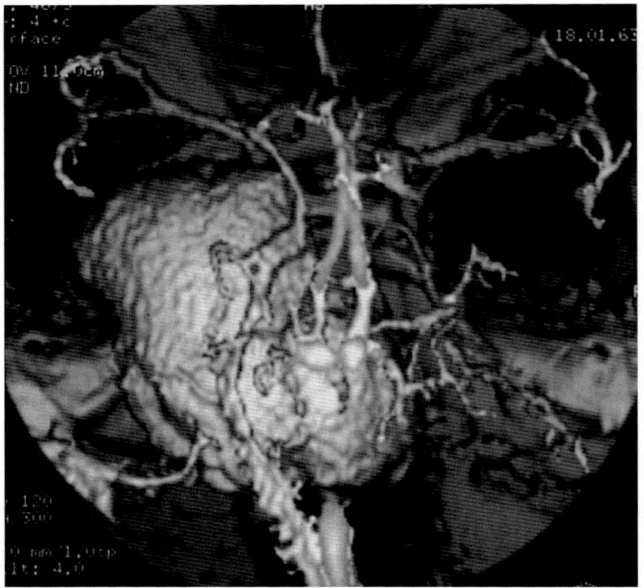

FIG. 7. Spiral three-dimensional computed tomography scan of a trigeminal schwannoma involving the petroclival region. This technique provides excellent spatial information about the tumor's relation to the skull base and surrounding vessels.

Magnetic resonance imaging demonstrates the relationship between tumor and surrounding vascular and neural tissues (Fig. 8). Magnetic resonance angiography depicts the involvement of major arterial and venous vessels, making cerebral angiography obsolete in individual cases (Fig. 9). Cerebral angiography demonstrates tumor vascularization and the displacement and involvement of important vessels, and provides the necessary information for preoperative embolization.

Once radiologic investigations have depicted both the extension of the lesion and the involvement of normal surrounding structures, the surgical strategy can be precisely planned.

PETROCLIVAL APPROACHES

Skull base tumors arising from the petroclival region may result in destruction of bony structures and compression of the brainstem. Tumor extension into the middle and posterior fossae frequently occurs, and involvement of the cavernous sinus is not unusual. Different approaches to the petroclival region have been described that consider the major extension of the lesion. A number of reports have ap-

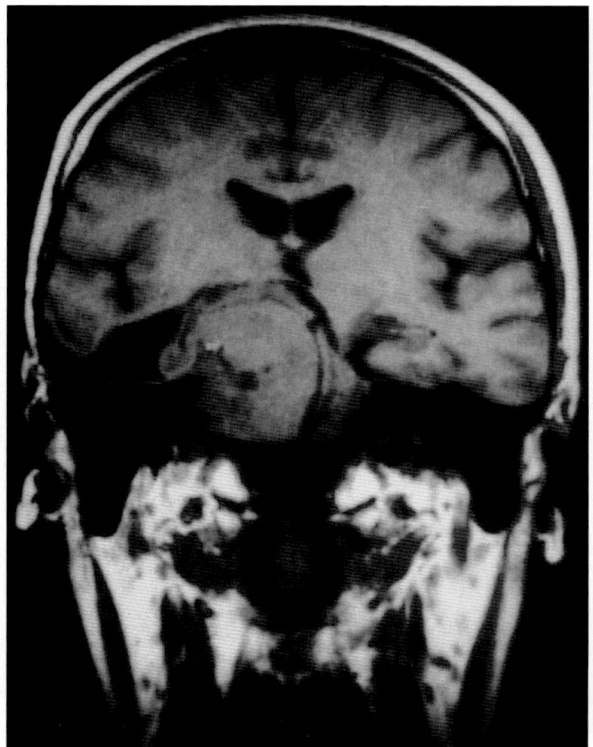
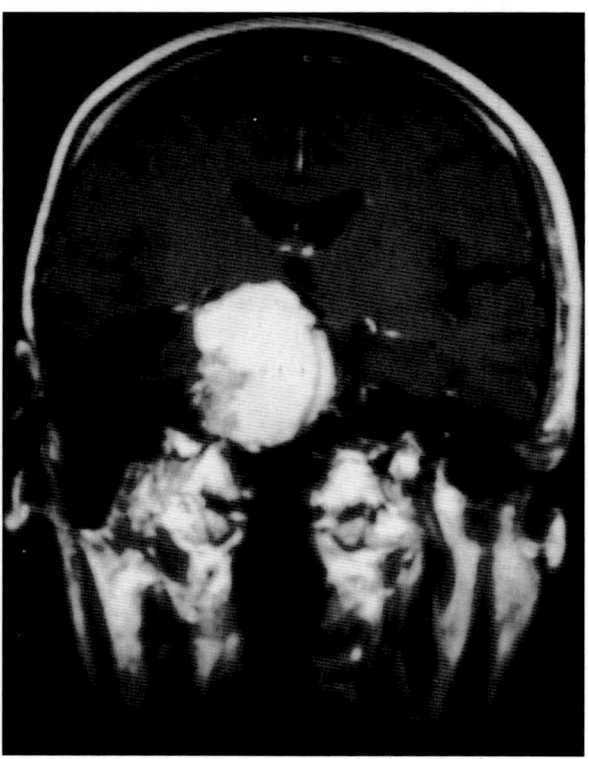

FIG. 8. Coronal magnetic resonance images before **(A)** and after **(B)** intravenous contrast injection, demonstrating the relation between tumor and surrounding brain tissue and vessels. Note the involvement of the basilar artery in this case.

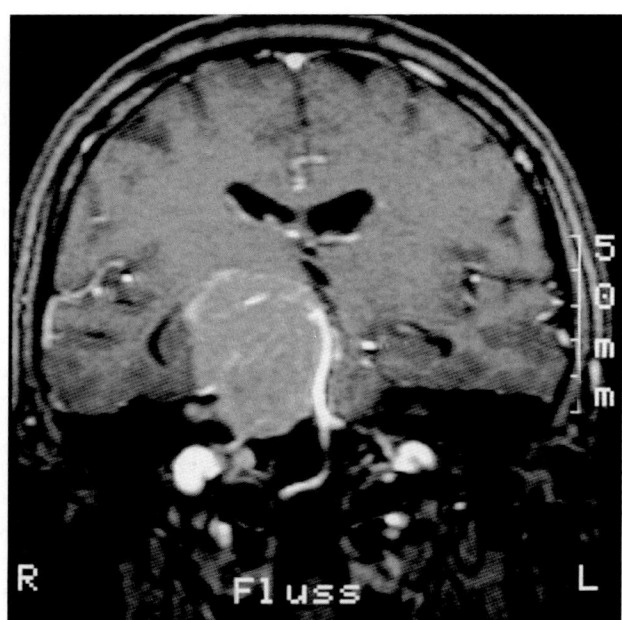

FIG. 9. Magnetic resonance angiogram of the patient in Fig. 8.

peared indicating improvements in tumor resection and postoperative outcome (1,8,12–14,16,21,23,25–30).

For didactic purposes, access to the petroclival region may be divided into four major approaches (31,32):

1. Middle fossa approaches
   a. Primary extradural (extended middle fossa)
   b. Primary intradural (subtemporal transtentorial)
2. Posterior fossa approaches
   a. Primary extradural (presigmoid)
   b. Primary intradural (retrosigmoid)

All these approaches can be combined with the others to enlarge the exposure. For most petroclival cases, the authors use the *combined subtemporal transtentorial–presigmoid approach*. These approaches are described in the following sections.

Posterior Fossa Primary Extradural–Presigmoid Approach

Indications

The *presigmoid approach* is the authors' approach of choice for most petroclival lesions. It is used in combination with a subtemporal approach. The major indications are lesions centered in the lateral incisural space extending infratentorially to the upper and mid-clivus, and lesions situated in the anterior part of the posterior pyramis extending supratentorially to the middle fossa. Frequent lesions include petroclival meningiomas, and large, dumbbell-shaped trigeminal schwannomas. Vascular processes such as aneurysms of the upper and middle basilar artery can also be accessed with this exposure.

The major advantages of the presigmoid approach are less brain retraction and the shorter route to the petrous apex provided by the bone removal, and the multiangle approach to the petroclival area that is afforded. The major disadvantages are the potential for hearing and facial damage during pyramidal bone drilling, and the possibility of vascular injuries, particularly to the vein of Labbé. For processes reaching the lower clivus and foramen magnum, the presigmoid approach can be combined with the retrosigmoid approach.

The *combined supratentorial–infratentorial approach with division of the sigmoid sinus* gives the same large exposure as the presigmoid approach combined with the retrosigmoid route. The main advantage of the transsigmoid approach is that the vein of Labbé is retracted upward along with the transverse sinus. This avoids the stretching and possible rupture of the vein, which may occur in the presigmoid approach when the vein is tethered to the transverse sinus during upward retraction of the temporal lobe. A major disadvantage of the transsigmoid approach compared with the presigmoid method is that transection of the sigmoid sinus may not be tolerated by a number of patients.

Operative Technique

Patient Position

The authors perform the presigmoid approach with the patient in semisitting position, and the head turned 60 degrees toward the side of the lesion and slightly anteflected. The legs are elevated to the level of the right cardiac atrium, and the head is fixed in place with Mayfield pins. Some surgeons prefer to operate with the patient in either the supine or the park-bench position.

Anesthesia and Monitoring

Intravenous anesthesia with isoflurane is induced. Prophylactic antibiotic is administered, and treatment with dexamethasone is initiated to reduce the risk of postoperative edema. Sensory evoked potentials are monitored continuously in the median nerve. Preoperative flexion–extension radiographs of the cervical spine are made to rule out craniocervical instability. All body parts subject to pressure are supported with cushions.

Major additional precautions during semisitting surgery include monitoring for air embolism using electrocardiography, oximetry, capnometry, precordial Doppler ultrasonography, catheterization of the right atrium, and central venous catheterization. Hearing is monitored by measurement of brainstem auditory evoked potentials. Subdermal needle electrodes are implanted for continuous electromyographic monitoring of the orbicular muscles of the eye and mouth.

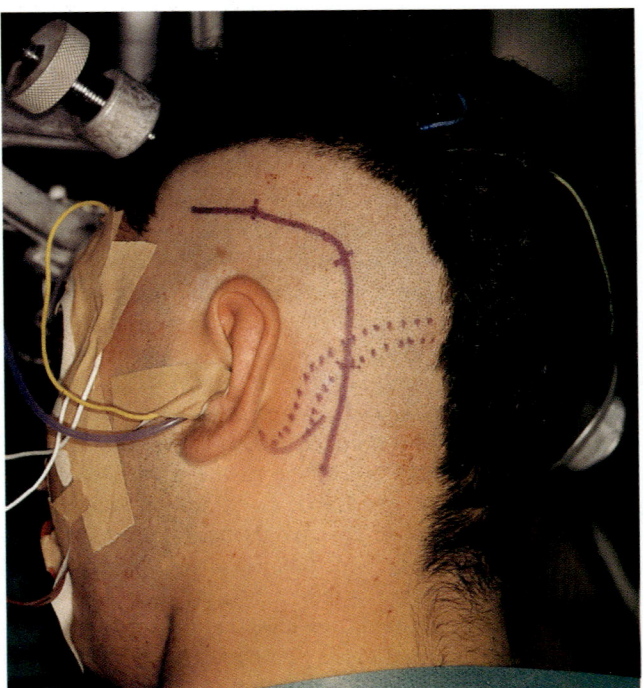

FIG. 10. Patient in semisitting position. The scalp is shaved, and the skin marked for the incision.

Skin Incision and Craniotomy

Part of the temporal, occipital, and suboccipital region of the scalp is shaved, and the skin is marked for the incision (Fig. 10). A curvilinear skin incision starting 2 cm above the upper part of the auricle is carried backward along the temporal line, and is curved downward in a linear fashion to the suboccipital area about 3 cm behind the ear, extending 2 cm under the mastoid tip.

The skin flap is reflected forward to the level of the external auditory canal. The temporalis muscle is cut in the area below the fascia insertion at the bone and reflected downward. The muscles over the mastoid and occipital bone are swept downward using subperiosteal dissection.

The first bur hole is placed at the region of the asterion, exposing the transition border of the transverse to sigmoid sinuses. The dura is slightly detached from the bone in the area around the bur hole using the dissectors. A temporal and suboccipital craniotomy is done with a high-speed craniotome, exposing the transverse sinus. The bone flap is elevated carefully, taking care to free dural adhesions along the transverse sinus. Small sinus lacerations are packed with fibrin sponge.

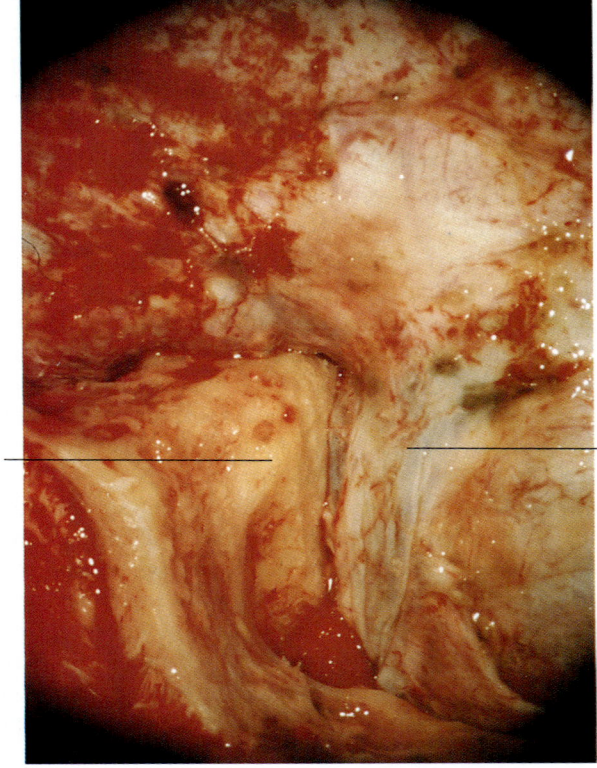

Labyrinth block — Sigmoid sinus

FIG. 11. Intraoperative photograph after the craniotomy flap is removed and the mastoid is drilled. The dura anterior to the sigmoid sinus is exposed (Trautmann's triangle).

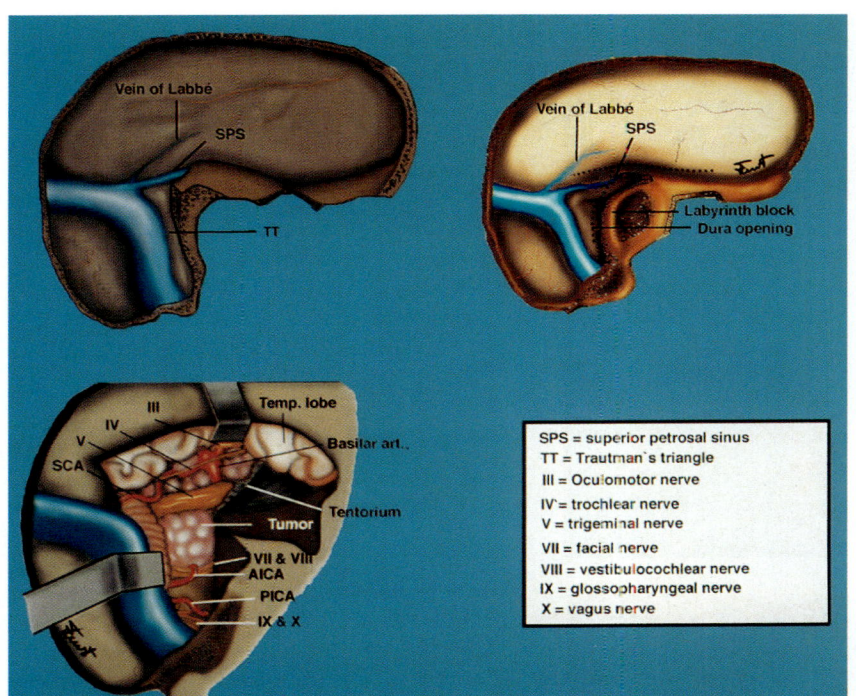

FIG. 12. Artist's depiction of the combined subtemporal–presigmoid approach. The dura is opened in a T-shaped fashion with division of the superior petrosal sinus. The temporal lobe is then retracted upward and the cerebellum backward.

Petrous Bone Drilling

From now until the dura is closed, the operation is conducted using the operating microscope. Using a high-speed air drill, a mastoidectomy is done with exposure of the sigmoid sinus as low as the jugular bulb (Fig. 11). The posterior wall of the petrous pyramid is drilled away in a lateromedial direction as far anterior as possible without opening the posterior semicircular canal or the fallopian canal. The distance between the posterior semicircular canal and the anterior border of the sigmoid sinus varies from a few millimeters to 1 cm. In cases of preoperative hearing loss, a wider exposure can be done with resection of the labyrinth. Care should be taken not to injure the facial nerve.

In most petroclival lesions, there is no need to open the fallopian canal or reroute the facial nerve.

Dural Opening

After the drilling procedure is completed, the exposure reveals the temporal, presigmoid, and retrosigmoid dura, and the transverse, sigmoid, and superior petrosal sinuses. The dura is then cut over the transverse sinus toward the temporal dura while preserving the junction of the vein of Labbé with the transverse sinus. The infratentorial dura is opened anterior to the sigmoid sinus in Trautmann's triangle. The lateral cerebellomedullary cistern is opened, and cerebrospinal fluid (CSF) is withdrawn to provide more space.

The posterior temporal lobe is retracted superiorly, and the cerebellum is held backward. The superior petrosal sinus is ligated and divided (Fig. 12).

Division of Tentorium

The tentorium is cut in a lateromedial direction anterior to the transverse sinus (and the vein of Labbé) and parallel to the petrous ridge (Fig. 13). The incision is extended through the medial tentorial edge behind the area in which the trochlear nerve penetrates the tentorium. Care is taken not to injure the trochlear nerve running close to the tentorial edge. Tentorial sinuses may sometimes bleed significantly and should be packed with fibrin sponges. No bipolar coagulation is used to stop bleeding because of risk of injury to the trochlear nerve.

Brain Retraction and Tumor Exposure

The cerebellum is then gently retracted posteriorly along with the sigmoid sinus and the edge of the divided tentorium. The tumor is exposed in its full extension along with the cranial nerves and vessels in the cerebellopontine angle (Fig. 14). Tumor is removed using the cavitron and microsurgical techniques. The dissection of tumor away from the vessels and nerves is carried out respecting the arachnoid planes. The combined presigmoid approach allows complete tumor resection in most cases, with preservation of normal struc-

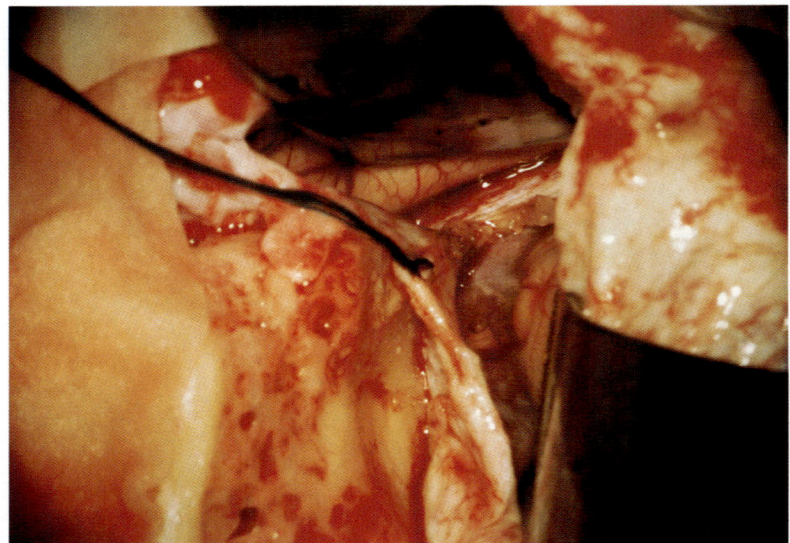
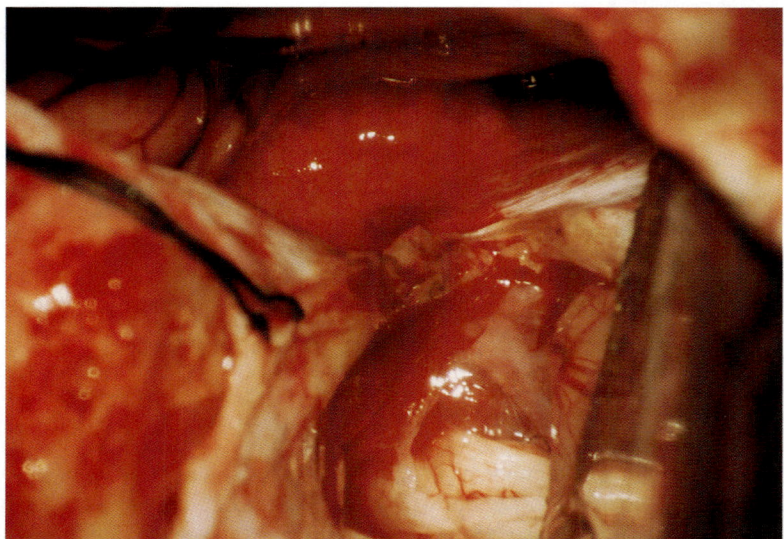
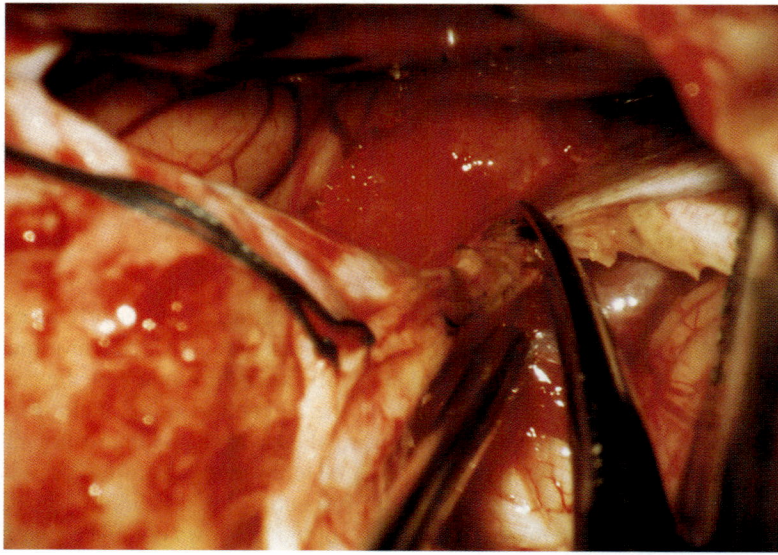

FIG. 13. After division of the superior petrosal sinus **(A)**, the temporal lobe and cerebellum are retracted, exposing the tumor **(B)**. The tentorium is then transected in lateromedial direction **(C)**.

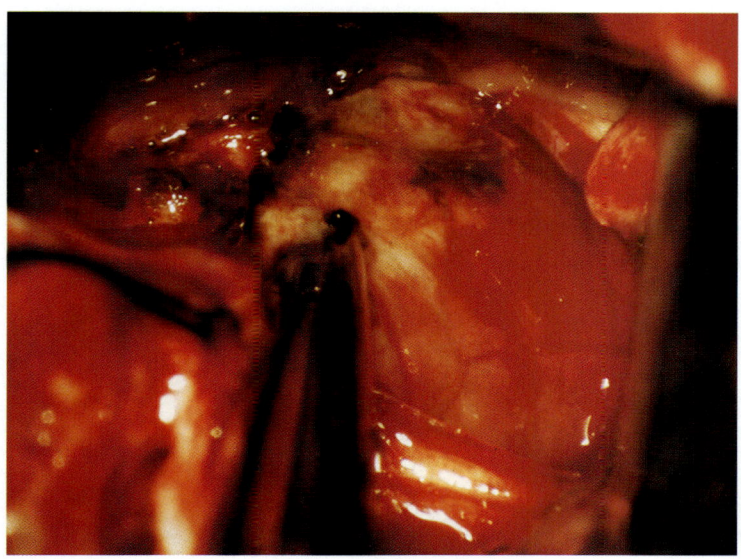

FIG. 14. The tumor is now exposed supratentorially and infratentorially in a single compartment.

tures (Fig. 15). However, particularly in meningiomas, if the arachnoid sheath surrounding nerves and vessels is absent or the brainstem pia mater is infiltrated, no attempt at radical surgical removal is made because of the risk of severe postoperative deficits.

The presigmoid approach has also been used for aneurysms of the middle basilar trunk. This approach provides good exposure of the middle and lower basilar artery from the vertebrobasilar junction to the basilar trunk above the anterior inferior cerebellar artery origins (4). The surgeon works between the cranial nerves V and the VII to VIII complex, or between the latter and the lower cranial nerves. There is enough space for temporary clipping if necessary.

Technical Aspects of Tumor Resection

Meningiomas. Resection of petroclival meningiomas includes alternating intratumoral decompression using the ultrasonic aspirator, bipolar coagulation, and microscissors, with dissection of the tumors from the surrounding structures (see Figs. 13–15). To minimize the risk to neurovascular structures, the dissection is carried out outside the arachnoid. In small petroclival meningiomas, cranial nerves VII and VIII are usually easily identifiable in the posterior aspect of the tumor. In large meningiomas, cranial nerves VII through XII may be engulfed by the tumor, and careful microsurgical dissection is necessary to preserve function.

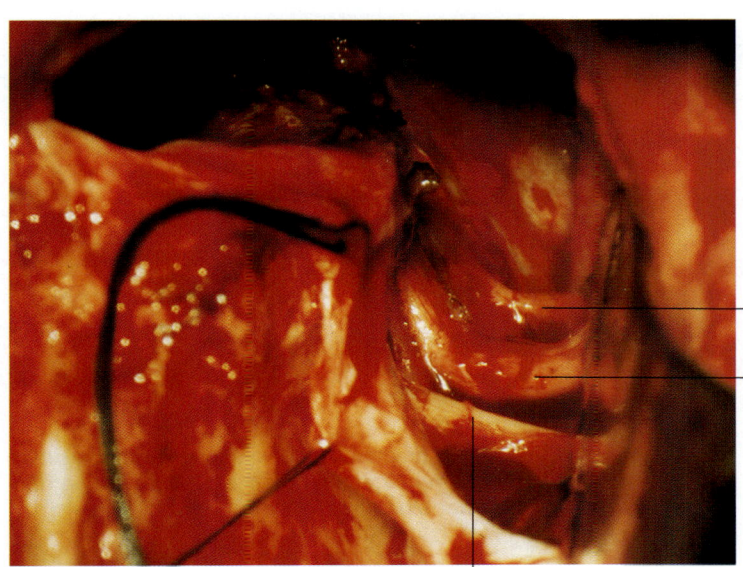

— Abducent nerve
— Trigeminal nerve

VII-VIII nerves

FIG. 15. Intraoperative photograph showing complete tumor resection with preserved cranial nerves.

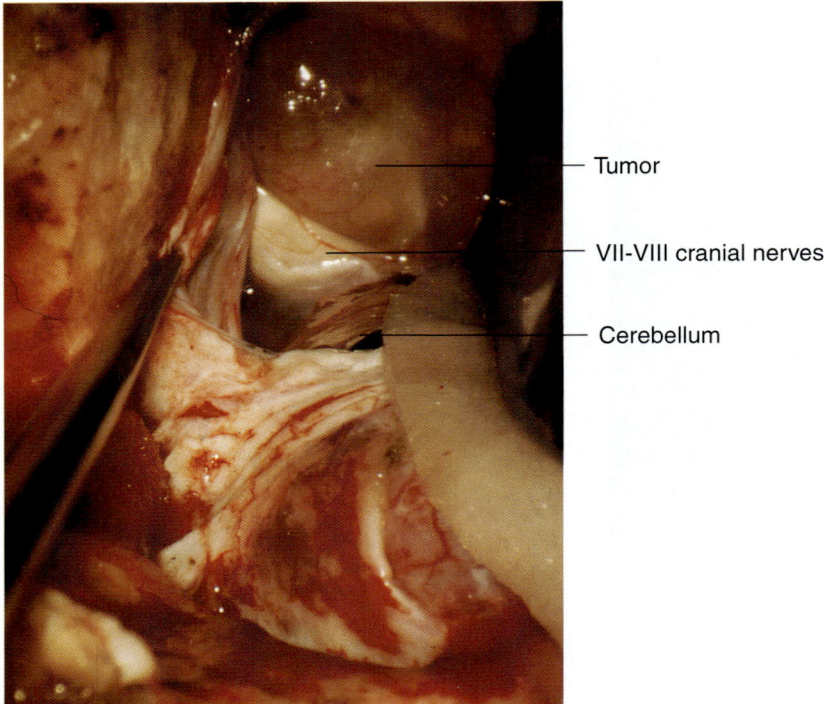

FIG. 16. Intraoperative photograph of a trigeminal schwannoma exposed using the combined subtemporal–presigmoid approach. Cranial nerves VII and VIII are displaced downward by the tumor.

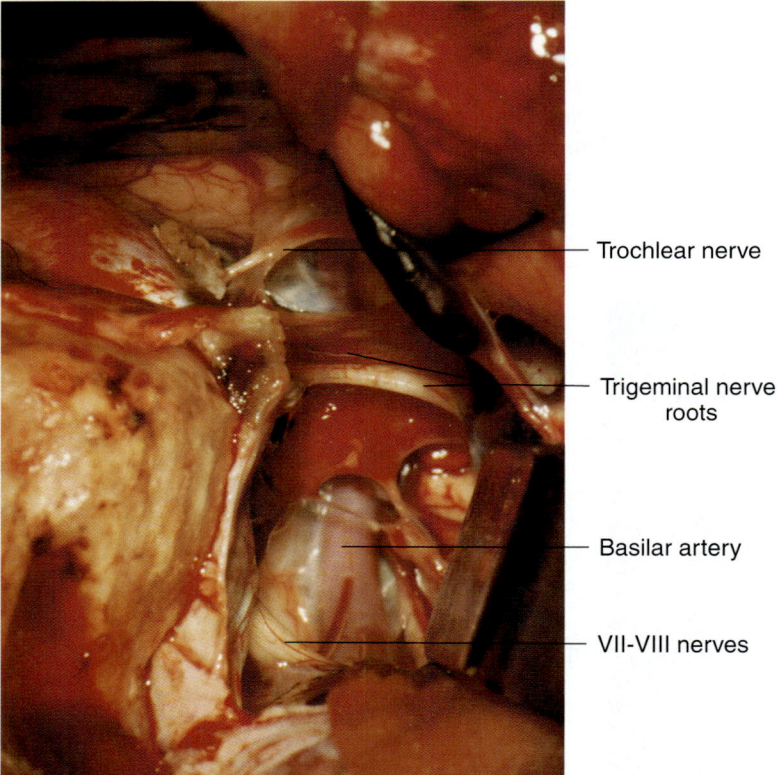

FIG. 17. Complete tumor resection with preservation of some trigeminal roots and surrounding neurovascular structures.

Trigeminal Schwannomas. Trigeminal schwannomas have been classified into four major types, depending on the major tumor extension (2). Dumbbell-shaped trigeminal schwannomas extending into the middle and posterior fossae are best resected by the presigmoid approach. The tumor is exposed as described previously (Fig. 16). It is then debulked and separated from the stretched fascicles of the trigeminal nerve. These tumors frequently have a good arachnoid plane, and it is usually possible to resect it and preserve most nerve fascicles (Fig. 17). Resection of the nerve fascicles results in postoperative numbness and disabling keratitis. If the tumor enters the cavernous sinus, every attempt should be made to remove it through the posterior approach. It is also essential to open Meckel's cave to achieve a radical resection.

Hemostasis and Closure

After tumor removal is completed and before the dura is closed, the jugular vein is compressed to elicit possible venous bleeding that may not be obvious in the semisitting position. Any venous bleeding should be stopped by bipolar coagulation, or packing with fibrin sponge or Surgicel. Once the hemostasis is secured, the dura is closed in watertight fashion. When the dural defect cannot be closed primarily, a dural reconstruction is done and lumbar spinal drainage is used for 5 to 7 days. A compressive dressing is applied for 1 week.

Posterior Fossa Primary Intradural Approach

Indications

The retrosigmoid approach is used only in cases of petroclival meningiomas with major extension into the posterior fossa and little involvement of the supratentorial surface of the tentorium, or in cases of large tumors in older patients, in which the only aim is brainstem decompression.

Operative Technique

The authors operate with the patient in the semisitting position, as described previously. The head is moved anteriorly and turned 30 degrees toward the side of lesion. After the skin incision is done approximately 3 cm behind the ear and the neck muscles are detached and retracted, suboccipital craniectomy or craniotomy is performed, exposing the margins of the transverse and sigmoid sinuses. The dura is opened some millimeters away and along the transverse and sigmoid sinus.

The inferior border of the cerebellum is elevated as a first step, and the cerebellomedullary cisterns are opened to allow CSF drainage. The cerebellum is now relaxed and can be easily retracted medially without major compression. This

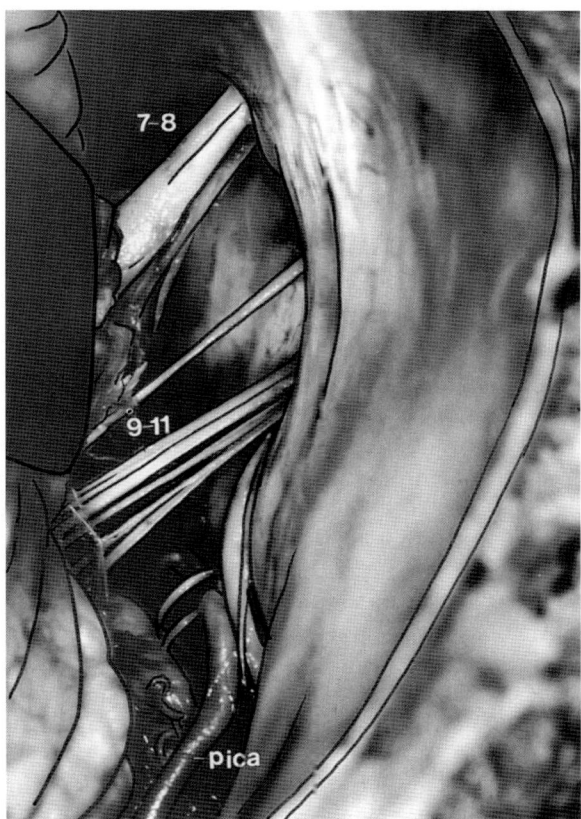

FIG. 18. Cadaver dissection showing a view of the lower cerebellopontine angle from the retrosigmoid approach. The cerebellum is held with a retractor. Cranial nerves VII and VIII are seen between the internal auditory meatus and the brainstem. The lower cranial nerves are seen between the jugular foramen and the brainstem.

approach allows visualization of cranial nerve V through the lower cranial nerves, depending on tumor size and extension (Fig. 18).

Petroclival meningiomas usually displace cranial nerves V, VII, and VIII dorsally and must be removed between the cranial nerves. The technique of arachnoid sheath dissection is used for tumor resection.

Epidermoid tumors may fill the entire cerebellopontine angle and even extend to the contralateral side, caudally to the foramen magnum, and cranially to the middle fossa. The cerebellopontine angle is divided into four floors, based on the cranial nerves: the first floor lies between the tentorium and cranial nerve V; the second floor between cranial nerve V and the complex of nerves VII and VIII; the third floor between the complex of nerves VII and VIII and the caudal cranial nerves; and the fourth floor below the caudal cranial nerves. The tumor is removed between these floors, mostly between the second and the third floors. In 40 cases of cerebellopontine angle epidermoids, 75% of the tumors were completely removed, but in 25% of the cases, very adherent tumor capsule could not be resected. An attempt to remove the capsule in these cases may produce severe, permanent neurologic deficits.

Middle Fossa Extradural Approach

Indications

This approach is mostly indicated for extradural processes involving the petroclival region, such as chordomas and chondrosarcomas.

Operative Technique

The patient's head is turned 90 degrees, positioned parallel to a horizontal line and slightly extended. A temporal craniotomy anterior to the ear and above the zygoma is performed. The dura is elevated from the floor of the middle fossa until the arcuate eminence and the greater petrosal nerve are visualized. Identification of the internal auditory canal involves drilling along the greater petrosal nerve, which indicates the geniculate ganglion. At this point, the drilling is turned medially to expose the labyrinthine portion of the facial nerve up to the fundus of the internal auditory canal (see Fig. 3). Another technique to locate the internal auditory canal is to subtend an angle of 60 degrees from the plane of the superior semicircular canal.

To reach the petroclival region, parts of the petrous apex are drilled away: between the trigeminal nerve anteriorly, the carotid artery and cochlea laterally, and the labyrinth block posteriorly (Kawase's approach). The bone removal is extended to the lateral side of the clivus, exposing the inferior petrosal sinus. The width of the bone resection from the trigeminal impression to the posterior wall of the internal auditory canal averages 13 mm (17). The dura is then opened anterior to cranial nerves VII and VIII.

The view can be widened by dividing the tentorium. The dural leaflets of the tentorium are retracted with sutures. This approach gives a view of cranial nerves III to VIII, the basilar artery, the posterior cerebral artery, the superior cerebellar artery, and the anterior inferior cerebellar artery (see later). The exposure, however, is small and may require significant temporal lobe retraction. Another disadvantage is the relatively high risk of facial nerve injury.

Middle Fossa Intradural (Transtentorial) Approach

Indications

This approach is mainly indicated for petroclival lesions with extension intradurally and brainstem displacement, such as meningiomas, schwannomas (cranial nerve VII), and epidermoid cysts. It may also be indicated for aneurysms of the basilar tip. Advantages of this approach include a more anterior angle and widened visualization of the interpeduncular area, the basilar apex and upper trunk, the ventral lateral brainstem, and the upper petroclival area. The disadvantage lies in the potential for injury to important bridging veins running from the temporal lobe to the base of the skull.

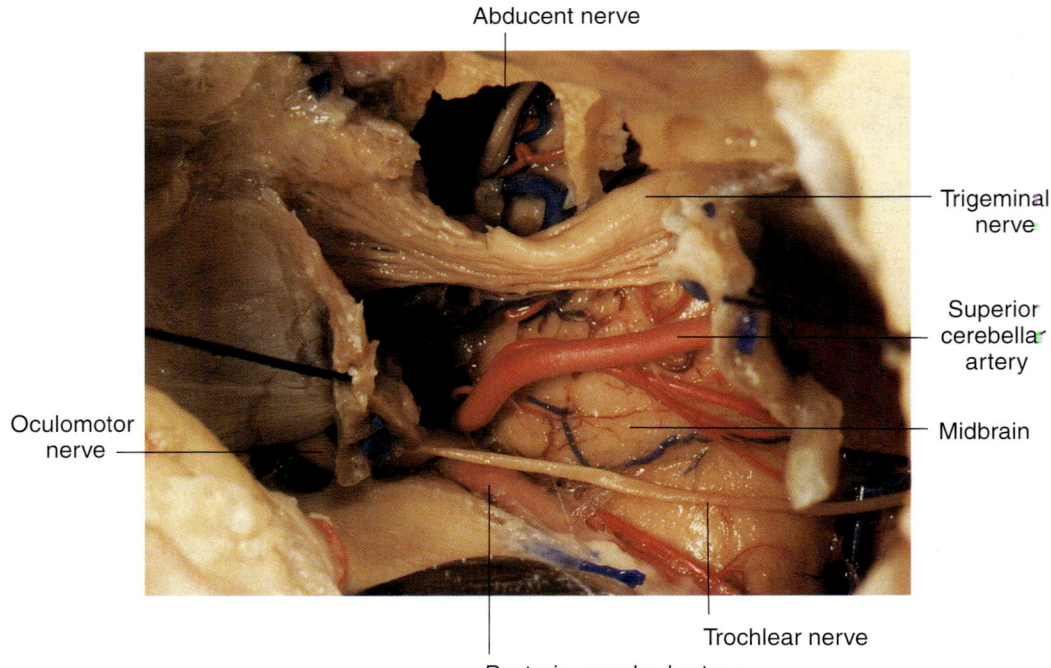

FIG. 19. Cadaver dissection of the middle fossa approach after drilling the petrous apex and division of the tentorium, exposing the region's anatomy.

Operative Technique

The head is positioned as described previously for the middle fossa approach, with the difference that the head is turned to form an angle of 15 degrees with the horizontal line (with the nose elevated). The craniotomy is done above and anterior to the ear. The zygomatic arch may be divided and reflected inferiorly with the attached muscle and fascia to allow for a low craniotomy and less temporal lobe retraction.

After the dura has been opened, the temporal lobe is gently elevated to visualize the tentorial edge. The tentorium is elevated to show the course of the trochlear nerve running into the dural tunnel at the tentorial edge (see Fig. 2). The tentorium is then divided 1 to 2 cm posterior to the entry point of cranial nerve IV. The dural tunnel of the trochlear nerve is opened, freeing the nerve. One of the key steps in the subtemporal transtentorial approach is the dissection of the trochlear nerve from the edge of the tentorium. The superior petrosal sinus can be divided after double clipping, bipolar coagulation, or packing with Surgicel. The tentorial flaps are then widely reflected, which provides visualization of the interpeduncular and prepontine cisterns between cranial nerves IV and V (Fig. 19). Temporal lobe retraction exposes the basilar artery apex and the oculomotor nerve.

The dura around the petrous bone can be resected to perform a partial petrosectomy by drilling part of the petrous apex at Kawase's triangle. Care should be taken not to injure the carotid artery and the cochlea.

MANAGEMENT OF COMPLICATIONS

Major complications of petroclival surgery include cranial nerve injury, vascular injury, and CSF leakage. The anterior approaches may be complicated by injury to the vein of Labbé, temporal lobe, and facial nerve. The posterior approaches may be complicated by injury to the labyrinth block, sinus thrombosis, and CSF leakage.

Cerebrospinal fluid leakage is avoided by watertight dural closure, or dural reconstruction and placement of lumbar drainage for about 1 week. The mastoid air cells are closed with muscle fragments and fibrin glue.

Thrombosis of the transverse or sigmoid sinus is a life-threatening complication that must be immediately recognized and treated (1). This complication can be prevented by avoiding severe sinus compression during the surgery.

Injury to the labyrinth has been related to postoperative hearing loss. However, labyrinth injury does not invariably result in complete hearing loss (33). Once part of the labyrinth is injured, suction of its contents should be avoided and the opening area immediately closed with muscle fascia and fibrin glue.

Review of the literature revealed that in most series, complete tumor removal was achieved in 70% of cases. Indeed, approximately 30% of meningiomas were not resectable. Incomplete tumor removal and surgical morbidity have been largely related to absence of the arachnoid sheath because of tumor infiltration, which may result in rupture of the pia and pial vessels of the brainstem with consequent brainstem infarction. Awareness of these risks and the surgical limitations is essential for management of petroclival lesions.

CASE REPORTS

CASE 1: PETROCLIVAL MENINGIOMA

A 56-year-old man presented with a 2-year history of progressive hearing loss and unsteady gait. Neurologic examination demonstrated a decreased hearing of 30 dB at 1 to 3 kHz, slight facial weakness, and diminished sensation on the face. The gait was unsteady with a broad base. CT and MRI scans showed a large petroclival mass extending to the middle and posterior fossae and compressing the brainstem (Fig. 20).

Through a combined supratentorial–presigmoid approach, the tumor was exposed and completely resected. At discharge from the hospital, no additional deficits were found. Postoperative CT showed total tumor resection (Fig. 21).

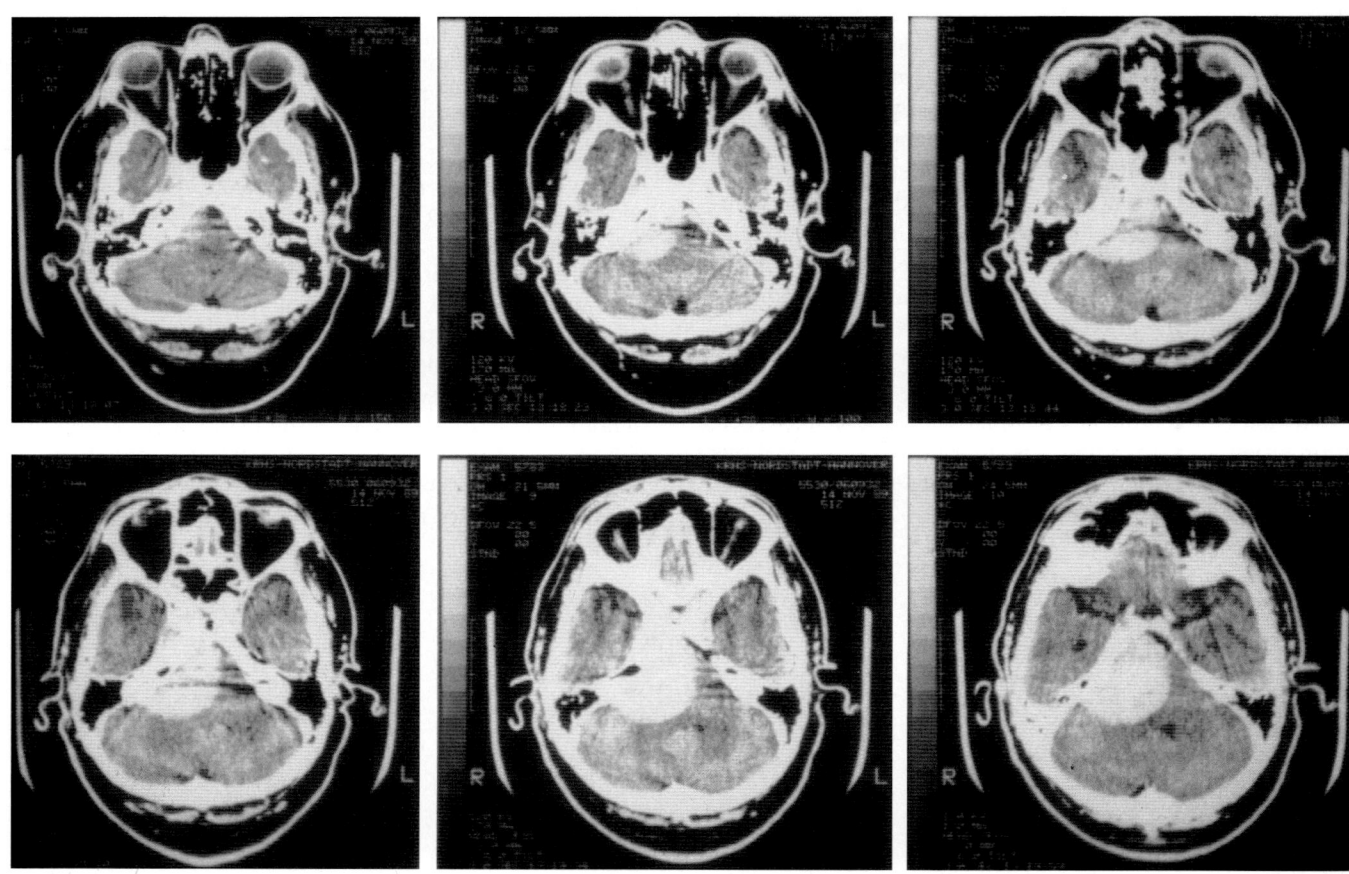

FIG. 20. Case 1. Serial enhanced computed tomography scan of a large petroclival meningioma.

CASE 1 (Continued)

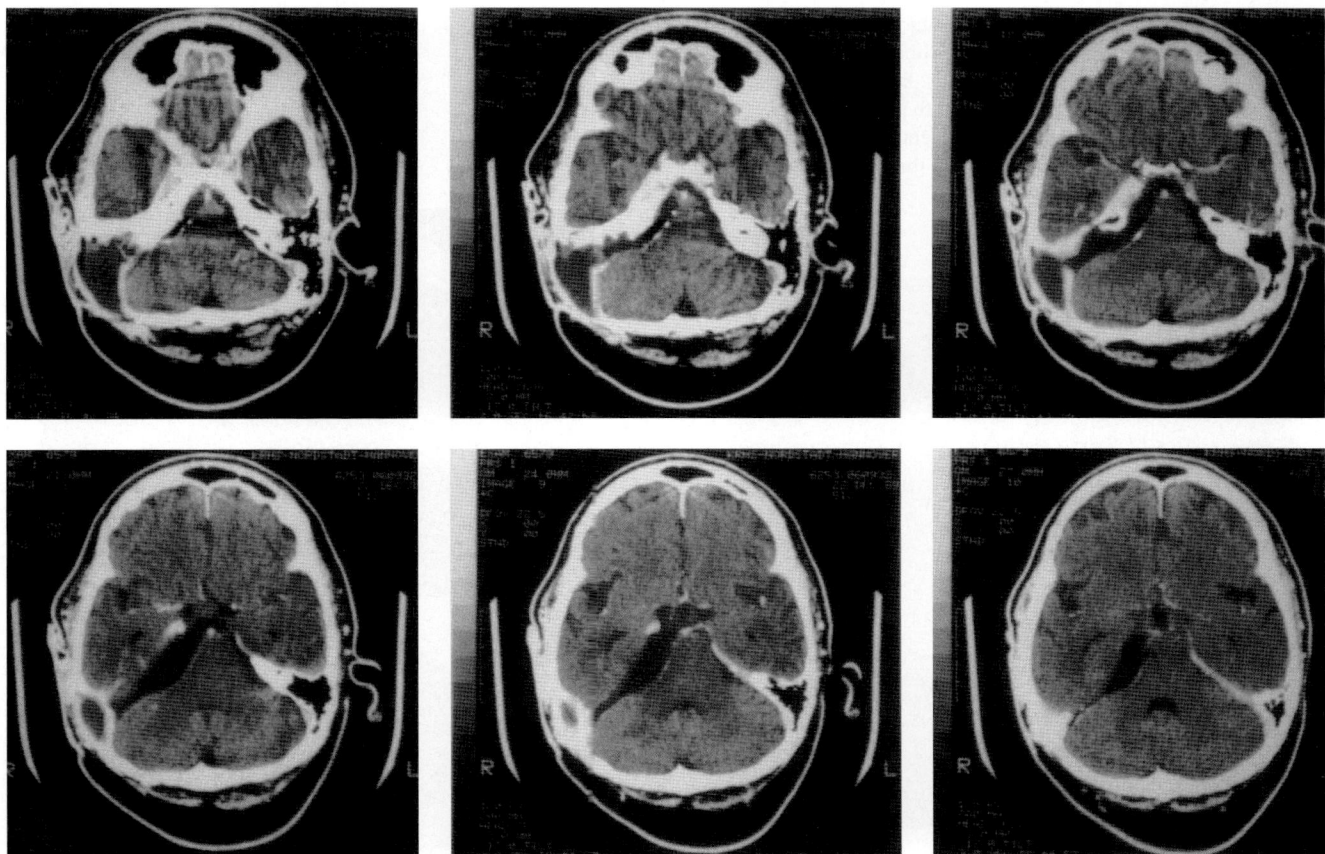

FIG. 21. Case 1. Serial enhanced computed tomography scan after tumor resection by the combined subtemporal–presigmoid approach.

CASE 2: TRIGEMINAL SCHWANNOMA

This 31-year-old man presented with a 2-year history of numbness of the left hemiface, and progressive headache and hearing loss of 1 year's duration. MRI showed a large, dumbbell-shaped tumor with compression of the brainstem and involvement of the cavernous sinus (Fig. 22). By a combined subtemporal–presigmoid approach, the lesion was resected with preservation of most trigeminal fascicles. The postoperative outcome was uneventful. Immediate postoperative CT depicted the amount of bone resection and tumor removal (Fig. 23).

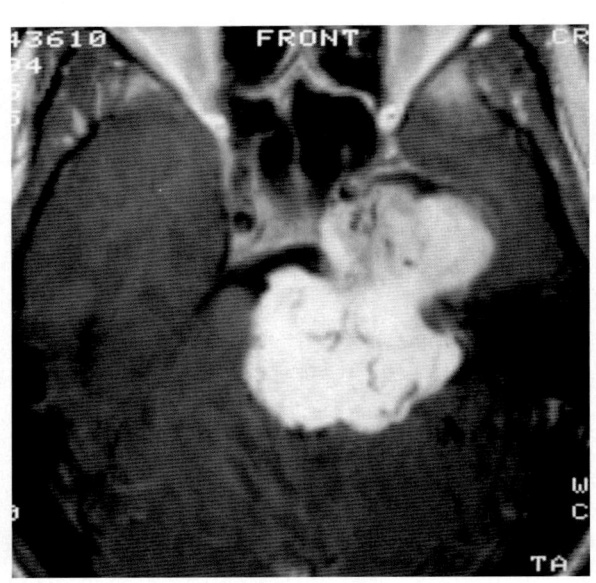

FIG. 22. Case 2. Enhanced magnetic resonance image of a large, dumbbell-shaped trigeminal schwannoma extending into the middle and posterior fossae.

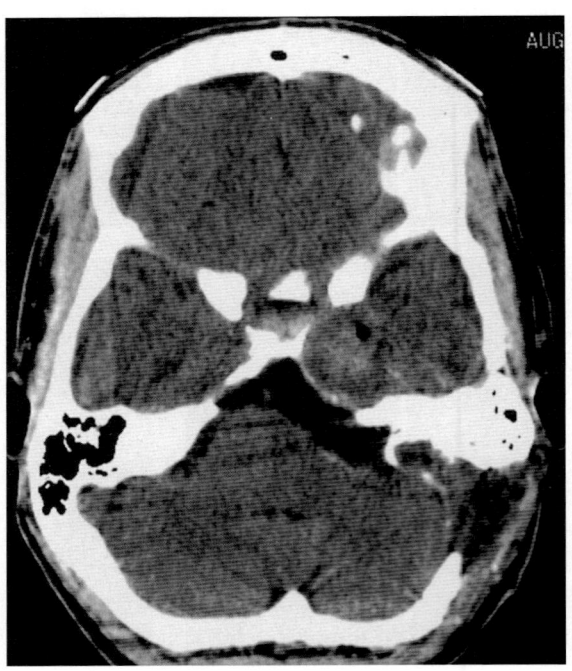

FIG. 23. Case 2. Computed tomography scan after tumor resection.

CASE 3: PETROCLIVAL CHORDOMA

This 48-year-old man had been operated on twice for a clivus chordoma before he was referred to our department with a tumor recurrence. The patient had complete deficit of cranial nerves VI through VIII on the left side. Preoperative MRI showed large tumor extension in the left petroclival area up to the foramen magnum (Fig. 24). By a combined presigmoid–transpetrosal (translabyrinthine, transcochlear) approach, the lesion was radically resected. Postoperative CT showed the degree of tumor and bone resection (Fig. 25). A 3-year follow-up did not show tumor recurrence.

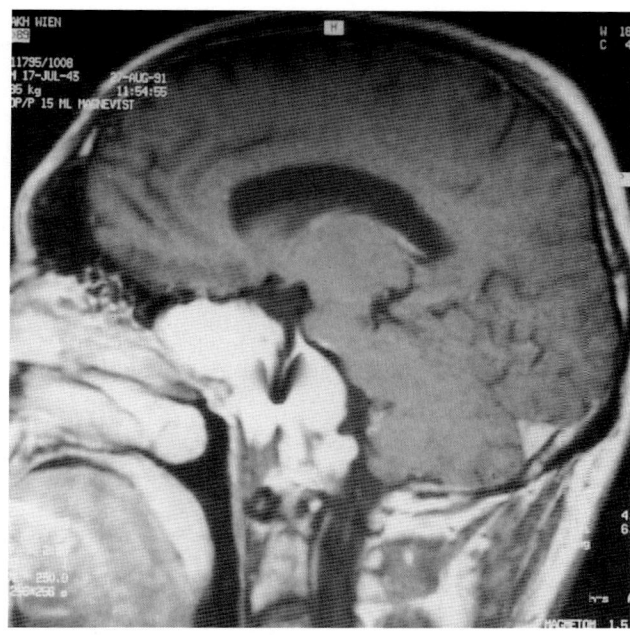

FIG. 24. Case 3. Sagittal magnetic resonance image of a large chordoma of the clivus extending from the middle fossa up to the lower clivus.

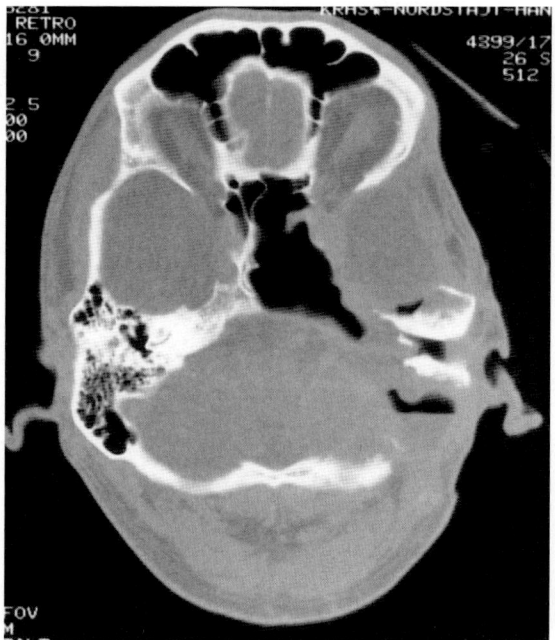
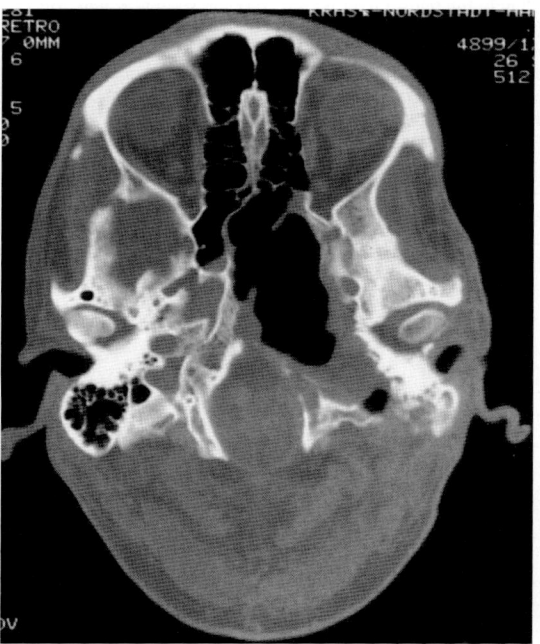

FIG. 25. Case 3. **A,B:** Postoperative computed tomography scan with bone algorithms showing degree of bone resection after radical tumor removal

ACKNOWLEDGMENTS

The authors thank Mr. Stefan Brinkmann for preparing the photographic material and Mrs. Marianne Faust for the illustrations.

REFERENCES

1. Samii M, Tatagiba M. Experience with 36 surgical cases of petroclival meningiomas. *Acta Neurochir (Wien)* 1992;118:27–32.
2. Samii M, Migliori M, Tatagiba M, Babu R. Surgical treatment of trigeminal schwannomas. *J Neurosurg* 1995;82:711–718.
3. Weber AL, Liebsch NJ, Sanchez R, Sweriduk SJ. Chordomas of the skull base: radiologic and clinical evaluation. *Neuroimaging Clin North Am* 1994;4:515–527.
4. Martin N. Vascular lesions. In: Samii M, Cheatham M, Becker D, eds. *Atlas of cranial base surgery*. Philadelphia: WB Saunders, 1995:201–211.
5. Castellano F, Ruggiero G. Meningiomas of the posterior fossa. *Acta Radiol (Suppl)* 1953;104:1–177.
6. Guthrie B, Ebersold M, Scheithauer B. Neoplasms of the intracranial meninges. In: Youmans JR, ed. *Neurological surgery*. Vol. 5. 3rd ed. Philadelphia: WB Saunders, 1990:3250–3315.
7. Yasargil M, Mortara R, Curcic M. Meningiomas of basal posterior cranial fossa. *Adv Tech Stand Neurosurg* 1980;7:3–115.
8. Al Mefty O, Ayoubi S, Smith RR. The petrosal approach: indications, technique, and results. *Acta Neurochir Suppl (Wien)* 1991;53:166–170.
9. Arriaga MA, Brackmann DE, Hitselberger WE. Extended middle fossa resection of petroclival and cavernous sinus neoplasms. *Laryngoscope* 1993;103:693–698.
10. Canalis RF, Black K, Martin N, Becker D. Extended retrolabyrinthine transtentorial approach to petroclival lesions. *Laryngoscope* 1991;101:6–13.
11. Hakuba A, Liu S, Nishimura S. The orbitozygomatic infratemporal approach: a new surgical technique. *Surg Neurol* 1986;26:271–276.
12. Kawase T, Shiobara R, Toya S. Middle fossa transpetrosal–transtentorial approaches for petroclival meningiomas: selective pyramid resection and radicality. *Acta Neurochir (Wien)* 1994;129:113–120.
13. King WA, Black KL, Martin NA, Canalis RF, Becker DP. The petrosal approach with hearing preservation. *J Neurosurg* 1993;79:508–514.
14. Samii M, Ammirati M. The combined supra-infratentorial pre-sigmoid sinus avenue to the petro-clival region: surgical technique and clinical applications. *Acta Neurochir (Wien)* 1988;95:6–12.
15. Sanna M, Mazzoni A, Saleh EA, Taibah AK, Russo A. Lateral approaches to the median skull base through the petrous bone: the system of the modified transcochlear approach. *J Laryngol Otol* 1994;108:1036–1044.
16. Sekhar LN, Pomeranz S, Sen CN. Extradural petrous bone and petroclival neoplasms. *Acta Neurochir Suppl (Wien)* 1991;53:183–192.
17. Tedeschi H, Rhoton AJ. Lateral approaches to the petroclival region. *Surg Neurol* 1994;41:180–216.
18. Thedinger BA, Glasscock ME, Cueva RA. Transcochlear transtentorial approach for removal of large cerebellopontine angle meningiomas. *Am J Otol* 1992;13:408–415.
19. Rhoton AJ, Tedeschi H. Lateral approaches to the cerebellopontine angle and petroclival region (honored guest lecture). *Clin Neurosurg* 1994;41:517–545.
20. Day JD, Fukushima T, Giannotta SL. Microanatomical study of the extradural middle fossa approach to the petroclival and posterior cavernous sinus region: description of the rhomboid construct. *Neurosurgery* 1994;34:1009–1016.
21. Miller CG, Van Lovereu HR, Keller JT, Pensak M, El-Kalliny M, Tew JJ. Transpetrosal approach: surgical anatomy and technique. *Neurosurgery* 1993;33:461–469.
22. Shao K, Tatagiba M, Samii M. Surgical management of high jugular bulb in acoustic neurinoma via retrosigmoid approach. *Neurosurgery* 1993;32:32–37.
23. Spetzler RF, Hamilton MG, Daspit CP. Petroclival lesions. *Clin Neurosurg* 1994;41:62–82.
24. Samii M, Tatagiba M, Piquer J, Carvalho G. Surgical treatment of epidermoid cysts of the cerebellopontine angle. *J Neurosurg*, 1996;84:14–19.
25. Samii M, Ammirati M, Mahran A, Bini W, Sepehrnia A. Surgery of petroclival meningiomas: report of 24 cases. *Neurosurgery* 1989;24:12–17.
26. Al Mefty O, Fox JL, Smith RR. Petrosal approach for petroclival meningiomas. *Neurosurgery* 1988;22:510–517.
27. Bricolo AP, Turazzi S, Talacchi A, Cristofori L. Microsurgical removal of petroclival meningiomas: a report of 33 patients. *Neurosurgery* 1992;31:813–828.
28. Cantore G, Delfini R, Ciappetta P. Surgical treatment of petroclival meningiomas: experience with 16 cases. *Surg Neurol* 1994;42:105–111.
29. Kawase T, Shiobara R, Toya S. Anterior transpetrosal–transtentorial approach for sphenopetroclival meningiomas: surgical method and results in 10 patients. *Neurosurgery* 1991;28:869–875.
30. Pensak ML, Van LH, Tew JJ, Keith RW. Transpetrosal access to meningiomas juxtaposing the temporal bone. *Laryngoscope* 1994;104:814–820.
31. Samii M, Tatagiba M. Neurosurgical aspects of tumors of the base of the skull. In: Youmans J, ed. *Neurological surgery*. Philadelphia: WB Saunders, 1996:3024–3040.
32. Samii M, Ammirati M. *Surgery of skull base meningiomas*. Berlin: Springer-Verlag, 1992:87–96.
33. Tatagiba M, Samii M, Matthies M, El Azm M, Schönmayr R. The significance for postoperative hearing of preserving the labyrinth in acoustic neurinoma surgery. *J Neurosurg* 1992;77:677–684.

/ # CHAPTER 23

Evaluation and Management of Vestibular Schwannomas

Hilary A. Brodie and Pamela Bohrer

In the early 1800s, Jean Cruveilhier presented a fascinating yet tragic account of a young woman with an acoustic neuroma. He carefully documented her progressive symptoms, both localized and generalized. The local symptoms resulted from direct tumor pressure and included progressive hearing loss, trigeminal neuralgia, and facial spasms. The generalized symptoms were caused by the increased intracranial pressure, and included headaches, blindness, hyposmia, and dysgeusia. She lived with these symptoms from age 19 until her death at age 26 years. Cruveilhier subsequently performed a postmortem examination and provided a remarkable description of a large acoustic neuroma: a firm, benign lesion arising from the internal auditory canal. It had eroded the temporal bone and compressed the surrounding nervous tissue, but true invasion was not seen. This detailed account is the first well documented case of the clinical and pathologic findings of a cerebellopontine angle (CPA) lesion.

It was Harvey Cushing, in the early 1900s, who brought focused attention to CPA lesions and took the first large steps toward successful surgical removal of these tumors (1). He emphasized early detection through high clinical suspicion, careful history taking, and thorough physical examination. However, surgical techniques of the time were poorly suited to dealing with lesions in the CPA, and his surgical results were relatively poor. To minimize the high morbidity associated with total tumor removal, he advocated debulking and partial tumor excision. Indeed, this tactic lowered morbidity rates, but tumor recurrence was common.

The modern era of surgical removal for CPA lesions began in the 1960s, with the work of William House. Before that time, mortality and morbidity rates were quite high using the suboccipital approach. House and Hitselberger advocated the use of the operating microscope and described and refined the translabyrinthine and middle fossa approaches to the CPA (2,3). Using these techniques, they achieved total tumor excision with acceptable morbidity and mortality. During this same time, the suboccipital approach was being refined, with the aid of the operating microscope, by the neurosurgical community. Today, the multidisciplinary skull base team is well versed in a variety of surgical approaches and tailors the surgical planning for each individual patient. Mortality rates have dropped to 1% in large series, and morbidity has been steadily decreasing.

The most common lesion in the CPA is an acoustic neuroma, or, more properly renamed, a vestibular schwannoma. In a large series of 1,354 lesions reported by Brackmann and Bartels in 1980, 91% of the tumors were vestibular schwannomas, 3% were meningiomas, 2% were primary cholesteatomas, and the remaining 4% were of widely varied histologic types (4). Magnetic resonance imaging (MRI) has significantly improved the preoperative evaluation of tumor type.

Magnetic resonance imaging has also enabled the detection of CPA tumors at a much earlier stage. Lesions of only a few millimeters in size, at a time when symptoms may be limited to mild hearing loss or even simply unilateral tinnitus, are being identified with MRI with gadolinium enhancement. In the modern era, the goal is early detection of vestibular schwannomas while patients are manifesting symptoms limited to unilateral hearing loss and tinnitus with mild unsteadiness, and before facial and trigeminal symptoms, hydrocephalus, and mass effects from very large tumors appear.

The emphasis on early detection and treatment of CPA lesions while small results from the fact that the morbidity of microsurgical excision is directly correlated to the size of the lesion. Unfortunately, microsurgical tumor excision can produce the same neurologic defects as the enlarging tumor.

H. A. Brodie: Department of Otolaryngology, University of California, Davis Medical Center, Sacramento, California 95817.
P. Bohrer: Department of Otolaryngology, Kaiser Permanente Medical Group, Santa Rosa, California 95403.

The following sections review the clinical presentation, diagnosis, treatment options, and microsurgical techniques for vestibular schwannomas. The challenge for the modern skull base team is to achieve total tumor extirpation with maximal preservation of function.

CLINICAL PRESENTATION

Hearing Loss

Vestibular schwannomas are varied in their presentation. Typically, patients present with a gradual, progressive, unilateral or asymmetric high-frequency sensorineural hearing loss, often with associated tinnitus. The rate of progression of hearing loss ranges from sudden onset to progressive over many years. Ten to 22% of patients with vestibular schwannoma present with sudden-onset sensorineural hearing loss (5–8). If questioned closely, up to 26% of patients report having had an episode of transient hearing loss at some point in their history (9). However, the overall incidence of vestibular schwannoma in patients with sudden sensorineural hearing loss is low. In one series of 836 patients with sudden sensorineural hearing loss, the incidence of vestibular schwannoma was 1.5% (10). In general, in patients with vestibular schwannoma there is no improvement in hearing thresholds after the acute loss, but there are subsets of patients who demonstrate fluctuating thresholds or recovery of hearing loss (6). In one series of 133 patients, 17 patients (13%) had a sudden sensorineural hearing loss, of whom 23% (4/17) recovered auditory function before resection of the vestibular schwannoma (6). Presentations suggestive of Meniere's syndrome occur in approximately 3% of patients with vestibular schwannoma (11). One case report describes a patient with recovery of hearing thresholds to normal levels on four separate occasions after steroid therapy. The patient had a 1.5-cm vestibular schwannoma (8).

As imaging techniques improve and MRI scans are obtained more readily, the incidence of vestibular schwannoma detected in patients with normal hearing is increasing. Five to 15% of patients with vestibular schwannoma have normal pure tone thresholds (9,12,13). Many of these tumors have been incidental findings. One report describes 10 patients with vestibular schwannoma and normal hearing thresholds (7). The most common presenting complaint among these patients was subjective hearing loss accompanied by tinnitus. Vertigo and dizziness, without any cochlear symptoms, were also frequently encountered. The average duration of hearing loss before the diagnosis of a vestibular schwannoma is approximately 4 years (9).

Given the significant variability in otologic presentation of patients with vestibular schwannomas and the relatively low incidence of vestibular schwannoma in patients with asymmetric sensorineural hearing loss, an efficient and cost-effective algorithm must be used to identify patients early in their clinical course, and to minimize false-negative workups

Tinnitus

Tinnitus associated with vestibular schwannoma is usually high pitched, continuous, and unilateral or asymmetric. However, as with hearing loss, the tinnitus also may be variable. Tinnitus is usually mild to moderate in severity and rarely incapacitating. Aside from the tendency to localize to one ear, there is nothing characteristic about the tinnitus to indicate an underlying vestibular schwannoma. The incidence of tinnitus ranges in the literature from 53% to 70% (14–17).

Vertigo

The actual perception of motion, or true vertigo, is much less common in patients with vestibular schwannoma than is disequilibrium. When present, disequilibrium tends to be mild to moderate in severity. The disequilibrium is rarely incapacitating, except in very large tumors with cerebellar and brainstem compression. The incidence of vertigo varies widely in the literature, from 18% to 58% (9,14–17). The incidence of vestibular dysfunction is a function of tumor size. Selesnick et al. demonstrated that vertigo was much more common in patients with smaller tumors, whereas disequilibrium was more prevalent in patients with larger tumors (9). They reported a 27% incidence of vertigo in patients with tumors less than 1 cm in size, as contrasted to a 19% incidence of vertigo in patients with tumors 1 to 3 cm in size. The incidence of vertigo decreased to 10% of patients with tumors greater than 3 cm in size. The incidence of disequilibrium with vestibular schwannomas less than 1 cm, tumors 1 to 3 cm, and tumors greater than 3 cm was 37%, 47%, and 71%, respectively (9). The incidence of cerebellar symptoms in the older literature ranges from 65% to 85% (14–16). More recent reports with a greater proportion of smaller tumors reflect a lower incidence of disequilibrium of 45% to 48% (9,18).

Trigeminal Nerve Dysfunction

Involvement of the trigeminal nerve may manifest as hypesthesia, paresthesia, or, rarely, anesthesia, typically in the mid-facial region. Historically, the incidence of trigeminal nerve involvement was quite common, with approximately 50% of patients manifesting symptoms of trigeminal nerve involvement, and 88% demonstrating evidences of trigeminal dysfunction on physical examination (15–17). The incidence of trigeminal nerve involvement is clearly proportional to the tumor size. Thomsen and Tos reported an incidence of trigeminal nerve involvement in 14% of patients with vestibular schwannomas less than 4 cm in size, and in 53% of patients with tumors greater than 4 cm in size (18).

Headache

In older series, headache was a common complaint of patients with vestibular schwannomas. The incidence of headache ranged from 65% to 85% (14–16). The incidence of headache in more recent studies reveals a lower incidence of 19% to 38% (9,19). The incidence of headache also is proportional to tumor size. In their series of patients with vestibular schwannomas less than 1 cm in size, Selesnick et al. reported no patients complaining of headache (9). Twenty percent of patients with tumors between 1 and 3 cm in size complained of headaches, and 43% patients with tumors greater than 3 cm in size experienced headaches.

Facial Nerve Dysfunction

Facial paresis is in general a late sequela of vestibular schwannomas. The weakness is typically gradual in onset and may be preceded by facial twitching, most commonly in the zygomatic branch distribution. Early series report a 15% incidence of symptomatic facial nerve involvement, with up to 65% of patients demonstrating subtle facial nerve involvement on physical examination (1,15,16). The incidence of facial nerve dysfunction in more recent series is significantly lower, at 10% (9,19). Sensory fibers are less resistant to the effects of compression and, consequently, manifest earlier clinically. This is the basis of Hitselberger's sign, which is a hypesthesia of the concha or external auditory canal (20,21). Hitselberger reported the presence of hypesthesia in 85% of patients with vestibular schwannomas. Another manifestation of sensory fiber dysfunction in the facial nerve is aching in the region of the mastoid. This symptom has been reported to occur in 25% of patients with vestibular schwannoma (22).

DIAGNOSTIC TESTING

Audiogram

The classic audiologic presentation of a patient with a vestibular schwannoma is a unilateral or asymmetric sensorineural hearing loss. The frequency pattern of loss is relatively nondiagnostic. Fifty-three to 66% of patients demonstrate a high-frequency sensorineural hearing loss, with most of the remainder typically manifesting a flat loss across all frequencies or profound loss (11,23–25). U-shaped or low-tone patterns of loss are less common (11,23). The severity of hearing loss is a poor indicator of tumor size (11). Deterioration of speech discrimination is typically disproportionate to the amount of threshold impairment, although the overall positive predictive value of speech discrimination remains low. Approximately 70% of patients with vestibular schwannoma have speech discrimination abilities of 60% or worse (11). Stapedial reflexes can provide additional support for a diagnosis of a cerebellopontine tumor. Absent stapedial reflex, elevated thresholds, or stapedial reflex decay are present in 75% to 98% of patients with vestibular schwannoma (11,26,27). Despite the relatively high sensitivity of acoustic reflex testing for retrocochlear disease, the test is of limited overall value because of its lack of specificity. Thomsen et al., in 1983, were unable to demonstrate a significant difference in reflex decay in patients with vestibular schwannomas, and in those patients who were being evaluated for the presence of a vestibular schwannoma but were later found to be negative (27). The most specific stapedial reflex abnormality in retrocochlear disease is absent reflexes across all frequencies (11,28).

Electronystagmography

Vestibular testing with electronystagmography (ENG) is in general a sensitive test for demonstrating vestibular disease in patients with retrocochlear lesions, but it lacks specificity and is of questionable value. One use of ENG is to determine whether the inferior or superior vestibular nerve is the site of origin for the vestibular schwannoma. This information is useful when approaching an intracanalicular tumor with a goal of hearing preservation. Caloric testing reveals the status of the horizontal semicircular canal and the superior vestibular nerve. Consequently, normal caloric testing results suggest that the inferior vestibular nerve is the site of origin. An abnormal caloric test result is less useful because, even if the tumor originates in the inferior vestibular nerve, the tumor compression of the superior vestibular nerve within the internal auditory canal may still yield an abnormal test result. If the ENG reveals a normal caloric, suggesting an inferior vestibular nerve site of origin, some surgeons prefer to approach these tumors through a suboccipital, as opposed to a middle cranial fossa, approach because of the position of the tumor relative to the facial nerve. Odkvist reviewed the ENG results of 78 patients with vestibular schwannomas (29). Fifty-eight percent manifested spontaneous nystagmus; 43% had positional nystagmus and 88% demonstrated caloric asymmetry (29).

Auditory Brainstem Response

Auditory brainstem response testing (ABR) has been an effective screening tool for retrocochlear lesions since the late 1970s. It is a sensitive test for retrocochlear disease, with a sensitivity of 90% to 100% (11,30–33). ABR is an excellent test to identify larger vestibular schwannomas but is less effective in demonstrating intracanalicular tumors or CPA meningiomas. The sensitivity of ABR in detecting small intracanalicular tumors drops to 63% to 67% (34,35). Another limitation of the ABR is detecting nonacoustic CPA tumors. The false-negative rate is 25% with CPA meningiomas. The specificity of ABR testing ranges from 54% to 78% (33,36,37). Because of the relatively low incidence of vestibular schwannomas, the probability of vestibular schwannoma in a patient with an abnormal ABR result is only 4% to 18% (33,38,39).

Cerebellopontine Angle Imaging

Before the availability of gadolinium-enhanced MRI, computed tomography (CT) scanning with air contrast cisternography was the gold standard for the diagnosis of CPA tumors. Contrast-enhanced CT scanning is a relatively sensitive test for CPA tumors. The region of lower sensitivity is small intracanalicular tumors; air cisternography is often required to identify these more occult lesions. However, the morbidity of adding air cisternography is quite high (40,41). Smith et al. report that 80% of patients are symptomatic after the procedure, and 62% require 3 or more days to return to normal health (41).

Today, MRI of the internal auditory canal and CPA with T1-weighted gadolinium enhancement has replaced the CT scan with air contrast cisternography as the gold standard in the diagnosis of vestibular schwannomas. MRI often demonstrates lesions for which conventional assessment provided ambiguous or negative results (42). MRI is also helpful in differentiating vestibular schwannomas from meningiomas (43). Meningiomas are typically sessile with a broad contact against the petrous apex, which is contrasted to the globular shape of vestibular schwannomas. Meningiomas may demonstrate hyperostosis of adjacent bone and may contain areas of calcification. Meningiomas are often eccentric to the internal auditory canal and are less likely to erode the internal auditory canal (43). A "dural tail" is often associated with meningioma but is not pathognomonic in that these dural tails have also been reported to occur with vestibular schwannomas (44,45). MRI, using a T2-weighted, fast spin-echo protocol, significantly improves the spatial resolution of the internal auditory canal and CPA. This technique has been advocated as a first-line investigation to rule out vestibular schwannomas without the need for gadolinium enhancement (46). When an equivocal T2-weighted, fast spin-echo image is obtained, the recommendation is to proceed with a T1-weighted, gadolinium-enhanced axial sequence.

Summary of Evaluation Algorithm

Patients presenting with a history of explained unilateral or asymmetric sensorineural hearing loss, sudden sensorineural hearing loss, or unexplained, persistent, unilateral tinnitus are evaluated directly with MRI. The imaging includes a gadolinium-enhanced, T1-weighted sequence and a T2-weighted, fast spin-echo sequence. ENG, ABR, electrocochleography, and audiologic site of lesion testing are not performed. Low-risk patients with mild asymmetric hearing or with a reasonable explanation for the hearing loss or tinnitus are evaluated either with an ABR or a screening T2-weighted, fast spin-echo MRI. This screening MRI can be performed at a cost similar to that of an ABR.

Patients in whom MRI cannot be obtained because of morbid obesity or retained magnetic metal are evaluated with ABR and, if abnormal, a contrast-enhanced CT scan is obtained. Air cisternography can be performed if there is a high index of suspicion and the initial CT scan does not reveal a CPA tumor.

TREATMENT OPTIONS

The treatment options for CPA tumors include surgical resection, radiation therapy, and, in elderly or high–surgical-risk patients, observation with sequential MRI.

Observation with sequential MRI is considered in patients with a vestibular schwannoma in an only hearing ear and in patients with advanced age and limited life expectancy, or significant cardiovascular, pulmonary, or other systemic disease. For such patients, the nonsurgical option of watchful waiting is a viable alternative.

A 1994 study reviewed the natural history of vestibular schwannomas in 51 patients with unilateral vestibular schwannomas who were followed by serial scanning for an average of 2.6 years (range, 0.5–11 years) (47). Thirty-nine patients (78% of the study group) demonstrated slow tumor growth rates of less than 0.2 cm per year. Of these, 16 had no growth of their tumor during the study period. One patient in the slow-growth group showed no change in tumor size for 6 years; however, the tumor then doubled in size over a 2-year period. This was the only exception to the observation that if tumor growth was demonstrated to be slow at the beginning of the study, it remained slow. Twelve patients (24%) eventually required microsurgical or radiosurgical treatment. This study suggests that up to 75% of patients who are poor surgical candidates may be successfully treated with watchful waiting. Because the follow-up period was short (an average of 2.6 years), it is recommended that MRI scans be performed 6 and 12 months after diagnosis, and then yearly, if a pattern of slow growth is established.

Since the late 1980s, there has been a surge of interest in stereotactic radiation therapy for the treatment of vestibular schwannomas. The therapy uses a focused beam of radiation to kill tumor cells while attempting to preserve the adjacent structures. Radiosurgery avoids much of the morbidity such as prolonged hospitalization, loss of productivity, cerebrospinal fluid (CSF) leaks, and wound infections associated with surgical resection of vestibular schwannomas. However, the structures adjacent to the tumors do not escape free of injury. Facial nerve paresis or complete paralysis occurs in 10% to 32% of patients, and maintenance of useful preoperative hearing is reported to occur in 50% of patients (48–52). Facial numbness occurs in 19% to 34% of patients. Other cranial nerve deficits are uncommon. Hydrocephalus requiring shunt placement occurs in 3%. It is interesting to note that the status of the hearing continues to change up to 2 years after radiosurgery. Initial hearing preservation rates are excellent, but by 2 years have dropped to 50%. The effects on neural tissue, vasculature, and presumably also on the tumor, are slowly progressive, and extended follow-up periods are necessary to evaluate long-term results. These results compare favorably with perioperative complication rates for microsurgery. There is a trend toward decreasing the radiation dose to decrease morbidity (51,53). Once again, long-term tumor control rates are not available.

The reluctance to support radiation therapy for a wide range of patients stems from the uncertainty regarding long-term tumor control. The longest available follow-up suggests a recurrence rate of approximately 17% (48). There is also the disturbing experience that when surgical excision is required postradiation because of continued tumor growth, there is an increased severity of postoperative deficits (54)

Selection of Surgical Approach

The choice of approach to resection of vestibular schwannomas and other CPA tumors is guided by the degree of residual hearing, hearing status in the contralateral ear, location of the tumor, size of the tumor, cell type, and age of the patient.

The first factor considered is the status of the patient's hearing. In choosing a hearing conservation approach (i.e., middle cranial fossa or retrosigmoid), the authors usually adhere to the 50:50 rule: less than 50 dB pure tone thresholds and better than 50% discrimination. The lack of consistency on the definition of useful hearing and the variability of the subjective appreciation of various levels of hearing loss by patients lead to controversy in applying this definition of useful hearing in the selection of approach. Patients with good hearing in the contralateral ear and less than 50% discrimination in the affected ear do not wear a hearing aid on the affected side because of the distortion. In addition, they do not maintain the ability to localize sound with greater than a 30-dB asymmetry between the two ears. Another factor on the audiogram that should be taken into account is the degree of "roll-over," which is common with these retrocochlear lesions. Roll-over is the phenomenon of diminished discrimination with increased sound intensity. Therefore, if a patient has a 40-dB hearing loss with 60% discrimination and severe roll-over, once adequately amplified, his or her discrimination will significantly deteriorate. The patient will be left with unusable hearing. There are clear exceptions to application of the 50:50 rule. In patients with poor hearing in the contralateral ear or neurofibromatosis, in which bilateral disease is common, every effort is made to preserve any residual cochlear function.

The second factor in choosing an approach is the location of the tumor. If the tumor extends into the lateral one third of the internal auditory canal and does not protrude greater than 0.5 cm into the CPA, and hearing conservation is indicated, the authors choose a middle fossa approach. The retrosigmoid approach can safely access only the medial two thirds of the internal auditory canal without damaging the labyrinth. Blevins and Jackler demonstrated that in the typical surgical exposure using a retrosigmoid approach, an average of 3.0 mm (range, 1.1–5.3 mm) must be left unexposed to avoid injury to the labyrinth (55). If the tumor is more medial in the internal auditory canal, either the middle fossa or retrosigmoid approach is appropriate. In tumors extending greater than 5 mm into the CPA and if hearing conservation is indicated, the retrosigmoid approach is used. Some authors advocate an extended middle fossa approach for tumors extending greater than 1 cm into the CPA (56–58). They use a wider resection of the petrous ridge and division of the superior petrosal sinus, yielding a modest exposure of the CPA. Jackler and Pitts point out that this approach for larger tumors provides insufficient exposure of the inferior aspect of the CPA and requires vigorous and prolonged temporal lobe retraction, increasing the potential for postoperative neurologic deficits (59). Consequently, the current authors limit their use of this approach to tumors protruding less than 5 mm into the CPA.

The third factor to be considered is the tumor size. Large tumors can be accessed by either the retrosigmoid or translabyrinthine approach. The decision on approach for vestibular schwannomas greater than 2.5 cm no longer takes into account attempts at hearing preservation, given the very poor prognosis for hearing conservation, unless it is an only hearing ear. In patients with contracted mastoid cavities, high jugular bulbs, or a history of chronic otitis media, the retrosigmoid approach is chosen. In large tumors with significant inferior extension, the retrosigmoid approach is also preferred. In the absence of these factors, the translabyrinthine approach is used. The translabyrinthine approach is also used in patients with smaller tumors and no salvageable hearing.

Vestibular schwannomas account for 85% to 95% of CPA tumors. However, when a CPA tumor of other origin is suspected on the preoperative evaluation, the surgical algorithm is modified. Preservation of useful hearing with vestibular schwannomas greater than 2 cm is rare, whereas with larger meningiomas and epidermoids, preservation of auditory function can occasionally be achieved. Consequently, tumors other than vestibular schwannomas are accessed by a retrosigmoid approach.

Another factor guiding the management of vestibular

schwannomas is the patient's age. In general, the middle fossa approach is avoided in patients older than 60 years of age because of the more tenuous nature of the temporal lobe dura. Elderly patients are placed at increased risk of temporal lobe injury as well as postoperative CSF fistula with the middle fossa approach. In general, elderly patients are not treated surgically or with stereotaxic radiosurgery unless the tumors are demonstrated with sequential MRI scans to be growing at a rate significant enough to interfere with the patient's projected longevity. The translabyrinthine approach is the preferred procedure in the elderly patient.

The indications for the use of stereotaxic radiosurgery remain controversial. The authors' current indications for stereotaxic radiosurgery are limited to patients who are poor surgical candidates because of underlying medical conditions. As newer protocols yield improved tumor control and reduced cranial nerve involvement, and longer-term follow-up data become available, the indications for the use of stereotaxic radiosurgery may broaden significantly.

The differences in complication rates between the various approaches also influence the choice of procedure. Informed patient input and choice of approach can only take place after a thorough discussion of the complication rates.

Complications

The surgical mortality rate before the popularization of microsurgical technique in vestibular schwannoma resection by William House was 10% to 20%. Current techniques have lowered the mortality rate to 1% to 2%. The occurrence of severe complications resulting in mortality is influenced by factors such as tumor size and complexity, patient age, and underlying medical conditions, as opposed to the surgical approach (59). With the significant reduction in mortality, much more attention has been focused on the differential morbidity from the different approaches.

Facial paralysis is one of the most dreaded of the complications from the patient's perspective. The incidence of this disfiguring complication has dropped significantly with the onset of facial nerve monitoring (60–63). Comparing results from various centers using the different approaches has been hampered by the lack of standardization in evaluation of postoperative facial function. The House-Brackmann grading system is an excellent attempt at standardization; however, subjective variations between centers interfere with the effectiveness of this tool (64). Most large series report a 95% or greater postoperative anatomic preservation of the facial nerve regardless of the surgical approach. The percentage of patients with House-Brackmann grade I or II facial function, 1 year after surgery, ranges from 70% to 90%. These statistics are easily skewed by the percentage of large tumors in the series. The incidence of normal function decreases with tumor size (65). It has been argued that the translabyrinthine approach can improve facial nerve preservation because the nerve is identified before tumor dissection. However, empirically, there is no apparent difference in long-term facial nerve outcomes using the different approaches (63).

Cerebrospinal Fluid Fistula

The incidence of CSF fistula varies considerably throughout the literature and has decreased since the late 1970s with the improvements in closure techniques. There does not appear to be a significant difference in the incidences of CSF fistula between the retrosigmoid and translabyrinthine approaches reported since the late 1970s. However, this remains controversial, with advocates of both approaches arguing lower rates of CSF fistula. The incidence of CSF fistula after the retrosigmoid and translabyrinthine approaches ranges from 7% to 21% (66–72). CSF fistula occurs significantly less frequently with the middle cranial fossa approach, with a rate of 4% to 6% (73,74).

Two thirds of CSF fistulas close with medical management and lumbar drains without the need for surgical intervention (75,76). Medical management consists of bed rest, elevation of the head of the bed 30 degrees, and stool softeners. Pressure dressings are reapplied to patients with CSF leaks after translabyrinthine approaches and to patients with CSF collections below the skin flap after any of the approaches. Lumbar drains are typically left in place for 5 days. Fistulas persisting for greater than 7 to 10 days are reexplored and the fistula closed. There is no difference in the incidences of persistent fistula requiring surgical closure after a translabyrinthine or retrosigmoid approach (77).

Various modifications of the standard approaches have effectively reduced the frequency of postoperative fistula. Removal of the ear canal and tympanic membrane, as performed in the transotic approach described by Fisch, allows for excellent exposure of the eustachian tube. Using this exposure, the middle ear mucosa is removed, the eustachian tube mucosa is inverted, and the orifice of the eustachian tube is securely sealed. This modification has been reported to decrease the incidence of CSF fistula to as low as 2% (78). The authors include this additional step in their translabyrinthine approach.

The frequency of CSF fistula can be diminished by careful inspection of the temporal bone for exposed air cells. Symon and Pell reported a reduction in the incidence of CSF fistula from 16% to 5% by packing air cells with bone dust and Surgicel soaked with fibrin glue (79). Sealing of air cells with ionomeric bone cement has also been reported to reduce significantly the incidence of CSF fistula (80). Regardless of whether bone wax or one of these other materials is used to seal the exposed air cells, the key factor in minimizing postoperative CSF fistula is the identification of exposed air cells. The angle of view, using the operating microscope, frequently misses exposed air cells with the retrosigmoid approach. Improved detection and sealing of these air cells can be achieved using 30-degree endoscopes, thereby reducing the incidence of postoperative CSF fistula.

Headache

Persistent, severe, postoperative headache occurs more frequently after vestibular schwannoma removal using the retrosigmoid approach. Harner et al. reported postoperative headache in 23% of patients at 3 months, 16% at 1 year, and 9% at 2 years (81). One of the factors that contributes to the pathophysiology of postoperative headache is the resection of the bone window. The absent bone window allows adhesions to develop between the dura and the prior muscle attachments to the skull base. This potential relationship to postoperative headache has been addressed by replacing the bone window with bone chips, methylmethacrylate, calcium phosphate cement, or other synthetic materials (82–84). Harner et al. reduced their incidence of postoperative headache from 17% to 4% by performing a methylmethacrylate cranioplasty (84).

TRANSLABYRINTHINE APPROACH

Removal of vestibular schwannomas by a translabyrinthine approach was developed and popularized by William House in the early 1960s (3). This technique has grown in acceptance because of its many advantages. The main advantage is excellent access to the CPA without retraction of the cerebellum. The translabyrinthine approach provides easy identification of the facial nerve in a constant location before tumor dissection. The approach minimizes the risk of recurrence of tumor as a result of residual tumor in the lateral aspect of the internal auditory canal. Using the current techniques of eustachian tube ablation, the risk of CSF fistula is less than with the retrosigmoid approach. One of the most significant advantages of the translabyrinthine approach is the reduction of postoperative headache, as discussed previously. The obvious disadvantage of the translabyrinthine approach is the obligate sacrifice of hearing. Other limitations of the approach include the reduced exposure in patients with a high jugular bulb or significantly contracted mastoid air cell system.

Preparation

At the outset of the procedure, the MRI scan is hung in the view box and the name of the patient and the site of the lesion are verified. Perioperative antibiotics are not routinely administered. Dexamethasone 0.1 mg/kg body weight is administered intravenously every 8 hours for 48 hours, with the first dose given before surgery. General anesthesia is induced and maintained by tracheal intubation after the administration of a short-acting muscle relaxant. No further muscle relaxants are used for the remainder of the procedure. The patient is placed supine on the operating table with the head turned away from the surgeon approximately 45 degrees. The patient's head is placed in Mayfield tongs with the neck slightly extended. The patient's hair is shaved 3 cm above the auricle and 6 cm posteriorly. The ear canal is injected with 2 ml of 1% lidocaine with epinephrine (1:100,000) in a four-quadrant block. The ear is also injected postauricularly. Two monopolar electromyography needle electrodes are inserted into the orbicularis oris and a second set into the orbicularis oculi. A fifth electrode is placed in the skin over the sternum as a ground. The electrodes are secured with tape. The left lower quadrant of the abdomen or the periumbilical area is prepared and draped for harvesting of the abdominal fat graft. If prior abdominal scars are available, these may be used instead. The entire postauricular region, auricle, external auditory canal, and preauricular skin is cleaned with a standard povidone–iodine preparation. This is followed by the application of benzoin, which is allowed to dry. In addition to the normal draping, an Iodoban plastic drape is used to cover the entire surgical field.

Procedure

A curved postauricular incision is made from the mastoid tip up to a point 1 cm above the auricle. Posteriorly, the incision is placed 3 cm posterior to the postauricular crease (Fig. 1). The incision is carried down through the skin and subcutaneous tissue, but not through the periosteum overlying the mastoid cortex. The postauricular skin flap is elevated forward up to the skin of the external auditory canal. An incision is made through the periosteum 2 cm posteriorly along the inferior temporal line. A second incision 1.5 cm inferior to the inferior temporal line is created parallel to this initial incision. The two parallel incisions are connected posteriorly with a perpendicular incision, creating an anteriorly pedicled periosteal flap attached to the external auditory canal (see Fig. 1). The periosteal flap is elevated up to the external auditory canal. The external auditory canal is then transected medial to the attachment of the periosteal flap (Fig. 2). After sectioning of the anterior canal wall, the plane of dissection is carried laterally between the parotid gland and the cartilaginous canal. The auricle is reflected anteriorly. The skin of the lateral portion of the external auditory canal is dissected off of the cartilage and everted out of the external auditory canal. The cartilage is then excised. The excess canal skin is excised and the remaining skin closed with 3-0 Vicryl suture. The second layer of closure is provided by the periosteal flap, which is reflected medial to the external auditory canal and sutured anterior, inferior, and superior to the opening into the canal (see Fig. 2). A moist sponge is placed

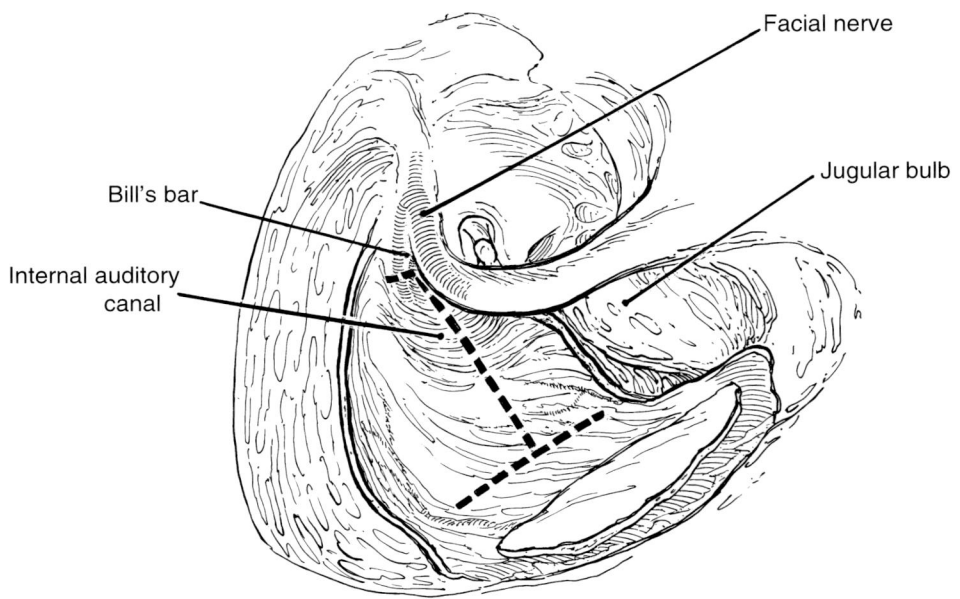

FIG. 8. After exposure of the posterior fossa dura and complete removal of the bone covering the skeletonized portion of the internal auditory canal, dural incisions are created. At the lateral aspect of the internal auditory canal, the facial nerve is separated from the superior vestibular nerve by the vertical crest, or "Bill's bar."

been completed, to minimize inadvertent injury to the underlying structures. The distal portion of the internal auditory canal is skeletonized as it projects laterally.

The final area of bony dissection is superior to the lateral portion of the internal auditory canal in the region of the intralabyrinthine portion of the facial nerve. The facial nerve exits the lateral portion of the internal auditory canal superior and slightly anterior to the superior vestibular nerve. The two nerves are separated by a bony septum, the vertical crest or "Bill's bar" (Fig. 8). It is at this point that the facial nerve enters the intralabyrinthine portion of the fallopian canal, the narrowest section of the pathway. To decrease the incidence of delayed postoperative facial paresis, this intralabyrinthine portion of the facial nerve is decompressed.

The remaining eggshell of bone covering the dura between the lateral sinus and porus acusticus is removed with a Duckbill elevator. To facilitate removal of bone covering the dura between the sinus and porus acusticus, the lateral sinus is gently compressed. This maneuver improves the exposure for drilling and also increases the anteroposterior dimension of the eventual window to the CPA. A Greenberg retractor is occasionally used to aid in the retraction. The bone covering the posterior fossa dura anterior to the lateral sinus is removed superiorly up until the superior petrosal sinus. An eggshell sheet of bone is left intact over the middle fossa dura. If additional superior exposure is required, this remaining sheet of tegmen can be removed and the temporal lobe dura retracted superiorly. All of the remaining bone covering the posterior 210 degrees of the internal auditory canal is elevated off the dura and removed. The entire wound and mastoid cavity are thoroughly irrigated with bacitracin solution to decrease the risk of postoperative infection and minimize subsequent CSF contamination with bone dust.

An incision is made in the dura extending from the sigmoid sinus to the porus acusticus with Jacobson scissors (see Fig. 8). The dura is elevated with a sharp hook to minimize the risk of injury to an underlying vessel. The undersurface of the dura is inspected as the dura is cut to avoid injury to any underlying vascular structures. The edges of the dura are cauterized using bipolar cautery. The dura is quite thick in the region around the porus acusticus, and these fibers are also severed.

The facial nerve is most easily identified in a relatively constant location in the intralabyrinthine segment of the fallopian canal. Verification of the position of the facial nerve is aided by stimulation of the nerve with the nerve probe set at 0.05 mA. Stimulation at this point in the procedure also verifies that the facial nerve monitor system is functioning properly. Once the facial nerve is clearly delineated, the superior vestibular nerve is sharply dissected away from the facial nerve with a tab or sickle knife. The tumor in the internal auditory canal is dissected off the facial nerve (Fig. 9). Typically, the facial nerve splays out anterior to the tumor as it is reflected anteriorly around the anterior lip of the porus acusticus. Adhesions to the nerve are dissected sharply with a round knife or scissors. Bipolar cautery is minimized in

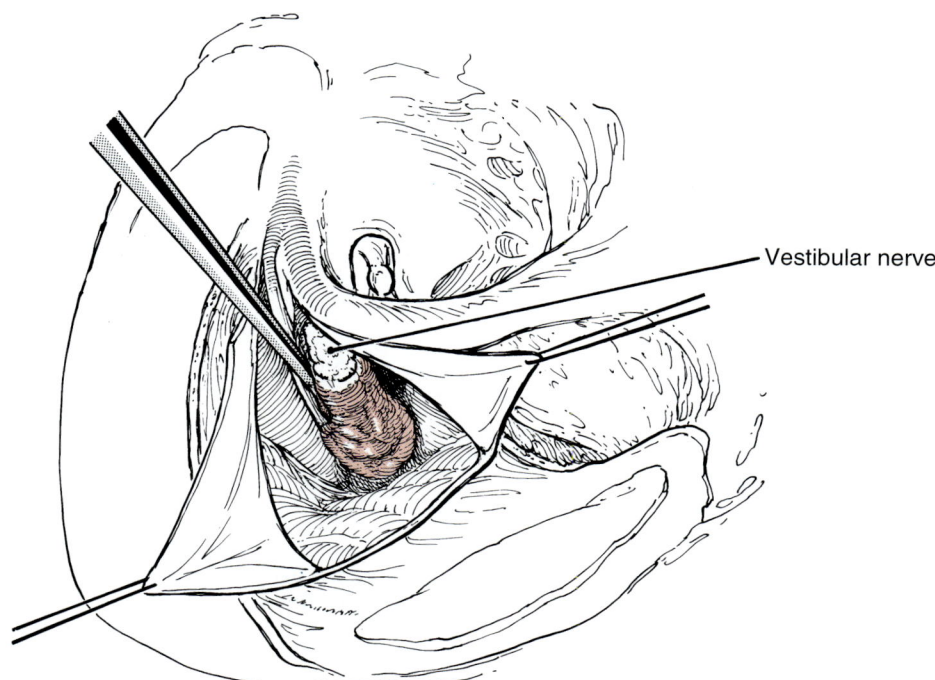

FIG. 9. The vestibular schwannoma is visualized within the internal auditory canal extending into the cerebellopontine angle. The distal free end of the vestibular nerve and tumor are dissected out of the internal auditory canal and off of the facial nerve.

controlling hemorrhage adjacent to the nerve; cottonoids or epinephrine-soaked Gelfoam is the first-line method for hemostasis adjacent to the nerve. Moist cottonoids are placed over the cerebellum. Once the tumor in the internal auditory canal is separated from the facial nerve, a piece is sent to pathology for frozen-section examination. The centers of small tumors are debulked with forceps, bipolar cautery, and suction. In larger tumors, intracapsular debulking is accomplished with the addition of the Cavitron ultrasonic aspirator. In larger tumors, additional exposure may be required in the CPA. This can be achieved with gentle retraction of the cerebellum posteriorly 1 to 2 cm. Retraction of the cerebellum can be minimized by draining CSF from the cisterna magna as well as by the infusion of intravenous mannitol. If CSF does not flow readily from the CPA after incision of the overlying dura, the inferior aspect of the cerebellum is elevated and the arachnoid over the cisterna magna is incised.

Once most of the intracapsular tumor mass is debulked, the tumor capsule is dissected off the remainder of the course of the facial nerve and brainstem. Small penetrating branches of the anterior internal carotid artery are cauterized with the bipolar cautery in the capsule of the tumor and incised with microscissors. Vessels coursing over the capsule, but not penetrating, are dissected free. A loop of anterior inferior cerebellar artery usually courses between cranial nerves VII and VIII. Cranial nerve VIII is identified and cauterized with bipolar cautery as it exits the tumor. The nerve is severed with microscissors. At the conclusion of the resection, cranial nerves V, VII, VIII, IX, X, and XI usually are visualized (Fig. 10).

Closure

The mucosa of the middle ear and protympanum is removed. The mucosa, lining the eustachian tube, is inverted as distally as possible. A small piece of temporalis muscle is harvested and inserted into the eustachian tube, filling the entire lumen. The long process of the incus is snipped and the incus is inserted into the eustachian tube, wedging it into place. A small piece of temporalis fascia is then placed over the incus and eustachian tube. The flaps of posterior fossa dura are reapproximated and a large piece of temporalis fascia is placed over the dura and draped over the facial nerve as it proceeds laterally in the internal auditory canal. The abdominal fat graft is trimmed to fill the entire mastoid cavity and middle ear cleft. The cavity should be mildly overpacked.

The mastoid periosteum is sutured with 3-0 Vicryl suture, forming a watertight closure. The skin is closed with 4-0 nylon suture. No drains are used for the mastoid wound. A pressure dressing is applied and left in place for 5 days. The abdominal fat graft site is closed with a deep closure of interrupted 3-0 Vicryl suture and a 4-0 nylon suture skin closure. The abdominal wound is drained with a Penrose drain and a pressure dressing applied.

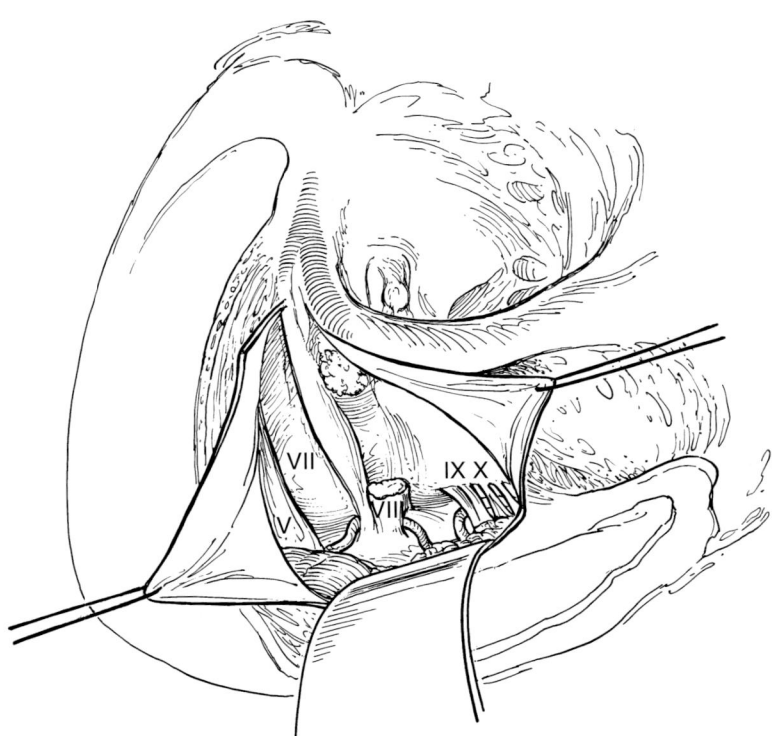

FIG. 10. The vestibular schwannoma has been resected. The facial nerve is visualized extending from the brainstem into the intralabyrinthine portion of the fallopian canal. The vestibular nerves have been resected with the tumor and the lower cranial nerves are visualized entering the jugular foramen.

Postoperative Care

Overnight, the patient is monitored in the intensive care unit and typically transferred out of intensive care on the first postoperative day. The patient is maintained on dexamethasone (0.1 mg/kg body weight) for 48 hours after surgery. Perioperative antibiotics are not routinely administered. The patient is maintained on Colace to minimize straining with bowel movements. A combination of metoclopramide and droperidol or ondansetron is used for nausea. Diazepam is used to control vertigo on a PRN basis. The head of the bed is elevated 30 degrees at all times. The physical therapist trained in techniques of vestibular rehabilitation begins working with the patient before discharge from the hospital and continues therapy after discharge as needed. If a patient has a postoperative facial palsy, an eye humidification chamber is applied. Lacrilube eye ointment is used at night and Celluvisc eye drops are applied every 2 hours while awake. This regimen continues at home until the facial palsy has resolved.

TRANSOTIC APPROACH

The initial exposure for the transotic approach, as described by Fisch, includes resection and two-layer closure of the external auditory canal, resection of the tympanic membrane and ossicles, and enclosure of the eustachian tube. The authors use this initial exposure in the translabyrinthine approach as well, to reduce the incidence of postoperative CSF fistula. This portion of the technique is described in the previous section. The transotic approach is an extension beyond the translabyrinthine technique. The entire translabyrinthine approach is completed before the transotic portion. The additional exposure of the transotic approach is achieved by drilling through the cochlea, skeletonizing the external auditory canal anteriorly. The bone between the external auditory canal posteriorly and the carotid artery anteriorly is removed with a cutting bur, followed by a coarse diamond bur (Fig. 11). The hypotympanic bone superior to the jugular bulb and posterior to the carotid artery is removed. Additional bone removal in the region of the retrofacial air cell track results in a bridge of suspended bone encasing the descending portion of the facial nerve (see Fig. 11). As in all of the approaches, the direction of bur rotation is away from the facial nerve to avoid inadvertent injury to the nerve. The dura is not incised until all of the bony work is completed and the bony cavity is copiously irrigated with bacitracin solution. The thin eggshell of bone covering the internal auditory canal is removed with a microraspatory or small round knife. An incision in the dura is created to extend from anterior to the sigmoid sinus through the posterior ring of fibrous tissue of the porus acusticus, as was described for the translabyrinthine approach. In addition, the fibrous ring of the porus acusticus is severed anteriorly and the dura is cut anteroinferior to the internal auditory canal. The dural edges are reflected and secured with 4-0 silk sutures.

This technique allows 300 degrees of exposure of the internal auditory canal. The anterosuperior wall of the internal auditory canal is the only segment to remain. Dissection anterior to the internal auditory canal allows for visualization of the facial nerve as it is splayed anteriorly before entering

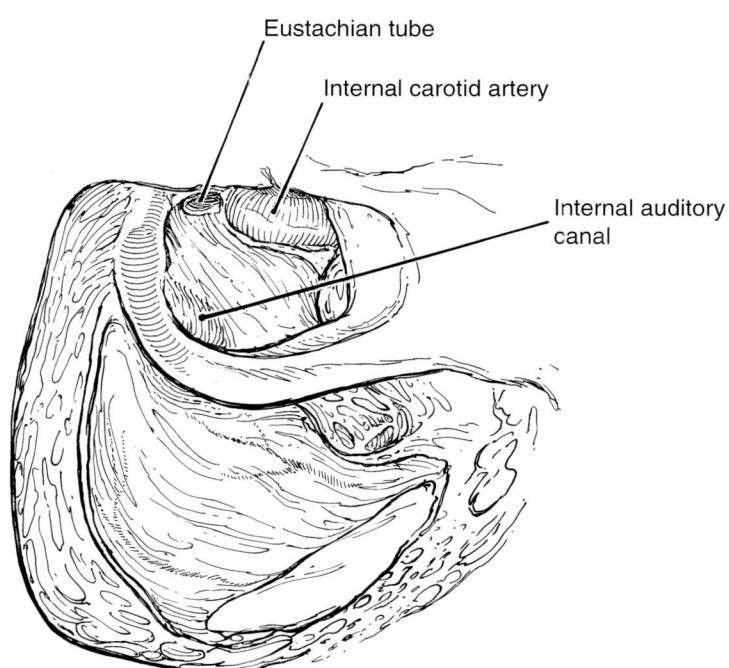

FIG. 11. The cochlea is removed, skeletonizing the internal carotid artery anteriorly, the jugular bulb inferiorly, and the internal auditory canal posteriorly and superiorly. Only a thin sheet of bone remains over the facial nerve to protect it from the shaft of the bur. The internal auditory canal is skeletonized 300 degrees around the circumference of the internal auditory canal, leaving only a small segment of bone in the anterosuperior wall of the internal auditory canal.

the porus acusticus. Tumor dissection is performed in a way similar to the technique described for the translabyrinthine approach. The technique differs in the increased exposure anteriorly and the visualization of the facial nerve as it is splayed over the anterior capsule of the tumor.

After completion of tumor removal, the facial nerve is stimulated at the brainstem. If good stimulation occurs with 0.05 mA, the prognosis for normal postoperative facial function is excellent.

Closure for the transotic approach is the same as that used for the translabyrinthine approach. A large piece of temporalis fascia is placed over the exposed area of dura and dural defect. A second, smaller piece of fascia is placed anterior to the facial nerve over the dural defect. After inversion of the eustachian tube mucosa into the eustachian tube, muscle is inserted into the orifice. The muscle is wedged in place with the modified incus. A third piece of temporalis fascia is then placed over the protympanum, covering the eustachian tube orifice. An abdominal fat graft is divided into two pieces. The first piece is wedged firmly under the bony canal of the facial nerve and used to obliterate the medial portion of the mastoid cavity. The second piece of abdominal fat is then placed lateral to the first graft and obliterates the remainder of the cavity. Again, the cavity is slightly overfilled to minimize dead space and potential CSF leakage into the cavity. The skin is closed in two layers and a pressure dressing is applied for 5 days.

RETROSIGMOID APPROACH

The retrosigmoid approach to the posterior cranial fossa is the latest of numerous modifications of the classic suboccipital approach originally popularized by Harvey Cushing (1).

The approach was modified by Dandy in 1941, with a significant reduction in mortality and morbidity (85). The approach traditionally used a sitting position and a large bone window extending from the midline to the sigmoid sinus, and necessitated partial cerebellar resection. With the advent of the operating microscope and accompanying improvement in microsurgical technique, improved results were obtainable with less morbidity and smaller craniotomies. The suboccipital approach is augmented by the "transmeatal" opening of the internal auditory canal to gain access to the intracanalicular portion of the tumor. In some temporal bones, the anatomic configuration of the labyrinth and canal makes it impossible to expose the most lateral portion of the tumor without entering the labyrinth (55). Failure to access and resect tumor in the lateral aspect of the internal auditory canal may result in recurrent tumor.

Preparation

The preparation for the retrosigmoid approach is similar to that described for the translabyrinthine approach. At the outset of the procedure, the MRI scan is hung in the view box and the name of the patient and the site of the lesion are verified. Perioperative antibiotics are not routinely administered. Dexamethasone 0.1 mg/kg body weight is administered intravenously every 8 hours for 48 hours, with the first dose given before surgery. General anesthesia is induced and maintained by tracheal intubation after the administration of a short-acting muscle relaxant. No further muscle relaxants are used for the remainder of the procedure.

The first important step in the suboccipital approach is surgical positioning, because an oblique line of sight from a

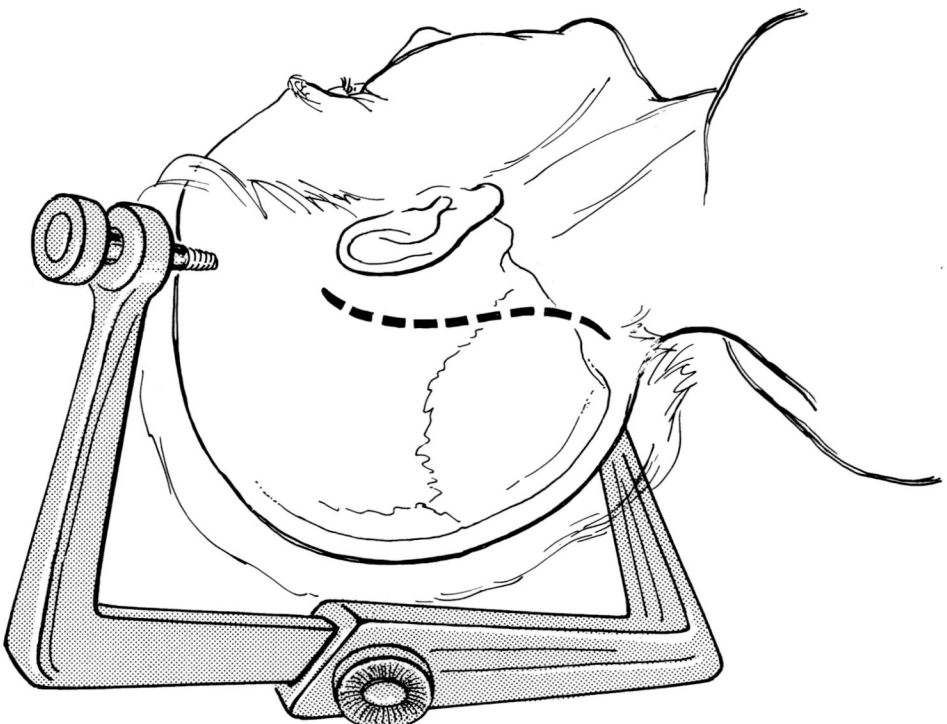

FIG. 12. The patient is placed in the three-quarters lateral position with the head placed in Mayfield tongs. A "lazy-S" incision is created four fingerbreadths behind the postauricular crease.

posterior lateral viewpoint is necessary for adequate exposure of the CPA. The patient is placed in the three-quarters lateral, or park bench position, with the head in pinions (Fig. 12). Care is taken to cushion and support the upper leg and arm to prevent pressure sores. A roll is placed under the dependent axilla, and an eggcrate or similar mattress pad is suggested. The patient should be firmly secured to the table so that it may be rotated toward and away from the surgeon. This is achieved with straps across the shoulders, hips, and legs. The shoulder is gently depressed using tape extending from the shoulder to the foot of the bed. The Mayfield head rest with pinions is engaged with the dual pins placed on the occiput, and the single pin on the forehead. The spine is maintained in a straight line; there is no lateral twisting of the head. A 4-cm rim of hair is shaved above and behind the ear. The facial and auditory function monitors are then positioned, before sterile preparation.

Procedure

The surgical incision is a "lazy-S" configuration four fingerbreadths behind the postauricular crease, extending below the bony occiput into the upper neck (see Fig. 12). After the subcutaneous layer has been divided, a small amount of undermining is performed, in anticipation of a two-layer closure (Fig. 13). The insertions of the neck musculature are freed from the skull with electrocautery and reflected inferiorly. Dissection proceeds onto the inferior surface of the occiput; the periosteum is elevated off the lateral mastoid and occiput, along with the muscular attachments. Self-retaining retractors are inserted, one in the skin, and one in the muscular layer.

A craniotomy is then created with the sigmoid sinus as its anterior border and the transverse sinus as its superior border, measuring approximately 4 × 4 cm in extent (Fig. 14). Either a craniotomy or craniectomy may be performed. If a craniotome is used to create a bone flap, it is still prudent to use a bur when removing bone over the sigmoid sinus (Fig. 15). This allows careful dissection of the delicate dural sinus and emissary vein with less risk of bleeding, and easier exposure when bleeding occurs. Mastoid air cells are usually encountered lateral or anterior to the sigmoid sinus. They should not be avoided because of a concern over CSF leak, because the sinus must be well exposed to gain adequate anterior exposure. The air cells are occluded with bone wax at the end of the procedure. Once the bone has been removed, the dura is opened. The dural incision forms an anteriorly pedicled dural flap (Fig. 16). The corners of the dural flaps are retracted with silk stitches. A moist cottonoid pledget is placed over the cerebellum and a flat blade retractor is used gently to retract the cerebellum. The arachnoid tissue is incised and decompression of the posterior fossa is achieved at the cisterna magna inferiorly or at the CPA cistern. CSF is

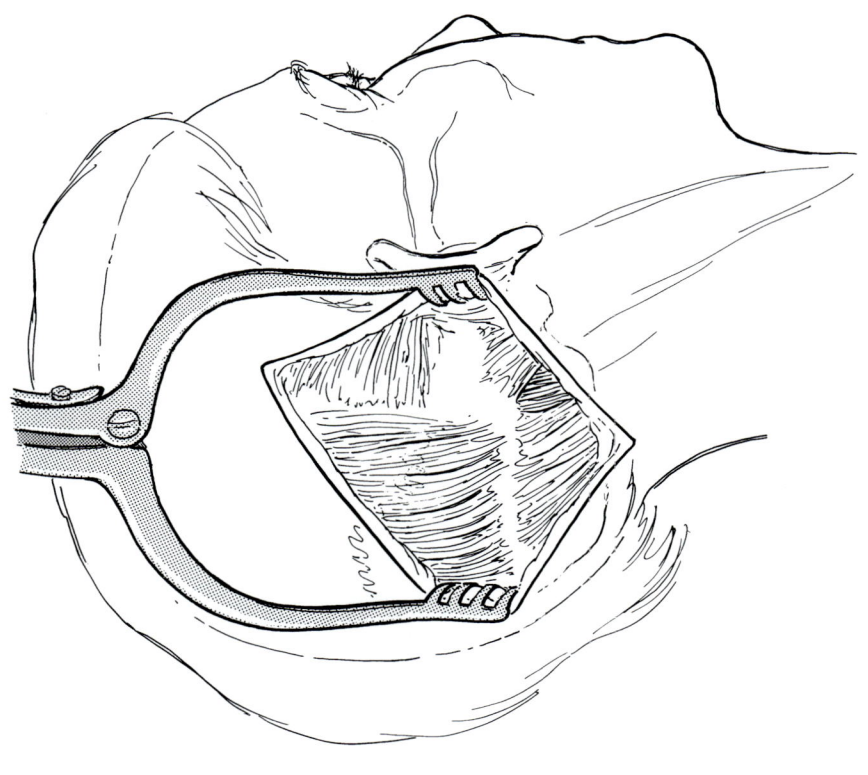

FIG. 13. The skin and subcutaneous tissue flaps are elevated and retracted with a self-retaining retractor.

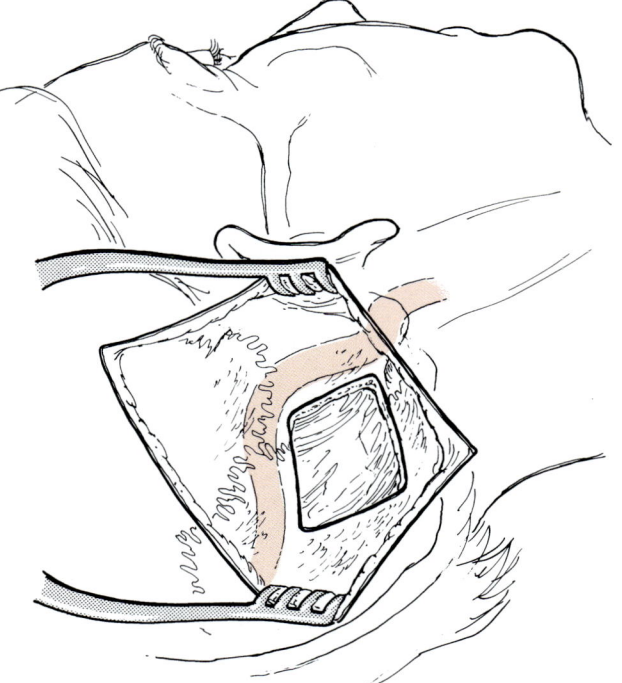

FIG. 14. A 4 × 4 cm craniotomy is created with the sigmoid sinus as the anterior border and the transverse sinus as the superior border.

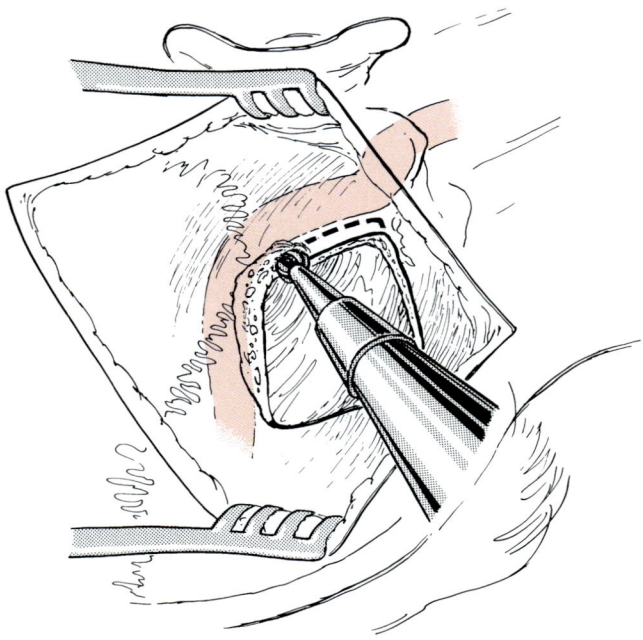

FIG. 15. The transverse sinus and sigmoid sinus are skeletonized using large cutting and coarse diamond burs.

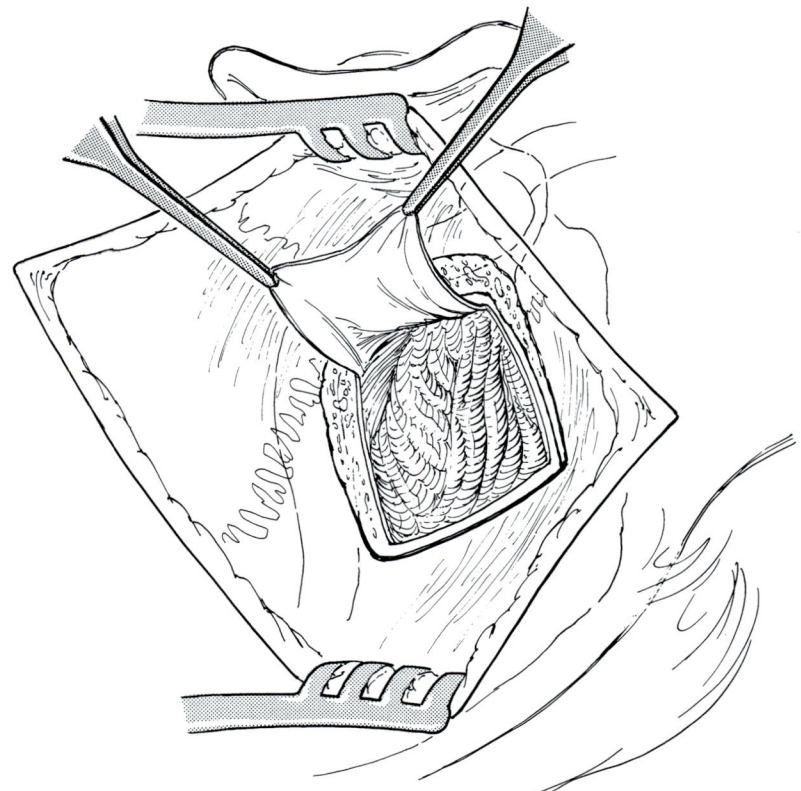

FIG. 16. Dural incisions form an anteriorly pedicled dural flap that is secured with silk suture.

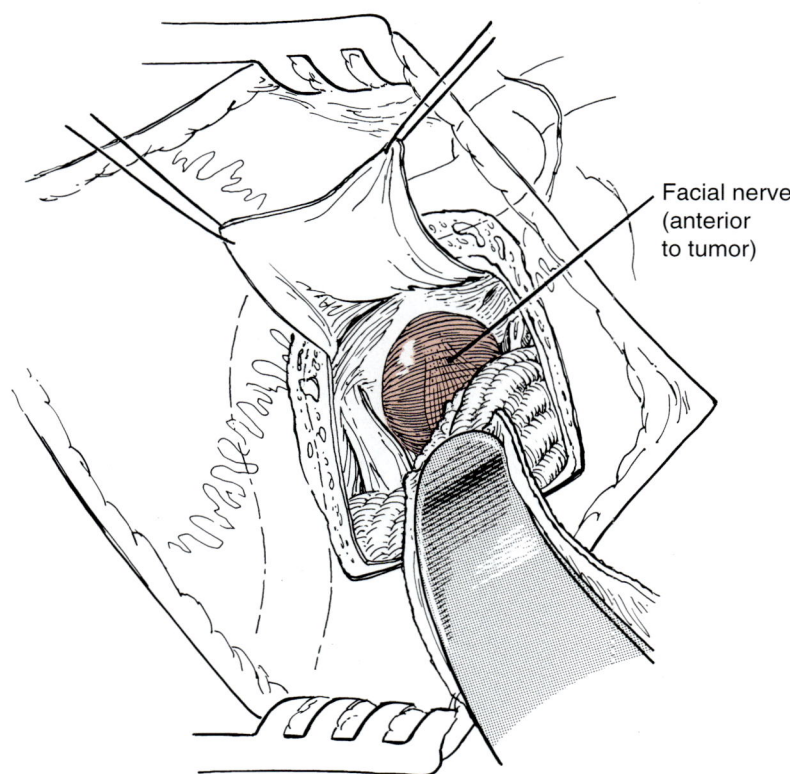

FIG. 17. After the lysis of arachnoid adhesions, the flat-blade retractor is advanced into the cerebellopontine angle. The tumor is visualized in the cerebellopontine angle obscuring the view of the porus acusticus. The facial nerve is depicted splayed out over the anterior surface of the tumor.

aspirated until adequate working space is exposed. Some surgeons choose to use mannitol to enhance intracranial decompression; this is usually administered in a dose of 1 gm/kg body weight intravenously before opening the dura. Arachnoid adhesions between the cerebellum and dura are lysed, and the flat-blade retractor is advanced into the CPA. When the tumor (or the audiovestibular nerve complex) can be well visualized, the retractor is stabilized, using a large, saline-soaked cottonoid to protect the cerebellum (Fig. 17).

With small tumors, several landmarks may be visible at this time. Cranial nerves VII and VIII are seen passing from the brainstem into the internal auditory canal. Superior to this, the trigeminal nerve may be seen, with the abducens and trochlear nerves anteriorly. Inferiorly, cranial nerves IX, X, and XI create a fan-shaped formation before they pass into the jugular formation, and are covered by an arachnoid sheath. Larger tumors often obscure these landmarks and require debulking before all of these structures can be identified. Once adequate exposure of the posterior face of the petrous bone and the operculum is achieved, the dura overlying the internal auditory canal is incised, elevated, and reflected as superiorly and inferiorly based flaps (Fig. 18).

Before exposure of the internal auditory canal, tumors greater than 1.5 cm, measured from the porus acusticus, are debulked with a Cavitron ultrasonic aspirator (Fig. 19). Tumor debulking remains within the confines of the capsule to avoid inadvertent injury to surrounding structures. Smaller tumors are debulked with bipolar cautery and cup forceps. A biopsy is obtained at this point in the procedure and sent for frozen-section histologic examination.

Bone removal is then performed with a 3- or 4-mm coarse diamond bur and copious suction–irrigation. In hearing conservation procedures, it is imperative to avoid entering the posterior semicircular canal and vestibule. One important landmark is the operculum, a bony projection along the posterior face of the petrous bone at which point the endolymphatic duct enters the bone (Fig. 20). Remaining medial and anterior to the endolymphatic duct and following it through its "inverted J"-shaped course reduces the risk of inadvertent entry into the vestibule and posterior semicircular canal. As the bony dissection proceeds, care is taken to identify the "blue lines" of these structures before their damage. In general, up to 7 mm of bone can be removed safely from the medial aspect of the internal auditory canal. The anatomy of the labyrinth and degree of lateral extension of the tumor may prohibit hearing conservation. Often, undesirable anatomy and very lateral tumor extension can be assessed before surgery on the gadolinium-enhanced MRI. In situations in which patients have no usable hearing or extremely poor prognostic factors for useful hearing conservation, wider bone removal is performed. If the most lateral extent of tumor cannot be accessed without labyrinthine injury because of the anatomic relationships, the hearing is sacrificed.

As the internal auditory canal is skeletonized along its entire length, an eggshell thickness of bone is left over the dura. This final layer of bone is removed by careful dissection with

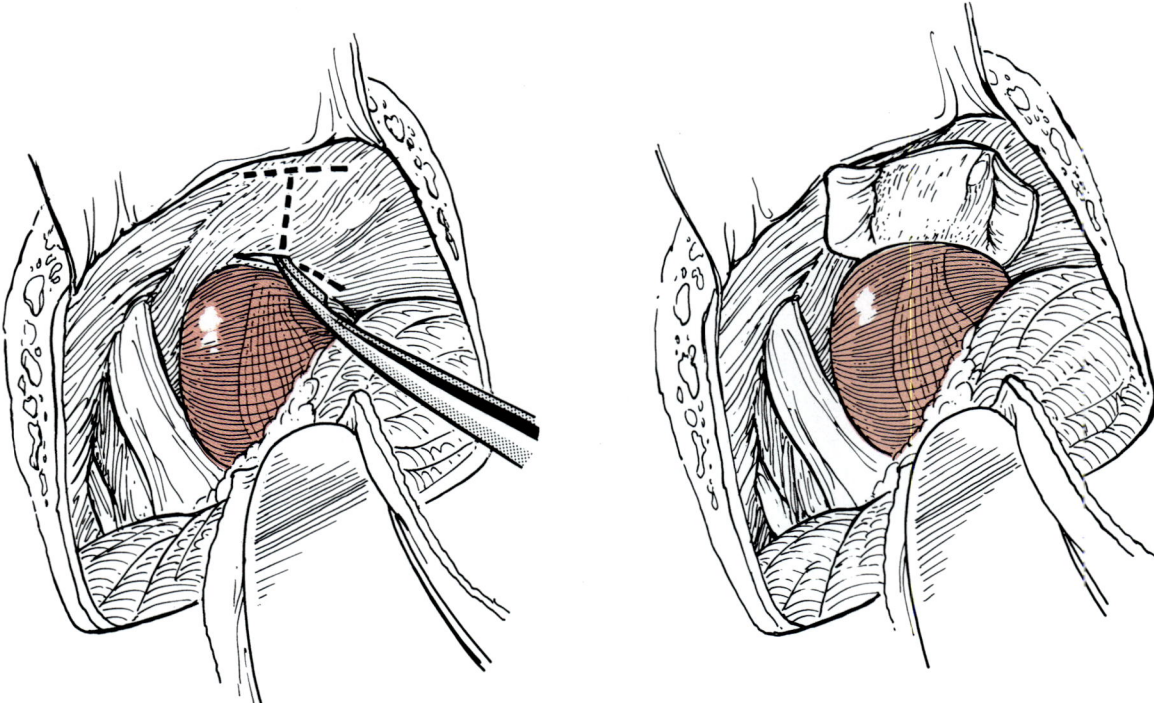

FIG. 18. Incisions are created in the dura over the petrous bone, creating superiorly and inferiorly based flaps.

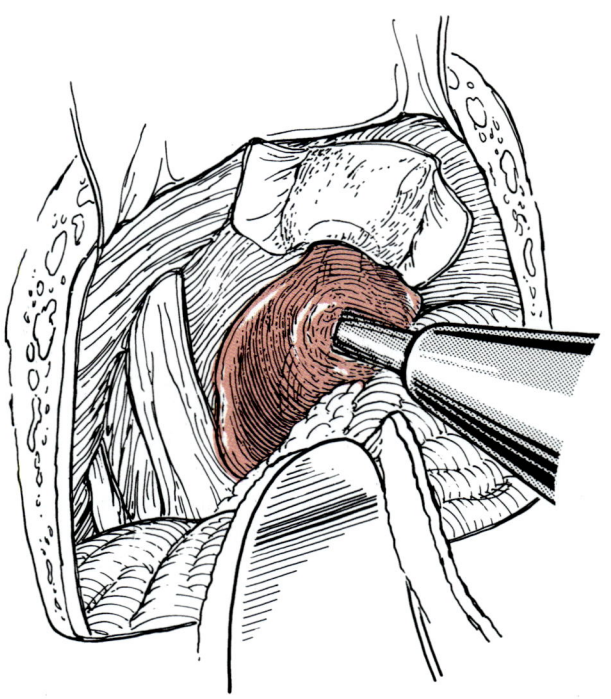

FIG. 19. The Cavitron ultrasonic aspirator is used to debulk the intracapsular tumor in the cerebellopontine angle.

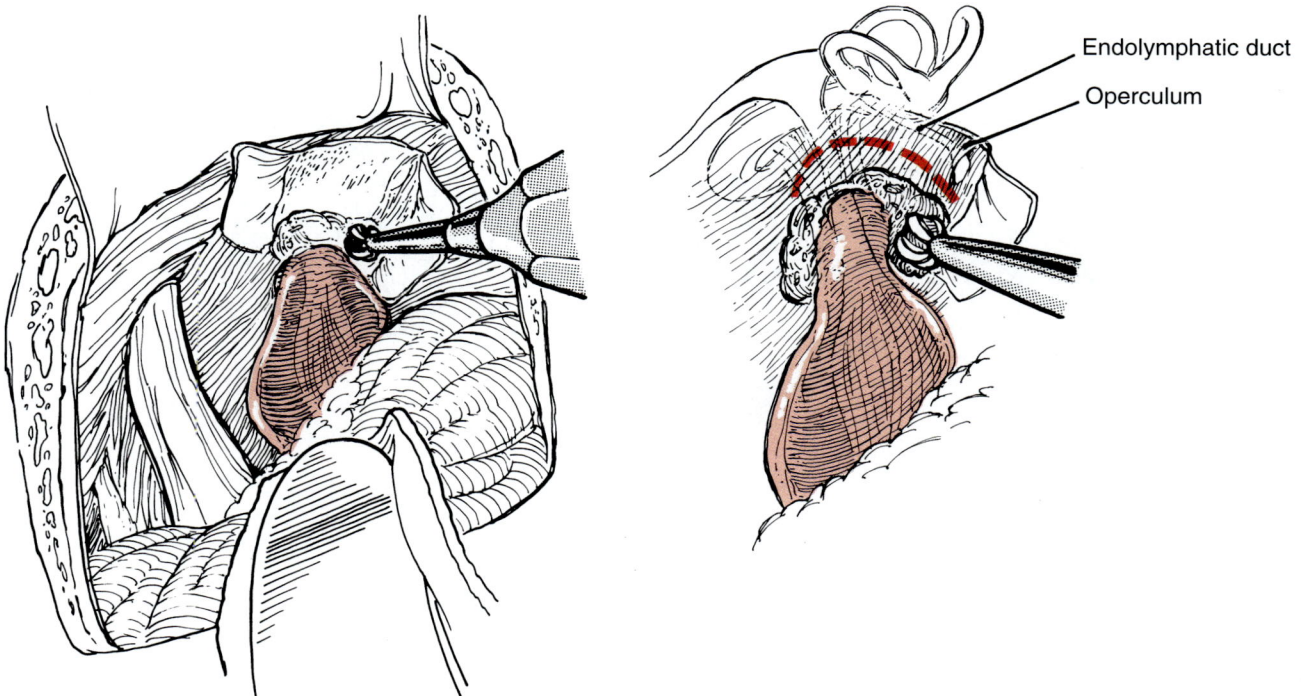

FIG. 20. The internal auditory canal is skeletonized using the operculum and endolymphatic duct as landmarks. Dissection of bone is performed medial and anterior to the endolymphatic duct to avoid inadvertent entry into the vestibule and posterior semicircular canal. In general, up to 7 mm of bone can be removed safely from the medial aspect of the internal auditory canal.

a diamond bur. The area is then copiously irrigated to remove all bone dust.

At the lateral extent of the internal auditory canal, "Bill's bar" is identified, which delineates the superior vestibular and facial nerves. The location of the facial nerve is ascertained by stimulation. The dura of the internal auditory canal is incised along the edges of the canal. The superior vestibular nerve is removed from its attachments to the labyrinth, and retracted medially. Dissection of tumor and vestibular nerve then proceeds in a lateral to medial direction along the length of the canal (Fig. 21). At this point, the location of the facial nerve has been verified. It typically is displaced anteriorly and splayed over the anterior surface of the tumor capsule as it exits the porus.

After removal of the intracanalicular portion of the tumor, the cerebellopontine component of the tumor is debulked. Depending on the extent of tumor, debulking is performed with cup forceps and bipolar cautery or the Cavitron ultrasonic aspirator. As the contents of the tumor are excised, the capsule is rolled inward and dissected off of the underlying facial and cochlear nerves. As debulking progresses, the brainstem origination of cranial nerves VII and VIII is identified and the tumor dissected off of the brainstem.

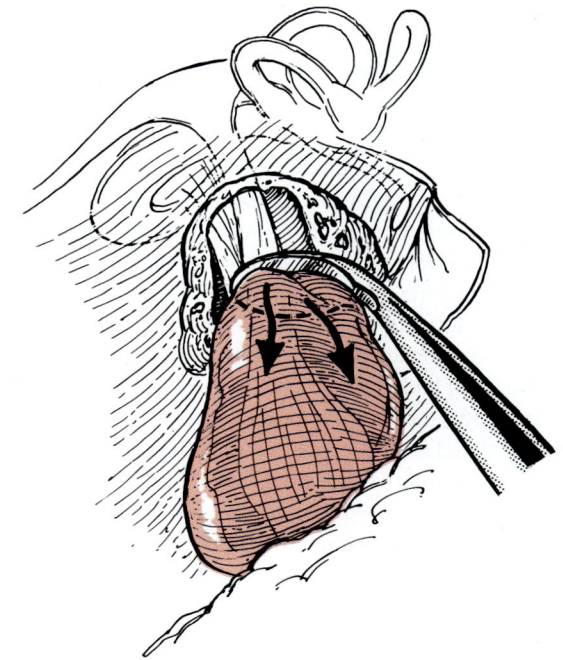

FIG. 21. The vestibular nerves and intracanalicular tumor are dissected off of the facial and cochlear nerves.

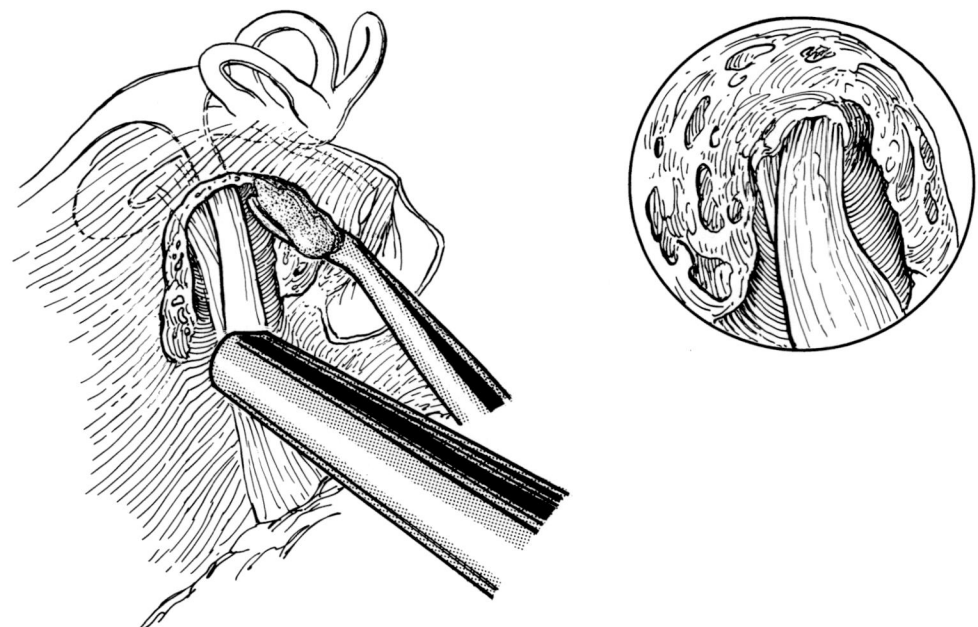

FIG. 22. Endoscopy is performed with a 30-degree, 2.7-mm ridged endoscope to inspect carefully the bone edges around the internal auditory canal. All visualized air cells are sealed with bone wax.

Closure

After completion of tumor removal, a careful check is performed to ensure hemostasis. Valsalva maneuvers and irrigation are used to identify sites of bleeding and bipolar cautery and hemostatic agents such as Surgicel or Avitene are used as necessary.

Bone wax is carefully placed into all air cells around the internal auditory canal and the mastoid air cells at the edge of the craniotomy to prevent CSF leak through the mastoid and middle ear. A continuous sheet of the bone wax reduces the risk of gaps allowing penetration of CSF into air cells (Fig. 22). It is often difficult to see the entire face of bone around the internal auditory canal to inspect for exposed air cells because of the angle of exposure. Consequently, a 30-degree, 2.7-mm rigid endoscope is used to inspect the bone and ensure that the air cells are sealed (see Fig. 22).

The dura that had originally been on the face of the petrous apex, overlying the internal auditory canal, is reflected into the surgical defect. A piece of temporalis fascia is then placed over the internal auditory canal. The large, anteriorly based dural flap is closed with a watertight closure, if possible, using 4-0 silk. The craniotomy bone flap is secured into position with nylon sutures from the bone flap to the edges of the craniotomy. The bone chips that were saved in normal saline are placed around the remaining exposed perimeter (Fig. 23). The attachments of the neck musculature are reat-

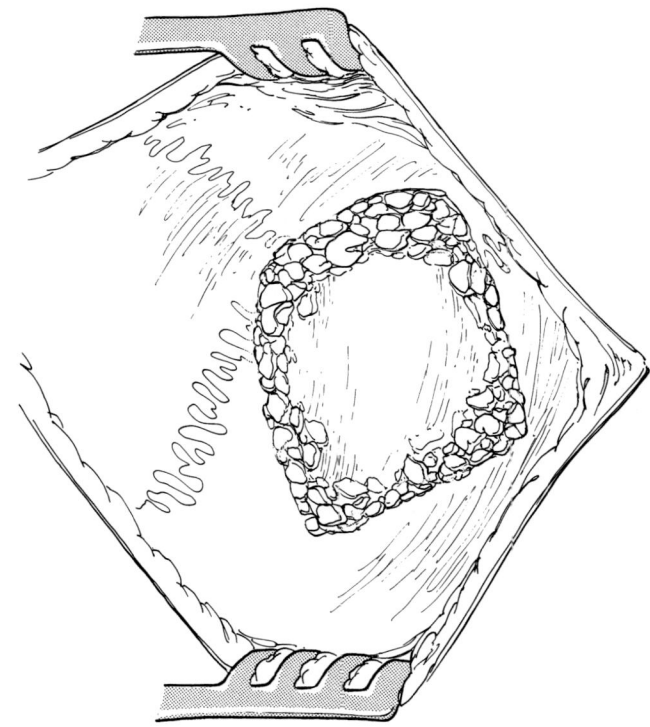

FIG. 23. The craniotomy bone flap and bone chips are replaced into the craniotomy defect before wound closure.

tached to the skull by suspension sutures, which pass through holes at the edge of the craniotomy. The skin is closed in three layers: galea, subcutaneous, and skin. A pressure dressing is applied, and left in position for 48 hours.

Postoperative Care

The postoperative management is the same as with the translabyrinthine approach, as outline previously.

MIDDLE FOSSA APPROACH

The middle fossa approach to the internal auditory canal was first described by Parry in 1904 (86). It was not until the 1960s, after the advent of the operating microscope, that William House popularized this approach for resection of vestibular schwannomas. The approach is ideal for small intracanalicular tumors. However, it was not until the development of gadolinium-enhanced MRI that small intracanalicular tumors were frequently identified. Consequently, since the mid-1980s, the frequency of middle fossa approaches has increased significantly. The middle fossa approach is primarily used in candidates for hearing preservation, for intracanalicular lesions that extend no more than 5 mm into the CPA (see section on Selection of Surgical Approach). Elderly patients are poor candidates for middle fossa surgery because of the more tenuous nature of their dura, and because retraction of the temporal lobe is more likely to cause postoperative seizures. A relative contraindication to this approach is a tumor originating from the inferior vestibular nerve. The tumor location is inferred from ENG findings (further discussion of this issue is found in the Diagnostic Testing section). The reason a tumor on the inferior vestibular nerve is more difficult to approach through the middle fossa is because the facial nerve is between the surgeon and the tumor. This makes tumor dissection with cranial nerve preservation more difficult.

Preparation

In the middle fossa approach, the surgeon is positioned at the vertex of the patient's head, facing down the long axis of the table. The patient is positioned supine, with the head turned so the affected ear is upward. If there is concern that torsion of the neck is excessive, the three-quarters lateral position (described for the suboccipital approach) may be used. The Mayfield head rest with pinions affords stability and accessibility. It is engaged with the dual pins on the contralateral occiput, and the single pin on the ipsilateral supraorbital rim. The scalp is shaved from the ipsilateral mid-pupillary line, to the vertex, and extending to the occipital condyle. In this fashion, almost half of the scalp is exposed. Facial and auditory monitoring devices are placed, and sterile preparation is performed. Mannitol is useful to decrease intracranial pressure and should be administered intravenously at the beginning of the craniotomy (1 g/kg body weight).

Procedure

The "lazy-S" skin incision extends from the preauricular crease to the vertex, first extending anteriorly, then posteriorly (Fig. 24). The skin flaps are undermined in the plane above the temporalis fascia, and held with Weitlander self-retaining retractors. The temporalis fascia is reflected inferiorly (see Fig. 24). The temporalis muscle is split vertically and elevated off of the squamosal portion of the temporal bone with a wide periosteal elevator. Dissection should extend underneath the zygomatic arch to allow adequate exposure for the craniotomy. The self-retaining retractors are adjusted to hold both muscle and skin.

A bone window is created with a 5- or 6-mm cutting bur and suction irrigation. This bone window is 4 × 4 cm in size and is set at the level of the zygomatic root (Fig. 25). Two thirds of the window is anterior to the vertical plane of the external auditory canal, and one third of the window is posterior to the canal. This relationship is important because it is usually the anterior extent of the exposure that is most difficult. The cutting bur is used to remove the bone around the edges of the bone flap until only a thin membrane of bone remains. Using a coarse diamond bur, dura is exposed around the perimeter of the bone flap. The window of bone is then elevated with the joker, and the dura tethered to the undersurface of the edges of the craniotomy is dissected free (Fig. 26). At the time the bone flap is removed, it is convenient to create holes in the edge of the flap and the craniotomy that will be used to suture the flap into position at the end of the procedure. A rongeur is used to remove the bone at the inferior edge of the craniotomy to the level of the middle fossa floor (Fig. 27). This allows for the optimal surgical line of site with minimal temporal lobe retraction.

The House-Urban middle fossa retractor is engaged with the prongs in the edge of the craniotomy. The blade is gradually advanced as the dura is elevated off the floor of the middle fossa (Fig. 28). It is common to encounter dural venous bleeding at the anterior extent of the dissection. This can usually be controlled with a hemostatic agent such as Surgicel. The landmarks in the middle fossa are the middle meningeal artery at the foramen spinosum, the greater superficial petrosal nerve at the facial hiatus, and the arcuate eminence (see Fig. 28). The geniculate ganglion may be exposed without a bony covering on the floor of the middle fossa, so care should be exercised during dural elevation. When these landmarks have been identified, the retractor blade is stabilized.

The landmark for the superior semicircular canal is the

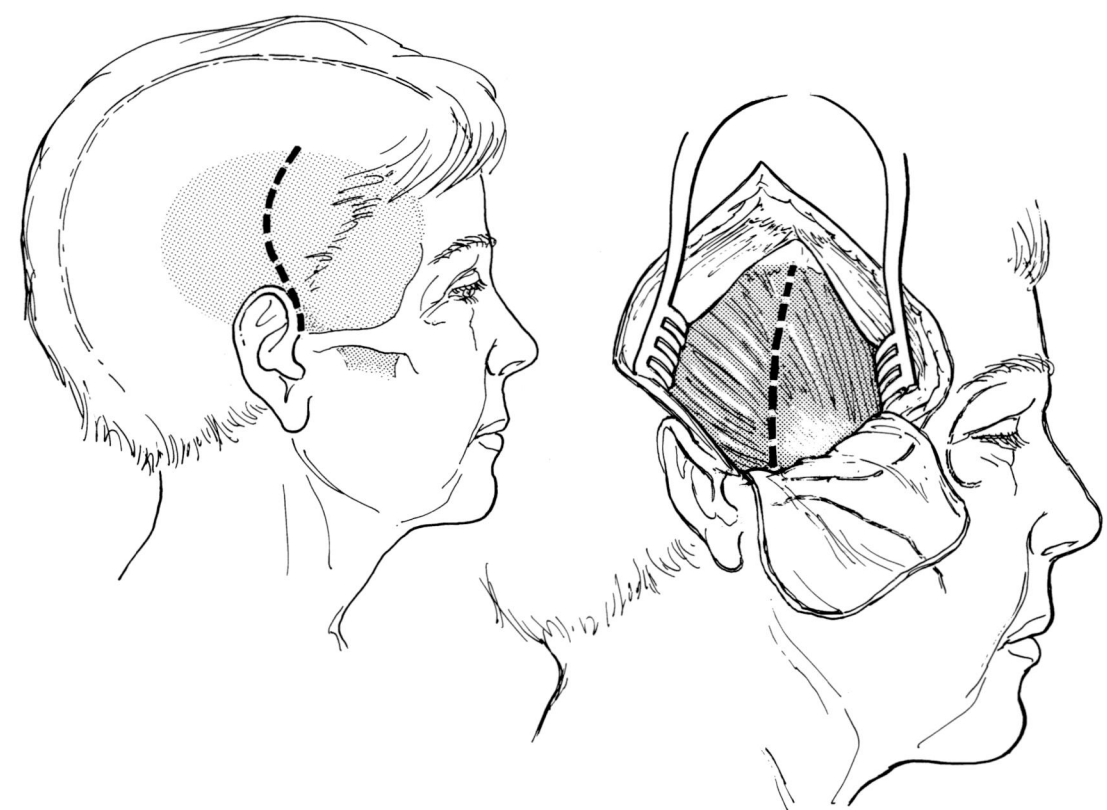

FIG. 24. A "lazy-S" skin incision extends from the preauricular crease toward the vertex. The incision is carried down to the temporalis fascia, which is elevated and reflected inferiorly. The temporalis muscle is split vertically, anterior to the plane of the external auditory canal.

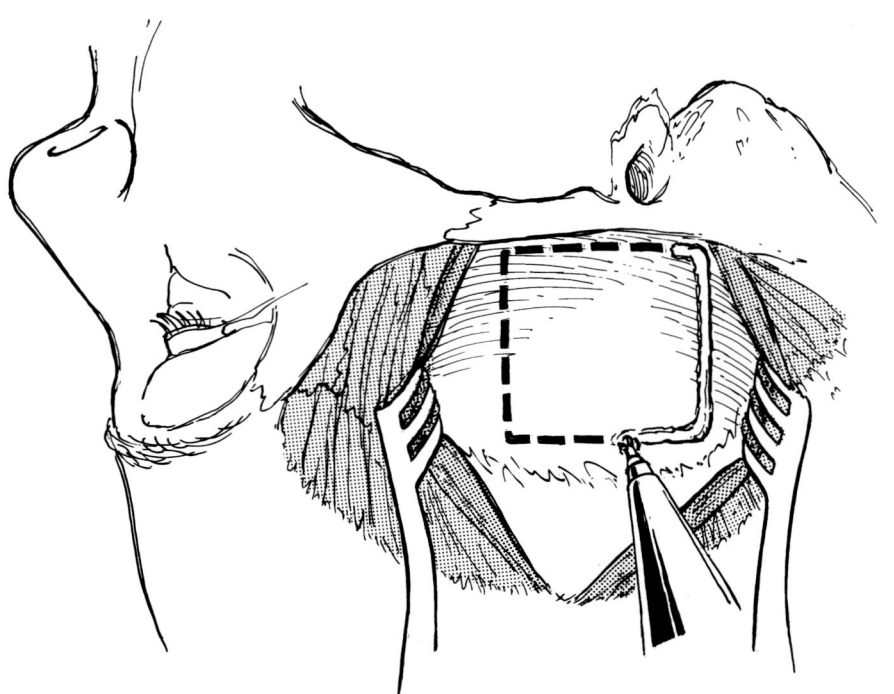

FIG. 25. A 4 × 4 cm window is created in the squamosal portion of the temporal bone. Two thirds of the window is anterior to the vertical plane of the external auditory canal, and one third is posterior to the canal.

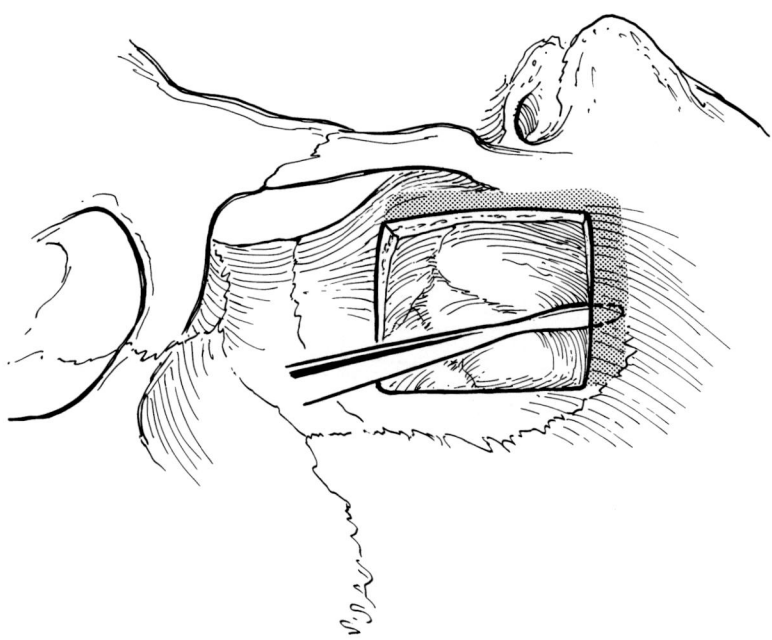

FIG. 26. Dura tethered to the undersurface of the edges of the craniotomy is dissected free around the perimeter of the window.

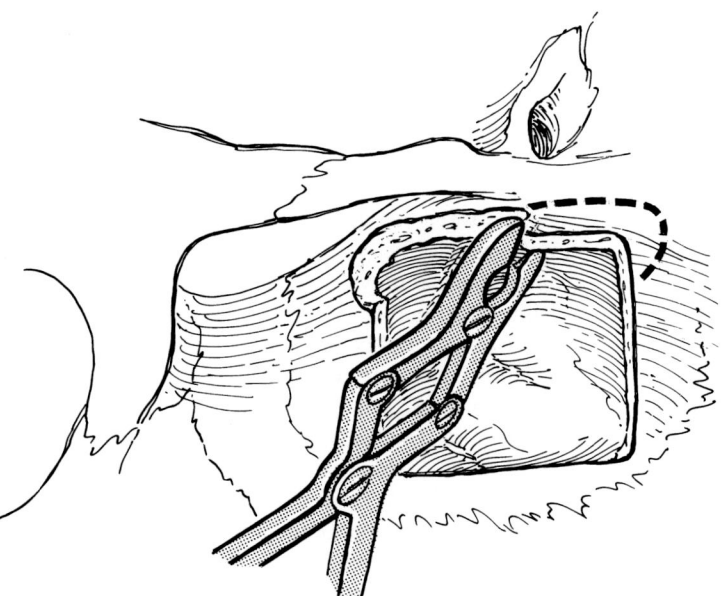

FIG. 27. Bone rongeurs are used to remove the remaining portion of the squamosal bone down to the level of the tegmen. Removal of this lip of bone provides an optimal surgical line of site with minimal temporal bone retraction.

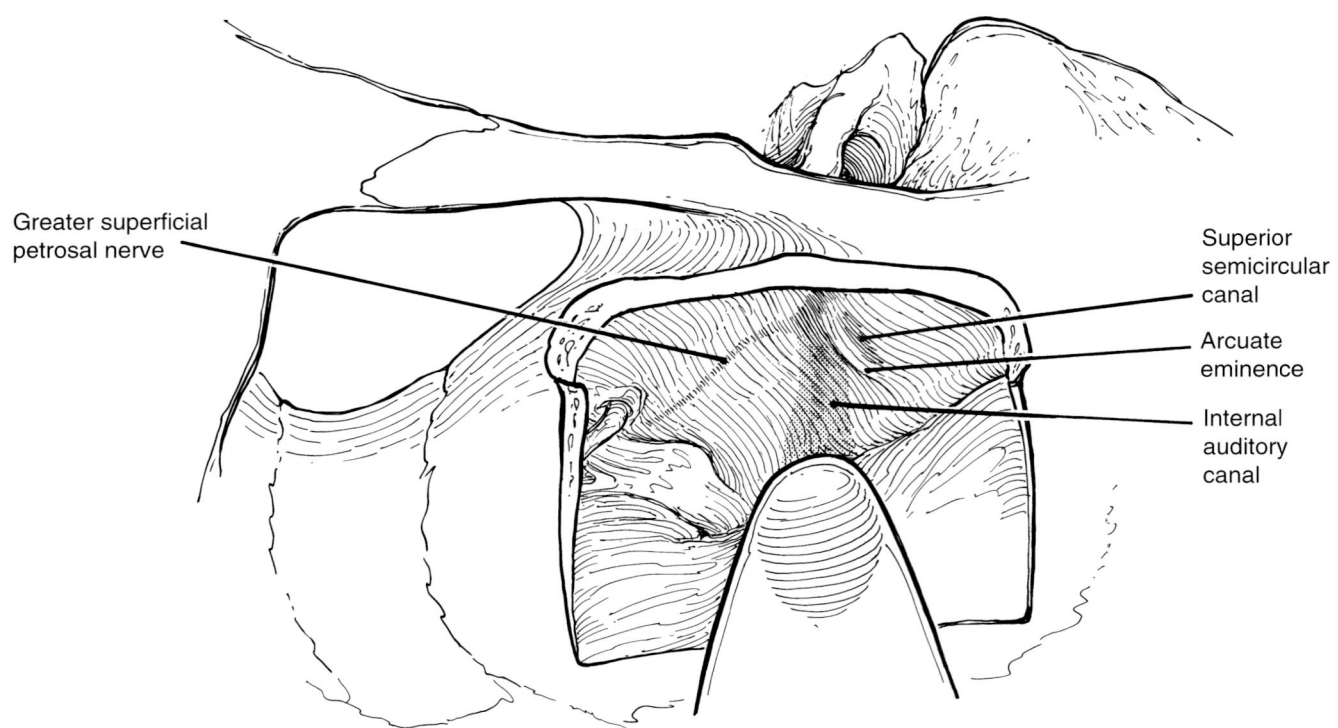

FIG. 28. Dura of the middle cranial fossa is elevated off the petrous bone. The locations of the greater superficial petrosal nerve, internal auditory canal, and superior semicircular canal have been ghosted in this illustration.

arcuate eminence (see Fig. 28), but the precise location of the canal does not uniformly correspond with the arcuate eminence. A coronal CT scan may be helpful in ascertaining the relationship between the two. It will show the contours of the middle fossa floor as they relate to the superior semicircular canal and the distance between the superior semicircular canal and the floor of the middle fossa. The canal may have very little bone coverage and can be seen as a blue line after simple dural elevation, or there may be a large number of air cells between the canal and the surface of the tegmen. If the superior semicircular canal cannot be located by drilling over the arcuate eminence, two other methods may be considered. First, the tegmen tympani may be opened, exposing the ossicles. The location of the superior semicircular canal can be established by the spatial relationships (Fig. 29). Second, the greater superficial petrosal nerve can be followed retrograde back through the facial hiatus to the geniculate ganglion. The intralabyrinthine portion of the facial nerve passes between the cochlea and the ampulla of the superior semicircular canal.

The bone over the superior semicircular canal is removed using suction irrigation and diamond burs. A 4-mm bur is a good choice for the initial dissection. A light medial-to-lateral stroke is used until the blue line of the superior canal is identified. After the superior canal has been identified, dissection proceeds along the "meatal plane," which is the bone within a 60-degree angle from the blue line of the superior canal (Fig. 30). Drilling within the confines of this plane reduces the risk of inadvertent injury to the cochlea. Note that much wider drilling may be performed medially, whereas at the lateral extent of the internal auditory canal, there is very little space between the cochlea and ampulla of the superior semicircular canal. The bur should hug the line of the superior canal as bone removal progresses. The dissection will appear quite deep before the internal auditory canal is encountered. Bone should be removed 180 degrees around the internal auditory canal, from the lateral aspect of the meatus to the porus acusticus. An eggshell thickness of bone should be left on the dura. The last steps are in exposure of the canal is careful removal of this bone and copious irrigation to remove bone dust (Fig. 31).

At the most lateral extent of the internal auditory canal the vertical crest or "Bill's bar" is identified, with the facial nerve anteriorly and the superior vestibular nerve posteriorly (see Fig. 31). The location of the facial nerve is confirmed by electrical stimulation set at 0.05 mA. The dura of the internal auditory canal is incised in a longitudinal fashion, along the posterior edge, away from the facial nerve. Under direct visualization, the dura is reflected. At this point the tumor and facial nerve should be visible. Cranial nerve VII is expected to be anterior or superior to the body of the tumor, and its location must be confirmed before tumor dissection. The superior vestibular nerve is then removed from its lateral attachment to the labyrinth and is retracted medially. Careful

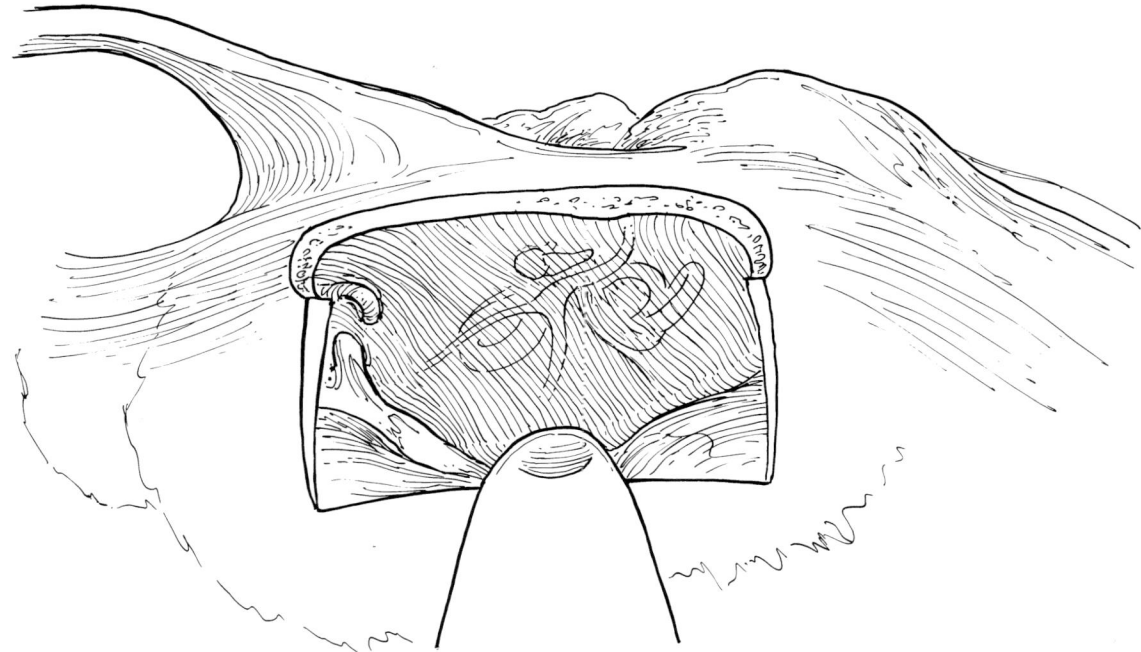

FIG. 29. The tegmen tympani has been removed, exposing the underlying attic containing the head of the malleus and body of the incus. These additional landmarks can be helpful when the arcuate eminence is not appreciated and the superior semicircular canal has not been located.

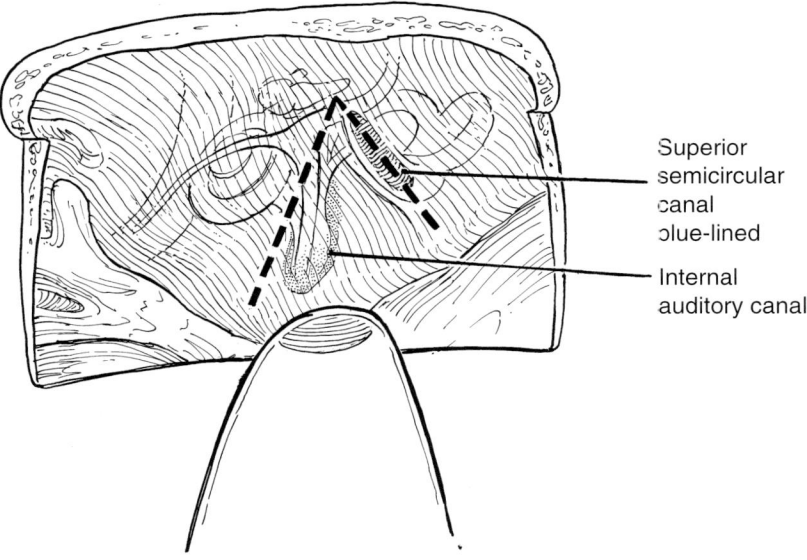

FIG. 30. Once the "blue line" of the superior semicircular canal has been identified, dissection proceeds over the meatal plane superior to the internal auditory canal. The internal auditory canal lies within a 60-degree angle from the blue-lined semicircular canal.

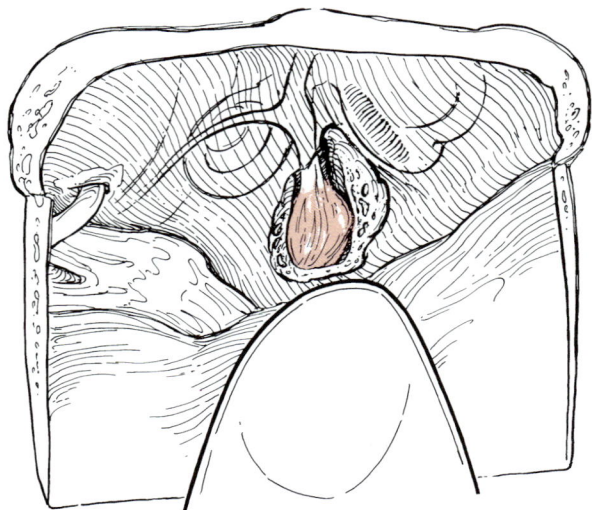

FIG. 31. The internal auditory canal is skeletonized around the superior 180 degrees of its circumference. In the lateral aspect of the internal auditory canal, "Bill's bar" separates the facial nerve anteriorly from the vestibular nerve posteriorly.

dissection then removes the vestibular nerve and tumor from the facial and cochlear nerves, in a lateral-to-medial direction.

Closure

After complete removal of the tumor, hemostasis is secured. Bone wax is used to fill exposed air cells. A piece of temporalis muscle is placed in the bony defect, and the pedicled temporalis fascia flap is reflected over the floor of the middle cranial fossa. The temporal lobe is released, compressing the fascia over the bony defect. The extradural nature of the surgery together with the reexpansion of the temporal lobe explain the relatively low incidence of postoperative CSF fistulas. The bone flap is secured to the edges of the craniotomy with silk sutures. The temporalis muscle is closed superiorly, leaving a gap inferiorly where the temporalis fascia is passing. The skin is closed in two layers. Fine nylon is recommended in the non–hair-bearing skin of the preauricular area. A pressure dressing is applied and left in position for 48 hours.

SUMMARY

Tremendous progress has occurred in the diagnosis and management of vestibular schwannomas over the past century. The advent of the operating microscope, improved microsurgical techniques, and the development of MRI has dramatically changed the focus of the management of these tumors. Focus has shifted from mortality to morbidity. Early detection, facial nerve preservation, and hearing conservation are the main areas of advancement. Four surgical techniques—translabyrinthine, transotic, retrosigmoid, and middle fossa—have evolved in the treatment of vestibular schwannomas. The differential indications, complications, and advantages have been reviewed. All of these techniques play an important role in the overall management of CPA tumors.

REFERENCES

1. Cushing, H. *Tumors of the nervus acusticus and the syndrome of the cerebellopontile angle*. Philadelphia: WB Saunders, 1917.
2. House WF. Exposure of the internal auditory canal and its contents through the middle cranial fossa. *Laryngoscope* 1961;71:1363–1385.
3. House WF. Evolution of the transtemporal bone removal of acoustic tumors. *Archives of Otolaryngology* 1964;80:731–742.
4. Brackmann DE, Bartels LJ. Rare tumors of the cerebellopontine angle. *Otolaryngol Head Neck Surg* 1980;88:555–559
5. Pensak ML, Glasscock ME, Josey AF, Jackson CG, Gulya AJ. Sudden hearing loss and cerebellopontine angle tumors. *Laryngoscope* 1985;95:1188–1193.
6. Berg HM, Cohen NL, Hammerschlag PE, Waltzman SB. Acoustic neuroma presenting as sudden hearing loss with recovery. *Otolaryngol Head Neck Surg* 1986;94:15–22.
7. Ogawa K, Kanzaki J, Ogawa S, Tsuchihashi N, Inoue Y. Acoustic neuromas presenting as sudden hearing loss *Acta Otolaryngol Suppl (Stockh)* 1991;487:138–143.
8. Berenholz LP, Eriksen C, Hirsh FA. Recovery from repeated sudden hearing loss with corticosteroid use in the presence of an acoustic neuroma. *Ann Otol Rhinol Laryngol* 1992;101:827–831.
9. Selesnick SH, Jackler RK, Pitts LW. The changing clinical presentation of acoustic tumors in the MRI era. *Laryngoscope* 1993;103:431–436.
10. Saunders JE, Luxford WM, Devgan KK, Fetterman BL. Sudden hearing loss in acoustic neuroma patients. *Otolaryngol Head Neck Surg* 1995;113:23–31.
11. Portmann M, Dauman R, Duriez F, Portmann D, Dhillon R. Modern diagnostic strategy for acoustic neuromas. *Arch Otorhinolaryngol* 1989;246:286–291.
12. Beck HJ, Beatty CW, Harner SG, Ilstrup DM. Acoustic neuromas with normal pure tone hearing levels. *Otolaryngol Head Neck Surg* 1986;94:96–103.
13. Selesnick SH, Jackler RK. Atypical hearing loss in acoustic neuroma patients. *Laryngoscope* 1993;103:437–441.
14. Olsen A, Horrax G. The symptomatology of acoustic tumors with special reference to atypical features. *J Neurosurg* 1944;1:371–378.
15. Edwards CH, Patterson JH. A review of the symptoms and signs of acoustic neurofibromata. *Brain* 1951;74:144–190.
16. Erickson LS, Sorenson GD, Mcgavran MH. A review of 140 acoustic neurinomas (neurilemmoma). *Laryngoscope* 1965;75:601–627.
17. Selesnick SH, Jackler RK. Clinical manifestations and audiologic diagnosis of acoustic neuromas. *Otolaryngol Clin North Am* 1992;25:521–551.
18. Thomsen J, Tos M. Acoustic neuroma: clinical aspects, audiovestibular assessment, diagnostic delay, and growth rate. *Am J Otol* 1990;11:12–19.
19. Harner SG, Laws ER. Diagnosis of acoustic neurinoma. *Neurosurgery* 1981;9:373–379.
20. Hitselberger WE, House WF. Acoustic neuroma diagnosis: external auditory canal hypesthesia as an early sign. *Archives of Otolaryngology* 1966; 83:218–221.
21. Hitselberger WE. External auditory canal hypesthesia. *Ann Surg* 1966;32:741–743.
22. Leonetti JP. The diagnosis and management of acoustic neuromas: contemporary practice guidelines. *Compr Ther* 1995;21:68–73.
23. Johnson EW. Auditory test results in 500 cases of acoustic neuroma. *Archives of Otolaryngology* 1977;103:152–158.
24. Brunas RL, Ylikoski J, Morra B. Pure tone auciogram configurations in acoustic tumor patients. *Rev Laryngol Otol Rhinol (Bord)* 1984;105:113–116.
25. Moffat DA, Hardy DG, Baguley DM. Strategy and benefits of acoustic neuroma searching. *J Laryngol Otol* 1989;103:51–59.

26. Kanzaki J, Ogawa K, Ogawa S, Yamamoto M, Ikeda S, O-Uchi T. Audiological findings in acoustic neuroma. *Acta Otolaryngol Suppl (Stockh)* 1991;487:125–132.
27. Thomsen J, Terkildsen K, Tos M. Acoustic neuromas: progression of hearing impairment and function of the eighth cranial nerve. *Am J Otol* 1983;5:20–33.
28. Clemis JD. Acoustic reflex testing in otoneurology. *Otolaryngol Head Neck Surg* 1984;92:141–144.
29. Odkvist LM. Otoneurological diagnostics in posterior fossa lesions. *Acta Otolaryngol Suppl (Stockh)* 1988;452:12–15.
30. Clemis JD, Mc Gee T. Brain stem electric response audiometry in the differential diagnosis of acoustic tumors. *Laryngoscope* 1979;89:31–42.
31. Legatt AD, Pedley TA, Emerson RG, Stein BM, Abramson M. Normal brain-stem auditory evoked potentials with abnormal latency-intensity studies in patients with acoustic neuromas. *Arch Neurol* 1988;45:1326–1330.
32. Josey AF, Glasscock ME, Musiek FE. Correlation of ABR and medical imaging in patients with cerebellopontine angle tumors. *Am J Otol* 1988;9[Suppl]:12–16.
33. Kotlarz JP, Eby TL, Borton TE. Analysis of the efficiency of retrocochlear screening. *Laryngoscope* 1992;102:1108–1112.
34. Wilson DF, Hodgson RS, Gustafson MF, Hogue S, Mills L. The sensitivity of auditory brainstem response testing in small acoustic neuromas. *Laryngoscope* 1992;102:961–964.
35. Levine SC, Antonelli PJ, Le CT, Haines SJ. Relative value of diagnostic tests for small acoustic neuromas. *Am J Otol* 1991;12:341–346.
36. Swan IR. Diagnostic vetting of individuals with asymmetric sensorineural hearing impairments. *J Laryngol Otol* 1989;103:823–826.
37. Harder H. Audiovestibular tests in the diagnosis of cerebellopontine angle tumours. *Acta Otolaryngol Suppl (Stockh)* 1988;452:5–11.
38. Weiss MH, Kisiel DL, Bhatia P. Predictive value of brainstem evoked response in the diagnosis of acoustic neuroma. *Otolaryngol Head Neck Surg* 1990;103:583–585.
39. Gstoettner W, Neuwirth-Riedl K, Swoboda H, Mostbeck W, Burian M. Specificity of auditory brainstem response audiometry criteria in acoustic neuroma screening as a function of deviations of reference values in patients with cochlear hearing loss. *Eur Arch Otorhinolaryngol* 1992;249:253–256.
40. Greenberger R, Khangure MS, Chakera TM. The morbidity of CT air meatography: a follow-up of 84 patients. *Clin Radiol* 1987;38:535–536.
41. Smith IM, Turnbull LW, Sellar RJ, Murray JA. CT air meatography: review of side effects in 60 patients. *J Laryngol Otol* 1989;103:173–174.
42. Saeed SR, Woolford TJ, Ramsden RT, Lye RH. Magnetic resonance imaging: a cost-effective first line investigation in the detection of vestibular schwannomas. *Br J Neurosurg* 1995;9:497–503.
43. Lalwani AK, Jackler RK. Preoperative differentiation between meningioma of the cerebellopontine angle and acoustic neuroma using MRI. *Otolaryngol Head Neck Surg* 1993;109:88–95.
44. Lunardi P, Mastronardi L, Nardacci B, Acqui M, Fortuna A. "Dural tail" adjacent to acoustic neuroma on MRI: a case report. *Neuroradiology* 1993;35:270–271.
45. Kutcher TJ, Brown DC, Maurer PK, Ghaed VN. Dural tail adjacent to acoustic neuroma: MR features. *J Comput Assist Tomogr* 1991;15:669–670.
46. Phelps PD. Fast spin echo MRI in otology. *J Laryngol Otol* 1994;108:383–394.
47. Strasnick B, Glasscock ME, Haynes D, McMenomey SO, Minor LB. The natural history of untreated acoustic neuromas. *Laryngoscope* 1994;104:1115–1119.
48. Noren G, Greitz D, Hirsch A, Lax I. Gamma knife surgery in acoustic tumours. *Acta Neurochir Suppl (Wien)* 1993;58:104–107.
49. Lunsford LD, Kondziolka DS, Flickinger JC. Radiosurgery of tumors of the cerebellopontine angle. *Clin Neurosurg* 1994;41:168–184.
50. Pollock BE, Lunsford LD, Kondziolka D, et al. Outcome analysis of acoustic neuroma management: a comparison of microsurgery and stereotactic radiosurgery. *Neurosurgery* 1995;36:215–224.
51. Hirato M, Inoue H, Nakamura M, et al. Gamma knife radiosurgery for acoustic schwannoma: early effects and preservation of hearing. *Neurol Med Chir (Tokyo)* 1995;35:737–741.
52. Foote RL, Coffey RJ, Swanson JW, et al. Stereotactic radiosurgery using the gamma knife for acoustic neuromas. *Int J Radiol Oncol Biol Phys* 1995;32:1153–1160.
53. Flickinger JC, Lunsford LD, Linskey ME, Duma CM, Kondziolka D. Gamma knife radiosurgery for acoustic tumors: multivariate analysis of four year results. *Radiother Oncol* 1993;27:91–98.
54. Slattery WH, Brackmann DE. Results of surgery following stereotactic irradiation for acoustic neuromas. *Am J Otol* 1995;16:315–319.
55. Blevins NH, Jackler RK. Exposure of the lateral extremity of the internal auditory canal through the retrosigmoid approach: a radioanatomic study. *Otolaryngol Head Neck Surg* 1994;111:81–90.
56. Wigand ME, Haid T, Berg M. The enlarged middle cranial fossa approach for surgery of the temporal bone and of the cerebellopontine angle. *Arch Otorhinolaryngol* 1989;246:299–302.
57. Rosomoff HL. The subtemporal transtentorial approach to the cerebellopontine angle. *Laryngoscope* 1971;81:1448–1454.
58. Kanzaki J, Kawase T, Sano K, Shiobara R, Toya S. A modified extended middle cranial fossa approach for acoustic tumors. *Arch Otorhinolaryngol* 1977;217:119–121.
59. Jackler RK, Pitts LH. Selection of surgical approach to acoustic neuroma. *Otolaryngol Clin North Am* 1992;25:361–387.
60. Harner SG, Daube JR, Ebersold MJ, Beatty CW. Improved preservation of facial nerve function with use of electrical monitoring during removal of acoustic neuromas. *Mayo Clin Proc* 1987;62:92–102.
61. Harner SG, Daube JR, Beatty CW, Ebersold MJ. Intraoperative monitoring of the facial nerve. *Laryngoscope* 1988;98:209–212.
62. Jellinek DA, Tan LC, Symon L. The impact of continuous electrophysiological monitoring on preservation of the facial nerve during acoustic tumour surgery. *Br J Neurosurg* 1991;5:19–24.
63. Lalwani AK, Butt FY, Jackler RK, Pitts LH, Yingling CD. Facial nerve outcome after acoustic neuroma surgery: a study from the era of cranial nerve monitoring. *Otolaryngol Head Neck Surg* 1994;111:561–570.
64. House JW, Brackmann DE. Facial nerve grading system. *Otolaryngol Head Neck Surg* 1985;93:146–147.
65. Uziel A, Benezech J, Frerebeau P. Intraoperative facial nerve monitoring in posterior fossa acoustic neuroma surgery. *Otolaryngol Head Neck Surg* 1993;108:126–134.
66. Harner SG, Ebersold MJ. Management of acoustic neuromas, 1978–1983. *J Neurosurg* 1985;63:175–179.
67. Robson AK, Clarke PM, Dilkes M, Maw AR. Transmastoid extracranial repair of CSF leaks following acoustic neuroma resection. *J Laryngol Otol* 1989;103:842–844.
68. Hardy DG, Macfarlane R, Baguley D, Moffat DA. Surgery for acoustic neurinoma. An analysis of 100 translabyrinthine operations. *J Neurosurg* 1989;71:799–804.
69. Bryce GE, Nedzelski JM, Rowed DW, Rappaport JM. Cerebrospinal fluid leaks and meningitis in acoustic neuroma surgery. *Otolaryngol Head Neck Surg* 1991;104:81–87.
70. Cohen NL. Retrosigmoid approach for acoustic tumor removal. *Otolaryngol Clin North Am* 1992;25:295–310.
71. Rodgers GK, Luxford WM. Factors affecting the development of cerebrospinal fluid leak and meningitis after translabyrinthine acoustic tumor surgery. *Laryngoscope* 1993;103:959–962.
72. Hoffman RA. Cerebrospinal fluid leak following acoustic neuroma removal. *Laryngoscope* 1994;104:40–58.
73. Gantz BJ, Parnes LS, Harker LA, McCabe BF. Middle cranial fossa acoustic neuroma excision: results and complications. *Ann Otol Rhinol Laryngol* 1986;95:454–459.
74. Shelton C, Brackmann DE, House WF, Hitselberger WE. Middle fossa acoustic tumor surgery: results in 106 cases. *Laryngoscope* 1989;99:405–408.
75. Tos M, Thomsen J. Cerebrospinal fluid leak after translabyrinthine surgery for acoustic neuroma. *Laryngoscope* 1985;95:351–354.
76. Cohen NL. Retrosigmoid approach for acoustic tumor removal. *Otolaryngol Clin North Am* 1992;25:295–310.
77. Hoffman RA. Cerebrospinal fluid leak following acoustic neuroma removal. *Laryngoscope* 1994;104:40–58.
78. Chen JM, Fisch U. The transotic approach in acoustic neuroma surgery. *J Otolaryngol* 1993;22:331–336.
79. Symon L, Pell MF. Cerebrospinal fluid rhinorrhea following acoustic neurinoma surgery: technical note. *J Neurosurg* 1991;74:152–153.
80. Ramsden RT, Herdman RC, Lye RH. Ionomeric bone cement in neurotological surgery. *J Laryngol Otol* 1992;106:949–953.
81. Harner SG, Beatty CW, Ebersold MJ. Headache after acoustic neuroma excision. *Am J Otol* 1993;14:552–555.
82. Schessel DA, Rowed DW, Nedzelski JM, Feghali JG. Postoperative pain following excision of acoustic neuroma by the suboccipital ap-

proach: observations on possible cause and potential amelioration. *Am J Otol* 1993;14:491–494.
83. Kamerer DB, Hirsch BE, Snyderman CH, Costantino P, Friedman CD. Hydroxyapatite cement: a new method for achieving watertight closure in transtemporal surgery. *Am J Otol* 1994;15:47–49.
84. Harner SG, Beatty CW, Ebersold MJ. Impact of cranioplasty on headache after acoustic neuroma removal. *Neurosurgery* 1995;36: 1097–1099.
85. Dandy WE. Results of removal of acoustic tumors by the unilateral approach. *Arch Surg* 1941;42:1026.
86. Parry RH. A case of tinnitus and vertigo treated by division of the auditory nerve. *J Laryngol Otol* 1904;19:402.

CHAPTER 24

Approaches to Jugulotympanic Paragangliomas

Rick A. Friedman and Derald E. Brackmann

BACKGROUND

The first descriptions of "swellings" or "ganglions" associated with the tympanic nerve appeared in the middle and late 1800s (1,2). It was not until 1941 that, in his address to the American Association of Anatomists, Guild described the "presence of a previously unrecognized structure" that he called the "glomus jugularis" or jugular body (3). In his first report, he described glomus formations along the course of Jacobson's nerve from its beginning near the adventitia of the jugular bulb, to the cochlear promontory. Soon thereafter, he noted these formations along the course of Arnold's nerve from the skull base into the mastoid canaliculus and fallopian canal.

In Guild's report of 1953, he made several more observations about the glomus bodies of the temporal bone. He found the average number of glomus formations, which measured approximately 0.5 × 0.25 mm in size, was 2.82 per ear, with the largest number appearing in midlife and a marked decrease in number after the age of 60 years. He found no racial or gender differences in the number or size of glomus formations. Although he found these glomus formations along the entire course of both Jacobson's and Arnold's nerves, he found that most were within the adventitia of the jugular bulb in the jugular fossa.

The first clinical description of a "carotid body tumor of the middle ear and mastoid" came in 1945 (4). Rosenwasser described a 36-year-old man with a "growth" in the external canal of the left ear and deafness. The tumor had eroded a significant amount of the mastoid bone and had exposed the facial nerve. The tumor bled significantly when manipulated. After pathologic review, Rosenwasser proposed that this tumor may have arisen from the glomus jugularis described by Guild 4 years earlier.

A variety of terms have been used to describe glomus formations and their tumorous counterparts. Lattes and Waltner, in 1949, attempted to clarify the nomenclature and wrote of Guild's "glomus jugularis": "The correct Latin diction should be glomus jugulare, and not glomus jugularis, because the Latin noun glomus is neuter (5)." He proposed the term "nonchromaffin paraganglioma," indicating that these structures and their tumors arise from paraganglionic tissue. Unlike the chromaffin paraganglia associated with the adrenal medulla, these nonchromaffin paraganglia had no affinity for dichromate stains. Despite these debates, several reports of "glomus jugularis" tumors appeared in the literature over the next few decades (6,7). By 1965, approximately 200 cases had been described (7).

BIOLOGY

The chief cells, the principal cells of paraganglionic tissue, are derived from the neural crest and migrate in close association with the ganglia of the sympathetic nervous system (8). The term "glomus" was applied because of an original belief that the chief cell was derived from specialized pericytes, as seen in true arteriovenous (glomus) complexes (8). This theory is no longer thought to be true, and hence the correct term is "paraganglia." Tumors of the paraganglia, paragangliomas, can be divided into two main groups, adrenal and extraadrenal (9) (Table 1). Adrenal paragangliomas are also known as pheochromocytomas. Extraadrenal paragangliomas are associated with sympathetic ganglia in the abdomen, chest, retroperitoneum, and mediastinum. Classification of paragangliomas of the head and neck (branchiomeric) is based on their anatomic location and includes carotid body, jugulotympanic, vagal, laryngeal, nasal, and orbital paragangliomas. The most common location in

---

R. A. Friedman: House Ear Clinic, Inc., Los Angeles, California 90057.

D. E. Brackmann: Department of Otolaryngology, Head and Neck Surgery, University of Southern California, Los Angeles, and House Ear Clinic, Inc., Los Angeles, California 90057.

the head and neck is the carotid body, followed by those of the jugulotympanic region (10).

Le Compte, in 1949, was one of the first to suggest catecholamine secretion by paraganglion cells (11). Initially, jugulotympanic paragangliomas, as well as the other branchiomeric paragangliomas, were thought not to be producers of catecholamines based on their failure to react with dichromate salts. Although once thought to indicate the presence of catecholamines in a tissue, this reaction has proven to be an insensitive measure of catecholamine presence and has been replaced by formaldehyde-induced fluorescence microscopy (12). Electron microscopic data have clearly demonstrated dense secretory granules known to contain catecholamines in the cytoplasm of chief cells. Chief cells have since been classified as members of the diffuse neuroendocrine system, a system of neuropeptide- and catecholamine-secreting cells (8). Immunohistochemical studies corroborate this by demonstrating chief cell staining for chromogranin, synaptophysin, neuron-specific enolase, neurofilaments, and a variety of neuropeptides (10).

Paragangliomas display a characteristic histologic pattern (Fig. 1). Light microscopy demonstrates clusters of chief cells (*Zellballen*) and sustentacular cells, with abundant small blood vessels and unmyelinated nerve fibers presumably derived from the glossopharyngeal nerve (10,13).

The main focus of this chapter is the management of paragangliomas arising in the temporal bone, the so-called jugulotympanic paragangliomas. This group of paragangliomas includes those of the jugular bulb region (jugulare) and the tympanic cavity (tympanicum). These tumors are considered the most common tumors of the middle ear and the second most common tumors of the temporal bone, after acoustic neuromas. Most of these tumors arise in the jugular bulb (10).

TABLE 1. *Paraganglioma classification scheme*

Adrenal
    Pheochromocytoma
Extraadrenal
    Branchiomeric
        Aorticopulmonary
        Coronary
        Intercarotid
        Jugulotympanic
        Laryngeal
        Orbital
        Pulmonary
        Subclavian
    Intravagal
    Aorticosympathetic
    Visceroautonomic

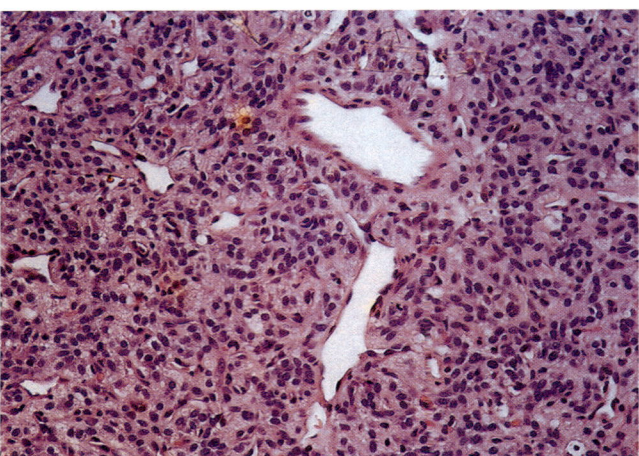

FIG. 1. Histologic slide demonstrating clusters of cells (*Zellballen*) separated by a fibrovascular stroma.

CLINICAL CHARACTERISTICS

Paragangliomas appear to be most common in whites, although there is no clear-cut racial predilection (13). These tumors occur more commonly in women and, although they have been described in patients as young as 6 months and as old as 88 years, they are typically identified in the fourth or fifth decades of life (8,13,14).

Multiple or synchronous tumors occur in 3% to 10% of patients (13,15,16). The most common combination noted in one series included a tympanicum tumor associated with an ipsilateral carotid body tumor (15). A hereditary component to some tumors has been described with an autosomal dominant mode of transmission (17). These patients display a much higher incidence of synchronous paragangliomas (25–35%). Furthermore, they are frequently associated with other tumors, both benign and malignant, most notably, pheochromocytomas (17).

Paragangliomas demonstrate a slow and insidious pattern of growth (13,14,18). The time to onset of symptoms depends on the site of origin of the tumor. However, there are typically few symptoms until the lesion is far advanced (18). The signs and symptoms have been placed into three groups based on the tumor characteristics and location (14):

1. Those due to the presence of tumor in the middle ear—conductive hearing loss, aural polyp, and aural discharge.
2. Those due to the vascularity of the tumor—pulsatile tinnitus, aural bleeding, and a positive Brown's or Aquino's sign (18,19) (the former consists of cessation of tumor pulsation and tumor blanching with positive pressure on pneumotoscopy, and the latter consists of cessation of tumor pulsation with ipsilateral carotid artery compression).

TABLE 2. *Presenting symptoms in 73 patients with tympanicum tumors studied at the House Ear Clinic, Inc.*

Symptom	Percentage
Pulsatile tinnitus	50
Hearing loss	30
Otalgia	7
Aural fullness	4
Otorrhea	3
Other	3
Asymptomatic	3

From ref. 20, with permission.

3. Those that suggest tumor extension to vital structures—sensorineural hearing loss, vertigo, aural pain, and cranial neuropathy.

Otologic symptoms are by far the most common presenting complaints and consist of pulsatile tinnitus and conductive hearing loss (13,16,18,20,21) (Tables 2, 3). Tympanicum tumors present earlier than those of the jugular bulb region because of earlier involvement of the umbo with resultant transmission of pulsations and subsequent conductive hearing loss (21).

Paragangliomas rarely metastasize (3–4%) and most often spread along paths of least resistance (13,22,23). They tend to migrate through the temporal bone by vascular channels, naturally occurring fissures, foramina, and, most important, along air cell tracts (14,24). Spector et al. have described two "dangerous triangles" that may allow tumors access to the intracranial cavity (14).

The first triangle is located in the protympanum and is bounded by the eustachian tube and tensor tympani muscle above, the great vessels below, and the cochlea behind. Tumors in this area can follow the peritubal air cells that lead directly to the petrous apex, they can grow into the nasopharynx through the eustachian tube, or they can follow the petrous carotid artery into the middle cranial fossa and cavernous sinus.

The second triangle, the hypotympanic, is in the area of the great venous sinuses and includes the jugular bulb, the inferior petrosal sinus, the sigmoid sinus, and the jugular vein. This pathway provides access to the skull base and its foramina, the carotid artery, and the various venous channels.

Paragangliomas can also invade the mesotympanum extensively, enveloping, but rarely destroying the ossicular chain, and, as stated previously, erode through the tympanic membrane and into the external auditory canal (18,21,24) (Fig. 2). Rarely, a tumor in the middle ear invades the otic capsule through the round window, leading to sensorineural hearing loss.

Neurologic deficits are the second major group of symptoms and signs, often appearing after considerable tumor growth. The incidence of cranial nerve involvement by tumor is approximately 37%, and that of intracranial extension is 15% (25). Medial and posterior extension of the tumor into the mastoid through the facial recess and retrofacial air cell tract may result in envelopment of the facial nerve in its horizontal and vertical segments (25). Facial paralysis has been noted in 21% to 66% of patients, usually several years after initial symptom onset (18,25).

Tumors originating in the jugular bulb, or those from the middle ear that extend inferiorly to involve this region, make

TABLE 3. *Presenting symptoms and signs in 52 patients with jugulare tumors studied at the House Ear Clinic, Inc.*

Symptoms and signs	Percentage
Pulsatile tinnitus	98
Hearing loss	63
Otalgia	12
Hoarseness	28
Dysphagia	17
Dizziness	21
Middle ear mass	94
External auditory canal mass	6
Neck mass	4
Facial hypesthesia	14
Decreased gag reflex	23
Vocal cord paresis	34
Trapezius/sternocleidomastoid muscle weakness	18
Tongue deviation	20

From ref. 16, with permission.

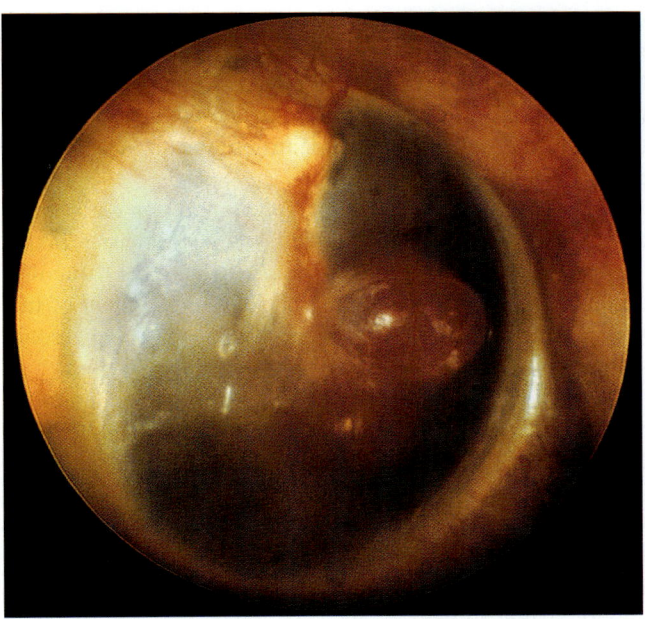

FIG. 2. Tympanicum tumor protruding through an intact tympanic membrane.

themselves apparent by their compression of cranial nerves IX, X, XI, and XII, either at the jugular foramen and hypoglossal canals (Vernet's and Collet-Sicard syndromes), or in the carotid sheath after extension into the parapharyngeal space. Involvement of the internal carotid artery either in the neck or in the petrous portion of the temporal bone can lead to Horner's syndrome by involvement of the sympathetic plexus (25). Spector et al. found posterior fossa extension in 50% of patients with jugular foramen syndrome and in 75% of patients with hypoglossal nerve involvement (25). Horner's syndrome was associated with a 50% incidence of middle cranial fossa invasion.

RADIOLOGIC DIAGNOSIS

Radiologic evaluation is essential for the proper diagnosis and management of jugulotympanic paragangliomas. Techniques such as plain films of the mastoid and polytomography have been supplanted by high-resolution computed tomography (HRCT) and magnetic resonance imaging (MRI). Furthermore, unless the tumor is embolized or envelopes much of the internal carotid artery, HRCT and MRI obviate the need for angiography.

The CT appearance of paragangliomas is highly variable. HRCT scans in the axial and coronal planes, including soft tissue and bone algorithms, provide information critical to the differential diagnosis and approach to management of these tumors (26–28). HRCT supplements clinical otoscopy in defining the extent of tumor beyond the microscopically visible limits of the tympanic annulus, and it aids in the differentiation of tumors from vascular anomalies. Furthermore, HRCT helps to define the extent of involvement of the temporal bone by the tumor and can assist in identifying intracranial extension. Last, HRCT with contrast helps to differentiate paragangliomas from other benign and malignant tumors of the skull base, and identifies synchronous tumors of the skull base and neck.

Because tympanicum tumors typically present early, they often appear as well circumscribed, soft tissue masses in the middle ear without bony erosion (29) (Figs. 3, 4). Jugulotympanic paragangliomas often display involvement of the hypotympanum and erosion of the jugular plate and carotid spine (24).

More extensive bone destruction is associated with tumors of the jugular bulb, which demonstrate an irregular or "motheaten" pattern of erosion of the jugulocarotid spine, the jugular foramen, or the hypoglossal canal (Fig. 5). HRCT demonstrates destruction of the pars nervosa medially and involvement of the inferior petrosal sinus along the petrooccipital suture (see Fig. 5). Although tumor may involve the hypotympanic air cells extensively, the hard bone of the otic capsule is often spared.

Magnetic resonance imaging is superior to HRCT in its ability to characterize the vascular nature of tumors involving the jugular bulb and skull base without the use of contrast

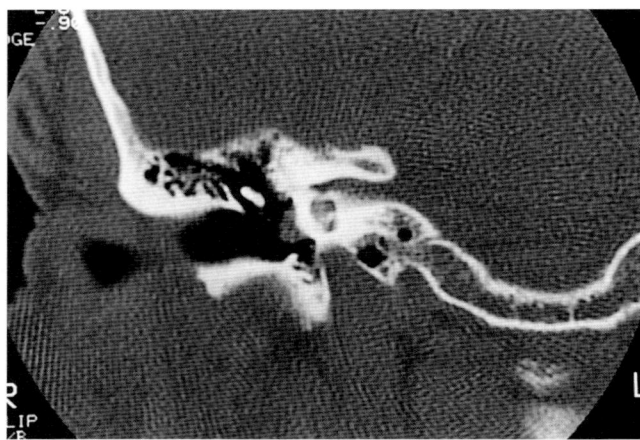

FIG. 3. Noncontrast coronal high-resolution computed tomography scan demonstrating a paraganglioma limited to the promontory.

and without the artifact from the petrous bone typically seen on CT (30). MRI displays the important relations of the tumor to the surrounding great vessels, including venous invasion (Fig. 6). T1-weighted images, with and without contrast, display the highly vascular nature of the tumor matrix, and T2-weighted images provide excellent soft tissue contrast (Fig. 7). For lesions larger than 2 cm, T2-weighted images often display the "salt-and-pepper" appearance characteristic of paragangliomas (30).

Stagnant blood in the jugular foramen can be mistaken for tumor, as can postenhancement images (30). Differentiation of these two entities can often be facilitated by magnetic resonance venography and HRCT (31). Magnetic resonance angiography, although helpful in the differential diagnosis of pulsatile tinnitus, does not reliably demonstrate the tumor vascularity seen on conventional angiography (32).

Detection of multicentric or metastatic lesions has been facilitated by radionuclide scintigraphy with indium-111–

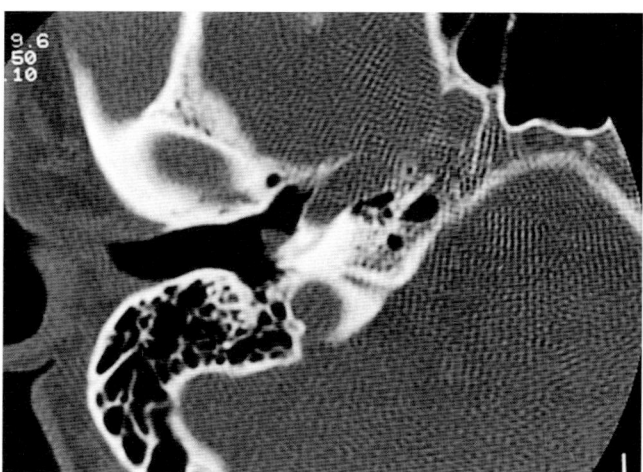

FIG. 4. Axial high-resolution computed tomography scan of the tumor shown in Fig. 3. Note the intact jugular plate in the hypotympanum.

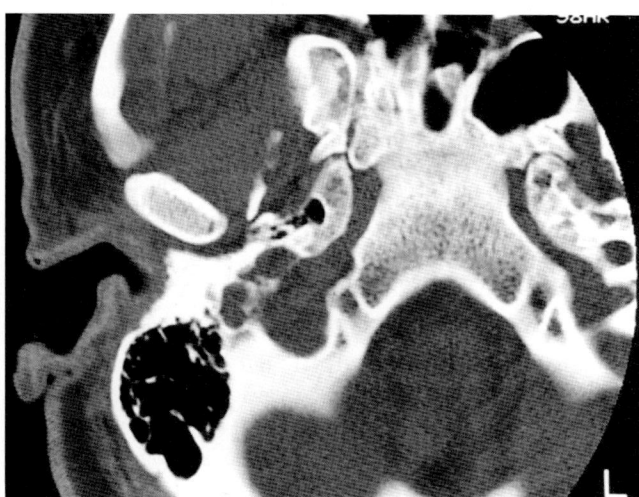

FIG. 5. Noncontrast axial high-resolution computed tomography scan displaying a "moth-eaten" pattern of destruction of the jugular foramen and extension of the tumor along the petrooccipital suture within the inferior petrosal sinus.

octreotide (33). Although it is useful in cases with high risk of multicentricity, such as hereditary tumors, the authors do not routinely screen patients before surgery.

PERIOPERATIVE MANAGEMENT

Secretion

Although all glomus tumors have the potential for catecholamine secretion, clinically significant secretion is identified in only 1% to 3% (34,35). Norepinephrine is the most commonly secreted substance, although dopamine secretion has been reported (34). Glomus tumors lack the ability to convert norepinephrine to epinephrine. Thus, if high levels of the latter are detected in the patient's serum, a search should be made for a concomitant pheochromocytoma (34).

The evaluation of a patient with a paraganglioma should include detecting the symptoms and signs of catecholamine secretion, which include the following: headaches, pallor, excessive perspiration, palpitations, hypertension, nausea, and orthostatic changes in blood pressure. Clinical suspicion of catecholamine secretion can be verified by measuring serum catecholamine levels and 24-hour urinary metanephrines (normetanephrine and metanephrine) and vanillylmandelic acid (34). Preoperative screening is essential in tumors originating from the jugular bulb. There is little evidence for secretion of catecholamines by tympanicum tumors, and routine screening for these tumors is unnecessary (20).

Management of patients with secreting tumors includes perioperative blood pressure management with α-blocking agents, including phentolamine and phenoxybenzamine, and intraoperative invasive hemodynamic monitoring (34).

Embolization and Assessment of Collateral Circulation

Although preoperative arteriography has largely been supplanted by noninvasive imaging, it continues to play a role in the embolization of large tumors involving the jugular foramen and skull base. The authors have found preoperative embolization of selected tumors significantly reduces operating time and intraoperative blood loss (36). The embolization is typically performed 24 to 48 hours before surgery.

For tumors abutting the internal carotid artery, it is often necessary to assess the cross-perfusion from the contralateral vessels when the potential for carotid sacrifice exists. Cross-compression angiography, measurement of stump pressures, oculoplethysmography, and balloon occlusion testing are all

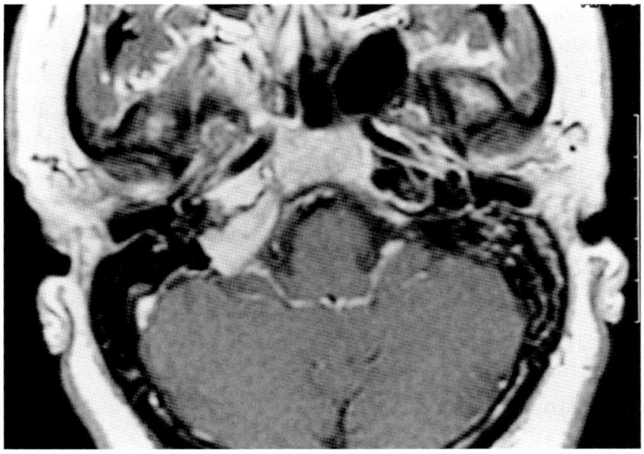

FIG. 6. Gadolinium-enhanced, T1-weighted axial magnetic resonance image demonstrating tumor involvement of the right inferior petrosal sinus up to the petroclival junction.

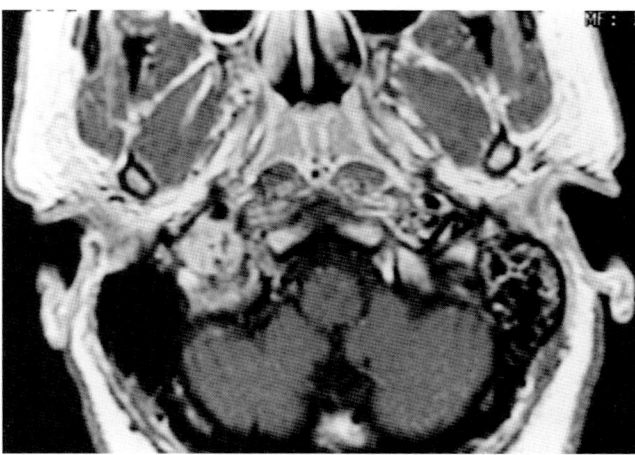

FIG. 7. Gadolinium-enhanced axial T1-weighted magnetic resonance image revealing several flow voids in this vascular tumor in the right jugular foramen.

methods of assessing the risk of cerebrovascular accident after carotid occlusion. Many of these studies have proven to be unreliable predictors of postoperative morbidity (37). ^{99m}Tc-hexamethylpropyleneamine oxime (HMPAO) cerebral perfusion single-photon emission CT imaging or xenon CT studies offer a more precise assessment of collateral blood flow and the risk of subsequent cerebrovascular accident (38–40). Patients requiring sacrifice of an extensively involved internal carotid artery and who perform well on these studies can be managed by preoperative permanent balloon occlusion (41). Those patients who fail the preoperative perfusion studies may require revascularization at the time of resection.

DIFFERENTIAL DIAGNOSIS

When considering the differential diagnosis of paragangliomas, two different presentations must be considered: (a) intratympanic vascular masses, and (b) lesions of the skull base causing caudal cranial nerve deficits. Radiographic imaging is an essential aid to the differential diagnosis, with HRCT the preferred modality for the former and MRI for the latter.

Vascular anomalies of the middle ear may present in a fashion identical to that of an intratympanic paraganglioma. The principal anomalies include the aberrant or laterally displaced internal carotid artery, the dehiscent or high-riding jugular bulb, and the congenital or acquired intratympanic carotid artery aneurysm (42–47).

The aberrant internal carotid artery can be distinguished by HRCT (48). HRCT displays the four features that establish the diagnosis: (a) enlargement of the inferior tympanic canaliculus by the aberrant vessel at its entry into the middle ear, (b) an enhancing mass in the hypotympanum, (c) absence of the vertical segment of the internal carotid canal, and (d) absence of the bony covering of the internal carotid artery (44). Aberrant internal carotid arteries are most frequently identified in women (90%) and in right ears (75%) (43,44).

The high-riding jugular bulb is the most common vascular anomaly of the middle ear and is readily recognized on HRCT (43). It is defined as a jugular bulb extending above the inferior tympanic annulus and is present in approximately 6% of patients.

Intratympanic carotid aneurysms are rare. They are thought to arise from congenital arterial anomalies, although posttraumatic and postinfectious aneurysms have been described (45–47).

These anomalies can often be differentiated from tumors by a careful microscopic examination. However, radiographic imaging is essential to their delineation. Ill-advised biopsy procedures performed on aberrant vessels have resulted in massive hemorrhage and hemiplegia (44,45).

The differential diagnosis of jugular foramen masses includes a variety of benign and malignant neoplasms and is beyond the scope of this chapter. In brief, schwannomas of cranial nerves IX, X, XI, and XII, and meningiomas can all present with caudal cranial nerve deficits. A variety of primary and metastatic lesions of the skull base can also lead to caudal cranial nerve deficits. Here, too, radiography is essential to the differential diagnosis.

TABLE 4. *Classification scheme devised by Antonio De la Cruz MD*

Anatomic classification	Surgical approach
Tympanic	Transcanal
Tympanomastoid	Mastoid–extended facial recess
Jugular bulb	Mastoid–neck (possible limited facial nerve rerouting)
Carotid artery	Infratemporal fossa
Transdural	Infratemporal fossa/intracranial

TUMOR CLASSIFICATION AND SELECTION OF SURGICAL APPROACH

Numerous classification schemes have been devised for the clinical characterization of paragangliomas. These schemes are largely based on anatomic location and tumor extent. The classification described by Antonio De la Cruz has been extremely useful in the treatment planning of these tumors. In this classification scheme, tumors are described by their anatomic extent, and each group of tumors has a corresponding operative approach (Table 4).

Tympanic tumors are those arising in the middle ear and confined entirely to the mesotympanum. The complete extent of the tumor is visible through the tympanic membrane; hence, tumor excision can be performed through a transcanal approach. In contrast, a *tympanomastoid* tumor arises from the middle ear but has extended into the posterior tympanum or the hypotympanum beyond the visible confines of the tympanic annulus. Radiographically, these tumors do not involve the jugular bulb, and they can be excised through a mastoid–extended facial recess approach.

Jugular bulb tumors are confined to this region and may extend to the middle ear and mastoid. They do not involve the carotid artery or the intracranial compartment. These tumors are excised through the mastoid–neck approach. Large tumors may require limited rerouting of the facial nerve to the second genu, as described in the section on Surgical Approaches. *Carotid artery* and *transdural* tumors are far more extensive and require an infratemporal fossa approach and excision of the intracranial component.

SURGICAL APPROACHES

Transcanal Approach

The transcanal approach is used for intratympanic paragangliomas limited to the mesotympanum (21). Although the entire extent of the tumor is visible microscopically,

HRCT scan is a useful adjunct for distinguishing the other vascular lesions of the middle ear described previously.

The tympanomeatal flap is incised with the inferior incision extending farther anterior than usual to allow exposure of the hypotympanum (Fig. 8). The tumor is identified on the promontory. The inferior tympanic branch of the ascending pharyngeal artery is often seen supplying the tumor. This vessel may be controlled with bipolar cautery or occlusion with a small piece of oxidized cellulose placed into the inferior tympanic canaliculus. Unipolar cautery should not be used on the cochlear promontory because this may result in sensorineural hearing loss.

The tumor can now be removed with a cupped forceps, and further bleeding, usually from small caroticotympanic arteriolar branches, can be controlled with Gelfoam. The tympanomeatal flap is replaced and the ear is lightly packed with Gelfoam or ointment. These patients are often ready for discharge a few hours after surgery. Accurate preoperative assessment of tumor extent is critical to the successful removal through the transcanal approach.

Mastoid–Extended Facial Recess Approach

The mastoid–extended facial recess approach is used for tympanomastoid tumors (21) (Fig. 9). Preoperative HRCT is essential to the surgical planning with this approach (20). Patient preparation and draping are identical to that for a routine tympanoplasty with mastoidectomy. A wide postauricular shave is performed, and an incision is made approximately 1 cm posterior to the postauricular crease. After complete mastoidectomy, the facial recess is opened in the usual fashion, using the chorda tympani, the facial nerve, and the fossa incudis as landmarks. The extended facial recess is performed by severing the chorda tympani nerve and following the tympanic annulus into the hypotympanum. This approach allows complete exposure of the middle ear and hypotympanum from a posterior direction without the need for a tympanomeatal flap. After identification of the tumor, bipolar cautery is used to shrink the tumor and control the feeding vessels. The tumor is removed with cupped forceps. Tumor involving the incus and stapes can be stripped free with the forceps. After complete tumor removal, any further bleeding can be controlled with Surgicel or Gelfoam.

Tumor extension into the retrofacial air cell tracts can be managed by direct exposure in the mastoid. Using a cutting bur, the air cells inferior to the posterior semicircular canal, medial to the facial nerve, and superior to the jugular bulb can be removed. A thin layer of bone surrounding the facial nerve should remain for support. Tumor in this area can then be removed using a mastoid curette.

Extensive tumor involvement in the middle ear may necessitate removal of the malleus, incus, or tympanic membrane. In these circumstances, a tympanoplasty and ossicular reconstruction can be performed in the same sitting. At the conclusion of the procedure, a mastoid dressing is applied, and the patient can be discharged on the first postoperative morning.

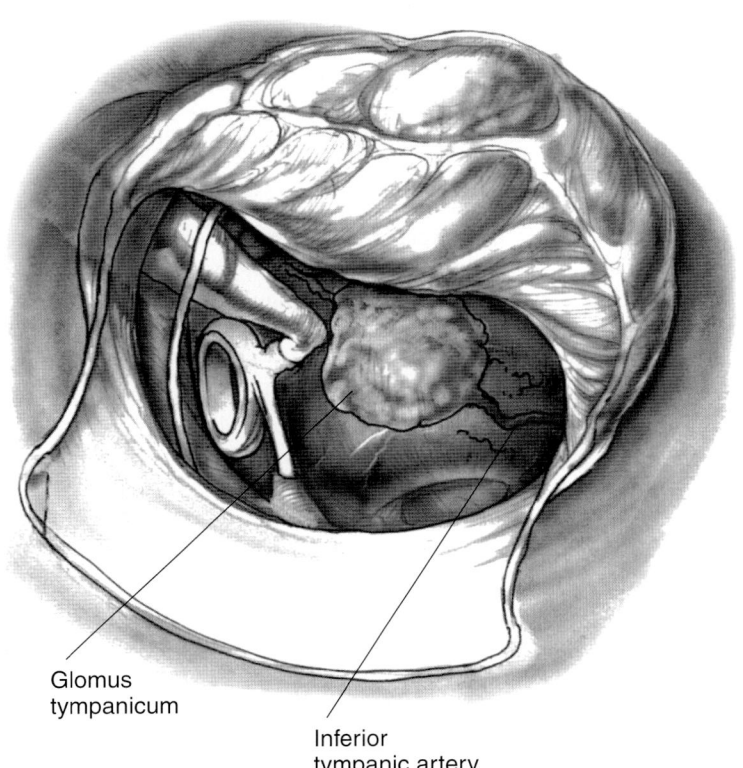

FIG. 8. Transcanal exposure of a tympanicum tumor limited to the promontory.

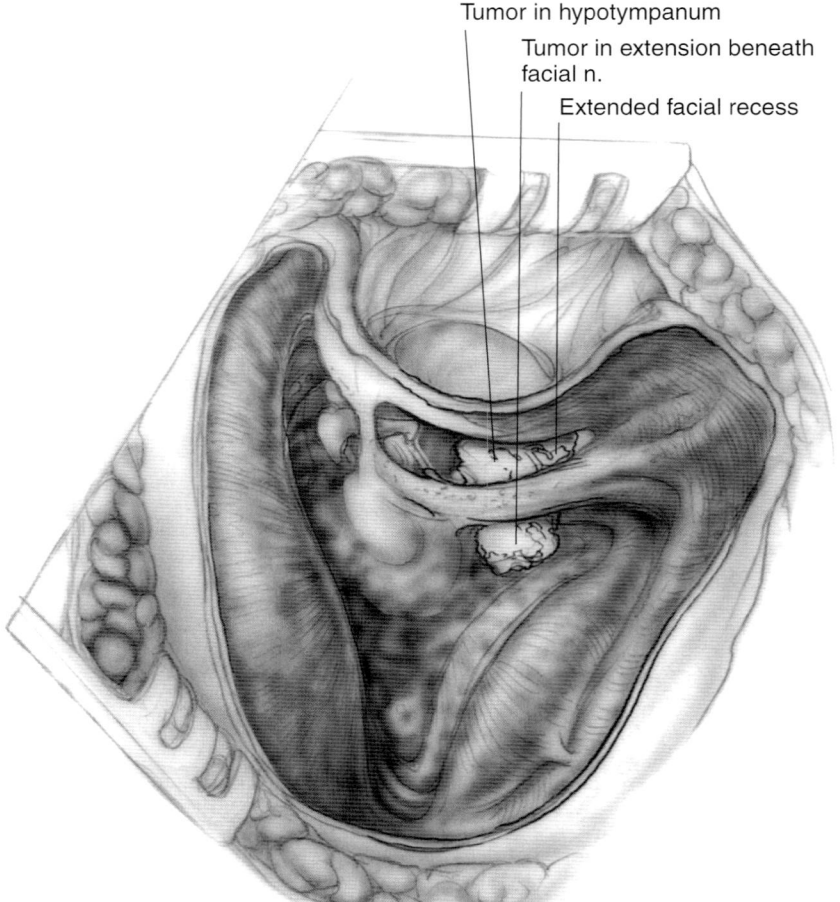

FIG. 9. Extended facial recess exposure of a tympanicum tumor that has extended into the hypotympanum. The retrofacial air cells have been removed to expose tumor medial to the facial nerve.

Mastoid–Neck Approach

The mastoid–neck approach is used for small jugulare tumors that do not involve the carotid artery or the posterior cranial fossa (49). Intraoperative electromyographic cranial nerve monitoring is an essential adjunct to this approach. Continuous intraoperative facial nerve monitoring is routinely used. Additional monitoring of cranial nerves IX, X, and XI by electrodes in the lateral pharyngeal wall, the vocalis muscle, and the trapezius muscle, respectively, can be used to assist in nerve preservation. This approach begins in the same fashion as the mastoid–extended facial recess approach (see Fig. 9).

The periosteum of the digastric is exposed posteriorly toward the occiput and anteriorly toward the stylomastoid foramen. Skeletonization of the digastric muscle facilitates amputation of the mastoid tip. The postauricular incision is carried down into the neck in a favorable neck crease, allowing exposure of the sternocleidomastoid muscle (SCM) and, ultimately, the great vessels and the lower cranial nerves. The SCM is dissected free of the mastoid tip by grasping the tip lateral to the digastric muscle with a Kocher clamp, rotating the tip posteriorly, and sharply dissecting the SCM attachments off the mastoid periosteum with a curved Mayo scissors. The posterior belly of the digastric is dissected free and reflected anteriorly to allow exposure of the great vessels and the lower cranial nerves. The internal jugular vein is isolated and ligated with multiple 2-0 silk sutures. The vein is then freed from inferior to superior over the transverse process of the first cervical vertebra and under the spinal accessory nerve into the jugular foramen. Blunt and sharp dissection in this area allows preservation of cranial nerves IX, X, and XI when they are not infiltrated by tumor.

Exposure of the sigmoid sinus and jugular bulb is completed using diamond burs, with care taken to preserve bone over the proximal sigmoid sinus to facilitate extraluminal packing. Although limited tumors do not involve the medial wall of the jugular bulb, these tumors arise from the adventitia and require resection of the lateral bulb in continuity with the tumor. Before opening the sigmoid sinus, it is packed extraluminally under the bone preserved proximally. The sinus is opened just distal to the packing. Despite the extraluminal packing proximally and the ligation of the jugular vein in the neck, brisk bleeding from the inferior petrosal sinus and the condylar vein often ensues. Oxidized cellulose is gently but firmly packed into the jugular bulb in an effort to occlude the inferior petrosal sinus and the condylar vein while avoiding compression and subsequent injury to the lower cranial nerves on the medial aspect of the jugular foramen. Overly vigorous packing of the inferior petrosal sinus can lead to damage to the glossopharyngeal nerve in the pars nervosa, leading to potential postoperative aspiration.

The tumor is now ready for complete removal. Bipolar cautery is useful for hemostasis and shrinkage of the tumor. After tumor removal, residual bleeding can be controlled with oxidized cellulose packing. If tumor extirpation required removal of the tympanic membrane or ossicles, these can be repaired as described previously (Fig. 10).

After surgery, these patients are managed in an intensive care setting for 24 hours to allow early identification of lower cranial neuropathy or postoperative hemorrhage. The patients are often ready for discharge on the third or fourth postoperative day.

Preoperative radiographic assessment is essential for this approach. The mastoid–neck approach is too limited for the removal of tumors involving the petrous carotid artery.

Mastoid–Neck Approach with Limited Facial Nerve Rerouting

For slightly larger tumors of the jugular bulb not involving the carotid artery or posterior cranial fossa, limited rerouting of the facial nerve to the second genu can facilitate removal with no added morbidity (49,50). After decompression of the vertical segment of the facial nerve, the eggshell of bone remaining is removed. The facial nerve is dissected free of its fibrous attachments within the canal from the second genu to the level of stylomastoid foramen. The periosteum at the foramen is preserved such that after mobilization of the posterior belly of the digastric, the muscle and the soft tissue surrounding the stylomastoid foramen are reflected anteriorly as a whole, preserving the blood supply in this region. A suture placed through the periosteum allows anterior displacement of the nerve without tension (Fig. 11). This modification allows complete removal of the air cells in the retrofacial area inferior to the posterior semicircular canal.

Infratemporal Fossa Approach

The development of the infratemporal fossa approach to large skull base tumors has contributed greatly to their safe surgical removal (51). Removal of the external auditory canal and rerouting of the facial nerve allows complete exposure of tumors involving the internal carotid artery. There are eight distinct steps in the infratemporal fossa exposure: (a) patient preparation, (b) management of the ear canal and tympanic ring, (c) mastoidectomy, (d) initial preparation of the jugular vein and neck exposure, (e) transposition of the facial nerve, (f) completion of the neck exposure and identification of the lower cranial nerves and skull base carotid artery, (g) tumor removal and intracranial extension, and (h) wound closure (49). Continuous facial nerve monitoring and electromyographic monitoring of the lower cranial nerves are used as previously described.

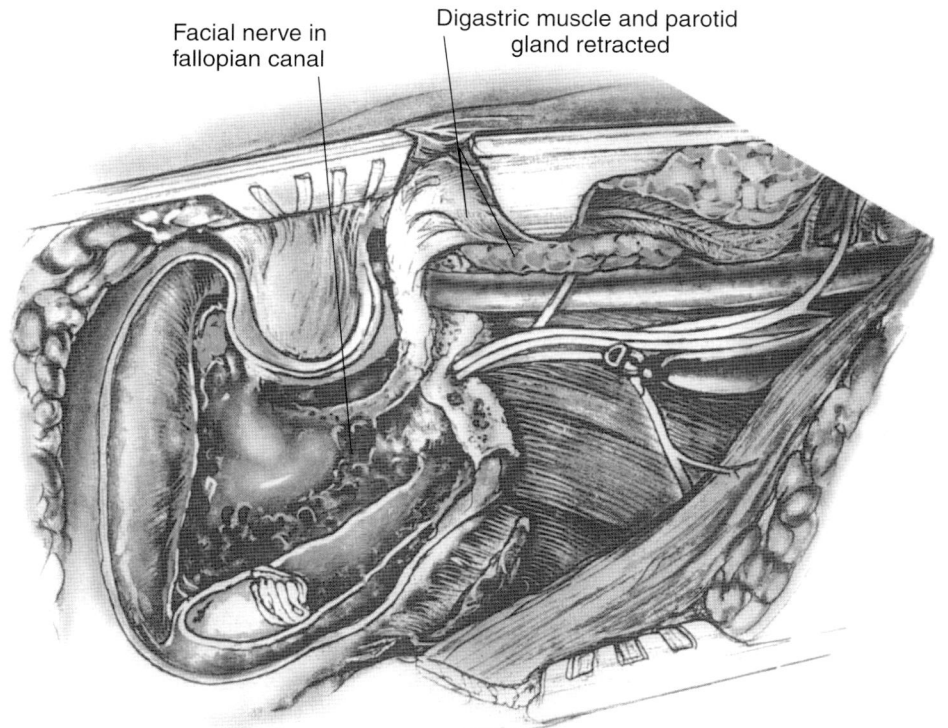

FIG. 10. Completed mastoid–neck approach demonstrating resected jugular bulb.

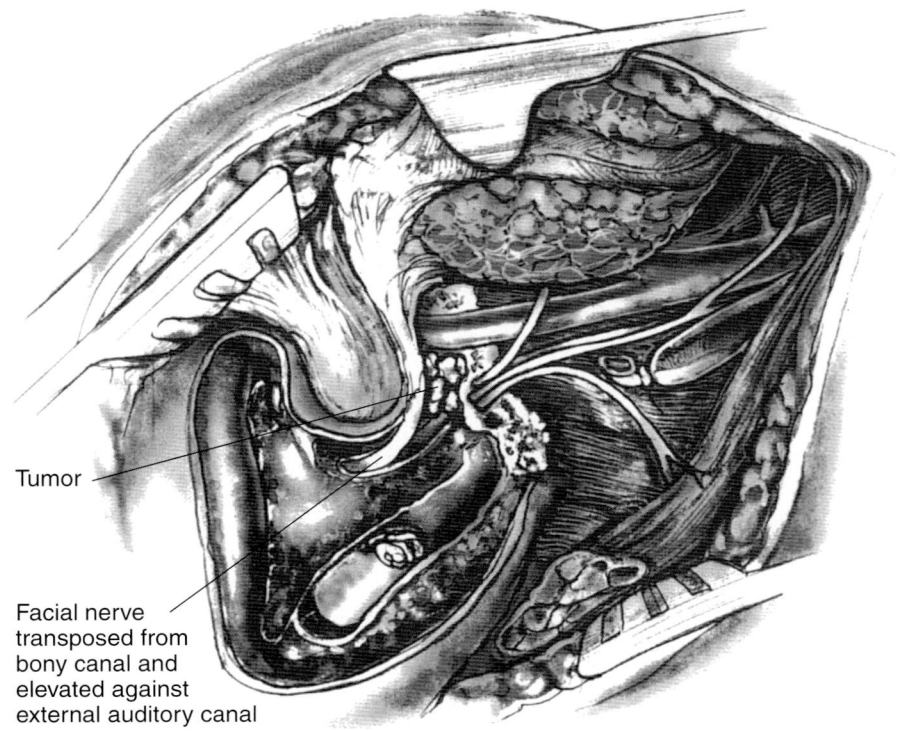

FIG. 11. Mastoid–neck approach with limited rerouting of the facial nerve for larger tumors of the jugular bulb.

A wide shave is performed in the preoperative waiting area. The area is prepared and draped such that wide exposure of the postauricular area and complete ipsilateral neck is facilitated. A large, postauricular C-shaped incision is made that is extended into the neck within a neck crease two fingerbreadths below the angle of the mandible. The ear is dissected forward and the ear canal is transected just medial to the bony–cartilaginous junction. The cartilage around the meatus is removed to facilitate eversion of a cuff of ear canal skin. The everted skin is closed with several interrupted 4-0 nylon sutures (Fig. 12). An anteriorly based mastoid periosteal flap is elevated and transposed anteriorly medial to the ear canal, providing another layer of closure (Fig. 13). After this soft tissue work, a mastoidectomy with an extended facial recess is performed to allow separation of the incudostapedial joint. The posterior external auditory canal with its overlying skin can now be safely removed using a rongeur and large cutting bur. The remaining skin, the tympanic membrane, and the malleus and incus are removed. The facial nerve can now be skeletonized from the geniculate ganglion to the stylomastoid foramen, leaving a thin eggshell covering. Caution must be exercised in the region of the oval window to avoid stapedial injury and subsequent sensorineural hearing loss. Using a combination of cutting and diamond burs, the bone of the tympanic ring is removed superiorly, anteriorly, posteriorly, and inferiorly. The facial nerve must be kept in view to avoid injury to its anterior surface. Complete bone removal in this way allows identification of the jugular bulb, the petrous carotid artery, and the temporomandibular joint (Fig. 14).

The postauricular incision can now be carried into the neck as described, allowing exposure of the SCM. The mastoid tip is removed as illustrated previously, and the internal jugular vein, internal and external carotid arteries, and cranial nerves IX, X, XI, and XII are identified and preserved. Ligatures are placed around the internal carotid artery and the jugular bulb for identification and vascular control. The posterior belly of the digastric is dissected free from the digastric groove.

The next step involves transposition of the entire facial nerve to the geniculate ganglion using a modification of the approach originally described by Fisch (50,51). The facial nerve is not dissected out to the pes anserinus as previously described; rather, the tail of the parotid is separated from its fibrous attachments to the SCM. The posterior belly of the digastric is dissected forward in continuity with the periosteum of the stylomastoid foramen. The eggshell of bone is removed from the entire facial nerve using a Rosen needle or sickle knife. The fibrovascular attachments of the facial nerve within its canal are sharply dissected and the nerve elevated to the second genu. The tympanic segment is elevated more readily because it does not have the fibrovascular attachments. The entire nerve is transposed forward along with the posterior belly of the digastric and the parotid tail. A large silk suture is placed through the stylomastoid perios-

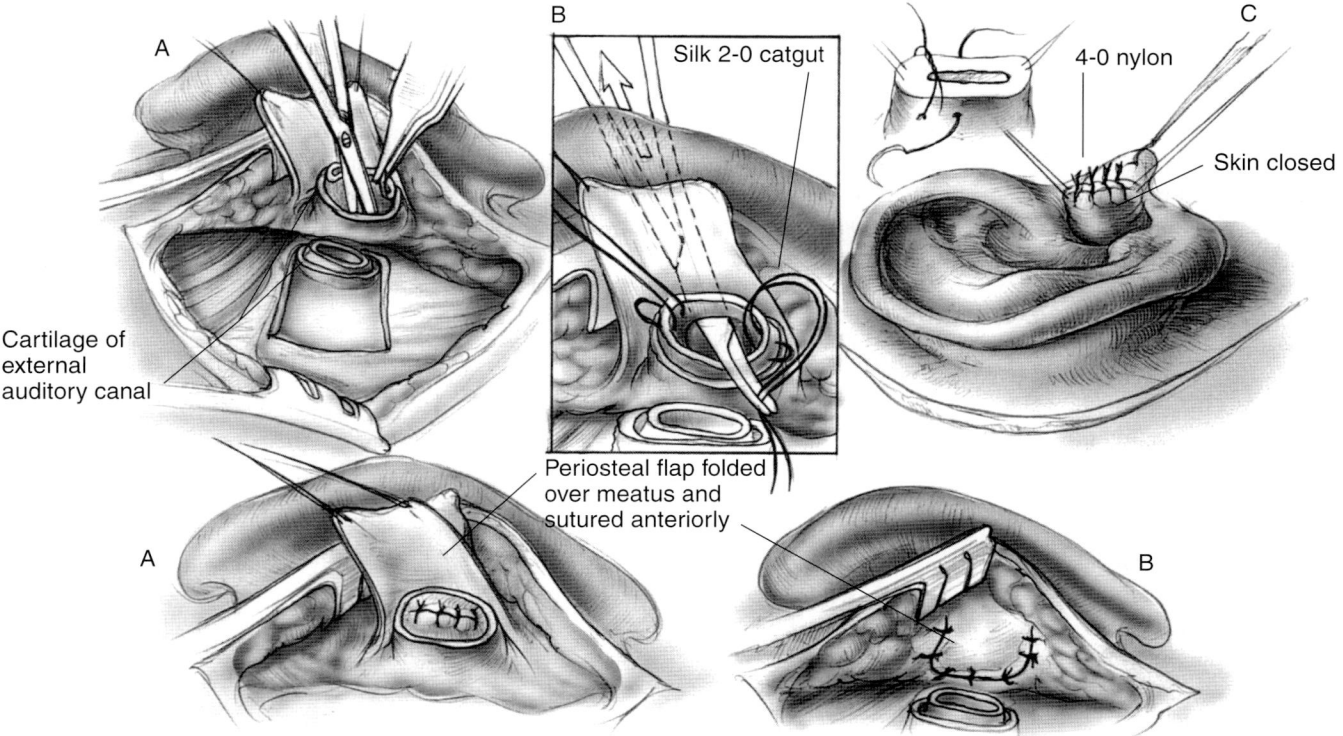

FIG. 12. A: Postauricular approach demonstrating preservation of an anteriorly based periosteal flap, and dissection of lateral canal skin from cartilage. **B:** Everting stitches placed superiorly and inferiorly that are grasped with a hemostat through the ear canal and brought out laterally. **C:** Complete closure of the everted canal skin.

FIG. 13. A,B: The anteriorly based mastoid periosteal flap is folded anteriorly and sutured in place, providing another layer of closure medial to the everted canal skin.

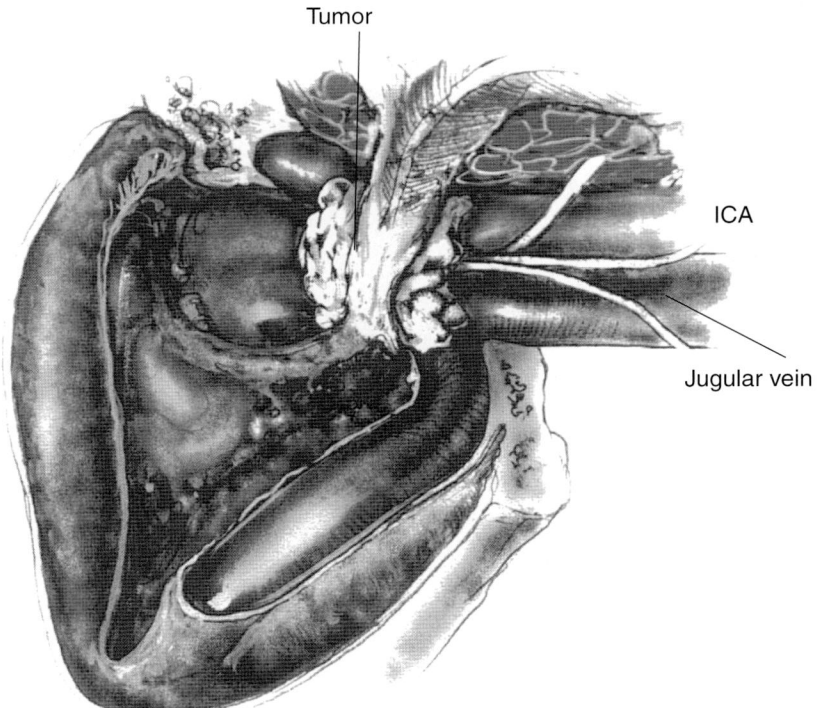

FIG. 14. Completed dissection. The facial nerve has been skeletonized, the tympanic ring has been removed, and the great vessels are exposed.

teum to the soft tissue surrounding the zygomatic root (Fig. 15). The use of continuous facial nerve monitoring during rerouting has dramatically improved postoperative facial nerve function (52).

A large Perkins retractor is placed beneath the mandibular angle, and the entire mandible is retracted anteriorly. The exposure offered by this maneuver obviates the need to resect the mandibular condyles, even with large tumors that extend into the infratemporal fossa. Attention is now directed to the sigmoid sinus, jugular bulb, and petrous carotid artery. Using diamond burs, the bone over these structures is removed, preserving a bony shelf over the proximal sigmoid sinus.

The jugular vein and external carotid artery are now doubly ligated proximally and distally in the neck. If the tumor extends intradurally, the proximal sigmoid sinus is doubly ligated with silk sutures passed through openings in the dura with an aneurysm suture passer (Fig. 16). If the tumor is extradural, the sigmoid sinus is packed extraluminally with oxidized cellulose, using the shelf of bone left remaining proximally. The jugular vein is then dissected from inferior to superior under the spinal accessory nerve to the level of the jugular bulb. Tumor is freed from the carotid artery and bleeding from the caroticotympanic vessels is controlled with bipolar cautery. If the tumor intimately involves the carotid artery, a small portion is left attached until the conclusion of the procedure. Delaying this subadventitial dissection allows complete exposure and direct repair of small entry sites into the carotid artery in the areas of the caroticotympanic branches (Fig. 17). The tumor is dissected superiorly off of the lower cranial nerves in continuity with the jugular bulb. Oxidized cellulose is used to pack the inferior petrosal sinus and condylar vein.

The management of intracranial tumor extension depends on the size and location of the tumor, and the status of the patient. Small intracranial tumor extensions are removed with the jugular bulb because this is typically the site of dural penetration. The decision to remove large intracranial extensions is based on the hemodynamic status of the patient. Blood loss in excess of 3 liters usually prompts a second-stage approach to total tumor removal. More often, the intraoperative blood loss is less than 3 liters, and the authors proceed with total tumor removal in a single stage.

Removal of the intracranial portion is facilitated by the earlier steps in the procedure, which have significantly devascularized the remnant. The remaining vessels can be cauterized discretely and the tumor removed from the posterior fossa (Fig. 18). Closure is accomplished by closure of the eustachian tube with oxidized cellulose and a temporalis muscle plug. The dural defect is approximated as closely as possible, and thin strips of abdominal fat are used to plug the remaining dural dehiscences and the lateral soft tissue defect. The wound is closed over a Penrose drain, and a pressure dressing is applied.

Lateral skull base defects from paraganglioma removal are rarely large enough to require regional or free flap coverage. Larger dural defects can be managed with a variety of local grafts and flaps, including temporalis fascia grafts, temporoparietal fascial flaps, or temporalis muscle flaps (53). Regional and free flaps are reserved for large lateral skull base defects in previously irradiated fields.

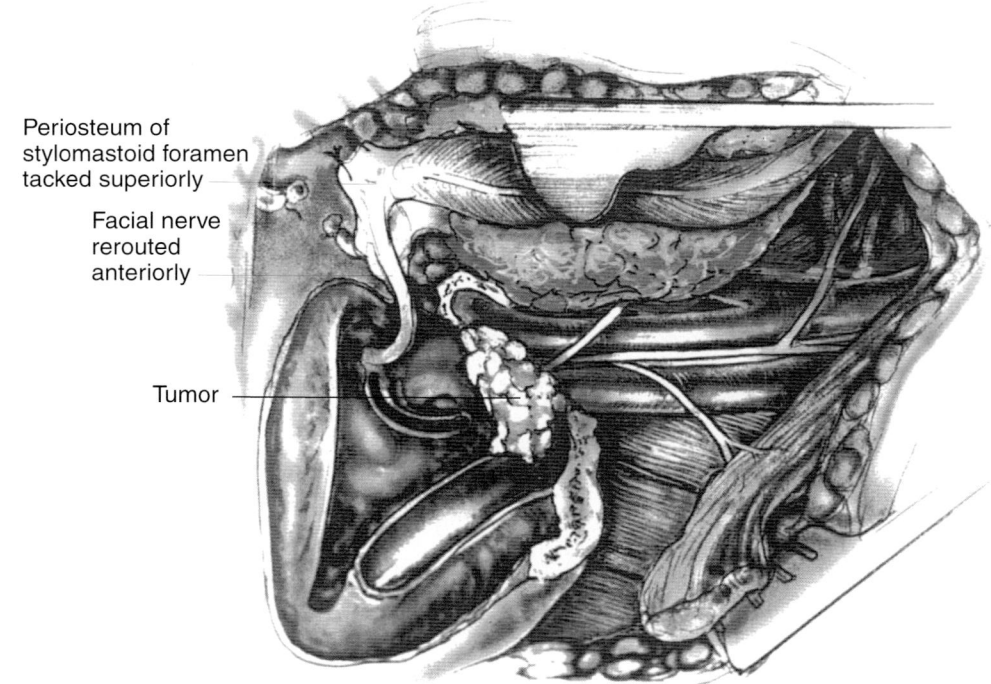

FIG. 15. The facial nerve has been transposed to the first genu and the periosteum of the stylomastoid foramen has been sutured anteriorly to support the nerve without tension.

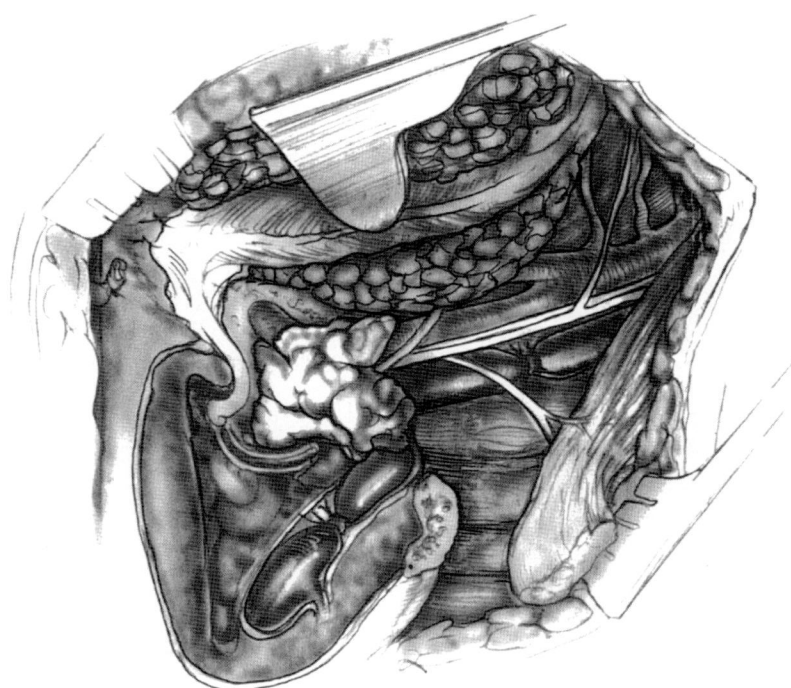

FIG. 16. The jugular vein and sigmoid sinus are doubly ligated. If the tumor is completely extradural, the sigmoid sinus is packed extraluminally in its more proximal course.

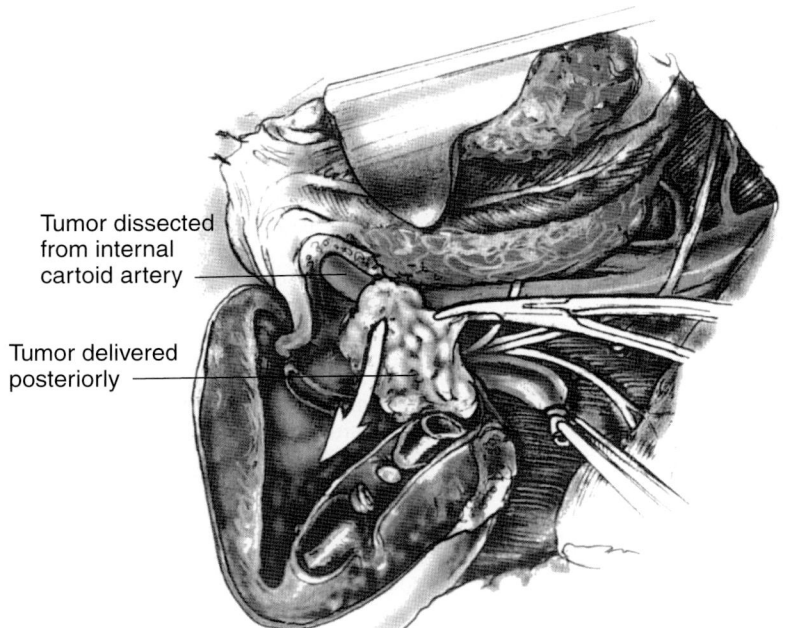

FIG. 17. The remaining piece of tumor is removed from the petrous carotid artery. The caroticotympanic branches can be closed at this time with vascular sutures.

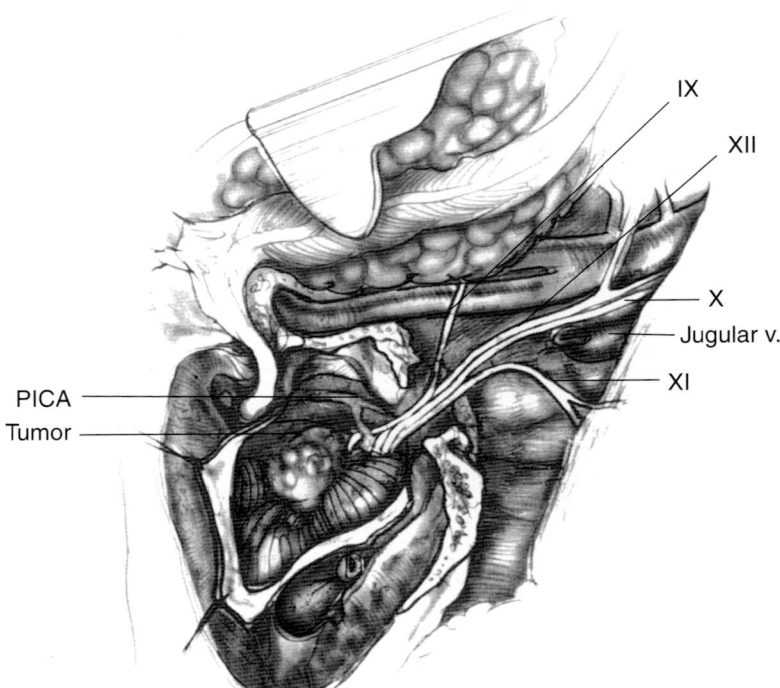

FIG. 18. The devascularized intracranial portion can now be removed. The feeding vessels are controlled with bipolar cautery.

If cerebrospinal fluid (CSF) is encountered, continuous lumbar drainage is placed for approximately 5 days after surgery. Once the epidural catheter is placed through the L4-5 interspace, intravenous tubing is attached in reverse direction through an intravenous infusion pump (54). The pump is set at 10 ml/hour and a continuous slow flow of CSF is withdrawn.

RESULTS

Tympanicum Tumors

O'Leary et al. reviewed 64 cases of tympanicum tumors treated at the House Ear Clinic between 1957 and 1990 (20). Eighty percent of these tumors were removed through a mastoid–extended facial recess approach. The preoperative mean air–bone gap was reduced from 10 dB to a postoperative mean of 4 dB. There were only five complications, including two tympanic membrane ruptures, one cholesteatoma, and one transient facial palsy that resolved to a House grade II/VI after decompression.

Jugulare Tumors

Green et al. reviewed the surgical outcome in 52 previously untreated jugulare tumors managed at the House Ear Clinic between 1980 and 1991 (16). The surgical approach most commonly used was the infratemporal fossa approach (83%). Twenty-nine percent of the tumors extended intradurally, and 21% involved the internal carotid artery. Complete surgical removal was possible in 85%, and there were no surgical mortalities. Of the eight patients with incomplete removal, three had involvement of the internal carotid artery and five had significant intraoperative blood loss prohibiting complete tumor removal in a single stage.

Postoperative complications are infrequent (Table 5). Long-term facial nerve function was good (House grade I/VI or II/VI) in 95% of the patients treated. Approximately 19% of the patients required vocal cord augmentation, and four required enteric feeding because of aspiration. No patient required immediate postoperative tracheotomy and, overall, 85% of the patients were able to resume their preoperative level of activity.

TABLE 5. *Postoperative complications in 52 patients with jugulare tumors studied at the House Ear Clinic, Inc.*

Complication	Percentage
Pneumonia	6
Stroke	0
Cerebrospinal fluid leak	4
Meningitis	4
Aspiration	4
Pulmonary embolus	2
Wound infection	6
Seroma	4

From ref. 16, with permission.

COMPLICATIONS

Tympanicum Tumors

The complications of tympanicum tumor removal are similar to those of tympanomastoid surgery for chronic ear disease. Tympanic membrane perforation, facial nerve injury, cholesteatoma, and bleeding are managed as they would be in all tympanomastoid surgery.

Jugulare Tumors

As described in the Results section, postoperative complications are infrequent (see Table 5). Intraoperative complications can be classified as cranial nerve, carotid artery, and intracranial injury. Continuous intraoperative facial nerve monitoring and modifications to facial nerve rerouting have led to improved postoperative results (16,52). Direct infiltration of the facial nerve requires excision and grafting. The authors have rarely found the need for tracheotomy or gastrostomy (<4%). Early vocal cord augmentation is recommended for new vagal paralyses, especially in the setting of glossopharyngeal nerve dysfunction (55).

The risk of vascular injury can be ascertained before surgery with the appropriate imaging studies. Although preoperative embolization diminishes intraoperative blood loss, the possibility of significant blood loss must be anticipated. The authors' patients are counseled on the utility of autologous donation in the weeks before surgery.

Intracranial removal of paragangliomas must be coordinated with a neurosurgeon. The possibility for intracranial hemorrhage, meningitis, or a CSF leak must be anticipated and may require neurosurgical management.

RADIATION THERAPY

The role of radiation therapy in the treatment of jugulotympanic paragangliomas is controversial. Many reports have appeared in the old and more recent literature reporting tumor control rates of 70% to 90% with radiation as primary, adjunctive, or salvage therapy (56–58). The doses given in these studies are between 3,500 and 5,000 cGy. The primary effect of radiation therapy appears to be on the vascular and stromal elements of the tumor, with little effect on the tumor cells (59). Viable tumor cells remain after radiation, and tumors have been known to recrudesce after more than a decade (58). With the advent of microsurgical techniques, the authors have identified few specific indications for radiation therapy. This form of treatment is recommended for elderly patients with symptomatic tumors or for patients who are unsuitable for or unwilling to undergo surgical resection.

CONCLUSIONS

Jugulotympanic paragangliomas are the most common tumors of the middle ear and the second most common tumors of the temporal bone. The diagnosis and management of these tumors have been facilitated by modern imaging techniques. Microsurgical techniques with electromyographic cranial nerve monitoring, coupled with the multitude of reconstructive options, make surgical excision the preferred method of treatment.

ACKNOWLEDGMENT

The authors thank Karen I. Berliner, Ph.D. for her editorial assistance.

REFERENCES

1. Valentin G. Ueber eine gangliose Anschwellung in der Jacobsonchen Anastomose des Menschen. *Archiv Fur Anatomie Physiologie Und Wissenchaftliche Medicin* 1840;89:287.
2. Krause W. Die Glandula Tympanica des Menschen. *Zentralblatt Fur Die Medicinischen Wissenchaften* 1878;16:737.
3. Guild SR. The glomus jugulare, a nonchromaffin paraganglion, in man. *Ann Otol Rhinol Laryngol* 1953;62:1045.
4. Rosenwasser H. Carotid body tumor of the middle ear and mastoid. *Archives of Otolaryngology* 1945;41:64.
5. Lattes R, Waltner JG. Nonchromaffin paragangliomas of the middle ear. *Cancer* 1949;2:447.
6. Winship T, Klopp CT, Jenkins WH. Glomus-jugularis tumors. *Cancer* 1948;1:441.
7. Steinberg N, Holz WG. Glomus jugularis tumors. *Archives of Otolaryngology* 1965;82:367.
8. Gulya AJ. The glomus tumor and its biology. *Laryngoscope* 1993;103[Suppl 60]:3.
9. Glenner GG, Grimley PM. Tumors of the extra-adrenal paraganglion system (including chemoreceptors). In: *Atlas of tumor pathology.* 2nd series, fascicle 9. Washington, DC: Armed Forces Institute of Pathology, 1974;1.
10. Wenig BM. Neoplasms of the ear. In: Wenig BM, ed. *Atlas of head and neck pathology.* Philadelphia: WB Saunders, 1993:368.
11. LeCompte PM. Tumors of the carotid body. *Am J Pathol* 1948;24:305.
12. Grimley PM, Glenner GG. Histology and ultrastructure of carotid body paragangliomas. *Cancer* 1967;20:1473.
13. Alford BR, Guilford FR. A comprehensive study of tumors of the glomus jugulare. *Laryngoscope* 1962;72:765.
14. Spector GJ, Sobol S, Thawley SE, Maisel RH, Ogura JH. Glomus jugulare tumors of the temporal bone: patterns of invasion in the temporal bone. *Laryngoscope* 1979;89:1628.
15. Spector GJ, Ciralsky R, Maisel RH, Ogura JH. Multiple glomus tumors in the head and neck. *Laryngoscope* 1975;85:1066.
16. Green JD, Brackmann DE, Nguyen CD, Arriaga MA, Telischi FF, De la Cruz A. Surgical management of previously untreated glomus jugulare tumors. *Laryngoscope* 1994;104:917.
17. Parkin JL. Familial multiple glomus tumors and pheochromocytomas. *Annals of Otology, Rhinology and Laryngology* 1981;90:60.
18. Brown LA. Glomus jugulare tumor of the middle ear: clinical aspects. *Laryngoscope* 1953;63:281.
19. Aquino J. Glomus jugulare tumors. *Archives of Otolaryngology* 1957;65:263.
20. O'Leary MJ, Shelton C, Giddings NA, Kwartler J, Brackmann DE. Glomus tympanicum tumors: a clinical perspective. *Laryngoscope* 1991;101:1038.
21. House WF, Glasscock ME. Glomus tympanicum tumors. *Archives of Otolaryngology* 1968;87:550.
22. El Fiky FM, Paparella MM. A metastatic glomus jugulare tumor. *Am J Otol* 1984;5:197.

23. Druck NS, Spector GJ, Ciralsky RH, Ogura JH. Malignant glomus vagale. *Archives of Otolaryngology* 1976;102:634.
24. Wright JW, Wright JW, Hicks GW. Radiologic appearance of glomus tumors. *Laryngoscope* 1979;89:1620.
25. Spector GJ, Gado M, Ciralsky R, Ogura JH, Maisel RH. Neurologic implications of glomus tumors in the head and neck. *Laryngoscope* 1975;85:1387.
26. Lo WWM, Horn KL, Carberry JN, et al. Intratemporal vascular tumors: evaluation with CT. *Radiology* 1986;159:181.
27. Lo WWM, Shelton C, Waluch V, et al. Intratemporal vascular tumors: detection with CT and MR Imaging. *Radiology* 1989;171:443.
28. Lo WWM, Solti-Bohman LG, Lambert PR. High-resolution CT in the evaluation of glomus tumors of the temporal bone. *Radiology* 1984;150:737.
29. Som PM, Reede DL, Bergeron T, Parisier SC, Shugar JMA, Cohen NL. Computed tomography of glomus tympanicum tumors. *J Comput Assist Tomogr* 1983;7:14.
30. Olsen WL, Dillon WP, Kelly WM, Norman D, Brant-Zawadzki M, Newton TH. MR imaging of paragangliomas. *AJNR Am J Neuroradiol* 1987;148:201.
31. Vogl TJ, Juergens M, Balzer JO, et al. Glomus tumors of the skull base: combined use of MR angiography and spin-echo imaging. *Radiology* 1994;192:103.
32. Rodgers GK, Applegate L, De la Cruz A, Lo W. Magnetic resonance angiography: analysis of vascular lesions of the temporal bone and skull base. *Am J Otol* 1993;14:56.
33. Kwekkeboom DJ, Van Urk H, Pawn BKH, et al. Octreotide scintigraphy for the detection of paragangliomas. *J Nucl Med* 1993;34:873.
34. Schwaber MK, Glasscock ME, Jackson CG, Nissen AJ, Smith PG. diagnosis and management of catecholamine secreting glomus tumors. *Laryngoscope* 1984;94:1008.
35. Cantrell RW, Kaplan MJ, Winn HR, Atuk NO, Jahrsdoerfer RA. Catecholamine-secreting infratemporal fossa paraganglioma. *Ann Otol Rhinol Laryngol* 1984;93:583.
36. Murphy TP, Brackmann DE. Effects of preoperative embolization on glomus jugulare tumors. *Laryngoscope* 1989;99:1244.
37. McIvor NP, Willinsky RA, TerBrugge KG, Rutka JA, Freeman JL. Validity of test occlusion studies prior to internal carotid artery sacrifice. *Head Neck* 1994;16:11.
38. Peterman SB, Taylor A, Hoffman JC. Improved detection of cerebral hypoperfusion with internal carotid balloon test occlusion and 99mTc-HMPAO cerebral perfusion SPECT imaging. *AJNR Am J Neuroradiol* 1991;12:1035.
39. Monsein LH, Jeffery PJ, van Heerden BB, et al. assessing adequacy of collateral circulation during balloon test occlusion of the internal carotid artery with ^{99m}Tc-HMPAO SPECT. *AJNR Am J Neuroradiol* 1991;12:1045.
40. de Vries EJ, Sekhar LN, Horton JA, et al. A new method to predict safe resection of the internal carotid artery. *Laryngoscope* 1990;100:85.
41. Andrews JC, Valvanis A, Fisch U. Management of the internal carotid artery in surgery of the skull base. *Laryngoscope* 1989;99:1224.
42. Sinnreich AI, Parisier SC, Cohen NL, Berzeby M. Arterial malformations of the middle ear. *Otolaryngol Head Neck Surg* 1984;92:194.
43. Glasscock ME, Dickins JRE, Jackson CG, Wiet RJ. Vascular anomalies of the middle ear. *Laryngoscope* 1980;90:77.
44. McElveen JT, Lo WWM, El Gabri TH, Nigri P. Aberrant internal carotid artery: classic findings on computed tomography. *Otolaryngol Head Neck Surg* 1986;94:616.
45. Conley J, Hildyard V. Aneurysm of the internal carotid artery presenting in the middle ear. *Archives of Otolaryngology* 1969;90:61.
46. Goodman RS, Cohen NL. Aberrant internal carotid artery in the middle ear. *Annals of Otology, Rhinology and Laryngology* 1981;90:67.
47. Stallings JO, McCabe BF. Congenital middle ear aneurysm of internal carotid. *Archives of Otolaryngology* 1969;90:65.
48. Lo WWM, Solti-Bohman LG, McElveen JT. Aberrant carotid artery: radiologic diagnosis with emphasis on high-resolution computed tomography. *Radiographics* 1985;5:985.
49. Brackmann DE, Arriaga MA. Surgery for glomus tumors. In: Brackmann DE, Shelton C, Arriaga MA, eds. *Otologic surgery*. Philadelphia: WB Saunders, 1994:579.
50. Brackmann DE. The facial nerve in the infratemporal approach. *Otolaryngol Head Neck Surg* 1987;97:15.
51. Fisch U. Infratemporal fossa approach for glomus tumors of the temporal bone. *Ann Otol Rhinol Laryngol* 1982;91:474.
52. Leonetti JP, Brackmann DE, Prass RL. Improved preservation of facial nerve function in the infratemporal approach to the skull base. *Otolaryngol Head Neck Surg* 1989;101:74.
53. Netterville JL, Civantos FJ. Defect reconstruction following neurotologic skull base surgery. *Laryngoscope* 1993;103[Suppl 60]:55.
54. Brackmann DE, Rodgers GK. Management of postoperative cerebrospinal fluid leaks. In: Brackmann DE, Shelton C, Arriaga MA, eds. *Otologic surgery*. Philadelphia: WB Saunders 1994:701.
55. Netterville JL, Civantos FJ. Rehabilitation of cranial nerve deficits after neurotologic skull base surgery. *Laryngoscope* 1993;103[Suppl 60]:45.
56. Mendenhall WM, Parsons JT, Stringer SP, Cassisi NJ, Singleton GT, Million RR. Radiotherapy in the management of temporal bone chemodectoma. *Skull Base Surgery* 1995;5:83.
57. de Jong AL, Coker NJ, Jenkins HA, Goepfert H, Alford BR. Radiation therapy in the management of paragangliomas of the temporal bone. *Am J Otol* 1995;16:283.
58. Cole JM, Beiler D. Long-term results of treatment for glomus jugulare and glomus vagale tumors with radiotherapy. *Laryngoscope* 1994;104:1461.
59. Brackmann DE, House WF, Terry R, Scanlan RL. Glomus jugulare tumors: effect of irradiation. *Ophthalmology and Otolaryngology* 1972;76:1423.

SECTION IV
Midline Approaches

CHAPTER 25

Extreme Lateral Transcondylar Approach to the Craniocervical Junction

Chandranath Sen and Peter J. Catalano

Tumors arising ventral and ventrolateral to the brainstem and the cervicomedullary junction pose some special problems for the neurosurgeon, including difficulty of access and involvement of the vertebral artery and lower cranial nerves, either by the tumor itself or the path of the surgical approach. Some of these tumors may also invade extradural tissues. Most of the tumors, either benign (e.g., meningiomas, schwannomas, glomus tumors) or locally aggressive (e.g., chordomas and chondrosarcomas), are amenable to radical resection, which provides the best chance for long-term control or cure. Aneurysms arising from the vertebral artery and vertebrobasilar junction may also present surgical difficulties.

A standard lateral suboccipital approach may not be adequate to achieve a radical tumor resection or safely clip an aneurysm with full visualization. A more lateral approach, along with control and mobilization of the vertebral artery as it enters the dura, with or without some resection of the occipital condyle, allows better visibility anterior to the brainstem and favorably influences the safety and completeness of the operation.

ANATOMIC CONSIDERATIONS

The Bony Anatomy

The shape of the bony foramen magnum can be round or oval, and thus the surface in front of the brainstem may be deep or shallow, depending on this shape. The occipital condyles form the anterolateral margins of the foramen magnum and are directed anteromedially, whereas the articular surfaces point anterolaterally. The hypoglossal canals run in the medial third of the condyles and a large condylar emissary vein exits posteriorly, joining the jugular bulb with the extracranial venous system. The shape of the foramen magnum determines how much of an obstacle the occipital condyle poses to surgical access of the area anterior to the brainstem. The occipital condyle is more of a hindrance in a deep and oval foramen magnum than a shallow one. This in turn determines the trajectory of the surgical approach—whether a lateral or a posterolateral approach with or without partial condyle resection is needed for the lesion.

The Vertebral Artery

The third portion of the vertebral artery begins at the foramen transversarium of C2 and ends where it enters the dura. Within the foramen transversarium of C2, the artery turns laterally and posteriorly and exits C2 at a different plane than the one at which it enters. The artery ascends to enter the transverse foramen of C1, after which it turns sharply backward, traveling along the upper surface of the C1 posterior arch. It curves around the occiput–C1 articulation and enters the dura on the lateral surface of the thecal sac. Between C2 and C1, as well as above C1, the artery may be redundant to a variable extent. This fact should be taken into account during surgery to avoid inadvertent injury to the artery. Up to the point where the artery enters the dura, it is surrounded by a periosteal and venous sheath. Below C1, the artery is crossed on its lateral surface from posterior to anterior by the ventral ramus of the C2 nerve root. Above C1, the artery closely adheres to the occiput–C1 joint capsule as it goes around to enter the dura. The artery pierces the dura in an oblique fashion, and this must be noted while the dura is being opened in this area.

C. Sen: Department of Neurosurgery, Mount Sinai Medical Center, New York, New York 10029.
P. J. Catalano: Department of Otolaryngology, Mount Sinai Medical Center, New York, New York 10029.

The Cranial Nerves

Because the jugular and hypoglossal foramina are immediately above the occipital condyle, cranial nerves IX to XII are often either directly involved by the tumor or in the field of the surgical approach. Within the jugular foramen, cranial nerves IX, X, and XII are medial to the jugular bulb. The inferior petrosal sinus joins the jugular bulb from a medial direction, and may enter by traveling in between the cranial nerves. This may be a troublesome source of bleeding in dealing with tumors in this area, and requires careful packing to avoid injuring the nerves. Cranial nerve XII exits separately inferior and medial to the jugular foramen. Within the bony canal, cranial nerve XII travels upward and laterally, whereas cranial nerves IX, X, and XI travel inferiorly and laterally. This relationship is important in dealing with extradural tumors. The hypoglossal nerve is accompanied by an emissary vein and a branch of the ascending pharyngeal artery.

PRINCIPLES OF THE SURGICAL APPROACH

1. Control and mobilization of the vertebral artery is a key step in the approach to lesions at the anterior surface of the foramen magnum.
2. To accomplish control and mobilization, the artery needs to be circumferentially freed from the dura at its entry.
3. Because the vertebral artery enters the dura close to the posterior edge of the occipital condyle and C1 lateral mass, some amount of bone removal from the condyle facilitates freeing up the vessel.
4. Extradural tumors that have invaded the condyle and are in the hypoglossal and jugular foramina require resection of the entire condyle and the diseased bone.
5. If the lower cranial nerves are involved by the tumor, they should be dissected from a normal to the abnormal area in their respective foramina, and this means exposing them proximally and distally.

PREOPERATIVE EVALUATION

A detailed neurologic evaluation is an essential baseline. Special attention is directed to the status of lower cranial nerve function because this is the most common cause of surgical morbidity. High-resolution computed tomography (CT) and magnetic resonance imaging (MRI) demonstrate, respectively, the bony and soft tissue relations of the lesion. Arteriography is performed to assess the relations between the vertebral arteries, tumor vascularity, and the status of the sigmoid sinus and jugular bulb. Improvements in MRI capabilities make it possible to assess MR angiograms stereoscopically, giving excellent three-dimensional visualization of the tumor and its surroundings. The shape of the foramen magnum as seen on CT scan can be useful in determining the directions of the approach and whether and how much removal of the occipital condyle may be necessary for adequate visualization.

THE SURGICAL APPROACH (1,2)

Position

Proper positioning is an important aspect of foramen magnum tumor surgery. Flexion and extension of the head on the spine causes changes in the dimensions of the foramen magnum. Thus, when there is a tumor impinging on the brainstem, there can be further compromise of neural function because of improper positioning. Rotation of the head on the spine leads to distortion of the vertebral artery anatomy at the occiput–C1-2 areas. Therefore, for tumors in this region, the patient is positioned in full lateral decubitus with the head and neck in a neutral position (Fig. 1). Somatosensory evoked potentials are monitored during positioning as well as during surgery.

Soft Tissue Dissection and Vertebral Artery Exposure

Usually, a C-shaped incision (see Fig. 12a) is used behind the ear such that the incision reaches the midpoint between the inion and the mastoid. If an occipitocervical fusion is planned, as might be necessary when the entire occipital condyle is resected, an inverted horseshoe incision is made (see Fig. 1). This is made with one of the limbs along the midline and the other limb at the side of the neck. The horizontal limb is at the level of the upper border of the ear. Muscle dissection in the posterior cervical triangle is preferably performed in anatomic layers, detaching each muscle from its cephalic attachment and reflecting it inferiorly (Fig. 2). This type of muscle dissection has two main benefits: it maintains the surgeon's orientation to the area of the approach during isolation and control of the vertebral artery; and it clears away the muscles from a wide arc so that the surgeon may view the area from a lateral and a medial trajectory instead of being restricted to only one line of view.

The transverse process of C1 and the muscles attached to it (i.e., levator scapulae, superior and inferior oblique) form an important landmark for the third segment of the vertebral artery. The internal jugular vein is in front of the transverse process of C1 and the accessory nerve curves around lateral to the vein in this area before entering the sternocleidomastoid muscle. The vertebral artery can be isolated for proximal control below or above C1, depending on the level of the lesion. If the inferior border of the inferior oblique muscle is followed anteriorly between the transverse process of C1 and the lateral mass of C2, the ventral ramus of the C2 root is seen crossing the vertebral artery. The portion of the artery above C1 is deep to the superior oblique muscle. The vertebral artery is surrounded by a plexus of veins that can be left

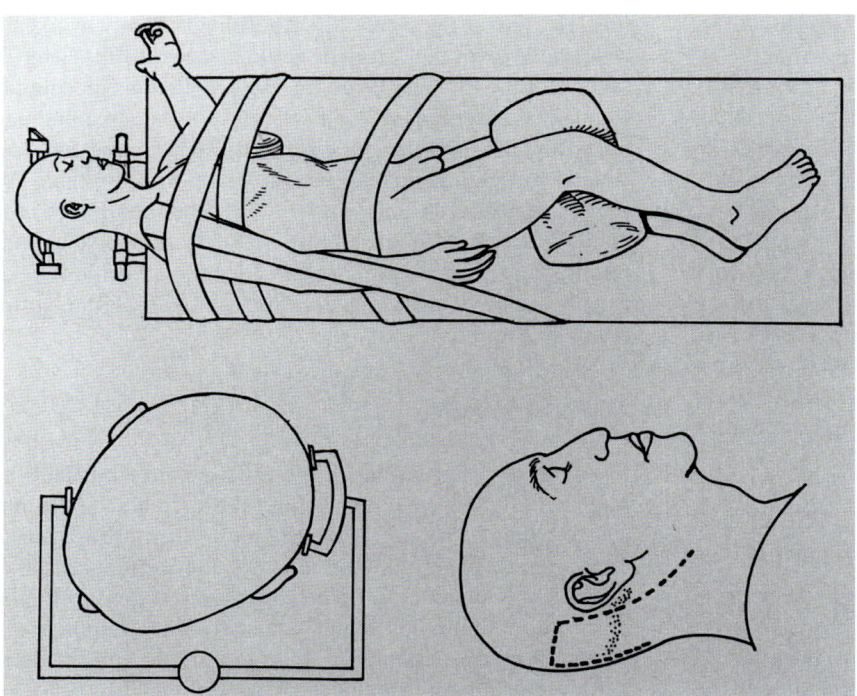

FIG. 1. The patient is positioned in a lateral decubitus position with the head fixed in a three-point head rest in a neutral position without rotation or flexion. The inverted horseshoe incision is shown.

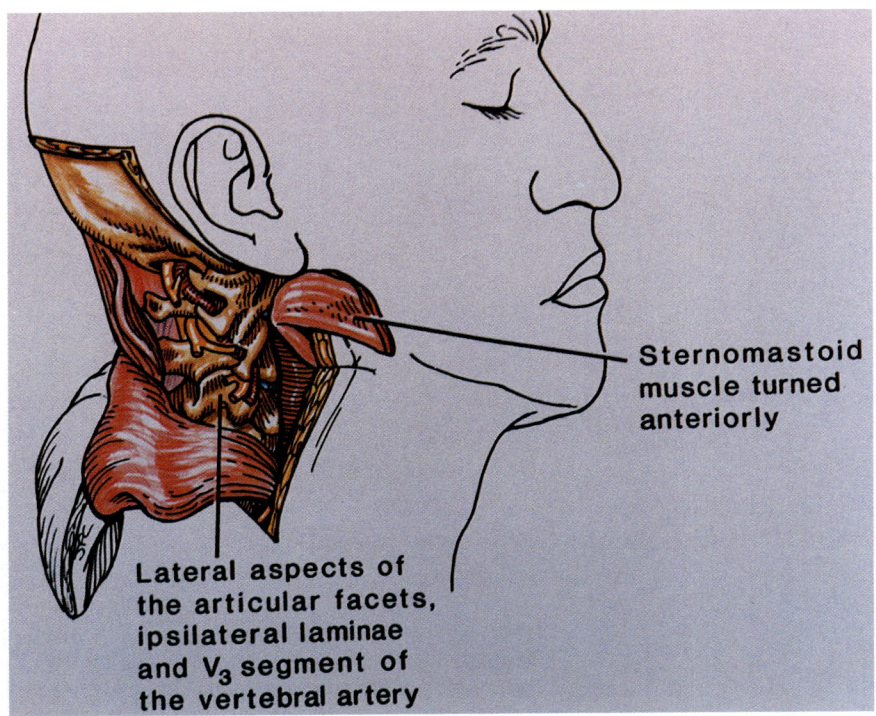

FIG. 2. The lateral view illustrates the muscle dissection in layers. The muscles are detached from their attachments to the occiput and C1 and reflected anteroinferiorly or posteroinferiorly.

intact if mobilization of the artery is not necessary. However, if the artery needs to be mobilized and displaced from its position, the venous plexus is stripped from the artery that is needed; otherwise, the venous bleeding can be troublesome. A rubber vessel loop passed around the artery provides an atraumatic handle on the vessel. Because the artery is thin walled, isolation and manipulation of the artery is preferably performed under magnification. The artery is intimately related to the occiput–C1 joint capsule and must be carefully freed from this for circumferential control. If access to the anterior aspect of C1 is also required, the vertebral artery is freed up from the foramen transversarium of C1 and the transverse process is then rongeured away so that the artery can be displaced out and posteriorly, providing clear access to the area in front.

Bony Exposure

The extent of the bony exposure is determined by the size and location of the lesion. If the tumor in the posterior fossa is large, a large craniectomy that extends up to the sigmoid and transverse sinuses is performed. The sigmoid sinus is completely unroofed down to the jugular bulb (Fig. 3). Tumor extension into the jugular foramen can be accessed by this exposure. Collaboration with an otologist is helpful for the temporal bone drilling. Tumors that are at the foramen magnum or lower do not require such extensive posterior fossa exposure. Hemilaminectomy of C1 may be necessary for low-lying tumors. After the vertebral artery has been fully exposed as needed, the bone in front of it, which is the posterior part of the condyle, is carefully drilled away to gain room in front of the artery as well as access to the anterior surface of the foramen magnum (Fig. 4). Venous bleeding is frequently encountered while working in this area and can arise from the condylar emissary vein. Packing with Surgicel usually suffices, along with careful elevation of the head. For purely intradural lesions, usually less than one third of the condyle needs to be drilled away for access. However, extradural tumors like chordomas and chondrosarcomas invading the condyle may necessitate removal of the entire condyle (Fig. 5).

Tumor Removal

The dura is opened medial to the sigmoid sinus and the jugular bulb and caudally, behind the vertebral artery entrance. After inspecting inside the dura, the dura is incised circumferentially around the vertebral artery entrance so that the artery is completely freed to be moved anteriorly and posteriorly, facilitating its dissection from the tumor or exposure of the aneurysm (Fig. 6). For intradural tumors, standard microsurgical techniques are used to debulk the tumor progressively and then dissect it off the brainstem, cranial nerves, and blood vessels. Extradural tumors may invade the dura and extend inside. Removal of the extradural tumor requires drilling of the temporal bone so that all the soft portion of the tumor and the infiltrated bone is removed. The jugular and hypoglossal canals may need to be skeletonized while carefully protecting the cranial nerves. Before entering the jugular bulb, the sigmoid sinus and the internal jugular

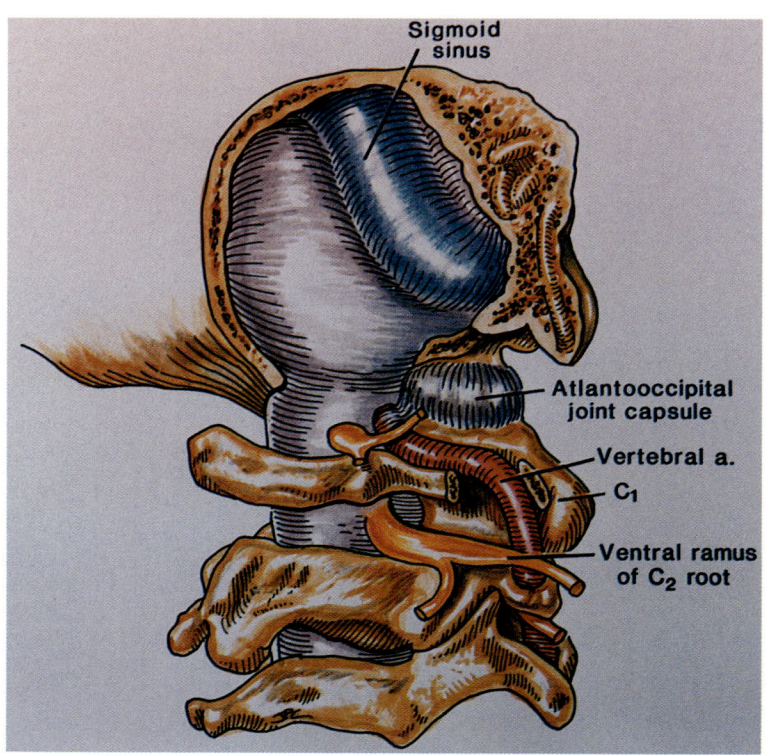

FIG. 3. A suboccipital craniectomy and a mastoidectomy have been performed. Only the posterior portion of the sigmoid sinus is usually unroofed unless the tumor extends into the jugular foramen, in which case the entire sigmoid sinus is unroofed.

EXTREME LATERAL TRANSCONDYLAR APPROACH / 495

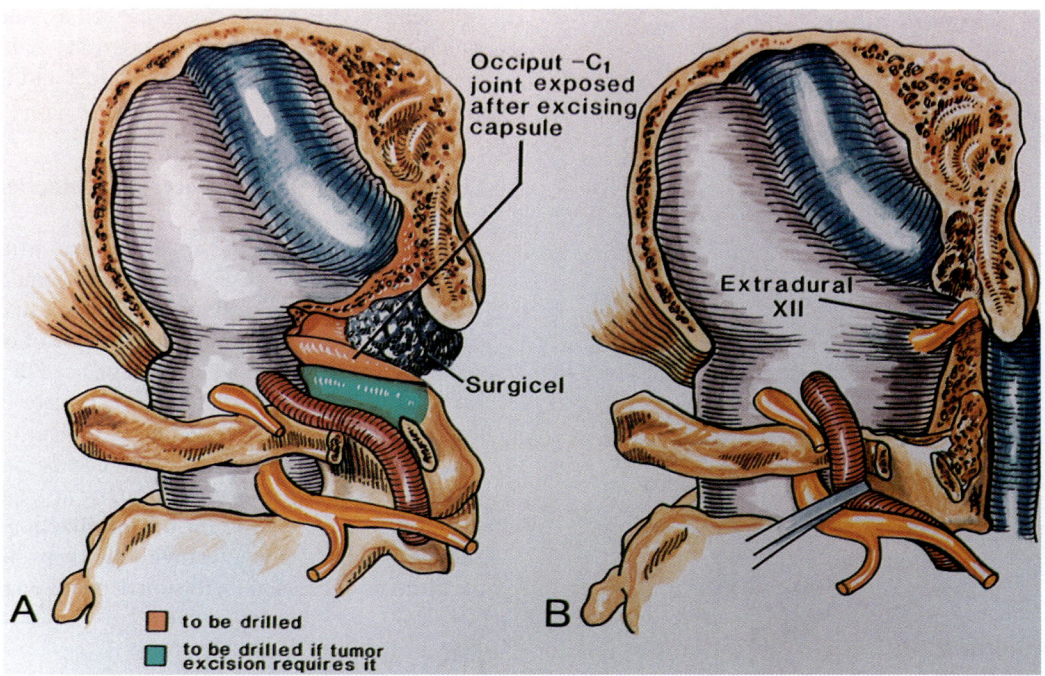

FIG. 4. A: A portion of the joint capsule of the occipital condyle and C1 is excised in preparation for the drilling. **B:** Most of the occipital condyle has been drilled away before opening the dura. The extradural cranial nerve XII has been exposed. The extent of drilling is tailored to the individual case. If the tumor is extradural, at the level of C1 the vertebral artery is displaced from the foramen transversarium of C1 and reflected posteriorly to improve the access to the anterior part of C1.

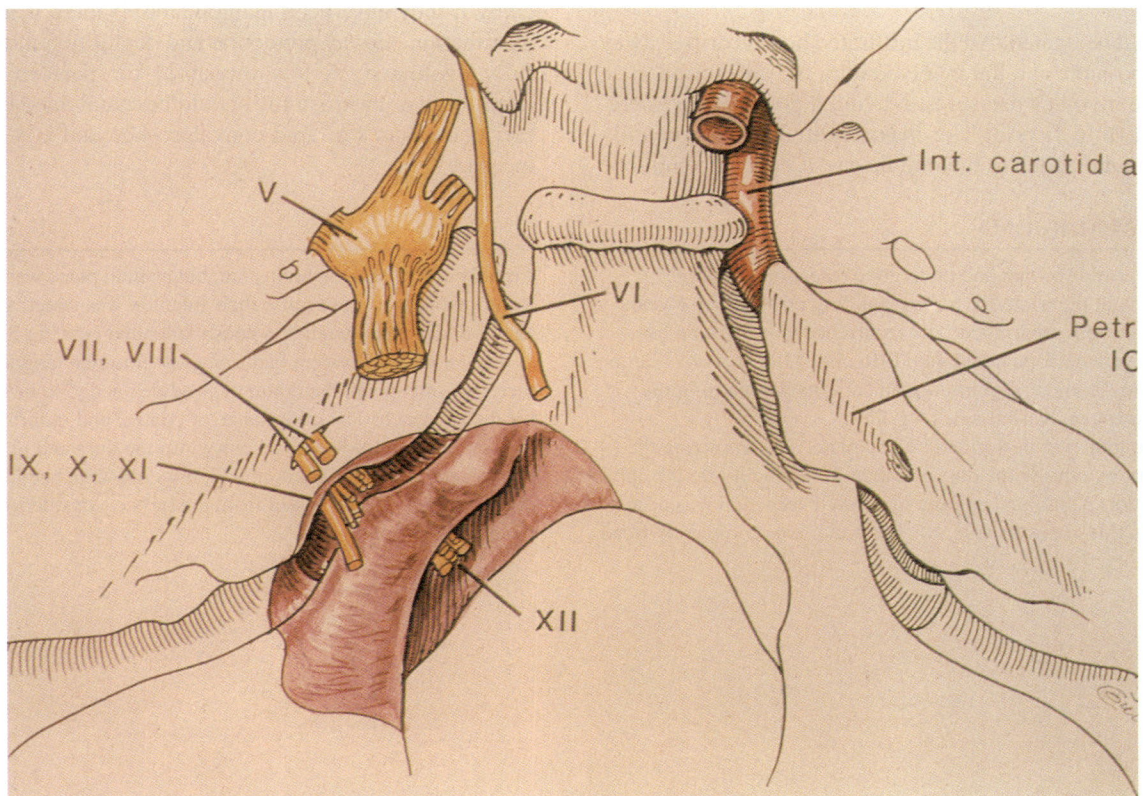

FIG. 5. A view of the interior of the skull at the foramen magnum region. The shaded area indicates the region of the condyle drilled away by this approach.

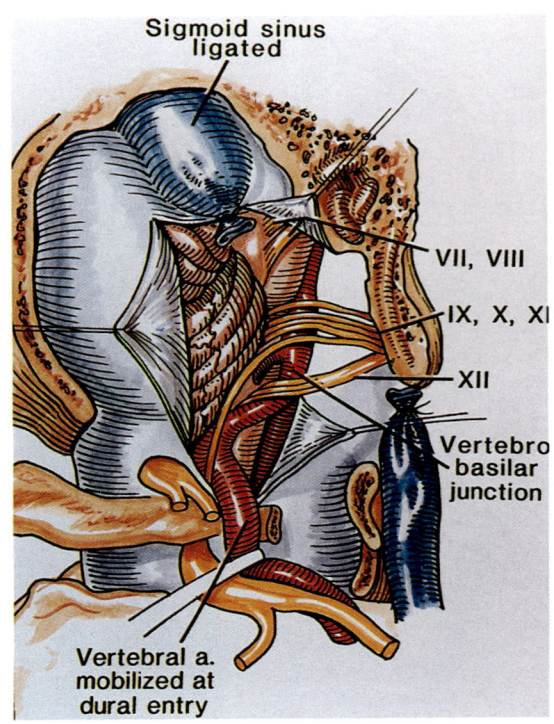

FIG. 6. Diagram showing that the internal jugular vein and the sigmoid sinus have been ligated and the infralabyrinthine bone and the occipital condyle have been drilled away to access the jugular foramen and foramen magnum.

vein should be ligated. All the infiltrated bone is drilled away as far as possible and the involved dura is also excised.

Closure involves measures to avoid a postoperative cerebrospinal fluid fistula. The mastoid air cells are heavily waxed and the aditus to the middle ear, if opened, should be well sealed. The dura is closed as well as possible, although watertight closure is almost impossible. A piece of autologous fat is placed over the dural defect and the muscles are closed in layers.

Stabilization of the Craniocervical Junction

If the remainder of the craniocervical articulation is normal, partial condyle resection does not render the joint unstable. Complete removal of the condyle usually warrants an occipitocervical fusion. Several methods of occipitocervical stabilization are available and can be used despite the posterior fossa craniectomy. Titanium hardware is preferable so that MRI is possible to monitor the patient for tumor recurrence. The stabilization procedure can be performed at the same sitting as the tumor removal, or at a later stage. Even though hardware is used for the stabilization, there must be enough bone laid in contact with the bony surfaces because the ultimate success of the fusion depends on the bony union.

POSTOPERATIVE CARE

A lumbar spinal drain is inserted the day after the operation and is kept in place for 5 days to minimize the development of a cerebrospinal fluid fistula or a pseudomeningocele. The function of the lower cranial nerves must be closely monitored in the early postoperative period, especially if they have been manipulated. If there is any sign of dysfunction, airway protection and deglutition must be carefully evaluated. A low threshold for performing a tracheostomy or gastrostomy should be maintained because either one ensures a rapid convalescence and is a temporary measure.

CASE 1: MENINGIOMA

This 68-year-old woman had undergone resection of a large meningioma in the posterior fossa extending down to C1 4 years before her current recurrence. The recurrence was detected because of severe neck pain and gait difficulty. MRI showed a large tumor in the foramen magnum region completely encasing the vertebral artery on her left side (Fig. 7).

The operation was performed by completely skeletonizing the vertebral artery outside the dura and then following it into the dura and the tumor. A minimal amount of condyle resection was necessary to gain this exposure (Fig. 8). The tumor was completely freed from the artery and the brainstem, but a small piece was left on the lower cranial nerves because their function was intact, and at her age a sudden palsy would be poorly tolerated (see Fig 8B,C).

Comment: This patient had a shallow foramen magnum and therefore only a small amount of condyle needed to be resected for the approach. The importance of control and mobilization of the vertebral artery before its entry into the dura and at its dural entry is evident here. Without this, it would have been very difficult to dissect out the vessel from the tumor, considering its complete encasement.

CASE 1 (Continued)

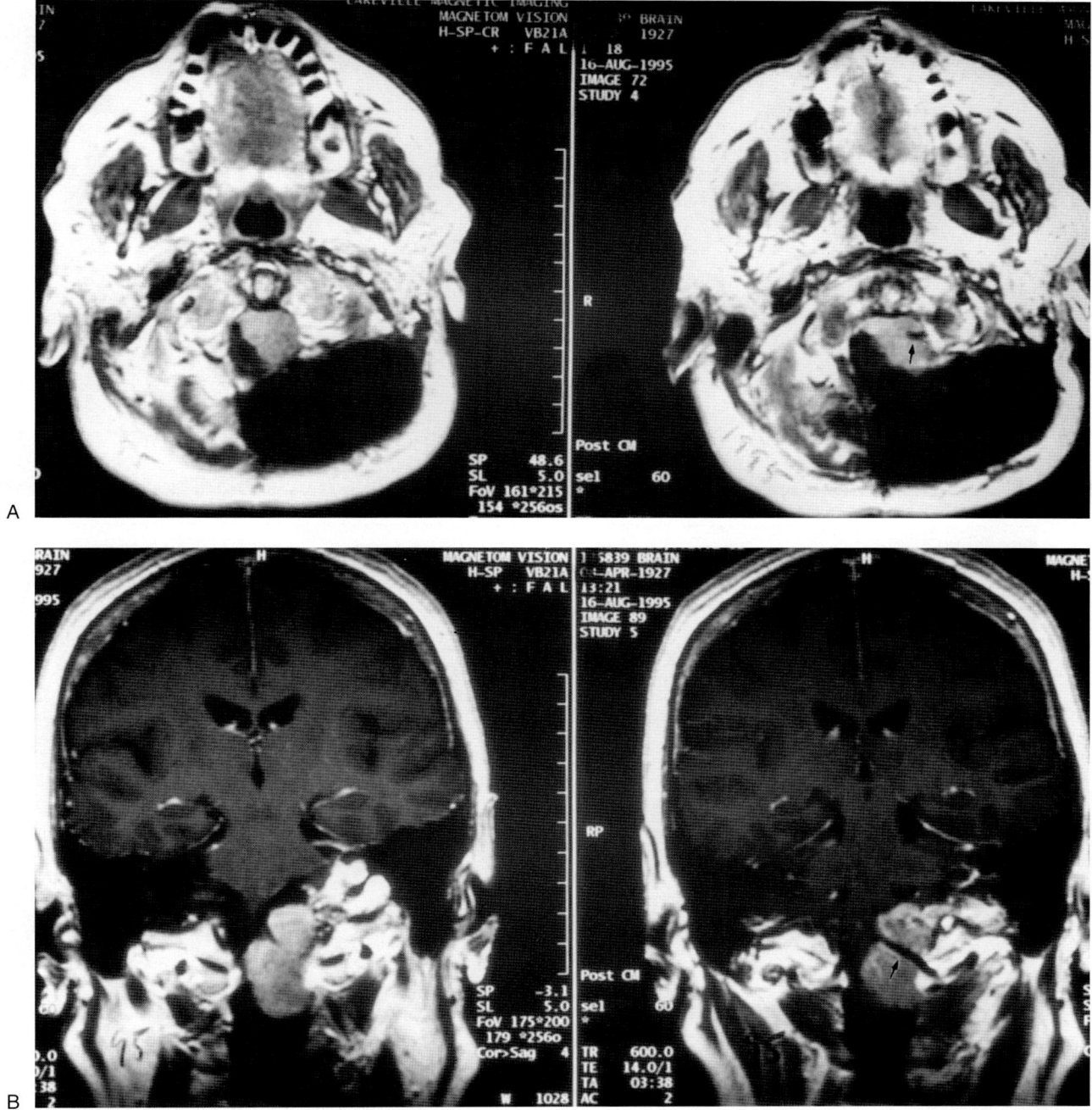

FIG. 7. Case 1. Axial **(A)** and coronal **(B)** magnetic resonance images of recurrent meningioma after administration of gadolinium show the tumor in the anterior intradural space; the vertebral artery is in the tumor (*arrow*) as soon as it enters the dura.

CASE 1 (Continued)

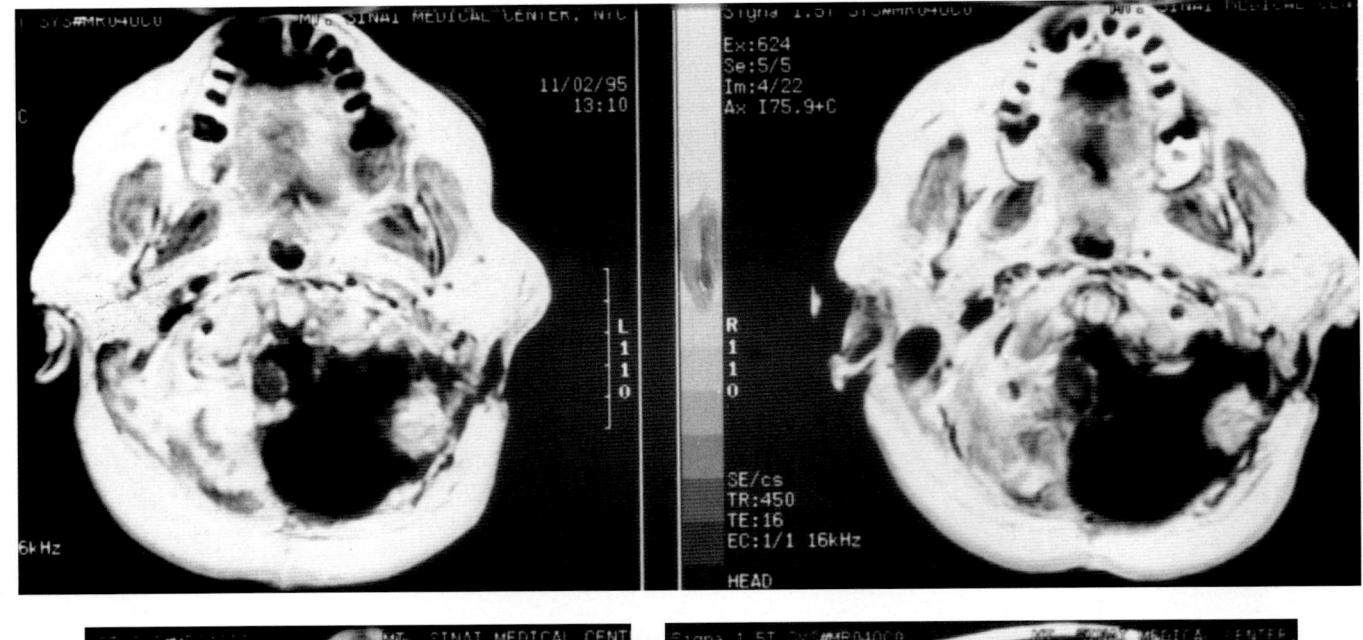

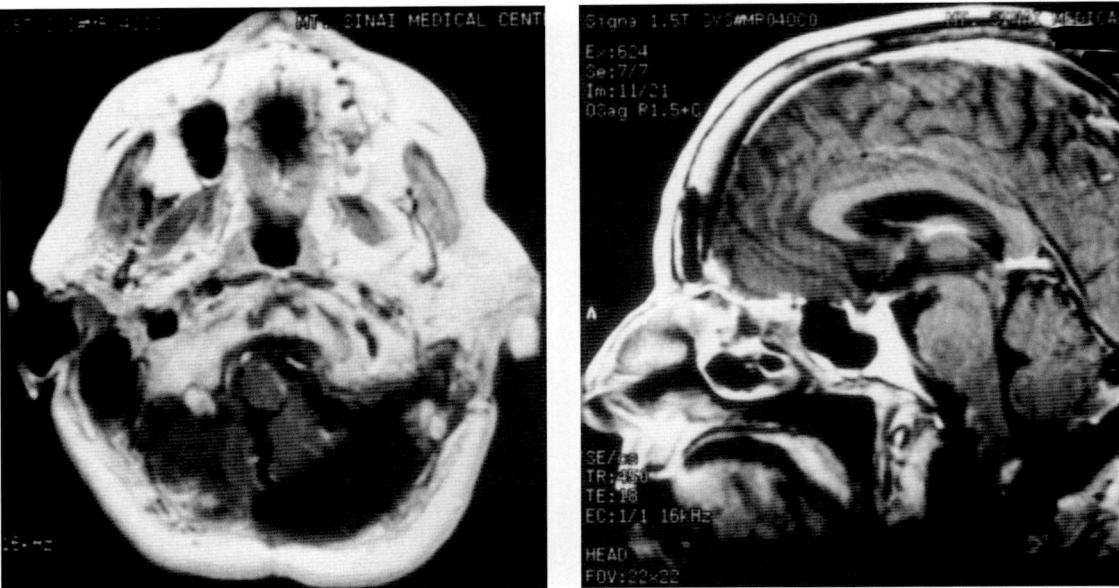

FIG. 8. Case 1 **A:** Postoperative magnetic resonance image showing that only a minimum amount of condyle was resected for the approach. **B,C:** Except for a small amount of tumor left on the lower cranial nerves, excellent tumor removal was achieved despite encasement of the vertebral artery.

CASE 2: GLOMUS JUGULARE TUMOR

This 38-year-old woman had symptoms for 3 years before her admission. These involved atrophy of the left side of the tongue, hoarseness of voice, and decreased hearing. MRI showed an extensive tumor in the clivus, posterior cavernous sinus, jugular foramen, and neck (Fig. 9). The angiographic appearance was that of a glomus tumor, and the external carotid artery feeders were embolized.

The operation was performed in two stages because of the tumor's size and multiple cranial nerve involvement. At the first operation, the temporal bone was partially drilled away to unroof the internal auditory canal, and the cochlea was drilled away to expose the genu of the petrous internal carotid artery. The vertebral artery was displaced posteriorly from the foramen transversarium of C1 up to its entry into the dura (Fig. 10). This considerably im-

CASE 2: (Continued)

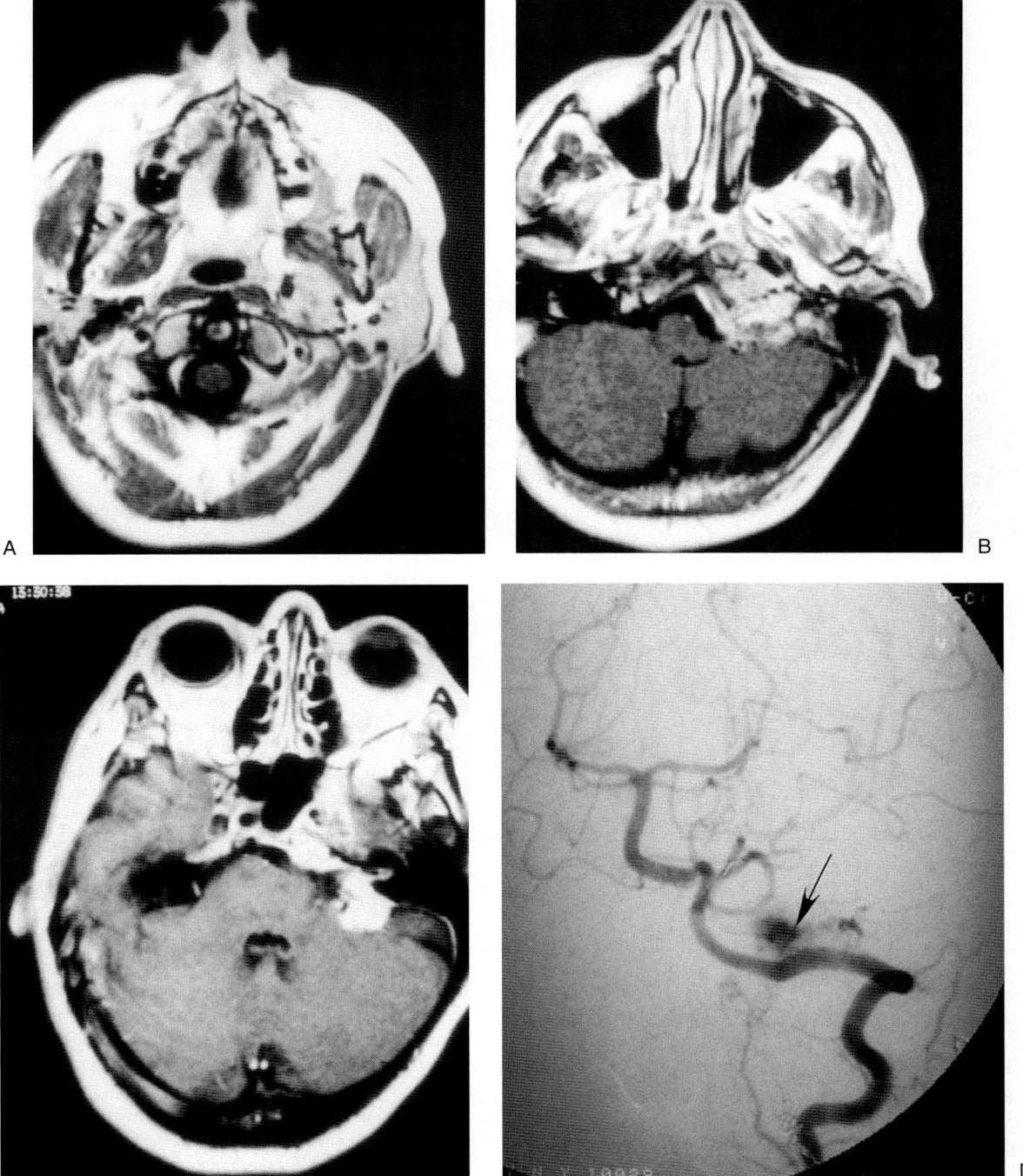

FIG. 9. Case 2. **A–C:** Glomus tumor extending from C2 to the posterior cavernous sinus, and into the internal auditory canal. **D:** Although the external carotid feeders had been embolized, the supply from the vertebral artery and internal carotid artery could not be occluded before surgery. By following the vertebral artery from the normal area at C1 into the tumor, the blood supply (*arrow*) could be directly interrupted.

CASE 2: (Continued)

proved access to the portion of the tumor that was coming down from the jugular foramen. A portion of the occipital condyle was drilled away to access the tumor in the hypoglossal canal. All the tumor that was caudal to the internal auditory canal was removed at this stage. At the second stage, the tentorium was divided and, through a combined subtemporal and posterior fossa approach, the tumor from the upper clivus and posterior cavernous sinus was removed.

Comment: The tumor followed the venous channels all the way up to the posterior cavernous sinus. It also extended into the clivus and petrous segment of the internal carotid artery. Taking the vertebral artery out of the C1 transverse foramen and moving it posteriorly provided additional room and permitted less facial nerve mobilization, so excellent tumor removal was achieved without any facial nerve morbidity. Because the tumor rose up to the posterior cavernous sinus, the operation was performed in two stages.

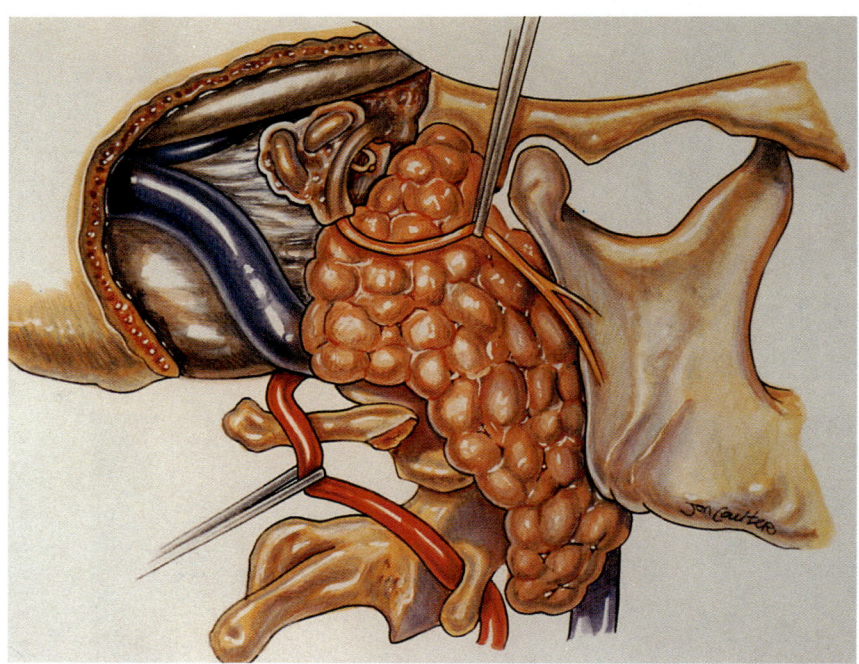

FIG. 10. Case 2. Posterior mobilization of the vertebral artery from the foramen transversarium of C1 and partial drilling of the occipital condyle improves the access to the tumor, reducing the amount of facial nerve mobilization.

CASE 3: CHORDOMA

This 66-year-old man was evaluated for difficulty swallowing and unsteadiness of gait. More recently, he complained of severe pain in his occiput and posterior neck. On examination, the right half of his tongue was atrophied and his gag reflex was diminished. He had a conductive hearing loss on audiometric evaluation. CT and MRI showed a large tumor in the clivus, foramen magnum, and C1 with severe brainstem compression (Fig. 11). Angiography showed distortion of the vertebral arteries and good communication of the transverse sinuses at the torcular.

The operation was performed in two stages (Fig. 12). At the first operation, the exposure was carried out. This included temporal and posterior fossa craniotomies, closure of the external ear canal, mastoidectomy, and labyrinthectomy. The petrous internal carotid artery was exposed through the cochlea, the jugular bulb was fully skeletonized, and the vertebral artery was taken out of the C1 foramen transversarium and followed to its dural entry. An elective tracheostomy and percutaneous gastrostomy was performed in view of his preoperative deficits and anticipated cranial nerve problems after surgery. The tumor resection, which was done at the second stage, was carried out through both intradural and extradural routes. The jugular bulb and the lower cranial nerves were skeletonized and the invaded dura was excised. The involved bone was drilled away, including the occipital condyle and part of the lateral mass and anterior arch of C1. An occipitocervical fusion with titanium instrumentation was performed after the tumor resection (Fig. 13).

Comment: Hearing on the right side was sacrificed because of the large size of the tumor. The entire occipital condyle and part of the lateral mass of C1 and its anterior arch were resected. The occipitocervical fusion was performed to reestablish the stability of the craniovertebral junction.

CASE 3: (Continued)

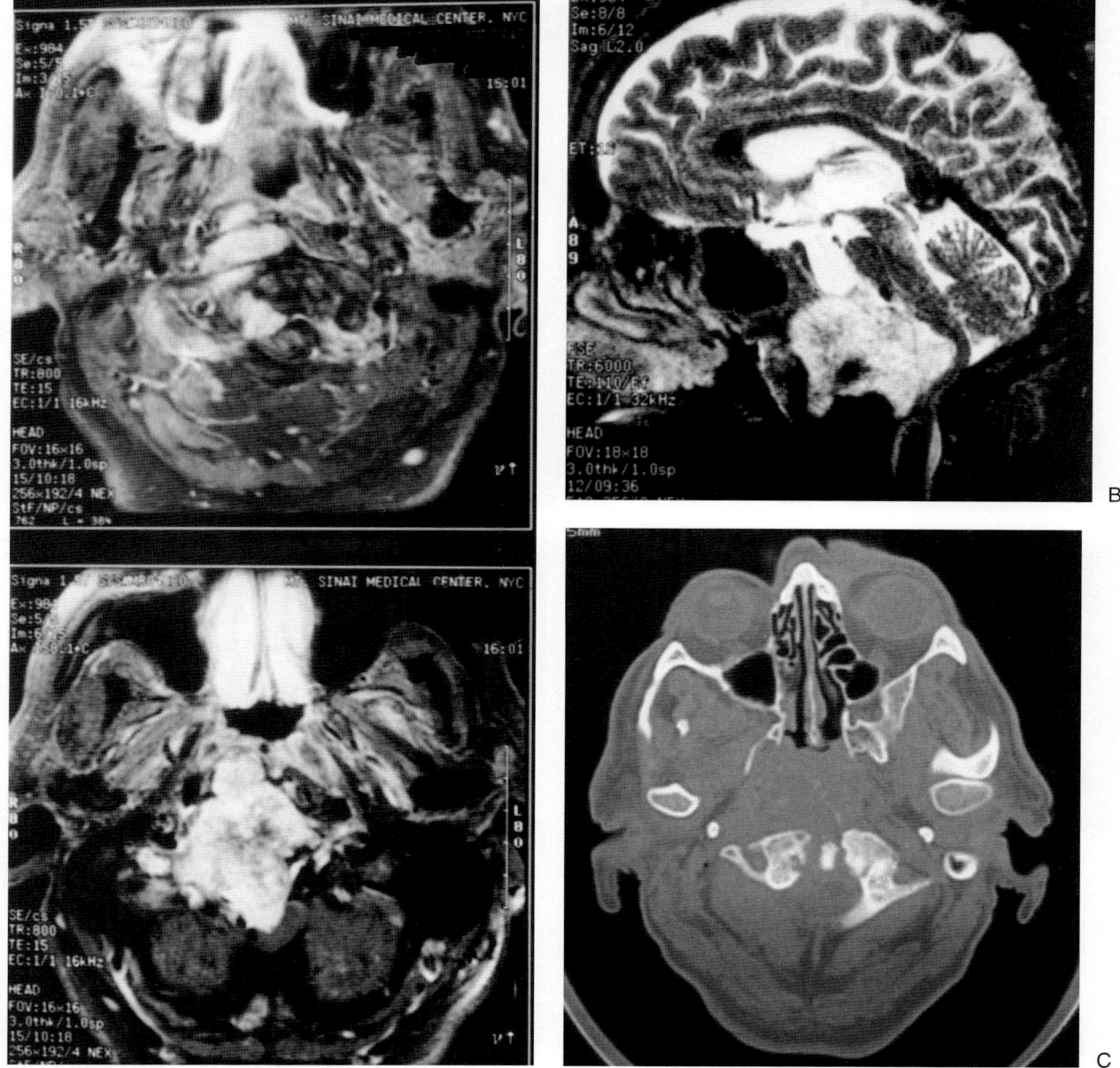

FIG. 11. Case 3. **A–C:** Preoperative magnetic resonance imaging and computed tomography (CT) show a chordoma extending intradurally as well as extradurally, involving the carotid and vertebral arteries on the right side. It severely indents the brainstem and reaches across the midline. CT shows that the right lateral mass of C1 is also invaded.

502 / CHAPTER 25

CASE 3: (Continued)

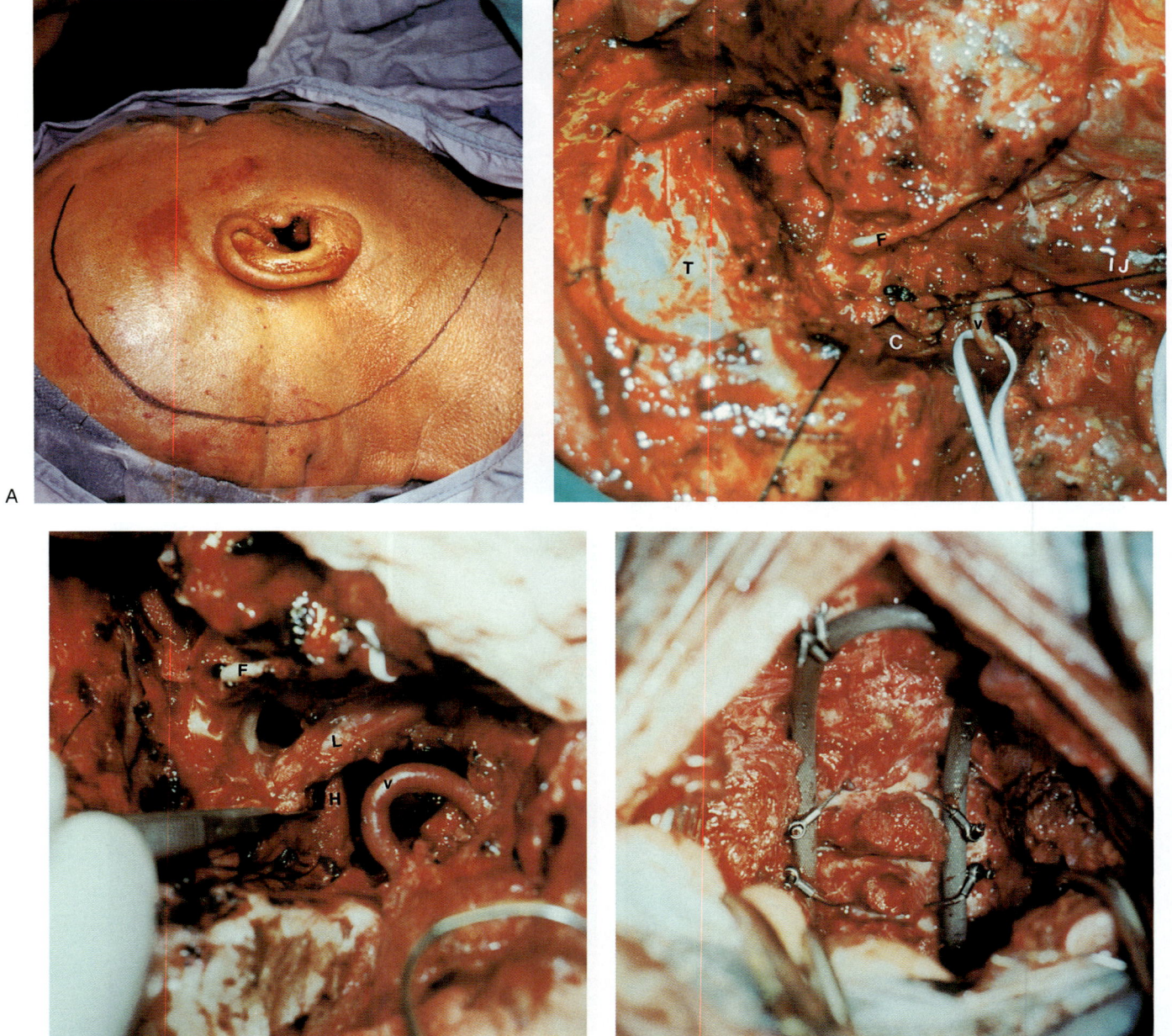

FIG. 12. Case 3. **A,B:** A large incision is used to provide access to the middle fossa, posterior fossa, and the neck. The external auditory canal was transected and closed. In **(B)**, the exposure is shown with the vertex to the viewer's left and nose to the top. *T*, temporal dura; *F*, vertical portion of cranial nerve VII; *C*, cerebellum seen after the dura was opened; *V*, vertebral artery at C1; *IJ*, internal jugular vein. **C:** After the second stage, the tumor has been resected and the orientation is the same as in **(B)**. *F*, vertical portion of cranial nerve VII; *L*, cranial nerves IX, X, and XI at the jugular foramen and below; *H*, cranial nerve XII in the hypoglossal canal; *V*, vertebral artery at C1. **D:** Occiput-to-C4 fusion with titanium hardware.

CASE 3: (Continued)

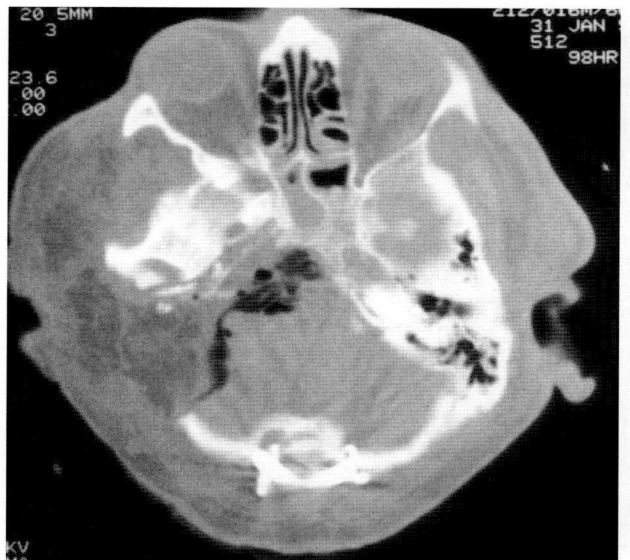
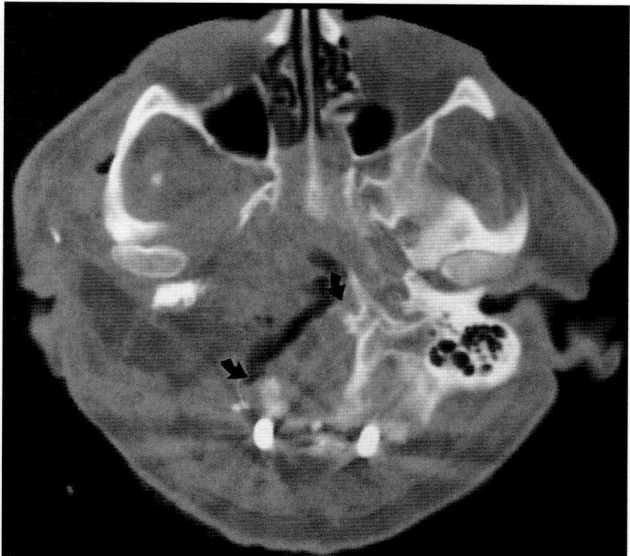

FIG. 13. Case 3. **A–C:** Postoperative computed tomography scan and cervical spine film showing the extent of bony resection through the combined approaches. The occipital condyle and anterior part of the lower clivus have been drilled away (*arrows*). Stabilization with internal hardware is needed in such extensive bony resection.

DISCUSSION

Among intradural tumors, meningiomas, schwannomas, and glomus tumors, whereas among extradural tumors, chordomas and chondrosarcomas comprise the majority found at the craniovertebral junction. There are several special problems posed by tumors in this region. These are access to the ventral area of the lower clivus and cervicomedullary junction, involvement of the vertebral artery on one or both sides, involvement of the lower cranial nerves, and invasion of extradural soft tissues and bone.

The problem of access is also common to aneurysms of the vertebral artery and vertebrobasilar junction. For many of the intradural tumors, the standard retrosigmoid approach usually suffices, but truly ventral tumors are inadequately resected by this approach. In addition, involvement of the extradural tissues cannot be addressed by the standard approaches because of the limitation of the jugular bulb, the occipital condyle, and the vertebral artery within the foramen transversarium of C1.

The concept of a laterally directed approach with partial resection of the occipital condyle to improve visibility to the

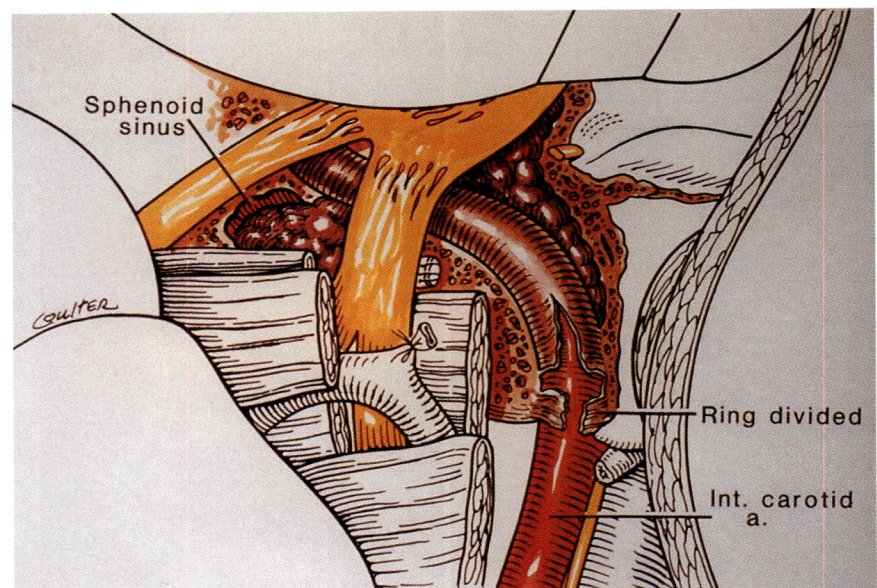
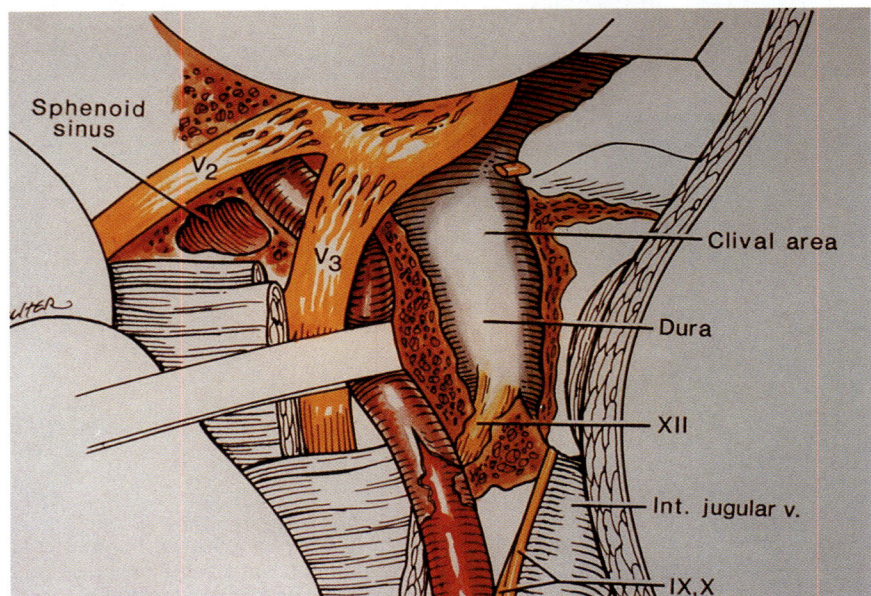
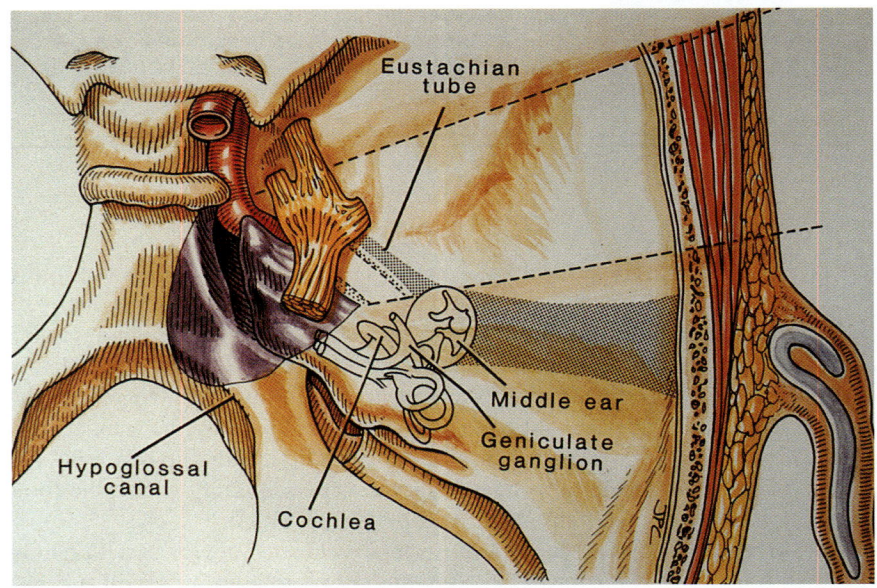

FIG. 14. A,B: The subtemporal and preauricular infratemporal approach through the left side of the head is shown. The petrous internal carotid artery is exposed and mobilized laterally to provide access to the clivus and petrous apex. **C:** An axial diagram showing the route of access anterior to the important temporal bone structures; shading indicates the area of the clivus that can be approached this way. Comparing this figure with Fig. 5, note how the approaches can be combined such that the inner ear structures are not damaged while accessing the area anterior to the craniocervical junction.

anterior surface of the foramen magnum was perhaps initially described by George et al. (1,2). A closer appreciation of the local anatomy shows the intimate relation of the vertebral artery to this region (3,4). The vessel closely skirts the occiput–C1 joint as it turns around this structure to enter the foramen magnum. It is adherent to the joint capsule in this course, and enters the dura obliquely just behind this articulation. Therefore, mobilization of the artery involves displacing it from the transverse foramen of C1, freeing it up from the joint capsule of atlantooccipital joint, and freeing it up circumferentially from the dural attachment, where it enters the dura. This opens up the passage to the ventral area for a variety of tumors. A laterally placed skin incision and lateral detachment of the muscles, moving them medially, removes any soft tissue bulk from the path of vision (5,6,7).

For purely intradural tumors, the amount of occipital condyle that may need to be resected to have enough room in front of the vertebral artery varies from minimal to none. In this situation, only a short portion of the extradural vertebral artery above C1 needs to be exposed. The limited condylar resection not only allows the surgeon to get in front of the artery, but improves the exposure to the anterior aspect of the foramen magnum (8). During resection of large glomus jugulare tumors, exposure and mobilization of the vertebral artery from the foramen transversarium of C1 improves access to the extracranial part of the tumor and can reduce the degree of facial nerve mobilization required (9). Chordomas and chondrosarcomas are predominantly extradural tumors, and therefore the operative approach should be directed primarily to this compartment. Such tumors may be extensive and also may have intradural extensions; therefore, a combination of approaches, either simultaneously or in a staged fashion, may be necessary. It is not sufficient simply to remove the soft portion of the tumor; the approach or combination of approaches must allow access to the involved bone, which needs to be drilled away, and the invaded dura should be resected if possible.

For a more extensive extradural access, the additional approaches that may be considered depend on the status of the patient's hearing (10). If the hearing is intact, a subtemporal preauricular infratemporal approach can be performed as a first stage to come in front of the ear, freeing up the internal carotid artery in the petrous bone and drilling away the involved bone in front of the labyrinth and cochlea (11) (Fig. 14). The subsequent operation can be done as described previously, coming from behind the inner ear. The infralabyrinthine bone drilling allows access to the jugular and hypoglossal canals. If no hearing is present or hearing is sacrificed, the temporal bone may be drilled away from behind and clear access is obtained from the vertebral artery to the carotid artery, and the in-depth exposure can be taken across the midline.

If the entire condyle is resected, which sometimes includes the articular mass of C1, a stabilization procedure is necessary. This can be performed either at the same sitting or at a separated stage. A midline posterior incision is necessary for this procedure. Titanium hardware should be used to allow MRI scanning because regular follow-up imaging of these tumors is needed.

Thus, there are several advantages to using the extreme lateral approach: (a) simultaneous lateral and posterolateral avenues of exposure are obtained on the lesion at the lower clivus, C1, and C2, allowing radical tumor resection; (b) the approach does not traverse contaminated areas such as the pharynx or the paranasal sinuses; (c) it permits excellent control and mobilization of the vertebral artery to allow its safe dissection from the tumor or elimination of the aneurysm; and (d) this operation can be combined with other approaches to enhance the completeness of tumor resection and is equally useful for intradural and extradural tumors.

REFERENCES

1. George B, Dematons C, Cophignon J. Lateral approach to the anterior portion of the foramen magnum. *Surg Neurol* 1988;29:484–490.
2. George B, Lot G, Velut S, Gelbert F, Mourier KF. Tumors of the foramen magnum. *Neurochirurgie* 1993;39[Suppl 1]:1–89.
3. de Oliveira E, Rhoton AL Jr, Peace D. Microsurgical anatomy of the region of the foramen magnum. *Surg Neurol* 1985;24:293–352.
4. Lang J, Kessler B. About the suboccipital part of the vertebral artery and the neighbouring bone-joint and nerve relationships. *Skull Base Surgery* 1991;1:64–72.
5. Sen C, Sekhar LN. An extreme lateral approach to intradural lesions of the cervical spine and foramen magnum. *Neurosurgery* 1990;27:197–204.
6. Sen C, Sekhar LN. Surgical management of anteriorly placed lesions of the craniocervical junction: an alternative approach. *Acta Neurochir (Wien)* 1991;108:70–77.
7. Babu RP, Sekhar LN, Wright DC. Extreme lateral transcondylar approach: technical improvements and lessons learned. *J Neurosurg* 1994;81:49–59.
8. Spetzler RF, Grahm TW. The far lateral approach to the inferior clivus and the upper cervical region: technical note. *BNI Quarterly* 1990;6:35–38.
9. Patel SJ, Sekhar LN, Cass SP, Hirsch BE. Combined approaches for resection of extensive glomus jugulare tumors. *J Neurosurg* 1994;80:1026–1038.
10. Fisch U. Infratemporal fossa approach for extensive tumors of the temporal bone and base of the skull. In: Silverstein H, Norrell H, eds. *Neurological surgery of the ear*. Birmingham, AL: Aesculapius Publishing Co., 1977:34–53.
11. Sekhar LN, Schramm VL Jr, Jones NF. Subtemporal and preauricular infratemporal fossa approach to large lateral and posterior skull base neoplasms. *J Neurosurg* 1987;67:488–499.

CHAPTER 26

Transoral Approach to the Clivus and Upper Cervical Spine

Paul J. Donald

ANATOMY

The anatomy of the elements of the occipitoatlantoaxial complex is covered superficially in a number of chapters or in depth in a few of the chapters (see Chapters 2, 25, and 27). For an exposition of anatomy of those key areas such as the vertebral artery, the reader is directed to those sections.

Embryologically, the occipital bone takes its origin in the most rostral three or four sclerotomes that form on the ventromedial surface of the primitive notochord (1,2). They fuse cranially with the chondrocranial anlage to the basiocciput to form the occipital bone (Fig. 1). The spinal sclerotomes that will become the provertebrae have a relatively loose cellular dorsal half and a more dense ventral half. The clear dorsal half of one spinal sclerotome fuses with the adjacent ventral half to form a provertebra. An intervertebral disk, which forms from a primordium called the intervertebral fissure, develops between each pair.

The atlas does not develop according to this schema followed by the other provertebrae. The dense caudal half of the first spinal sclerotome unites with the clear half of that adjacent to it, but the clear cranial half of the proatlantal sclerotome remains attached. Because the atlas does not form a body, the embryologic tissue otherwise destined to form it is the primordium of the dens. The dens then fuses with its base in the body of the axis. The tip of the odontoid process is thought to take origin in the clear cranial half of the proatlantal sclerotome. An early ossification site at the odontoid tip occurs that occasionally fails to fuse with the rest of the dens and is called the "ossiculum terminale." (3) This may be mistaken in some patients for a fracture. The final developmental quirk of the atlas that distinguishes it from the rest of the spine is that a portion of the anterior arch of this bone

P. J. Donald: Department of Otolaryngology—Head and Neck Surgery, and Center for Skull Base Surgery, University of California, Davis Medical Center, Sacramento, California 95817.

appears to develop from a condensation of sclerotomal mesenchyme ventral to it that is mostly destined to form the hypochondrial bow (4).

The Atlas

From this complex and confusing origin, the first cervical vertebra that supports the head and articulates with it through the occipital condyles takes its formation. Figure 2 illustrates the salient anatomic features of the atlas. Unlike the other cervical vertebrae, the atlas is essentially an osseous ring with a posterior tubercle on the dorsal part of the arch that corresponds to the spinous process of the vertebrae below it. The lack of this process permits free movement of the cranium on the spine. The dorsal superior part of this arch provides a groove for the attachment of the posterior atlantooccipital membrane. The inferior aspect has a groove for the posterior atlantoaxial membrane. The atlas does not possess a vertebral body, and the main bulk of the vertebra is made up by the lateral masses. The concave superior condylar facets articulate with the convexly shaped occipital condyles above and bear the weight of the cranium. The inferior facets of the lateral mass articulate with the axis. Projecting laterally from the lateral masses are the transverse processes, which have a foramen transversarium through which passes the vertebral artery. The artery curls around behind the lateral mass in a groove on the superior surface of the atlas, and then curves in a medial and upward direction to gain entry into the skull (see Chapter 27). The dorsal ramus of the first spinal nerve (the lesser occipital nerve) passes through this same groove with the artery.

The anterior arch of the atlas is relatively short, comprising only one fifth of its circumference. The anterior face of the arch has a tubercle to which the longus colli muscles are attached. The inner surface has a smooth articular facet for the dens, and posteriorly the attachment for the transverse at-

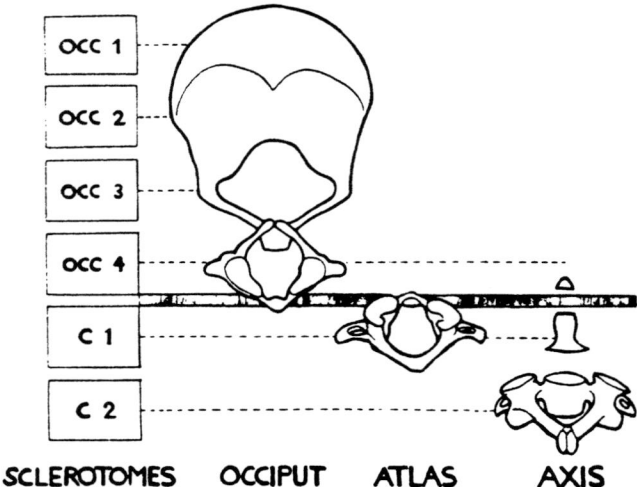

FIG. 1. Embryologic development of the craniocervical junction according to List. The occipital bone and condyles are seen from below. The axis and atlas are seen from above. (From ref. 4, with permission.)

lantal ligament that runs around the posterior surface of the dens. The anterior superior surface of the anterior arch has an attachment for the atlantooccipital membrane and inferiorly the insertion of the atlantoaxial ligament.

The Axis

The axis forms the pivot or swivel point of the head and atlas onto the spine (Fig. 3). The odontoid process is a substantial peglike process projecting superiorly from the body at the apex to accept the apical dental ligament. A smooth facet anteriorly articulates with a corresponding facet on the posterior surface of the anterior arch of the atlas. A shallow groove on the posterior surface accommodates the transverse ligament of the atlas. Rough surfaces on the lateral aspects are for attachment of the alar ligaments. The dens projects from the vertebral body, which has a curious inferior dip that overlaps the body of the third cervical vertebra and provides a further attachment for the longus colli muscle. The laminae, transverse processes, and pedicles are thick and strong. The superior facets are directed more horizontally and the inferior facets directed in the same oblique direction as the rest of the cervical vertebrae.

The Craniocervical Junction

The bony articulation of the occiput–atlas and axis has been already alluded to. The ligamentous attachments are multiple and complex, providing strength and flexibility to this complex. The atlantooccipital capsular ligaments that surround the condylar attachments are thin and loose. Anteriorly, the anterior atlantooccipital ligament connects the anterior aspect of the occipital bone at the foramen magnum with the cranial aspect of the anterior arch of the atlas (Fig. 4A). A thickening of the ligament connects the anterior tubercle of the atlas to the occiput above. Two lateral atlantooccipital ligaments connect the transverse processes to the occiput above. These strong ligaments reinforce the weaker capsular ligaments

On the posterior surface (see Fig. 4B), a much thinner, broad, flat posterior atlantooccipital ligament forms an attachment between the cranial surface of the posterior arch of the atlas and occiput above. There are dehiscences bilaterally to admit the vertebral arteries. The inner surface of the posterior ligament is in intimate contact with the spinal cord dura.

The ligaments on the anterior aspect of the atlas are much more complex (see Fig. 4C). Directly opposite the chordal dura anteriorly is the tectorial membrane, which is the superior extension of the posterior longitudinal ligament of the spinal canal inferiorly. Although adherent to the posterior surface of the vertebral body of the axis, it is free over the transverse ligament of the atlas and broadens as it ascends into the intracranial surface of the occipital bone just inside the foramen magnum. It is inserted into the bone and blends with the dura of this aspect of the cranial base. Anterior to the tectorial membrane is the transverse ligament, which overlies the dens. It has two lateral components that connect one tubercle of the anterior atlas at one extremity of the anterior arch of the atlas to its fellow on the opposite side. A central slip of the ligament extends superiorly to the lip of the foramen magnum and is intimately associated with the tectorial membrane. An inferior slip descends and inserts on the axis. Together, these ligaments form a continuous cross-shaped configuration. Laterally, the dens is connected to the inner surfaces of the occipital condyles by the thick, tough alar ligaments that take the form of check ligaments, preventing overrotation of the head and atlas around the atlantoaxial axis. The alar ligaments blend laterally with the anterior atlantooccipital ligament.

The atlas and axis are bound together by the anterior atlantoaxial membrane, which is a continuation of the anterior longitudinal ligament of the spine. It is thick and strong, and further reinforced by a central ligamentous thickening that connects the anterior tubercles of the atlas and axis and continues on to the undersurface of the occiput. In contrast, the posterior atlantoaxial membrane, which connects the laminae of C2 to the arch of C1, is somewhat thinner and more loosely constructed. It is the superior substitute of the ligamentum flavum.

The final ligament stabilizing the cervical spine and indirectly the craniocervical junction is the ligamentum nuchae. It connects the external occipital protuberance to the atlas and the spinous processes of the cervical vertebrae all the way to C7. It divides the posterior cervical muscles in the midline and is a midline source of attachment of the trapezius muscle.

The rectus capitis minor originates on the occiput and inserts into the posterior tubercle of the atlas. From a similar

Text continues on page 513

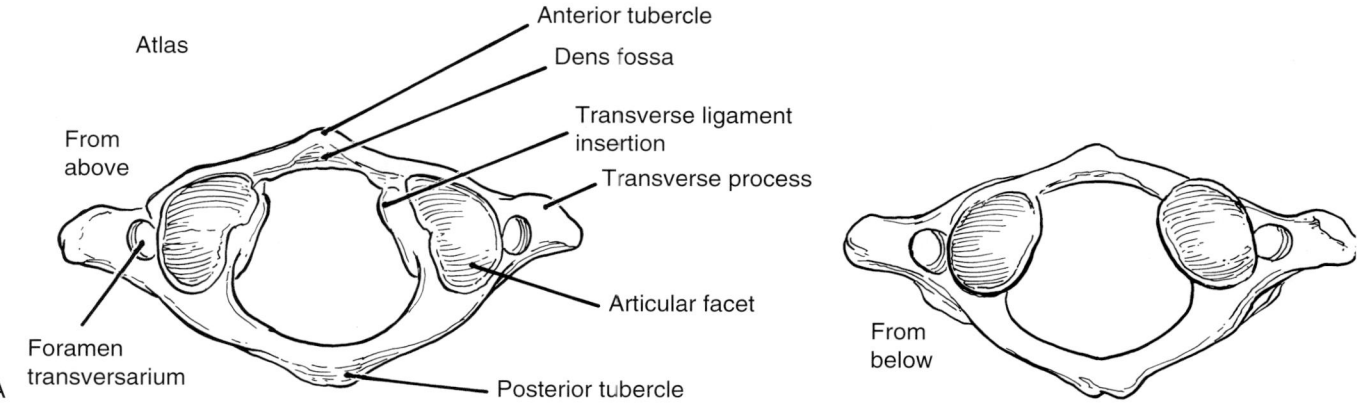

FIG. 2. A: The atlas from above. **B:** The atlas from below.

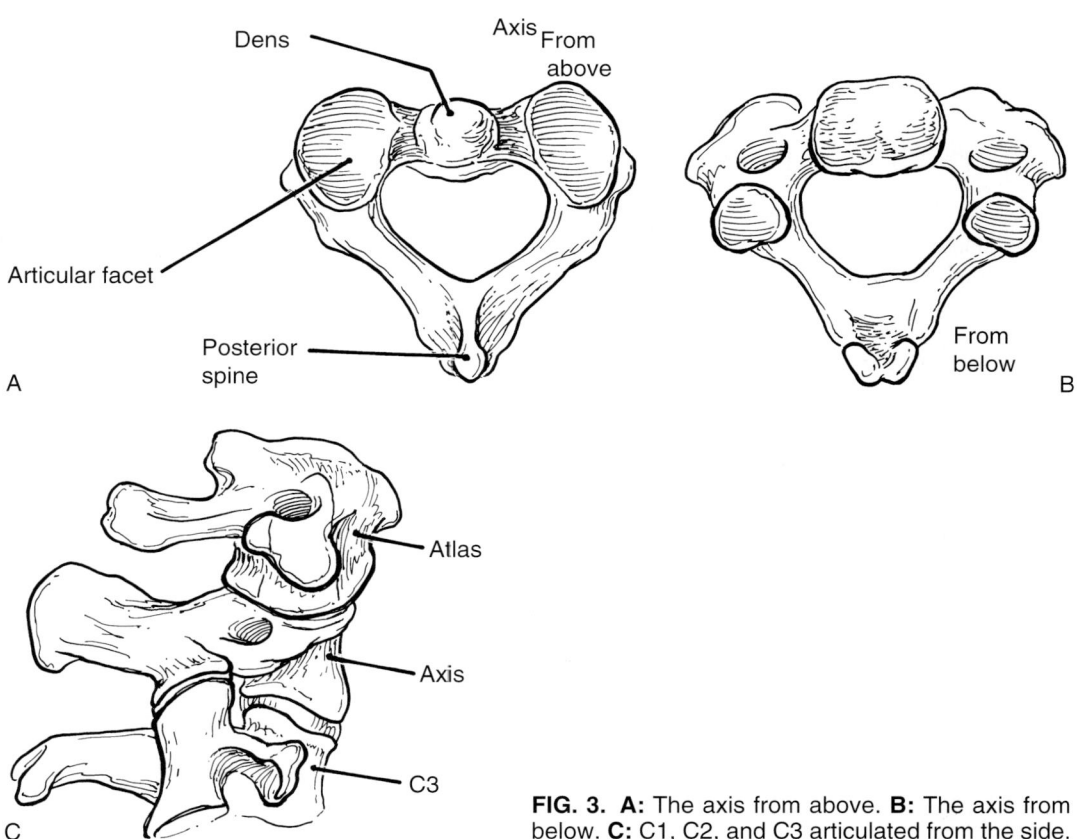

FIG. 3. A: The axis from above. **B:** The axis from below. **C:** C1, C2, and C3 articulated from the side.

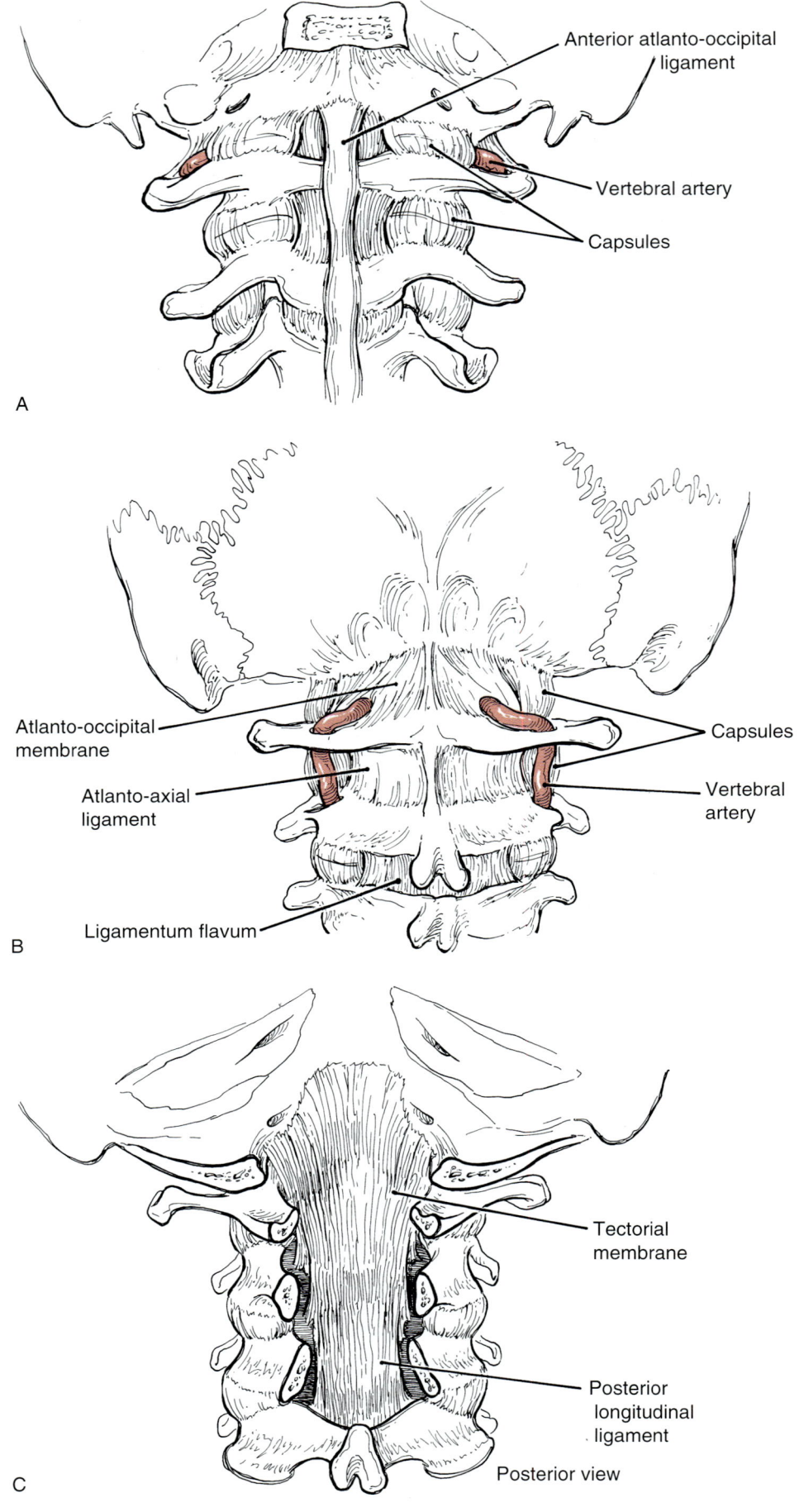

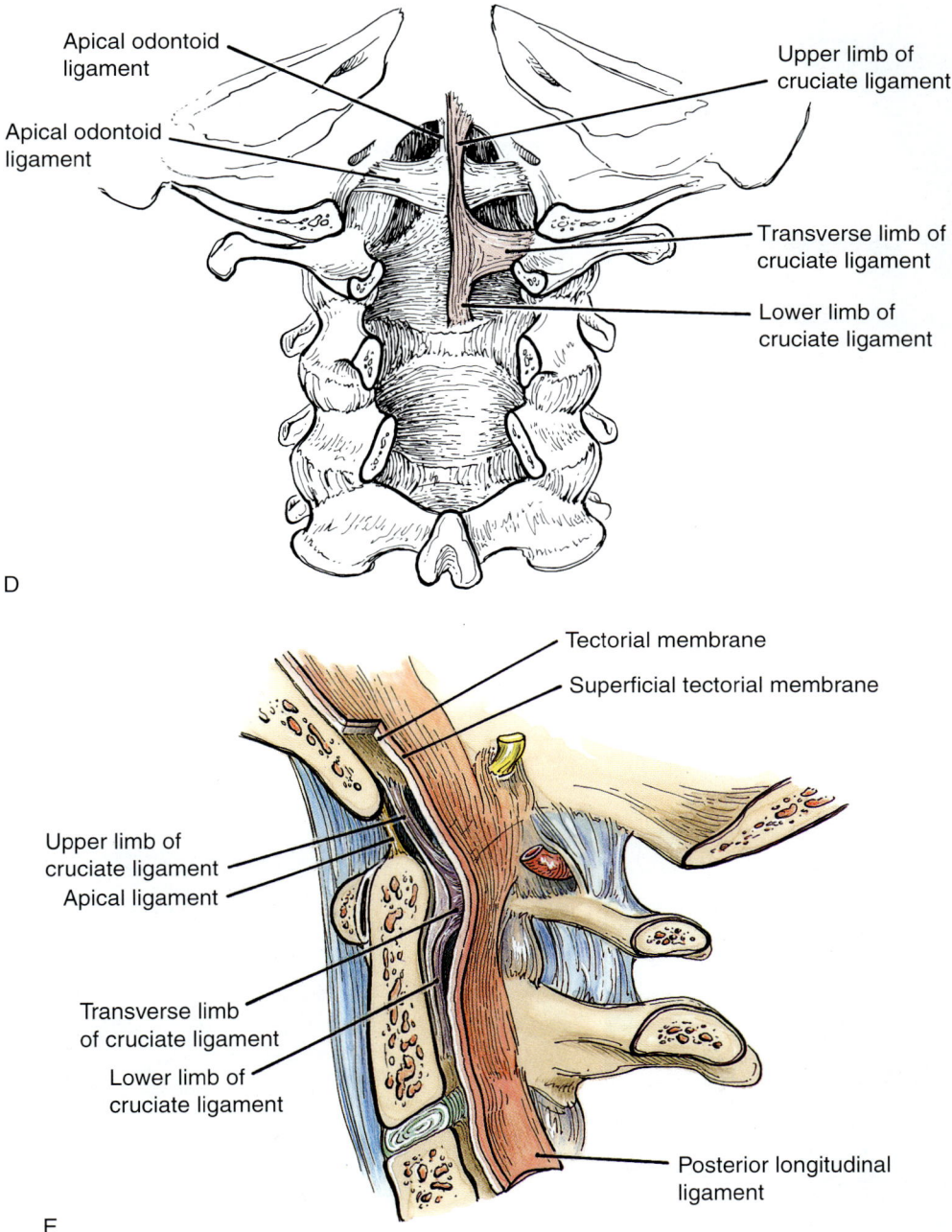

FIG. 4. A: Anterior view of the craniocervical junction. **B:** Posterior view of the craniocervical junction. **C:** Posterior view of the craniocervical junction with the laminae and spinal cord removed, showing tectorial membrane. **D:** Same view with tectorial membrane removed. **E:** Craniocervical junction from three-quarter view.

512 / CHAPTER 26

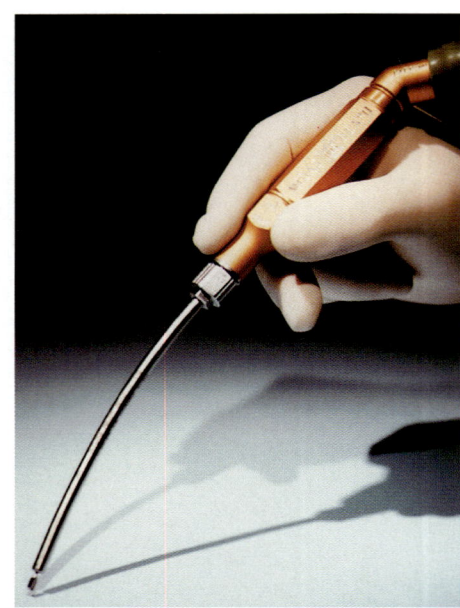
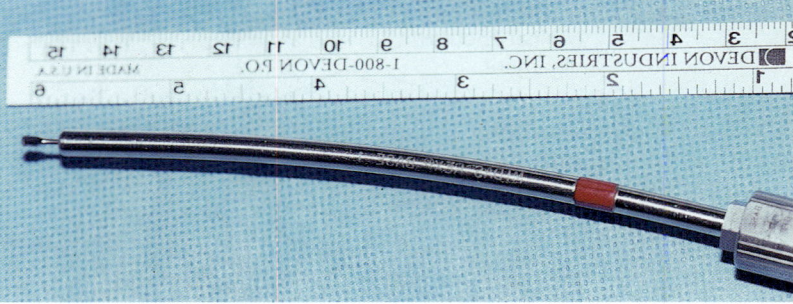

FIG. 5. Midas Rex TAC attachment. This is an innovative instrument that enables a deep dissection in confined exposures, permitting easy bone removal in the transoropharyngeal approach to the clivus. **A:** Photograph of instrument showing curved shaft. **B:** Close-up view.

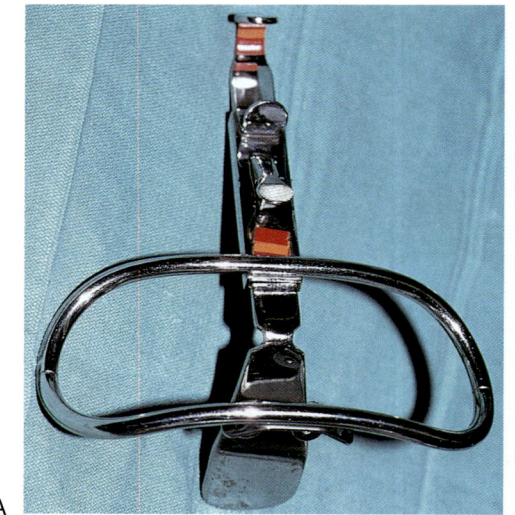
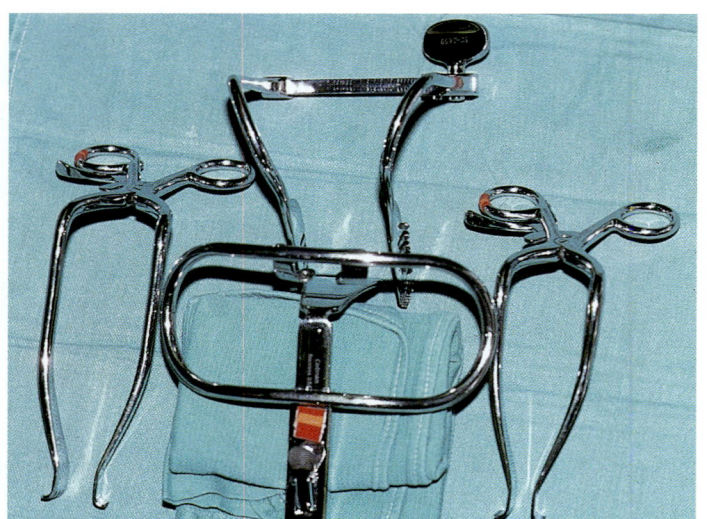

FIG. 6. The Crockard instrument set. **A:** Mouth gag. **B:** Mouth gag blades and self-retaining retractors.

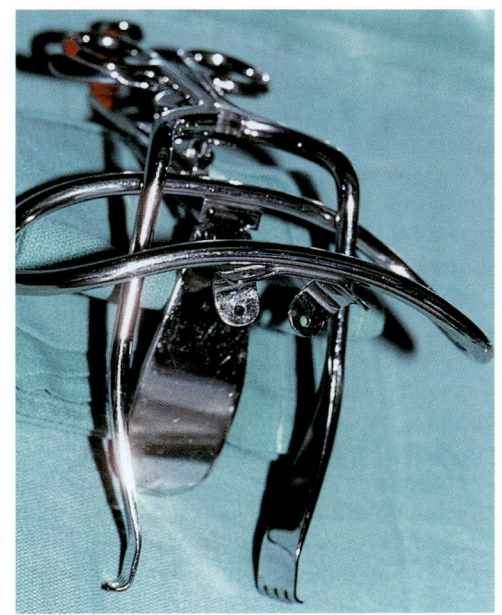
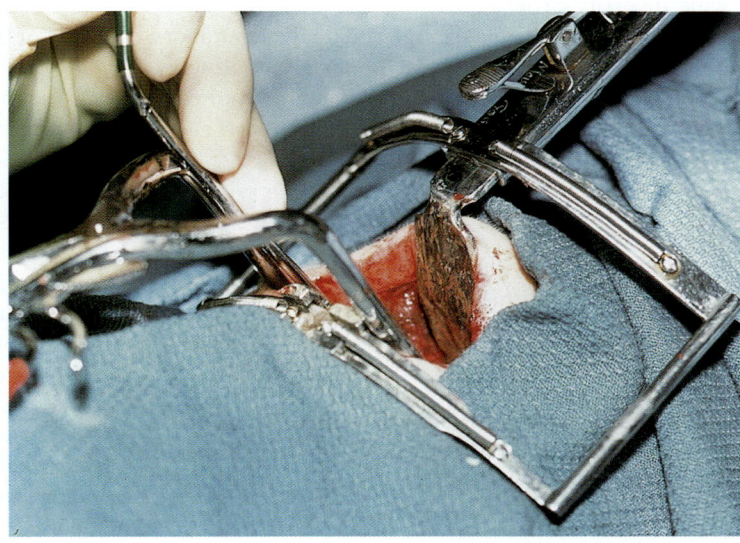

FIG. 6. *Continued.* **C:** Crockard self-retaining retractors and mouth gag articulated. **D:** Dingman mouth gag and Crockard retractors in a patient.

origin, the rectus capitis major inserts into the spinous process of the axis, as does the inferior oblique muscle. The superior oblique inserts into the transverse process of C2. The overlying posterior cervical muscles further stabilize the spine.

The upper cervical spine, especially the region of C1 and C2 and the lower clivus, occupies an anatomically central position, and by virtue of this location is difficult to access through most approaches. The oral cavity and oropharynx provide the most direct route to this otherwise surgically obscure area. The lesions requiring resection or structures needing correction are only 1 to 2 cm from the epithelial incision used to gain the exposure. Concern regarding oral contamination of the wound, especially if dura is exposed, is usually unfounded, especially in the face of vigorous antisepsis in the mouth and systemic coverage with antibiotics. One of the major impediments to effective surgery in this area has been the lack of appropriate surgical instrumentation. With an increasing interest in skull base surgery, more instruments are being developed to facilitate an easier and more effective dissection. Especially important has been the introduction of the Midas Rex drill, and in particular the TAC attachment (Fig. 5). The curved carrier tube protects the soft tissues from the rotating shaft that carries the small match-head cutting bur. The high speed of the bur reduces chatter and shortens dissecting time. The curve of the shaft removes it as a visual obstruction and permits a clear view of the bur at all times. The Crockard instrument set has a unique series of self-retaining retractors that produce maximal exposure in this restricted area (Fig. 6). The Raveh dissecting instruments are both long and strong, and allow the operator's hand to be outside the mouth while the working end can be constantly seen, even while working in the depths of the resection cavity (Fig. 7). The Cob elevator used in orthopedic surgery is sturdy and very effective in elevating the periosteum from the clivus and cervical bodies. An adaptation by the author allows the hand to be removed from the line of sight (Fig. 8).

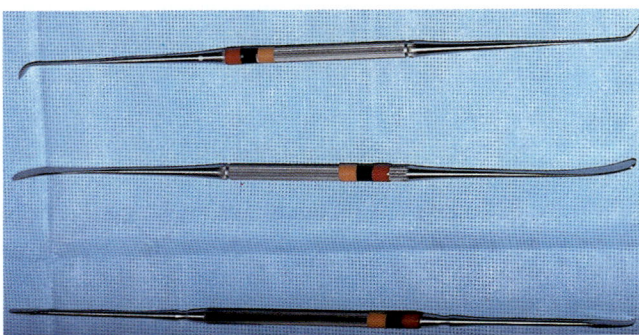

FIG. 7. Raveh skull base dissectors.

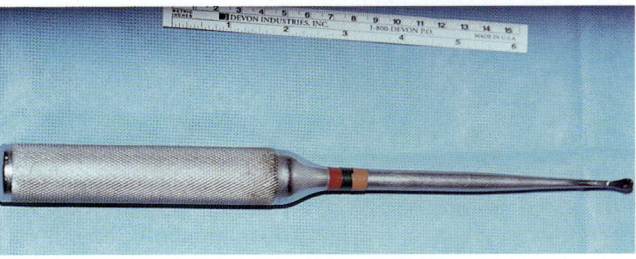

FIG. 8. Cob clival periosteal elevator.

PATHOLOGY

A wide diversity of lesions afflict this area and include congenital anomalies, trauma, benign and malignant tumors, inflammatory conditions, and those of uncertain etiology. Their common denominator is the production of cord compression or spinal instability.

Congenital

Congenital anomalies include basilar impression syndrome, odontoid malformations, and a group of cranial anomalies of the posterior skull base. Their common denominator is the resultant brainstem and upper cord compression. Basilar impression, although uncommon, is one of the more usual indications for odontectomy. This may also need to be combined with a craniectomy to provide adequate brainstem decompression. Basilar impression is the "pushing up" or invagination of the normally convex occipital bone by the upper cervical spine. This results in an impingement of the odontoid onto the undersurface of the brainstem as well as an infolding of the occipital bone, adding further compression to this structure (Fig. 9). This lesion can either be congenital or acquired. A number of congenital syndromes, albeit often very rare, carry with them the problem of basilar impression. Hajdu-Cheney syndrome or acroosteolysis combines dolichocephaly, an unusual protuberance of the squamous part of the occipital bone (bathrocephaly), and progressive basilar invagination with characteristic unusual facies and extremity abnormalities (4), including dissolution of the terminal phalanges. Cloverleaf skull or

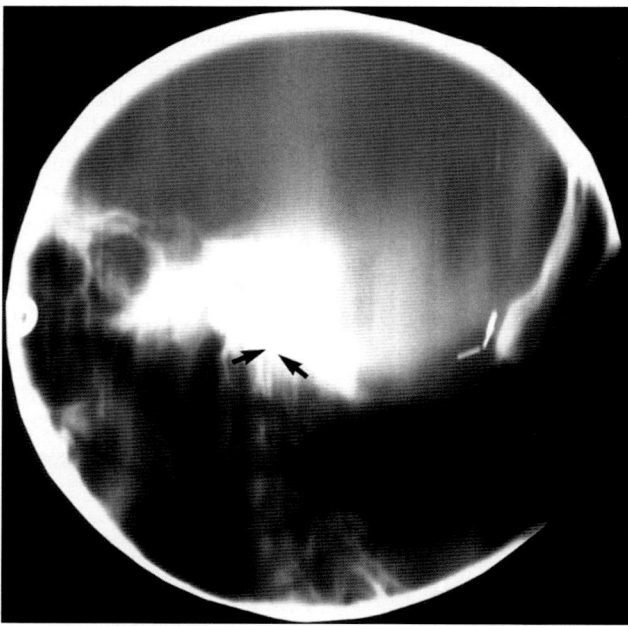

FIG. 9. Lateral radiograph of basilar impression syndrome. Note prior craniectomy. Odontoid is anterior to the craniectomy and is compressing the brainstem through a crumbling clivus. *Arrows* indicate site of odontoid.

Klieblättschadel is another rare genetic syndrome in which thanatophoric dwarfism and multiple extremity anomalies are combined with a bizarre trilobed skull (5). These anomalies of the calvarium, with petrous tips that are level with the floor of a posterior cranial fossa markedly reduced in height, are coupled with basilar impression. Sjögren-Larsson syndrome and pyknodysostosis are further rare syndromes that may be associated with basilar impression; the latter disorder was the putative affliction of the famous Impressionist Toulouse-Lautrec (6). Achondroplastic dwarfism has a number of associated cranial anomalies, one of which may be basilar impression.

Acquired disorders of the cranial bones such as osteomalacia, osteogenesis imperfecta, cretinism, and rickets cause bone softening. This produces a malleability of the bone that may lead to progressive invagination of the occiput as the weight of the cranium and its contents impinges on the upper cervical spine (7). Gardner contends that all basilar impression is acquired in that all the congenital syndromes are without basilar impression until the weight of the head begins to be imposed on the cervical spine as the person assumes the upright position (8).

Congenital anomalies of the odontoid are associated with a number of disorders, including Morquio's syndrome (mucopolysaccharidosis type IVB), Aarskog's syndrome, Dyggve-Melchior-Clausen syndrome, pseudoachondroplasia, cartilage-hair hypoplasia, congenital spondyloepiphysial dysplasia, and spondylometaphysial dysplasia (9). Morquio's syndrome has multiple spinal anomalies including severe kyphoscoliosis and shortened cervical vertebrae. The odontoid may be hypoplastic, absent, or anomalously formed, causing upper cord compression. In Aarskog's syndrome (facial-digital-genital syndrome), the posterior arch of C1 may be unfused and ascend with the articulated odontoid into the foramen magnum on cranial extension. Dyggve-Melchior-Clausen syndrome is also associated with dwarfism. There is instability of the atlantoaxial joint that can lead to cord compression. Although the appearance of these patients resembles that of Morquio's syndrome, they have no mucopolysacchariduria or corneal clouding, but have microcephaly and mental retardation. Although the remaining disorders mentioned previously may be accompanied by odontoid malformations, the dens is usually hypoplastic in nature and predisposes the patient more to instability than impingement of this structure against the brainstem.

Traumatic

The traumatic lesion most commonly requiring this exposure is the odontoid fracture, but it is rarely seen. This is an uncommon injury and may also be seen as part of a "hangman's fracture," a fracture–dislocation of C2 on C3. If the dens is fractured, the craniocervical junction may be destabilized and the cord acutely compressed. These fractures are most often the result of automobile accidents in the young

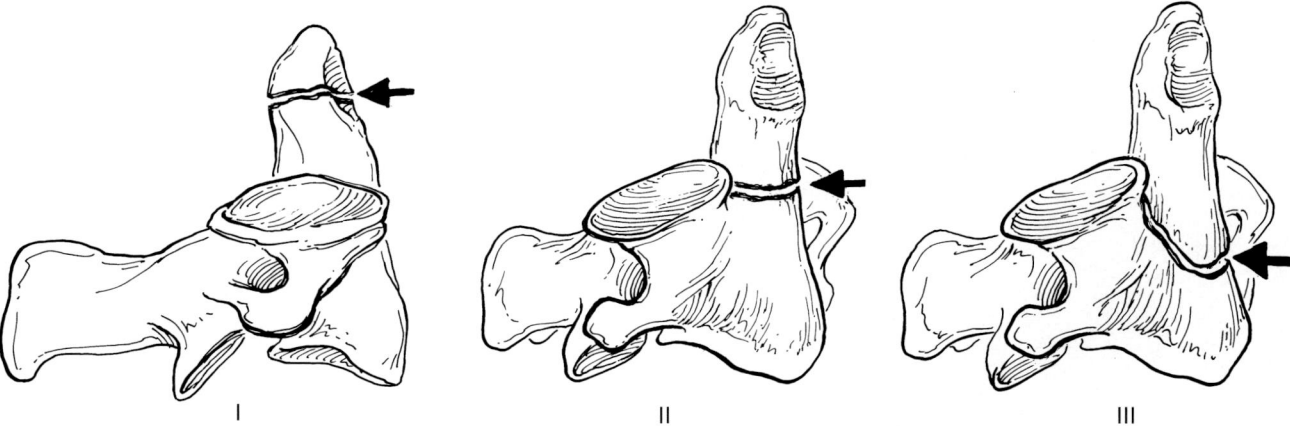

FIG. 10. Three types of odontoid fracture.

and falls in the elderly, and may be asymptomatic or present with cord compression.

There are three types of odontoid fractures (10) (Fig. 10). Type I is a fracture of the odontoid tip and may be confused with the congenital anomaly of os odontoideum. The anomaly is differentiated by its characteristic radiographic appearance of a diamond-shaped image with smooth sides (Fig. 11). The fracture looks like a normal tip with a separating line between it and the remainder of the dens. Type II fractures are those that go through the base of the process, and the mechanism of fracture commonly places the dens anteriorly onto the body of C2. The type III fracture goes through the odontoid and enters the marrow space of the body of C2. These fractures usually stabilize and are treated only with analgesics and immobilization. When combined with a C2-3 fracture–dislocation, the type III fracture is very unstable and difficult to treat (11,12).

If the odontoid fractures are displaced, they are slightly more commonly flexion in type with displacement of the tip anteriorly. Occasionally, a posterior fracture occurs with the head forced back against the upper end of the spine, which may result in instant death from respiratory arrest. When force is applied anteriorly, a fracture of the atlantal ring may in turn fracture the odontoid posteriorly. Force from behind can fracture the odontoid by the sudden impaction transferred by the transverse atlantal ligament. The eventual position of the odontoid may be related more to the subsequent motion of the patient's head after the fracture rather than to the mechanism of injury. In addition, degrees of displacement may be entirely unrelated to spinal stability. Neurologic symptoms are less likely to develop with anterior displacements than with those that occur in a posterior direction (11,13,14) (Table 1). In Dunn and Seljeskog's (13) series of 110 odontoid fractures, only 20% of patients with no subluxation had neurologic deficits.

Most odontoid fractures are reduced by traction and immobilization. Only selected, symptomatic fractures in which the odontoid remains displaced require resection. Type I fractures usually require collar immobilization or simply analgesics. In Dunn and Seljeskog's (13) series, 14 patients were treated with open reduction and internal fixation and 80 patients with external fixation. No patients with a type III injury had a nonunion. A nonunion occurred in 70% of posterior dislocations of the type II variety. A similar experience was noted by Altholl and Bardholm (15). Of the 48 fractures with a nonunion, 41 had successful bone healing. It appears from the literature that the posterior dislocations do better with an open operation. The transoral approach for upper

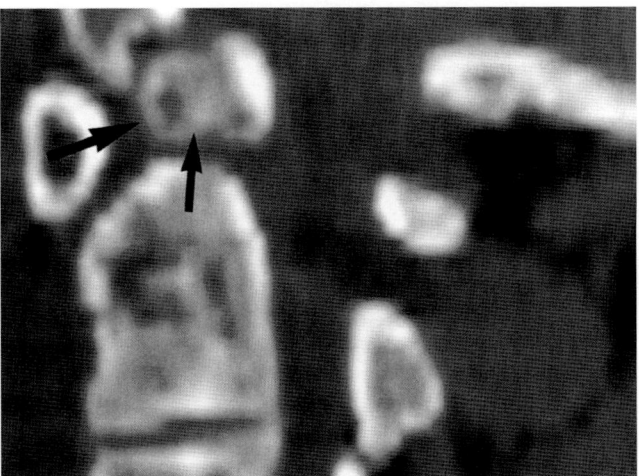

FIG. 11. Lateral computed tomography scan of os odontoideum. *Arrows* indicate separate ossification site at tip of dens.

TABLE 1. *Facial subluxation related to neurologic deficit (110 patients)*

Neurologic deficit	No. of patients with subluxation of odontoid fractures		
	None	Anterior	Posterior
Present	5	5	15
Absent	33	37	15
Total	38	42	30

From ref. 10, with permission.

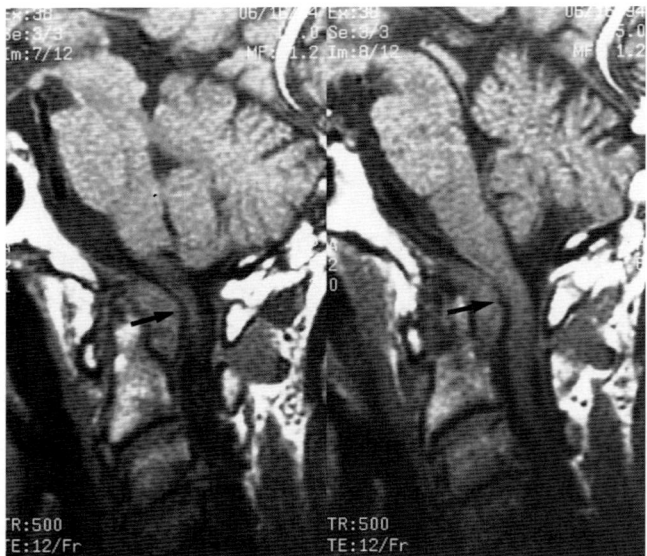

FIG. 12. Arthritic pannus compressing upper cervical cord.

cord or brainstem compression is reserved for those cases in which the dens does not relocate after traction or a posterior approach for relocation and fusion.

Inflammatory

The principal inflammatory condition of concern here is the pannus, secondary to rheumatoid arthritis. Unfortunately, many of these patients have been severely debilitated by the systemic effects of this disorder. Peripheral joints are commonly badly afflicted before upper cervical cord symptoms become manifest. The pannus is an infiltration of a vascular granulation tissue, chronic inflammatory cells, and fibroblasts that covers the joint surfaces. The pannus produces cytokines (granulocyte–macrophage colony-stimulating factor) and tumor necrosis factor-α that result in the stimulation of polymorphonuclear leukocytes and dissolution of articular cartilage. In peripheral joints, this process is seen as an irregular, deforming bulge of the skin overlying the affected joint. The joints have a tendency to sublux, and fibrosis causes joint fusion. At the top of the cervical spine, the pannus may produce an atlantoaxial subluxation and compression of the upper cervical spinal cord by pushing the transverse ligament against the dura, thus indenting the cord (Fig. 12). In addition, joint degeneration and migration of the odontoid superior form a type of acquired basilar impression (Fig. 13).

Neoplastic

A variety of tumors can begin in the craniocervical junction. They may be either benign or malignant, and the malignancies may be either primary or secondary (Fig. 14). The importance of a biopsy cannot be overstressed because of the frequency of uncommon and rare lesions at this site. Sufficient tissue must be harvested to perform electron microscopy and special stains. The most common epithelial lesion is squamous cell carcinoma, and the most common bony lesion, although uncommon in general, is chordoma. Squamous cell carcinomas are usually of nasopharyngeal or oropharyngeal origin. Fortunately, the stout pharyngobasilar fascia provides a formidable barrier to tumor penetration. Tumors of nasopharyngeal origin have more of a propensity

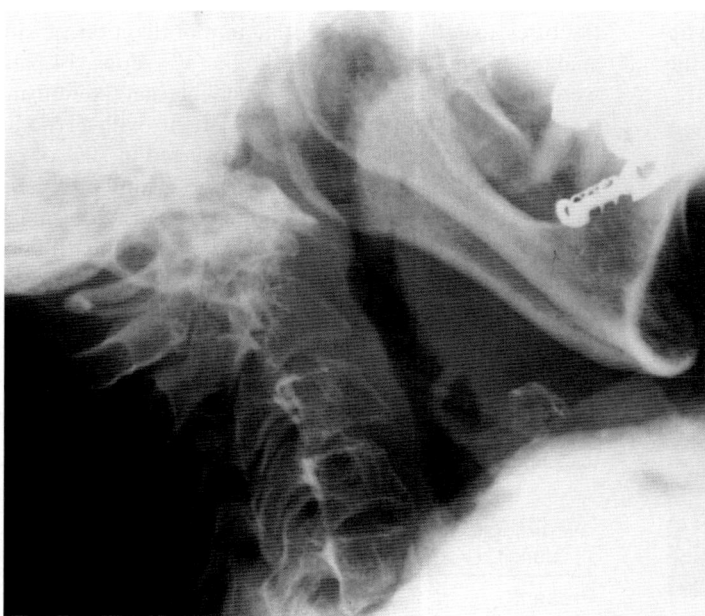
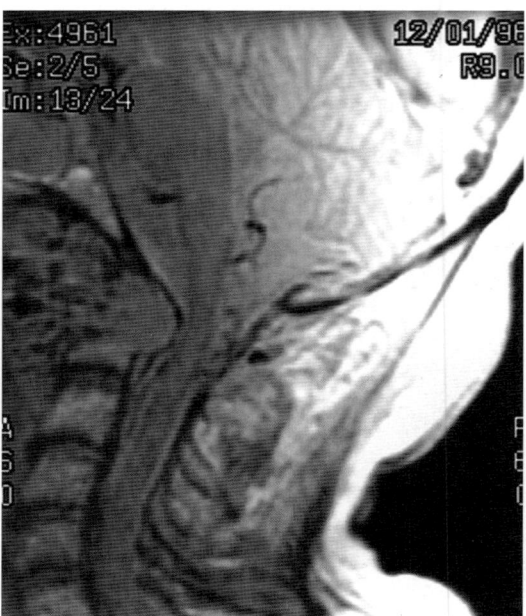

FIG. 13. **A:** Lateral radiograph of elderly woman showing migration of the upper cervical spine with subluxation at C1 and C2. **B:** Lateral magnetic resonance image showing upper cord compression.

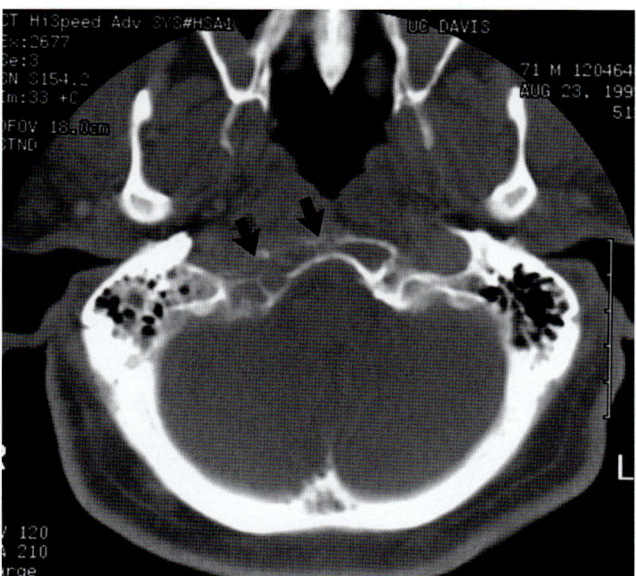

FIG. 14. Axial computed tomography scan showing prostate carcinoma metastatic to the clivus.

to invade clival bone than those of the oropharynx do the cervical spine (Figs. 15, 16). Squamous tumors extend laterally along the eustachian tube or under the skull base, which may carry them out of reach of the transoropharyngeal approach. Squamous cell carcinomas primary to the posterior wall of the oropharynx are rarely amenable to this approach because complete tumor resection with adequate margins is difficult to impossible unless the lesion is very small.

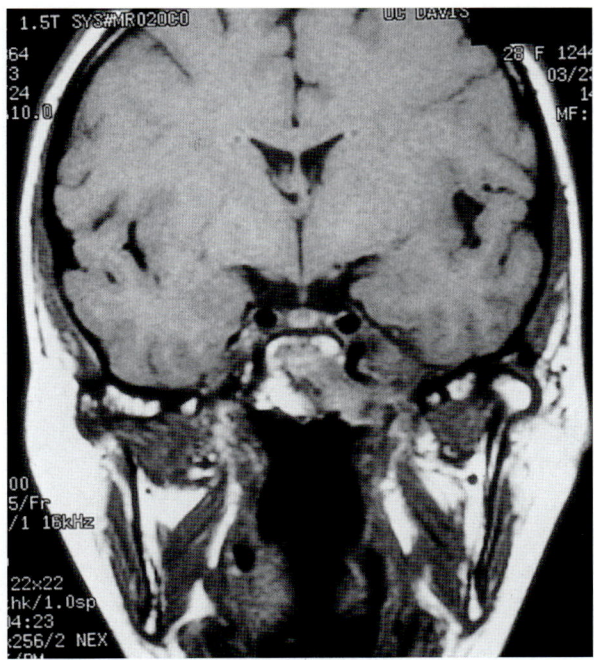

FIG. 15. Coronal magnetic resonance image of nasopharyngeal carcinoma with invasion of clival bone and extension into cavernous sinus.

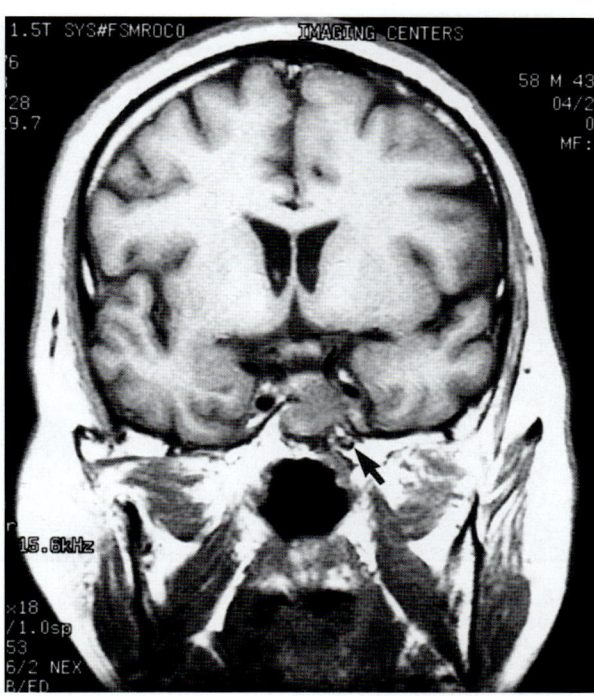

FIG. 16. Coronal magnetic resonance image showing extension of a carcinoma of the nasopharynx through foramen lacerum.

Chordoma is an enigmatic lesion thought to originate in primitive notochordal remnants and characterized histologically by a fat-filled, foamy-appearing cell described as a "physaliferous cell" (Fig. 17) (see also Chapter 3). In the skull base, this tumor uncommonly metastasizes. (In a review by Chambers and Schwinn [16], 30% of chordomas metastasized within 3 to 4 years of diagnosis, but only 7% of these primaries originated in the skull base.) In behavior, they are a sort of transition-type tumor, similar to the ameloblastoma of the jaws and inverting papilloma of the nose and paranasal sinuses. Radiographic examination reveals a soft tissue density replacing clival bone with occa-

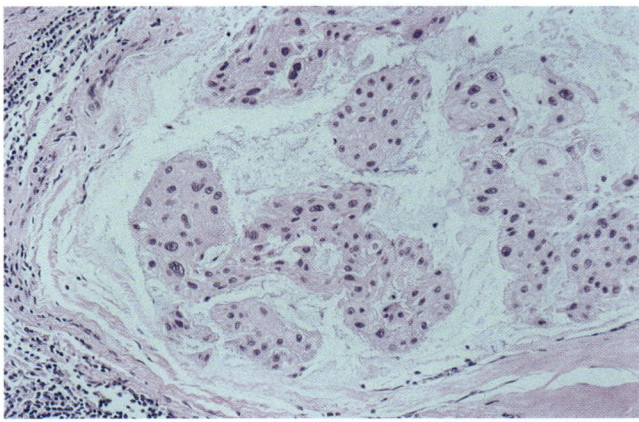

FIG. 17. Chordoma of clivus demonstrating the characteristic physaliferous cell. (Hematoxylin and eosin; original magnification 400×).

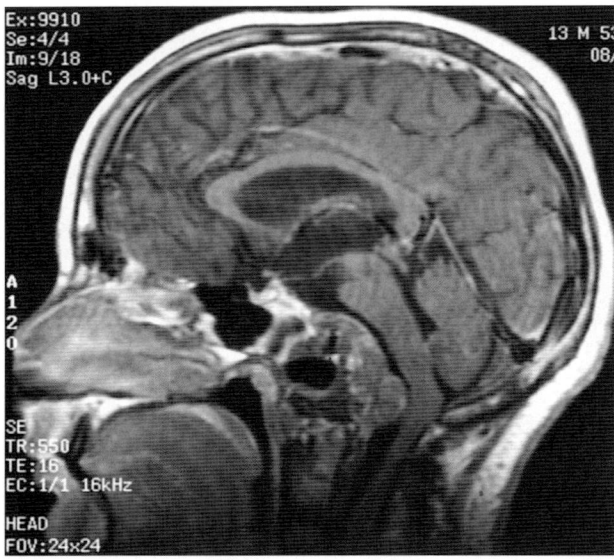

FIG. 18. Lateral magnetic resonance image showing extensive clival chordoma from the posterior clinoid processes to C2, with brainstem compression.

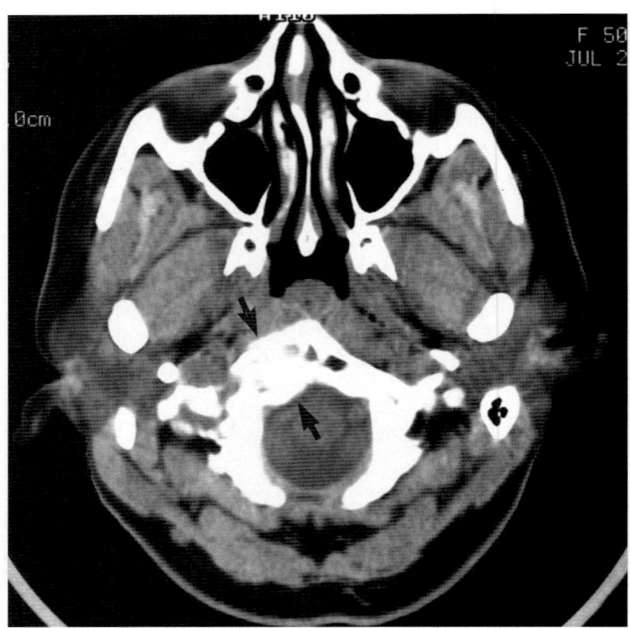

FIG. 20. Axial computed tomography scan showing fibrous dysplasia of clivus (*arrows*).

sional focal areas of calcification, although not as commonly seen at this site as in those tumors involving the vertebrae (Fig. 18). If the tumor is completely resected with a narrow margin of uninvolved tissue, it will not recur. The problem with clival and C1 chordoma is the difficulty of adequate exposure and access to effect total tumor removal. The tumor freely erodes bone, may invade adjacent soft tissue, and may become attached to dura. Transdural spread is most often the result of prior surgery with breaching of the dura and incomplete removal. The tumor is slow growing and relatively resistant to radiation therapy. In contrast to squamous cell carcinoma and most other epithelial neoplasms, which are white and hard, chordomas are gray and soft. Neither type is encapsulated, and both readily invade adjacent tissue.

A biologic behavior similar to that of chordoma is seen in chondroma and chondrosarcoma. In these tumors of cartilaginous origin, the malignant variety is far more common

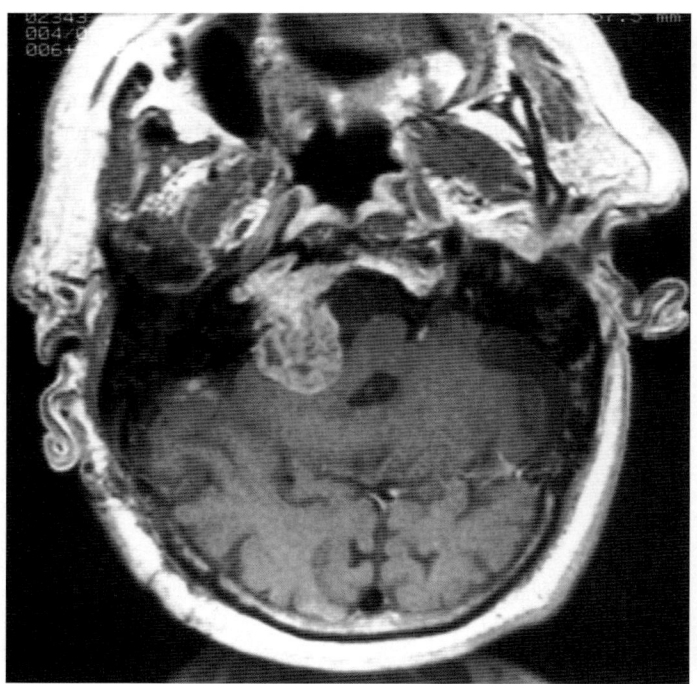
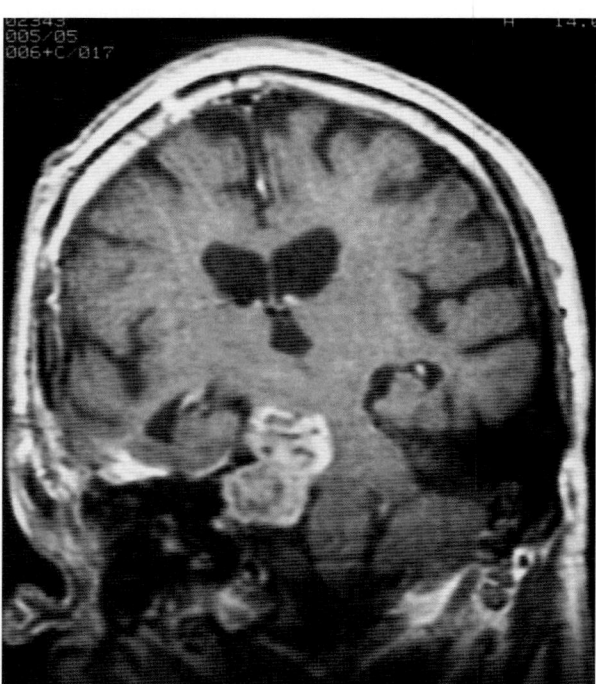

FIG. 19. Magnetic resonance images of elderly man with chondrosarcoma of clivus. **A:** Axial view. **B:** Coronal view.

than the benign. Grossly, the tumor is firm to hard, white, tan, or grayish-blue and usually seen under an intact mucosa. Radiographically, they present a variable picture of radiolucency, radiodensity, and focal calcification. Local irregular bone destruction is obvious (Fig. 19). Histologically, the chondroma resembles normal cartilage but may be more cellular, although the cells have a normal configuration. There may be foci of ossification, thereby qualifying them as osteochondromas. The chondrosarcomas are highly cellular, and these cells are irregular, pleomorphic, with hyperchromatic and occasional multiple nuclei, but with infrequent appearance of mitotic figures (17). Histologically, the lesion is sometimes difficult to differentiate from a chondroid chordoma. They rarely metastasize and are radioinsensitive.

Secondary malignancies such as those originating in the prostate or kidney or from cutaneous melanoma may show up as a lytic lesion in the clivus. A computed tomography (CT) scan of the head and neck stimulated by the patient's complaint of occipital or posterior neck pain may reveal such a finding as the only initial manifestation of an otherwise occult primary malignancy. The importance of biopsy is paramount (see Chapter 3). Meningiomas can invade the clivus from the cranial side and can have significant osseous involvement. Neurologic symptoms occur as the tumor compresses the brainstem or migrates through the foramen magnum (18). A number of other disparate lesions may present as clival masses. Fibrous dysplasia (Fig. 20) and nonspecific inflammation resembling the Tolosa-Hunt syndrome (Fig. 21) may present with clival erosions as their primary objective findings.

CLINICAL PRESENTATION

Lesions in the clivus may be purely incidental findings on a CT scan or routine head film, with little or no clinical manifestations. Odontoid lesions and disease of the atlantooccipital or atlantoaxial axis are usually symptomatic.

Clival lesions may simply present as a history of posterior cervical pain or occipital cephalgia. One patient in the author's experience presented with a 5-year history of postauricular pain over the mastoid process (Fig. 22). Encroachment on the hypoglossal canal may produce paresis or paralysis of cranial nerve XII, resulting in slurred speech and oral dysphagia. These symptoms often tend to be transient because the patient usually rapidly accommodates to unilateral lingual paralysis. Further expansion into the skull base laterally produces the jugular foramen syndrome with compromise of cranial nerves IX, X, and XI. This well known constellation of symptoms, consisting of shoulder weakness secondary to sternocleidomastoid and trapezius paralysis, and hoarseness, aspiration, and pharyngeal dysphagia resulting from vagal paralysis, with the dysphagia additionally aggravated by glossopharyngeal paralysis, can be severely debilitating. The presence of a nasopharyngeal mass may cause nasal obstruction and eustachian tube dysfunction, the latter producing a middle ear effusion. The second most common symptom after a mass in the neck in the manifestations of nasopharyngeal carcinoma is a conductive hearing loss sec-

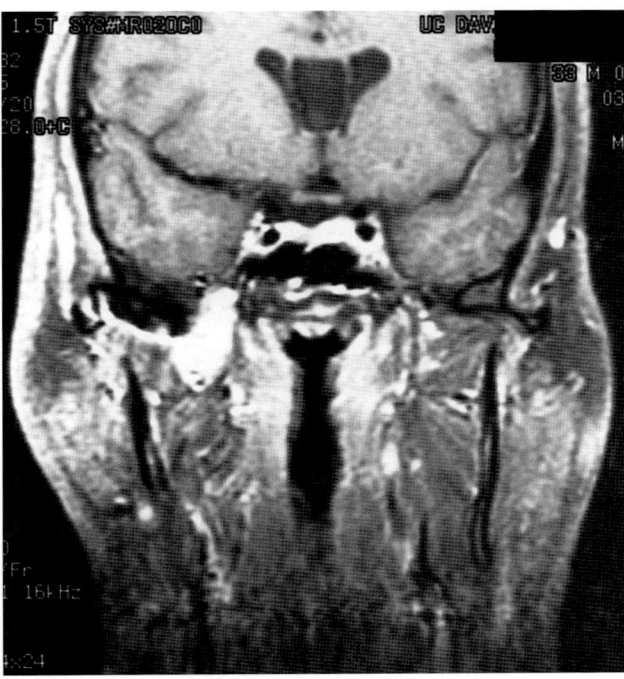

FIG. 21. Computed tomography scan of Tolosa-Hunt syndrome showing invasion of clivus extending into the cavernous sinus.

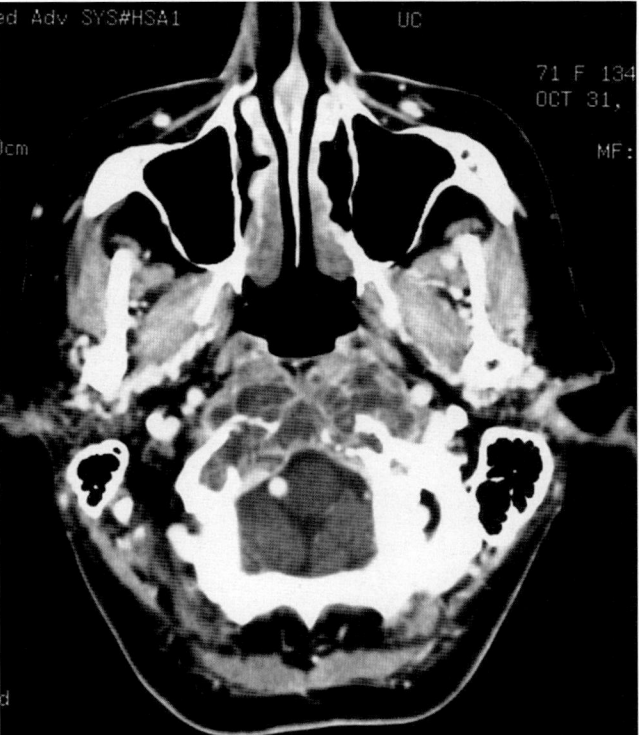

FIG. 22. Computed tomography scan of elderly woman with erosive lesion of clivus producing postauricular pain (see text). Biopsy revealed clival chordoma.

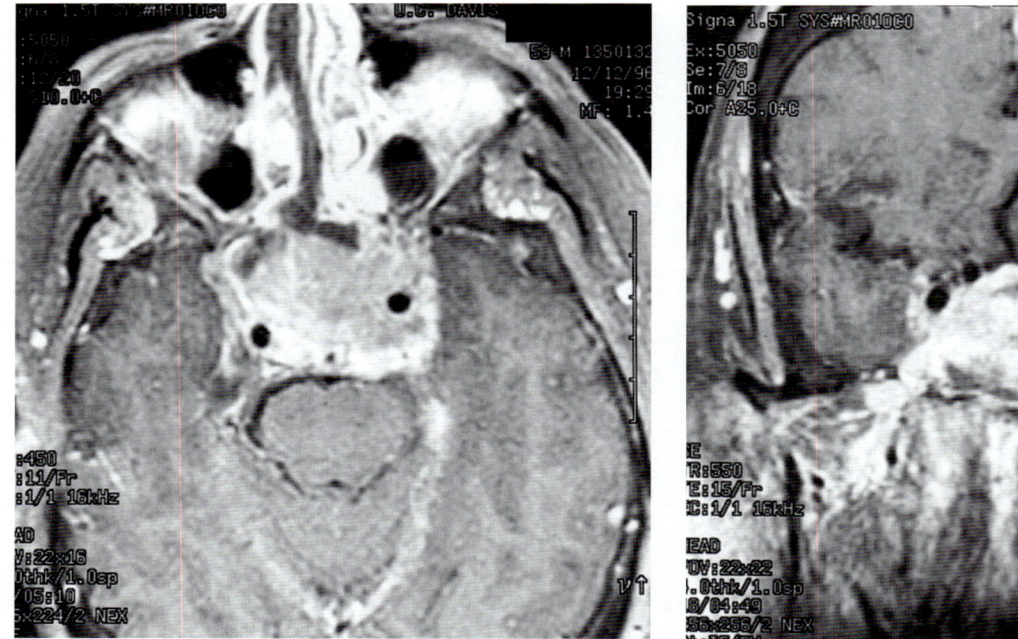

FIG. 23. Magnetic resonance images of massive prolactinoma in a late middle-aged man. He presented with massive epistaxis, visual disturbance, and semicoma. These symptoms were preceded by months of nasal obstruction. **A:** Axial view. **B:** Coronal view.

ondary to this effusion. If a nasopharyngeal mass is of clival origin, ulceration of the mucosa is very uncommon and bleeding rarely a presenting symptom. Mucosal malignancies such as nasopharyngeal carcinoma are commonly ulcerative, and bleeding, although rarely massive, is a frequent symptom. Lesions such as large pituitary tumors (Fig. 23) and nasopharyngeal angiofibromas (Fig. 24), although not originating in the clivus, may spread to it, causing erosion and presenting not only with nasal obstruction but massive, life-threatening epistaxis. Posterior extension of clival tu-

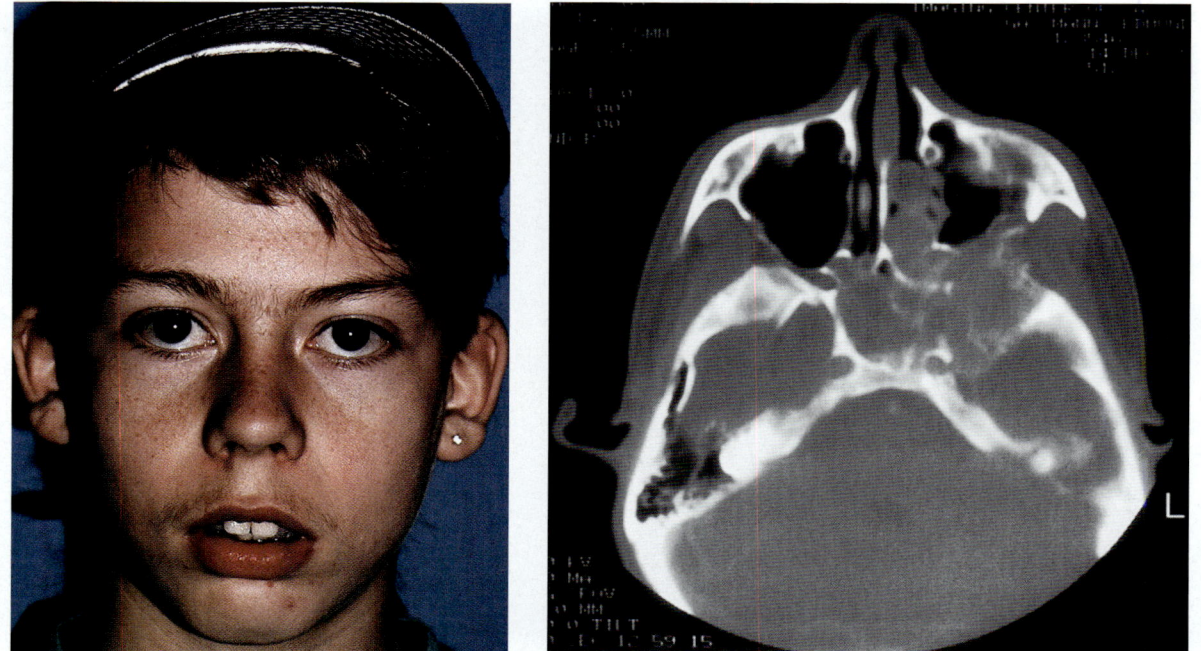

FIG. 24. A: Preoperative photograph of 13-year-old with nasal obstruction, epistaxis, proptosis, and bulging in left cheek secondary to a massive angiofibroma. **B:** Magnetic resonance image showing tumor invading middle cranial fossa and cavernous sinus.

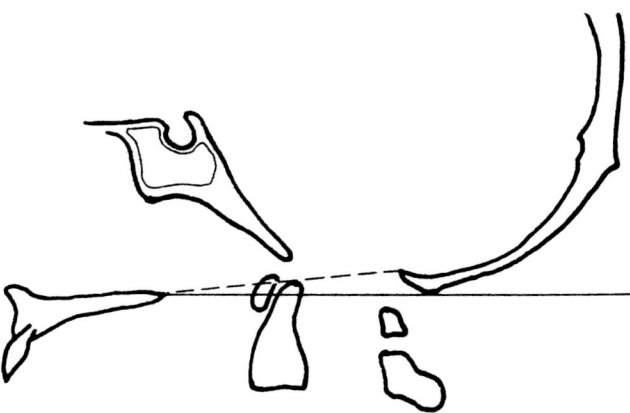

FIG. 25. McGregor's line (*solid line*) compared with Chamberlain's line (*dotted line*).

mors may cause brainstem compression. Early symptoms may be simply suboccipital pain and vague dysesthesia in the arms. The syndrome is often initially misdiagnosed as degenerative disease of the spine (18). Upper extremity weakness and gait disturbance may occur, as well as cranial nerve XI palsy, as lower clival compression progresses. In the upper and middle clivus, cranial nerve VI disturbance, vertigo, ataxia, syncopal episodes, and even hydrocephalus may develop.

Basilar impression syndrome produces brainstem compression and may result in the cerebromedullary syndrome with ataxia, vertigo, oscillopsia, and vertical nystagmus. Lower cranial nerve involvement may also be present (3,19,20).

Pressure against the pons can produce sudden cardiorespiratory arrest. One patient in the author's experience (21) experienced repeated cardiorespiratory arrests requiring cardiopulmonary resuscitation, finally relieved temporarily by traction using Crutchfield tongs and permanently by odontectomy and spinal fusion (see Fig. 9). Compression in the atlantoaxial area can result in lower limb paralysis, upper limb paresthesia, weakness, and complete tetraparesis.

Radiographic evaluation can provide useful information in the diagnosis and estimate of severity of basilar impression syndrome. A lateral skull CT or plain film can portray the position of the odontoid tip relative to the skull base. Chamberlain's line (22) connects the dorsal lip of the foramen magnum to the posterior termination of the hard palate (Fig. 25). The tip of the odontoid process should be below that line. Because the dorsal lip may be difficult to visualize, McGregor (23) defined another line that connects a point at the inferior convexity of the occiput to the distal tip of the hard palate. McGregor calculated that the odontoid should project no more than 4 to 5 mm above this line (see Fig. 25). Fischgold's line is also a useful measurement (24). This is produced on a posteroanterior film. The mastoid tip of one side is connected to that of the opposite side, and the line thus produced should pass through the atlantooccipital joint and the tip of the dens (Fig. 26, dotted line). Metzger's line connects each digastric groove, and if the condyles or dens reach this point, this is a definite sign of basilar impression (24) (see Fig. 26, solid line.) Current magnetic resonance imaging technology has rendered these measurements less important than formerly in that soft tissue compression can be so precisely displayed. It is important at this juncture to clarify the distinction between platybasia (a term used often in the past as a synonym for basilar invagination) and the often separate entity of basilar impression. "Platybasia" refers to an obtuse angle between the floor of the anterior cranial fossa and the midplane of the clivus. The Boogard and Mc Rae angles describe this abnormality (Fig. 27). The Boogaard angle (25) is at the point that connects the standard cephalometric line S-N with a line passing from point S to the cranial portion of the distal tip of the clivus (normal = 120–140 degrees). The McRae (26) angle is similar and is at the point that connects a line that runs along the anterior cranial fossa floor from the point N to the tip of the anterior clinoid process and a line from the tip of the anterior clinoid to the upper surface of the distal clival tip (normal = 118–147 degrees). An increase above normal limits indicates platybasia, but, as previously mentioned, not necessarily basilar impression.

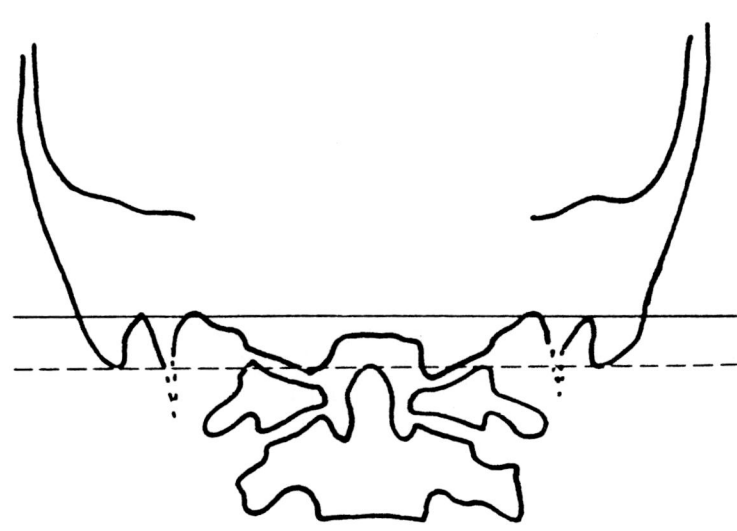

FIG. 26. Fischgold's line (*dotted line*) and Metzger's line (*solid line*).

Odontoid fractures, especially with posterior dislocation, can result in a cardiorespiratory arrest and sudden death (7,13). Severe posterior neck pain made much worse with coughing or stooping, upper limb paresthesia and weakness, lower extremity weakness or paralysis, or complete tetraparesis may result.

OPERATIVE TECHNIQUE

Preparation

The patient is operated on in the supine position. A C-arm fluoroscope should be put into position before the start of the surgical sterile preparation of the patient. The apparatus is at times a cumbersome nuisance but provides immediate information regarding surgical orientation. The fluoroscope is not essential in all cases, and spot films can be taken instead with a mobile machine during the course of the procedure. Spinal cord monitoring is wise during the procedure, especially when any spinal or atlantooccipital instability is anticipated.

Head position during the conduct of the operation is extremely important, as is the maintenance of its stability. Unlike many of the interdisciplinary procedures involving head and neck surgery and neurosurgery, in which stabilizing cranial pins are avoided to permit free movement of the head necessary for optimal visualization during the subcranial portion of the surgery, these operations need fixation. The head is manipulated into the surgically most advantageous position while the electrical activity of the spinal cord is carefully monitored. For the transoropharyngeal approach, the best position is with as much head extension as possible.

Before surgery, the extent of jaw opening is assessed, as is the size of the oral cavity and the oropharyngeal isthmus. In patients with rheumatoid arthritis, involvement of the temporomandibular joint with disease is not uncommon. Restriction of jaw motion may require surgical mobilization of the joint (21) or an approach using a median labial mandibuloglossoptomy (Fig. 28).

A tracheostomy is often done, for a number of reasons. With elimination of the endotracheal tube from the oral cavity, more room can be obtained and the pervasive concern regarding tube compression can be avoided. The tube also acts as a source of bacterial contamination because it is rarely inserted under sterile technique. The presence of the tube also adds to the pressure on the tongue already created by the blade of the mouth gag, leading to the possibility of increased postoperative lingual swelling. Most important, postoperative tongue edema with airway compromise and the necessity for sputum expectoration after coughing in the face of the pharyngeal closure are the major postoperative reasons for tracheostomy. Often the patient is stabilized in a halo brace. These patients not uncommonly have both dysphagia and aspiration. Airway protection in the early postoperative days is afforded by the tracheostomy.

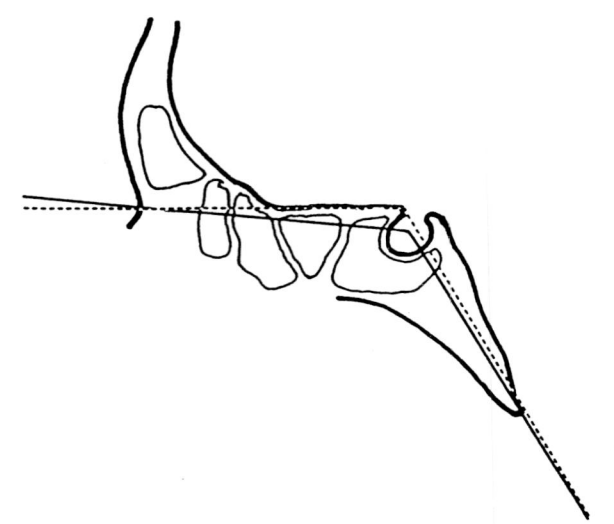

FIG. 27. Boogard line (*solid line*) and McRae line (*dotted line*).

Eye protection is best served by the use of Frost stitches (see Chapter 10). Corneal shields are adequate for short cases, but for a procedure going beyond 3 or 4 hours, these sutures will prevent any corneal irritation that may result from prolonged use of the shields.

A lumbar subarachnoid drain is placed, as in most skull base cases, at any time when dural resection is anticipated. Many of the transoropharyngeal procedures are done extradurally because the lesion is one of bone and adjacent muscle and mucosa. If a dural resection is anticipated, intraoperative cerebrospinal fluid (CSF) drainage, usually extended 2 to 3 days after surgery, is routine.

The surgical sterile preparation includes the head and neck and any anticipated donor sites, such as the thigh for a fascia lata graft and the abdomen for fat grafting. The patient is encouraged to brush his or her teeth vigorously for some days in anticipation of the surgery. Obviously, all grossly infected teeth or gums must be remediated before surgery. Povidone–iodine-soaked sponges are placed in the mouth at the time of the sterile preparation.

Operative Procedure

In most cases, excellent exposure is obtained through the oral cavity. The Crockard or Dingman mouth gag is placed to retract the tongue and cheeks and prop open the mouth. Care is taken to protect the tongue tip from compression against the teeth. After the gag has been in place for 5 minutes or so, maximal jaw opening can be achieved with a couple of additional opening "clicks" of the gag as relaxation and stretching of the perioral tissues and jaw musculature proceeds.

Injection of the posterior pharyngeal wall, the soft palate, and the hard palate is done with 0.5% lidocaine in 1/100,000 or 1/200,000 epinephrine. The hard palate injection is done only if superior extension is required. The initial injection is in the proposed incision line, and a further infusion is made over the areas of planned soft tissue elevation. The incisions

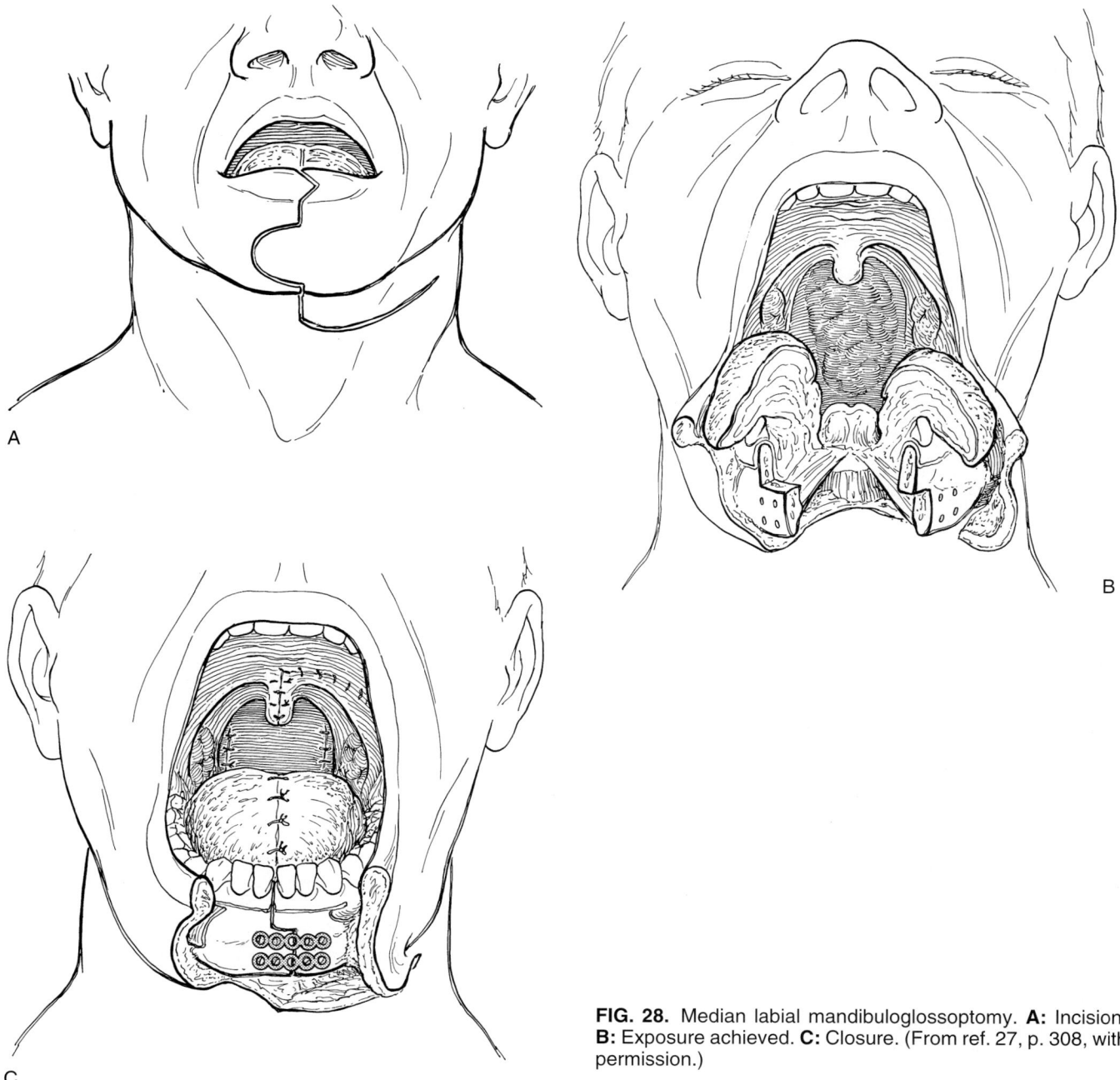

FIG. 28. Median labial mandibuloglossoptomy. A: Incision. B: Exposure achieved. C: Closure. (From ref. 27, p. 308, with permission.)

are made in the palate first (Fig. 29). A midline incision in the soft palate, splitting the uvula in the midline, is the first step and may be all that is required to provide adequate exposure of the clivus. If exposure of the sphenoid clivus and the floor of the sphenoid sinus is needed, an exposure through the hard palate is often required. An incision in the palatal mucosa from the junction of the soft to hard palate is made laterally to approximately 3 to 5 mm from the necks of the teeth. This is carried around the anterior aspect of the hard palate just posterior to the incisive foramen to the other side, and carried down to about the level of the first molar tooth on the opposing side. The hard palatal mucoperiosteum is dissected to the junction of the hard and soft palate. The greater palatine neurovascular bundle on the side of greatest exposure is isolated, and a ligature slid around it and tied (Fig. 30). The insertions of the soft palate muscles on the posterior projection of the hard palate are dissected away. On the side of lesser involvement, this is done submucosally if possible to avoid a T-shaped incision that is prone to wound breakdown and subsequent fistulization. The self-retaining retractor is inserted, exposing the entire nasopharyngeal and oropharyngeal walls from the posterior nasal septum to the level of C3 and even C4. The posterior pharyngeal wall is clearly seen and a lateral incision is made from the mucosa

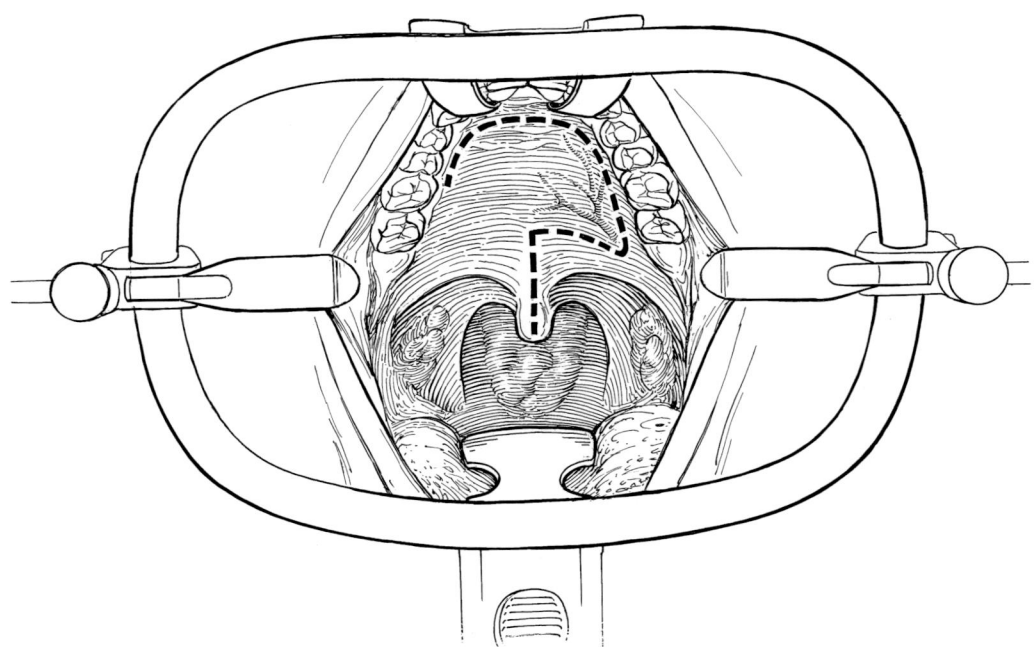

FIG. 29. Outline of soft and hard palate incisions.

through the superior constrictor muscle to the alar fascia. The incision is made as far lateral in the pharynx as possible, just medial to the posterior pillar of the tonsil, and extends from the nasopharynx to the level of the tip of the epiglottis. Care is taken to avoid accidental incision of the ascending pharyngeal artery. The alar fascia is identified as a glistening, white, fibrous layer on the outer aspect of the constrictor muscle, yet anterior to the cervical prevertebral fascia. In the oropharynx, the muscle is clearly and easily identifiable and the alar fascia is obvious. In the nasopharynx, the muscle becomes tendinous and inserts into the pharyngeal tubercles of the clivus. The right-angled scissors dissect the muscle layer from the incision to the opposite lateral pharyngeal wall (Fig. 31). Hemostasis is ensured with the suction cautery. Once the wound is dry, a parallel incision is created on the opposite side and of the same length as its fellow. Hemostasis is again established. The two incisions are connected superiorly, with this incision placed in such a fashion that closure near the nasopharynx can easily be effected at the end of the operation. This incision is usually located just behind the choanae. Sharp dissection connects the free retropharyngeal plane into the nasopharynx to create an inferiorly based posterior pharyngeal flap, as first described for this operation by Crumley and Gutin (27). The flap is dissected inferiorly, folded on itself, and temporarily tamped into the hypopharynx. The author has found that the flap can be secured in this position throughout the remainder of the procedure by placing a suture at each corner of the flap superiorly, running the suture through a small square of lead, and stuffing the lead into the hypopharynx (Fig. 32).

A drill is now used to remove enough palatal bone to achieve the required exposure of the upper clivus. This exposure may extend as far anteriorly as the cribriform plate, if so desired. The nasal mucoperiosteum of the posterior nasal floor is rather delicate and difficult to preserve; however, the septal mucoperiosteum over the vomer is much tougher. Once sufficient palate is removed, the inferior aspect of the

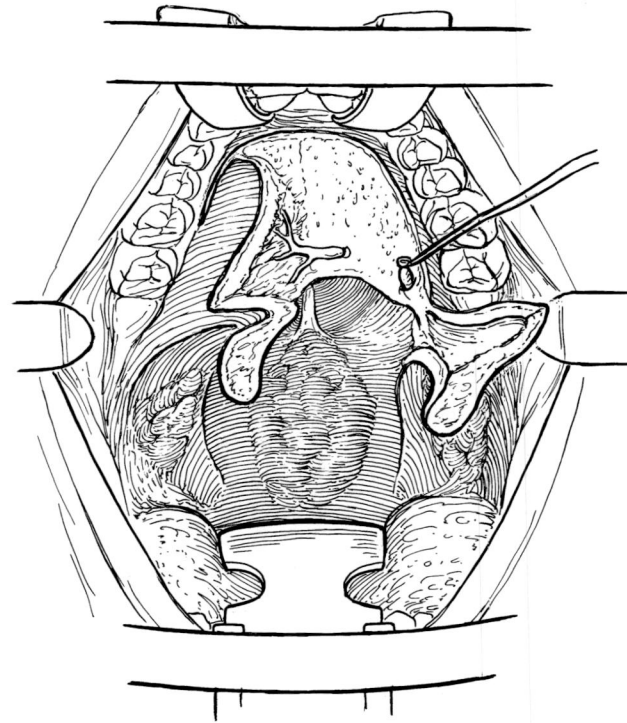

FIG. 30. Palatal incisions made and greater palatine neurovascular bundle ligated.

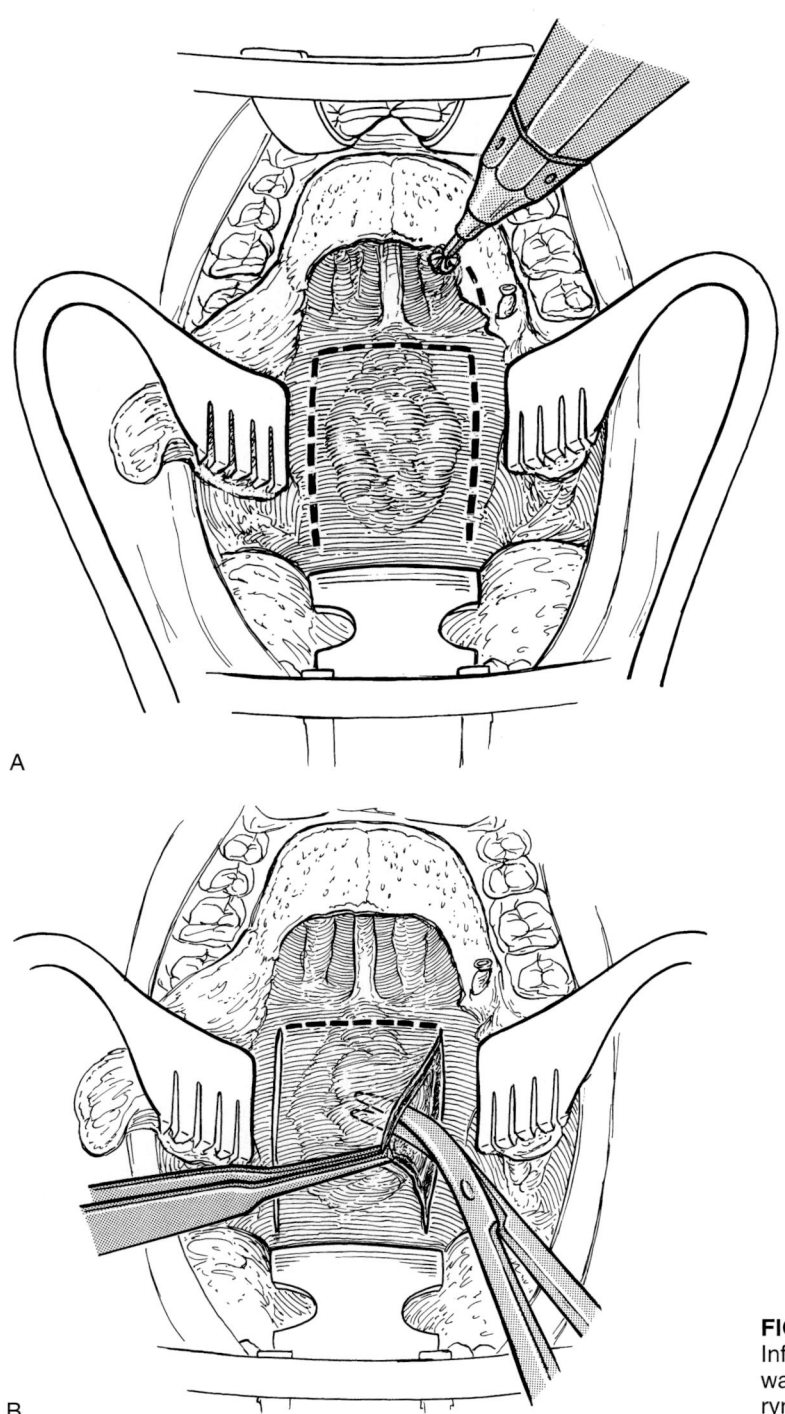

FIG. 31. A: Crockard self-retaining retractor inserted. Inferior-based pharyngeal flap on posterior pharyngeal wall outlined. **B:** Lateral incision made with superior pharyngeal constrictor in the plane of the alar fascia.

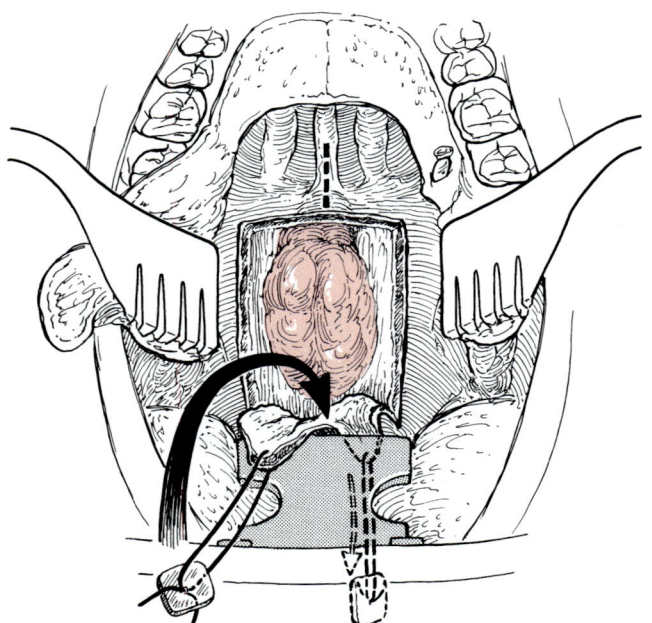

FIG. 32. The pharyngeal flap has sutures with small squares of lead placed on its distal end, then stuffed into the hypopharynx to stabilize the flap during subsequent dissection.

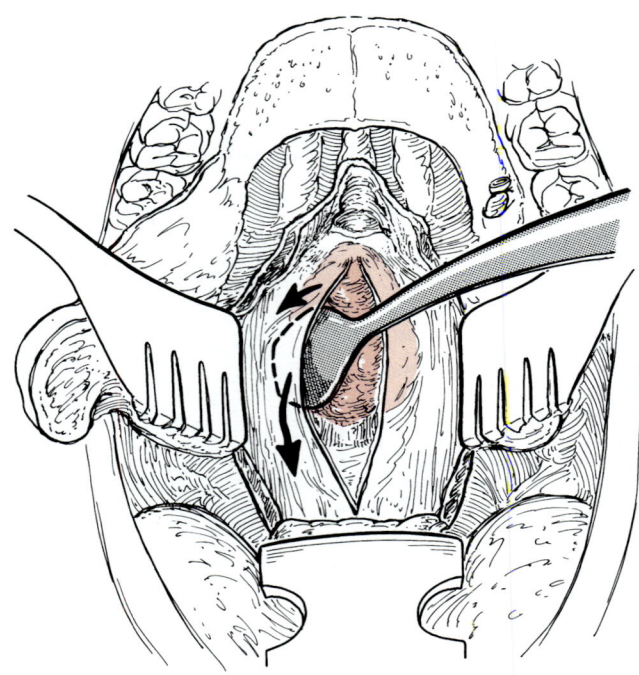

FIG. 34. The heavy elevator is used to dissect the tough soft tissues off the clivus and cervical spine. The Crockard retractor is then reapplied to give enhanced exposure of the tumor and surrounding bone.

nasal septum becomes obvious. It is split on the choanal side right up to the sphenoid rostrum, and dissection of the septal mucoperiosteal leaves is carried up this high and the posterior septal bone removed (Fig. 33). The Crockard palatal retractor is now inserted.

The midline posterior septal incision becomes continuous with a midline incision through the tough, tendinous tissue over the clivus and the prevertebral fascia and muscles of the

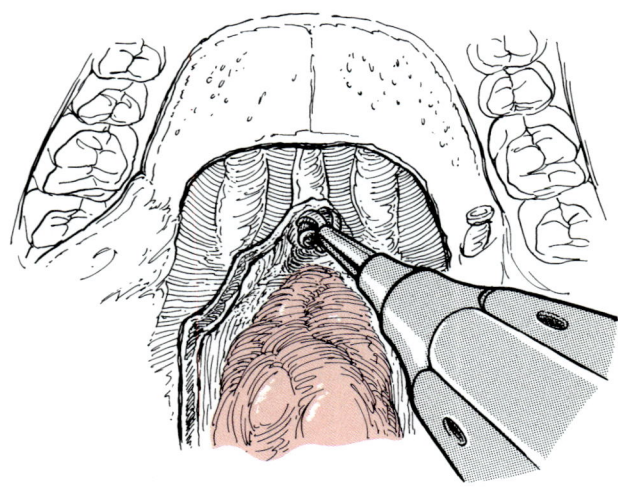

FIG. 33. The palate is drilled away to an amount sufficient to provide adequate exposure of the clival involvement by tumor. The posterior septum is removed to expose the sphenoid contribution to the clivus.

upper cervical spine. The heavy elevator is now used to dissect this soft tissue over the clivus and upper two or three cervical vertebrae (Fig. 34). The Crockard retractor is reapplied and the soft tissue held in place, exposing the site of proposed bony resection or tumor.

If such exigencies as a very small oropharynx, severe trismus, or severe microgenia and retrognathia are present, or if exposure to the C4 to C6 level is also required, additional exposure may be gained by using the median labial mandibuloglossoptomy originally described by Trotter (28–30). A skin incision through the middle of the lip, using a dart in the vermilion descending vertically to the chin button, circling the chin and into the submental area, is created (see Fig. 28A). The mandible is exposed in the midline and a stairstep incision is etched in the symphysis. Drill holes for two parallel plates are placed to secure the bone at the end of the case (see Fig. 28B). Care is taken that the uppermost plate screw holes are below the roots of the incisor teeth, which are generally double the crown length of the tooth. A saw cut begins between the central incisor teeth either with a fine saw blade or the Midas Rex B5 cutting tool, assiduously avoiding the lamina dura of either tooth. Once the saw cut has bisected the mandible, the anterior floor of the mouth tissues is cut in the midline and the tongue is split down the midline raphe to the hyoid bone. With improved exposure inferiorly, the pharyngeal flap can be dissected to the postcricoid area, providing the improved access desired. At the end of the resection, the mandible is secured by two plates (see Fig. 31C). This exposure is rarely needed.

Once the paraspinous tissues have been retracted, drilling of clival and spinal bone may ensue to expose or provide access to tumor or the odontoid. The curved drill of the TAC attachment of the Midas Rex is ideal for this dissection (Fig. 35). Coupled with continuous suction irrigation, bone removal is fast, efficient, and safe.

Tumor Excision

Most tumors addressed by this approach are chordomas and chondrosarcomas (see Fig. 22). The author has also encountered fibrous dysplasia, nonspecific fibrogranulomatous lesions similar to those of Tolosa-Hunt syndrome (see Fig. 21), and metastatic carcinoma (see Fig. 14).

Often the tumor is present under the periosteum. Additional exposure is gained by progressive resection of bone with the cutting drill. Long dissection instruments developed by Raveh and the author are long enough for this task and remove the hand from obscuring the view. In removing a chordoma, great care is exercised to avoid penetrating the dura (Fig. 36). Although every attempt is made to remove the entire tumor, local recurrences unfortunately are common and, if intradural, exceedingly difficult to eliminate. Fortunately, the anterior longitudinal ligament provides some barrier to penetration during tumor dissection.

Lateral extension of neoplasm at the skull base toward the hypoglossal canal is a serious impediment to complete excision, and a second staged operation such as a lateral approach may be needed for complete tumor removal. Superior resection can be carried into the sphenoid sinus and up to the sella turcica.

Surgical stabilization of the spine may be necessary for a few weeks after surgery.

Odontectomy

Removal of the dens is done in some cases of fracture, but most commonly for brainstem and upper cervical cord compression from an arthritic pannus (see Fig. 13). It is also done for decompression in basilar impression syndrome (see Fig. 9).

The exposure almost never requires the median labial mandibuloglossoptomy. Removal of palatal bone is minimal or not necessary. Exposure is from the lower clivus to the level of C2. In basilar impression syndrome, cases of other congenital spinal anomalies, and even in rheumatoid arthritis, where collapse of the spinal bodies is not uncommon, landmarks are often difficult to define. Identification of the arch of C1 is sometimes problematic and the frequent use of the fluoroscope is encouraged to register position.

An exposure similar to that described for tumor is done, but usually only a soft palatal split is required, without the necessity of removing hard palatal bone. Once identified, the anterior arch of C1 is removed with the drill (Fig. 37). In basilar impression, the bony distortion is often so great that the lower clivus must be excised before the odontoid can be reached. The occipital clivus in these cases is often crumbly and weak. It and the arch of C1 are removed until the pe-

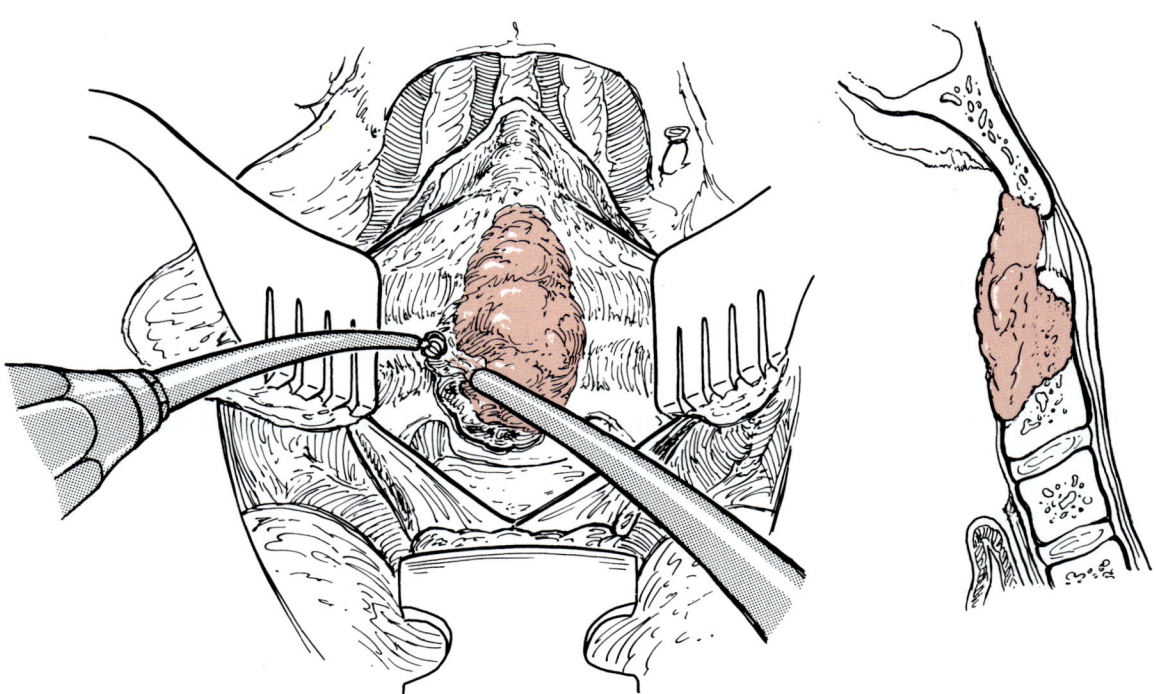

FIG. 35. The curved Midas Rex TAC attachment is used to remove bone from the clivus and cervical spinous bodies to expose the limits of tumor.

528 / Chapter 26

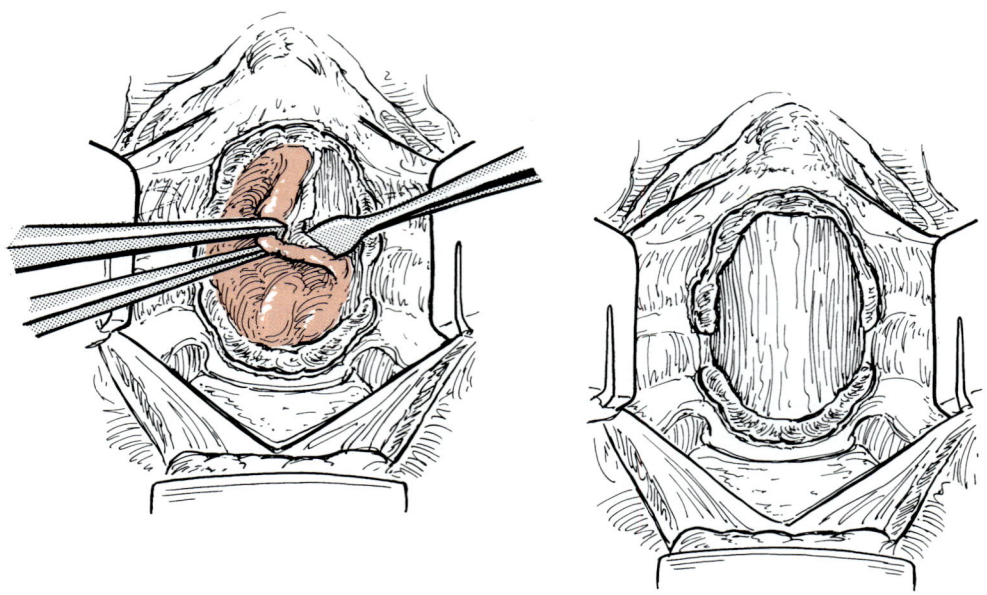

FIG. 36. Tumor is removed completely and great care is taken to avoid injury to the dura.

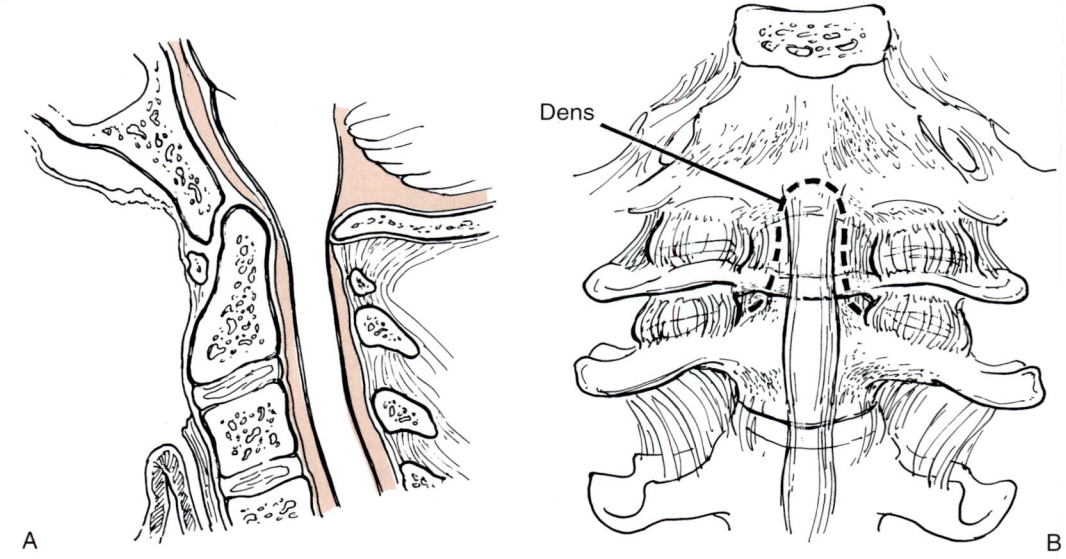

FIG. 37. A: Diagram of basilar impression. **B:** The areas of the C1 arch and adjacent clivus to be resected are marked out.

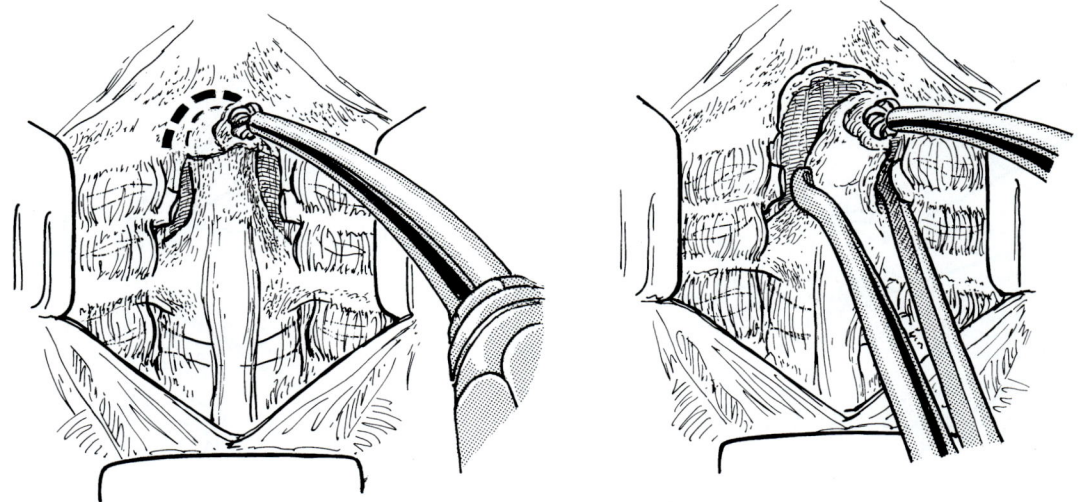

FIG. 38. A: Arch of C1 and adjacent clivus drilled away with cutting bur, exposing deformed dens. **B:** Dens grasped with Crockard instrument and removed with drill.

riosteum over the odontoid is reached. The odontoid is grasped with the Crockard forceps and the dens drilled away (Fig. 38).

In cases of rheumatoid arthritis, although the dens is often deformed, there is no migration of the spine. The pannus projects against the brainstem. The C1 arch and only a small portion of the clivus need resection (Fig. 39). Once the ligament is reached, much inflammatory reaction is present and the pannus becomes obvious, requiring sharp dissection (Fig. 40). Excessive vigor in this endeavor may lead to a breach in the transverse ligament and laceration of dura. This must be avoided, if possible, because dural leaks here are difficult to repair. Checking depth of dissection with the fluoroscope is very helpful.

Closure

Once the resection is finished, any dural disruption is repaired by suturing a fascia graft augmented by fibrin glue. The dead space created by the resection must be obliterated. Surgicel is often placed against the dura and the defect filled with Gelfoam. The defect may be filled with cancellous bone from the hip.

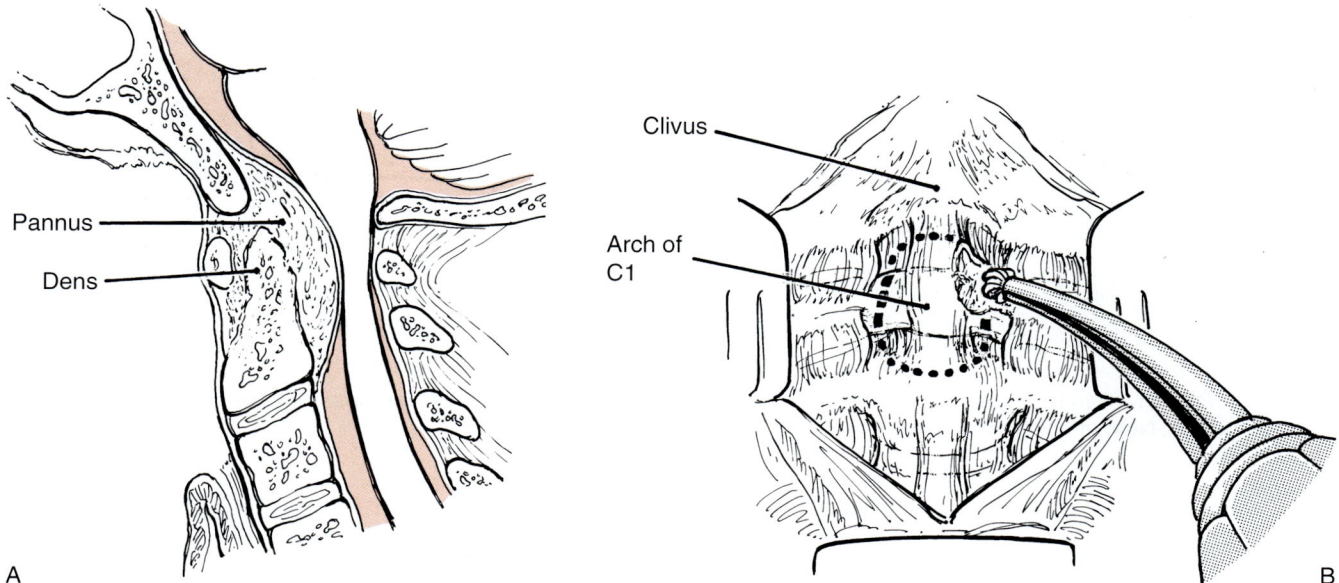

FIG. 39. A: Pannus surrounds deformed dens in a patient with rheumatoid arthritis. **B:** Area of bone removal outlined.

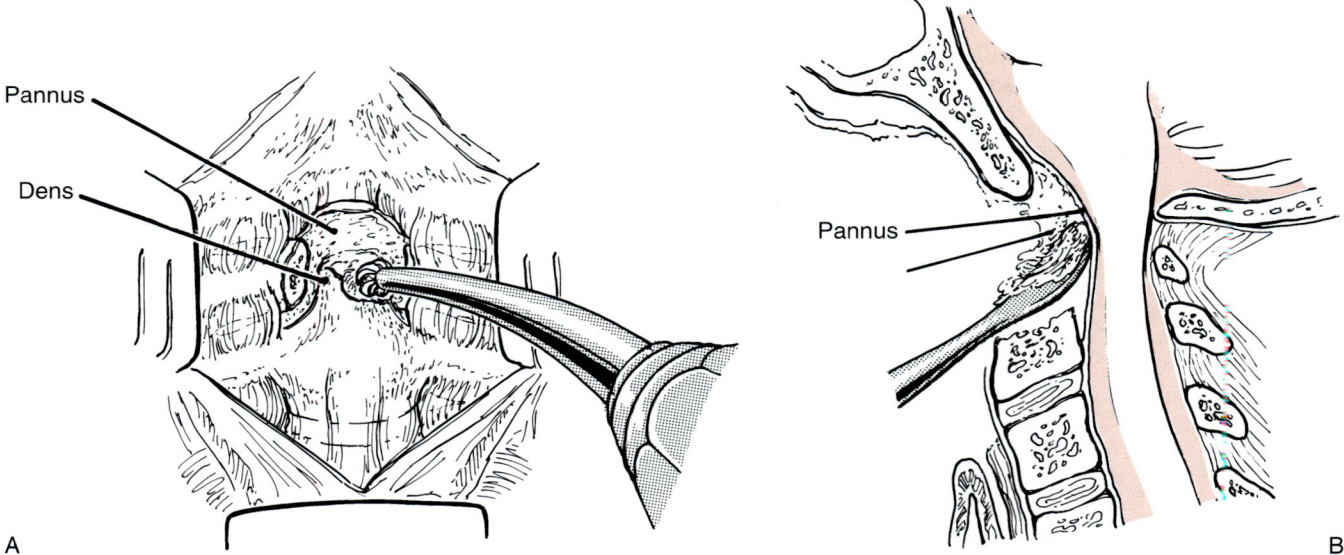

FIG. 40. A: Midas Rex drill used to excise arch of C1 and small amount of clivus. **B:** Sharp dissection is needed to remove pannus.

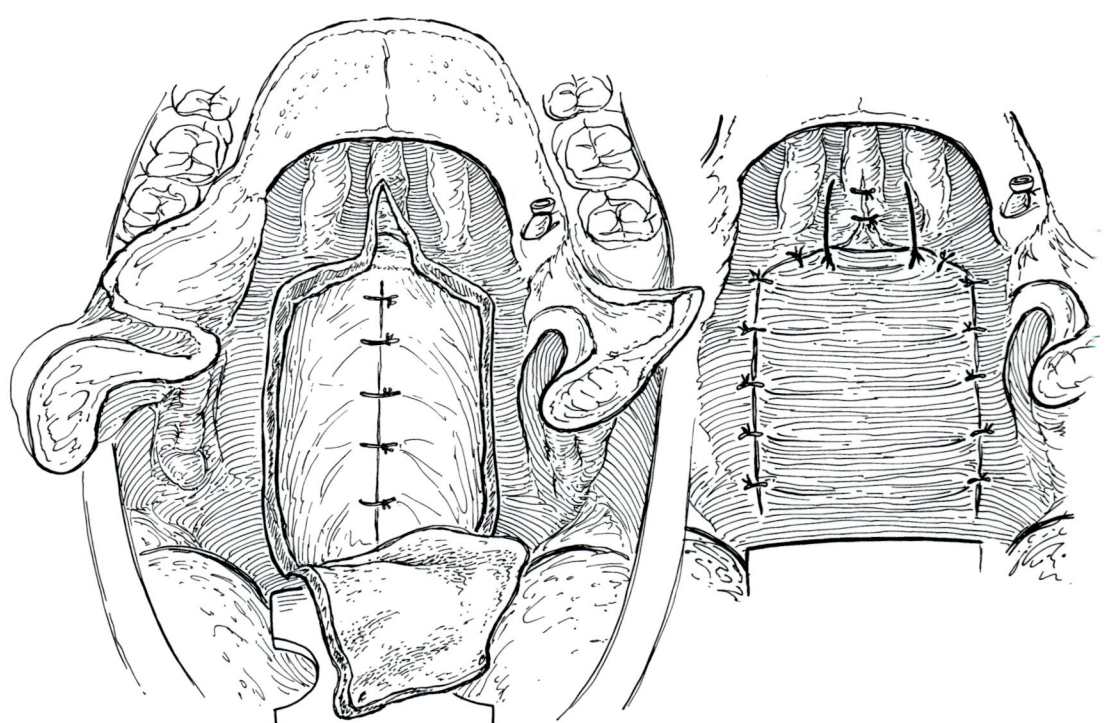

FIG. 41. Paraspinous muscles and connective tissue approximated in midline. *Inset:* Pharyngeal closure. Note bridging sutures in choanal mucoperiosteum.

The paraspinous muscles and connective tissue are approximated in the midline with absorbable sutures (Fig. 41). This closure is not as tidy over the clivus as it is over the cervical spine. The pharyngeal flap is retrieved from the hypopharynx, the lead weight keepers removed, and the flap restored to its original position. Lateral sutures are placed with little difficulty, but the uppermost ones in the transverse incision in the nasopharynx are harder to secure. The nasopharyngeal mucosa is more friable than that of the oropharynx, so that bridging sutures to the mucoperiosteum of the choanal vault may be necessary to anchor the upper portion of the flap.

To avoid fistulization, it is essential to close the soft palate in three layers. The nasopharyngeal side of the palate is closed initially with interrupted absorbable sutures from the posterior nasal septum to the tip of the uvula. The palatal muscle and the oral mucosa are closed with four horizontal mattress sutures in a fashion similar to the closure of a cleft palate. More accurate approximation of the oral mucosa is done with fine suture material (Fig. 42).

The tough mucoperiosteum of the hard palate is secured with a few interrupted sutures. The anteriormost part of the wound is often difficult to close because the tissue is thin and attenuated and the angle makes suturing mechanically difficult. Because the bony resection is designed to come short of the mucosal incision, sufficient overlap of mucoperiosteum prevents fistula formation.

Closure of the median labial mandibuloglossoptomy is relatively simple. The deep tongue musculature is approximated with 3-0 absorbable sutures and the mucosal surface with 4-0 sutures. The mandibular split is repaired with low-profile titanium plates and screws. Skin and mucosal closure are meticulous to avoid deforming scars. It is essential to accurately approximate the white roll of the lower lip because this is the keystone to good aesthetic repair. Interrupted sutures in the skin produce a much better scar than a running closure.

The tracheostomy is maintained after surgery until the pharyngeal and palatal wounds have healed. No pharyngeal diversion is necessary and nasogastric tube feeding is avoided. Oral alimentation can often resume in about 5 days. If complications preclude oral feedings, then a nasogastric tube is placed, taking great care to avoid disruption of the palatal and pharyngeal wounds. If necessary, fiberoptic control can be used.

In most cases, the atlantooccipital junction is unstable and later upper cervical fixation through a posterior approach will be necessary. In the intervening period, the patient's spine is stabilized with halo-type fixation.

COMPLICATIONS

This surgery is more difficult in the elderly than the young. Elderly patients with rheumatoid arthritis of the severity requiring odontectomy are often functioning marginally. They are more prone to complications of aspiration and dysphagia in the early postoperative period, and are slow to recover because of their diminished mobility.

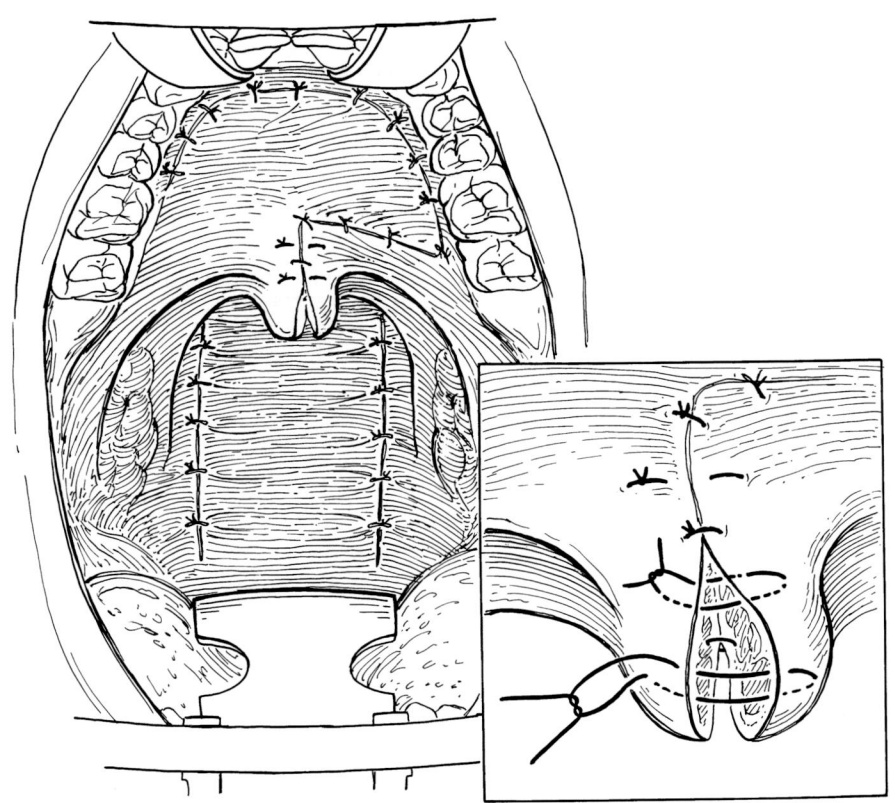

FIG. 42. Closure of soft palate is carefully done in three layers: the nasal mucosa, horizontal mattress sutures in the soft palatal mucosa, and a simple suture in the oral side

Tongue swelling is common immediately after surgery, and resolves spontaneously within a few days. The temptation to use systemic steroids should be suppressed because of the inhibitory effect of these medications on wound healing.

Wound complications include CSF leak, wound infection, and wound breakdown. CSF leakage may stop with lumbar drainage, semi-Fowler's position, and cessation of oral alimentation. If the drainage has not stopped in 3 to 5 days, re-suturing of the dura must be done. Wound infection is fortunately very uncommon. Some of the sutures must be released (one of the virtues of placing interrupted sutures at the time of closure) to drain any purulent collection. Appropriate antibiotic therapy is instituted and the patient taken off oral alimentation until the wound is clean and granulating.

Palatal dehiscence is probably the most common complication. If a T-type incision is required for exposure, breakdown at the trifurcation occurs almost 50% of the time. The patient is often distressed at the nasal regurgitation on swallowing and the air escape during speech, creating a denasal quality to the voice. The use of a dental obturator is encouraged and closure of the fistula delayed until wound epithelialization and maturation is completed. This may be as long as 6 to 12 months.

REFERENCES

1. Sperber GH. Craniofacial embryology. In: *The cranial base*. Chicago: Year Book, 1976:78–87.
2. Prader A. Die frubembrymal Entwicklung der menschlichen Zwischenwirbelscheibe. *Acta Anat* 1947;3:68–83.
3. List CF. Neurologic syndromes accompanying developmental anomalies of the occipital bone: atlas and axis. *AMA Archives of Neurology and Psychiatry* 1941;45:577–616.
4. Gorlin RJ, Cohen MM, Lenin LS, eds. *Syndromes of the head and neck*. 3rd ed. New York: Oxford University Press, 1990:258–260.
5. Salmon MA, Lindenbaum RH, eds. *Developmental defects and syndromes*. Exeter, United Kingdom: M&M Publishers, 1978:32–34.
6. Maroteaux P, Lamy M. The malady of Toulouse Lautrec. *JAMA* 1965;191:715–717.
7. Bertrand G. Anomalies of the craniovertebral junction. In: Youmans JR, ed. *Neurological surgery*. Vol. 3. 2nd ed. Philadelphia: WB Saunders, 1982:1482–1508.
8. Gardner WJ. Anomalies of the craniovertebral junction. In: Youmans JR, ed. *Neurological surgery*. Vol. 1. Philadelphia: WB Saunders, 1973:628–644.
9. Sperber GH. *Craniofacial embryology*. In: The cranial base. Chicago: Year Book, 1976:110–113.
10. Anderson LD, D'Alonzo RT. Fractures of the odontoid process of the axis. *J Bone Joint Surg Am* 1974;56:1663–1674.
11. Clark K. Injuries of the spinal cord. In: Youmans JR, ed. *Neurological surgery*. Vol. 4. 2nd ed. Philadelphia: WB Saunders, 1982:2318–2337.
12. Larson SL. Post traumatic spinal instability. In: Pitts LH, Wagner FC, eds. *Craniospinal trauma*. New York: Thieme Medical Publishers, 1990:159–185.
13. Dunn ME, Seljeskog EL. Experience in the management of odontoid process injuries: an analysis of 128 cases. *Neurosurgery* 1986;18:306–310.
14. Hadley MN, Browner C, Sonntag VKH. Axis fractures: a comprehensive review of management and treatment in 107 cases. *Neurosurgery* 1985;17:281–290.
15. Altholl B, Bardholm P. Fracture of the odontoid process: a clinical and radiographic study. *Acta Orthop Scand Suppl* 19xx;177:61–95.
16. Chambers PW, Schwinn CP. Chordoma: a clinicopathological study of metastasis. *Am J Pathol* 1979;72:765–776.
17. Barnes LB, Pul LR, Verbin RS, Goodman MA, Appel BN. Diseases of the bones and joints. In: Barnes LB, ed. *Surgical pathology of the head and neck*. Vol. 2. New York: Marcel Dekker, Inc., 1985:957–962.
18. Samii M, Ammirate M. Meningiomas involving the lower clivus and the foramen magnum. In: Samii M, ed. *Surgery of skull base meningiomas*. New York: Springer-Verlag 1992:61–67.
19. Garcin R, Oeconomos D. *Les aspects neurologigues des malformations congénitales de la charnière cranionachidienne*. Paris: Masson, 1953.
20. Wallin DG. The osodontoideum, separate odontoid process. *J Bone Joint Surg Am* 1963;45:1459–1471.
21. Donald PJ, Bernstein LB. Transpalatal excision of the odontoid process. *Transactions of the American Academy of Ophthalmology and Otolaryngology* 1978;86:729–731.
22. Chamberlain WE. Basilar impression (platybasia). *Yale J Biol Med* 1939;11:487–496.
23. McGregor MB. The significance of certain measurements of the skull in the diagnosis of basilar impression. *Br J Radiol* 1948;21:171–181.
24. Fischgold H, Metzger J. Etude radiotomographique de l'impression basilaire. *Rev Rhum* 1952;3:261–264.
25. Boogaard JA. Basilar impression: its causes and consequences. *Ned Tijdschr Geneeskd* 1865;2:81–108.
26. McRae DL. Bone abnormalities in the origin of the foramen magnum: correlations of the anatomic and neurological findings. *Acta Radiol* 1953;40:335–354.
27. Crumley RL, Gutin PH. Surgical access for clivus chordoma. *Archives of Otolaryngology* 1980;106:1–5.
28. Trotter W. Operation for malignant disease of the pharynx. *Br J Surg* 1929;16:485.
29. Donald PJ. Infratemporal fossa and skull base surgery. In: Donald PJ, ed. *Head and neck cancer: management of the difficult case*. Philadelphia: WB Saunders, 1984:277–312.
30. Martin H, Tollefson HR, Gerold FP. Median labial mandibular glossoptomy. *Am J Surg* 1961;102:753–759.

CHAPTER 27

Management of the Vertebral Artery

Bernard George

The vertebral artery (VA) is the most important vascular structure in the vicinity of the craniocervical junction. At this level, its course is complex and may present several variations and anomalies. The VA may be directly involved by different lesions, mostly tumors. Control of the VA allows for the safe and adequate treatment of these lesions, as well as permitting the preservation of VA flow. Moreover, controlling the VA may improve the access to different parts of the skull base, such as the foramen magnum (FM) or the jugular foramen.

HISTORICAL DATA

As early as 1888, Matas (1) reported surgical treatments for distal VA posttraumatic aneurysms. In 1917, a route to the C1-2 segment of the VA was described by Henry (2), who concluded that "it was a cure for which there is no disease." Since then, many reports on cervical VA surgery have been published (3–5), but most relate to the two proximal VA segments. Although many pathologic processes, including occlusive vascular disease, craniocervical junction malformations, vascular malformations, and FM or jugular foramen tumors have been treated (3,6–16), distal VA exposure is rarely considered. The deep location of the VA and the danger of bleeding from the perivertebral venous plexus explain why this exposure is usually considered difficult and hazardous.

ANATOMIC DATA

The VA segments close to the skull base are the third (suboccipital segment), extending from the transverse foramen of C2 to the FM dura, and the fourth (intracranial segment), running from the FM to the vertebrobasilar junction.

B. George: Department of Neurosurgery, Hôpital Lariboisière, 75475 Paris, France.

Course

Third Segment

The VA comes out the transverse foramen of C2 in a posterolateral direction, immediately turns vertically, and courses through the transverse foramen of the atlas. Inside this foramen, the VA curves medially and posteriorly to reach the VA groove lying behind the lateral mass of the atlas. At the end of this groove, the VA runs in an oblique superior and anteromedial direction toward the FM dura (17).

Fourth Segment

After piercing the FM dura, the VA proceeds in the same superior and anteromedial direction in the subarachnoid space to reach the lateral side of the medulla oblongata (MO). It then passes around the MO and joins the contralateral VA in front of the MO at approximately the level of the pontomedullary junction, to form the basilar artery.

Relationships

In the third segment, the VA is surrounded by a venous plexus, and it is noteworthy that both the VA and its venous plexus are enclosed in a continuous periosteal sheath. This periosteal sheath is continuous with the periosteum of the transverse foramina of C1 and C2, with the deep aponeurosis of the muscles between these transverse foramina, with the posterior atlantooccipital membrane that arches over the VA groove of the atlas, and with the FM dura mater. There, the VA and its periosteal sheath invaginate the FM dura before perforating it, making a double sleeve of periosteum and dura around the VA of 3 to 5 mm. Intracranially, the VA wall is directly in contact with the cerebrospinal fluid. There are no more satellite veins or periosteal sheath.

Between C1 and C2, the VA is crossed by the ventral ramus of the second cervical spinal nerve root. Above C1, the first cervical spinal nerve root, which pierces the dura with the VA or separately, runs along the posteroinferior aspect of the VA and merges under it posteriorly in the middle of the groove. Intracranially, the VA proceeds under the arch made by the first two digits of the dentate ligaments, and successively courses ventral to the rootlets of cranial nerves XII, X, and IX. The spinal part of cranial nerve XI ascends in the spinal canal posterior to the dentate ligaments, crosses the posterior aspect of the VA, and finally joins its cranial part below the cranial nerve IX and X rootlets.

Branches

Along the suboccipital VA segment, there are usually no important branches. The anterior meningeal artery arises at the C2-3 level (18). Radiculomuscular branches originate between C1 and C2, at the outlet of the transverse foramen of the atlas and at both ends of the VA groove. The intracranial VA segment gives rise to the anterior spinal artery and to the posteroinferior cerebellar artery (PICA), which, respectively, arise from its first few millimeters and at the level of the lateral aspect of the MO (15 mm in average from the dura perforation). Branches of various size and number supplying the MO may arise either directly from the VA or from the PICA (Fig. 1).

Variations and Anomalies

Size

Vertebral artery diameter varies greatly from large to very small (2–8 mm). A small VA is termed hypoplastic when it joins the opposite VA, and atretic if not (see Fig. 1). In general, a small VA is inversely related to a large contralateral one; the former is called the minor VA and the latter the dominant VA. VA of equal size on both sides are observed in 40%. Bilateral small VA are uncommon and suggest the presence of a persistent congenital anastomosis between the basilar trunk or the VA and the internal carotid artery (19). In descending order of frequency, those connections are the trigeminal, otic, hypoglossal, and proatlantal arteries. The two caudal ones are connected with the VA; the hypoglossal artery is intracranial and the proatlantal is extracranial. The proatlantal artery may join the VA with either the external or the internal carotid artery (19–22).

Course

Occasionally, the VA may enter the dura mater at the C1-2 level. In fact, there is a VA duplication with an atretic branch that follows the normal extracranial course, and a normal-sized branch that takes the abnormal intradural course (23–26).

The VA course is also modified by craniocervical junction malformations such as malposition, segmentation, fusion, or agenesis of different bone elements (27–30).

Above the posterior arch of the atlas, calcification or ossi-

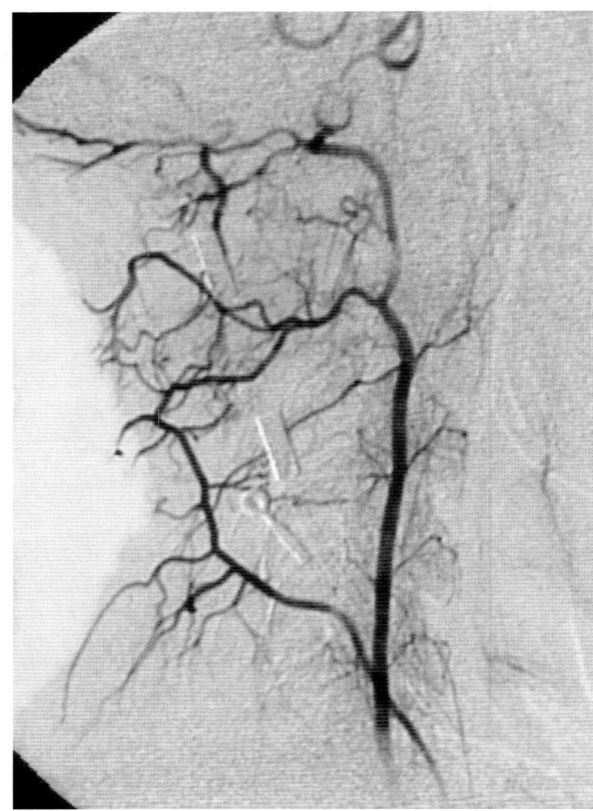

FIG. 1. Atretic vertebral artery ending at the occipital artery, with very small connection with the posteroinferior cerebellar artery. Note all the vascular branches connecting with branches of the external carotid artery and ascending cervical artery.

fication of the posterior atlantooccipital membrane may turn the VA groove into a bony tunnel (31), raising some difficulties for VA exposure.

Branches

In addition to persistent congenital anastomosis between the VA and the carotid artery, variations in the origin of the PICA and the anterior spinal artery may be observed. The site of origin of the PICA is extracranial in about 20%, arising mostly from the VA above the posterior arch of the atlas or between C1 and C2 (32–34), and rarely from the external carotid artery. Intracranially, the PICA may arise anywhere along the VA or from the basilar trunk (by a common trunk with the anteroinferior cerebellar artery). The origin of the anterior spinal artery may be located on either side of the dura; when the origin is extradural, it pierces the dura with or without the VA.

Dynamic Changes

The suboccipital VA segment has a particular course, showing a double bayonet shape and a horizontal "U" shape on lateral and anteroposterior angiographic views, respectively. This course allows VA flow to be preserved during head movements. Moreover, the VA wall is untethered to the periosteal sleeve, whereas the periosteal sheath is fixed at each transverse foramen. At the FM level, the VA wall is adherent to the periosteal sheath in continuity with the dura mater. Therefore, this is the only fixed point of the VA during head movements. The two parts (above C1 and between C1 and C2) of the suboccipital VA segment are stretched during extension and rotation toward the opposite side but are compressed during flexion and ipsilateral rotation.

Therefore, the course of the VA and its anatomic relationships with the periosteal sheath have many consequences for VA surgery.

Initially, these factors influence the surgical positioning of the patient. In the anterolateral approach (ALA), the patient is supine with the head extended and rotated to the opposite side. In this position, because only the atlas follows head rotation, while the axis does not, the two VA parts (above C1 and between C1 and C2) are stretched and almost parallel with the posterior arch of the atlas between them (Fig. 2).

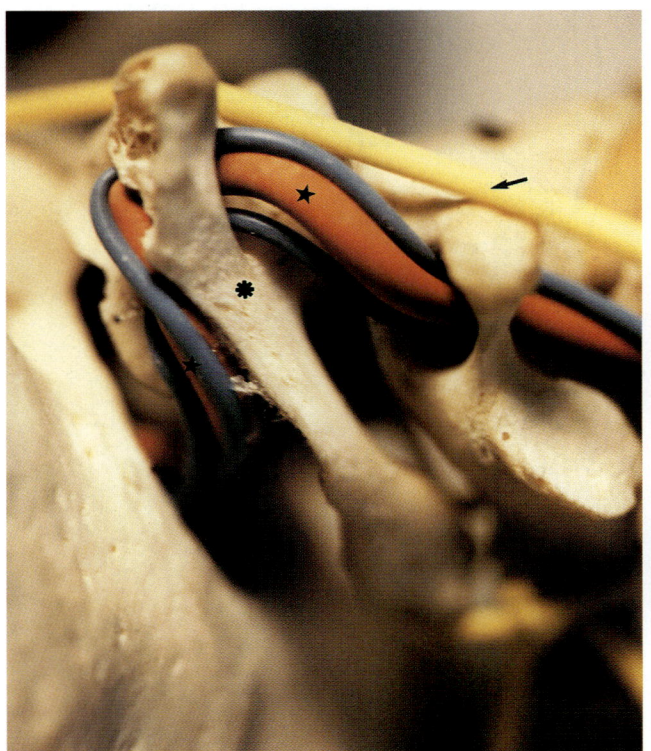

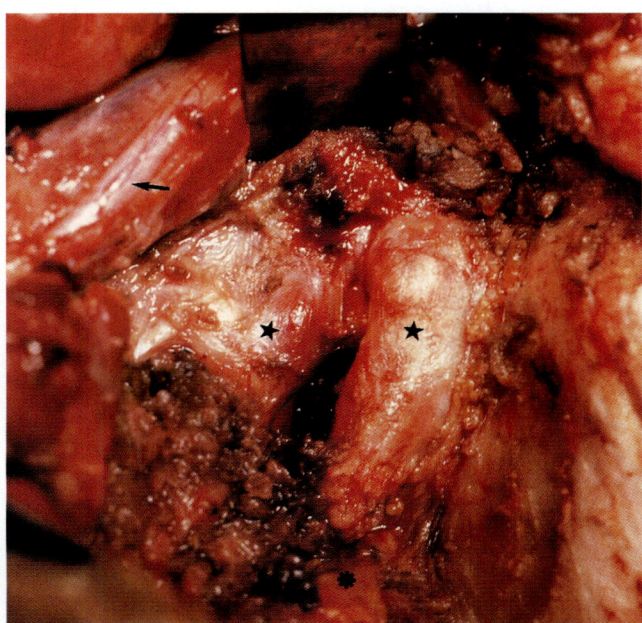

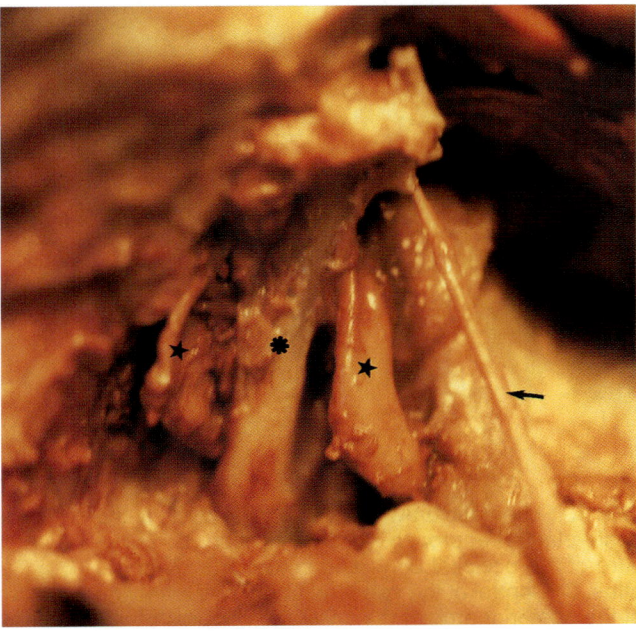

FIG. 2. Dynamic changes of the vertebral artery (VA) during contralateral rotation of the head. **A:** Dry bone with the VA (*red bundle*), the venous plexus (*blue bundle*), and the accessory nerve (*yellow bundle*). **B:** Cadaver view. **C:** Surgical view. *Asterisk*, posterior arch of atlas; *star*, VA; *arrow*, accessory nerve.

There are several anatomic and radiologic reports in the literature on changes in VA diameter during head movements. Some of them, especially the anatomic ones, demonstrate VA occlusion during extension and contralateral rotation of the head (35–38). In living patients, it occurs rarely unless there is a pathologic condition that worsens the VA stretch. These pathologic conditions include osteophytes, fibrous bands, nerve compression, bony malformations, or tumors. In fact, this is seldom observed on the third VA segment. In the author's experience, there have been only two cases of intermittent VA compression during head movement due to craniocervical junction malformation.

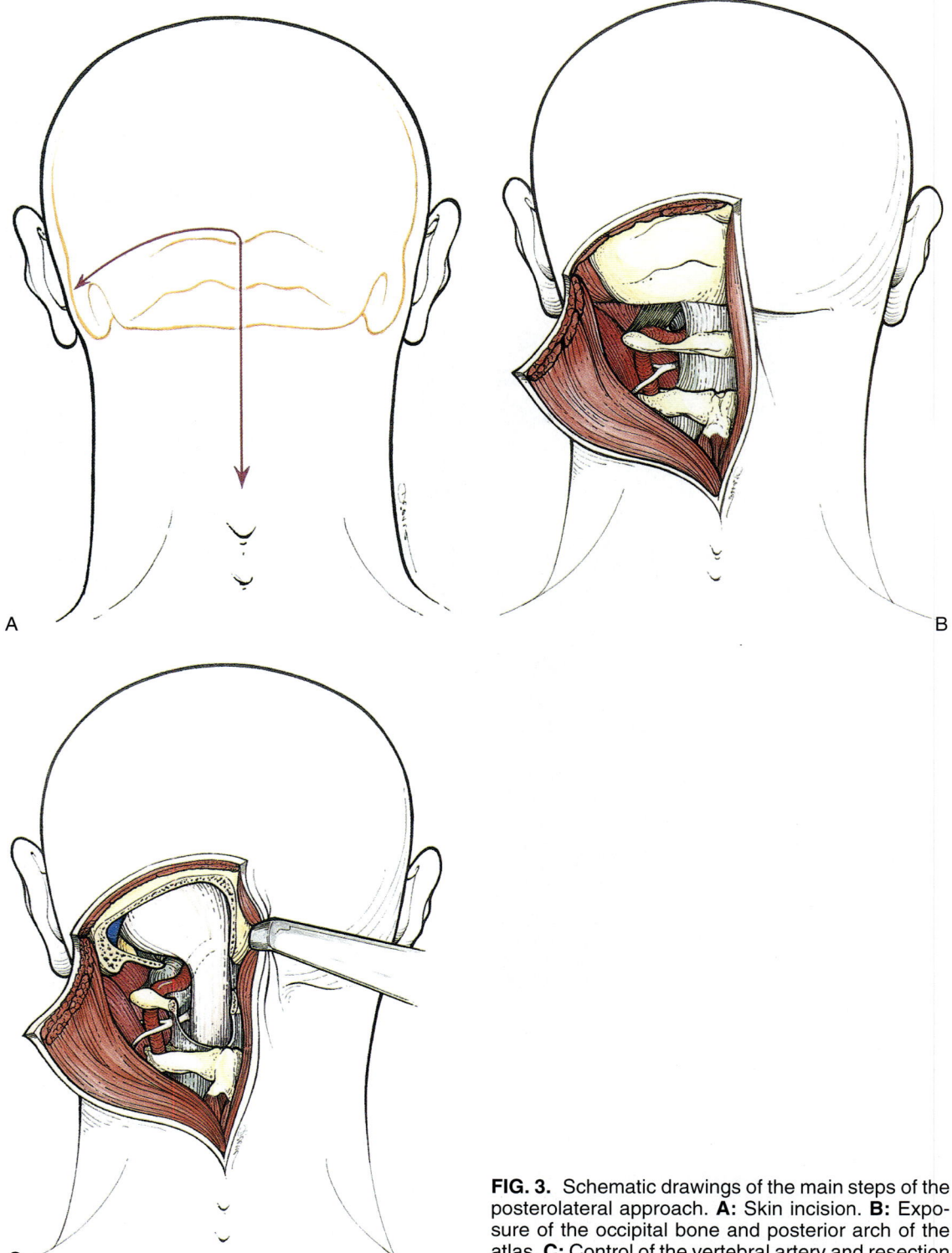

FIG. 3. Schematic drawings of the main steps of the posterolateral approach. **A:** Skin incision. **B:** Exposure of the occipital bone and posterior arch of the atlas. **C:** Control of the vertebral artery and resection of the posterior arch of the atlas and occipital bone.

The VA's course also allows the surgeon to pull a few millimeters of the artery out of the transverse foramen after opening the periosteal sheath. This provides more VA length between the two transverse foramina, making it easier to apply clips when performing an anastomosis.

Finally, the adherence between the dura, periosteal sheath, and the VA wall at the FM level makes dissection of the VA very difficult. It is in general much safer to cut dural and periosteal sheaths 2 or 3 mm around the VA.

EXPOSURE

The lateral location of the VA along its entire course makes its surgical exposure easier using the lateral approaches. The medial approaches, either anterior (the transoral approach) or posterior (the standard posterior approach), are too limited laterally to reach the VA.

The lateral approaches include two main routes, posterolateral and anterolateral, according to the VA side approached.

The Posterolateral Approach

The patient is placed in a sitting, prone, or lateral position (3,9,39) (Fig. 3). The incision begins on the midline, ascends vertically up to the occipital protuberance, bends laterally along the occipital crest, and descends toward the mastoid process. The laminae of C2, the posterior arch of the atlas, and the occipital bone are exposed initially. The exposure is then extended subperiosteally up to the transverse processes of C2 and C1. The C1-2 VA segment is identified following the C2 spinal nerve root, which divides in ventral and dorsal rami running on either side of the VA. These rami of the C2 spinal nerve root are very good landmarks because they are in direct contact with the periosteal sheath. The VA segment above C1 is exposed in its groove lying on the posterior arch of the atlas. The medial end of this groove is clearly identified by the marked increase in height of the posterior arch of the atlas. The safest way to proceed is to split the periosteum on the inferior aspect of the posterior arch from the midline toward the transverse process; then, the exposure is extended

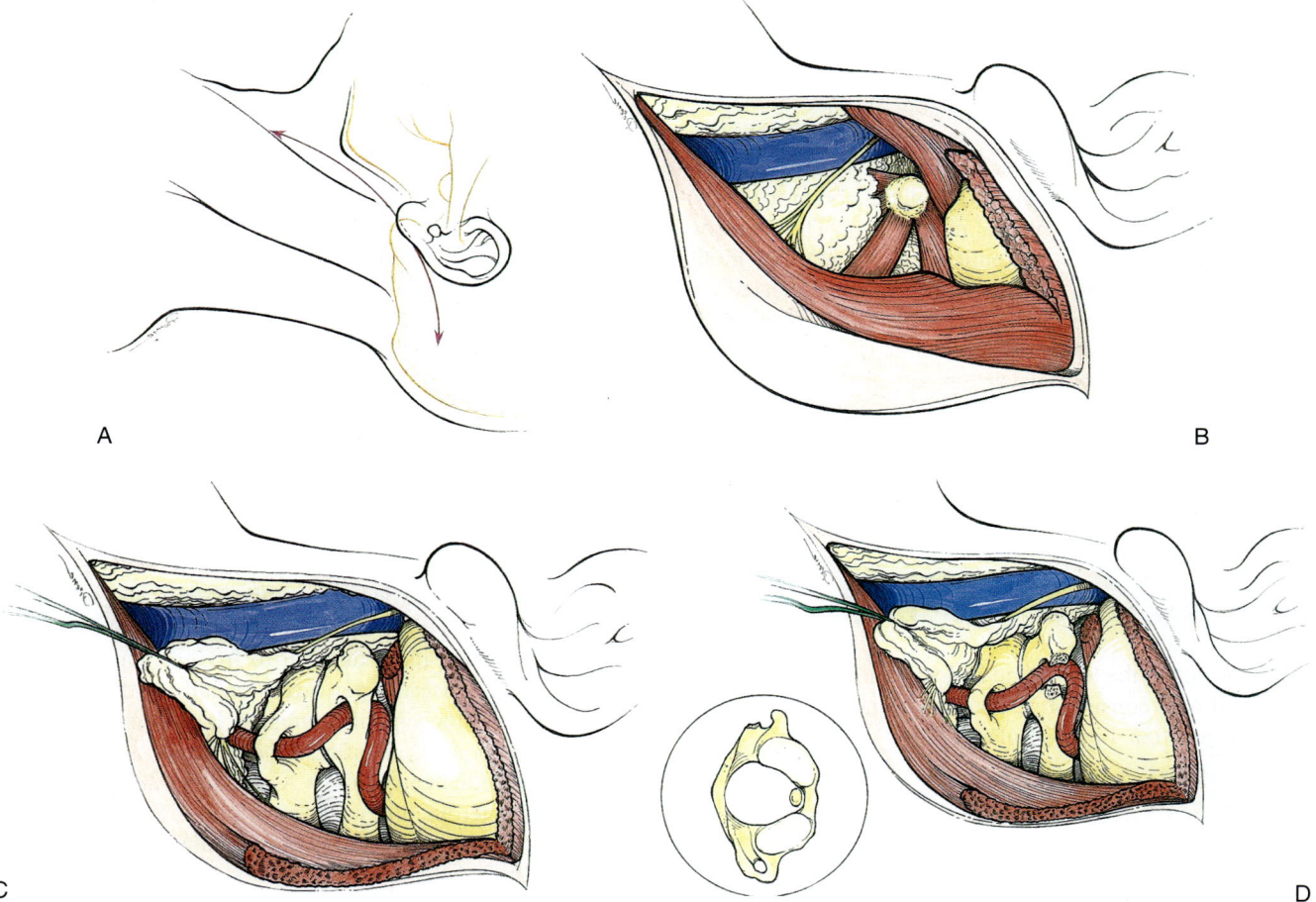

FIG. 4. Schematic drawings of the main steps of the anterolateral approach. **A:** Skin incision. **B:** Opening of the plane between the sternocleidomastoid muscle and the internal jugular vein with identification and mobilization of the accessory nerve. **C:** Resection of the muscles inserted on the transverse process of the atlas, exposing the vertebral artery (VA) between C1 and C2, and above C1. **D:** Opening of the transverse process of the atlas. (*Continued.*)

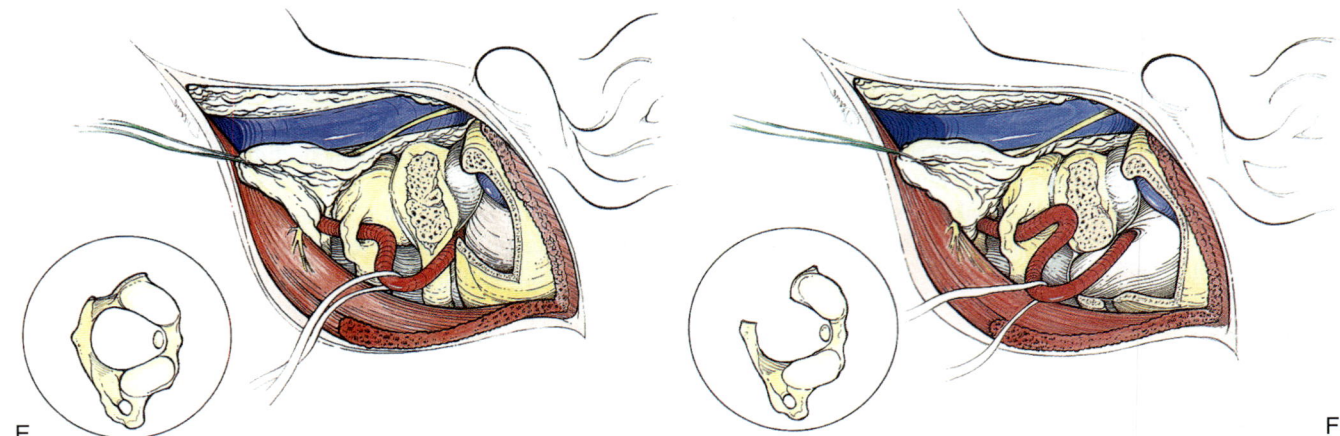

FIG. 4. *Continued.* **E:** Complete resection of the transverse process of the atlas with VA transposition. **F:** Resection of the posterior arch of the atlas and occipital bone up to the sigmoid sinus.

toward the superior aspect of the posterior arch of atlas. If necessary, the C1 transverse foramen is opened.

Anterolateral Approach

The patient is placed in a supine position with the head slightly extended and rotated to the opposite side (3,9,13) (Fig. 4). The skin incision is made along the anterior edge of the upper part of the sternocleidomastoid muscle (SCM), extended over the mastoid process, and then taken approximately along the occipital crest. The dissection proceeds between the SCM and the internal jugular vein. The accessory nerve (cranial nerve XI) is identified at its junction with the SCM and dissected up to the skull base. Cranial nerve XI is usually retracted inferiorly and medially by the fatty sheath covering the depth of the field, which is freed and wrapped around the nerve. The transverse process of the atlas is then clearly visible and the oblique muscles inserted on it are cut, exposing the two VA segments. The C1-2 VA segment is crossed by the ventral ramus of the C2 spinal nerve root. The C1 spinal nerve root merges under the VA in the groove of the atlas.

VERTEBRAL ARTERY MANAGEMENT

According to the lesion and its location, VA management differs. It may consist of VA control alone, or mobilization and transposition, or revascularization.

Control

At the least, all VA management requires VA control, and in many cases, VA control alone is enough.

The key points in VA control are, first, to stay outside the periosteal sheath as long as possible and, second, to obtain adequate VA control proximal and distal to the lesion. The VA segments exposed must be long enough to be able to clip the artery if necessary. In general, it is necessary to control the VA up to the next proximal and distal transverse processes or up to the FM dura.

C1-2 Segment

The landmark for the C1-C2 segment is the ventral ramus of the C2 spinal nerve root, which crosses the C1-2 segment just before the VA periosteal sheath. The C2 spinal nerve root often needs to be divided. Because the distal branches have already been cut subcutaneously during the skin incision, this adds no sensory deficit. The numerous anastomoses and the overlapping cutaneous territories of the superficial cervical plexus explain why the long-term results of C2 spinal nerve root division are limited to hypesthesia of the earlobe and a small area of the jaw angle. To obtain complete control of this segment, dissection must be done all around the VA with control of the radiculomuscular branch, which usually arises from the posteromedial aspect.

Segment Above C1

The groove of the atlas must be subperiosteally exposed to preserve the VA periosteal sheath. Freeing the inferior aspect of the VA periosteal sheath from the groove usually is easy. It is much more difficult to free the superior aspect, however, because the periosteal sheath is adherent to the posterior atlantooccipital membrane. It is even more difficult if that membrane is calcified or ossified.

At the medial end of the VA groove of the atlas, the VA proceeds anteromedially and superiorly toward the FM dura mater. There are often radiculomuscular branches at both ends of the VA groove (9,11–14,40–42) (Fig. 5).

The C1 spinal nerve root, which is always very small, is often cut inadvertently without serious consequences.

Some difficulties may arise when there is an extracranial origin of the PICA or the anterior spinal artery. These must be identified and dissected along their course up to the dura.

Intracranial Segment

Intracranially, the difficulties arise from the lower cranial nerves crossing the posterior aspect of the VA. The VA has thus to be controlled as it passes between the network of cranial nerve rootlets. To enlarge the operative field and obtain a wider angle that allows control of the distal VA, the bone opening must be widened laterally. The occipital bone is resected up to the sigmoid sinus, therefore including a partial mastoidectomy. The lateral wall of the FM above the VA (i.e., the condyle and jugular tubercle) also has to be partially drilled. This drilling is extended up to the vicinity of the condylar and jugular foramina. It is often useful to check the intradural space while drilling extradurally to control the location of the condylar and jugular foramina and avoid any nerve injury. At its maximum, drilling can be done completely around cranial nerve XII or nerves IX, X, and XI, which permits extradural access to the lower part of the clivus.

Mobilization or Transposition

The VA may be displaced to reach different structures. Obviously, mobilization and transposition require previous complete control of the VA and cutting of all collateral branches (9,11–14,40–42) (see Fig. 5; Fig. 6).

Mobilization or transposition is performed to improve access to the FM or jugular foramen or to facilitate tumor resection close to the VA.

Mobilization concerns the VA segment above C1 and may be either in a superior or inferior direction. The VA and its periosteal sheath must be completely freed from the C1 transverse foramen to the FM dura.

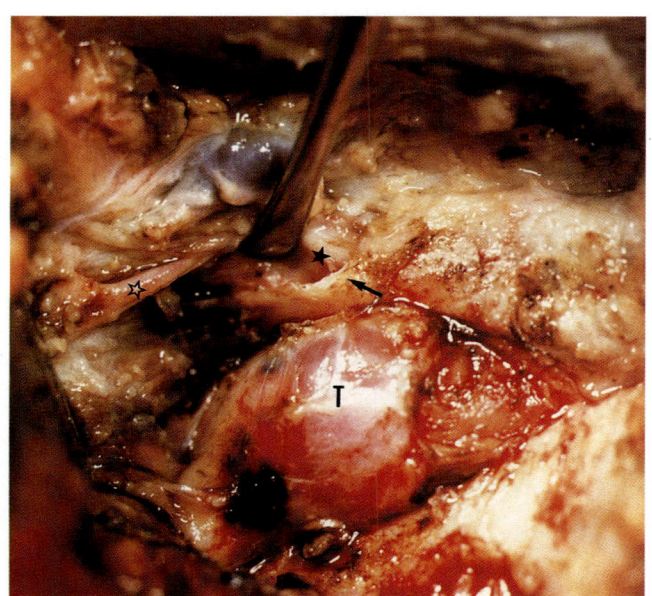

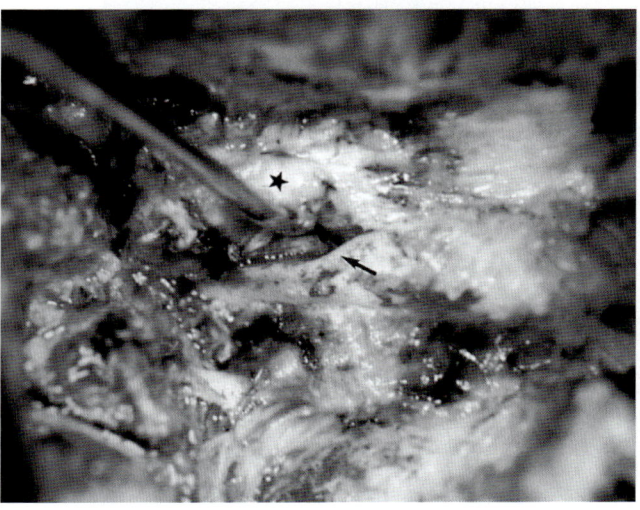

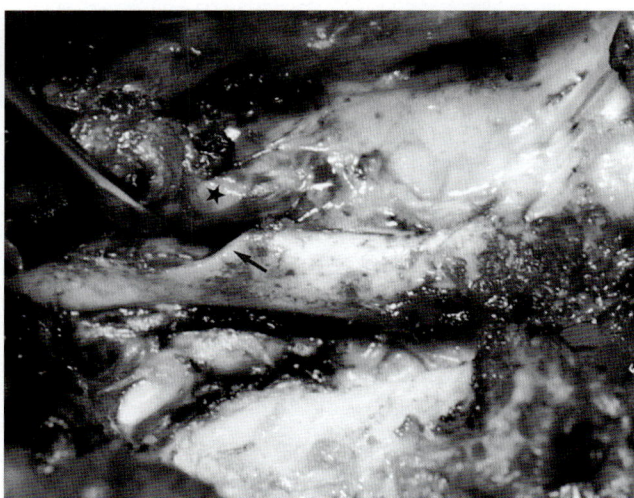

FIG. 5. Three examples of control and mobilization of the vertebral artery (VA) above C1 through PLA. **A:** Extradural extension of a neurinoma (*T*) and the C1 nerve root (*open star*). **A–C:** Notice the change in the height of the posterior arch of the atlas at the medial end of the VA groove (*arrow*). *Black star*, VA.

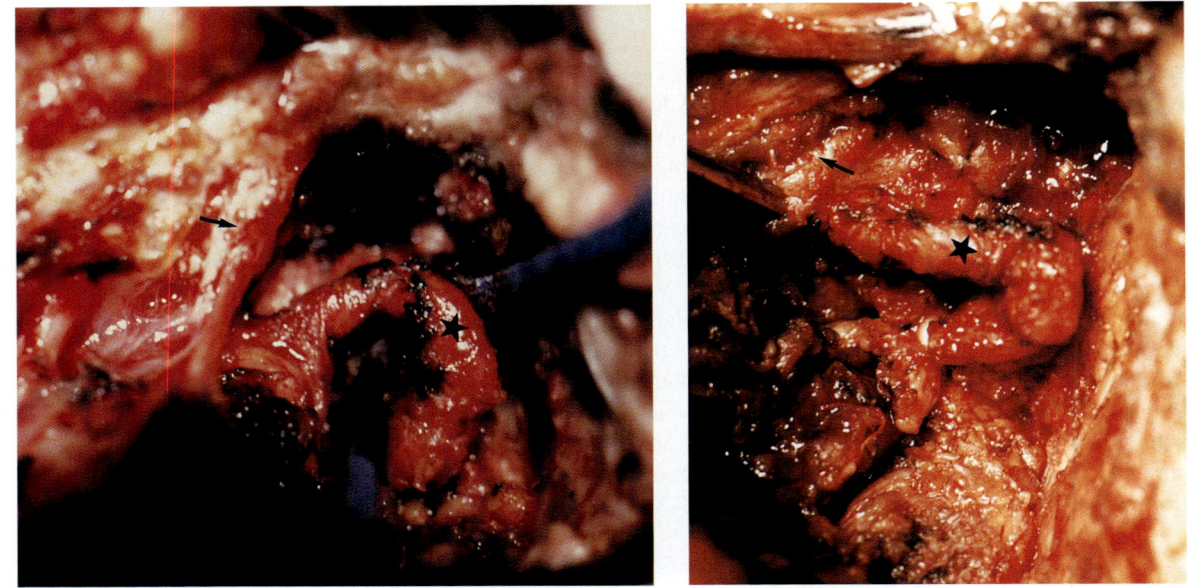

FIG. 6. Two examples of transposition of the vertebral artery (VA) after resection of the transverse process of the atlas. **A:** Chordoma. **B:** Aneurysmal cyst. *Star*, VA; *arrow*, accessory nerve.

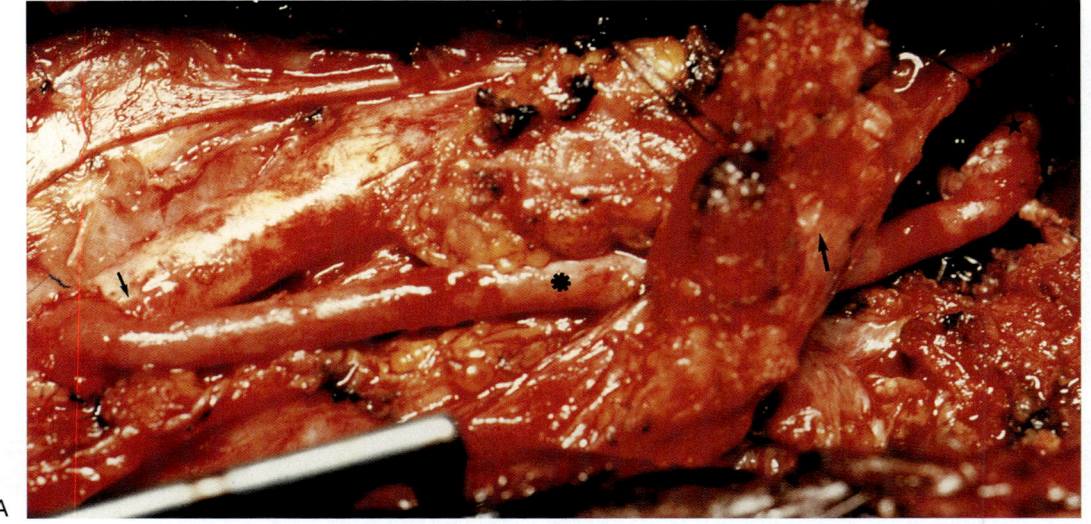

FIG. 7. Revascularization. **A:** Saphenous vein graft (*asterisk*) bypassing the common carotid artery (*small arrow*) and the vertebral artery (VA) between C1 and C2 (*star*). Notice the accessory nerve wrapped in the fatty sheath (*arrow*).

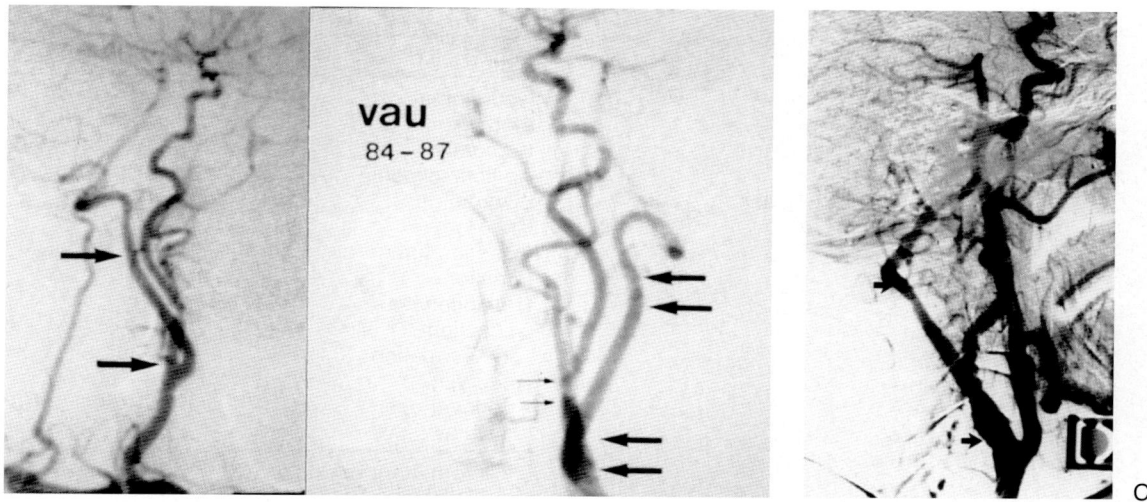

FIG. 7. *Continued.* **B:** Angiographic control of a bypass between the common carotid artery and the VA between C1 and C2. **C:** Angiographic control of a bypass between the carotid bifurcation and the VA above C1.

Transposition applies to the whole suboccipital segment from C2 to the FM dural penetration; consequently, it requires the opening of the C1 transverse foramen. After controlling the two parts of the suboccipital segment on each side of the C1 transverse foramen, the periosteal sheath is followed inside the foramen, splitting the periosteum from the bone. Then, the transverse foramen is unroofed, biting its external wall progressively using the Kerrison rongeur. To achieve the transposition, the medial wall must also be resected to provide space in the concavity of the VA loop and allow the VA to be pulled without damaging the periosteal sheath.

Revascularization

Occlusion of a dominant VA may lead to vertebrobasilar insufficiency (3,6–10,14) (Fig. 7). To restore adequate flow and pressure, revascularization of the VA is necessary. This is usually achieved by common carotid-to-distal VA venous bypass grafting. The usual site of graft implantation is the C1-2 VA segment, and occasionally the VA segment above C1 or even the intracranial VA segment. In general, an end-to-side anastomosis between the saphenous vein graft and the distal VA is used; an end-to-end anastomosis is reserved for situations in which a proximal temporary clip cannot be placed. Complete exposure and control of the VA is essential to perform such an anastomosis. This is obtained by opening the VA periosteal sheath and coagulating the perivertebral venous plexus.

PATHOLOGY

Vertebral artery management is required in two different circumstances: when the VA is directly involved by the pathologic process, and when the VA precludes access to the pathologic process. In addition, VA exposure helps to control the vascular supply to some vascular lesions (3,14,41,43,44), or allows a VA revascularization procedure to be performed.

Vertebral Artery Involvement

Many pathologic processes involve the VA, including tumors, infection, bone malformations, and traumatic lesions.

Tumors

Many tumoral types grow close to the VA (Fig. 8); they sometimes even encase the VA with or without invading its periosteal sheath. It is never possible to determine radiologically whether the periosteal sheath is invaded. Therefore, the VA must always be controlled proximal and distal to the tumor (or at least proximal, if distal control appears difficult). Then, the dissection proceeds along the VA, trying to stay outside the periosteal sheath as long as possible. Usually, a good plane can be developed between the tumor and the periosteal sheath, avoiding any troublesome bleeding from the perivertebral venous plexus. Venous bleeding caused by small tears of the sheath can be stopped by direct bipolar coagulation of the sheath, applying the bipolar forceps on each side of the laceration. In most benign tumors and in many malignant ones, preservation of the periosteal sheath is possible even if the VA segment involved supplies the tumor. The feeding branches can be coagulated and divided outside the periosteal sheath. In the rare instances in which the periosteal sheath is invaded by the tumor, proximal control of the VA allows coagulation or packing of the perivertebral venous plexus and dissection of the tumor from

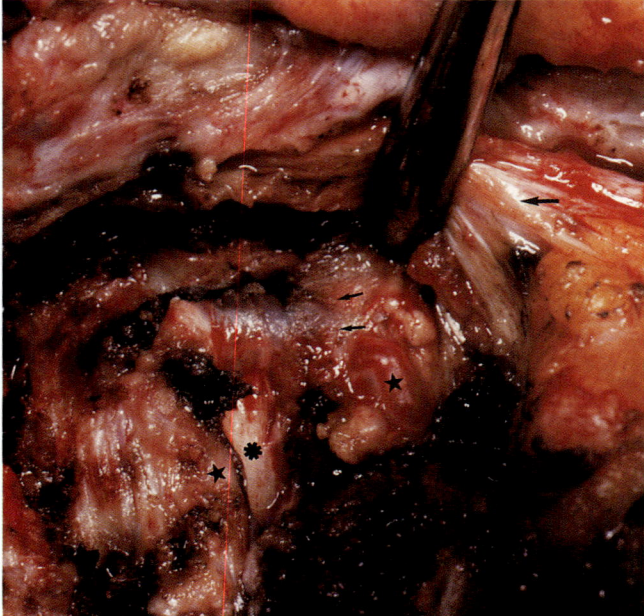

FIG. 8. Histiocytosis with invasion of the periosteal sheath of the vertebral artery (*star*). *Asterisk* indicates posterior arch of the atlas; *small arrows* indicate the tumor inside the periosteal sheath; *arrow* indicates the accessory nerve.

TABLE 1. *Lesions involving the vertebral artery*

Lesion	Total	Stenosis	Occlusion
Neurinoma	18	3	—
Meningioma	5	2	—
Sarcoma	5	3	3 perioperative
Angiomyolipoma	1	—	—
Lymphoma	1	—	1
Chordoma	12	—	—
Osseous tumor	13	3	1
Infection	2	—	1
Craniocervical junction malformation	2	—	2[a]
Aneurysm	8[b]	—	—
Arteriovenous fistula	2	—	—

[a] Intermittent occlusion.
[b] Six intracranial and two extracranial.

the wall of the artery. However, in some sarcomas, and particularly in recurrent ones, no plane can be found between the tumor and the wall of the VA, which makes it necessary to sacrifice the VA. Resection of the VA may also be necessary in some malignant tumors to achieve a radical removal. This situation must be anticipated, and the patient's tolerance of VA occlusion must be assessed by preoperative balloon occlusion testing. The occluding balloon must be applied precisely at the designated level of surgical ligation. A balloon placed too far from the tumor may spare some collateral branches that could feed the VA distally. Ideally, the occlusion test is performed proximal and distal to the tumor. Most of the time, the VA occlusion test is perfectly tolerated and no revascularization is necessary. In the author's series of 156 tumors involving the cervical VA, the VA was sacrificed in 5 cases without complications, and a revascularization was performed only once, in the case of an osteoblastoma in a 6-year-old boy that involved both VA and that had already been operated on in another center.

Table 1 gives the distribution of tumors involving the VA, the number of patients who had surgical VA occlusion, and the number of patients with preoperative VA stenosis or occlusion.

The most common tumor involving the VA is neurinoma of the C1 or C2 spinal nerve root (42). Neurinomas often have an extradural component and are distinguished by multiplicity and bilaterality owing to a frequent association with neurofibromatosis (see Fig. 5A; Fig. 9). Meningiomas of the craniocervical junction usually are intradural, but occasionally are either entirely extradural or both intradural and extradural (39,40,41,43) (Fig. 10). In a series of 42 meningiomas of the FM region, the author observed 1 extradural and 4 intradural–extradural cases. Similarly, in a French cooperative study, the author's team collected 106 meningiomas that included 4 extradural and 11 intradural–extradural occurrences (40). Meningiomas with an extradural component often behave very aggressively and may invade the bone and cervical soft tissues, including the VA. Malignant tumors are frequently characterized by invasiveness, but meningioma is the only benign tumor that may have this invasive feature; this is explained by the continuity between the dura and periosteum. Among nonosseous tumors, the author observed a few cases of sarcomas (rhabdomyosarcomas and undifferentiated sarcomas) and one case of angiomyolipoma (Fig. 11).

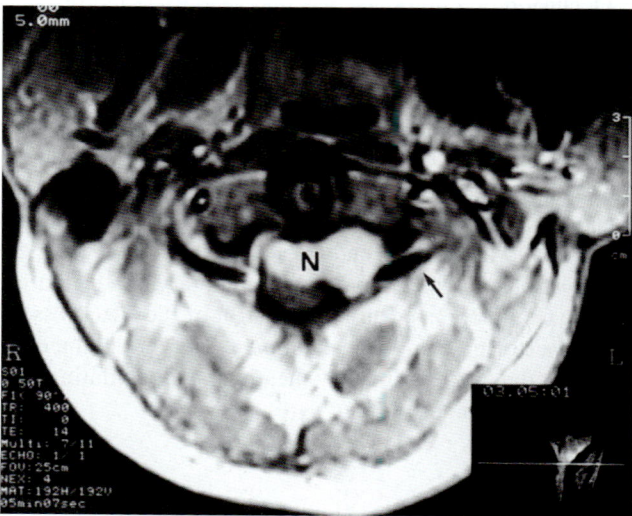

FIG. 9. Intradural–extradural neurinoma (*N*) in contact with the vertebral artery (*arrow*).

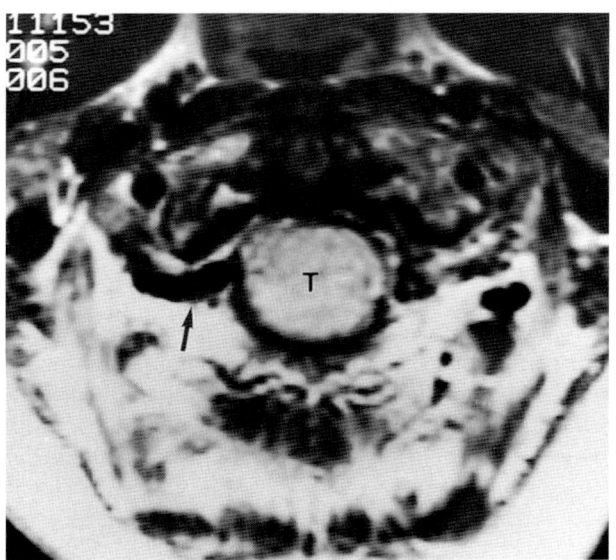
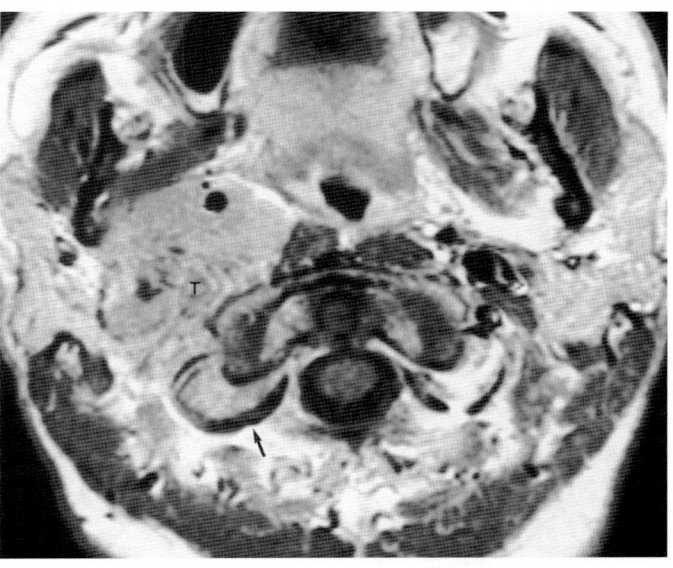

FIG. 10. Two examples of meningioma involving the vertebral artery (VA). **A:** Intradural foramen magnum meningioma. **B:** Extradural meningioma with cervical extension. *T*, tumor; *arrow*, VA.

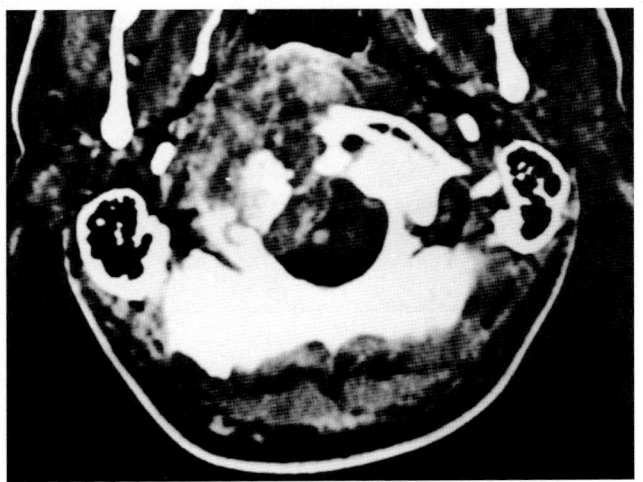

FIG. 11. Nonosseous tumors involving the vertebral artery. **A:** Sarcoma. **B:** Neurinoma. **C:** Angiomyolipoma.

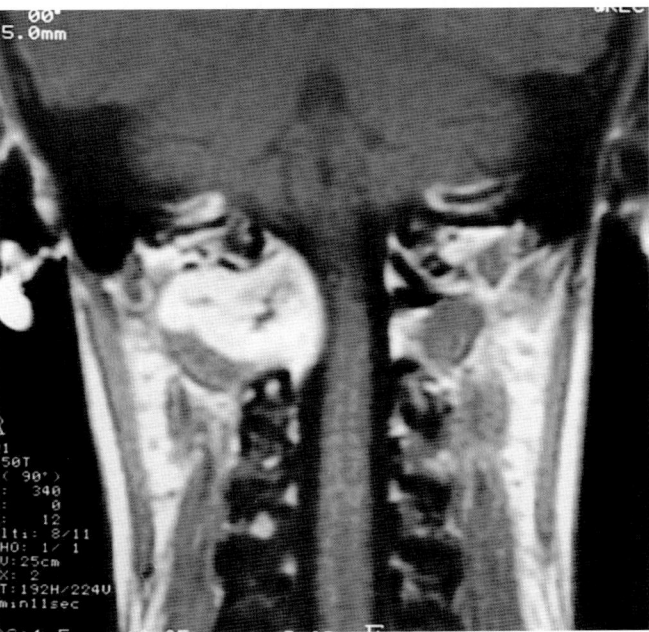
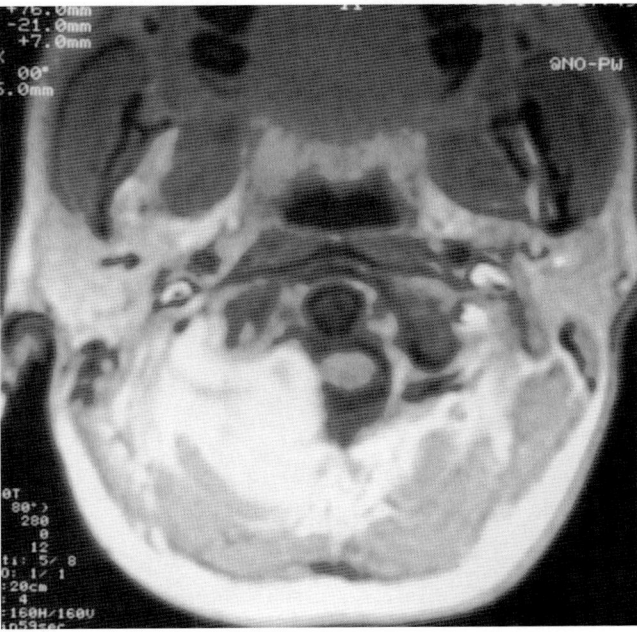

There are many types of osseous tumors, but metastasis from carcinoma is the most common (Fig. 12). Chordomas usually develop on the midline, but in the author's experience, they can also present with lateral (and sometimes bilateral) extension with VA encasement; this was observed in 12 cases (Fig. 13).

Vertebral artery stenosis or occlusion produced by tumoral compression is rare, and induced ischemic manifestations are exceptional (14,26). In the author's series, occlusion was noticed in 2 cases (one osteochondroma and one Hodgkin's disease) and stenosis was observed in 11 cases. They were never associated with any ischemic symptoms. The slow growth of tumors always permits the development of collateral flow to compensate for VA occlusion. The only ischemic event seen was an embolism in the posterior cerebral artery after VA occlusion by a low-grade chondrosarcoma of the lower part of the neck.

Nontumoral Processes

Nontumoral processes at the C2-1 and FM levels can induce permanent or intermittent VA compression. Intermittent VA compression may be symptomatic during head and neck movements, usually rotation. To consider a process compressing the VA as the cause of clinical symptoms, the

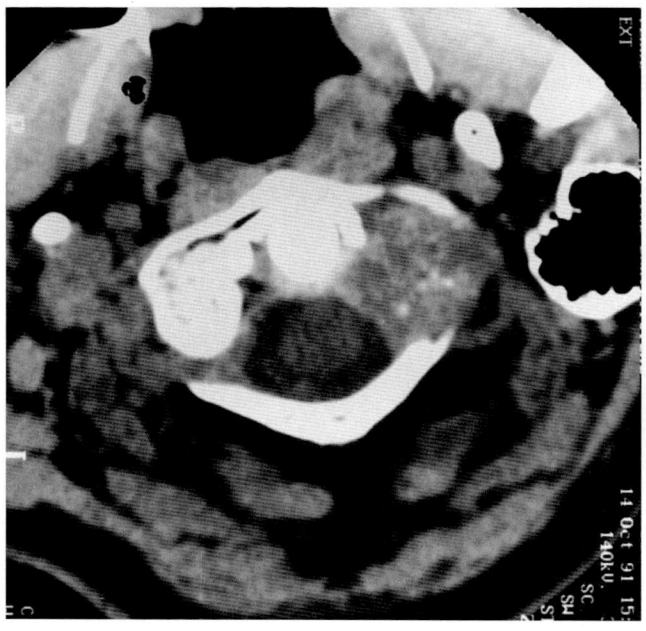

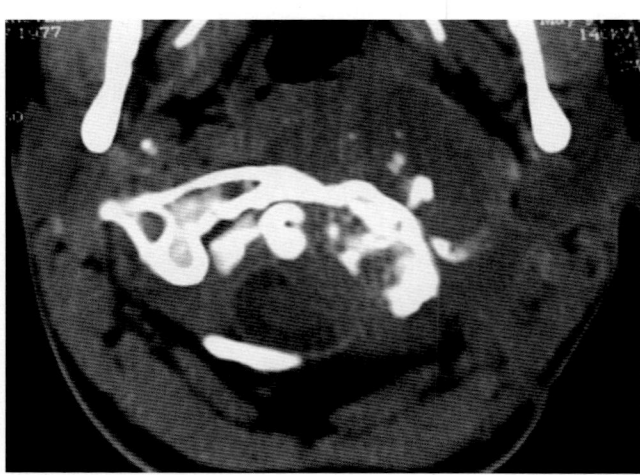

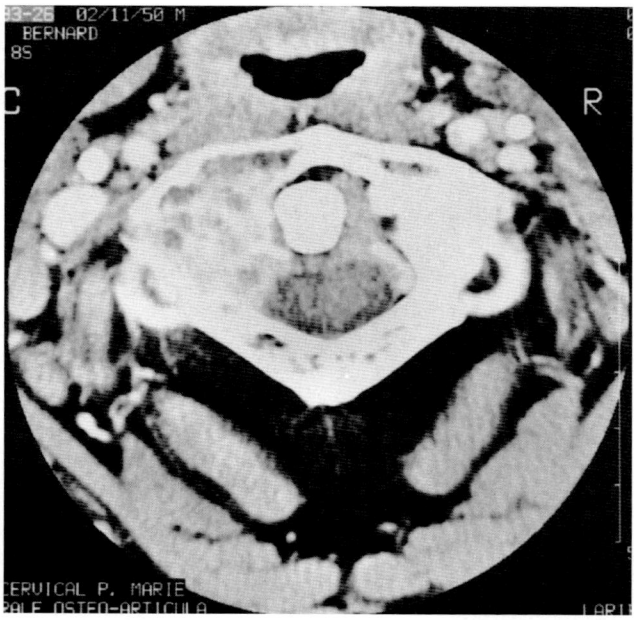

FIG. 12. Osseous tumors involving the vertebral artery. **A:** Metastasis. **B:** Histiocytosis (see Fig. 8). **C:** Aneurysmal cyst (see Fig. 6B).

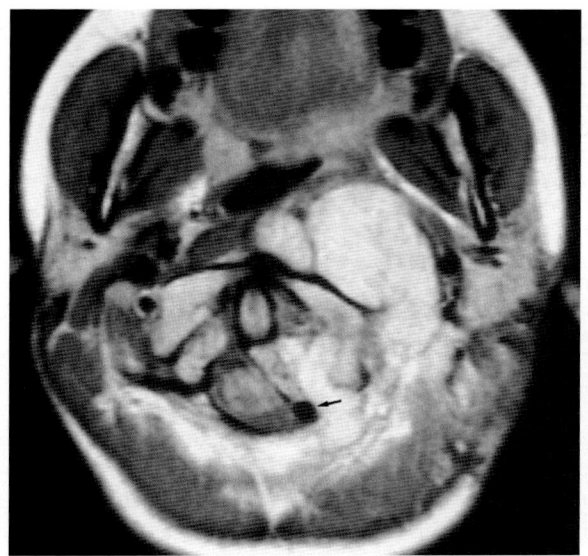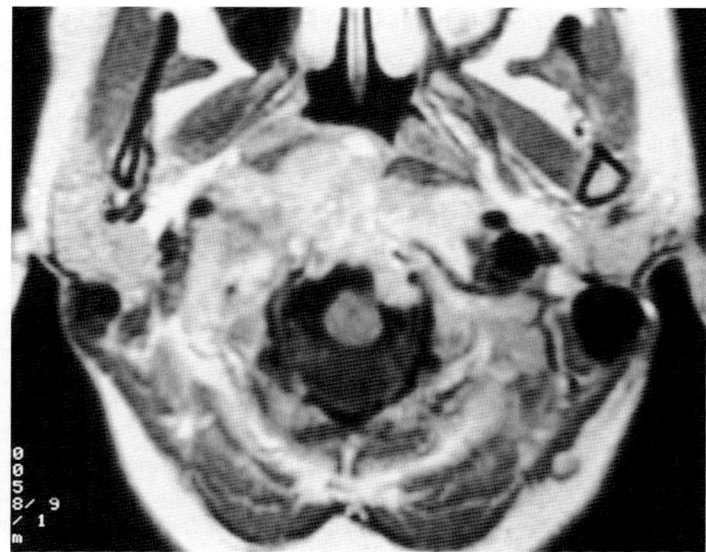

FIG. 13. Unilateral (A) and bilateral (B) chordomas involving the vertebral artery (arrow).

same movement carried out during angiography must produce a severe VA compression associated with the usual clinical symptoms. The author observed two such cases, including a bilateral one, that were both related to a craniocervical junction malformation: a C1-2 fusion in one case and a supplementary condyle in the other.

In the case of the C1-2 fusion, the patient could not rotate her head to either side without experiencing vertigo and often fainting. On angiography, there was a complete blockage of contrast in both VA at the C1 level during rotation toward the opposite side. Surgery using the bilateral posterolateral approach (PLA) revealed a tortuous course of both VA along C1-2. The transverse foramina of C1 and C2 were opened on both sides, and all the fibrous bands crossing the VA were resected from C2 to the FM. The laminae of C2 were completely fused with the posterior arch of C1, making it impossible for the atlas to rotate with the head. After surgical decompression, the patient could move her head in every direction without clinical symptoms, and angiography showed an almost normal VA diameter along its entire course and on both sides in any head position.

The second case was a 12-year-old girl with a supplementary condyle. She presented with occasional posterior headaches and stiffness, followed one day by a sudden and transitory coma after physical exercise. The author did not dare perform angiography in different head positions because three-dimensional computed tomography obviously demonstrated the dominant VA traveling around the supplementary condyle. Surgery using unilateral PLA showed a stretched VA around the abnormal bony piece, which was extensively drilled. Because there was some doubt about the stability of the craniocervical junction, a fusion was done using iliac bone grafts placed between the occipital bone and the posterior arches of C1 and C2.

In the author's personal series, there was also a case of tuberculosis involving C1 and C2 inducing a VA occlusion on one side and a severe stenosis on the other (3). This patient presented with repeated transient ischemic deficits in the vertebrobasilar system that disappeared totally after medical therapy. Both VA repermeabilized completely without any surgical treatment.

Vertebral artery compression may also be due to neural elements, as in the case reported by Carney at the C1-2 level (6). In the author's material, there is one asymptomatic case probably due to the second cervical spinal nerve root (3).

The author's team also has dealt with three cases of acute VA injury. Two cases occurred during posterior fossa opening with inadvertent VA laceration. The exposure was enlarged laterally to control and temporarily clip the VA proximal and distal to the tear. Then, in one case, the repair was done with simple stitches, and in the other case with a small venous patch. The third case was an extradural hematoma of the posterior fossa with a fracture of the occipital bone. A piece of bone was displaced inferiorly, compressing the VA. The VA had to be exposed in its groove above C1 before the bony compression could safely be released. The periosteal sheath was opened but the arterial wall itself was intact. In all three cases, the follow-up was uneventful.

To release VA compression, the PLA or ALA can be used according to the extent of the lesion (39,40). The PLA is preferred when the lesion has an intradural extension and when the extradural component is rather limited. On the contrary, the ALA is the better choice if the extraspinal–extracranial part is large, and especially if it extends toward the retropharyngeal space. A lesion of limited size in the bone or the extradural space near the VA can be exposed by any of the approaches. When the lesion is bilateral, the PLA can be done on both sides by the same incision, whereas two ALA have to be done separately or require separate incisions.

Vertebral Artery Obstructing Surgical Access

Control of the VA helps in getting access to different neighboring regions, including the FM, upper cervical, and jugular foramen regions (Tables 2, 3).

Foramen Magnum Region

The VA is the key point in the approach to tumors of the FM region (Fig. 14). Control of the VA gives access to the FM lateral wall, including the jugular tubercle, condyle, lateral mass of the atlas, and the C1-2 joint. Mobilization of the VA upward or downward allows the surgeon to drill the bony structures located below or above, respectively. Consequently, it is very important before surgery to define the location of the tumor with regard to the VA. Using the PLA, drilling allows access to the subarachnoid spaces lateral and anterior to the neuraxis (3,39,40,41,43–46). In most cases, these spaces are naturally enlarged by the tumor, which displaces the MO and spinal cord in the direction opposite to tumoral growth. Usually, drilling does not need to extend beyond the medial third of the bony structures. Lateral tumors displace the neuraxis toward the opposite side, enlarging the subarachnoid space naturally. In anterior tumors, the neuraxis is shifted posteriorly and must be circumvented; therefore, more drilling of the FM lateral wall is needed to reach anterior tumors without retraction of neural structures. Dural opening must also be done according to the relationship between the tumor and the VA. The dura is cut vertically with a horizontal contraincision toward the VA above or below it, or even on both sides (Fig. 15).

The relationship between FM tumors and the VA improves anticipation of the location of the lower cranial nerves. In tumors located below the VA, the nerves are always displaced upward with the VA, whereas in those located above the VA, displacement of the nerves is unpredictable. Therefore, in the former case, the nerves are always found on the superior pole of the tumor; in the latter case, they must be searched for all around the tumor.

The lower third of the clivus is usually included in the FM region. In some cases, the PLA can be used to resect tumors extending up to the clivus. Removal can be done using the space made by the tumor and starting inferiorly. For this purpose, it is often useful to combine the PLA with a retrosigmoid approach or, occasionally, with a presigmoid or transsigmoid approach (retrolabyrinthine or translabyrinthine route).

With the ALA, the posterior arch of the atlas, the mastoid process, and the occipital bone can be exposed posteriorly. Again, mobilization of the VA then gives access to the jugular tubercle and condyle above the VA, and to the lateral mass of the atlas below it (3,10,39,40). Moreover, if the VA is transposed posteriorly and medially, the surgeon can reach the odontoid, C1-2 facet joint, anterior arch of the atlas, and tip of the clivus. Therefore, drilling of the bone at this corresponding level exposes the dura in front of the medulla or upper spinal cord. In most of the author's cases, this exposure was facilitated by the tumor itself, which invaded or even destroyed the bony structures.

As a general principle, the PLA is used for intradural processes and the ALA for osseous or extradural ones. Table 4 lists the lesions for which these two surgical approaches were respectively used. However, in some extradural lesions, the PLA was chosen (see Table 4). For instance, small, bilateral extradural tumors like neurinomas were always removed by PLA. One case of synovial cyst on the anterior midline, extradural but protruding intradurally, was resected by PLA; the transoral approach could have been an alternative, but it involves greater risks of postoperative instability.

TABLE 3. *Osseous tumors and lesions contiguous to the vertebral artery*

Osseous tumors (no.)	Osseous lesions (no.)
Chordoma (12)	Infection (2)
Metastasis (8)	Synovial cyst (1)
Fibrous dysplasia (3)	Craniocervical junction malformation (4)
Osteochondroma (1)	
Osteoid osteoma (2)	
Plasmacytoma (1)	
Histiocytosis (1)	
Sarcoma (5)	
Aneurysmal cyst (1)	

TABLE 2. *Nonosseous tumors contiguous to the vertebral artery*

Tumor	Total	Intradural	Intradural–extradural	Extradural
Meningioma	41	36	4	1
Neurinoma	23	6	8	9
Hemangioblastoma	2	2	—	—
Epidermoid cyst	3	3	—	—
Melanoma	1	1	—	—
Angiomyolipoma	1	—	—	1
Lymphoma	1	—	—	1
Ependymoma	2	2	—	—
Jugular foramen tumors				
Paraganglioma	8	—	6	2
Neurinoma	6	—	5	1
Meningioma	4	—	4	—

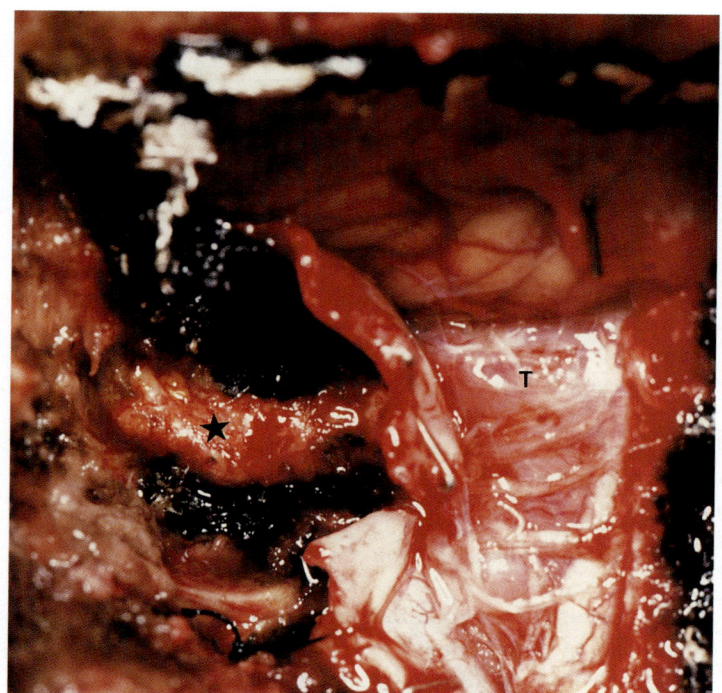
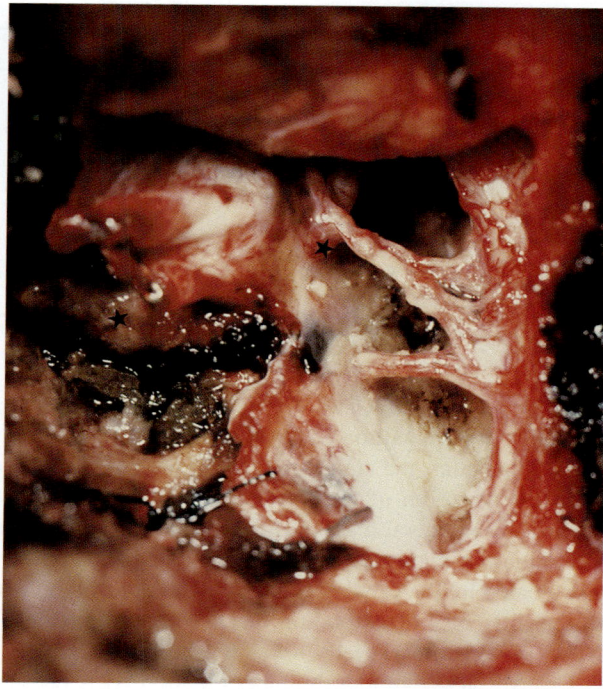

FIG. 14. Intraoperative view of exposure **(A)** and resection **(B)** of a meningioma using the posterolateral approach. *T*, tumor; *star*, vertebral artery.

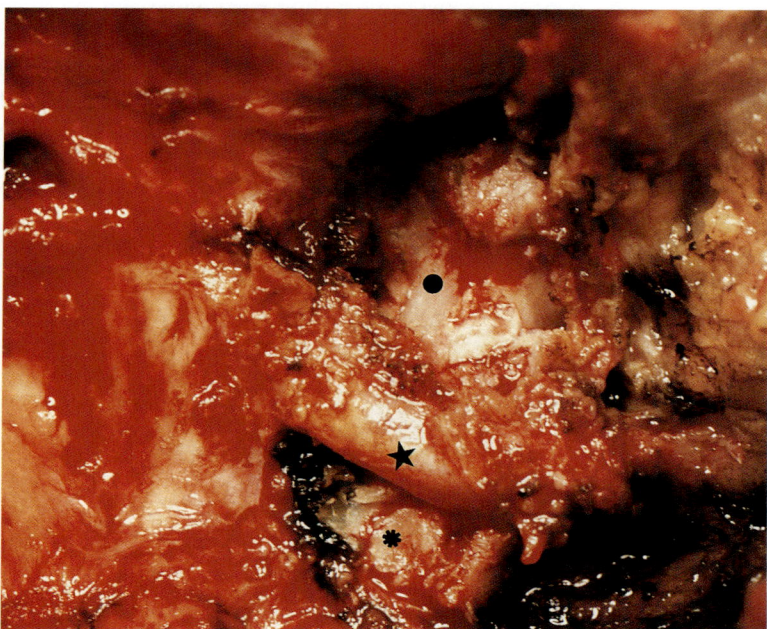
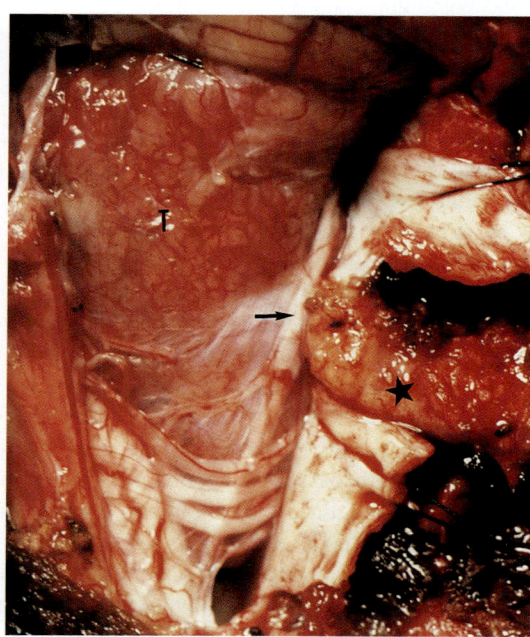

FIG. 15. Posterolateral approach for a meningioma with extension on both sides of the vertebral artery (VA). **A:** Extradural exposure with some drilling of the condyle (*circle*) and of the lateral mass of the atlas (*asterisk*). **B:** Intradural exposure. Note the dural incision on both sides of the VA. *T*, tumor; *star*, VA; *arrow*, cranial nerve XI.

TABLE 4. *Indications for surgical approaches*

Lesion	Total	Posterolateral approach	Anterolateral approach
Foramen magnum area			
Intradural tumors	50	50	—
Intradural–extradural tumors	12	12	—
Extradural tumors	12	1	11
Osseous tumors	22	4	18
Chordoma	12	—	12 (3[a])
Osseous lesions	7[b]	5 (1[a])	1
Jugular foramen area			
Jugular foramen tumors	18	3	15

[a] Bilateral approach.
[b] One case (tuberculosis) treated medically.

Similarly, for a small osteoid osteoma medial to the lateral mass of the atlas, the author's team chose the PLA with upward mobilization of the VA, rather than the ALA with drilling of the lateral mass of the atlas. Bone malformations like odontoid malposition or supplementary condyle were also treated by PLA owing to their bilateral development or to the difficulty of extending the head as required in the ALA. However, no strictly intradural lesion was treated by the ALA. Large extradural tumors required ALA on one or even both sides if they had extensive bilateral extension, as was the case in three cases of chordoma. Therefore, there are no absolute criteria for one or the other technique. They must be discussed after a precise radiologic work-up that establishes the tumor's size and location in relation to the dura and the VA (40).

Upper Cervical Spine

Using the ALA, the anterior aspect of the upper cervical spine (above C3) can be exposed (3,10,11,12) (Fig. 16). The opening between the jugular vein and the SCM is extended downward. The prevertebral muscles (longus colli and anterior rectus) covering the lateral aspect of the vertebral bodies of C2 and C3 are resected, exposing the transverse processes. Before this, the sympathetic trunk must be identified under the prevertebral aponeurosis and retracted medially with all the neurovascular elements (carotid artery, jugular vein, and vagus nerve); to do so, the sympathetic trunk's anastomosis with the cervical spinal nerve roots must be divided. This may induce a transient and always very limited Homer's syndrome if the main trunk of the sympathetic chain was preserved. Next, the transverse foramina of C2 and C3 are opened, taking care to preserve the VA periosteal sheath. The course of the VA changes abruptly at the outlet of the C3 foramen, running posteriorly and superiorly and thus becoming more remote from the lateral side of the vertebral bodies. The VA may then be pulled out of the transverse foramina or kept in place, protected by a spatula, to work on the cervical bodies. This approach permits resection of a bone tumor, oblique drilling of the cervical bodies (47), access to the anterior aspect of the spinal cord, and removal of anterior extradural tumors like neurinomas, meningiomas, or chordomas.

Jugular Foramen Region

Coronal computed tomography or magnetic resonance imaging clearly shows the transverse process of the atlas projecting exactly below the jugular foramen (Fig. 17). Therefore, proceeding successively along the lateral mass of the atlas, the condyle, and the jugular tubercle, the surgeon can reach the lower part of the jugular foramen. This permits the jugular foramen to be opened without any petrous bone drilling (Fig. 18). The approach is similar to the ALA in its first steps, using the same patient positioning and the same skin incision. The VA is exposed from C2 to the FM dura. The internal jugular vein and the accessory nerve are also identified. Then, the vagus (X), glossopharyngeal (IX), and hypoglossal (XII) nerves are dissected as much as possible

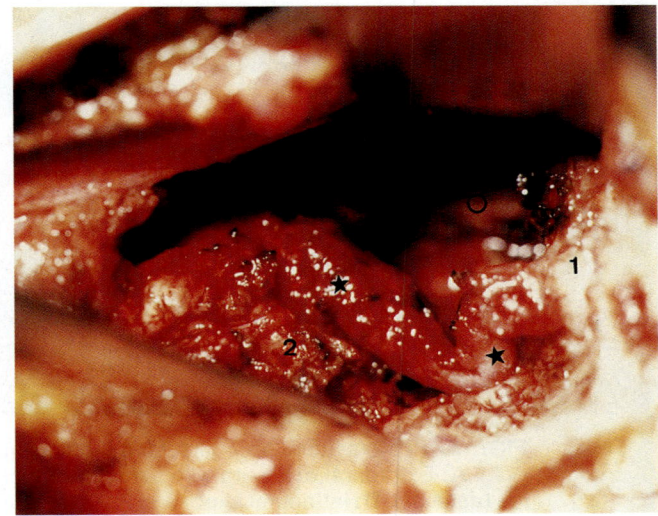

FIG. 16. Intraoperative view after removal of a meningioma at the C1-2 level using the anterolateral approach. *Stars*, vertebral artery; *1*, transverse process of atlas; *2*, transverse process of axis; *circle*, dura mater.

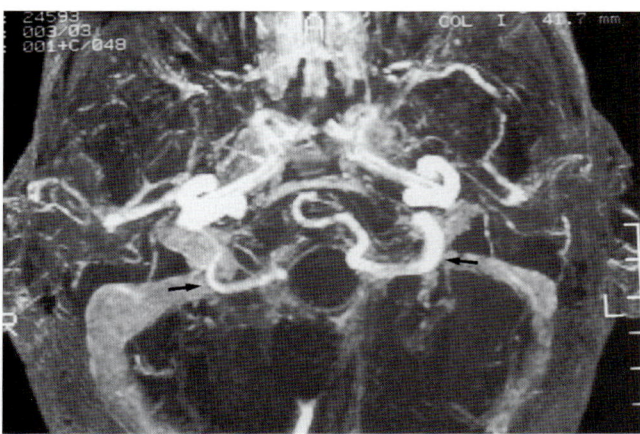

FIG. 17. Magnetic resonance angiogram showing the superimposition of the loop of the vertebral artery in the transverse process of the atlas and the jugular bulb in the jugular foramen (*arrow*).

up to the skull base. The mastoid process is partially resected to expose the sigmoid sinus. At this stage, the tip of the C1 transverse process, which is always much bigger than the other transverse processes, obstructs the route to the jugular foramen. To enlarge the access, the mastoid process and the petrous bone must be drilled more extensively, and thus an infratemporal approach is performed. This permits the opening of the superior and lateral aspects of the jugular foramen. However, if the C1 transverse process is resected, the inferior and posterior sides of the jugular foramen may be exposed and drilled. To do so, the C1 transverse process must be completely removed, leaving bone only on the medial side. Sometimes, the space gained by the C1 transverse process resection is not sufficient, and the VA must be transposed. This juxtacondylar route to the jugular foramen (48) is mainly useful to resect tumors located in the jugular foramen without extension to the petrous bone; this is especially the case in neurinomas and meningiomas, and occasionally

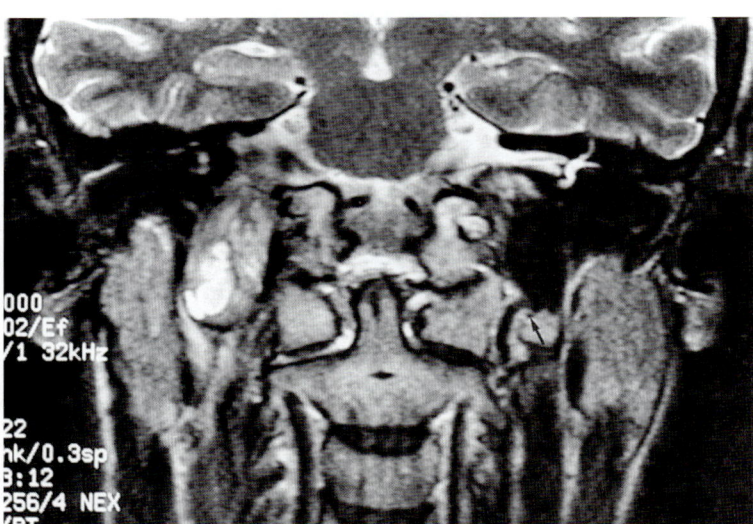

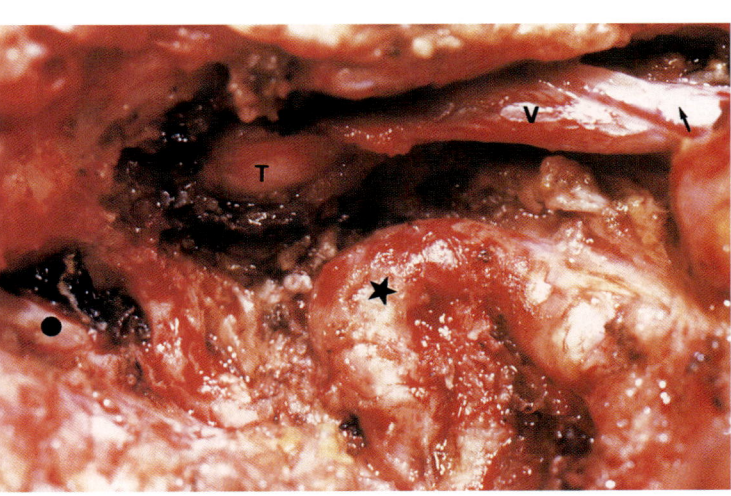

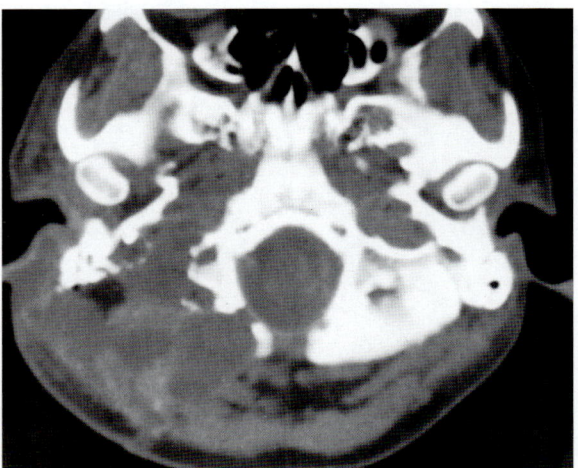

FIG. 18. Jugular foramen neurinoma. **A:** Coronal magnetic resonance image. Note the vertebral artery (VA) in the transverse process of the atlas and the jugular vein (*arrows*). **B:** Intraoperative view of the same case. **C:** Postoperative computed tomography scan control. *Star*, VA; *T*, tumor; *V*, internal jugular vein; *arrow*, accessory nerve; *circle*, sigmoid sinus.

in paragangliomas. However, paragangliomas usually arise from the middle ear promontory and the dome of the jugular foramen and therefore invade the petrous bone, which has to be drilled. For paragangliomas, the juxtacondylar approach is used as a complement to the standard infratemporal technique (49).

Vascular Control and Revascularization

Whatever the lesion and its relation with the VA may be, VA exposure and control may decrease its vascular supply. This is principally useful in vascular tumors like meningiomas or paragangliomas (Fig. 19). In these tumors, the vascular feeders may arise from branches of the ascending and deep cervical arteries and the external carotid artery, which are easily controlled through the ALA (or occasionally by embolization). Vascular feeders may also come from the VA itself, which shares with the ascending pharyngeal artery the vascular supply to the FM and jugular foramen regions. For example, anterior meningiomas of the FM are always mainly fed by the anterior meningeal artery, which branches from the second interspace radicular artery. Moreover, paragangliomas of the jugular foramen also are primarily supplied by the VA. Control of the VA combined with resection of the atlas transverse process not only enlarges the space to reach the posteromedial aspect of the jugular foramen but simultaneously divides all the tumoral feeders.

Surgical treatment of vascular malformations, when required, also needs VA control. Arteriovenous malformations

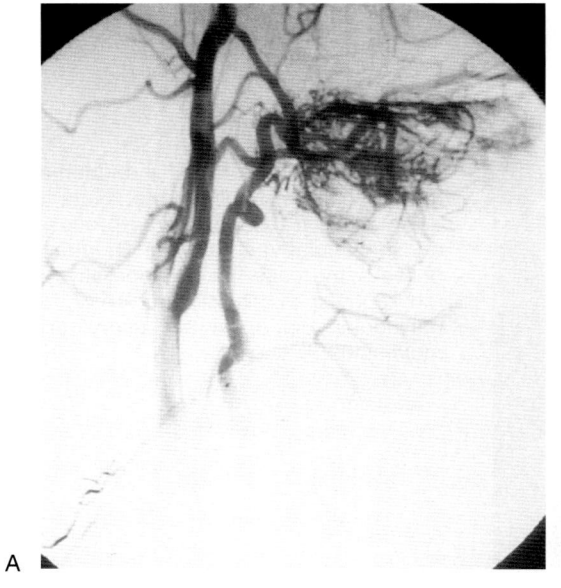
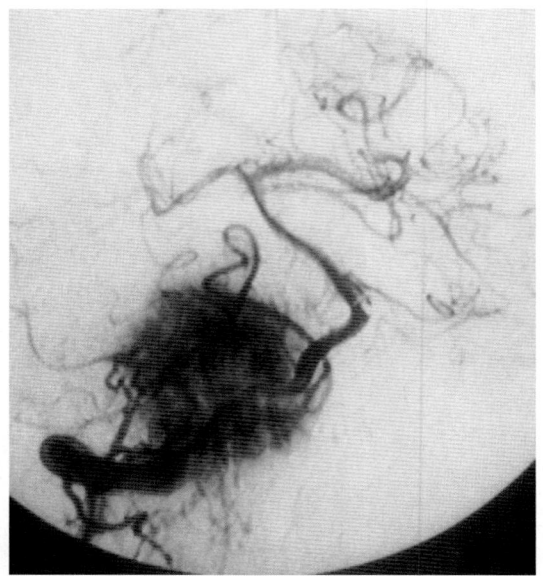
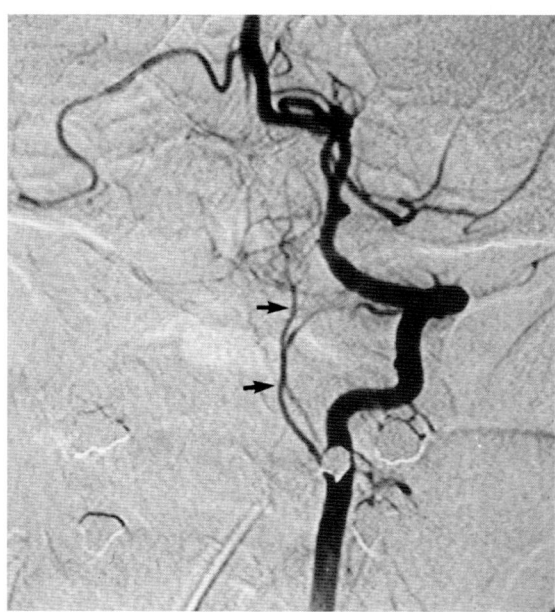

FIG. 19. Tumoral vascular supply from the vertebral artery. **A:** Angiomyolipoma (see Fig. 11C). **B:** Angioblastic meningioma. **C:** Meningioma fed by the anterior meningeal artery (*arrows*).

are essentially fistulas between the VA and neighboring veins, most commonly the perivertebral venous plexus and the jugular vein. Those fistulas often seem very complex on angiography, but usually are simple, unique fistulas that may be obliterated by endovascular techniques (3,50,51). Surgical treatment was, in the author's experience, very rarely required (2 of 41 cases of fistula above C2) (3,9). One case was a stab wound with a direct fistula between the VA and the internal jugular vein. The other was a posttraumatic (fall) aneurysm at the C1-2 level fed by the C2 radicular branch of the VA and the occipital artery and draining into the epidural venous plexus. Therefore, occlusion by embolization must always be attempted first, because even if it fails, it permits identification of the exact site of the fistula. Another type of arteriovenous malformation is angiodysplasia, which is a complex lesion involving the skin, muscle, bone, and sometimes the dura. It usually only results in cosmetic problems. Indications for treatment are limited because it often requires extensive resection of muscles and skin followed by plastic reconstruction. Cutaneous ulceration with bleeding is the only condition requiring surgery.

Aneurysms of the VA include different types of lesions, each one having a particular prognosis and requiring a specific treatment.

Vertebral artery aneurysms must be separated into extracranial and intracranial aneurysms, which have different origins and presentations. Extracranial aneurysms are caused by many pathologic processes, of which the dissecting hematoma is the most frequent (Table 5).

Dissecting hematoma most often induces tubular stenosis, but occasionally causes aneurysm. The two usual locations are the transversary canal inlet (C6) and the suboccipital segment (C2–FM).

Stenosis usually heals spontaneously in few weeks or months. On the contrary, aneurysms are very unlikely to decrease in size. Therefore, as with aneurysms of any other cause, the risk of embolism persists and must be prevented by surgical exclusion. Treatment is best achieved by a common carotid artery-to-VA bypass, distal to the aneurysm, using a saphenous vein graft. Direct repair is not recommended because the arterial wall is dysplastic and therefore difficult to suture. The author has treated two cases of aneurysm above C2. One was on the VA segment above C1, probably of congenital origin, and was treated by common carotid-to-distal VA bypass. The other one was a traumatic dissection on the C2 radicular branch with a 2-cm–diameter aneurysm draining slowly in the perivertebral venous plexus, and was treated by direct resection.

Intracranial aneurysms are of two main types, saccular and dissecting aneurysms. Intracranial dissecting aneurysms are recognized by the usual angiographic features of dissecting hematoma and by their usually more-or-less fusiform aspect. Their most common mode of presentation is not ischemia from embolism, as in extracranial aneurysms, but subarachnoid hemorrhage. Because of their high tendency to rebleed, they must be treated as soon as possible to exclude the arterial segment involved. This can be achieved surgically or by interventional radiologic means, either by proximal occlusion or by trapping of the involved arterial segment. Occlusion or trapping must be discussed according to the size of the VA and to the site of origin of the PICA and of branches to the medulla. In most of the author's cases, proximal occlusion with coil or balloon is the chosen treatment because fixing a distal coil is often hazardous. The balloon is placed distal to the PICA whenever possible. Obviously, definitive occlusion is performed only when the tolerance test with clinical and angiographic control in normal and hypotensive conditions is successful. In case of poor tolerance, the balloon is drawn back and placed more proximally. In the author's experience, it is always possible to find a place (even extracranial) where the occlusion is well tolerated.

Saccular aneurysms of the VA have the same presentation as aneurysms in other locations. However, VA aneurysms (like internal carotid artery aneurysms) are more commonly observed in women and are associated with fibromuscular dysplasia. Multiplicity is also a very common feature. Endovascular technique is the first choice if the angiographic appearance is suitable—that is, a narrow neck compared with the size of the aneurysm and the diameter of the parent vessel. Surgery was chosen in the author's experience when, with similar or lower risks, a major artery (VA or PICA) could be preserved by surgery but could not be by endovascular treatment. This is particularly true for VA–PICA junction aneurysms, where the endovascular material often cannot completely treat the lesion without stenosing or occluding the parent vessels.

For surgery, how distal the aneurysm is along the VA is the main point to consider. VA aneurysms proximal to the lateral side of the MO are easy to reach. On the contrary, distal aneurysms anterior to the MO raise much greater difficulties. In fact, the two most frequent locations are the VA–PICA junction and the VA–basilar junction. Aneurysms located on the intermediate segment are more likely to be dissecting aneurysms than saccular ones. The exposure is always done by the PLA with a variable degree of lateral enlargement. The more distal the aneurysm, the more lateral is the opening extension. For proximal aneurysms, the posterior arch is resected up to the lateral mass of the atlas, with little drilling of the condyle and lateral mass. For distal aneurysms, the VA is exposed up to the transverse foramen

TABLE 5. *Causes of extracranial vertebral artery aneurysms*

Dissecting hematoma
Fibromuscular dysplasia
Collagen diseases (Ehler-Danlos syndrome)
Neurofibromatosis
Atherosclerosis
Trauma
Radionecrosis

of the atlas and the bone opening is extended as far as the sigmoid sinus, with more drilling of the occipital condyle and lateral mass of the atlas. The dura is then opened by a paramedian vertical incision with three horizontal contraincisions: one at the lower and upper extremities and one toward the VA dural penetration. The dissection proceeds along the VA; with the PLA, the angle of work is quite lateral and there is no need to retract the neuraxis. Therefore, the main problem is the lower cranial nerves. VA–PICA aneurysms are most commonly located at the level at which the VA and the nerves cross, and thus nerve rootlets must be displaced superiorly or inferiorly to place the clip properly. To reach distal VA aneurysms, the surgeon must find the most appropriate access between the lower cranial nerves; the access is sometimes very easily found. However, in some cases, the surgeon has to deal with multiple rootlets and arterial branches; they must be dissected along their length from the brainstem to the jugular foramen so that they can be displaced upward or downward without stretching. Exposure of the aneurysmal neck may raise some difficulties in VA–PICA forms in separating it from the PICA origin, and in VA–basilar trunk junction aneurysm if they point inferolaterally over the distal VA, thus hiding the neck. It is often very useful to perform selective distal angiography to anticipate the anatomic disposition and clip position. Fenestrated clips are often used to pass around the cranial nerves or the PICA.

Revascularization has very limited indications because, as previously mentioned, VA occlusion is usually very well tolerated and compensated for by the contralateral VA and by extracranial as well as intracranial anastomoses (1,6–9,16). Moreover, the need to sacrifice one VA is very rare because in most lesions, separation with preservation of the VA can be achieved. Among the lesions observed at the skull base (above C2), there was only one case of aneurysm at the C1 level requiring carotid artery-to-VA bypass (1). In addition to this case, the author's team did 42 distal VA revascularizations for proximal lesions, mostly atherosclerotic occlusive disease (N = 37) and few cases of aneurysm (N = 1), arteriovenous fistula (N = 1), dissection (N = 1), and tumor (N = 1 bilateral; Table 6).

MORTALITY AND MORBIDITY

With regard only to the technical problem of VA management, mortality and morbidity are very limited. The surgical approach, particularly the ALA, may produce some nerve dysfunction. The C2 spinal nerve root may be cut either proximally near the C1-2 VA segment or distally at the level of its subcutaneous branches. The resulting sensory deficit is usually very mild and restricted to a small area around the jaw angle and the earlobe. The sympathetic chain dissected at the suboccipital level produces a Homer's syndrome that resolves in few weeks. Dissection and, moreover, retraction of cranial nerve XI may induce pain and stiffness of the SCM muscle that generally do not last more than 1 or 2 months. Motor deficit of the SCM and trapezius muscles means there was too strong retraction of cranial nerve XI if there was no particular involvement by the lesion. The author observed 4 cases of painful stiffness, all regressive, and 2 cases of mild muscular deficit in his series of 60 cases using the ALA.

Control, mobilization, and transposition of the VA should not result in any particular complications because either the VA flow is preserved or its occlusion is anticipated by a balloon occlusion test. The author never observed any unintentional occlusion, even after VA transposition.

The total resection rate is 98% in the series of benign tumors and 92% in the malignant ones (including chordomas).

Therefore, control of the VA is a safe and reliable technique that greatly increases the surgeon's possibilities at the level of the craniocervical junction and in contiguous areas where the VA is a key anatomic structure.

REFERENCES

1. Matas R. Traumatisms and traumatic aneurysms of the vertebral artery, and their surgical treatment with report of a cured cases. *Ann Surg* 1893;18:477.
2. Henry AK. Exposures of long bones and other surgical methods. Cited in the author's book: *Extensive exposures* (Wright 1927). Edinburgh: Livingstone, 1966:58.
3. George B, Laurian C. *The vertebral artery: pathology and surgery.* Springer-Verlag: Wien, New York, 1987:258.
4. Chiari, 1829. Cited by Chassaignac EPM. *Traité clinique et pratique d'opérations chirurgicales.* Vol. 1. Paris: Masson, 1861:334.
5. Maisonneuve JG, Favrot A. Observation de ligature de l'artère vertébrale. *Journal des Connaissances Médico-Chirurgicales* 1852;11(2):181.
6. Carney AL. Vertebral artery surgery: historical development, basic concepts of brain hemodynamics, and clinical experience of 102 cases. *Adv Neurol* 1981;30:249.
7. Clark K, Perry MU. Carotid vertebral anastomosis: an alternative technic for repair of the subclavian steal syndrome. *Ann Surg* 1956;1963:414.
8. Corkill G, French BH, Michas C, Cobb CA, Mims TJ. External carotid vertebral artery anastomosis for vertebro-basilar insufficiency. *Surg Neurol* 1977;7:109.
9. George B, Laurian C. Surgical possibilities on the third portion of the vertebral artery above C2. *Acta Neurochir (Wien)* 1979;28:263.
10. George B, Laurian C. Surgical approach to the whole length of the vertebral artery with special reference to the third portion. *Acta Neurochir (Wien)* 1980;51:259.
11. George B, Laurian C, Cophignon J, Rey A. Traitement des tumeurs en rapport avec l'artère vertébrale dans sa portion transversaire. *Neurochirurgie* 1982;28:173.
12. George B, Laurian C, Keravel Y, Cophignon J. Extra-dural and hourglass cervical neurinomas: the vertebral artery problem. *Neurosurgery* 1985;16:54.

TABLE 6. Vascular lesions of the vertebral artery

Lesion	Revascularization	Direct repair
Occlusion	30	—
Stenosis	7	—
Dissection	1	—
Aneurysm	2	1[a]
Arteriovenous fistula	1	1[b]
Tumor	1[c]	

[a] Plus arteriovenous fistula.
[b] Plus aneurysm.
[c] Bilateral revascularization.

13. George B, Dematons C, Cophignon J. Lateral approach to the anterior portion of the foramen magnum. *Surg Neurol* 1988;29:484.
14. George B, Laurian C. Impairment of VA flow caused by extrinsic lesions. *Neurosurgery* 1989;24:206.
15. Powers SR, Drislane TM, Nevins S. Intermittent vertebral artery compression: a new syndrome. *Surgery* 1961;49:257.
16. Spetzler RF, Hadley MN, Martin NA, et al. Vertebro-basilar insufficiency. Part 1: microsurgical treatment of extracranial vertebrobasilar disease. *J Neurosurg* 1987;66:648.
17. Francke JP, Dimarino V, Pannier M, Argenson C, Libersa C. Les arterès vertébrales: segments atlanto-axoidien V3 et intra-crânien V4 collatérales. *Anatomia Clinica* 1980;2:229.
18. Lasjaunias P, Moret J, Theron J. The so-called anterior meningeal artery of the cervical vertebral artery. *Neuroradiology* 1978;17:51.
19. Tasi FY, Mahon J, Woodruff JV, Roach JP. Congenital absence of bilateral vertebral arteries with occipital basilar anastomosis. *AJR Am J Roentgenol* 1975;124:281.
20. Lasjaunias P, Theron J, Moret J. The occipital artery: Normal anatomy, arteriographic aspects, embryological significance. *Neuroradiology* 1978;15:31.
21. Ritter VH, Grossman K, Basche S, Heerklotz I, Schiffmann R, Schumann E. Die perkutane transluminale Angioplastik (PTA) von Aortenbogenasten. *Fortschraft Rontgenstradiologie* 1982;136:365.
22. Rao TS, Sethi PK. Persistent Pro-atlantal artery with carotid vertebral anastomosis: case report. *J Neurosurg* 1975;43:499.
23. Hasegawa T, Kuboto T, Ito H, Yamamoto S. Symptomatic duplication of the vertebral artery. *Surg Neurol* 1983;20:244.
24. Lasjaunias P, Braun JP, Hasso AN, Moret J, Manelfe C. True and false fenestration of the vertebral artery. *J Neuroradiol* 1980;7:157.
25. Mizukami M, Tomita T, Mine T, Mihara K. By-pass anomaly of the vertebral artery associated with cerebral aneurysm and arteriovenous malformation. *J Neurosurg* 1972;37:204.
26. Rogers LA. Acute subdural hematoma and death following lateral cervical spinal puncture: case report. *J Neurosurg* 1983;58:284.
27. Djindjian R, Clay R, Hurth M, Vedrenne Cl. Etude clinique, artériographique et anatomique d'un cas de malformation de la charnière cervico-occipitale. *Presse Med* 1964;72:3013.
28. Djindjian R, Hurth M. L'artériographie vertébrale dans les malformations de la charnière cervico-occipitale. *Ann Radiol (Paris)* 1964;7:887.
29. Heerschaft H, Duus P. Die obstruierenden Erkrankungen der Arteria vertebralis in ihrer zervikalen Verlaufstrecke. *Folia Angiologica* 1972;20:22.
30. Janeway R, Toole JF, Leinbach LB, Miller HS. Vertebral artery obstruction with basilar impression: an intermittent phenomenon related to head turning. *Arch Neurol* 1966;15:211.
31. Radojevic S, Negovanovic B. La gouttière et les anneux osseux de l'artère vertébrale de l'atlas. *Acta Anat* 1963;55:186.
32. Lasjaunias P, Guilbert-Tranier F, Braun JP. The pharyngo-cerebellar artery or ascending pharyngeal artery origin of the PICA. *J Neuroradiol* 1981;8:317.
33. Franckhauser H, Kamano S, Hanmura T, Amano K, Hatnaka H. Abnormal origin of the PICA: case report. *J Neurosurg* 1979;51:569.
34. Margolis MT, Newton TH. Borderlands of the normal and abnormal PICA. *Acta Radiologica: Diagnosis* 1972;13:163.
35. Lazorthes G, Gouaze A, Santini JJ, Lazorthes Y, Laffont J. Le modelage du polygone de Willis: rôle des compressions des voies arteriélles d'apport dans les mouvements de la colonne cervicale et de l'extrémité céphalique. *Neurochirurgie* 1971;17:361.
36. Schneider RC, Gosch HH, Taren JA. Blood vessel trauma following head and neck injuries. *Clin Neurosurg* 1972;19:312.
37. Schneider RC, Crosby EC. Vascular insufficiency of brain stem and spinal cord in spinal trauma. *Neurology (Minneapolis)* 1959;9:643.
38. Toole JF, Tucker SH. Influence of head position upon cerebral circulation. *Arch Neurol* 1960;2:616.
39. George B, Lot G, Velut S. Tumors of the foramen magnum. *Neurochirurgie* 1993;39:1.
40. George B, Lot G. Anterolateral and posterolateral approaches to the foramen magnum: technical description and experience from 97 cases. *Skull Base Surgery* 1995;5:9.
41. George B, Lot G. Foramen magnum meningiomas: a review from personal experience of 37 cases and from a cooperative study of 106 cases. *Neurosurgery Quarterly* 1995;5:149.
42. George B, Lot G. Neurinomas of the two first cervical nerve roots: a series of 42 cases. *J Neurosurg* 1995;82:917.
43. George B. Meningiomas of the foramen magnum. In: Schmidek HH, ed. *Meningioma and their surgical management*. Philadelphia: WB Saunders, 1991:459.
44. Bertalanffy H, Seeger W. The dorsolateral, suboccipital, transcondylar approach to the lower clivus and anterior portion of the craniocervical junction. *Neurosurgery* 1991;29:815.
45. Spetzler RF, Graham TW. The far lateral approach to the inferior clivus and upper cervical region: technical note. *BNI Quarterly* 1990;6:35.
46. Sen C, Sekhar LN. An extreme lateral approach to intradural lesions of the cervical spine and foramen magnum. *Neurosurgery* 1990;27:197.
47. George B, Zerah M, Lot G, Hurth M. Oblique transcorporeal approach to anteriorly located lesions in the cervical spinal canal. *Acta Neurochir (Wien)* 1993;121:187.
48. George B, Lot G, Tran Ba Huy P. The juxta-condylar approach to the jugular foramen (without petrous bone drilling). *Surg Neurol* 1995;44:279.
49. Fisch U. Infratemporal fossa approach for glomus tumours of the temporal bone. *Ann Otol Rhinol Laryngol* 1982;91:474.
50. Reizine D, Laouti M, Guimaraens L, Riche MC, Merland JJ. Vertebral arteriovenous fistulas: clinical presentation, angiographical appearance and endovascular treatment. A review of twenty-five cases. *Ann Radiol (Paris)* 1985;28:425.
51. Vinchon M, Laurian C, George B, D'Arrigot G, Reizine D, Ayrnard A. Vertebral arteriovenous fistulas: a study of 49 cases and review of the literature. *Cardiovasc Surg* 1994;2:359.

CHAPTER 28

Lesions of the Sella Turcica

Andrew E. Sloan, Keith A. Black, and Donald P. Becker

The treatment of sellar lesions is one of the more challenging and satisfying aspects of skull base surgery. The wide variety of lesions that occur in this region and the complexity of their treatment necessitates a thorough understanding of sellar anatomy, as well as the clinical symptoms and diagnostic evaluation of the myriad disease processes involving the pituitary gland.

ANATOMY

Sphenoid Bone and Sella Turcica

The sphenoid bone is located at the base of the skull, posteroinferior to the anterior cranial fossa and anterior to the temporal and occipital bones (Fig. 1). The sella itself is a midline depression in the mid-portion of the sphenoid bone. It is bounded anteriorly and inferiorly by the sellar floor, anterolaterally by the anterior clinoid process, laterally by the cavernous sinuses, posteriorly by the dorsum sellae and the posterior clinoid processes, and superiorly by the diaphragma sellae. The floor of the sella is lined with an endocranial layer that is continuous with the diaphragma sellae superiorly, and contains the intercavernous or circular sinuses. These are highly variable, but typically develop in the anterosuperior and posterosuperior regions of the sella. The cavernous sinuses drain into the basilar venous plexus posterior to the dorsum sellae along the upper clivus, which joins the superior and inferior petrosal sinuses.

The sphenoid sinus is just anterior and inferior to the sella,

A. E. Sloan: Division of Neurosurgery, Wayne State University, Detroit Medical Center, and The Karmanos Cancer Institute, Detroit, Michigan 48201.
K. A. Black: Department of Surgery, Cedars-Sinai Medical Center, Los Angeles, California 90048.
D. P. Becker: Division of Neurosurgery, University of California, Los Angeles Medical Center, Los Angeles, California 90095-7039.

and is divided by one or more vertical septa that are often asymmetric (Fig. 2). The degree of pneumatization of the sphenoid sinus varies among individuals and is classified as conchal, parasellar, or sellar (1,2) (Fig. 3). The sellar type is well pneumatized beneath the entire sella, which bulges into the sinus and is found in 70% to 86% of adults. The presellar sphenoid sinus extends only to the mid-portion of the sella, has no sphenoid bulges, and is found in 11% to 24% of adults. The conchal sphenoid sinus has minimal pneumatization and at least 10 mm of bone between the undeveloped sphenoid sinus and the sella turcica. This configuration is common in prepubertal children, but occurs in only 3% of adults.

Nasal Cavity

The nasal cavity provides access to the sphenoid sinus for transsphenoidal approaches. The most important anatomic features for the surgeon are the medial structures comprising the anterior septum that support the nose. These consist of the septal cartilage ventrally and superiorly, the vomer posteriorly and inferiorly, and the perpendicular plate of the ethmoid (Fig. 4).

Pituitary Gland and Hypothalamus

The pituitary gland resides in the sella turcica and is attached to the hypothalamus by the pituitary stalk. The stalk enters the sella through an opening in the diaphragma sellae, a membrane of basilar dura stretched between the tuberculum sellae and the posterior clinoids that separates the cranium from the sella. A small outpouching of the arachnoid accompanies the stalk through the central opening in the diaphragma in about 50% of specimens, to form a small pituitary cistern anterosuperior to the adenohypophysis (3). This is a potential source of cerebrospinal fluid (CSF) leak in the transsphenoidal approach to sellar lesions.

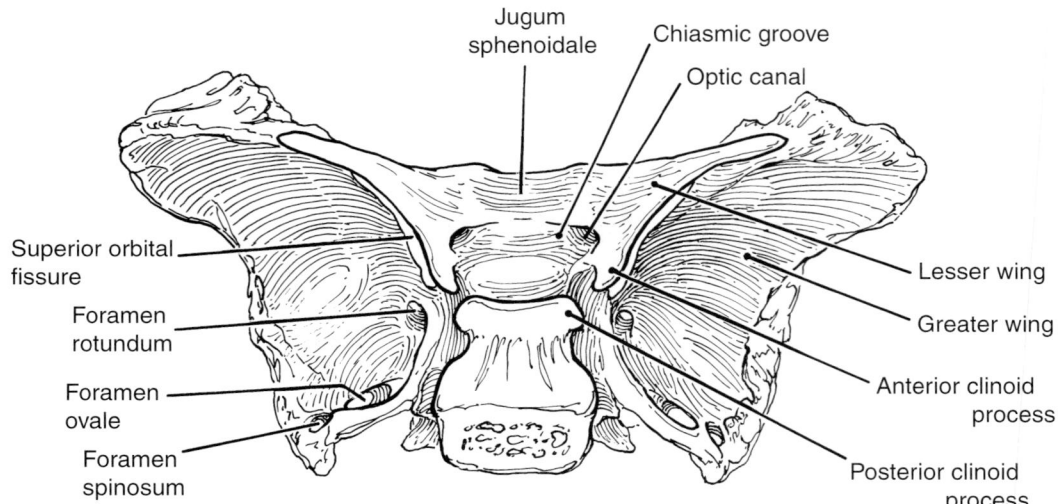

FIG. 1. Anatomy of the sphenoid bone.

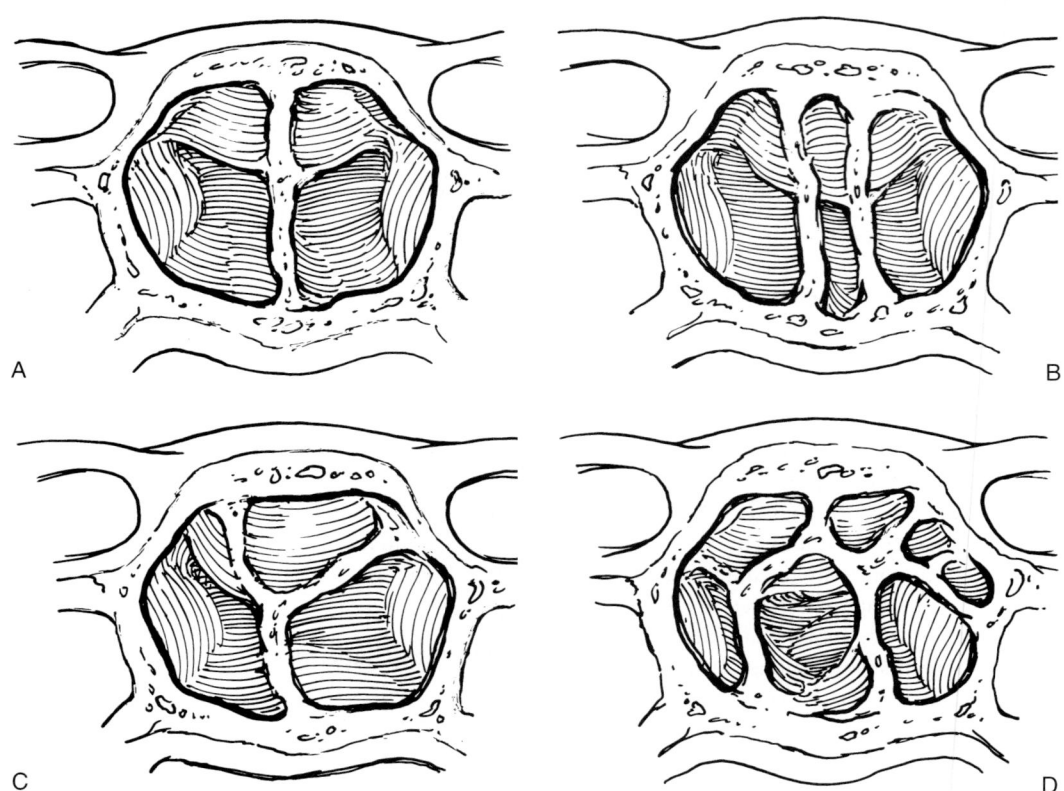

FIG. 2. Variations in the septation of the sphenoid sinus. **A:** Midline vertical septum. **B:** Dual vertical septum. **C:** Oblique. **D:** Honeycomb pattern.

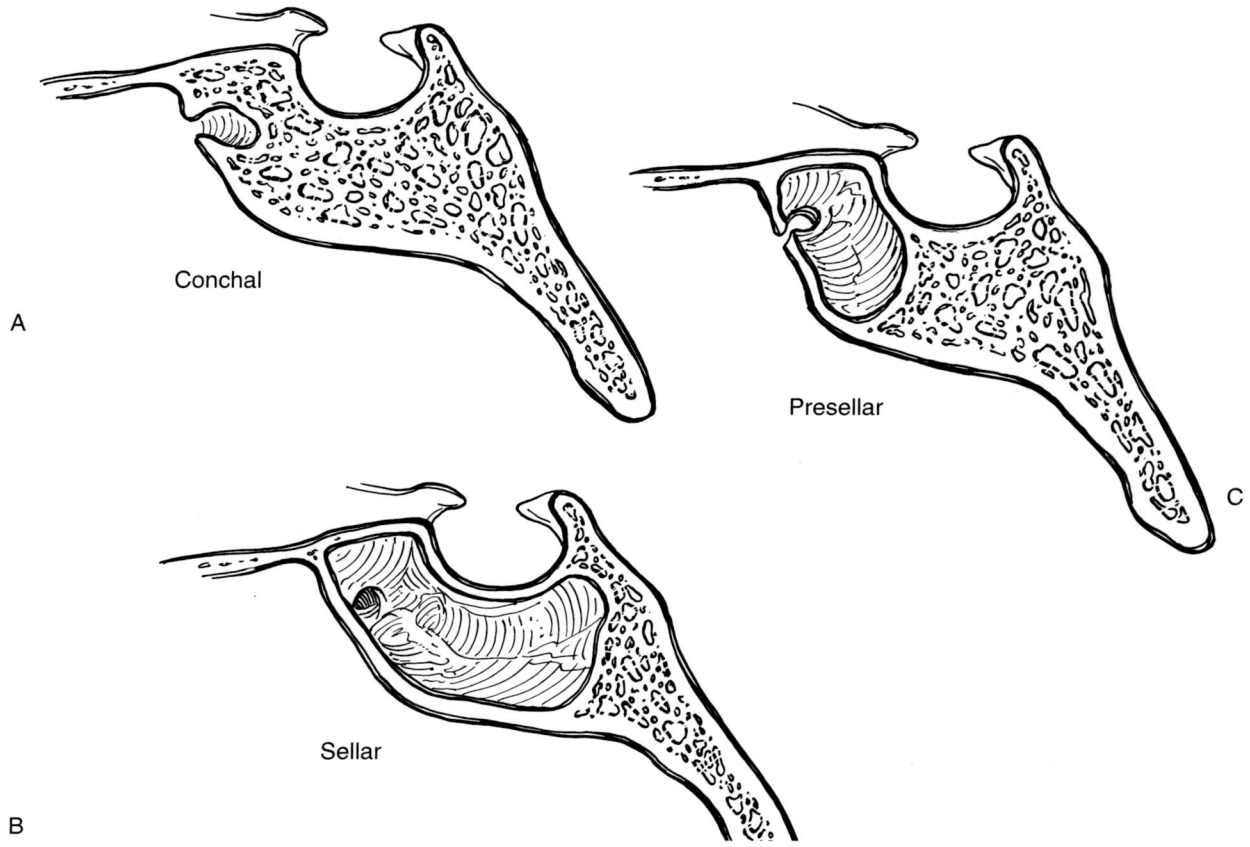

FIG. 3. Degree of pneumatization of sphenoid sinus. **A:** Chonchal. **B:** Presellar. **C:** Sellar.

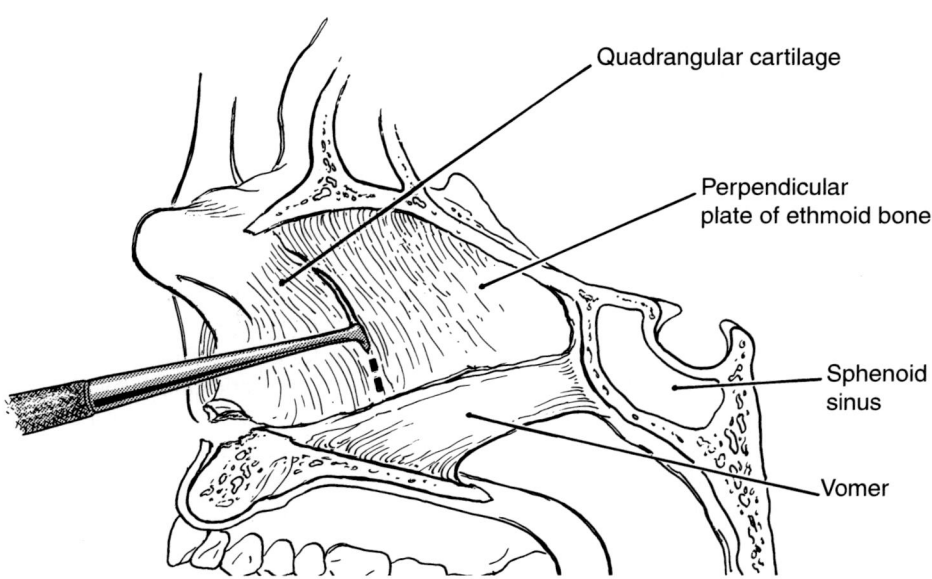

FIG. 4. Anatomy of the nasal septum: anatomic relationship between the vomer, perpendicular plate, and quadrangular cartilage.

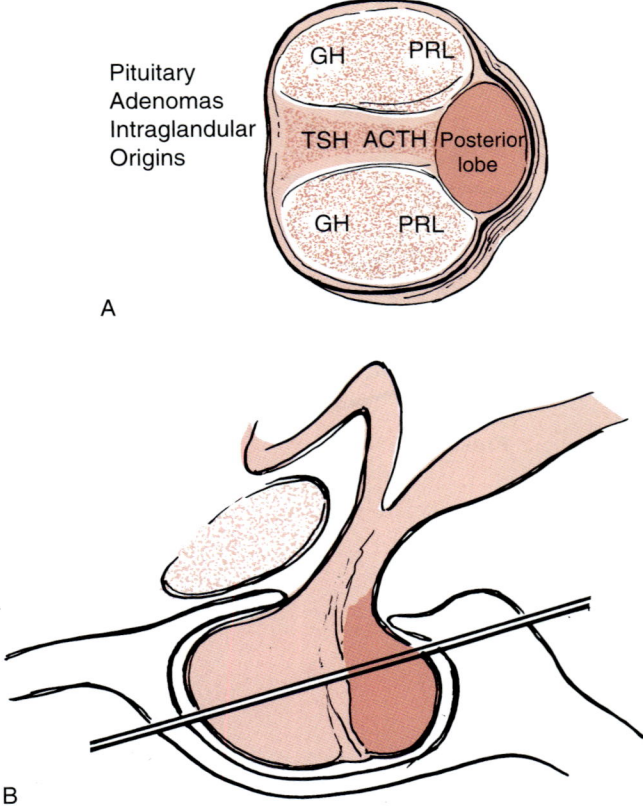

FIG. 5. A,B: Differential concentration of cell types in the pituitary gland.

The pituitary is composed of two lobes, distinct in embryologic origin, structure, and function, which come together during embryogenesis. The adenohypophysis is yellowish in color, and has a relatively firm consistency. It arises from the primitive stomodeum as Rathke's pouch, which grows toward the neural tube to form the craniopharyngeal duct. The anterior portion of Rathke's pouch develops into the pars distalis, the functional portion of the anterior pituitary. A thin sleeve of tissue derived from the adenohypophysis extends upward along the pituitary stalk to form the pars tuberalis, which rises a short distance above the diaphragma sellae. The posterior wall of Rathke's pouch develops into the intermediate lobe, a cystic structure, vestigial in function, lined by ciliated, mucus-producing adenohypophyseal cells. Although the adenohypophysis is uniform in structure, the cells are differentially concentrated in three regions. The cells in the central "mucoid wedge" produce thyroid-stimulating hormone (TSH) anteriorly and adrenocorticotropic hormone (ACTH) posteriorly, and are basophilic (Fig. 5). Some of these ACTH-producing cells invaginate the posterior pituitary with increasing age, a phenomenon known as "basophilic invasion." The cells of the lateral "acidophilic wings" produce primarily the peptide growth hormone anteriorly and prolactin posteriorly. Gonadotropic cells producing luteinizing hormone and follicle-stimulating hormone are located diffusely throughout the gland.

The adenohypophysis is vascularized predominately by the superior hypophyseal artery by way of the hypophyseal portal system (Fig. 6). This venous plexus originates in the anterior inferior portion of the hypothalamus and the floor of the third ventricle, where capillaries with a specialized fenestrated epithelium arise from branches of the superior hypophyseal arteries. These capillaries are associated with the terminals of the tuberoinfundibular neurons, which synthesize the hypothalamic-releasing hormones and secrete them into the capillary network. These vessels drain into the hypothalamic portal veins, which descend to the adenohypophysis along the anterior portion of the stalk, giving it a striated appearance. In the adenohypophysis, the portal veins develop into a second capillary network that supplies the secretory cells of the adenohypophysis and drains into the cavernous sinus.

The neurohypophysis, or posterior lobe, appears gray in color and has a soft, gelatinous consistency. It arises from the median eminence, a downpouching in the floor of the third ventricle. The upper portion becomes the pituitary stalk, whereas the distal end fuses anteriorly with the adenohypophysis and remnants of the craniopharyngeal duct and becomes the neurohypophysis. The stalk comprises unmyelinated axons from the tuberoinfundibular neurosecretory neurons of the supraoptic and paraventricular nuclei of the hypothalamus, which transport granules of vasopressin and oxytocin synthesized by these neurons to the posterior pituitary. These granules are stored in the nerve terminals of the neurohypophysis until released by action potentials generated in the cell bodies of the hypothalamic nuclei. The neurohypophysis is vascularized primarily by the inferior hypophyseal arteries, although the portal vessels also form some anastomoses with capillaries of the neurohypophysis.

Parasellar Structures

Parasellar structures include the optic nerve and chiasm; the internal carotid artery and its branches; the cavernous sinus and the cranial nerves contained within it; and the medial temporal lobes (Fig. 7). Symptoms and signs of sellar and parasellar lesions are often the result of involvement of these structures. The optic chiasm overlies the diaphragm in about 80% of people. The remainder are equally split between prefixed chiasms overlying the tuberculum sellae and postfixed chiasms overlying the dorsum sellae. The cavernous sinuses are lateral to the sella, and contain the carotid artery and the sixth cranial nerve suspended by fibrous trabecula. The third and fourth cranial nerves, and the ophthalmic and maxillary divisions of the trigeminal nerve, lie within the lateral walls of the cavernous sinus.

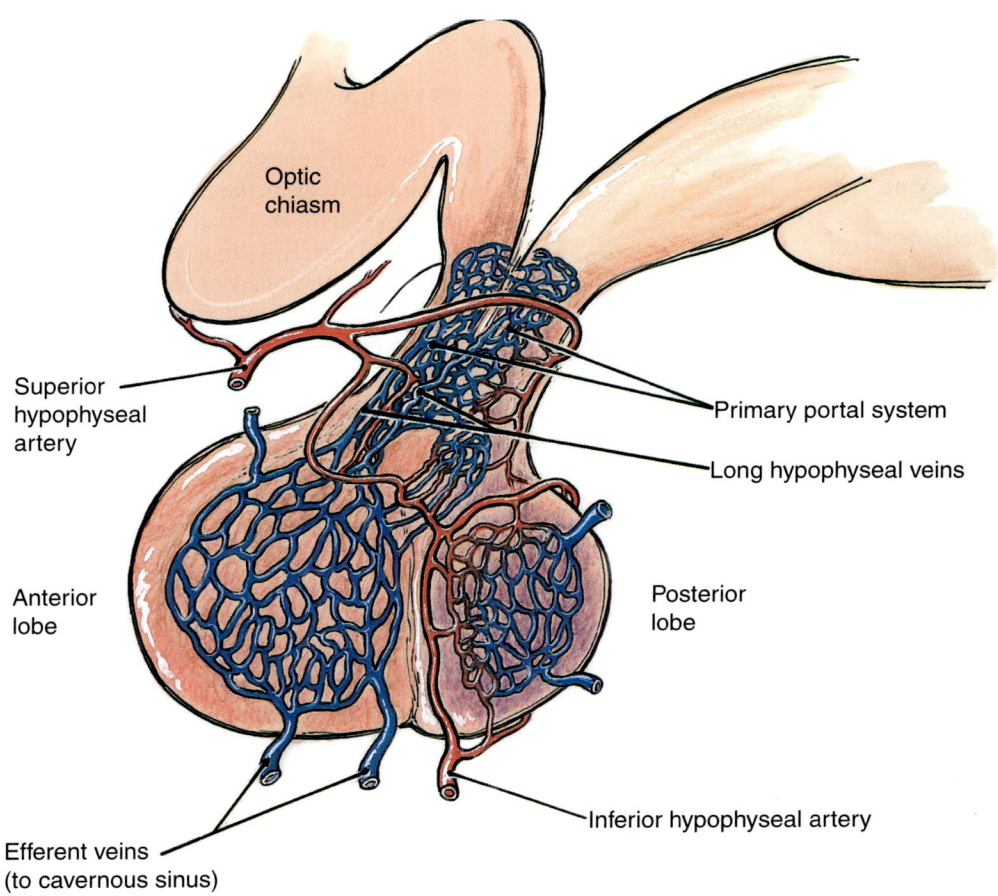

FIG. 6. Vascular supply of the infundibulum and pituitary gland.

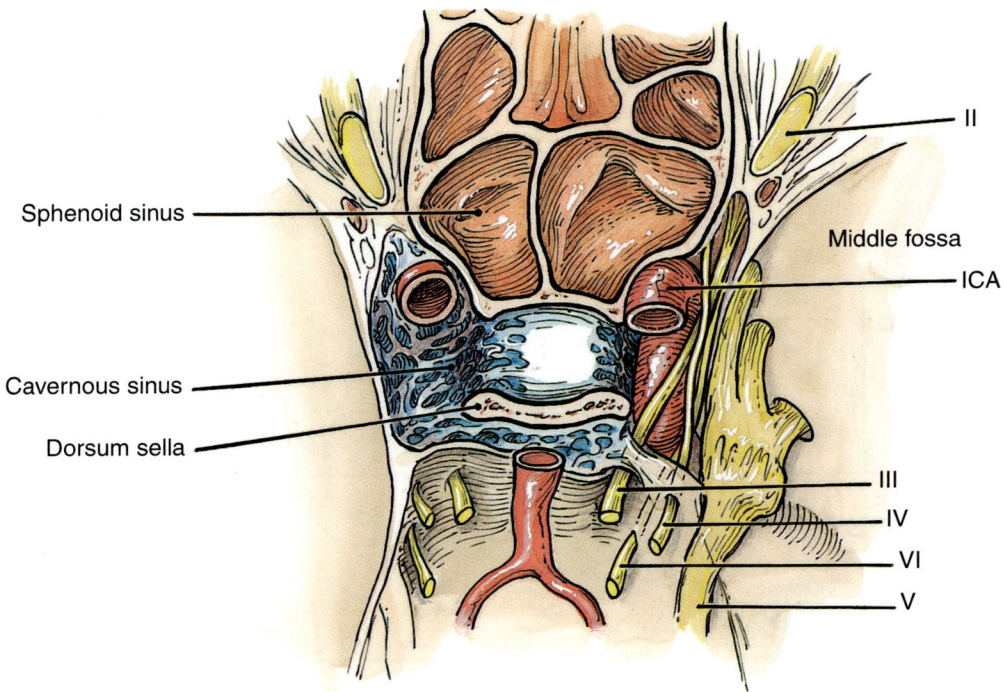

FIG. 7. Relationship of sellar and parasellar structures in cross-section.

TABLE 1. *Differential diagnosis of sellar and parasellar masses*

Neoplastic lesions
Pituitary neoplasms
    Pituitary adenomas
    Pituitary carcinomas
    Granular cell tumors
Nonpituitary neoplasms
    Craniopharyngiomas
    Meningiomas
    Chordomas
    Dermoid cysts
    Epidermoid cysts
    Germinomas
    Teratomas
    Lipomas
    Melanomas
    Metastases
Nonneoplastic lesions
Cysts
Rathke's cleft cysts
Mucoceles
Arachnoid cysts
Inflammatory and infectious lesions
Lymphocytic hypophysitis
Sarcoidosis
Giant cell granulomas
Langerhans' cell histiocytosis (histiocytosis X)
Abscesses
Vascular lesions
Aneurysms
Carotid cavernous fistulas
Cavernous angiomas

PATHOLOGY

The close apposition of neural, endocrine, vascular, and meningeal tissue in the confined region of the sella gives rise to a large number of pathologic entities. Many of these are listed in Table 1. A complete pathologic description of each of these lesions, many of which are rare, is beyond the scope of this chapter. The pituitary adenoma and the craniopharyngioma, the most common sellar lesions, are discussed in detail. Other common neoplastic, cystic, inflammatory, and infectious lesions are addressed only briefly.

Neoplastic Lesions

Pituitary Adenomas and Carcinomas

Pituitary adenomas are the most common sellar neoplasm, accounting for 15% of all intracranial tumors. The annual incidence of these lesions is about 15 per 100,000 population (4). It is likely, however, that these symptomatic adenomas represent only a fraction of the true incidence of these neoplasms, because their prevalence in unselected autopsies is 22.5% (5). The highest incidence occurs in the third to sixth decades of life. Statistically, there appears to be an increased incidence in premenopausal women, though many contend that this is merely because of the sensitivity of the menstrual cycle to the relatively minimal endocrinologic imbalances often produced by these neoplasms. The symptoms produced in men are far less conspicuous and often ignored.

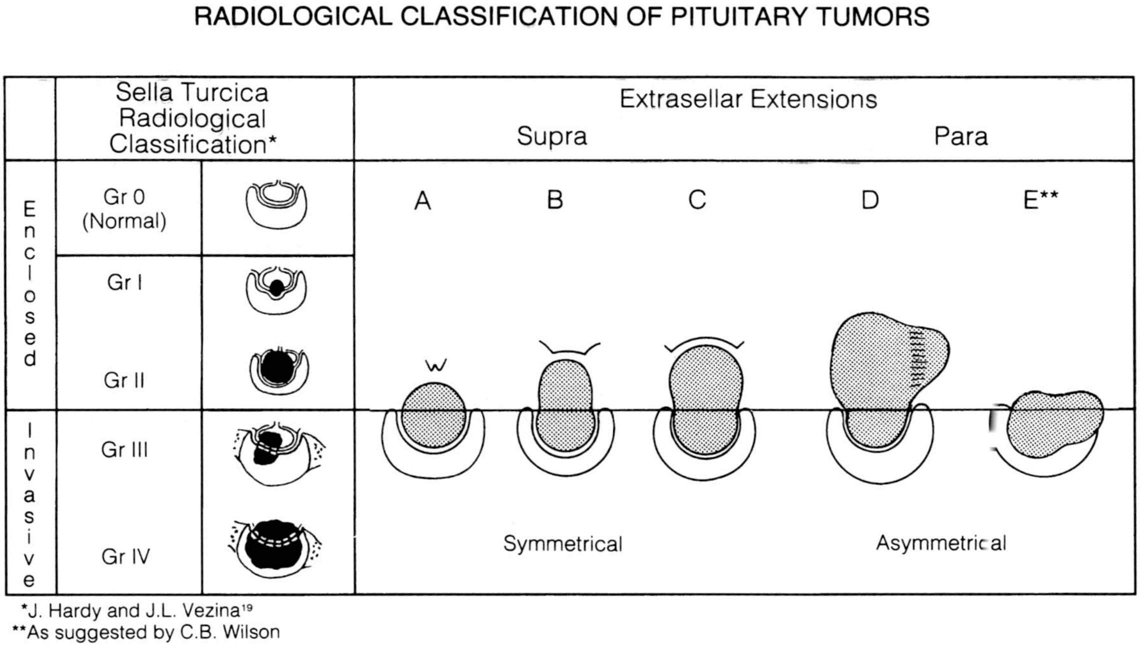

RADIOLOGICAL CLASSIFICATION OF PITUITARY TUMORS

	Sella Turcica Radiological Classification*		Extrasellar Extensions				
			Supra			Para	
			A	B	C	D	E**
Enclosed	Gr 0 (Normal)						
	Gr I						
	Gr II						
Invasive	Gr III						
	Gr IV		Symmetrical			Asymmetrical	

*J. Hardy and J.L. Vezina[19]
**As suggested by C.B. Wilson

FIG. 8. Radiologic classification of sellar neoplasms. (From ref. 59, with permission.)

Pituitary adenomas have been classified by radiologic appearance, clinical presentation, and pathologic characteristics. The radiologic classification, known as the Hardy classification, distinguishes adenomas based on size and gross pathoanatomic relationships (6) (Fig. 8; Table 2). Adenomas 10 mm or less in diameter are classified as microadenomas; those greater than 10 mm as macroadenomas. Other investigators have classified adenomas greater or equal to 40 mm in diameter, or ascending to within 5 mm of the foramen of Monroe as giant adenomas (7). Although the original classification was based on lateral skull tomograms, these have been supplanted by computed tomography (CT) and magnetic resonance imaging (MRI) without formally altering the classification scheme.

Microadenomas are classified as being grade O or I depending on the presence of sellar bulging. Macroadenomas are graded from II to IV based on the degree of sellar enlargement and destruction. Macroadenomas are further staged A to E according to the degree of suprasellar and extrasellar extension. This classification scheme has proven useful in surgical planning and correlates with operative risk and outcome (8).

Pituitary adenomas can be classified clinically in accordance with symptomatic endocrinologic activity. Endocrinologically active adenomas are those that produce and release endocrinologically active anterior pituitary hormones such as prolactin, growth hormone, ACTH, and TSH. These typically present with symptoms of endocrinopathy. In contrast, endocrinologically inactive adenomas either fail to produce hormone (i.e., null cell adenomas); produce hormone that is inadequately secreted (i.e., α-subunit only [9]) or biologically inactive (i.e., silent corticotropic adenomas); or fail to produce symptoms (i.e., follicle-stimulating hormone or luteinizing hormone in male patients).

Pathologic grading schemes for pituitary adenomas originally used cytoplasmic staining affinities to distinguish tumor subtypes. More recent studies have demonstrated, however, that cytoplasmic staining affinities correlate not only with the contents of the secretory granules, but with their density. The classification scheme currently in use uses immunohistochemistry, supported in some cases by ultrastructural morphology, to classify adenomas into 10 types based on the storage and secretion of granules filled with pituitary hormones (10) (Table 3).

The invasiveness of adenomas has been classified radiographically, surgically, and histologically. Although radiologic and gross surgical invasiveness appear to correlate with poor outcome, there appears to be no correlation between microscopic dural invasion, ploidy, mitotic index, and the aggressiveness of these neoplasms, which occasionally invade locally into bone, vessels, dura, or the brain (11).

TABLE 3. *Pathologic classification of pituitary adenomas*

Prolactin cell adenomas
Growth hormone cell adenomas
Mixed prolactin cell–growth hormone cell adenomas
Acidophilic stem cell adenomas
Mammosomatotropic cell adenomas
Corticotropic cell adenomas
Gonadotropic cell adenomas
Thyrotropic cell adenomas
Plurihormonal adenomas
Null cell adenomas

TABLE 2. *Classification of pituitary adenomas*

	Radiologic	Anatomic	Surgical
	Sella Turcica		
Grade 0	Intact, normal contour	**Micro**	**Enclosed**
Grade I	Intact, focal bulging		
Grade II	Intact, enlarged	**Macro**	
Grade III	Destroyed, partially		**Invasive**
Grade IV	Destroyed, totally		
(Grade V)	(Distant spread through cerebrospinal fluid or blood)		
	Extrasellar Extension		
	Suprasellar (symmetric)		
	A. Suprasellar cistern		
	B. Recesses third ventricle		
	C. Whole anterior third ventrical		
	Parasellar (asymetric)		
	D. Intracranial–intradural		
	Anterior		
	Midline		
	Posterior		
	E. Extracranial–extradural (lateral cavernous)		

From ref. 59, with permission.

Carcinoma of the pituitary is extremely rare, and impossible to diagnose based on histologic features alone. It is thought to arise from pituitary adenomas of all types and is defined as Hardy grade V by distant spread through blood or CSF. These tumors typically present with multiple local recurrences followed by metastatic dissemination to the subarachnoid space or extraneuronal sites such as bone, liver, lymph node, lung, or kidney.

Primary Neoplasms of the Posterior and Intermediate Lobes of the Pituitary

The neurohypophysis is rarely the site of clinically significant primary neoplasms. The most common of these is the granular cell tumor, also referred to as choristoma. The histogenesis of these lesions is uncertain, but they are found in 6.8% to 17% of pituitary glands of asymptomatic people at autopsy (12), and may also occur in the stalk. They most often present in the fifth decade of life. Gliomas, gangliocytomas, and hamartomas of the neurohypophysis are extremely rare (13).

Craniopharyngiomas

Craniopharyngiomas comprise 1% to 3% of intracranial tumors. They most commonly present as suprasellar masses, although approximately 20% are primarily intrasellar, and they are the most frequent parasellar lesions of children and adolescents and the second most common sellar lesions in adults. They are thought to be derived from cell rests of the intermediate lobe that arise from remnants of Rathke's pouch and are typically filled with a viscous fluid, rich in lipid and cholesterol, grossly resembling motor oil. They are frequently calcified and surrounded by intense gliotic reaction.

Meningiomas

Meningiomas are the third most common sellar lesions, comprising 1% to 3% of lesions in this region (14). Peak incidence of meningiomas is between 40 and 50 years of age, and women outnumber men by fourfold or more. Purely intrasellar meningiomas are rare (15). More commonly, meningiomas arising at the tuberculum sellae, medial sphenoid wing, olfactory groove, diaphragma sellae, or cavernous sinus invade the sellar and parasellar structures.

Chordomas

Chordomas are slowly growing, expansile, extradural neoplasms thought to arise from notochordal remnants. Median age at presentation is 45 years, and there is a slight male predominance. About 40% arise in the skull base, and of these, 33% involve the sellar or parasellar region (16). These tumors typically originate in the clivus and erode through the posterior clinoids and dorsum sellae into the sella and sphenoid sinus. Primary sellar lesions also occur (16,17). Metastatic dissemination is a late occurrence in 10% to 20% of cases.

Other Primary Neoplasms

Gliomas of the optic nerve and chiasm, germ cell tumors, and hamartomas also occur in the parasellar region and should be considered in the differential diagnosis of sellar lesions, particularly in children. Epidermoid and dermoid cysts comprise approximately 1% and 0.1%, respectively, of all intracranial neoplasms, and occasionally present as sellar lesions in adults.

Metastatic Neoplasms of the Sella

The sella is a common site of systemic metastasis. Gross evidence of sellar metastasis occurs in 1% to 10% of patients dying of systemic cancer (10), although microscopic analysis reveals an incidence approaching 27% (18,19). However, sellar metastases usually occur in the context of advanced systemic disease and are rarely symptomatic (20). The most common manifestation of metastatic disease is osseous involvement of the sella. Metastatic deposits also occur in the pituitary gland and neurohypophysis, but two thirds of these result from contiguous spread. Hematopoietic metastases commonly arise as meningeal lesions, particularly in non-Hodgkin's lymphoma (21).

Nonneoplastic Lesions

Cysts

Benign cysts of the pituitary are identified in 13% to 23% of routine autopsies (22). These include Rathke's cleft cysts, mucoceles, and arachnoid cleft cysts.

Rathke's cleft cysts are epithelial cysts derived from the remnants of Rathke's pouch. Although the involution of the craniopharyngeal duct is usually accompanied by the involution of Rathke's pouch, persistent, discontinuous, cystic remnants of the intermediate lobe are common. These usually are not large enough to be symptomatic. Those that are, presumably grow by progressive accumulation of their colloidal content. They are typically lined with cuboidal epithelium, but cysts lined with squamous epithelium indistinguishable from craniopharyngioma have also been described. They present over a wide range of ages and have no gender predilection.

Mucoceles are epithelial cysts arising from the paranasal sinuses. They are histologically indistinguishable from Rathke's cleft cysts, and differentiation relies on anatomic evidence of extension from a paranasal sinus obtained radiologically or at surgery.

Arachnoid cysts consist of distended areas of arachnoid filled with CSF that occasionally become symptomatic because of mass effect. They can be sellar, suprasellar, or both. Their pathogenesis is unclear: some believe them to be congenital, whereas others contend they are acquired.

Inflammatory and Infectious Lesions

Inflammatory Lesions

The most common inflammatory lesions of the pituitary are lymphocytic hypophysitis, Langerhans' cell histiocytosis, giant cell granuloma, and sarcoidosis. Lymphocytic hypophysitis is a destructive inflammatory process affecting the anterior pituitary that is presumed to be an autoimmune phenomenon. It occurs mainly in women, either during pregnancy or in the first postpartum year, and is often associated with autoimmune diseases of other endocrine glands. It also occurs in older patients of both genders (23).

Langerhans' cell histiocytosis, formerly known as histiocytosis X, consists of a group of poorly understood eosinophilic granulomatous disorders that may be localized or diffuse. Involvement of the central nervous system in patients with disseminated disease is not uncommon, although isolated lesions of the sella are extremely rare (13,24). These granulomas appear to have a predilection for the stalk and adenohypophysis; the posterior pituitary is usually spared.

Giant cell granuloma and sarcoidosis are also granulomatous lesions. Giant cell granulomas are noncaseating granulomas of the adenohypophysis and infundibular stalk. They are typically multiple and have neither a sexual predilection nor an association with pregnancy (25). Sarcoidosis of the central nervous system occurs in 5% of patients with systemic sarcoidosis. Although neuritis is the most common presentation, inflammation of both the anterior and posterior lobes of the pituitary, as well as the stalk and hypothalamus, also occurs in about 1% of patients (26).

Infectious Lesions

Infection of sellar structures occurs only rarely. Bacterial abscesses may arise hematogenously or by secondary extension from an anatomically contiguous focus. Acute sphenoid sinusitis or osteomyelitis are the most likely niduses for contiguous spread. The most frequent organisms are *Staphylococcus aureus*, *Streptococcus pneumoniae*, group A *Streptococcus*, and *Klebsiella* (27). There seems to be a predilection for abscesses to occur in the bed of a preexisting sellar lesion such as pituitary adenoma or craniopharyngioma (28). Tuberculosis, still endemic to certain areas, typically involves the sella in a dense, basilar meningitis, with or without arteritis. Intrasellar tuberculomas are usually associated with systemic tuberculosis and can result in pituitary destruction. Aspergillosis may also present with an inflammatory sellar mass (29), as can parasitic diseases such as cysticercosis (30) or echinococcosis (31).

Vascular Lesions

Aneurysms of the sellar region usually derive from the infraclinoid or intracavernous carotid artery. They are readily diagnosed by MRI and mentioned here merely as a diagnostic consideration to be excluded.

CLINICAL PRESENTATION

Patients with sellar lesions present with a myriad of symptoms and signs. These can be classified as general or specific.

General Symptoms and Signs

The general symptoms and signs produced by sellar lesions result from mass effect, which stretches or compresses the densely packed neurovascular structures of the sella. These structures include the internal carotid artery and its proximal branches; the optic nerve, chiasm, and tracts; the pituitary gland; the infundibular stalk; the hypothalamus; the cavernous sinus and the cranial nerves within; the frontal and medial temporal lobes; the pons and midbrain; and the ventricular system.

Visual Manifestations

The most common manifestation of sellar or parasellar lesions in adults is visual impairment. Chiasmal compression produces a deficit of the bilateral superior temporal visual quadrant initially, followed by involvement of the inferior temporal quadrant. A junctional scotoma consisting of ipsilateral central scotoma with a contralateral superior temporal quadrantanopsia may also be produced by involvement of optic nerve fibers crossing into the chiasm at acute angles (Von Willebrand's knee). Further compression may lead to irreversible chiasmal damage, resulting in total blindness. Isolated compression of the prechiasmal optic nerve results in an afferent pupillary defect known as Marcus Gunn's sign.

Hypothalamic and Pituitary Dysfunction

Compression of the hypothalamus may lead to dysregulation of pituitary secretion as well as a myriad of other physiologic processes regulated by the hypothalamus. These include water balance, body temperature, level of consciousness, and behavior.

Compression of the median eminence or infundibular stalk may result in the impairment of synthesis of hypophysiotropic hormones or their transport to the pituitary gland itself. This results in varying degrees of hypopituitarism as well as diabetes insipidus. By interfering with the transport of dopamine—the predominant prolactin-inhibiting factor—to the lactotrophs, stalk compression also produces a paradoxical mild to moderate hyperprolactinemia (typically

30–150 ng/ml). This may present as hypogonadism or galactorrhea in women or men.

Compression of the pituitary gland itself also commonly results in hypopituitarism. The clinical symptoms depend on the cell types affected, and the degree of hyposecretion. The gonadotrophs are the most vulnerable and are usually affected first, leading to amenorrhea or oligomenorrhea in women, gonadal atrophy in men, and loss of libido in both sexes. Thyrotrophs and somatotrophs are usually affected next. Corticotrophs have the greatest functional reserve, and addisonian symptoms of nausea, vomiting, and postural hypotension usually present only in severe panhypopituitarism.

Cavernous Sinus Involvement

Sellar lesions extending into the cavernous sinus may involve the third, fourth, and sixth cranial nerves, resulting in partial or complete ophthalmoplegia. This is more commonly found in meningiomas than pituitary adenomas or craniopharyngiomas. The oculomotor nerve is the most commonly affected nerve in the cavernous sinus, followed by the abducens and trochlear nerves. Involvement of the first two branches of the trigeminal nerve results in numbness or pain in these distributions.

Headache

Headache results from stretching or compressing the dura of the diaphragma sellae, tentorium, cavernous sinus, or the base of the skull, all of which are innervated by the first division of the trigeminal nerve. Other mechanisms by which sellar lesions produce headache are inflammation or pressure on other pain-sensitive dural structures, and elevated intracranial pressure due to mass effect or obstructive hydrocephalus.

Hydrocephalus

Sellar lesions with significant suprasellar extension may obstruct the foramen of Monro, producing unilateral or bilateral obstructive hydrocephalus. This may result in headache, papilledema, and decreased levels of consciousness. Stretching of the sixth cranial nerve may also produce an abducens palsy.

Cortical Involvement

Sellar lesions with significant suprasellar or parasellar extension may compress adjacent brain. Usually, slow-growing lesions reach large size before becoming symptomatic. Compression of the frontal lobes produces personality change and memory loss, whereas temporal compression or irritation may induce seizure.

Apoplexy

Pituitary apoplexy is a clinical manifestation of hemorrhage or infarction of a pituitary adenoma. The syndrome is characterized by the acute onset of severe headache and meningismus, often accompanied by nausea and vomiting. Partial or complete ophthalmoplegia is common, and a decreased level of consciousness may also occur. This clinical emergency results from the acute onset of mass effect on parasellar structures such as the optic chiasm or the cavernous sinus. This occurs in about 1% to 2% of pituitary adenomas and appears to be more frequent in clinically nonfunctional macroadenomas.

Specific Symptoms and Signs

Specific symptoms and signs may be diagnostic of certain endocrinologically active pituitary adenomas.

Prolactinomas

Prolactinomas account for about 30% to 40% of all pituitary adenomas and are the most commonly encountered endocrinologically active adenomas. They present differently in men and women. Women present threefold more frequently than men and complain of oligomenorrhea or amenorrhea, often with infertility and galactorrhea. They are typically 20 to 30 years of age and have microadenomas with moderately elevated prolactin levels (>200 ng/ml). In contrast, men typically present between 40 and 50 years of age, with general symptoms of mass effect. Men often harbor invasive macroadenomas with significantly higher prolactin levels. They often admit to decreased libido or impotence, but rarely present with this as a chief complaint. Galactorrhea also occurs occasionally in men.

Growth Hormone-Secreting Adenomas

Excess growth hormone due to pituitary adenoma results in giganticism if manifested in childhood before fusion of the epiphysis of the long bones. In adults, these tumors present with acromegaly, resulting in gross enlargement of soft tissues of the face and the extremities. Bone density also increases, resulting in degenerative joint disease, spinal stenosis, and compressive neuropathies. Acromegaly is also associated with systemic illness, including brittle diabetes, hypertension, severe atherosclerosis, and organomegaly. Poorly understood respiratory disease and cardiomyopathy result in decreased life expectancy for these patients.

Adrenocorticotropic Hormone-Secreting Adenomas

Hypercortisolism, or Cushing's syndrome, results in a myriad of clinical features, including moon facies, centripetal obesity, "buffalo hump," hirsutism, abdominal striae, poor wound healing, frequent infections, atrophy, weakness, acne, oligomenorrhea, amenorrhea, and behavioral changes. Associated metabolic disturbances include impaired glucose tolerance, hypertension, left ventricular hypertrophy, anasarca, hypokalemia, osteoporosis, erythrocytosis, immunosuppression, and eosinophilia. These conditions are severe and usually fatal if the condition is untreated.

Unlike the aforementioned endocrinopathies, which are essentially pathognomonic for pituitary adenomas, Cushing's syndrome has several possible etiologies. Cushing's disease, defined as hypercortisolism due to an ACTH-producing pituitary adenoma, accounts for only 60% of cases of Cushing's syndrome (32). Nearly 25% of cases of Cushing's syndrome result from primary cortisol hypersecretion by adrenal adenoma or carcinoma, whereas 15% of cases are due to ACTH secretion from ectopic sources, including bronchogenic carcinoma, carcinoid tumors, and pancreatic tumors (32,33). Iatrogenic and factitious hypercortisolism also occur.

Nelson's syndrome is an iatrogenic condition caused by unopposed growth of an ACTH-secreting pituitary adenoma after bilateral adrenalectomy. Patients typically are hyperpigmented, with characteristic copper-colored skin and advanced symptoms and signs of Cushing's disease. Often, they have manifestations of mass effect as well. The incidence of Nelson's syndrome has declined because of recognition of the pathophysiology of this morbid condition, as well as improved diagnosis and treatment of Cushing's disease.

Thyroid-Stimulating Hormone-Secreting Adenomas

Thyroid-stimulating hormone-secreting adenomas are extremely rare, accounting for less than 1% of pituitary adenomas (34). Patients present with clinical symptoms of hyperthyroidism, and typically have microadenomas (35). As with Cushing's syndrome, other etiologies must be excluded before making this diagnosis.

DIAGNOSTIC EVALUATION

Because of the close approximation of structures influencing neurologic, endocrine, and visual function in the sellar region, the evaluation of patients suspected of having a sellar mass is best approached as an interdisciplinary effort. Guided by findings obtained during the clinical evaluation, the diagnostic process begins with the determination of an anatomic diagnosis and an endocrine diagnosis.

Radiologic Evaluation

Magnetic Resonance Imaging

The superior anatomic resolution of gadolinium-enhanced MRI has made it the imaging modality of choice in the evaluation of sellar lesions. High-resolution, multiplanar MRI can routinely detect lesions as small as 3 mm in diameter. MRI also gives excellent resolution of the critical spatial relationships between the sellar lesion, normal gland, and surrounding cisterns and neurovascular structures. The relative positions of the carotid arteries, chiasm, infundibulum, pituitary remnant, hypothalamus, and the third ventricle relative to the lesion are particularly important. These features enable the clinician precisely to determine the location of the lesion, and thus facilitate the differential diagnosis. Moreover, the extent of suprasellar and parasellar extension, the relative position of the chiasm, and the degree of pneumatization of the sphenoid sinus are critical in planning the operative approach, if surgery is indicated.

The soft tissue imaging characteristics of MRI also help the clinician narrow down the diagnostic possibilities in the evaluation of sellar lesions. For example, the characteristic appearance of an aneurysm on MRI enables this diagnostic possibility to be immediately included or excluded in most cases. Likewise, the appearance of a "dural tail" may be strongly suggestive of a meningioma.

Computed Tomography

Although MRI provides better anatomic resolution of soft tissues, high-resolution CT, with or without image reconstruction, remains superior to MRI in the resolution of bony anatomy. Thin-section (1.5-mm) cuts with coronal and axial reconstruction are useful for evaluating the thickness of the sellar floor, the presence of hyperostosis or bony destruction, pneumatization of the sphenoid sinus, and the position of sphenoid septa. CT is also superior to MRI in detecting dystrophic calcification, making it valuable diagnostically as well as for planning the surgical approach. Contrast-enhanced CT is also critical in the evaluation of patients with contraindications to MRI imaging, such as the presence of ferromagnetic foreign bodies in the form of aneurysm clips, pacemakers, or cochlear implants.

Skull Radiography

Lateral skull radiography has been largely supplanted by MRI and CT. Although it does not provide additional information, it is more readily obtained than MRI or CT, and thus useful for specific indications. These include intraoperative imaging and the serial evaluation of pneumocephalus in the postoperative setting.

Angiography

Although angiography was once essential in the work-up of sellar lesions for evaluating mass effect and excluding the presence of sellar aneurysms, this function has been largely supplanted by MRI and magnetic resonance angiography.

Angiography is now indicated only rarely for the immobilization of particularly vascular lesions, and for petrosal sinus sampling in the evaluation of Cushing's syndrome.

Metrizamide Cisternography

Cisternography, once routinely used for imaging, has also been replaced by high-resolution CT and MRI. The only remaining indication for this technique is the evaluation of CSF rhinorrhea.

Ophthalmologic Evaluation

A complete neuroophthalmologic evaluation should be obtained in all patients with visual symptoms or signs, as well as any patient with lesions that have extrasellar extension. Visual acuity and perimetry are formally assessed, and the presence of optic atrophy and visual field deficits is documented. These examinations may then be performed serially to document the course of the disease and the response to treatment.

Endocrinologic Evaluation

Every patient with a suspected or known sellar lesion should have an initial endocrine screening examination. This should include measurements of baseline levels of plasma electrolytes and osmolarity as well as prolactin, growth hormone, cortisol, ACTH, luteinizing hormone, follicle-stimulating hormone, α-subunit, thyroxine, and TSH. This allows the clinician to evaluate the integrity of the various hypothalamic–pituitary–target organ axes. Further provocative testing or special hormone assays designed to diagnose particular endocrinopathies may then be indicated for further evaluation (36).

SURGICAL APPROACHES TO THE SELLA

Management options for sellar lesions include observation, surgery, pharmacologic treatment, and radiation therapy. The decision to operate should be based on the patient's clinical diagnosis, age, medical condition, and prognosis. In patients with endocrinopathies, the diagnosis can often be made based on history and clinical findings combined with laboratory and radiologic tests consistent with acromegaly, Cushing's disease, or marked hyperprolactinemia, as noted previously. In many cases, however, definitive diagnosis itself requires a surgical specimen.

Approaches to the sella can be classified as extracranial–extradural and transcranial–intradural. The choice of approach depends on the clinical diagnosis, the relationship between the lesion and the critical juxtasellar structures, and the goals of surgery (Fig. 9). In most cases, the transsphenoidal procedure, an extradural approach, is the treatment of choice because of its simplicity and safety. Transsphenoidal surgery offers excellent sellar exposure and enables the surgeon to remove the lesion while preserving normal gland, which is rarely possible with the transcranial approach. Transsphenoidal surgery is faster, with equal chiasmal decompression equal to, and endocrine preservation superior to, that obtained with transcranial surgery (8,37–40). Moreover, transsphenoidal surgery has a lower morbidity and mortality than transcranial surgery, and thus shortens hospital stays. Occasionally, however, other approaches are required for increased superior or lateral exposure, or for lesions with intradural extension. This section addresses the techniques of the surgical approaches and concentrates primarily on the transsphenoidal approach. The management of specific lesions is addressed in a later section.

Extracranial–Extradural Approaches

Transsphenoidal Approach

The transnasal, transsphenoidal (TNTS) approach to the sella was introduced in 1907 by Schloffer (41), and popularized by Hardy (6), and is regarded as the procedure of choice for midline lesions of the sella with limited lateral or posterior extension (42). The contraindications to the transsphenoidal approach are acute sinusitis; ectatic intrasellar "kissing" carotids; an "hourglass" configuration of tumor, with extensive suprasellar extension and a normal sella; a suprasellar mass too fibrous or calcified to collapse into the sella; and significant extension of the lesion into the subfrontal, retrochiasmatic, middle, or posterior fossae (Table 4). Rhinoplasty or previous transnasal surgery is not a contraindication to the transsphenoidal approach, nor is a conchal sphenoid sinus, which can be opened with a high-speed drill.

Before surgery, the patient is given a single dose of antibiotics (usually a first-generation cephalosporin) and intubated with an orotracheal tube placed on the left side of the mouth. Patients with neural or endocrine compromise are given high-dose corticosteroids (hydrocortisone, 100 mg). The patient is positioned in the supine position with the head in a donut, tilted 15 degrees to the right, and elevated 15 degrees above the heart (Fig. 10). The donut permits small ad-

TABLE 4. *Contraindications to the transsphenoidal approach*

Acute sinusitis
"Kissing" carotids
"Hourglass" tumor with normal sella and extensive suprasellar extension
Fibrous suprasellar mass
Extension into frontal, middle, or posterior fossa
Gross dural invasion

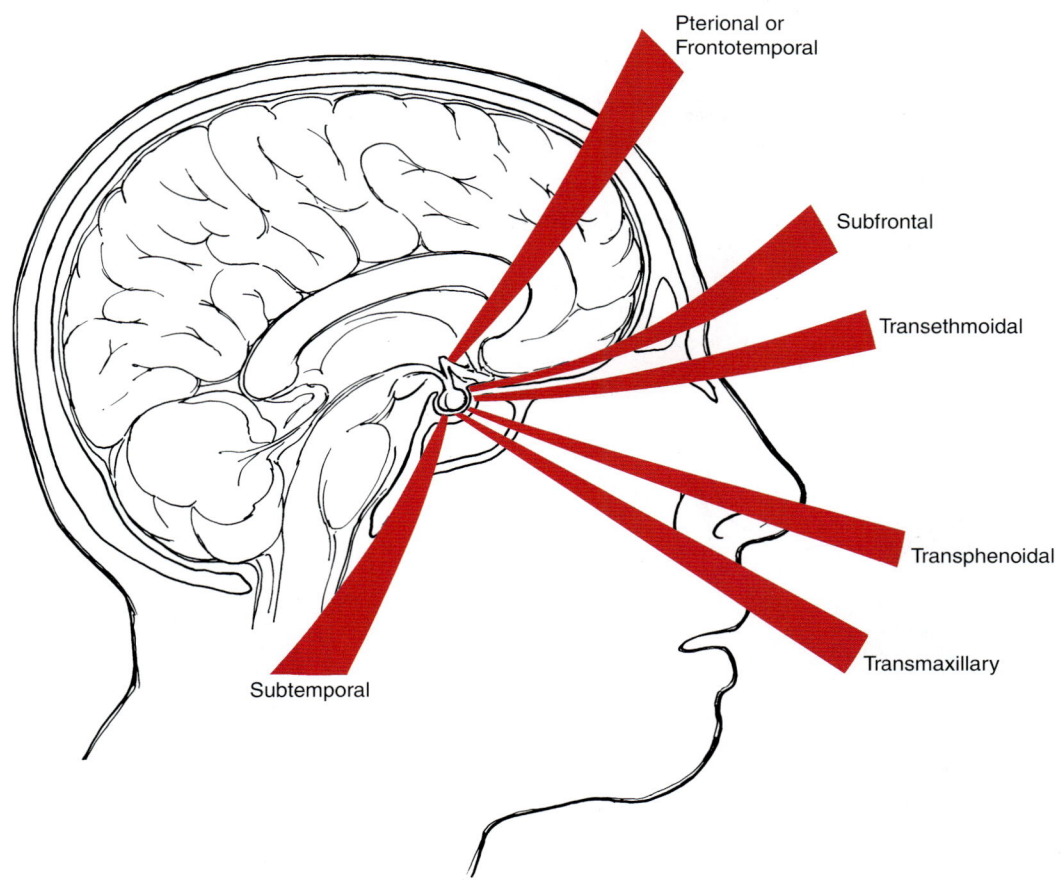

FIG. 9. Surgical approaches to the sella turcica.

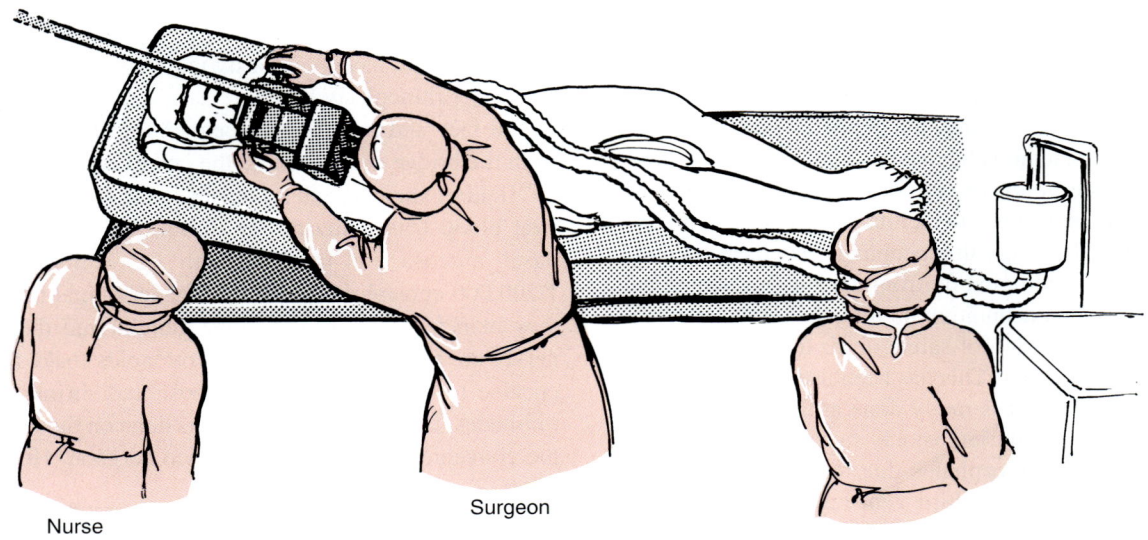

FIG. 10. Position of the patient and operating team for the transnasal–transsphenoidal approach.

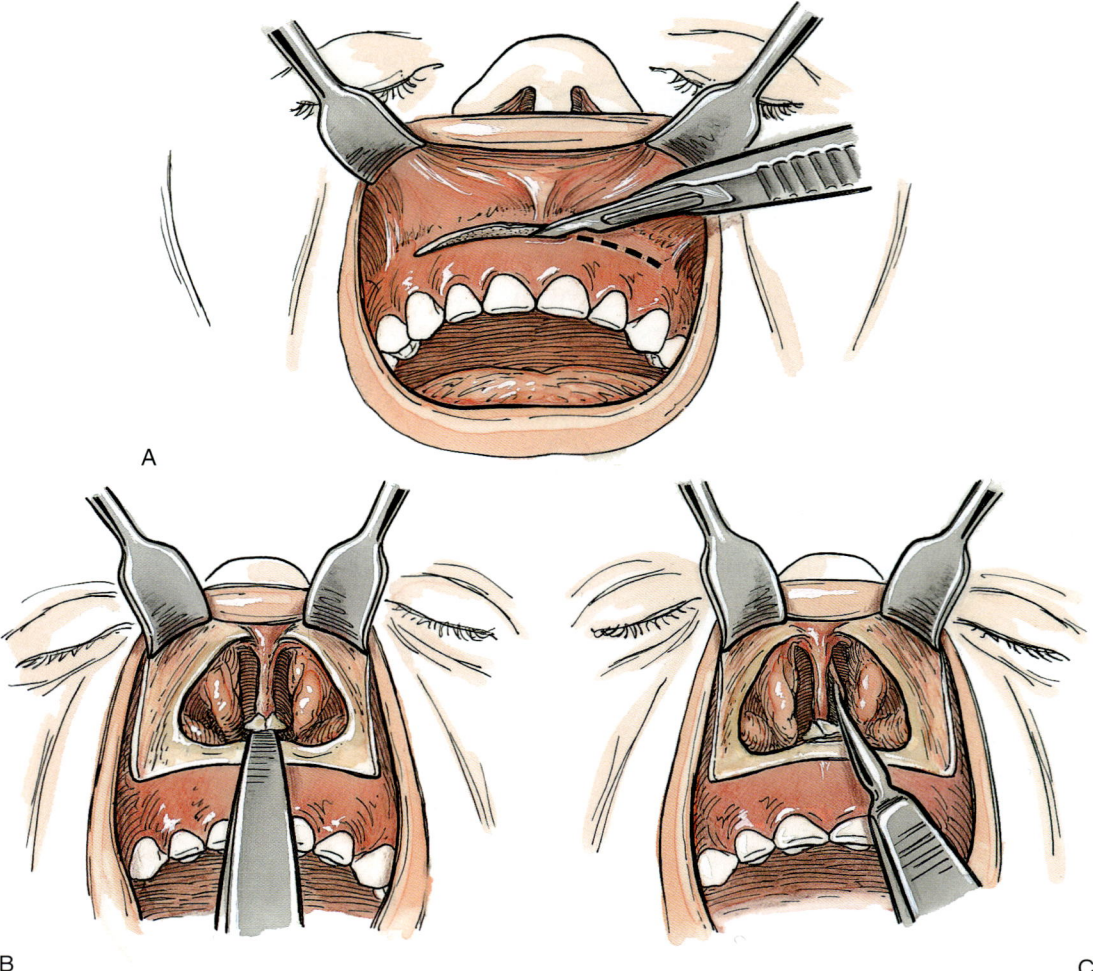

FIG. 11. Transsphenoidal approach to the sella turcica. **A:** The gingival mucosa is incised from canine to canine with a no. 15 blade. **B:** After dissection, the pyriform aperture is enlarged as required. **C,D:** The mucosa is elevated off the left side of the quadrangular cartilage ventral to the anterior boarder of the perpendicular plate. **E:** After freeing the quadrangular cartilage from the vomer and the perpendicular plate, the left anterior and inferior submucosal tunnels are sharply dissected, and the quadrangular cartilage is retracted to the right using the nasal speculum.

justments of the head to facilitate improved visualization. Further flexion of the head improves access to the posterior sella and clivus, whereas extension improves exposure of the tuberculum and planum sphenoidale. The left thigh is positioned on a bolster to expose the superolateral aspect of the leg from the hip to the knee to facilitate a graft of fat and fascia lata, if needed. In very thin people, it may rarely be necessary to remove additional fat from the anterior abdominal wall. A lumbar subarachnoid drain may also be inserted before surgery for injection of saline or air to aid in bringing down a suprasellar mass. This has been used extensively by some surgeons (43) but is rarely done at the authors' institution. Preoperative ventriculostomy may also be indicated for patients with hydrocephalus due to obstruction of the foramen of Monro or the third ventricle by a suprasellar mass. The fluoroscopy unit may also be used, although this is usually required only for patients with a conchal sphenoid sinus or patients lacking the usual anatomic landmarks, such as patients who have previously undergone transsphenoidal surgery or rhinoplasty.[1]

The face and mouth are prepared with povidone–iodine from the bridge of the nose to the jaw to create a "semisterile" field. A vaginal pack is inserted in the oropharynx to prevent blood from entering the throat, and the gingiva and nasal mucosa are injected with 0.5% lidocaine with 1/200,000 epinephrine using a 25-gauge spinal needle until they blanch. The sphenopalatine ganglia and the ethmoid nerves are blocked with 1×3 cm cottonoids soaked with 4% cocaine to vasoconstrict the mucosa and shrink the nasal turbinates. Usually, the dissection is done on the left side for the convenience of the right-handed surgeon. However, if

---

[1] **Editor's note:** *The transnasal portion of the operation is best done by an otolaryngologist and the intrasellar part by the neurologic surgeon. This is especially important when prior septal surgery or septorhinoplasty has been done, or if there is a significantly deviated septum.*

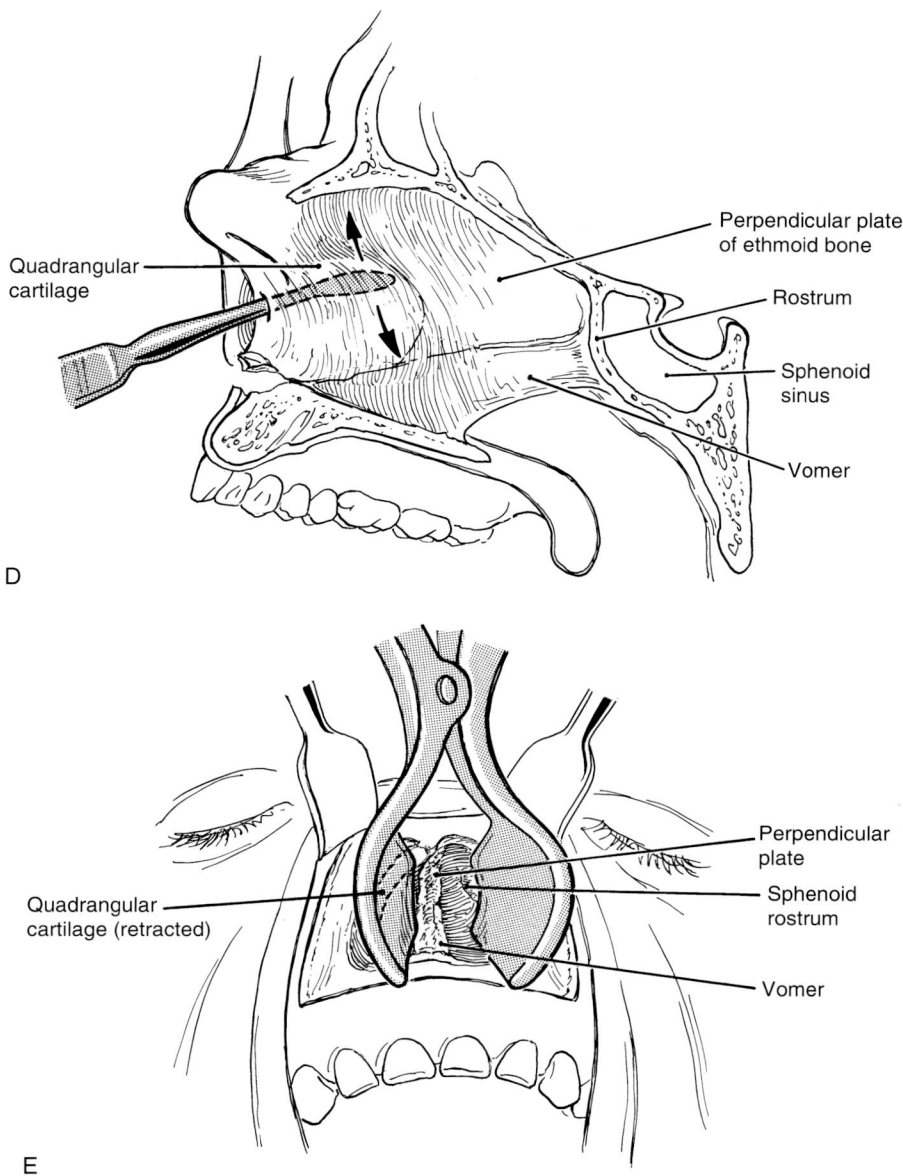

FIG. 11. *Continued.*

the septum is deviated significantly to the left, the right side should be used. Because the thigh is a sterile field, it is prepared separately. Two separate operative fields are maintained, each with a separate set of instruments that are not to be shared.

There are two variations of the transsphenoidal approach, the transseptal and the sublabial. The transseptal incision is quicker but gives a narrower exposure. It is useful when the nostril is large and the tumor is small. The sublabial incision, which the authors use exclusively, was introduced by Cushing and gives a wider exposure with better access to the superior aspect of the sella. Using a headlight for illumination, the gingival mucosa is incised from canine to canine down to the periosteum the maxilla (Fig. 11A). The mucoperiosteum is then dissected superiorly in a subperiosteal fashion to expose the pyriform aperture. The spine and any superomedial extension of the maxillary rostrum is then removed with a Kerrison rongeur as required to flatten the view of the floor of the nose (see Fig. 11B).

Bilateral inferior tunnels are made first. The mucosa is first dissected from the nasal floor up to the maxillary crest of the septum using Cottle, Woodson, and Freer elevators. Next, the quadrangular cartilage is exposed sharply in the midline by incising the mucosa with a no. 15 blade. The subperiosteal dissection then proceeds posteriorly and superiorly to free the quadrangular cartilage from the interdigitation of the septal perichondrium with the periosteum of the maxillary crest (see Fig. 11C). These connections are typically concentrated along the junctions between the crest, the vomer, and the perpendicular plate of the ethmoid. The mucoperichondrium of the septal cartilage is extended beyond its bony septal attachments. This creates an anterior submucosal tunnel. The connective tissue bands connecting the quadrangular cartilage to the superior vomer and the anterior perpendicular plates are then sharply dissected with a Freer knife (see Fig. 11D). The quadrangular cartilage is then retracted laterally to the right with the nasal speculum (see Fig. 11E). The contralateral nasal mucosa and superior aspect of the quadrangular cartilage remain intact. The mucosa of the nasal floor is elevated into the inferior meatus on each side. The perpendicular plate is fractured, removed, and saved for possible use during closure. As the final septal mucoperiosteal dissection proceeds over the vomer to the posterior termination of the nasal septum, nasal specula of increasing length are used for the exposure. Care is taken to provide wide access to the sphenoid rostrum superiorly. By preserving a small, short spike of vomer or ethmoid plate protruding from the maxillary crest, a guidepost is maintained to the midline of the nasal cavity.

The long Cottle speculum is now replaced by the Hardy retractor. Careful dissection of mucoperiosteum over the face of the sphenoid is carried down to the sphenoid sinus ostia exposes bilaterally. The ostia are opened with a Kerrison rongeur until the sphenoid face begins to change its attitude from a vertical to a horizontal plane (Fig. 12). The speculum is continuously readjusted with the help of the "persuader" to capture the sphenoid face mucosa precisely under the tips of the retractor and to prevent "ballooning" of the mucosa into the visual field. Placement of the speculum in the sphenoid sinus should be avoided because fractures may result in traction damage to the optic nerve or the carotid artery. The entire anterior wall of the sphenoid sinus is removed. In patients with a conchal sphenoid sinus, a high-speed drill is used to open the sphenoid bone using fluoroscopic monitoring. Fluoroscopy may also be useful in other patients whose bony anatomy has been similarly obscured by previous transsphenoidal surgery or rhinoplasty. The sphenoid sinus mucosa is then removed using a pituitary rongeur or Decker.

The bulge of the sella is readily appreciated, as is the floor of the optic canal and the bony prominence of the carotid arteries (Fig. 13). Often, expansile sellar masses erode through the sellar floor, and resection can begin after merely opening the anterior wall of the sphenoid sinus. The carotid arteries may erode through the bone as well, however, particularly in older, hypertensive patients. When the sellar wall is intact, it is perforated and removed using a small osteotome and Kerrison rongeurs. The sphenoid septa are also removed when present. The bony resection can be extended superiorly to the tuberculum when there is a large degree of suprasellar extension.

After the bony resection is complete, the dura is coagulated transversely with a bipolar cautery, then incised in a cruciate manner (Fig. 14). The intercavernous sinuses are often encountered at the superior and inferior margins of ex-

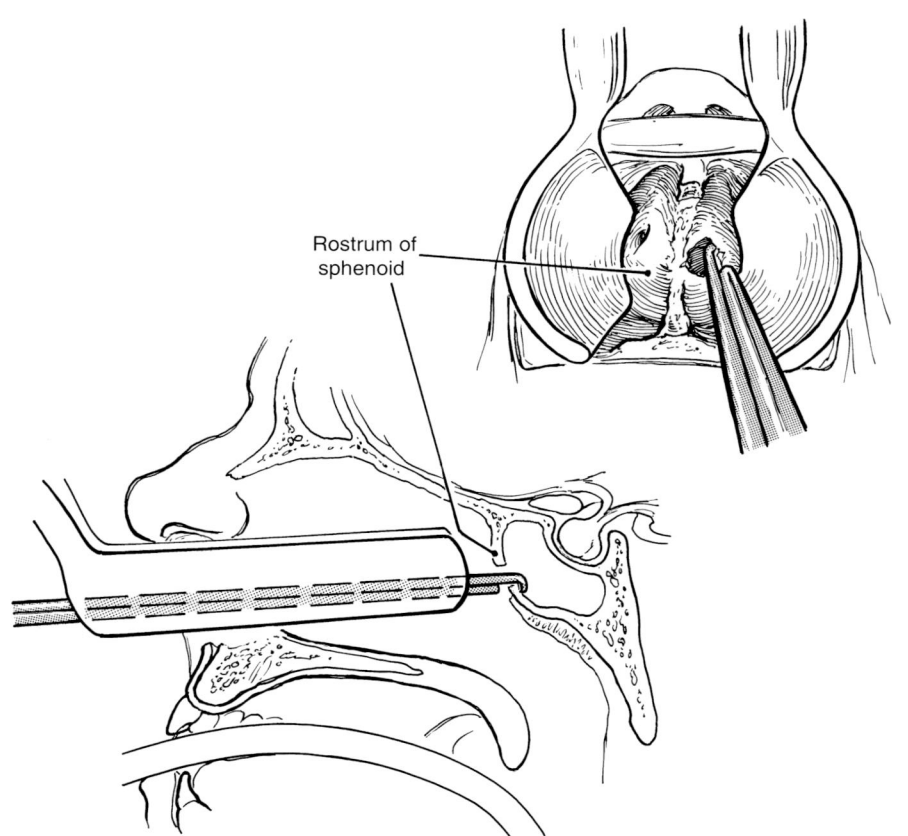

FIG. 12. The sphenoid ostia are identified and enlarged using a rongeur. The entire rostrum of the sphenoid is removed in this fashion.

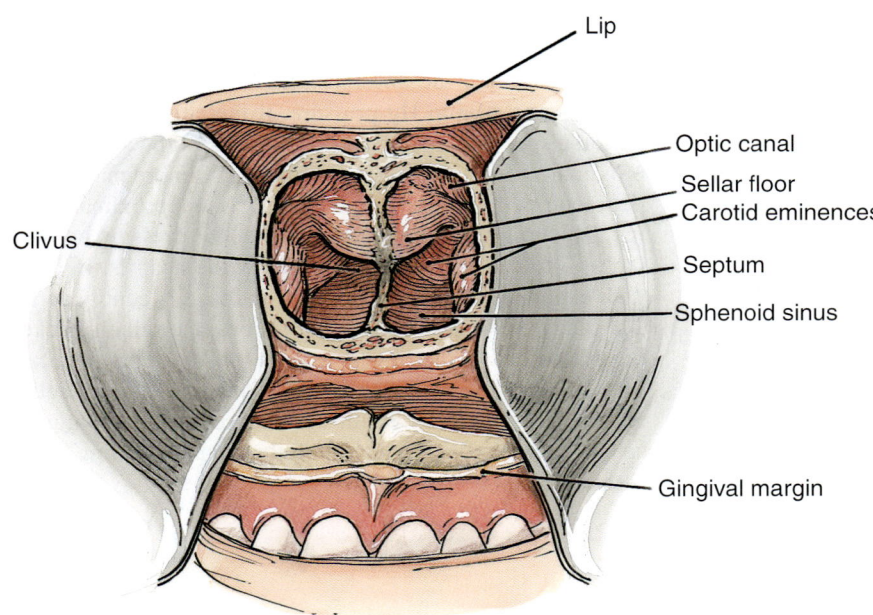

FIG. 13. Appearance of the sella after removal of the sphenoid rostrum.

posure, resulting in brisk bleeding. This is controlled by coagulating the leaves of the dura with a bipolar cautery.

Once access to the sella has been achieved, the lesion can be sampled for biopsy and gently resected using Hardy microinstruments, bayonetted ring curettes, and aspiration. Pituitary adenomas are nonencapsulated, soft, and gelatinous, with the consistency of jam, and are readily removed using this technique. Great care is taken to preserve the normal gland, which is often seen as orange-tinged tissue abutting the stalk or the posterior wall of the sella. Cystic lesions, such as craniopharyngiomas, are drained with a needle under direct visualization before resecting the solid portion of the mass. Intermittent Valsalva maneuver by the anesthesiologist or injection of saline or air through a lumbar drain expedites tumor removal by elevating the intracranial pressure, which forces the mass inferiorly. The integrity of the arachnoid is maintained, when possible, to avoid a CSF fistula.

When lesions involve only the sella or the medial cavernous sinus, the standard transsphenoidal approach is sufficient. However, when lesions extend more laterally into the cavernous sinus (Hardy grade D), exposure can be improved by enlarging the pyriform aperture or performing a medial maxillotomy contralateral to the invaded cavernous sinus (44). This allows the speculum and the resection itself to be directed laterally (Fig. 15). The medial wall of the cavernous sinus consists of a single thick layer, contiguous with the lateral layer of sellar dura. Neoplasms invading the medial cavernous sinus typically obliterate the venous sinuses and can be removed using fine ring curettes and microdissectors. These instruments can be passed around the carotid artery to

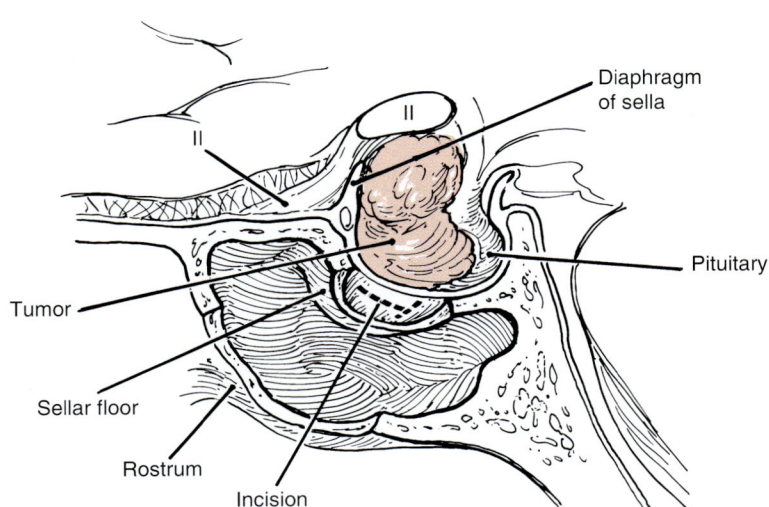

FIG. 14. After removing the sellar floor with rongeurs, the dura is opened in a cruciate fashion.

remove tumor that has extended laterally. Significant venous bleeding is usually not encountered until the patent portion of the cavernous sinus is exposed in the final phase of the resection, and is well controlled with Surgicel and direct pressure. Although this technique can often be used safely to resect neoplasm lateral to the carotid, narrowing of the caliber of the cavernous carotid on MRI suggests invasion of the vessel wall and is a relative contraindication to aggressive exploration using this technique.

After maximal resection has been completed, the sella and the pituitary gland itself are systematically inspected. If the tumor capsule prolapses into the sphenoid sinus, or there is a gross CSF leak visible, fascia lata, fat, and bone are used to reconstruct the sellar floor (Fig. 16). The fascia lata is placed in the sellar opening and sealed with fibrin glue after packing the sella with a small amount of fat or Surgicel. The fascia is then buttressed within the sella by the wedge of bony septum removed earlier. The integrity of the closure is then tested by having the anesthesiologist maintain a Valsalva maneuver at 40 mm Hg pressure. If the closure is satisfactory, the speculum is removed and the nasal mucosa is reapproximated and tamponaded using gauze impregnated with petroleum jelly. The gingival mucosa is reapproximated using 3-0 chromic suture, and a "mustache" dressing consisting of a folded gauze is placed below the nostrils. In cases with extensive CSF leaks, lumbar drainage is continued for 2 to 3 days. For large suprasellar lesions, the sella is packed regardless of whether a CSF leak is present. This is necessary because the resection may produce an "empty sella" secondarily. This may result in collapse of the diaphragma sellae and consequent traction on the chiasm, leading to decreased vision.

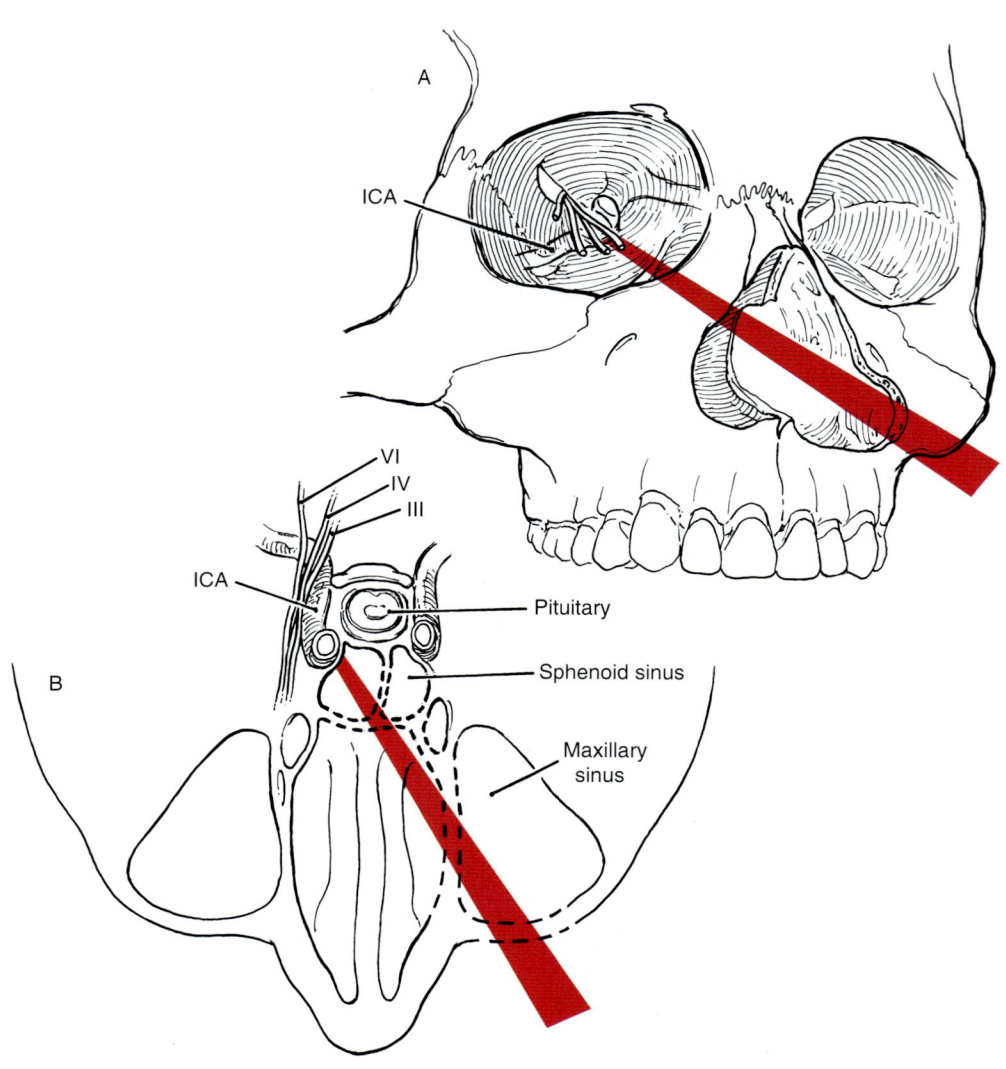

FIG. 15. The extended transsphenoidal approach for lesions extending lateral to the carotid artery (Hardy grade D). The pyriform aperture is enlarged contralateral to the lesion, facilitating improved lateral exposure of the neoplasm.

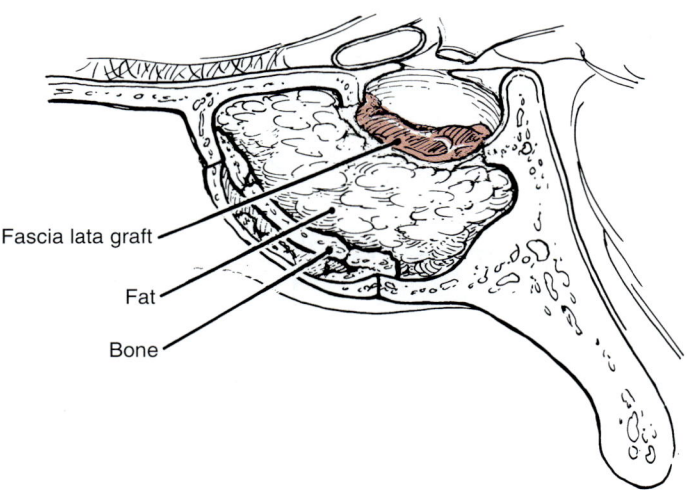

FIG. 16. Repair of cerebrospinal fluid (CSF) fistula. If a CSF leak is identified during surgery, it may be patched with fascia lata and held in place with Gelfoam or fat, tamponaded with bone.

After surgery, patients are managed in the neurosurgery step-down unit, where close attention is paid to the ophthalmologic examination and the detection of diabetes insipidus. New deficits are rare, and improvement in the visual field examination is sometimes noted early in the postoperative period. Diabetes insipidus usually does not appear before 12 to 24 hours after surgery, and polyuria is not treated unless the diagnosis of diabetes insipidus is clear: urine output greater than 300 ml/hour for 2 consecutive hours with a specific gravity less than 1.005, urine osmolarity of 50 to 150 mOsm/L, and a serum Na of at least 145 and rising. The patient is allowed to drink *ad libitum* and treated with aqueous DDAVP (vasopressin), 1 μg every 12 to 24 hours intravenously or subcutaneously as needed. In the immediate postoperative period, serum sodium and osmolarity and urine output are monitored closely. The patients are encouraged to ambulate the night of surgery, and the Foley catheter is removed after 24 hours unless diabetes insipidus makes this inconvenient. Intravenous antibiotics are continued until the nasal packing is removed on the third postoperative day, after which the patient undergoes a postoperative MRI. Patients without complications are routinely sent home on the second or third postoperative day on a tapering dose of steroids, with follow-up appointments for both the neurosurgery and endocrinology clinics.

The most frequent complications of the transsphenoidal approach are CSF leaks and damage to the carotid artery or cranial nerves. CSF leaks can usually be avoided using the techniques outlined previously. Persistent leaks are usually controlled with prolonged lumbar drainage and elevation of the head. Reoperation for repair of a CSF leak refractory to conservative management is sometimes required and is usually done using the TNTS approach. Tension pneumocephalus, a related complication, occurs because of continual accumulation of intracranial air through a dural tear with a ball-valve mechanism that prevents its egress. This is far more rare, but more deadly, and this possibility should be considered in patients whose postoperative mental status deteriorates, particularly when a lumbar drain is in place. After the lumbar drainage is discontinued, and the diagnosis is confirmed, the patient is placed on 100% oxygen. The pneumocephalus gradually resolves over several days. Tension pneumocephalus may also be decompressed with a spinal needle transnasally or transcranially in emergent circumstances.

Laceration of the intracavernous carotid is another rare but serious complication that occurs more frequently in cases requiring cavernous sinus exploration. Because of the narrowness of the field, temporary occlusion and primary repair of the carotid are impossible in the transsphenoidal approach. Lacerations are treated by holding direct pressure with Surgicel and cotton pledgets until the bleeding stops. An intraoperative angiogram should be obtained when possible to document patency of the carotid and rule out contrast extravasation. Follow-up angiograms should be obtained before discharge and at 3 months to rule out pseudoaneurysms. Cranial nerve palsies as well as lesions of the brainstem and hypothalamus are also possible, although rare. After ruling out hematoma or pneumocephalus, they are managed expectantly. Recovery is variable.

Because of the versatility and low morbidity of the TNTS approach, it can be used even in the presence of extensive suprasellar extension. When the lesion is soft (as pituitary adenomas usually are), the suprasellar mass often collapses into the sella, where it can be safely resected at the initial procedure. Occasionally, when the tumor does not descend immediately, the residual neoplasm may collapse further into the sella with time (Fig. 17), allowing the residual to be resected by repeat TNTS if further surgery is indicated.

Facial Degloving and Extended Maxillotomy Approaches

Lesions invading the superior clivus above the hard palate and medial to the carotid arteries, such as chordomas, medial chondrosarcomas, and juvenile angiofibromas can be approached using facial degloving or extended maxillotomy approaches either alone or in combination. These procedures are detailed in Chapters 11 and 12.

Transsphenoethmoidal Approach

The transsphenoethmoidal approach to the sella was introduced by Chiari (45). This option is discussed in detail in Chapter 14, and is covered here only briefly. The advantage of this approach over the transsphenoidal approach is the shorter operative distance to the sella (46). However, it requires a facial incision, provides a narrower axial exposure,

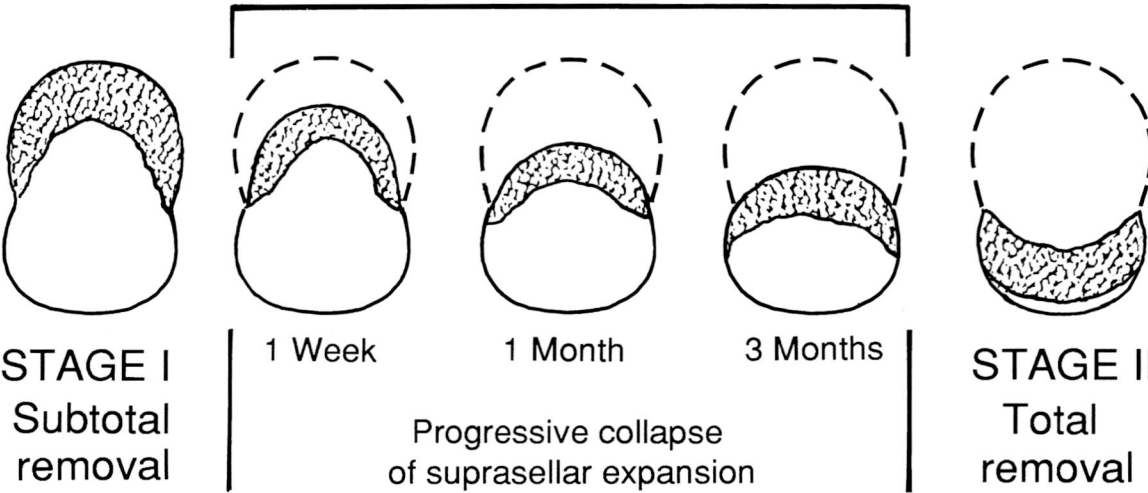

FIG. 17. Two-stage removal of pituitary macroadenoma with suprasellar extension. (Adapted from ref. 43, with permission).

and carries a risk of injury to the optic nerve. One version combines this with medial maxillectomy for improved axial exposure of the sella (47). However, this combination holds little benefit over maxillotomy with midface degloving, which has a lower risk and superior cosmesis.

A 3-cm incision is made along the medial border of the nose, beginning from the inferior margin of the eyebrow, and the lacrimal sac is retracted laterally. The anterior ethmoid artery is sacrificed, and the lamina papyracea over the lacrimal fossa is removed, as is the underlying middle turbinate. The ethmoid mucosa is removed to identify the sphenoid ostia. The anterior and posterior walls of the sphenoid are then removed to expose the sella. The operation then proceeds as in the standard TNTS approach.

Transcranial–Intradural Approaches

The indications for transcranial–intradural approaches to the sella consist primarily of patients for whom transsphenoidal surgery is contraindicated for reasons discussed previously. Lesions invading the cavernous sinus laterally, with secondary sellar invasion; lesions that frankly violate the dura; and residual suprasellar or lateral cavernous sinus lesions that could have been only partially resected from the transsphenoidal approach are additional indications for transcranial approaches. In addition, repair of CSF leaks may also require a transcranial approach.

There are several possible transcranial approaches to the sella turcica, but the most useful are the transbasal, pterional, and subtemporal approaches (see Fig. 9). The choice of approach is determined by the location of the lesion with respect to the sella, and to some extent by the personal preference of the surgeon. These approaches are described in other chapters (Chapters 20, 18, and 24, respectively), and are discussed briefly in the following sections specifically in terms of their utility for the resection of sellar and parasellar lesions.

Transbasal Approach

The transbasal approaches to the sella are versions of the anterior subcranial approach. A unilateral or bilateral frontal craniotomy is performed with or without orbitofrontal craniotomy. The tuberculum sellae is removed anterior to the chiasm with a high-speed drill (Fig. 18). This minimizes the effect of a prefixed chiasm, when present, and gives the surgeon an unobstructed view of the sella between the optic nerves with minimal brain retraction. In contrast to the other transcranial approaches, the pituitary stalk is easily identified and avoided, as are the carotid arteries and their branches. This approach is particularly useful for extradural lesions such as esthesioneuroblastomas and craniopharyngiomas, as well as for tuberculum sellae and olfactory groove meningiomas with secondary sellar involvement. There is a high risk of anosmia due to avulsion of the olfactory nerves with this approach, as well as a small risk of optic nerve or carotid injury. Frontal lobe swelling can usually be avoided by proper positioning, lumbar drainage, and minimizing brain retraction.

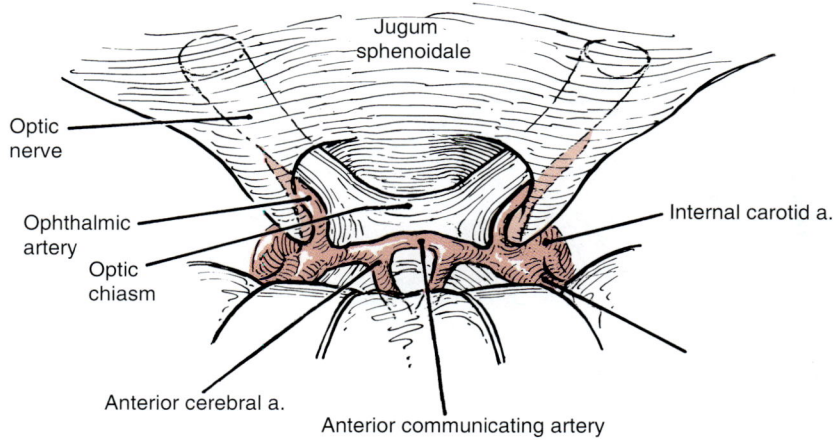

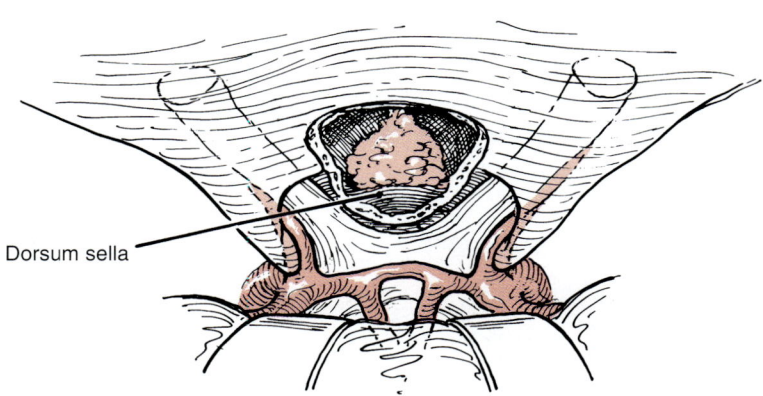

FIG. 18. The subfrontal approach to the sella turcica. The tuberculum sellae is removed with a high-speed drill to facilitate exposure of a suprasellar mass.

Pterional Approach

The pterional approach is the shortest route to the parasellar region. This is usually done on the side of either the greatest tumor extension, or the patient's worst vision. If neither of these are considerations, the craniotomy is done on the nondominant side. After performing a standard pterional craniotomy, the sphenoid ridge lateral to the superior orbital fissure is removed extradurally with a high-speed drill. The sylvian fissure is widely split and the frontal and temporal lobes are gently retracted to maximize exposure of the sellar region, and the anterior clinoid process is drilled away (Fig. 19). This gives excellent exposure of lateral parasellar lesions such as meningiomas or eccentric pituitary macroadenomas spilling into the middle fossa. Access to the sella itself, however, is somewhat impeded by the optic nerve, third cranial nerve, and carotid artery, which lie in the surgeon's line of sight. In addition, the contralateral optic nerve may be poorly visualized. The risks of this approach include damage to the carotid artery as well as the optic and third cranial nerves.

Subtemporal Approach

The subtemporal approach gives superior access to the posterior aspect of the sella, including the posterior clinoid process and the top of the clivus. It is most useful for lesions with retrochiasmatic extension such as chordomas and chondrosarcomas of the uppermost clivus, as well as meningiomas in that region. The approach begins with the standard pterional craniotomy. Aggressive temporal bone resection is used to minimize brain retraction. A zygomatic osteotomy may further enhance exposure. After opening the dura, the sylvian fissure is widely split, and the median temporal lobe is retracted laterally to reach the upper clivus and posterior clinoid process. The disadvantage of this approach is that the

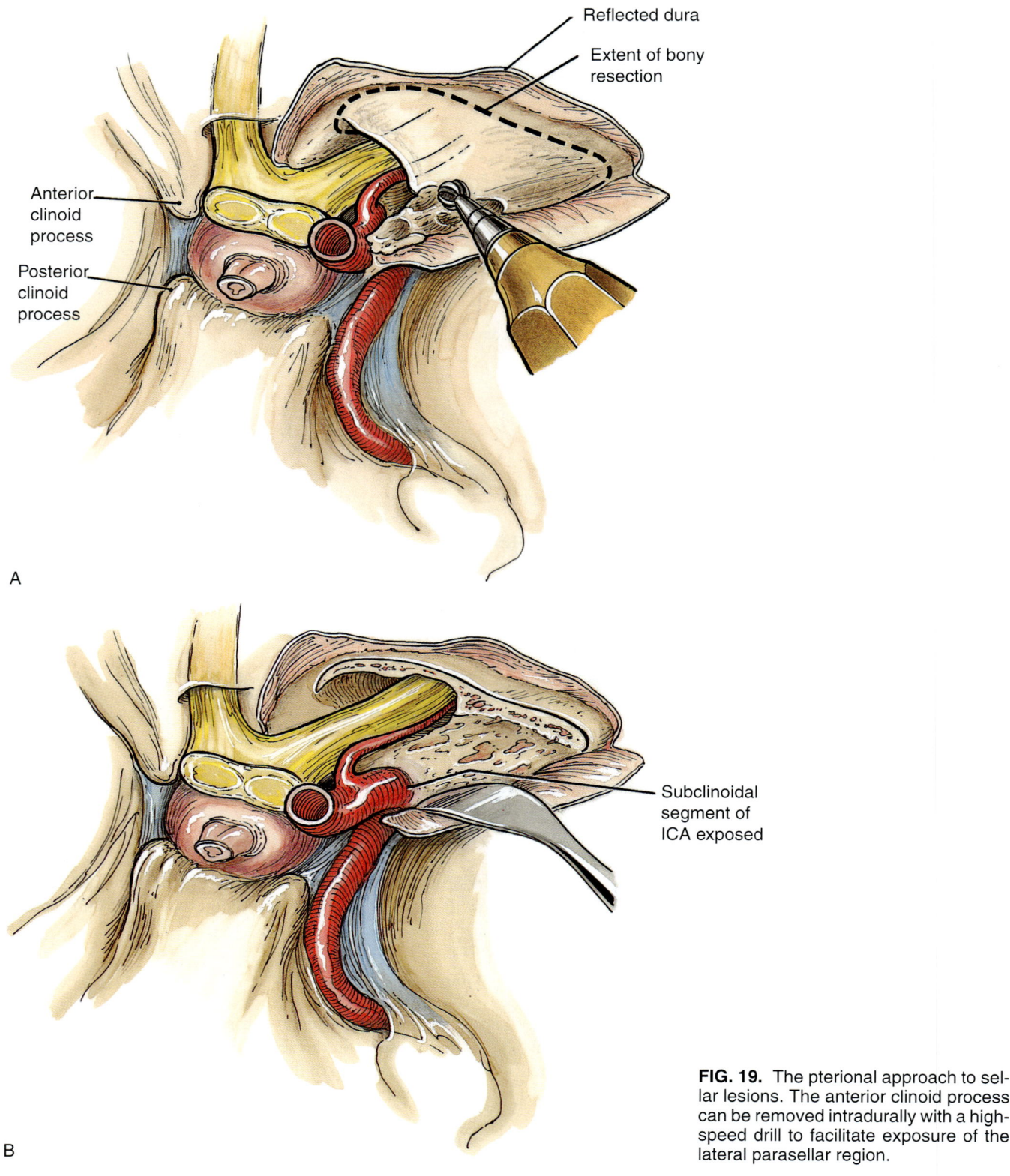

FIG. 19. The pterional approach to sellar lesions. The anterior clinoid process can be removed intradurally with a high-speed drill to facilitate exposure of the lateral parasellar region.

ipsilateral third and fourth cranial nerves are interposed between the surgeon's line of sight and the sella. In addition, visualization of the contralateral posterior cerebral artery (PCA) and superior cerebellar artery (SCA) is poor. The major risk of this approach is temporal lobe damage due to excessive retraction.

The aforementioned three approaches can also be combined.

Adjunctive Surgical Techniques: Frameless Stereotaxy

The authors have also employed frameless stereotactic devices extensively for complex cases. This has been useful for intraoperative determination of the trajectory required for resection of certain skull base lesions, allowing the exposure to be optimized. It is also useful for intraoperative confirmation of the limits of resection and for determining the proximity of critical neurovascular structures in regions with distorted anatomy. Although brain "shift" after the dura is opened (48) limits the accuracy of this technique for deep intraparenchymal lesions, this technique is accurate for localizing skull base lesions.

TREATMENT

Pituitary Adenomas

The goals of treatment for patients with pituitary adenomas are to remove the mass effect (if present) and to normalize or restore hormonal function. Endocrinologically inactive microadenomas are usually discovered incidentally and rarely require treatment. The treatment of endocrinologically active microadenomas depends on their endocrine activity. Pharmacologic therapy has proven useful for shrinking some of these adenomas and reducing excess hormone levels. However, none of these cytotoxic agents is curative, and symptoms usually resume shortly after the drug is discontinued. Surgery, particularly through the transsphenoidal approach, is effective and relatively benign, and remains the mainstay of therapy for most pituitary adenomas other than prolactinomas. Radiation therapy has a delayed effect and is complicated by damage to the optic nerves and hypothalamic–pituitary axis as well as by radiation necrosis. Impaired mental status and radiation-induced tumors have also been described. Focused-beam radiation therapy is useful in patients with recurrent or residual tumor, or poor operative candidates whose tumors cannot be controlled with medical therapy. The treatment of specific subtypes of pituitary adenoma is addressed in the following sections.

Prolactinomas

The treatment of prolactinomas remains controversial. Medical therapy with bromocriptine, an ergot derivative, not only shrinks the tumor but also decreases prolactin synthesis and release (49), and is considered first-line therapy for most prolactinomas. This produces relief of symptoms, including galactorrhea and amenorrhea, and can restore fertility. Although accelerated tumor growth can occur during pregnancy, this is rarely significant in microprolactinomas. There have been no teratogenic effects reported from use of bromocriptine to achieve conception. The drug can be discontinued during pregnancy, then reinstituted after delivery. Patients with microprolactinomas desiring fertility can also be treated with transsphenoidal surgery. Surgical cure and subsequent fertility has been reported in 83% of patients (50). Surgery is also indicated for patients with macroadenomas with persistent mass effect despite maximal tolerated dose of bromocriptine; patients who are noncompliant, have serious side effects from bromocriptine, or do not want to continue medical therapy; and women with macroprolactinomas desirous of pregnancy. Preoperative prolactin levels correlate both with tumor size and operative success: surgical cure is achieved in 70% of patients with preoperative prolactin levels of 200 to 500 ng/ml, and 14% of patients with prolactin levels over 1000 ng/ml (51).

Bromocriptine is useful for treatment of residual or recurrent prolactinomas in patients who are poor surgical candidates. One caveat is that bromocriptine induces tumor fibrosis, which makes resection difficult and reduces the surgical cure rate by approximately half (52,53). Radiation therapy is effective at relieving symptoms and reducing prolactin levels. However, because of the effectiveness of surgery and pharmacotherapy for this disorder, radiation therapy is rarely indicated. It is reserved for symptomatic patients with recurrent or residual tumor who are not surgical candidates and are unable or unwilling to control their tumor using bromocriptine.

Growth Hormone-Secreting Adenomas

Excess growth hormone secretion produces not only the visibly obvious deformities of giganticism or acromegaly but also results in severe, systemic metabolic effects that result in a significant decrease in life expectancy. These include atherosclerosis, cardiomyopathy, cerebrovascular disease, respiratory disease, and diseases of the muscles, joints, and peripheral nerves. Thus, the goals for managing growth hormone-secreting adenomas are normalization of growth hormone and somatomedin C levels, in addition to elimination of mass effect.

Two agents have been used for medical therapy of growth hormone-secreting adenomas: bromocriptine and somatostatin. Bromocriptine decreases growth hormone production in 74% of patients, but normalizes levels in only 20% (54). Shrinkage occurs only in isolated cases (55) and requires higher doses of bromocriptine than those used for prolactinomas. These tumors probably represent mixed prolactin cell/growth hormone cell adenomas.

More recently, octreotide, a somatostatin analog, has demonstrated its effectiveness in suppressing growth hormone levels to below 5 mg/ml in 50% of patients, and less than 2 mg/ml in 25% of patients (56). However, this drug must be given by subcutaneous injection two to three times per day, making it suitable only for intelligent, highly motivated patients who can administer the injections themselves. Because of the inconvenience and morbidity of medical treatment, and the effectiveness of surgery in curing most of these patients (57,58), pharmacologic therapy is reserved for patients who are poor surgical candidates or those with recurrent or residual disease who are unwilling or unable to undergo reoperation. Radiation therapy is reserved for patients in whom an endocrinologic cure cannot be achieved by surgery combined with medical therapy.

Adrenocorticotropic Hormone-Secreting Adenomas

In contrast to hyperprolactinomas, the endocrinopathy of Cushing's disease is life threatening. When untreated, the 5-year mortality rate is 50%; thus, the goal of therapy must be endocrinologic cure. Because most corticotropic adenomas are microadenomas, radiologic diagnosis by gadolinium-enhanced MRI is achieved in only 40% to 60% of cases. When a pituitary mass is noted by MRI of the sella, or suggested by diagnostic petrosal sinus sampling in the absence of pulmonary or adrenal lesions on radiologic examination of the thorax and abdomen, transsphenoidal surgery is almost always the treatment of choice. Tumor noted on MRI is usually easily found and resected, while sparing the normal gland. Systematic exploration and sectioning of the gland is indicated to locate radiographically occult adenomas. Usually, several deep vertical and horizontal incisions are made in the gland to find the abnormal tissue. This technique is often successful. When it is not, a total hypophysectomy is usually recommended for older adults, from whom consent should be obtained for this eventuality before surgery. Children and young adults in whom no tumor is found are treated conservatively with medical management and reimaging before further surgery or radiosurgery. However, hypophysectomy is sometimes required by the severity of the endocrinopathy. Resection of the central "mucoid wedge" has also been reported (46,59). Unilateral hypophysectomy is also an option in patients with occult ACTH-secreting adenomas that have been localized to one side by petrosal sinus sampling (35). Surgical cure has been reported in 90% of microadenomas and 65% of macroadenomas using this technique, with a recurrence rate of 8.5% (60). Successfully treated patients have had an immediate fall in blood cortisol levels with gradual resolution of cushingoid features.

In patients who are refractory to surgical cure, or who are poor operative candidates, pharmacologic treatment or radiation therapy can be used to achieve endocrinologic control. Medical therapy consists primarily of agents that pharmacologically block adrenal steroidogenesis. Ketoconazole is the most useful of these and has been used to stabilize severely ill patients as a preparation for surgery or radiation therapy (61). Other pharmacologic agents such as metyrapone (62), cyproheptadine, a serotonin inhibitor (63), aminoglutethemide, and mitotane (64) have been used to control serum cortisol levels with variable degrees of success.

The delayed effect of radiation therapy makes this modality inadequate as the primary treatment. However, radiation is reported to control disease in 50% to 70% of patients by 3 years (33,65). This makes it useful as adjuvant treatment when combined with pharmacologic treatment in patients who are poor operative candidates or have persistent or recurrent disease. Bilateral adrenalectomy is immediately effective in curing hypercortisolism, but because of the severe metabolic consequences and the possibility of inducing Nelson's syndrome in patients with occult pituitary adenomas, this procedure is reserved as a last resort in most patients.

Although pituitary adenomas producing Nelson's syndrome are usually macroadenomas and easily visualized, they are characteristically invasive and difficult to cure. Normalization of ACTH and hyperpigmentation occur in less than half the cases (66). Although data are sparse, there is some suggestion that radiation therapy may be somewhat helpful in patients with Nelson's syndrome.

Thyrotropic Adenomas

Thyrotropic adenomas are the least common adenomas, accounting for less than 1% of all pituitary adenomas. They can be microadenomas but often are invasive macroadenomas, particularly in patients who have undergone thyroid ablation. Surgical excision is the treatment of choice and can be achieved in most microadenomas. The surgical cure rate for invasive macroadenomas is only about 40% (67). Octreotide has been reported to reduce TSH levels but does not significantly reduce mass effect, and adjuvant radiation therapy should be used in these cases.

Endocrinologically Inactive Adenomas

Endocrinologically inactive adenomas consist of null cell adenomas and gonadotropin-producing adenomas, which do not produce symptoms of excess endocrine secretion. These collectively account for 25% of all pituitary adenomas. Patients typically present with macroadenomas with mass effect, although they may present with symptoms of mild hyperprolactinemia due to stalk compression. Symptoms of hypopituitarism are often more evident. The goal of surgery is reduction of mass effect, and the treatment of choice is surgery. Although gross total resection is the surgeon's intuitive goal, the fact that these tumors occur mainly in the elderly and are slow growing with a high incidence of cavernous sinus invasion suggest that therapy be individualized. The transsphenoidal approach is usually the procedure of choice, and near-total to gross-total resection can usually be achieved, although microscopic invasion is usually present (68). Vision improves or stabilizes in over 90% of these patients (69), and headache and cranial nerve palsies due to cavernous sinus compression often resolve. The patients presenting with panhypopituitarism seldom regain normal pituitary function (70), and they require long-term hormonal therapy. Bromocriptine may decrease prolactin levels through a direct effect on the hypothalamic–pituitary axis. However, it does not shrink these tumors and has no role in the treatment of mass effect. Adjuvant radiation therapy has been advocated by some. However, given the benign nature of these neoplasms, their slow growth rate, and the success of reoperative surgery, the authors prefer conservative management, or "watchful waiting," of any residual tumor. If the tumor grows, consideration is given to reoperation before instituting radiation therapy.

Giant Adenomas

The management of giant adenomas is both complex and controversial. These are usually a subset of endocrinologically inactive adenomas presenting with mass effect and obstructive hydrocephalus. Giant adenomas producing prolactin and other hormones have also been reported. Treatment is surgical, but these patients tend to do poorly with a high incidence of morbidity, and a 20% mortality rate (7,71). The pathophysiology of this phenomenon is unclear, but it is thought to be due to exacerbated hydrocephalus, seemingly related either to tumor swelling after an incomplete resection, or due to a traction effect on the third ventricle. These tumors should be managed conservatively, with debulking through a transsphenoidal approach. Ventriculostomy can be done before or during surgery if hydrocephalus is present. Complete resection is rarely required or achieved. Regional radiation therapy may be useful in poor operative candidates.

Apoplexy

Pituitary apoplexy is a clinical emergency requiring urgent surgical decompression of the sella and parasellar structures, usually through a transsphenoidal approach.

Pituitary Carcinoma

Pituitary carcinoma is rare, with less than 40 cases reported (72). They appear to arise from pituitary adenomas of all types, although endocrinologically active adenomas predominate. They typically present with multiple local recurrences followed by metastatic dissemination to the subarachnoid space or extraneuronal sites such as bone, liver, lymph node, lung, or kidney. This is usually accompanied by an escalation of histologic grade. The most symptomatic region is usually the sella, and the therapy is directed at control of the primary neoplasm. Aggressive reoperation is used with adjuvant radiation therapy and pharmacologic therapy as indicated by the characteristics of the original adenoma (66). In most cases, death from pituitary carcinoma results from a failure of local control with progressive local invasion, rather than from metastatic disease.

Tumors of the Posterior Pituitary

Granular cell tumors, or choristomas, are usually benign and asymptomatic, although malignant transformation has been reported. Symptomatic granular cell tumors most often present with visual disturbance, although hypopituitarism, hyperprolactinemia, precocious puberty, and acromegaly also occur. Diabetes insipidus is rare. Transsphenoidal surgery is usually indicated for diagnosis and resection. There is no evidence that these tumors are radiosensitive (13).

Management of metastatic lesions is more complex. Although most metastases to the neurohypophysis are asymptomatic, metastases to the stalk may present with hypopituitarism or mass effect (13). Treatment is palliative, and consists of surgery, radiation therapy, chemotherapy, or combinations of these modalities depending on the need for tissue confirmation, tumor type, and the medical condition of the patient. Usually, metastases are amenable to excision using the transsphenoidal approach if this is clinically indicated, and surgery can prolong survival.

Craniopharyngiomas

Craniopharyngiomas are among the most challenging tumors to treat. Although they are slow growing, benign, extraaxial neoplasms, some consider them malignant by virtue of location. Their tenacious attachment to pial vessels and critical neurovascular structures increases the morbidity of aggressive resection. Yet, the high recurrence rate and consequent morbidity after subtotal resection make this option equally distasteful.

The presenting symptoms depend on the size and location of the tumor. Craniopharyngiomas present with mass effect and symptoms of increased intracranial pressure in 80% of children, and with visual symptoms in 80% of adults. Endocrine dysfunction, including partial or complete hypopituitarism and diabetes insipidus, occurs in most patients of all ages, although it is usually not the presenting symptom.

Craniopharyngiomas are classified as endosellar, suprasellar, or intraventricular based on their position relative to the sella, chiasm, and third ventricle (73). Endosellar craniopharyngiomas are subdiaphragmatic and confined to the sella. They comprise 3% to 8% of craniopharyngiomas (74). Suprasellar craniopharyngiomas arise from the midportion of the stalk and typically enlarge beneath the third ventricle, elevating the third ventricular floor. Intraventricular craniopharyngiomas arise from the infundibulum. They invade the floor of the third ventricle and often extend into the interpeduncular fossa. The latter two types are considered retrochiasmatic craniopharyngiomas.

There is general agreement that surgery is the treatment of

choice for craniopharyngiomas. However, the choice of approaches, the extent of resection, and the use of adjuvant radiation therapy remain controversial. The difficulty is that these tumors recur unless gross total resection is achieved, and many believe that the initial operation represents the only opportunity for cure. However, the tumor capsule is tenaciously attached to vital structures such as the optic chiasm, optic tract, infundibulum, pituitary, hypothalamus, third ventricle, and the vessels that supply these critical structures. Despite advances in microsurgical technique, aggressive resection of these densely adherent tumors has resulted in a high rate of neurovascular and endocrine complications. Even in experienced hands, the mortality rate for primary craniopharyngiomas has been reported to be as high as 8% to 15%, with varying degrees of visual compromise in 50% to 60% of patients, and 80% of patients require postoperative endocrine replacement (75,76). This morbidity is thought to result from devascularization of critical structures due to aggressive resection of tumor capsule. Thus, it is preferable to leave densely adherent capsule attached to critical neurovascular structures rather than pursue more aggressive resection that may lead to unacceptable morbidity.

The choice of surgical approach depends on the location, shape, and size of the tumor. Endosellar lesions with an enlarged sella and a prominent cystic component can be safely approached through the transsphenoidal route. Because of their subdiaphragmatic position, these tumors are not attached to the hypothalamus or optic chiasm. After draining the cystic component under direct vision, the intracapsular contents are removed with a grasping forceps and curettes. The capsule collapses and can be detached from the undersurface of the diaphragma sellae. Normal preoperative pituitary function is a relative contraindication to the transsphenoidal approach because the gland is often situated anteriorly within the sella and damaged during tumor resection. The stalk can usually be preserved.

Suprasellar craniopharyngiomas are best resected using transcranial approaches. If hydrocephalus is present, ventricular drainage should be instituted before definitive therapy. The most useful approaches are the pterional and the subfrontal. Both have the advantage of allowing direct visualization of the optic nerve and chiasm. The pterional approach is the shortest and offers superior visualization of the retrochiasmatic region. The subfrontal approach provides better visualization of the optic pathways by way of the subchiasmatic pathway, as well as a midline route to the lamina terminalis. The opticocarotid pathway may also be useful. In addition, access to the sella can be achieved by removing the tuberculum sellae with a high-speed drill.

Intraventricular craniopharyngiomas are best approached by the subfrontal–lamina terminalis approach, the interhemispheric–transcallosal approach, or a combination of these. The subfrontal–lamina terminalis approach allows direct visualization of the chiasm and permits good access to the anterior third ventricle. However, this approach also carries the greatest risk of hypothalamic damage. The interhemispheric–transcallosal approach utilizes the foramina of Monro, which are usually enlarged due to hydrocephalus, to resect the intraventricular portion of the tumor. Alternately, if the foramina of Monro is not enlarged, the interforniceal approach may be used. Although the latter two approaches minimize the risk of devascularizing the hypothalamus, they carry the risk of bilateral forniceal damage and consequent memory impairment. Because these approaches give access only to intraventricular tumor, they are often combined with pterional or subfrontal approaches. The transcortical approach is associated with a high risk of hydrocephalus and postoperative seizures, in addition to the aforementioned risk of bilateral forniceal injury, and should be avoided except in cases of marked preoperative ventricular dilatation.

In all approaches, the presence of a subarachnoid plane facilitates complete resection and preservation of the normal vasculature. Electrocautery often disrupts this interface and should be avoided whenever possible. Although radiation therapy has been effective in reducing recurrence and increasing survival in some series with minimal morbidity (77), the risks of radiation therapy have prompted the authors to follow patients with serial examination and imaging studies, and individualize treatment of recurrence.

Meningiomas

Usually, parasellar meningiomas are large, and present predominantly with mass effect. Visual loss is the predominant symptom. Pituitary insufficiency is uncommon and usually mild. Because resection of parasellar meningiomas requires resection of the dura itself, an intradural approach is required for complete resection. The choice of approach is governed by the location and orientation of the lesion. Meningiomas of the tuberculum sellae, olfactory groove, and anterior clinoids are best approached through a subfrontal approach. Meningiomas of the medial sphenoid wing and cavernous sinus require a pterional approach, whereas retrochiasmal meningiomas are usually best resected using the subtemporal approach. The transsphenoidal approach may be indicated for diagnostic biopsy.

Chordomas

Chordomas of the sella typically present with symptoms of mass effect and hypopituitarism depending on their size and direction of growth. Occasional small tumors confined to the sella can be resected through the transsphenoidal approach alone. At the end of such an operation, the clivus should be drilled beyond the obvious tumor margin because of invasion within cancellous lumen. A tumor-free margin of well vascularized bone should be observed. The clival dura should be exposed and prolapse freely into the bony defect. However, most chordomas involve parasellar structures as well. Because gross total resection is associated with increased survival (16), such patients require a more extensive extradural or transcranial approach than can be achieved by the transsphenoidal approach alone. An extended transsphenoidal, transmaxillary, or transoral approach may be required to maximize exposure in these cases. There are some studies suggesting that adjuvant proton-beam radiation therapy may also prolong survival (78).

Nonneoplastic Cysts

Rathke's cleft cysts, mucoceles, and arachnoid cysts are the most common nonneoplastic cysts of the sella. They are usually asymptomatic. Occasionally, however, patients do present with symptoms of mass effect, hypopituitarism, or mild hyperprolactinemia due to stalk compression. Suprasellar extension may occasionally produce visual loss or hypothalamic dysfunction. Transsphenoidal decompression of the cyst, or marsupialization, without excision of the cyst wall is usually curative.

Inflammatory and Infectious Lesions

Inflammatory Lesions

Lymphocytic hypophysitis, Langerhans' cell histiocytosis, giant cell granuloma, and sarcoidosis are the most common inflammatory lesions of the sella turcica. These sellar lesions are often indistinguishable from pituitary adenoma on MRI. Transsphenoidal biopsy is required for diagnosis, but radical resection is rarely indicated. Lymphocytic hypophysitis typically presents with mass effect, symptoms of moderate hyperprolactinemia, and varying degrees of hypopituitarism, although diabetes insipidus is unusual. At surgery, the adenohypophysis is yellow, rubbery, and firm, and the inflammatory mass frequently extends into the suprasellar region. Patients are started on hormonal replacement and treated with steroids.

Langerhans' cell histiocytosis (histiocytosis X) of the sella usually presents with diabetes insipidus because of its preferential involvement of the stalk and posterior pituitary gland. Mild to moderate hypopituitarism may also be present. These lesions should be resected. Adjuvant radiation therapy has also been used (13).

Granulomatous lesions such as giant cell granuloma and sarcoidosis present with hypopituitarism and, occasionally, hyperprolactinemia. Sarcoidosis may also produce mass effect, diabetes insipidus, and even hypothalamic dysfunction. After biopsy to exclude infectious processes, they are treated conservatively with endocrine replacement, if required, and steroids.

Infectious Lesions

Abscesses of the pituitary typically present with symptoms of mass effect and moderate to severe hypopituitarism. In the setting of meningitis, this diagnosis should always be considered. The transsphenoidal approach is used to debulk and to obtain a diagnostic specimen for aerobic, anaerobic, acid-fast, and fungal cultures. Patients are then treated with the appropriate antibiotic, antituberculous, or antifungal agents.

Vascular Lesions

Aneurysms and carotid cavernous fistulas of the infraclinoid or cavernous carotid may present with a clinical picture indistinguishable from that of an endocrinologically inactive pituitary adenoma. Visual deficit, mild hyperprolactinemia, and hypopituitarism are common. Fortunately, the diagnosis is readily made by MRI, magnetic resonance angiography, or conventional angiography. The treatment of aneurysms and carotid–cavernous fistulas is beyond the scope of this chapter.

REFERENCES

1. Renn WH, Rhoton AL Jr. Microsurgical anatomy of the sellar region. *J Neurosurg* 1975;43:288–298.
2. Tindall GT, Barrow DL, eds. *Disorders of the pituitary.* St. Louis: Mosby, 1986.
3. Lang R. Anatomy of the sellar region. In: Samii M, Draf W, eds. *Surgery of the skull base: an interdisciplinary approach.* Berlin: Springer-Verlag, 1989:27–35.
4. Annegers JF, Coulam CB, Abboud CF, et al. Pituitary adenomas in Olmsted County, Minnesota, 1935–1977. *Mayo Clin Proc* 1978;53: 641–643.
5. Costello RT. Subclinical adenoma of the pituitary gland. *Am J Pathol* 1936;12:205–216.
6. Hardy J. Transsphenoidal microsurgery of the normal and pathologic pituitary. *Clin Neurosurg* 1969;16:185–217.
7. Symon L, Jakubowski J, Kendall B. Surgical treatment of giant pituitary adenomas. *J Neurol Neurosurg Psychiatry* 1979;42:973–982.
8. Wilson CB. Neurosurgical management of large and invasive pituitary tumors. In: Tindall GT, Collins R, eds. *Clinical management of pituitary disorders.* New York: Raven Press, 1979:334–342.
9. Ridgeway EC, Klibanski A, Ladenson PW, et al. Pure alpha-secreting adenomas. *N Engl J Med* 1981;304:1254–1259.
10. Kovacs K, Horvath E. Tumors of the pituitary gland. In: *Atlas of tumor pathology.* 2nd series, fascicle 21. Washington, DC: Armed Forces Institute of Pathology, 1986.
11. Scheithauer BW, Kovacs K, Laws ER Jr. The pathology of invasive pituitary tumors with special reference to their functional classification. *J Neurosurg* 1986;65:733–744.
12. Luse SA, Kernohan JW. Granular cell tumors of the stalk and posterior lobe of the pituitary gland. *Cancer* 1955;8:616–622.
13. Albrecht S, Bilbao JM, Kovacs K. Nonpituitary tumors of the sellar region. In: Melmed S, ed. *The pituitary.* New York: Blackwell Science, 1995:591–676.
14. Canbas B, Akar N, Ciplak G, et al. Tumors of the sellar-parasellar region: analysis of 238 cases. In: Samii M, ed. *Skull base surgery.* Basel: Karger, 1992:317–320.
15. Grisoli F, Vincentelli F, Raybaud C, et al. Intrasellar meningioma. *Surg Neurol* 1983;20:36–41.
16. Gay E, Sekhar LN, Rubinstein E, et al. Chordomas and chondrosarcomas of the cranial base: results and follow-up of 60 patients. *Neurosurgery* 1995;56:887–897.
17. Mathews W, Wilson CB. Ectopic intrasellar chordoma. *J Neurosurg* 1974;40:260–263.
18. Max MB, Deck MDF, Rottenberg DA. Pituitary metastasis: incidence in cancer patients and clinical differentiation from pituitary adenoma. *Neurology* 1981;31:998–1002.
19. Roessmann U, Kaufmann B, Friede RL. Metastatic lesions in the sella turcica and pituitary gland. *Cancer* 1970;25:478–480.

20. Branch CL, Laws ER. Metastatic tumors of the sella turcica masquerading as primary pituitary tumors. *J Clin Endocrinol Metab* 1987;65:469–474.
21. Buchmann E, Schweisinger G. Hypophyse und Hamoblastosen. *Zentralbl Neurochir* 1979;40:35–40.
22. Shanklin WM. On the presence of cysts in the human pituitary. *Anat Rec* 1949;104:379–407.
23. Lee JH, Laws ER Jr, Guthrie BL, et al. Lymphocytic hypophysitis: occurrence in two men. *Neurosurgery* 1994;34:159–163.
24. Nishio S, Mizuno J, Barrow DL, et al. Isolated histiocytosis X of the pituitary gland. *Neurosurgery* 1987:21:718–721.
25. Taylon C, Duff TA. Giant cell granuloma involving the pituitary gland. *J Neurosurg* 1980;52:584–587.
26. Stern BJ, Krumholtz A, Johns C, et al. Sarcoidosis and its neurological manifestations. *Arch Neurol* 1985;42:909–917.
27. Berger SA, Edberg SC, David G. Infectious disease in the sella turcica. *Rev Infect Dis* 1986;8:747–755.
28. Domingue JN, Wilson CB. Pituitary abscesses: report of seven cases and review of the literature. *J Neurosurg* 1977;46:601–608.
29. Ramos-Gabatin A, Jordan RM. Primary pituitary aspergillosis responding to transphenoidal surgery and combined therapy with amphotericin-B and 5-fluoro-cytosine: case report. *J Neurosurg* 1981;54:839–841.
30. Del Brutto OH, Guevar J, Sotelo J. Intrasellar cysticercosis. *J Neurosurg* 1988;69:58–60.
31. Osgen T, Bertan V, Kansu T, et al. Intrasellar hydatid cyst: case report. *Neurosurgery* 1984;60:647–648.
32. Martin JB. Management of hypersecretory pituitary adenomas. *Clin Neurosurg* 1980;27:99–247.
33. Orth DN, Liddle CW. Results of treatment in 108 patients with Cushing's syndrome. *N Engl J Med* 1971;285:243.
34. Wilson CB. Role of surgery in the management of pituitary tumors. *Neurosurg Clin North Am* 1990;1:139–159.
35. Benoit R, Pearson-Murphy BE, Robert F, et al. Hyperthyroidism due to a pituitary TSH secreting tumor with amenorrhea–galactorrhea. *Clin Endocrinol* 1980;12:11–14.
36. Melmed S, ed. *The pituitary*. New York: Blackwell Science, 1995.
37. Ciric I, Mikhael M, Stafford T, Lawson L, Grarces R. Transsphenoidal management of pituitary macroadenomas with long term follow-up results. *J Neurosurg* 1982; 59:395–401.
38. Cohen AR, Cooper PR, Kupersmith MJ, et al. Visual recovery after transsphenoidal removal of pituitary adenomas. *Neurosurgery* 1985; 17:446–452.
39. Nicola G. Transsphenoidal surgery for pituitary tumors with extrasellar extension. *Progress in Neurological Surgery* 1975;6:149–164.
40. Symon L, Jakubowski J. Transcranial management of pituitary tumors with extrasellar extension. *J Neurol Neurosurg Psychiatry* 1979;42:123.
41. Schloffer H. Erfulgreiche Operation eines Hypophysentumors suf Nasalm Wege. *Wien Klin Wochamschar* 1907;20:621.
42. Weiss MH. Transnasal transsphenoidal approach. In: Apuzzo MJ, ed. *Surgery of the third ventricle*. Baltimore: Williams & Wilkins, 1987: 476–494.
43. Hardy J. Transsphenoidal approach to the sella. In: Wilson CD, ed. *Neurosurgical procedures*. Baltimore: Williams & Wilkins, 1992: 21–40.
44. King WA, Becker DP. Transphenoidal resection of cavernous sinus tumors. In: Samii M, ed. *Skull base surgery*. Basel: Karger, 1992: 458–463.
45. Chiari O. Ueber eine Modifikation der Schloffer'schen Operation von Tumoren der Hypophyse. *Wien Klin Wochenschr* 1912;25:5–6.
46. Black PM, Zerevas NT. Surgical management of sellar and parasellar lesions. In: Schmidik R, Sweet R, eds. *Operative neurosurgical techniques*. 2nd ed. New York: Grune & Stratton, 1988:300–307.
47. Lalwani AK, Kaplan MJ, Gutin PH. The transphenoethmoid approach to the sphenoid sinus and clivus. *Neurosurgery* 1992;31:1008–1014.
48. Galfinos JG, Fitzpatrick BC, Smith LR, et al. Clinical use of a frameless stereotactic arm: results of 325 cases. *J Neurosurg* 1995;83:197–205.
49. Landolt AM. Prolactinomas: preoperative bromocriptine treatment. *Perspectives in Neurologic Surgery* 1990;1:105–115.
50. Laws ER Jr, Fode NC, Randal RV, et al. Pregnancy following transsphenoidal resection of prolactin-secreting pituitary tumors. *J Neurosurg* 1983;58:685–688.
51. Tindall GT, McLanahan CS, Christy JH. Transphenoidal microsurgery for pituitary tumors associated with hyperprolactinemia. *J Neurosurg* 1978;48:849–860.
52. Landolt AM, Keller PJ, Froesch ER, et al. Bromocriptine: does it jeopardize the result of later surgery for prolactinomas? *Lancet* 1982;2:657–652.
53. Landolt AM, Osterwalder V. Perivascular fibrosis in prolactinomas: is it increased by bromocriptine? *J Clin Endocrinol Metab* 1984;58:1179–1182.
54. Besser GM, Wass JAH, Thorner MO. Bromocriptine in the medical management of acromegaly. *Adv Biochem Psychopharmacol* 1980;23:191–198.
55. Oppizzi C, Luizzi A, Chiodini P, et al. Dopaminergic treatment of acromegaly: different effects of hormone secretion and tumor size. *J Clin Endocrinol Metab* 1984;58:988–992.
56. Ezzat S, Snyder PJ, Young WF, et al. Octreotide treatment of acromegaly: a randomized multicenter study. *Ann Intern Med* 1992; 117:711–718.
57. Laws ER Jr, Piepgras DG, Randall RV. Neurosurgical management of acromegaly: results in 82 patients treated between 1972 and 1977. *J Neurosurg* 1979;50:454–461.
58. Laws ER Jr, Randall RV, Abboud CF. Surgical treatment of acromegaly: results in 140 patients. In: Givens J, ed. *Hormone secreting pituitary tumors*. Chicago: Year Book, 1982:225–228.
59. Hardy J. *Atlas of transsphenoidal microsurgery in pituitary tumors*. New York: Igaku-Shoin, 1991.
60. Salassa RM, Laws ER Jr, Carpenter RC, et al. Transsphenoidal removal of pituitary microadenoma in Cushing's disease. *Mayo Clin Proc* 1978;53:24–28.
61. Sonino N, Boscaro M, Merola G, et al. Prolonged treatment of Cushing's disease by ketoconazole. *J Clin Endocrinol Metab* 1985;61:718–722.
62. Jeffcoate WJ, Rees LH, Tomlin S, et al. Metyrapone in long-term management of Cushing's disease. *Br Med J* 1977;2:215–217.
63. Krieger DT, Amorosa L, Linick F. Cyproheptadine-induced remission of Cushing's disease. *N Engl J Med* 1975;293:893–896.
64. Luton JP, Mahoudeau JA, Bouchard P, et al. Treatment of Cushing's disease by o,p'-DDD: survey of 62 cases. *N Engl J Med* 1979;300:459–464.
65. Edmonds MW, Simpson WJK, Meakin JW. External irradiation of the hypophysis for Cushing's disease. *Can Med Assoc J* 1972;107:860–862.
66. Thapar K, Smith M, Elliott E, et al. Corticotroph adenomas of the pituitary: long term results of operative treatment. *Endocrine Pathology* 1992;31:553–555.
67. Thapar K, Laws ER Jr. Pituitary tumors. In: Laws ER Jr, ed. *Brain tumors: basis for individual management*. Philadelphia: JB Lippincott, 1995:759–773.
68. Selman WR, Laws ER Jr, Scheithauer BW, et al. The occurrence of dural invasion in pituitary adenomas. *J Neurosurg* 1986;64:402–407.
69. Trautmann JC, Laws ER Jr. Visual status after transsphenoidal surgery at the Mayo Clinic, 1971–1982. *Am J Ophthalmol* 1983;96:200–208.
70. Nelson AT Jr, Tucker H St G, Becker DP. Residual anterior pituitary function following transsphenoidal resection of pituitary macroadenoma. *J Neurosurg* 1984;61:577–580.
71. Decker RE, Chalif DJ. Progressive coma after the transsphenoidal decompression of a pituitary adenoma with marked suprasellar extension. *Neurosurgery* 1991;28:154–158.
72. Pernicone PJ, Scheithauer BW. Invasive pituitary adenomas and pituitary carcinomas. In: Lloyd RV, ed. *Surgical pathology of the pituitary gland*. Philadelphia: WB Saunders, 1993:121–136.
73. Northfield DWC, Rathke-pouch tumors. *Brain* 1957;80:293–301.
74. Litofsky NS, Levy ML, Apuzzo MLJ. Craniopharyngioma. In: Apuzzo MLJ, ed. *Brain surgery: complication avoidance and management*. New York: Churchill Livingstone, 1993:313–378.
75. Yasargil MG, Curcic M, Kis M, et al. Total removal of craniopharyngiomas: approaches and long-term results in 144 patients. *J Neurosurg* 1990;73:3–11.
76. Baskin DS, Wilson CP. Surgical management of craniopharyngiomas: a review of 74 cases. *J Neurosurg* 1986;65:22–27.
77. Hug EB, Fitzek MM, Liebsch HJ, Muzenrider KJE. Locally challenging osteo- and chondrogenic tumors of the axial skeleton: results of combined proton and photon radiation therapy using three-dimensional treatment planning. *Int J Radiat Oncol Biol Phys* 1995;31:467–476.
78. Austin-Seymour M, Munzenrider J, Goitein M, et al. Fractionated proton radiation therapy of chordoma and lowgrade chordosarcoma of the base of the skull. *J Neurosurg* 1989;70:13–17.

SECTION V
Adjunctive Considerations

CHAPTER 29

Complications

Paul J. Donald

The initial reluctance to accept skull base surgery by the medical community was in part based on the fear that there would be an unacceptably high complication rate. This is especially because of the exposure of the delicate structures in the intracranial space to the sea of microbes that reside in the nose, paranasal sinuses, nasopharynx, and oral cavity. Table 1 is a compilation of reports of the most important complications in skull base surgery, cerebrospinal fluid (CSF) leak, and meningitis. Another deterrent was related in particular to malignant tumors and the notion that dural or brain involvement portended a hopeless prognosis.

Unfortunately, complications do indeed occur, and every chapter on surgical technique in this book has outlined what the complications are, and briefly how to manage them. The purpose of this chapter is to give a more detailed discussion of the prevention and management of each complication. In the instances when such problems and their solutions have been well described, the section is simply referred to and only briefly mentioned here.

The chapter first discusses how to prevent complications, and second, if they occur, how to treat them. The focus is directed toward the complications at the operative site, and little attention is given to other systemic complications such as pneumonia, cardiac decompensation, and the like, except when they arise directly as a result of another complication of the surgery such as cranial nerve compromise. Detailed accounts of these latter problems are found in Chapter 30, on postoperative management, and Chapter 8, on nursing care.

PREVENTION

Preoperative Preparation

The prevention of intraoperative and postoperative complications begins at the preoperative assessment. A thorough history and physical examination and a complete review of past records, radiographs, and pathology reports is essential. The initial encounter with the average skull base surgery patient takes about 45 to 60 minutes. As mentioned in Chapter 5, most patients have already received some form of prior therapy. It is essential to review all operative records and discharge summaries as well as the patient's and the family's own interpretation of these events.

As previously mentioned, not only are the pathology reports reviewed, but it is essential that the tissue block and histologic slides be reviewed by the skull base team's own head and neck pathologist.

The patient's intercurrent disease status must be carefully reviewed and the function of all organ systems optimized before surgery. Cardiac, pulmonary, renal, and hepatic function must be fine tuned for the rigors of skull base surgery. Moreover, if the patient's intercurrent disease processes are too severe, skull base surgery is contraindicated. The appropriateness of type and dosage of all medications is reviewed. A careful inquiry concerning the use of salicylates and other anticoagulant medications is made, and these medications stopped in sufficient time before surgery to prevent bleeding during surgery.

All radiographs are reviewed, keeping in mind the fact that these studies not infrequently inaccurately represent the extent of disease.

The patient is mentally prepared as best as possible before surgery. A relaxed, confident, reassured patient will do much better than a frightened one. A carefully coordinated, orderly surgical plan is conceptualized, bearing in mind the prevention of complications. The surgeons, anesthetists, and nurses must organize their efforts to have an effective therapeutic plan that ablates the disease but is continuously cognizant of the fine details that preclude the development of a complication.

Surgical Preparation

The prevention begins in the initial phases of surgical preparation. An early, quick start to the case goes a long way to ensuring a timely ending. Often, the longer the procedure

---

P. J. Donald: Department of Otolaryngology—Head and Neck Surgery, and Center for Skull Base Surgery, University of California, Davis Medical Center, Sacramento, California 95817.

TABLE 1. *Incidence of cerebrospinal fluid leak and meningitis after anterior approach skull base surgery*

Author	No. of cases	Cerebrospinal fluid leak (no. [%])	No. of meningitis cases — Early	Late	Total (%)
Bergermann et al. (2)	21	1 (5)	0	0	0
Schramm (3)	32	?	1	—	1 (3)
Ketcham et al. (4)	48	12 (25)	—	—	6 (12.5)
Schramm (5)	44	2 (3)	1	—	1 (3)
Deschler et al. (6)	53	6 (11)	1	—	1 (2)
Kraus et al. (7)	71	2 (2)	—	—	1 (1.2)
McCutcheon et al. (8)	38	2 (6)	0	0	0

drags on, the greater the risk of complications. A tracheostomy is done on almost all patients for a number of important reasons. The elimination of the endotracheal tube from the field provides an opportunity for excellent sterile preparation of the surgical field. Although the oral cavity has traditionally been considered to be a source of heavy bacterial contamination, a povidone–iodine surgical preparation can render it virtually sterile. The endotracheal tube is a continuous source of bacterial contamination because it is inserted in an unsterile fashion and extremely difficult to prepare. In addition, it brings the anesthetic hose connection in precariously close proximity to the surgical field. Any disconnection brings the potential for contamination. Airway control during the postoperative period in the skull base patient is most important, and may be necessitated by an intercurrent pulmonary problem or if a significant spell of coma ensues because of the central component of the procedure. A final important factor is the prevention of pneumocephalus. This may result as a consequence of grunting respirations during a comatose or semicomatose episode in the early postoperative period. In these patients, a ball valve type of action occurs at the site of dural or pericranial repair, trapping air and producing the pneumocephalus (Fig. 1).

The eyes must be protected throughout the procedure. Plastic corneal shields provide less-than-optimal protection for surgery prolonged beyond 4 to 5 hours. Much better protection is afforded by temporary tarsorrhaphy sutures. Details of their insertion are depicted in Fig. 2. It is essential to ensure that the eyelashes are not included within the eye. Placing the suture through the "gray line" at the site of exit of the meibomian glands prevents this.

The lumbar subarachnoid drain provides a mechanism for decompressing the brain to make it slack during surgery and to diminish the brain retraction that is so often the source of postoperative central complications. Although the drain is a potential source of infection, it is usually left in place for only 3 to 6 days and is rarely a site of bacterial contamination. In the author's series, the drain site has never been a cause for meningitis. During the postoperative period, the drain provides a method for maintaining a stable CSF pressure. This is helpful in the prevention of postoperative CSF leakage.

The use of a Mayfield horseshoe head rest provides an easy way to position the head, allowing maximal exposure of the surgical field. Careful padding of the rest (also see Chapter 8) and frequent change of head position during surgery prevent the development of pressure sores of the scalp. The author's team has not as yet encountered this complication in skull base surgery but has seen this occur in one head and neck oncologic patient who had a simultaneous bilateral neck dissection.

Intraoperative Management

Prophylaxis against complications begins with the initial incision. The operation should proceed with dispatch. The longer the patient remains under anesthesia, the more likely

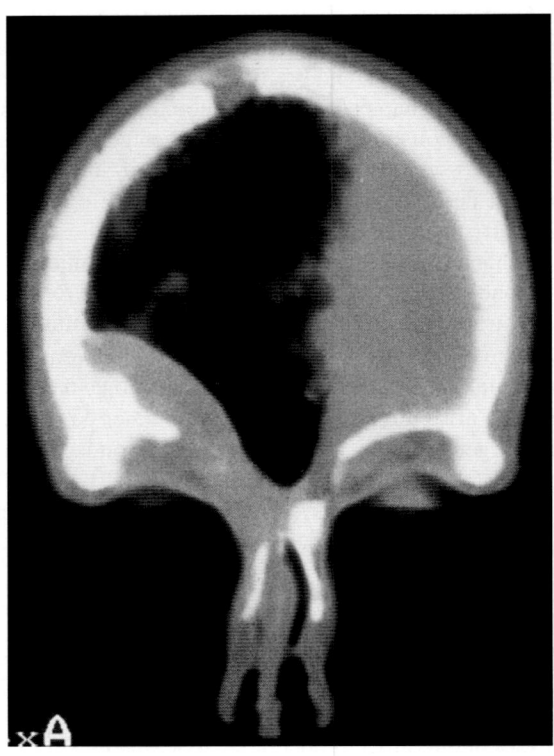

FIG. 1. Massive anterior cranial fossa pneumocephalus secondary to air grunted into the intracranial space through a ball valve defect in dura in a patient who had a period of postoperative coma.

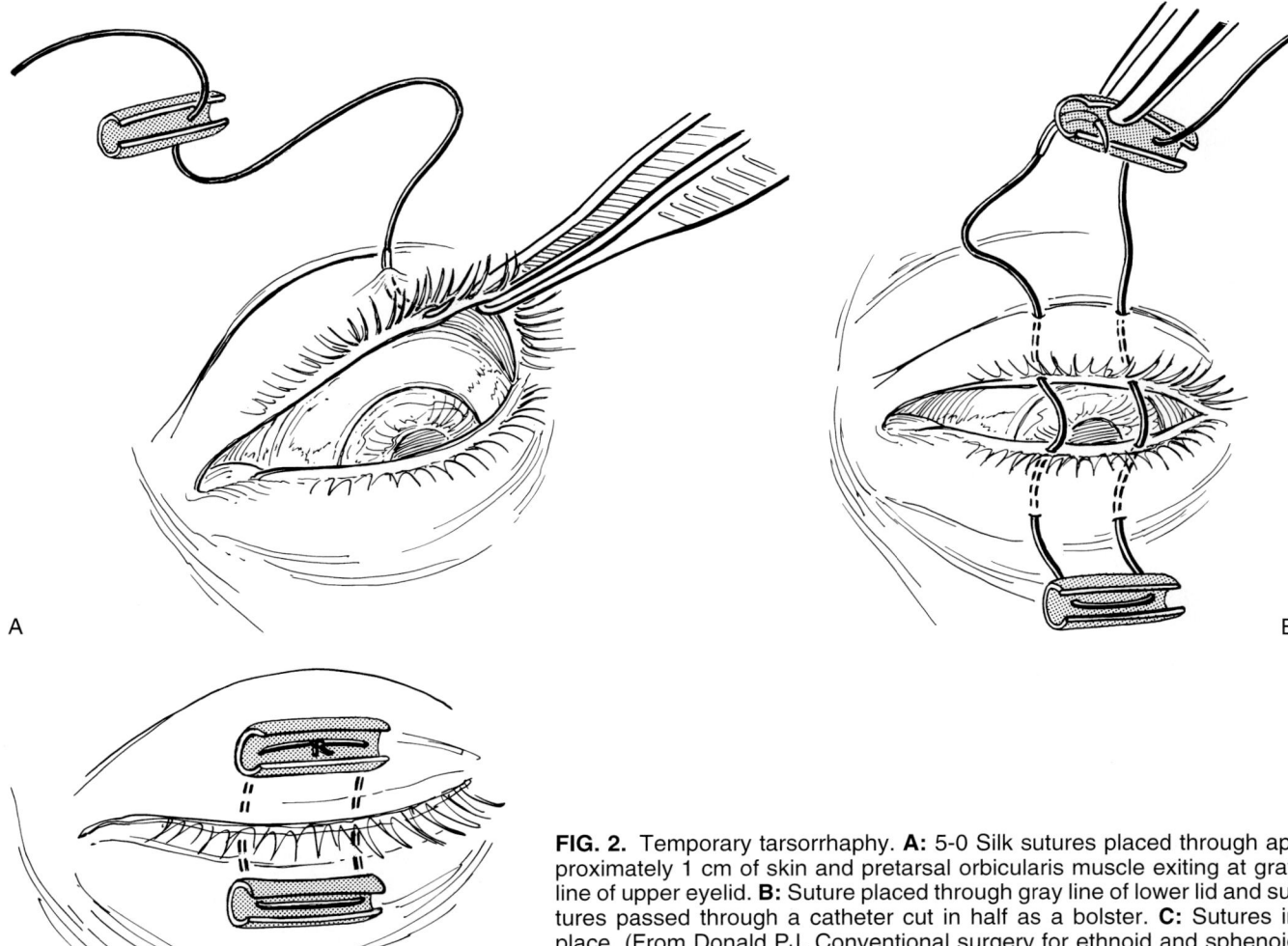

FIG. 2. Temporary tarsorrhaphy. **A:** 5-0 Silk sutures placed through approximately 1 cm of skin and pretarsal orbicularis muscle exiting at gray line of upper eyelid. **B:** Suture placed through gray line of lower lid and sutures passed through a catheter cut in half as a bolster. **C:** Sutures in place. (From Donald PJ. Conventional surgery for ethnoid and sphenoid sinusitis. In: Donald PJ, Gluckman JL, Rice DH, eds. *The sinuses.* New York: Raven Press, 1995:234.)

subsequent untoward postoperative events are to occur. Hemostasis with a system such as Rainey clips markedly reduces blood loss from the scalp incision. Attention to hemostasis in the neck and face is important. The bipolar cautery has gone a long way in reducing operative time in this regard. Major intraoperative bleeding may come from a hemorrhagic tumor such as an arteriovenous malformation, glomus tumor, or juvenile angiofibroma. Preoperative embolism of feeding vessels, especially with Gugliemi detachable coils or particulate materials, coupled with controlled hypotension and even temporary cardiac standstill with bypass, help to minimize blood loss.

Control of major supply vessels in the neck—namely, the internal and external carotid arteries and the internal jugular vein—is good prophylaxis against inadvertent vessel interruption intracranially. The placing of temporary, loose, rubber vascular loops around these vessels is worthwhile time spent (Fig. 3). Similarly, exposure of critical dural venous sinuses greatly aids more central control. It is important for both principal members of the surgical team to know how to achieve both intracranial and extracranial hemostasis. The head and neck surgeon must be facile with the bipolar cautery, bone wax, the use of thrombin-soaked Gelfoam pledgets and hemostatic gauze, and the application of pressure with cottonoid patties. Similarly, the neurosurgeon must acquire the skills of applying fine ties to vessels clamped in long, deep holes and the use of the hemostatic suture ligature.

Copious irrigation is necessary throughout the procedure to prevent the drying of tissues. Skin and muscle flap and areas of the wound not under direct surgical attention must be dressed with saline-soaked gauze. Brain protection and protection of cranial nerves is essential. All devitalized tissue must be removed because it will become a potential nidus for later infection.

The elimination of "time wasters" is essential. Factors such as waiting for equipment can be eliminated by judicious planning and timely anticipation. The premature use of the microscope must be guarded against in that a too narrowly focused attention may be directed before adequate exposure has been established by gross removal of bone or the dissection of soft tissue. This is especially true during mastoidectomy, clivectomy, and occipital bone and lateral upper cer-

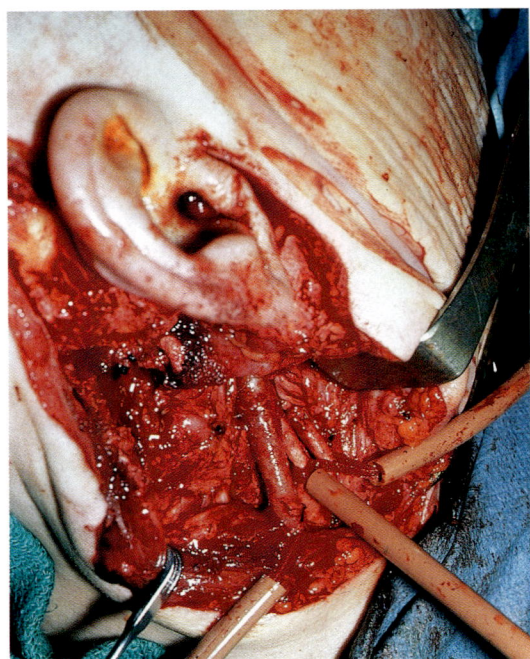

FIG. 3. Vessels in the neck are encircled by loosely applied, temporary rubber vascular loops to be tightened if sudden control of hemorrhage higher up is required.

vical spine resection. The rough work should proceed with dispatch, and the finely focused work done with the microscope at the end. The preoperative surgical plan should be followed and pushed ahead unless unexpected contingencies arise. Dawdling and unfocused activity because of indecision have no place at any time in surgery, and especially not during surgery involving the skull base.

Periodic assessment of the progress and details of the anesthesia are necessary. Estimates of blood loss, fluid administration, lumbar drainage, antibiotic prophylaxis, and overall patient homeostasis must be checked on a regular basis. The surgeon must encourage the anesthesiologist to monitor fluid administration carefully because fluid overload can lead to significant postoperative complications of edema, both central and peripheral, heart failure, and pulmonary edema. Peripheral nerve and central monitoring are checked periodically to ensure neurologic integrity.

Once the pathologic process initiating the surgery has been resolved and the wound copiously irrigated, the reconstruction begins. Modern reconstructive techniques are one of the major reasons that modern skull base surgery is so highly successful and relatively complication free.

Dural closure is done with the central goal of achieving a watertight seal. Separation of the upper aerodigestive tract from the subarachnoid space is the key procedure in successful reconstruction. However, this separation is not always possible, and if CSF leakage occurs in the postoperative period, the danger of meningitis is omnipresent. Resected dura may be successfully replaced with autograft fascia or lyophilized cadaver dura or even bovine peri-

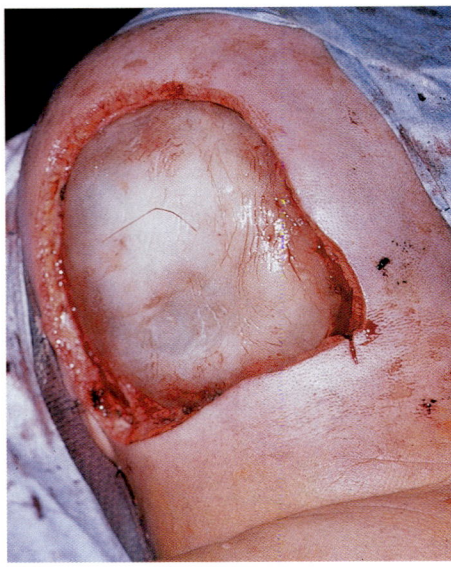

FIG. 4. Replacement with methylmethacrylate of a large segment of resected occipital calvarium infiltrated by tumor.

cardium. In areas where suture placement is difficult or impossible, tissue glue is used. The next layer comprises living tissue to reinforce the closure. Pericranium in the form of a vascularized flap is the most commonly used flap in anterior approaches. This is less feasible in the lateral and posterior approaches, and pedicled or free vascularized tissue is inter-

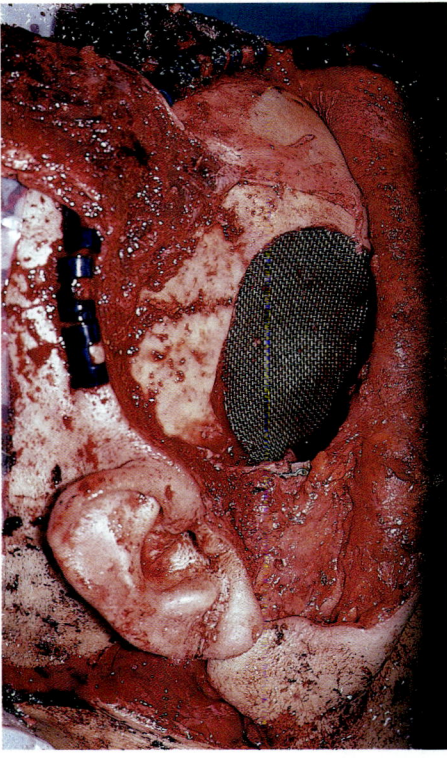

FIG. 5. Titanium mesh used to replace temporal bone squama when bone resection was necessary because of tumor invasion.

posed between the dural repair and the upper aerodigestive tract. Cranial bone is replaced when possible, but occasionally in large defects, calvarial replacement is done with allografts (Figs. 4, 5). Meticulous epithelial closure with adequate drainage finalizes the reconstruction. The issue of direct wound drainage is often controversial in that the head and neck surgeon prefers suction drainage in areas of large flap elevation and the neurosurgeon has an overriding fear of CSF fistula. Wound contingencies and the integrity of the dural closure must be balanced against each other.

The details of postoperative care are well described in Chapter 30 and receive no consideration here. The complications discussed are those linked directly to the surgical site. The management of more generalized problems is also dealt with in Chapter 30.

CEREBROSPINAL FLUID LEAKAGE

Next to sudden death and massive postoperative hemorrhage, the most dreaded complications are those secondary to CSF fistulization. There are really two forms of CSF fluid leakage: the hygroma and a true fistula. The fistula connects the subarachnoid space to either the cutaneous wound or to a previously made incision in the epithelium of the upper aerodigestive tract. The drainage can be direct or circuitous. The latter is often seen from the posterior or middle cranial fossa through the eustachian tube and into the pharynx. The hygroma is a collection of CSF that does not drain through the epithelium. The most common sites are under the scalp or neck.

If a CSF fistula occurs, it is initially managed conservatively with elevation of the head of the bed, fluid restriction, the use of stool softeners, and the withdrawal of 75 to 150 ml of CSF daily. The institution of prophylactic antibiotics to prevent meningitis is and has been highly controversial since the mid-1970s. The concern about the development of a resistant organism is balanced against the concern of potential bacterial contamination from the subcutaneous wound or upper aerodigestive tract. Because therapy will be short-lived, in that a failure to stop CSF drainage mandates early operative intervention, antibiotics should be used in most if not all cases. A combination that covers the wide spectrum of microorganisms that inhabit the upper aerodigestive tract is used. Anaerobic bacteria and gram-negative rods need to be covered, as well as *Staphylococcus aureus* and *Streptococcus pyogenes*. The author routinely uses a combination of Kefzol (cephazolin; Eli Lilly and Co., Indianapolis, IN) and Flagyl (metronidazole; Searle and Company, Chicago, IL) if the oral cavity or nasopharynx is in continuity with the intracranial defector, and Kefzol alone if these sites are not potential sources of contamination.

If in 3 to 5 days the leak has not stopped and the patient is stable, then the wound is reopened and the dural seal is reestablished. A hygroma may be watched for a longer time depending on its location. Collections under the scalp are needle aspirated and a pressure dressing applied. Often the collection resolves, but if not, then reoperation and surgical closure are done. Cervical hygromas are harder to apply pressure to, and reopening of the wound is often necessary to stem the leak (Fig. 6). The dural dehiscence is either sutured directly or reinforced with a temporalis fascia or fascia lata graft.

Cerebrospinal fluid leakage emanating from the eustachian tube is occasionally seen after acoustic neurinoma surgery. The wound is opened, absorbed or inadequate fat grafts replaced, a more complete fascial covering of the internal auditory canal done, and a more thorough bone waxing of the residual petrous air cells performed (see also Chapter 23). The eustachian tube mucosa must be elevated in the region of the protympanum, inverted into the bony portion of the tube, and plugged with bone paté or a bone plug.

When leakage occurs into the nose or sinus exenteration cavity, the location of the leak is carefully identified. The site

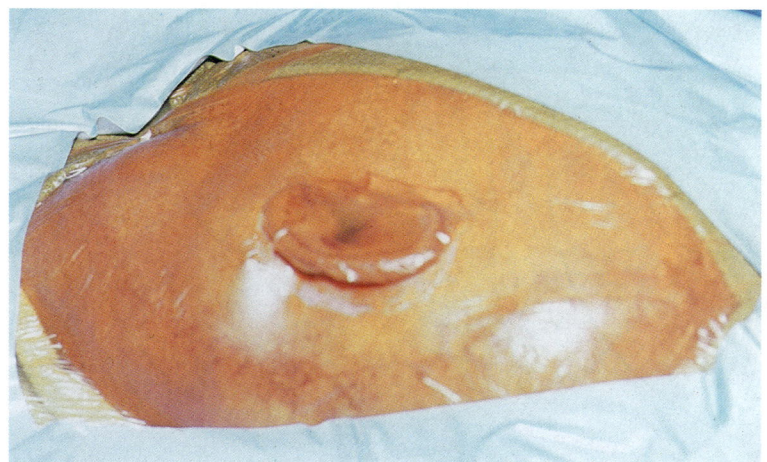
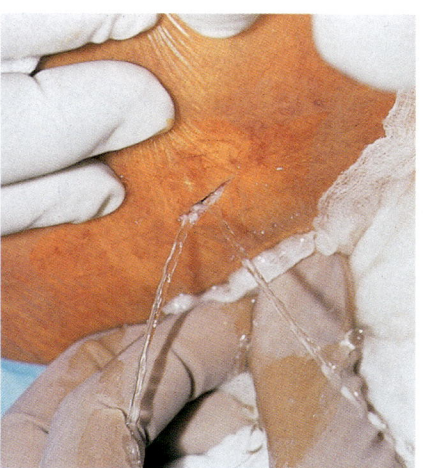

FIG. 6. Cervical hygroma secondary to cerebrospinal fluid (CSF) leak from posterior cranial fossa after resection of a massive glomus tumor. **A:** Hygroma in patient ready for surgery. **B:** CSF gushes out of wound when initial incision is made.

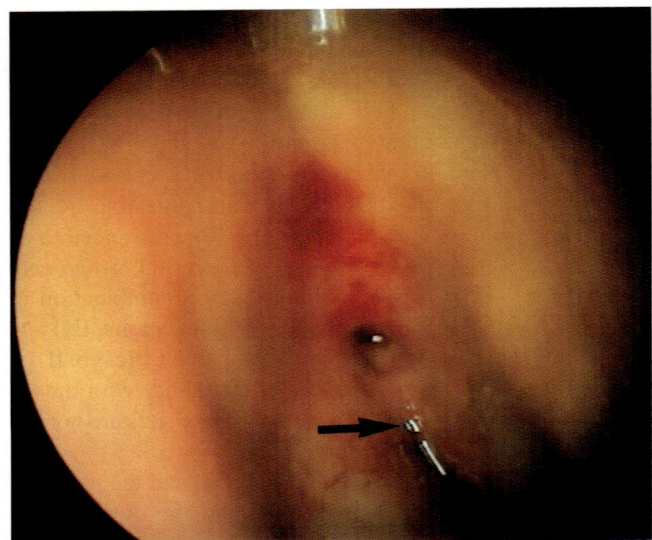

FIG. 7. Endoscopic view of cerebrospinal fluid (CSF) fistula demonstrating the drainage of fluorescein-stained CSF. *Arrow* points to leak. Note fluorescein staining to the sides.

of the leak usually can be demonstrated by instilling fluorescein into the subarachnoid space through the lumbar drain, then carefully visualizing the nasal cavity with a 0-degree sinus endoscope (Fig. 7). Once the site is identified, an intracranial or extracranial approach is planned, usually depending on the site and size. Extracranial approaches can be done endoscopically. Grafts of fascia or muscle can be inserted from below and covered with nasal septal flaps, if such a source of tissue can be obtained (1) (Fig. 8). The mucosal flap is packed into position with medicated gauze packing that is left in place for 1 week.

One patient in the author's experience was leaking into the exenteration cavity from the foramen rotundum. A small piece of fascia was placed into the intracranial side through the foramen and the bony hole obstructed by a cork of bone forced into the foramen, which stopped the leak.

In the author's series (2), as in others (3) (see Table 1), a CSF fistula is an unusual complication. With the exception of the early report by Ketcham et al. (4), done at a time before pericranial flaps were performed, the average CSF leak rate was reported to be approximately 7%. Compulsiveness in closing the dura in a watertight fashion, the double layer provided by the pericranial flap, and the use of the lumbar subarachnoid drain, all combine to prevent this complication.

CENTRAL NERVOUS SYSTEM INFECTION

Meningitis

The most common serious sequel to a CSF leak is meningitis. Meningitis is fortunately an uncommon complication. One of the initial deterrents to skull base surgery was the fear of this complication. In the early years of skull base surgery, a "Cushing's veil" (Fig. 9) was used as a barrier to infection. The veil consisted of a surgical towel soaked in an antibiotic solution and stapled to the scalp flap. This was alternately placed over the face or exposed dura and brain, depending on which part of the resection was being done. More recently, this has been abandoned by most, being perceived as more of a nuisance than a help.

Prevention, of course, is a vital element in avoiding this dire complication. This becomes increasingly difficult as the

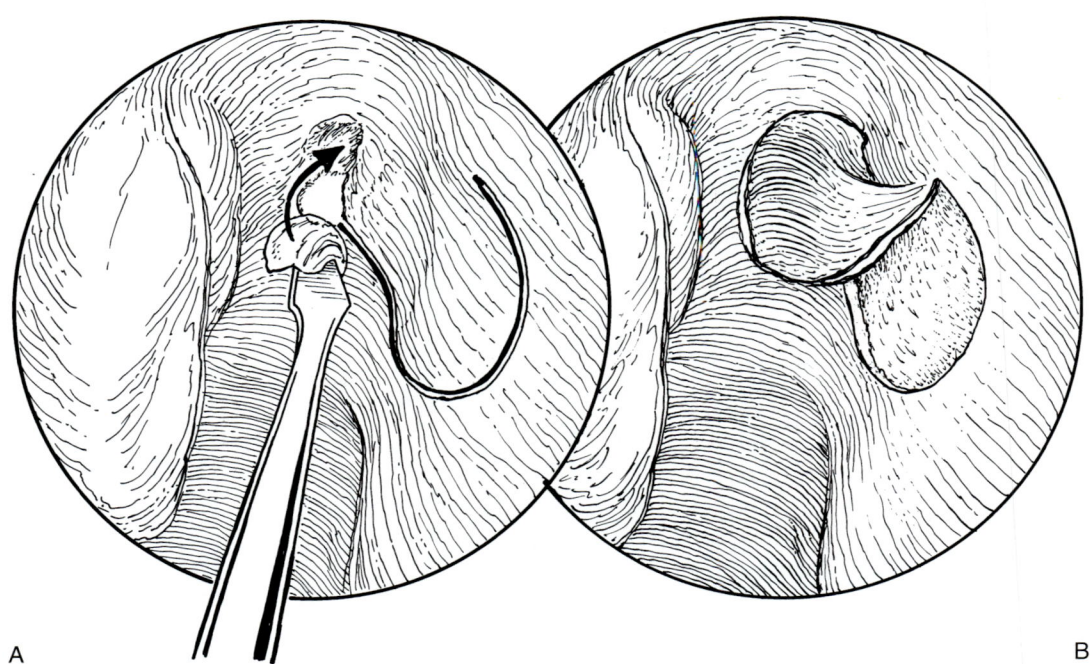

FIG. 8. **A:** Muscle or fascia placed in arch of dehiscence with septal flap outlined. **B:** Septal flap rotated into position.

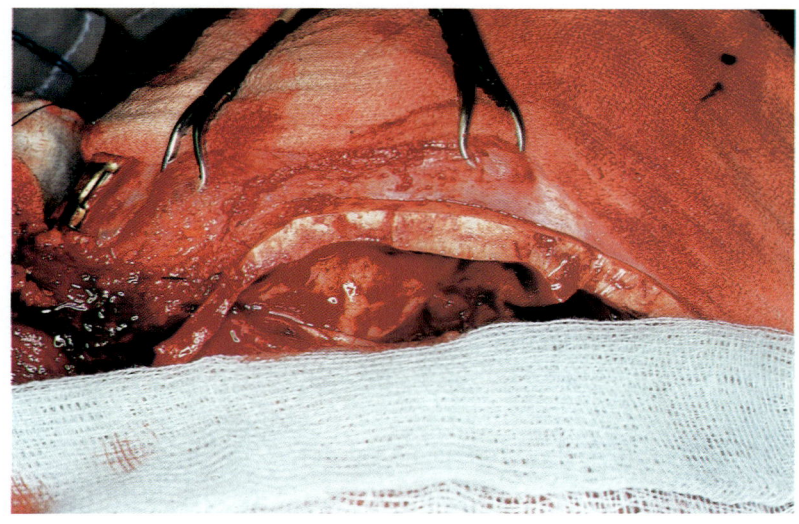

FIG. 9. Cushing's veil. An antibiotic-soaked towel or laparotomy pad clipped to the scalp flap was thought to improve sterility of the intracranial operative field.

number of team members and their various pieces of necessary equipment increases. Diligent antiseptic technique is vital, and breaks in technique are avoided at all costs. Because of these considerations, the use of a large operating theater is vital.

Cerebrospinal fluid from the lumbar drain is checked twice daily for the presence of leukocytes or bacteria. Body temperature and leukocytosis are carefully monitored. Any sudden change in the patient's general condition, a seizure, or change in mental status should raise the suspicion of meningitis. It may be mild and asymptomatic, manifested only by fever and leukocytosis, or the patient may be profoundly ill with sepsis and coma. The classic symptoms of a stiff neck, fever, and headache are often the only clinical presentation. Vomiting, lethargy, and focal signs are usually seen later. A leukocytosis of usually greater than 50,000 white blood cells with a 90% or greater predominance of polymorphonuclear lymphocytes, a depressed sugar level below 45 mg/ml, and an elevated protein above 45 mg/ml are the usual laboratory findings in the CSF.

Untreated bacterial meningitis is almost invariably fatal. The most common organism in the postoperative setting is the pneumococcus. Control of the infection with antibiotics followed by surgery to correct the leak once the patient is stable is the usual course of treatment. Penicillin or a penicillin-based drug is most commonly used in combination with a nonlactamase drug effective against *Hemophilus*. This is especially important in children. Ampicillin, chloramphenicol, cephalosporins, and aminoglycosides have all been used depending on the putative organism and corresponding sensitivities.

The patient in Fig. 10 had suffered a bout of meningitis after a fall. He had two prior operations for recurrences of an aggressive neurotropic carcinoma of the facial skin. His last procedure was a massive resection involving a lateral rhinectomy, with a middle fossa craniotomy, removal of the cavernous sinus and temporal lobe dura, and complete dissection of the petrous and intracranial internal carotid artery (see Chapter 15, Fig. 35). The area was reconstructed with a latissimus dorsi free vascularized flap (see Chapter 15, Fig. 41). One year later, a fall from a stool while inebriated resulted in a CSF rhinorrhea that was followed by meningitis. Once control of infection had been accomplished with an antibiotic, the CSF leak was sealed with a graft of fascia lata (see Fig. 10A–C).

Occasionally, aseptic meningitis may occur and be confused with the bacterial form. The clinical picture is not dissimilar to purulent meningitis, and the etiology is unknown. A reaction to intracranial blood and the products of blood breakdown has been thought to be the cause in many cases.

Brain Abscess

A dreaded complication of craniotomy is brain abscess. It is most commonly either the result of a postoperative meningitis or a nidus of necrotic material such as dead bone, fascia, or dura. This latter cause is more commonly associated with prior radiation therapy resulting in the reduced vascularity of tissues within the field. The use of well vascularized flaps of unirradiated tissue is vital in the reconstruction of these cases to provide maximal protection at the operative site from this complication.

Pathologically, a brain abscess can take many forms. The pus may be contained within a thick fibrous wall, confined by a thin wall, or surrounded only by edema (9). Most postoperative abscesses are surrounded by a zone of cerebral edema. The thick-walled abscesses are usually chronic in nature and centered around the nidus of infection. There is often a connection between the source of infection and the abscess by a stalk. This is especially important after skull base surgery because the connection to an area of necrotic tissue or an infected focus may be seen. Both aerobic and anaerobic organisms, common inhabitants of the upper aerodigestive tract, are often the organisms responsible.

Brain abscess is a complication with serious potential debilitating complications and even death. Judgment regarding the choice between surgical drainage or antibiotic therapy is

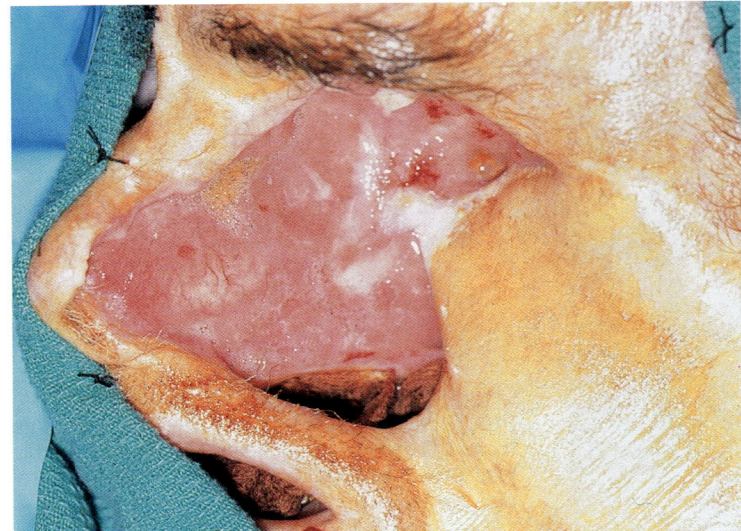
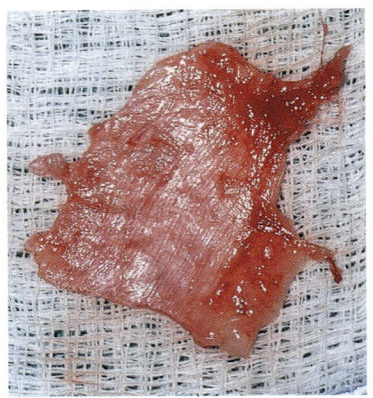
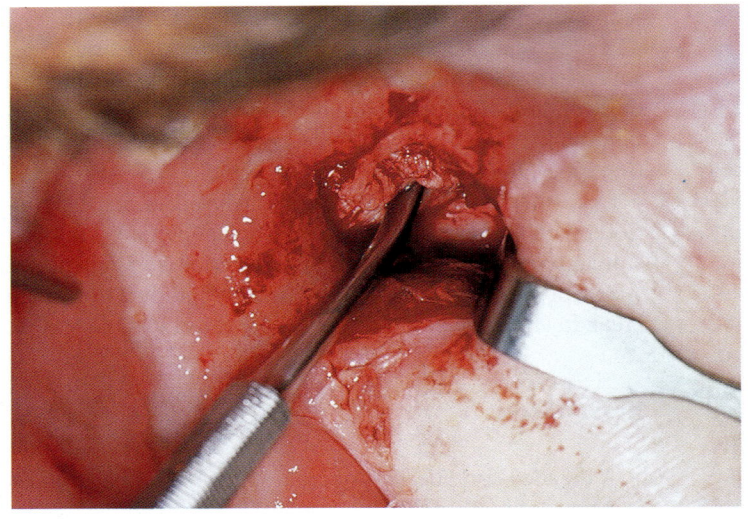

FIG. 10. Cerebrospinal fluid (CSF) leak stemmed by fascia lata graft in a patient whose leak developed after a fall 1 year after massive skull base resection. Patient contracted meningitis, and after antibiotic therapy the CSF fistula sealed. **A:** Area of leak in sphenoid sinus exposed. **B:** Fascia lata graft. **C:** Fascia applied to defect.

often very difficult and must be highly individualized. Chronic antibiotic therapy is usually used after surgical drainage. A deteriorating clinical picture or enlargement of the infected focus despite adequate dosage of antibiotics forces surgical drainage. If a focus of necrotic material such as sequestered osteoradionecrotic bone is the source of the infection, it must be removed.

Skrap et al. (10) describe successful drainage of nine brain abscesses treated from 1991 to 1995 by stereotactic puncture and drainage of pus. Postoperative antibiotics were used. There was only one recurrence at 2 months, and it was successfully treated by antibiotics and steroids. The efficacy of stereotactic drainage is also supported by data from Bucholz and Greco (11) and Shahzadi et al. (12).

PNEUMOCEPHALUS

Some degree of pneumocephalus is commonplace after skull base surgery. Despite attempts to eliminate intracranial dead space at the end of the procedure, some residual air is not uncommon. Posnick et al. (13) have shown that a substantial volume of air is common after forehead advancement for craniofacial dysmorphia. In all 23 patients in their series, complete absorption of air and obliteration of the space by expanding brain had occurred by 6 to 8 weeks. Intracranial air is worrisome, but usually asymptomatic. However, large volumes of air or a tension pneumocephalus can be life threatening. Tension pneumocephalus comes about by two mechanisms. Because normal intracranial pressure exceeds atmospheric pressure, there is a natural pressure gradient between the intracranial and extracranial spaces. According to Henry and Heathcote (14), there are two basic mechanisms that can cause tension pneumocephalus. The "ball valve" mechanism occurs when extracranial pressure is raised to exceed intracranial pressure by such mechanisms as coughing, straining, or grunting-type respirations. (A flap of dura or other tissue may flap shut when such pressure normalizes.) The "inverted bottle" mechanism results from fluid leaking from this area of higher intracranial pressure to the extracranial space and air bubbling into the intracranial space to replace this lost volume. A third mechanism is proposed by Campanelli and Odland (15). They posit that air already present in the intracranial subarachnoid space in the presence of a lumbar drain will cause a tension pneumocephalus based on the much greater difference in compliance of air versus fluid. The air may come from the diffusion of gases from the intravascular space. Once the air is present, a significant withdrawal of CSF by the drain results in enlargement of the gas bubble.

The most common symptoms are headache, nausea, and vomiting. In the early postoperative period, a change in consciousness is apparent. Seizures, meningismus, and hemiparesis or an obvious CSF leak may also be present (16). Most commonly, air is forced through a dural dehiscence into the subdural space, with compression of brain in the affected cranial fossa. This is seen most often in the anterior fossa cases, and in the author's experience occurred in two patients who had obtunded consciousness during the first few postoperative days and did not have a tracheostomy. During this time, grunting respirations blow air through the dehiscence into the intracranial compartment. A tracheostomy is done routinely on all the author's anterior fossa skull base patients to prevent this complication. The only two cases of pneumocephalus occurred in these patients who were not tracheostomized.

Management of the tension pneumocephalus is initially directed to prevent reversal of the pressure differential by implanting a tracheostomy and relieving the pressure of the air bubble by needle aspiration. The needle can be placed directly into the bubble or, if indicated, by needle ventriculostomy. Attention is then turned to the sealing of the dural leak. This usually requires a direct approach by reopening the craniotomy and sealing the dural dehiscence permitting the air entry. This is usually done with pericranial flaps and fascial grafts. In some resistant recurrent cases, a free flap of vascularized tissue may be required (17).

HEMORRHAGE

Bleeding can occur intracranially or extracranially. Despite the fact that the subcranial resection occurs in one of the most hemorrhagic areas of the body (i.e., the paranasal sinuses), postoperative bleeding is a rarity. With orbital exenteration, the ophthalmic artery and the ophthalmic veins are at risk but are almost never the source of this complication. The internal maxillary artery and its branches are a potential source of trouble, especially the internal maxillary. This artery may retract between the paired heads of the lateral pterygoid muscle and go into spasm, only to open up in the early postoperative period. The pterygoid plexus of veins is a lower-pressure system, but if the exenteration cavity is inadequately packed, it may bleed after surgery. Bleeding here may become quite troublesome during surgery and may require the liberal use of suture ligatures and hemostatic gauze packing to produce hemostasis and thus prevent postoperative hemorrhage.

If a portion of the greater palatine canal is preserved, the greater palatine artery may retract and bleed briskly. Bone may need to be removed and the canal exposed to ligate or coagulate this vessel. A small plug of bone may be thrust into the canal as an alternative method of achieving hemostasis.

Intracranial bleeding may be fatal. A change in level of consciousness in the absence of a temperature change or obvious CSF leak, especially in the early postoperative period, must alert the surgeon to the possibility of an intracranial hemorrhage. An emergency computed tomography scan is imperative to rule out an intracranial accumulation of blood. Immediate craniotomy should solve the problem. The presence of blood against brain tissue provides its own set of problems, even in the absence of an increase in intracranial pressure. Most of the bleeding, however, is in the extradural space, reflected by no apparent blood in the CSF from the lumbar drain.

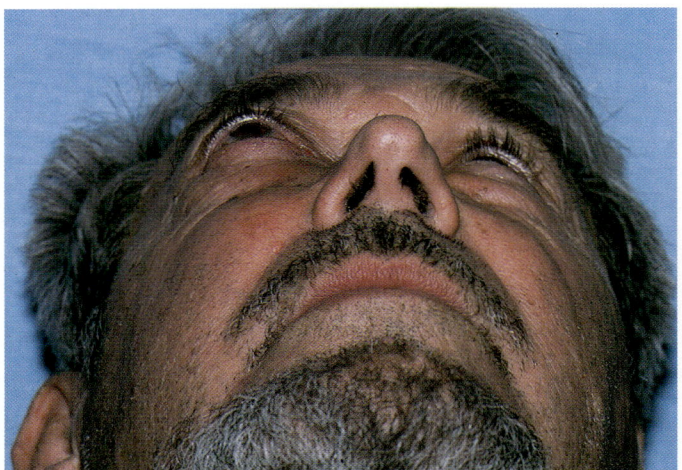
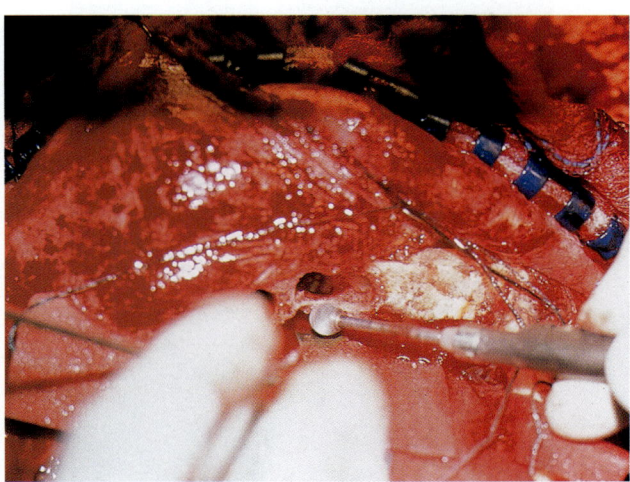

FIG. 11. Patient with a malignant melanoma invading the sphenoid sinus during resection of the lateral wall of the sinus. **A:** Base view of patient showing proptosis. **B:** Drilling in region of lateral wall of sphenoid sinus.

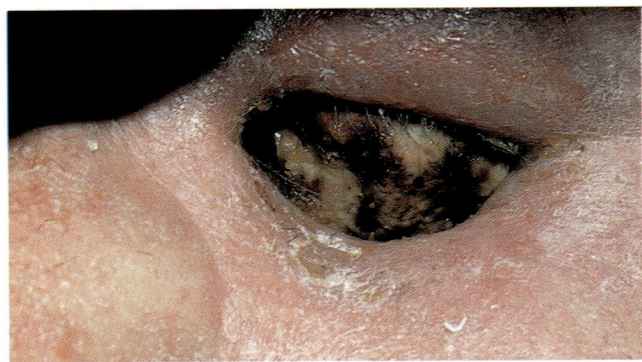

FIG. 12. Patient with a sloughing pericranial flap and necrotic prolapsed frontal lobe showing.

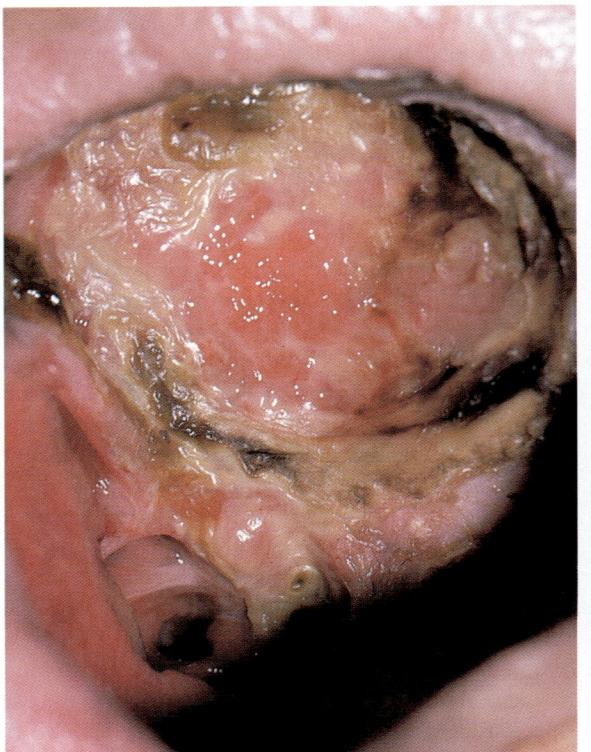

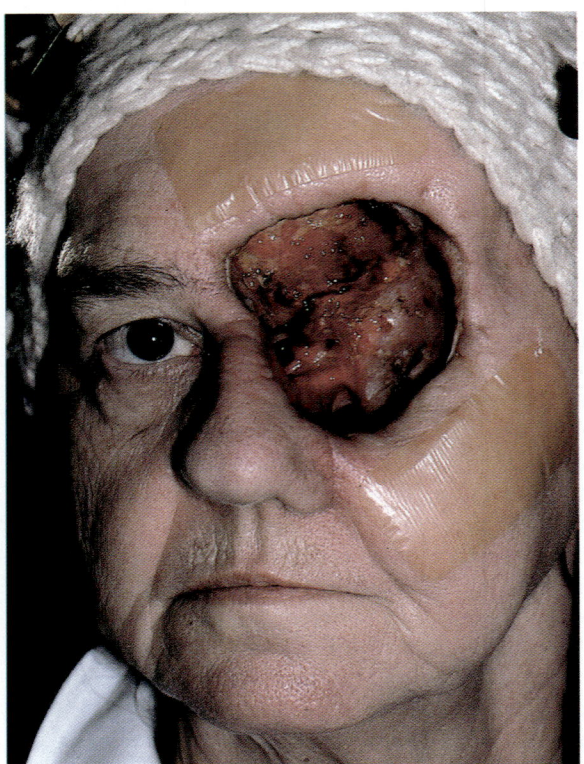

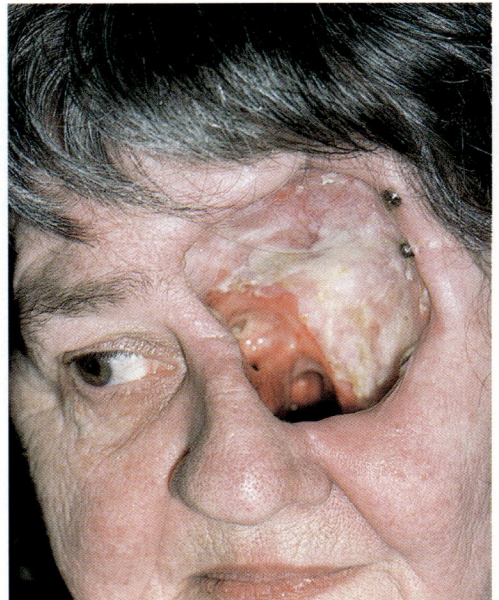

FIG. 13. A: Loss of split-thickness skin over pericranial flap. **B:** Six weeks later, reepithelialization had occurred. **C:** Two years later, with BUD interosseous implants (BUD Industries, Inc., Tonawanda, NY) in place.

Bleeding may occur from the free flap or myocutaneous flap, and a return to the operating room may be required. A massive hematoma occurred in one of the author's patients between the flap and the reconstructed dura. Exploration revealed the bleeding vessel and it was ligated. This was the only major flap bleed in the author's series. If a carotid artery graft is done, then bleeding can occur from an imperfect anastomosis. If the arterial graft is exposed to the upper aerodigestive tract, it may become necrotic and burst. This is more common in the patient who has been irradiated. The internal carotid may be exposed and go unnoticed during reconstruction, or the overlying protective tissue placed during reconstruction may necrose and expose the vessel. This is especially important in the petrous segment and cavernous sinus. The cavernous segment exposure may occur in the sphenoid sinus. The patient in Fig. 11 had this exposure and came to the clinic about 4 weeks after surgery with a pulsating internal carotid in the lateral sphenoid wall visible on endoscopy. He had already had a small herald bleed but refused intervention. After much importuning, 24 hours later he consented to vascular embolism but exsanguinated in the angiographic suite before an arterial catheter could be placed.

These two cases are the only severe hemorrhagic complications the author has encountered.

PERICRANIAL FLAP SLOUGH

This is a rare complication and has occurred only once in the author's experience. The patient in Fig. 12 continued to smoke throughout his postoperative course against the most stringent and insistent advice. Initially his skin graft sloughed and, in the ensuing 3 weeks, his pericranial flap gradually deteriorated. His frontal lobe began to herniate into the cavity. He remained asymptomatic, but continuing brain fungus and the fear of infection from his exenteration cavity necessitated amputation of necrotic brain and relining of the cavity by a radial forearm free flap.

Maceri (D. Maceri, *personal communication*, 1989) reports the case of a pericranial flap that died in the immediate postoperative period in a patient who had previously been heavily irradiated. This resulted in subsequent meningitis and marked prolongation of hospital stay. Patients who have had full-course irradiation to the donor site of a proposed pericranial flap should probably have the resection site reconstructed with a free revascularized flap. In addition, consideration should be given to the use of a galeal pericranial flap as described by Jackson et al. (18). The added vascularity of this flap may preclude sloughing.

Sometimes only the skin graft lining the cavity sloughs, but the pericranium maintains its viability. The patient in Fig. 13 had not been previously irradiated but had a grossly infected tumor at the time of her resection. With meticulous postoperative care, using frequent sterile saline irrigations and wet-to-dry dressing, she went on to complete healing of her cavity.

OSTEOMYELITIS

Osteomyelitis of the craniotomy flap is in general a rare occurrence. The author has had only two cases of major flap loss in his experience. One occurred in a patient who required resection for a frontal intracranial/extracranial meningioma. In addition to multiple prior resections, he had received prior full-course irradiation. A sinus tract developed onto the forehead skin. The necrotic bone flap was removed through a coronal skin flap and the skin allowed to heal. The area was subsequently reconstructed with a split calvarial graft. Radiation damage to the forehead skin and the underlying frontal bone is often the culprit in this complication. Healing is retarded and the bone flap is in jeopardy.

The second patient was 80 years of age and had a straightforward, otherwise uncomplicated anterior skull base resection for inverting papilloma. Despite warning, he performed vigorous postoperative nose blowing, propelling air and mucus under his forehead skin flap through the rhinotomy osteotomy. An abscess eventually developed over his frontal bone flap, leading to osteomyelitis of the craniotomy flap (Fig. 14). Removal of the bone flap was later done and cranioplasty delayed.

A second problem that may cause not only frontal bone osteomyelitis, but epidural and, more commonly, subdural abscess, arises from mismanagement of the frontal sinus. If the lining mucosa is violated, which commonly occurs during the frontal craniotomy, it must be properly managed or there is a high probability of the complication of mucopyocele occurring. Extensive research has shown that damaged frontal sinus mucosa does not regenerate in the same way as that lining the ethmoid or maxillary sinuses (19). These latter sinuses reproduce a mucosa that histologically and functionally resembles that of the preoperative state. Moreover, if the mucosa was chronically infected and adequate drainage and appropriate antibiotics have been administered, it regenerates into a more healthy state. Such is not the case in the frontal sinus. There is a tendency to reproduce a thickened mucosa, sometimes devoid of cilia, which possesses an unusual propensity to form cysts. Furthermore, there is only one point of egress from each frontal sinus, and it is very susceptible to stenosis when injured. The damaged frontal sinus tends to form mucoceles either from the obstructed frontonasal duct or *de novo* from injured mucosa. If the sinus is transgressed during craniotomy, especially when the floor and duct of the sinus need operative intervention, one of two management principles must prevail. Either adequate drainage of the sinus must be ensured (a difficult thing to achieve on a long-term basis), or the sinus eliminated. The sinus is most safely eliminated either by obliteration or by cranialization. The latter is the easiest procedure to do, especially in view of the fact that all vestiges of mucosa can be readily removed because of the excellent exposure afforded by the craniotomy. The principal steps are to remove the posterior wall of the sinus and then drill out all the mucosa of the anterior wall and floor. The mucosal removal must be com-

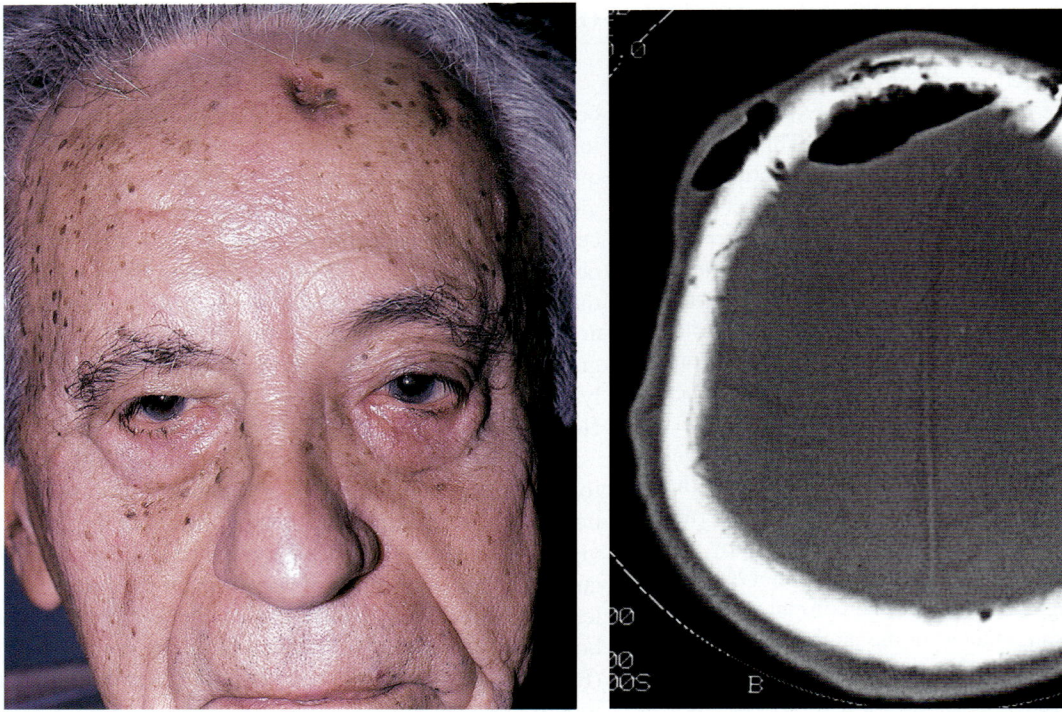

FIG. 14. Osteomyelitis of cranial bone flap. **A:** Depression in forehead over prior bur hole with a sinus tract. **B:** Computed tomography scan showing "moth-eaten" bone characteristic of osteomyelitis of cranial bone flap.

plete. Any remaining fragments will regenerate and be a significant source of infection. Because of the propensity for mucosal remnants to be retained in the small vascular pits that pockmark the sinuses' interior, drilling of the cavity is essential. The mucosa of the frontonasal duct is inverted on itself and the bone of the duct area lightly burred. The pericranial flap will lay directly over this area (20).

Osteomyelitis of the frontal bone is treated by bone flap excision. Reconstruction should be delayed until all traces of inflammatory resection have passed. A period of 12 months from bone removal to reconstruction provides ample opportunity for resolution and stabilization. Reconstruction is best done with split calvarial bone, but alloplasts such as cold-cure acrylic or hydroxyapetite may be used if the forehead skin appears sufficiently vigorous.

Minor degrees of bone exposure and small foci of osteomyelitis have occurred in four patients who had undergone the infratemporal fossa–middle fossa approach. These instances all occurred at the root of the zygoma or the adjacent squamosal temporal bone (Fig. 15). All four patients had re-

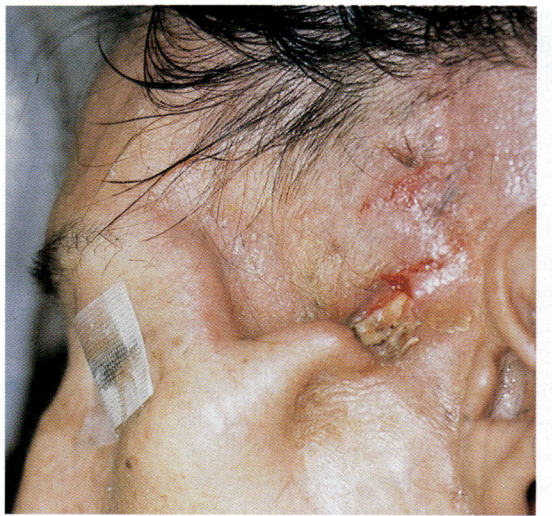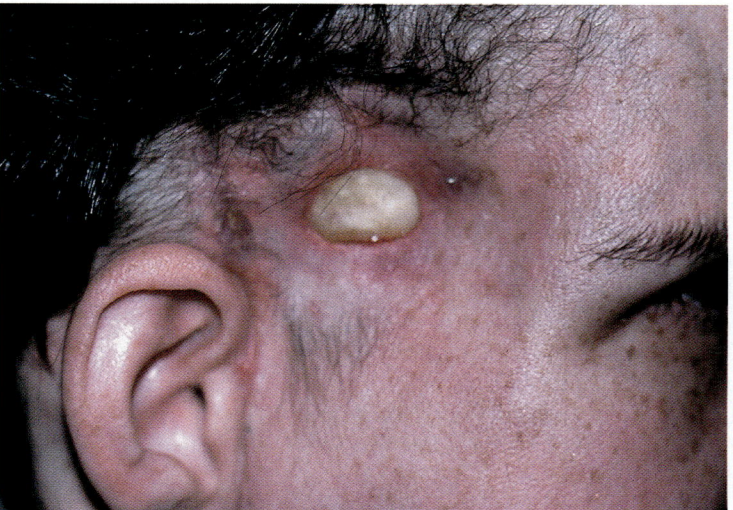

FIG. 15. Minor foci of osteomyelitis from bone exposure after the infratemporal fossa–middle fossa approach. **A:** Root of zygoma exposed. **B:** Squamous temporal bone exposure.

ceived radiation therapy at some time in the course of their treatment. In the author's earlier cases, an attempt was made to preserve the middle ear. This was often complicated by suppurative otitis media and adjacent wound infection despite the intraoperative placement of pneumatic ventilating tubes. This has become less frequent since the author's team began ablating the middle ear.

These areas are managed by conservative debridement and sterile wet-to-dry dressings to encourage granulation tissue formation, and then split-thickness skin grafting is done. Larger defects such as in Fig. 15B may need coverage with a flap such as the Oritcochea flap or flaps.

REFERENCES

1. Pearson BW. Cerebrospinal fluid rhinorrhea. In: Donald PJ, Gluckman JL, Rice DH, eds. *The sinuses.* New York: Raven Press, 1995:563–579.
2. Bergermann M, àWengen DF, Donald PJ. Management of inflammatory complications of skull base surgery. *Skull Base Surgery* 1993;3:7–10.
3. Schramm VL Jr. Anterior craniofacial resection. In: Sekhar LN, Schramm FL, eds. *Tumors of the cranial base.* Mount Kisco, NY: Futura Publishing Company, 1987:265–278.
4. Ketcham AS, Wilkins RH, Van Buren JM, Smith RR. A combined intracranial facial approach to the paranasal sinuses. *Am J Surg* 1963;106:698–703.
5. Schramm VL Jr. Anterior craniofacial resection. In: Jackson CG, ed. *Surgery of skull base tumors.* New York: Churchill Livingstone, 1997:67–83.
6. Deschler DG, Gutin PH, Kaplan MJ, Mamelak A, McDermott MW. *Complications of anterior skull base surgery.* Presented at the joint annual meeting of the German and North American Skull Base Societies, Lake Buena Vista, Florida, February 13, 1994.
7. Kraus DH, Shah JP, Arbit E, Galicich JH, Strong EW. *Complications of craniofacial resections for tumors involving the anterior skull base.* Presented at the 4th annual meeting of the North American Skull Base Society, Scottsdale, Arizona, February 14, 1993.
8. McCutcheon IE, Blacklock JB, Weber RS, Moser RP, Byers MS. *Transcranial resection of tumors of the paranasal sinuses.* Presented at the 4th annual meeting of the North American Skull Base Society, Scottsdale, Arizona, February 14, 1993.
9. Goodman SJ, Stern WE. Cranial and intracranial bacterial infections. In: Youmans JR, ed. *Neurological surgery.* 2nd ed. Vol. 6. Philadelphia: WB Saunders, 1982:3343–3355.
10. Skrap M, Milatini A, Vassallo A, Sidoti C. Stereotactic aspiration and drainage of brain abscesses: experience with 9 cases. *Minim Invasive Neurosurg* 1996;39:108–112.
11. Bucholz RD, Greco DJ. Image guided surgical techniques for infections and trauma of the central nervous system. *Neurosurg Clin North Am* 1996;7:187–200.
12. Shahzadi S, Lozano AM, Bernstein M, Guba A, Tasker RR. Stereotactic management of bacterial brain abscesses. *Can J Neurol Sci* 1996;23:34–39.
13. Posnick JC, Al-Qattan MM, Armstrong D. Monoblock and facial bipartition osteotomies for reconstruction of craniofacial malformations: a study of extradural dead space and morbidity. *Plast Reconstr Surg* 1996;97:1118–1128.
14. Henry AK, Heathcote RSA. The causation of intracranial aerocoele by brain-flap: an experimental proof. *Surg Gynecol Obstet* 1928;348:782–785.
15. Campanelli J, Odland R. Management of tension pneumocephalus caused by endoscopic sinus surgery. *Otolaryngol Head Neck Surg* 1997;116:247–250.
16. Markham JW. Pneumocephalus. In: Vinken PJ, Brayn GW, eds. *Handbook of clinical neurology.* Vol. 24. Amsterdam: North Holland Publishing Company, 1976:201–213.
17. Tokiyoshi K, Iwata Y, Mizuta T, Shimizu H, Nishioka K. Successful reconstruction of a skull base fracture with frontal lobe contusion by omental transplantation for recurrent posttraumatic tension pneumocephalus. *No Shinkei Geka* 1994;22:557–560.
18. Potparic Z, Fukuta K, Colen LB, Jackson IT, Carraway JH. Galeo-pericranial flaps in the forehead: a study of blood supply and volume. *British Journal of Plastic Surgery* 1996; 49(8):519–528.
19. Donald PJ. The tenacity of the frontal sinus mucosa. *Otolaryngol Head Neck Surg* 1979;87:557–566.
20. Donald PJ. Frontal sinus fractures. In: Donald PJ, Gluckman JL, Rice D, eds. *The sinuses.* New York: Raven Press, 1995:389–399.

CHAPTER 30

Postoperative Management

Bernard M. Lyons

The management of patients who have undergone skull base surgery can be complex and demanding. Just as the preoperative planning and surgical procedure are best undertaken using a multidisciplinary team approach, so the postoperative care should be coordinated by a dedicated skull base team. The surgery is often of long duration, and the possibility of life-threatening complications is high. This was demonstrated in many of the early craniofacial resection series (1,2). Many of these problems can be avoided by an experienced team. Familiarity with the particular surgical procedure, vigilance, and anticipation allow early detection of possible complications and thus prompt intervention.

The various surgical subspecialties should all be intimately involved in postoperative care, but a team leader should be designated to coordinate decision making (Table 1). Specialist nursing, as well as involvement of the various paramedical disciplines, including speech pathology, physiotherapy, dietetics, and occupational therapy, are essential to the smooth rehabilitation of these patients.

EARLY POSTOPERATIVE PERIOD

The first 2 weeks after skull base surgery is the most critical period and is when most of the life-threatening complications occur.

Recovery Room

Close monitoring in the recovery room in the first 1 to 2 hours is important because the patient's cardiovascular status may be quite labile. Hypovolemia and hypotension must be avoided to maintain adequate cerebral perfusion.

Rebound hypertension may be a problem if intraoperative hypotensive anesthetic techniques are used, and this may increase the risk of intracranial hemorrhage.

B. M. Lyons: Department of Otolaryngology—Head and Neck Surgery, St. Vincent's Hospital, and Royal Victorian Eye and Ear Hospital, Melbourne 3002, Australia.

Hypoxia must also be avoided, particularly in those patients who have undergone carotid artery intervention of any sort. Hypoxia, hypovolemia, and hypotension may be enough to precipitate cerebral infarction in a patient who has already experienced significant intraoperative cerebral ischemia. In those patients who do not have a tracheostomy, premature extubation may result in hypoventilation and possibly raised intracranial pressure (ICP) if respiratory obstruction occurs. It may be wiser to keep the patient intubated for 1 to 2 days if it is suspected that their conscious state will not allow adequate voluntary respiration. In most cases, however, it is preferable to have the patient breathing spontaneously to monitor better their neurologic status. Hypothermia can also be a significant problem after these often lengthy procedures. All of these factors should be closely controlled into the first 48 hours.

Intensive Care

After the patient has been sufficiently stabilized, he or she should be transferred to intensive care or to a head and neck or neurosurgical high-dependency nursing unit. Most patients have central venous and arterial lines. Lumbar spinal drains or, occasionally, ICP monitors require specialized nursing care.

Cardiorespiratory monitoring, as mentioned previously, is vital. Adequate respiration is maintained with an inspired oxygen concentration of 30%. The P_{CO_2} should be maintained at 28 to 30 mm Hg to prevent cerebral vasodilation. The patient should be kept recumbent at 30 to 45 degrees from the horizontal to decrease cerebral venous pressure.

A urinary catheter is usually *in situ* because of the length of the procedure, the need for osmolar diuretics, and the need to monitor urinary output, specific gravity, and osmolality. Intravenous fluids should be restricted to 1,500 to 2,000 ml of 4% dextrose and 20% normal saline every 24 hours. This prevents fluid overload and consequent cerebral edema and may reduce the risk of cerebrospinal fluid (CSF) leakage.

TABLE 1. *The skull base team*

Otolaryngology
Neurosurgery
Plastic surgery
Radiology
Nursing
Dental
Radiation oncology
Prosthetics
Physiotherapy
Social worker
Dietician
Occupational therapy

Frequent arterial blood gas and electrolyte estimations should be performed. Sodium aberrations may occur in the syndrome of inappropriate antidiuretic hormone secretion (SIADH) or diabetes insipidus. Hyperglycemia can occur particularly in patients receiving corticosteroids.

Neurologic Monitoring

The neurologic status of the patient is closely monitored in the first 48 hours, initially every 15 minutes for 4 hours, then at 30-minute intervals for 24 hours. It is essential to detect any early deterioration in neurologic signs to prevent an impending intracranial catastrophe. Therefore, a neurologic baseline must be established in the recovery room.

Cerebral edema or intracranial hemorrhage are the most common early problems and must be distinguished by computed tomography (CT) scan. Failure of the patient to regain consciousness when expected to in the recovery room may require immediate CT scanning or occasionally emergency evacuation of hematoma. CT scanning may also be required if the neurologic status deteriorates within the first few days. An early baseline CT scan is useful to assess the degree of pneumocephalus.

Cerebral edema can be an enormous problem, and measures must be taken to prevent its development. These begin during the operation with surgical techniques designed to minimize brain retraction and prevention of obstruction to venous drainage by good head positioning. Other measures are fluid restriction, intravenous dexamethasone, diuretics such as mannitol, and hyperventilation. These continue after surgery. ICP monitoring may occasionally be indicated in severe cases. ICP should be maintained at less than 20 mm Hg and can be measured by subarachnoid bolt or intraventricular catheter. Temporal lobe edema can be a big problem and lead to uncal herniation. In severe cases, temporal lobectomy may be indicated to reduce ICP if all other measures have failed and coning is imminent.

Other neurologic problems that can occur are CSF leak, meningitis, impaired brain function due to ablation of cerebral tissue or temporary neuronal dysfunction (especially the pituitary or hypothalamus), cranial nerve palsy, or epilepsy.

Epileptic seizures are important to detect because a postictal state may be misconstrued as a more ominous neurologic deterioration. All patients are maintained on anticonvulsants such as phenytoin for a minimum of 3 months.

Cerebrovascular events may also occur due to vasospasm, hypotension, embolus, or thrombosis. Pneumocephalus has occasionally been a problem in the author's experience (3) (Fig. 1). Most patients have some degree of intracranial air, but this will reabsorb over a period of weeks. Tension pneumocephalus can develop and lead to progressive obtundation of the patient, but will respond to aspiration through a bur hole. Pneumocephalus may be aggravated by excessive CSF drainage (4) or closed-nose swallowing with nasal packing *in situ*, a simulation of the Toynbee maneuver (5). Closed-nose swallowing initially results in increased nasopharyngeal pressure, which may promote the accumulation of intracranial air. Elective tracheostomy may prevent this problem in anterior craniofacial resection by diverting airflow away from the nasopharyngeal–intracranial interface.

In addition to the standard neurologic observations, the Glasgow Coma Scale (6) is used to record the neurologic status of the patient. This scale is based on eye opening and motor and verbal responses (Table 2). These three parameters are thought to give a more reliable and standardized assessment of the unconscious patient.

Cerebrospinal fluid lumbar drainage is often used. This serves two purposes: first, to allow intraoperative CSF removal to slacken the brain and minimize retraction, and second, to reduce the risk of postoperative CSF fistula, especially in anterior craniofacial resections. Lumbar spinal drainage is continued for up to 5 days. Close monitoring of the drains is essential. Maximum drainage of CSF is 5 to 10 ml/hour. This can be achieved at a constant rate by gravity positioning of the collecting burette with respect to the patient. A safer way to control flow is to drain 5 ml at the start of the hour and then leave the drain shut, or to regulate flow

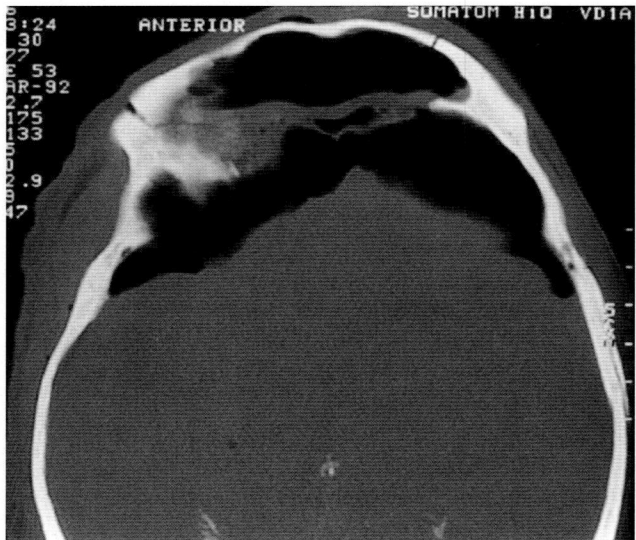

FIG. 1. Patient with marked pneumocephalus after anterior craniofacial resection. The pericranial flap is seen bridging the air space.

TABLE 2. *Glasgow Coma Scale*

Response	Score
Eyes	
Open	
Spontaneously	4
To verbal command	3
To pain	2
No response	1
Best motor response	
To verbal command	
Obeys	6
To painful stimulus	
Localizes pain	5
Flexion–withdrawal	4
Flexion–abnormal	3
Extension	2
No response	1
Best verbal response	
Oriented and converses	5
Disoriented and converses	4
Inappropriate words	3
Incomprehensible sounds	2
No response	1
Total	3–15

using an Imed pump as described by Swanson et al. (7). Patients should not be allowed to ambulate with an open spinal drain. Excessive CSF drainage may result in extradural hematoma (8) or aggravation of pneumocephalus, as previously mentioned. Daily CSF microcultures should be undertaken to check for developing meningitis. Antibiotic prophylaxis in the form of flucloxacillin is aimed at counteracting staphylococcal contamination of the indwelling catheter.

Antibiotic prophylaxis is usually administered to patients who undergo skull base surgery in any case. This is because of the long duration of the cases and the high risk of meningitis in anterior skull base cases, where the CSF may be exposed to the aerodigestive tract. Broad-spectrum antibiotics such as cefotaxime or ceftriaxone are given in combination with metronidazole on induction of anesthesia, and continued for 48 hours. Penicillin and chloramphenicol are also an effective and time-honored combination. If nasal packing is left *in situ*, antibiotics are continued until this is removed. Nasal packing is usually used in anterior craniofacial cases in the form of iodoform gauze. This is left *in situ* for 5 to 7 days, and reduces bleeding and promotes healthy, healed sinonasal cavities. It is usually best to remove the packs under general anesthesia. This also provides the opportunity to inspect and clean the cavity.

General Nursing Care

Tracheostomy may sometimes be performed to counteract airway edema, prevent aspiration, or divert the airway, as in anterior craniofacial resection. Frequent suctioning and adequate inspired air humidification should be ensured. The cuff pressure should be checked and deflated regularly to prevent complications such as subglottic stenosis.

Pressure care and skin care is important because these patients may be immobilized for long periods. Chest physiotherapy and incentive spirometry are instituted early on.

Deep-vein thrombosis prophylaxis is instituted in the form of antiembolic stockings, low-dose subcutaneous heparin (5,000 units twice daily), and early ambulation.

In the author's institution, a dry, nonstick dressing material (Telfa) is used along the suture line. Head bandaging is considered cumbersome, unattractive, and unnecessary. Occasionally, seromas develop under the scalp but they rarely require drainage. Drain tubes are avoided because they may promote CSF leak, and most subgaleal collections resolve spontaneously.

Intravenous fluids are maintained for 48 hours or until oral intake is instituted. It is usually unnecessary to feed a patient parenterally during this period. If it is anticipated that feeding will be delayed, then a percutaneous endoscopic gastrostomy is performed. Nasogastric tubes are avoided, particularly in anterior craniofacial cases, where they may ride up and impinge on the dural reconstruction. Attempts at nasogastric reinsertion can result in inadvertent intracranial placement. Gastric pH is monitored and antacids and intravenous ranitidine are used to guard against gastrointestinal hemorrhage.

Procedure-Specific Management

Certain aspects of postoperative management are determined by the type of surgical procedure performed. If microvascular free flaps have been used for reconstruction, then flap viability must be closely monitored. Free vascularized muscle flaps at the skull base provide a vital separation between the aerodigestive tract and the intracranial space. This is particularly important in patients who have been previously irradiated or in whom the carotid artery has been exposed or grafted. Flap necrosis in these situations may lead to meningitis or carotid blow-out and death. The flaps are monitored by direct observation, if visible. If the flap is buried, Doppler ultrasound monitoring of the vascular pedicle is performed or a sentinel portion of the flap is left at skin level. Arterial compromise is indicated by ischemia, and venous occlusion results in flap congestion. It is important to detect these changes early if the flap is to be salvageable. Intravenous rheologic agents may be necessary to guard against occlusion of the vessels.

In cases where carotid artery grafting or significant carotid manipulation has been performed, a carotid angiogram should be performed in the first 24 to 48 hours to ensure vessel patency. The possibility of false aneurysm formation also exists if the vessel has been traumatized.

Ocular management is important, particularly where facial paresis is expected. Reduced eye closure can lead to corneal ulceration. If this problem is thought to be temporary, it can be managed with ophthalmic ointments, lubricant drops, eye taping, or moisture chambers. Concomitant involvement of the ophthalmic division of the trigeminal nerve and the facial nerve requires more stringent measures for protection of the cornea, and a tarsorrhaphy should be performed (Fig. 2). Increasingly in situations where the facial nerve is thought to be permanently damaged, upper lid gold weight implantation is being performed as a primary procedure (9,10). Visual acuity should be monitored where dissection has occurred near the orbit or orbital apex. Edema and compression of the optic nerve can occur, and intraorbital hematoma can result in rapid loss of vision unless decompression and lateral canthotomy and cantholysis are performed. Patching of the eye may be necessary if significant diplopia is present.

Lateral skull base approaches in which the eustachian tube has been resected require appropriate management of the middle ear space. Some authors advocate obliteration of the middle ear in infratemporal fossa resections (11). It is this author's practice to insert a ventilation tube when the temporal bone is not directly involved with tumor. This allows maintenance of hearing. Long-term follow-up is required to detect middle ear complications such as atelectasis or cholesteatoma formation.

Particular problems can arise in surgery of the suprasellar or parasellar region and are usually related to fluid and electrolyte imbalance. Diabetes insipidus results in uncontrolled urine output and is associated with a urine specific gravity of less than 1.005. Serum and urine electrolytes and osmolalities are monitored and treatment commenced with intramuscular or intravenous vasopressin. When the situation stabilizes, intranasal DDAVP is instituted. SIADH can also occur after any intracranial procedure and, again, fluid and electrolyte balance must be closely monitored.

Patients with lower cranial nerve dysfunction usually are not fed enterally in the early postoperative period but may run into problems with aspiration pneumonia anyway because of inability to handle their own upper airway secretions. In this situation, early tracheostomy may need to be considered.

Ward Management

After the first 48 hours, or when the patient is hemodynamically and neurologically stable, he or she is transferred to the general ward. Most acute neurologic problems will have declared themselves, apart from an ongoing risk of meningitis, abscess formation, or CSF leak. CSF rhinorrhea or otorrhea should be checked for routinely. CSF can be distinguished from nasal secretions by electrophoresis to detect β-transferrin.

The emphasis at this stage should be on early ambulation and physiotherapy. Nutritional considerations also arise. Many patients are able to undertake oral feeding at this stage. Risks of salivary fistula, food contamination of free flap, or lower cranial nerve palsy may require alternative measures. Nasogastric tube placement should be avoided where there are defects in the anterior skull base or where free flaps are likely to be impinged on by the tube. Percutaneous endoscopic gastrostomy feeding or total parenteral nutrition should be considered in these cases. The problem is worse when cranial nerve paresis occurs. Posterior fossa surgery potentially involves the glossopharyngeal, vagus, and hypoglossal nerves. This results in reduced pharyngeal sensation, muscle tone, and coordination. All phases of the act of swallowing are interfered with, and aspiration of food and secretions can occur. Compounding this problem is the inability to produce an effective cough because of vocal cord paralysis. It must be said that patients who have preoperative evidence of lower cranial nerve palsy will cope much better because they have already adapted to the deficit over a period of time. Acute injury to the lower cranial nerves can result in significant and often long-term disability. In this situation, anticipation of the problem is important and early gastrostomy or jejunostomy is wise. Nasogastric tubes can compound the problem by promoting gastroesophageal reflux and laryngeal edema.

Tracheostomy should be considered to protect the airway but may cause additional problems by impairing laryngeal elevation on swallowing, reducing laryngeal reflexes and reducing cough effectiveness. The standard tracheostomy cuff does not always protect against aspiration. A modified type

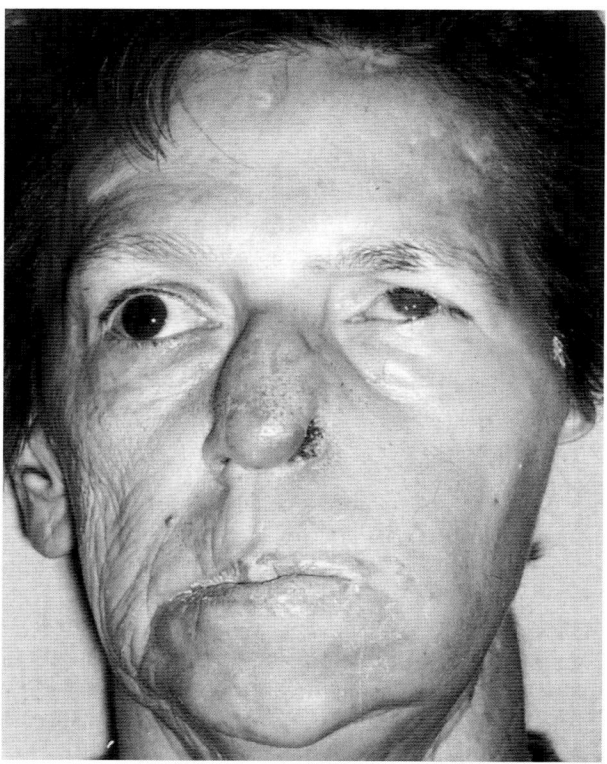

FIG. 2. Patient after surgery for posterior fossa meningioma. Left eye has undergone tarsorrhaphy because of combined facial and ophthalmic division paralysis.

of foam cuff tube may provide better protection. Decannulation is often a slow process, and swallowing rehabilitation may need to be continued long term. Gelfoam and Teflon injections have been used to improve laryngeal competence. Silastic medialization laryngoplasty, performed as a primary procedure, is thought to be a better option, may avoid the need for tracheostomy, and is potentially reversible if recovery occurs (12).

Wound complications are also likely to occur in this period. Seromas or subcutaneous CSF collections should resolve spontaneously. Abscesses may require drainage. Skin flap necrosis in anterior skull base surgery is rare but may occur when preoperative radiation therapy has been used or when a galeal component has been combined with a pericranial flap, resulting in impaired vascularity of the flap (13). It is the author's belief that pericranium alone provides adequate separation of the anterior cranial fossa from the nose, and avoids the possibility of scalp necrosis.

Severe hemorrhage may occur if carotid exposure develops because of flap necrosis or inadequate coverage. Emergency interventional radiology and balloon occlusion may be the only way to salvage this situation.

Trismus can occasionally occur with lateral procedures, especially if temporomandibular joint interference is combined with pterygoid muscle resection. This is best dealt with early, and distraction devices can be useful to counteract the trismus.

Nasal decrusting and saline irrigation is performed early in anterior skull base cases and may need to be continued long-term by the patient.

INTERMEDIATE POSTOPERATIVE PERIOD

This period extends from 2 weeks to 3 months postsurgery. Most patients will have been discharged from hospital, but delayed complications can still occur in this period. Admission to a rehabilitation unit may be necessary if there has been significant neurologic damage or swallowing problems. Patients are checked at frequent intervals in the outpatient clinic for delayed wound complications and nasal decrusting. CSF leaks can occur even at this time, especially in irradiated patients. If this occurs, a CT scan is prudent to rule out the development of hydrocephalus. Extrusion of free bone flaps (frontal or orbitozygomatic) can occur with associated osteomyelitis and extradural abscess (Fig. 3). This is more commonly seen in patients who have had prior radiation therapy. This is managed by drainage, debridement, and intravenous antibiotics.

Adjuvant therapy may need to be instituted in the form of external beam irradiation. It is important that this occurs in a timely, coordinated fashion, preferably before 6 weeks has transpired.

Nasolacrimal duct problems may occur even if the sac is marsupialized and stented after anterior craniofacial resections. Persistent epiphora can be readily dealt with by endoscopic dacryocystorhinotomy (Fig. 4).

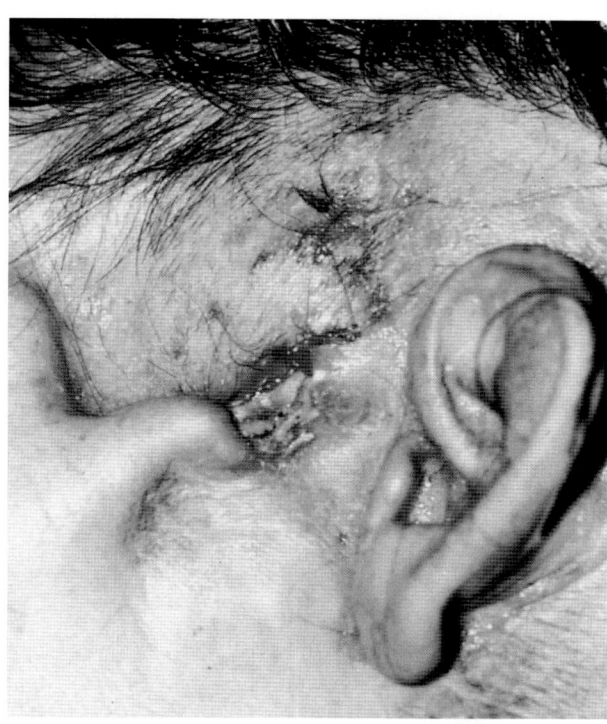

FIG. 3. Extrusion of zygomatic arch and skin necrosis after infratemporal fossa resection and radiation therapy.

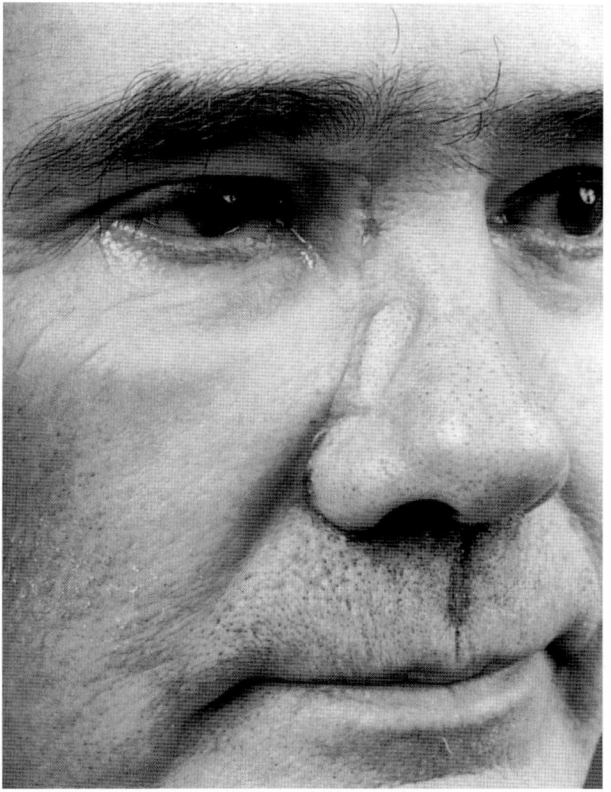

FIG. 4. Right epiphora after lateral rhinotomy and anterior craniofacial resection.

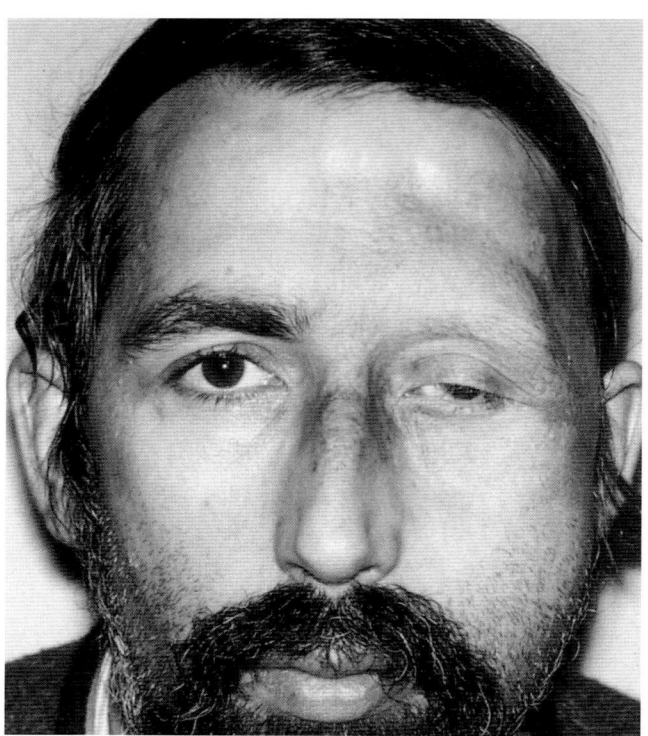

FIG. 5. Left frontalis paralysis and temporalis wasting after infratemporal fossa resection for meningioma.

LATE POSTOPERATIVE PERIOD

After 3 months, most skull base surgery patients have recovered from the surgery, completed their postoperative radiation therapy, and are looking to return to a more normal lifestyle. At this stage, the role of the team is mainly supportive. Many patients, although having come through the surgical process well, are left with significant psychosocial problems. Depression and anxiety are common. Patients are fearful about tumor recurrence and have self-doubts about their ability to return to the workforce after such major surgery. Most people, with encouragement and support from their skull base team and with vocational rehabilitation, can return to near-preoperative levels of performance.

Tumor follow-up is important, and patients are seen regularly for 3 years to detect clinical tumor recurrence. At 3 months, the author would ordinarily obtain a radiologic baseline, preferably with a magnetic resonance imaging (MRI) scan. This allows later tumor recurrence to be distinguished from postsurgical changes. Routine scans are then performed at 6-month intervals. Reconstruction plates can create streak artifact, which can make follow-up with CT scan difficult. The use of titanium plates or wire obviates the problems inherent in the use of steel for MRI follow-up.

Wound complications are very infrequent at this stage, but cosmetic factors may need to be addressed (Fig. 5). Enophthalmos may develop after extensive orbitomaxillary surgery and require augmentation bone grafting. Microvas-

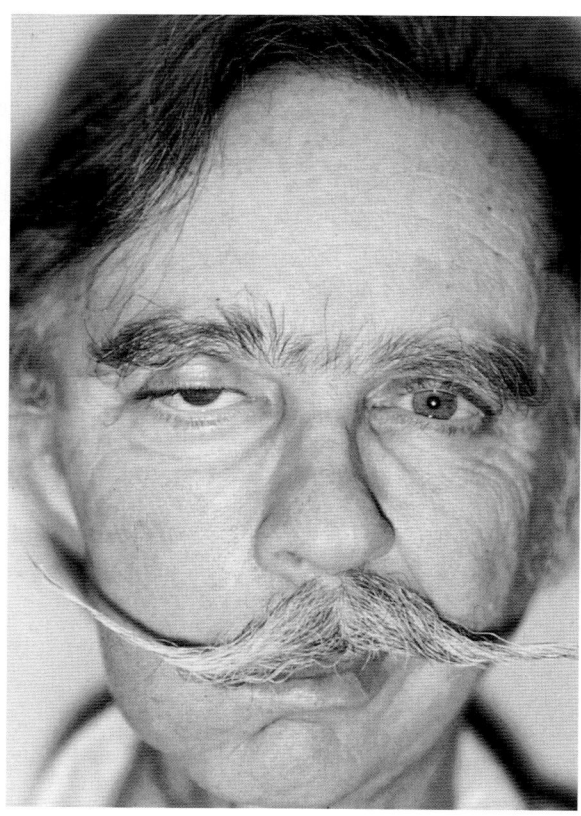
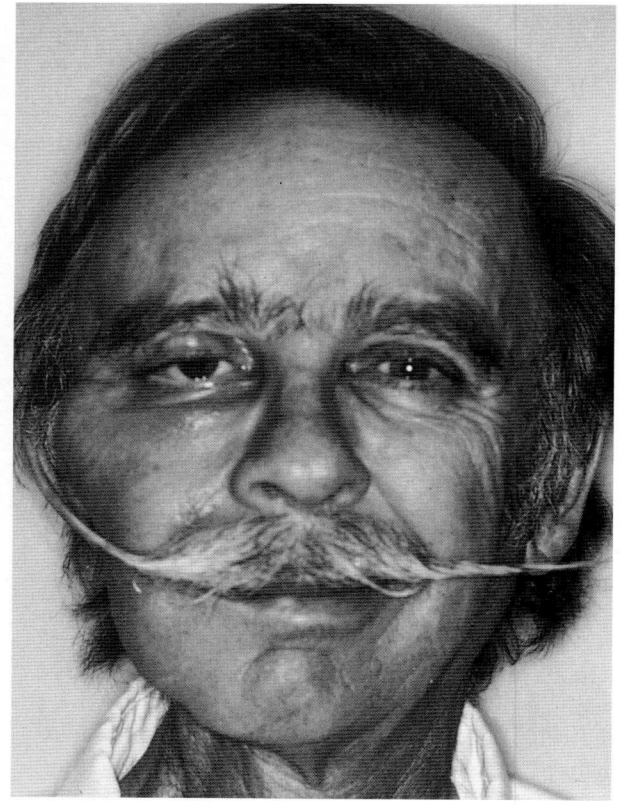

FIG. 6. A: Right facial nerve paralysis after radical parotidectomy. **B:** Patient after temporalis muscle sling and right upper eyelid gold weight for facial reanimation.

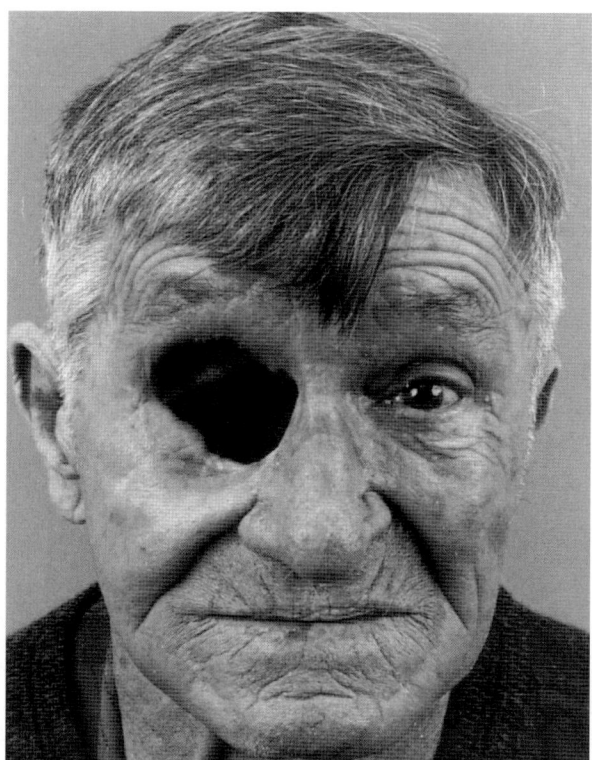
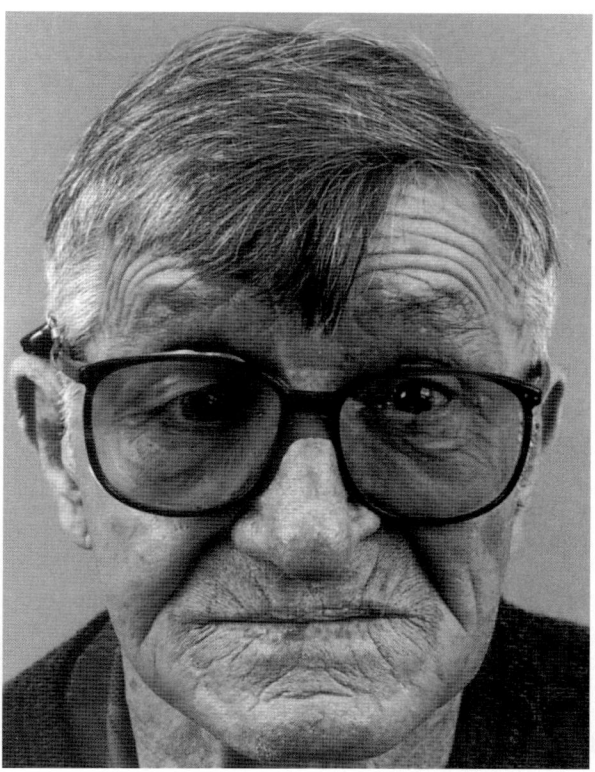

FIG. 7. A: Orbital exenteration defect after craniofacial resection or carcinoma of ethmoid sinus. **B:** Eyeglass-borne ocular prosthesis.

cular free flaps, in particular the muscle component, can atrophy and require revision. Failure of the facial nerve function to recover after 6 to 12 months may require facial reanimation or static sling procedures (Fig. 6). Likewise, troublesome diplopia can be corrected with lenses or extraocular muscle surgery. Prosthetic correction of orbital, auricular, or dental defects is normally instituted early in the postoperative period (Fig. 7). Refinements need to be made to these as wound contracture occurs. More definitive prostheses and further surgical procedures may be needed if osseointegration techniques are used. Osseointegrated implants are rapidly becoming the method of choice for securing prostheses.

Auditory rehabilitation has been ignored to a large extent in the past. Many patients with intact auditory nerve function and obliterated middle ear clefts have been left without hearing in that ear. It should be possible with adequate planning for these patients to be rehabilitated with an osseointegrated, bone-anchored hearing aid (14) (Fig. 8). In general, these produce superior sound characteristics to

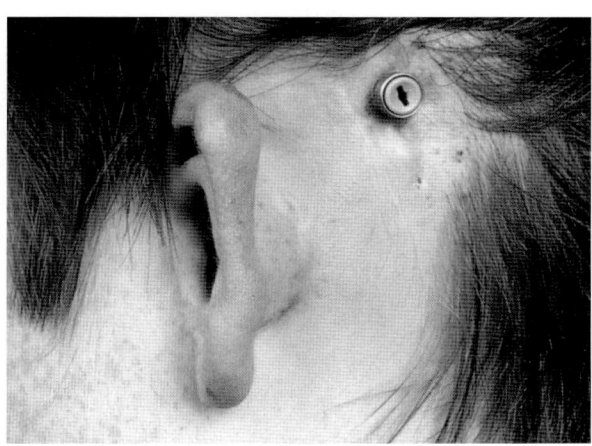
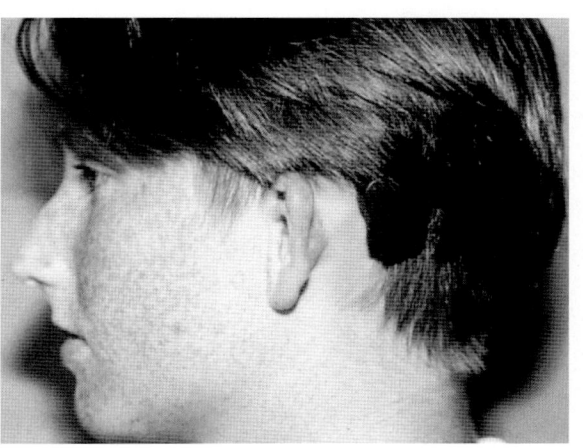

FIG. 8. A: Titanium fixture with abutment for bone-anchored hearing aid. **B:** Bone-anchored hearing aid *in situ*. (Photographs courtesy of Branemark Implant Unit, Alfred Hospital, Melbourne, Australia.)

conventional bone-conducting hearing aids. Patients with complete sensorineural hearing loss after skull base surgery, especially those with poor contralateral hearing, can now have a brainstem electrode implanted (15). This is particularly applicable in patients with bilateral acoustic neuromas. The auditory rehabilitation process in these cases is long-term.

An often neglected problem after anterior craniofacial resection is total anosmia. This can be a problem when combined with other cranial nerve deficits, and these patients should be advised to fit smoke detectors in their homes.

CONCLUSION

The postoperative management of skull base patients requires a coordinated team approach. If conducted in this manner, most problems can be anticipated and avoided. Care can be provided in a cost-effective, orderly sequence and ensure the timely return of the patient to his or her normal life circumstances.

REFERENCES

1. Ketcham AS, Wilkins RH, Van Buren JM, Smith RR. A combined intracranial facial approach to the paranasal sinuses. *Am J Surg* 1963;106:698–703.
2. Terz JJ, Alksne JF, Lawrence W. Craniofacial resection for tumours invading the pterygoid fossa. *Am J Surg* 1969;118:732–740.
3. Lyons BM, Sykes JM, Boggan JE, Donald PJ. Craniofacial resection for intracranial inverting papilloma with frontal sinus mucocoele. *Skull Base Surgery* 1992;2(2):92–97.
4. Effron MZ, Black O, Burns DS. Tension pneumocephalus complicating the treatment of postoperative CSF fistula. *J Neurosurg* 1964;21:275–278.
5. Perlman HB. Observations on the eustachian tube. *Archives of Otolaryngology* 1951;53:370–385.
6. Jennett B, Teasdale G. Aspects of coma after severe head injury. *Lancet* 1977:878–881.
7. Swanson SE, Chandler WF, Koron MJ, Bogdasarian RS. Flow regulated continuous spinal drainage in the management of cerebrospinal fluid fistulas. *Laryngoscope* 1985;95:104–106.
8. Graf CJ, Gross CE, Beck DW. Complications of spinal drainage in the management of cerebrospinal fluid fistula: report of three cases. *J Neurosurg* 1981;54:392–395.
9. May M. Gold weight and wire spring implants as an alternative to tarsorrhaphy. *Arch Otolaryngol Head Neck Surg* 1987;113:656–660.
10. Kartush JM, Linstrom CJ, McCann PM, Graham MD. Early gold weight eyelid implantation for facial paralysis. *Otolaryngol Head Neck Surg* 1990;103:1016–1023.
11. Fisch U, Fagan P, Valavanis A. The infratemporal approach to the lateral skull base. *Otolaryngol Clin North Am* 1984;17:513–544.
12. Netterville JL, Jackson CG, Civantos F. Thyroplasty in the functional rehabilitation of neurotologic skull base surgery patients. *Am J Otol* 1993;14:460–464.
13. Shah JP, Kraus DH, Arbit E, Galicich JH, Strong EW. Craniofacial resection for tumours involving the anterior skull base. *Otolaryngol Head Neck Surg* 1992;106:387–393.
14. Tjellstrom A, Hakansson B. The bone anchored hearing aid: design principles, indications and long term results. *Otolaryngol Clin North Am* 1995;28:53–72.
15. Briggs RJS, Brackman DE, Baser ME, Hitselberger MD. Comprehensive management of bilateral acoustic neuromas. Current perspectives. *Arch Otolaryngol Head Neck Surg* 1994;120:1307–1314.

CHAPTER 31

Free Flaps in Skull Base Surgery

Jonathan E. Aviv and Mark R. Sultan

The field of cranial base surgery, although originating in the 1960s, has been expanding greatly since the mid-1980s (1,2). There are several reasons for this expansion. First, diagnostic tools such as magnetic resonance imaging (MRI) and high-resolution computed tomography (CT) scanning have improved markedly (3–5). Second, advances in interventional neuroradiology have enhanced both the ability to map precisely the extent of neoplasms as well as the ability to decrease their vascularity through superselective embolization (6). Third, surgical approaches to the skull base through new transfacial and craniofacial incisions have greatly improved the head and neck surgeon's safe access to the skull base. As the techniques for diagnosis and extirpation of skull base lesions have become more sophisticated, tumors previously deemed "unresectable" are now being pursued vigorously. However, without an ability to definitively and reliably reconstruct defects resulting from the resection of skull base tumors, the oncologic strides made would not be realized. Fortunately, concomitant with advances in radiographic imaging and surgical approaches, there has been an equal interest and development of expertise in reconstructive microvascular surgery.

Clearly, not all cranial base defects require free tissue transfer for their closure. In many cases, local flaps such as temporalis muscle and fascia or pericranium can provide adequate vascularized tissue to reconstruct small defects of the anterior or posterior cranial fossae (7). However, for defects involving exposure of the paranasal sinuses, nasopharynx, oropharynx, or hypopharynx, local, regional, or pedicled flaps from the trunk are often insufficient to safely achieve the goals of the reconstructive effort.

J. E. Aviv: Department of Otolaryngology, Head and Neck Surgery, College of Physicians and Surgeons, Columbia University, and Columbia Presbyterian Medical Center, New York, New York 10032.

M. R. Sultan: Department of Surgery, St. Luke's/Roosevelt Hospital, New York, New York 10019.

HISTORY

The description of free flaps for use in skull base reconstruction began in the early 1970s with a report by McLean and Buncke describing the use of omentum to reconstruct a large scalp defect (8). Since then, studies describing the application of free flaps for skull base reconstruction have proliferated. With refinements in microvascular surgical techniques, variations in the use of muscle flaps—the rectus abdominis in particular—have been described that have increased the versatility of various donor sites for application to geometrically complex skull base defects. These variations include using free muscle with overlying skin, fat, and deepithelialized skin (9).

For complex defects of the cranial base that involve the midface, free latissimus dorsi flaps have been described (10,11), either alone or in combination with other subscapular system flaps (12).

In addition to muscle-only and myocutaneous free flaps, cutaneous free flaps have been advocated for skull base reconstruction (13–15).

PATIENT SELECTION FACTORS

Considerations such as age, cardiopulmonary status, nutritional status, and underlying competency of the immune system, although germane to free flap reconstruction in general, are particularly important in patients undergoing skull base tumor surgery.

In skull base cases where the primary tumor is not in the neck, the recipient vessels for a microvascular anastomosis are readily and easily found in the neck. Typically, branches of the external carotid arterial system, and the facial artery in particular, are readily accessible for the artery from the flap. The external jugular vein and its venous tributaries, such as the posterior facial vein, are extremely reliable recipient vessels for the venous anastomosis. In cases where the neck has been irradiated, the possible use of vein grafts needs to be considered because it has been demonstrated experimentally that radiation therapy may injure blood vessels, thereby increasing the chance for a failed microvascular anastomosis (16). The superficial temporal vessels may be considered as potential recipient vessels because of their proximity to the lateral skull base. However, the artery, and particularly the vein, may be of moderate caliber or poor quality, thus precluding reliable use. Because most of the commonly used free flaps in skull base reconstruction have long pedicles, the superficial temporal vessels can usually be avoided in preference to larger-caliber neck vessels without the need for vein grafts.

GOALS OF CRANIAL BASE RECONSTRUCTION

When faced with massive, composite defects of the craniofacial region, it is important to keep in mind the goals of the reconstructive effort. The primary goal is to seal the intradural space from the extradural space, thus preventing cerebrospinal fluid (CSF) leak, ascending infection, and fulminant meningitis.

The choices of tissue that can be used to restore form as well as function depend on a number of factors, including the nature of the defect, the underlying disease process, the available donor sites, and the preferences and skills of the reconstructive surgeon.

Local free grafts of dermis, fascia, or muscle may be satisfactory when applied to small defects. However, in irradiated, scarred recipient beds, or in chronically infected cavities with large defects, regional pedicled flaps or distant free flaps provide a greater volume of reliable tissue. The distinct advantage of free flaps is that they have independent vascularity and can be more accurately contoured to the defect. Also, the problem of gravitational pull from the donor site is avoided.

The ideal donor site for restoring form and function to craniofacial defects should offer a substantial amount of pliable tissue that has a long vascular pedicle with large-diameter vessels. In addition, two surgical teams should be able to work simultaneously: the oncologic team at the head, and the reconstructive team harvesting tissue from a donor site that will not functionally or cosmetically impair the patient. Although no single flap consistently meets all of these criteria, the latissimus dorsi, serratus anterior, radial forearm, rectus abdominis, and scapular system free flaps are among the most commonly chosen free flaps for skull base defect reconstruction because they often best fulfill the aforementioned criteria. Other, less commonly used free flaps for this purpose are the omental, gracilis, and deep circumflex iliac artery flaps.

RADIAL FOREARM FREE FLAP

For limited defects with complex geometry, thin, pliable tissue is required, and the fasciocutaneous radial forearm free flap is very useful.

Anatomy

The radial forearm flap is based on the radial artery and cephalic vein and can be designed to transfer the skin of the volar aspect of the forearm extending from the antecubital fossa to the level of the flexor retinaculum (13). In addition, one of the sensory nerves to the forearm, either the medial or lateral antebrachial cutaneous nerves, can be harvested as well, should a sensate flap be desired (14).

Vascularized bone can also be provided by this flap by inclusion of a cuff of the flexor pollicis longus over the radius. In a man, one third of the diameter of the radius with a length approaching 14 cm is available. However, the relatively high incidence of donor site morbidity, including pathologic fracture of the radius, coupled with the fact that better sources of vascularized bone exist, preclude its widespread use for this purpose (17).

Although the radial forearm free flap usually is not bulky enough when reconstructing large cranial base defects, it has been shown to be a very reliable method of reconstructing geometrically complex cranial base defects (15). Figures 1 through 7 illustrate the application of a radial forearm free flap in reconstructing a complicated, contained defect of the anterior cranial fossa.

CASE 1

A 64-year-old man had an adenoid cystic carcinoma of the ethmoid sinus that extended superiorly into the anterior cranial fossa. The patient had originally undergone a craniofacial resection and orbital exenteration and was to undergo a secondary cranioplasty. However, a nasocutaneous fistula as well as an extradural–cutaneous fistula developed in the patient (see Fig. 1), resulting in pneumocephalus (see Fig. 2) and severe headaches. Before the cranioplasty, the patient required closure of the communication between the orbital cavity, the nasal cavity, and the extradural space.

To secure such a reconstruction, a radial forearm free flap was planned (see Fig. 3). The skin paddle was designed with a central cutaneous portion with two "tabs" on either side of the central skin paddle (see Fig. 4). The purpose of this design modification was to tuck vascularized, deepithelialized tissue into the geometrically complex confines of the nasal and orbital cavities, thereby sealing the nose and orbit from intracranial exposure (see Figs. 5, 6). The donor vessels were tunneled subcutaneously under the skin of the cheek into the neck (see Fig. 4). The recipient vessels for the microvascular anastomoses were the external jugular vein and the facial artery.

After surgery, the patient did well with resolution of headache. With the patient's infection controlled, he subsequently underwent a cranioplasty with an acceptable cosmetic result 1 year after surgery (see Fig. 7).

CASE 1 (Continued)

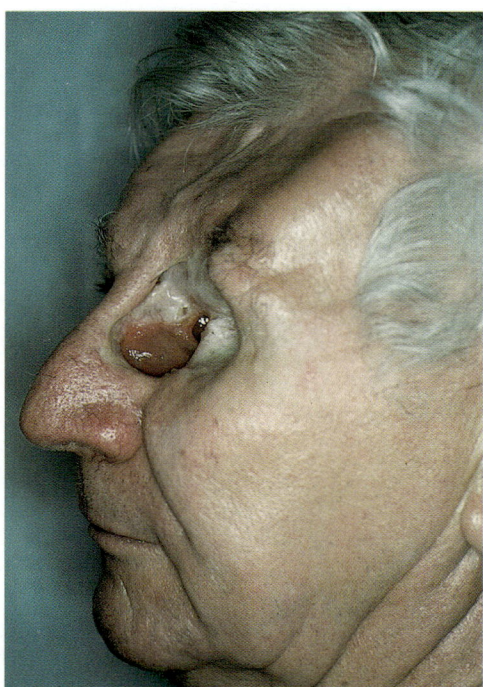

FIG. 1. Case 1. Preoperative lateral view of patient status resection of adenoid cystic carcinoma of ethmoid sinus that extended into the anterior cranial fossa.

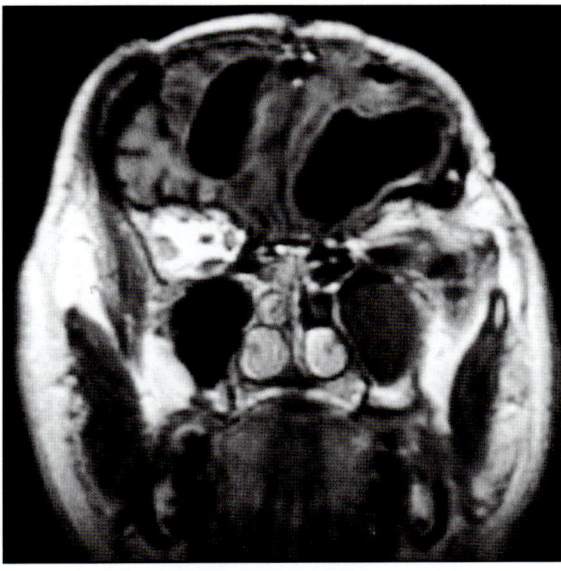

FIG. 2. Case 1. Magnetic resonance image demonstrating extensive pneumocephalus.

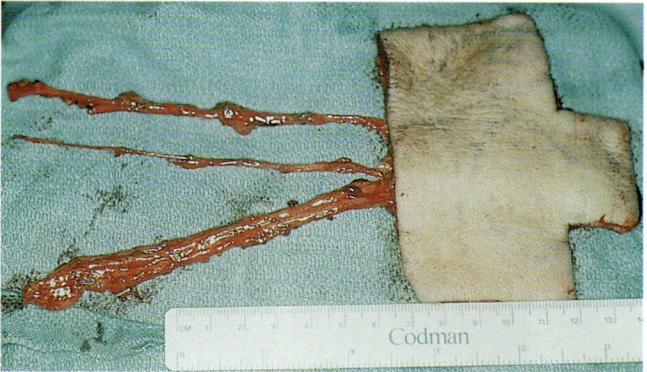

FIG. 3. Case 1. Harvested radial forearm free flap demonstrating the radial artery and its venae comitantes, the cephalic vein, and the lateral antebrachial cutaneous nerve.

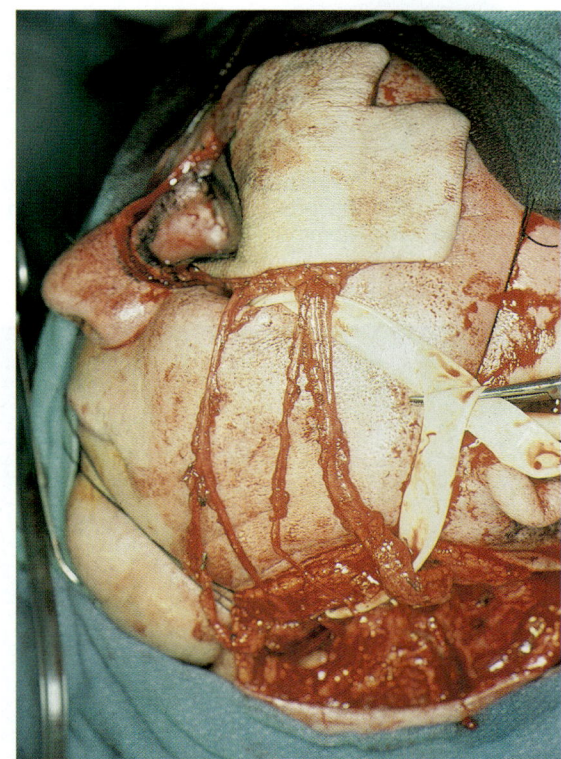

FIG. 4. Case 1. Radial forearm free flap being inset into nasal and orbital cavities. The neurovascular structures are shown along the cheek, directed toward the recipient vessels in the neck.

CASE 1 (Continued)

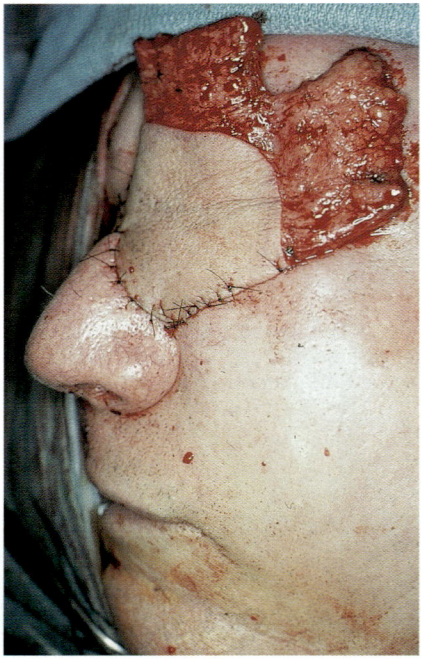

FIG. 5. Case 1. Deepithelializing portions of the radial forearm free flap allowed the nasal and orbital cavities to be sealed from intracranial communication.

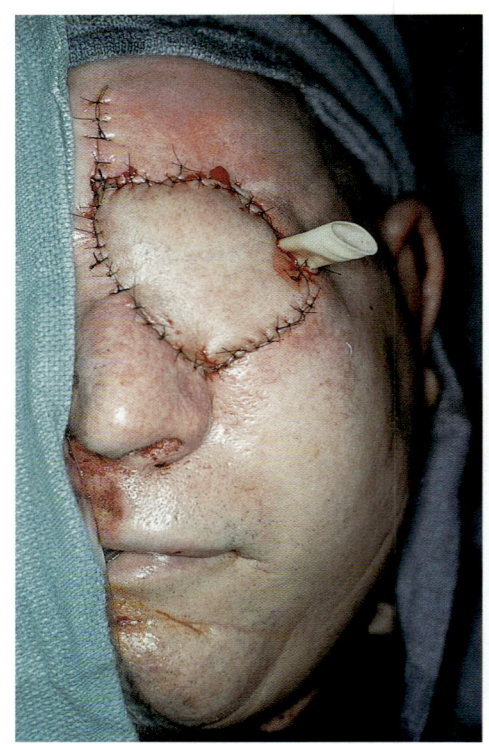

FIG. 6. Case 1. Immediate postoperative view.

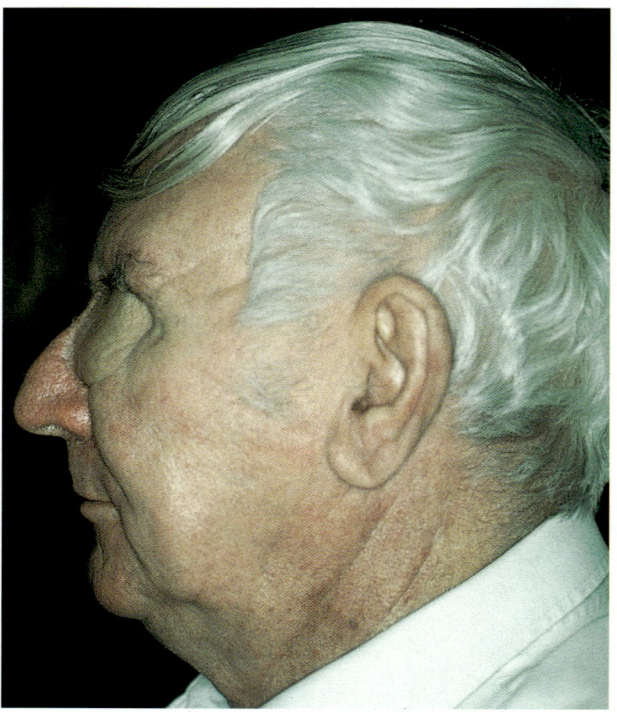

FIG. 7. Case 1. Patient about 12 months after surgery, free of headache and after cranioplasty.

Advantages

The advantages of the radial forearm free flap include the thin, pliable tissue it provides as well as the fact that its vascular pedicle is long and has a large diameter. The fact that the flap has sensate potential may be relevant only when reconstructing cranial base defects involving the nasopharynx.

Disadvantages

The greatest shortcoming of this flap is that its surface area is limited, which makes the flap unsuitable for resurfacing large defects.

RECTUS ABDOMINIS

The rectus abdominis free flap has emerged as the "workhorse" flap for reconstructing most extensive cranial base defects because it offers several distinct advantages over other soft tissue flaps (11). These include its long, large, and constant vascular pedicle, its large size, and low donor site morbidity. Furthermore, with the patient in the supine position, its distant location from the head and neck allows for simultaneous harvest as the skull base resection is being performed.

Anatomy

The blood supply to this flap is the deep inferior epigastric artery and vein, which enter the lateral border of the rectus muscle halfway between the pubis and umbilicus, just below the arcuate line (18). Although the superior epigastric vessels also supply the rectus abdominis muscle, the deep inferior epigastric vessels are a more reliable and accessible vascular supply for this free flap (19).

CASE 2

A 40-year-old diabetic woman weighing over 350 pounds had a recurrent meningioma of the frontal lobe resected and, after surgery, lost her frontal bone flap to infection (Fig. 8). Subsequently, CSF rhinorrhea, fulminant meningitis, and a large frontal lobe abscess developed in the patient (Fig. 9).

The patient was taken to the operating room to drain the abscess and to separate the nasal cavity from the dura and brain (Fig. 10). To cover the defect and to seal the intradural space from the extradural space, a large volume of vascularized tissue was required. Therefore, a rectus abdominis muscle free flap was harvested (Figs. 11, 12).

The muscle was placed carefully along the anterior cranial fossa and tacked into position (Fig. 13). The vascular pedicle was oriented along the preauricular region and anastomosed to recipient vessels in the neck (Fig. 14).

In closing the facial skin flap, a small portion of rectus muscle was left exposed in the preauricular region to monitor the flap. Within 72 hours after surgery, there was no further CSF leak and the patient ultimately recovered from her meningitis.

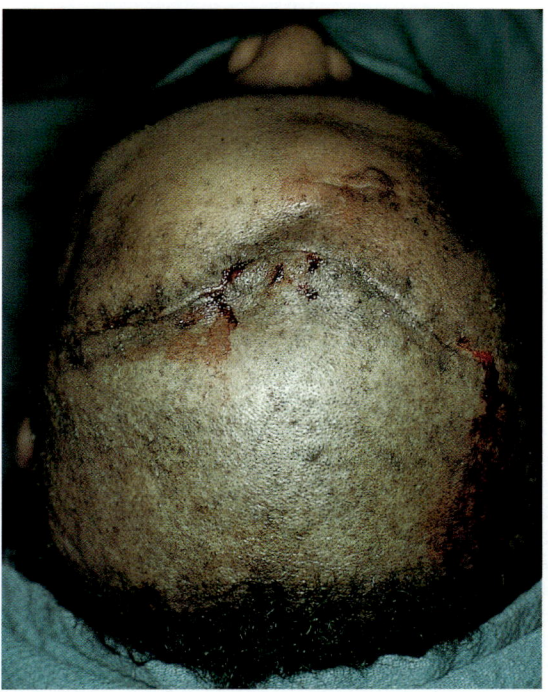

FIG. 8. Case 2. Preoperative view, from above, of diabetic patient who has lost her frontal bone flap secondary to infection.

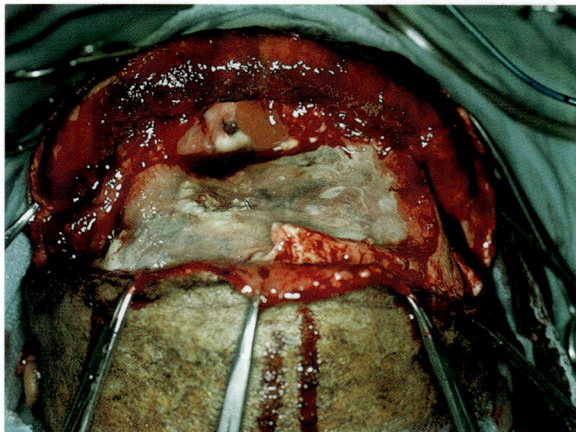

FIG. 9. Case 2. Forehead skin flap is elevated and what is being visualized is a sea of pus overlying, and adherent to, the dura of the frontal lobe. At the center of the wound is the superior aspect of the nasal cavity, which contains remnants of polypoid sinus mucosa.

CASE 2 (Continued)

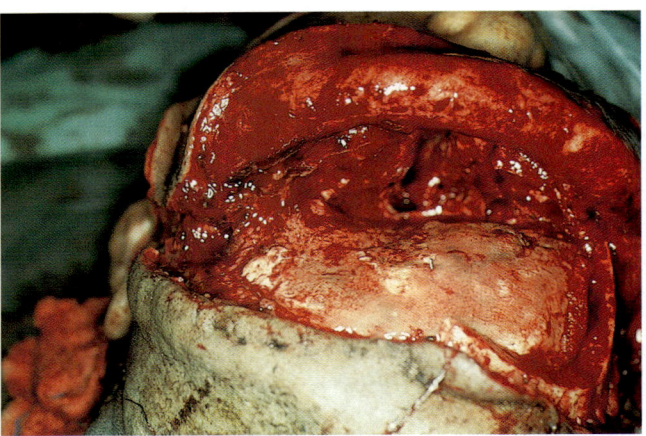

FIG. 10. Case 2. The sinus mucosa was completely removed and the infected material on the dura was carefully debrided, leaving a sizable dural defect.

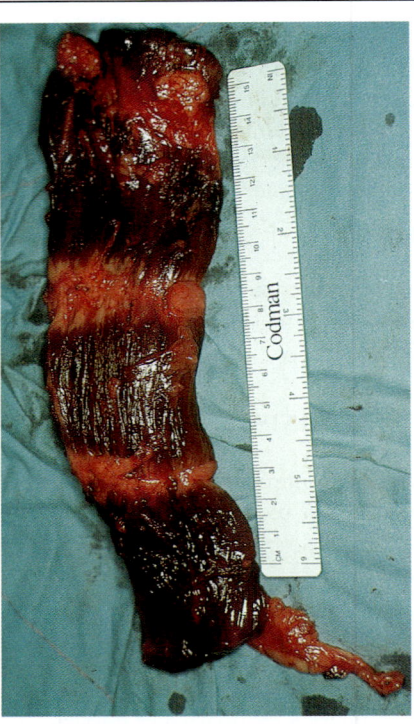

FIG. 12. Case 2. Rectus abdominis muscle harvested with the vascular pedicle exiting laterally.

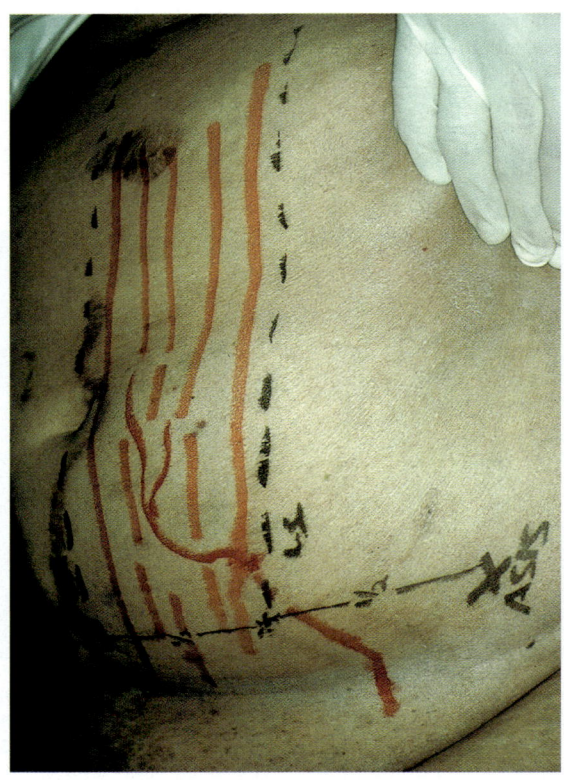

FIG. 11. Case 2. These are the landmarks of the anterior abdominal wall that allow an approximate mapping of the topographic anatomy of the rectus abdominis muscle. The rectus muscle is shown extending from the pubis to the inferior costal margin. Also shown is the linea alba, which represents the medial extent of the rectus muscle, extending from the pubis to the midline of the xiphoid process. The linea semilunaris, which represents the lateral extent of the rectus muscle, is located about halfway between the anterior superior iliac spine (ASIS) and the midline. Note also the arcuate line—below which the posterior rectus sheath is composed only of transversus abdominis aponeurosis. It is located roughly at the level of the ASIS.

CASE 2 (Continued)

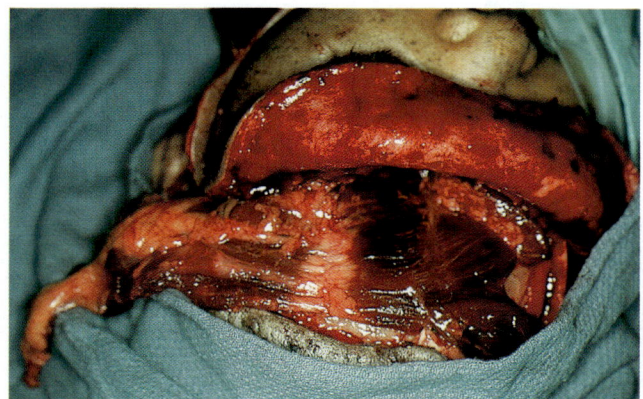

FIG. 13. Case 2. The rectus abdominis muscle free flap placed along the floor of the anterior cranial fossa.

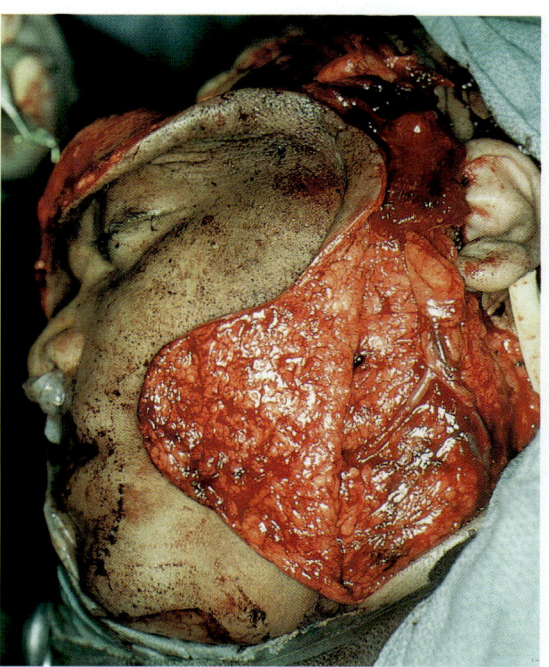

FIG. 14. Case 2. The vascular pedicle was brought along the preauricular region and anastomosed to recipient vessels in the neck.

CASE 3

A 64-year-old man had a recurrent squamous cell carcinoma of the orbital and nasal skin that grossly involved the eye, forehead, nasal dorsum, and underlying facial and frontal bones (Figs. 15, 16). An *en bloc* orbital exenteration was performed, including full-thickness loss of skin, muscle, and bone involving the nasal dorsum and forehead, as well as a portion of the dura of the frontal lobe (Figs. 17, 18). The reconstructive challenge included separation of the intracranial space from the nose and paranasal sinuses. A vascularized pericranial flap was used to patch the dura.

A free rectus muscle flap was used to reconstruct the anterior cranial base defect (Fig. 19), with the ipsilateral superficial temporal vessels serving as the recipient vessels. A split-thickness skin graft was placed over the rectus muscle (Fig. 20). After surgery, in the intensive care unit, the patient had an acute myocardial infarction and hypotension. The patient was immediately and successfully resuscitated with no loss of flap viability or development of CSF leak. On follow-up examinations, he did quite well, with primary healing of his wound (Figs. 21, 22).

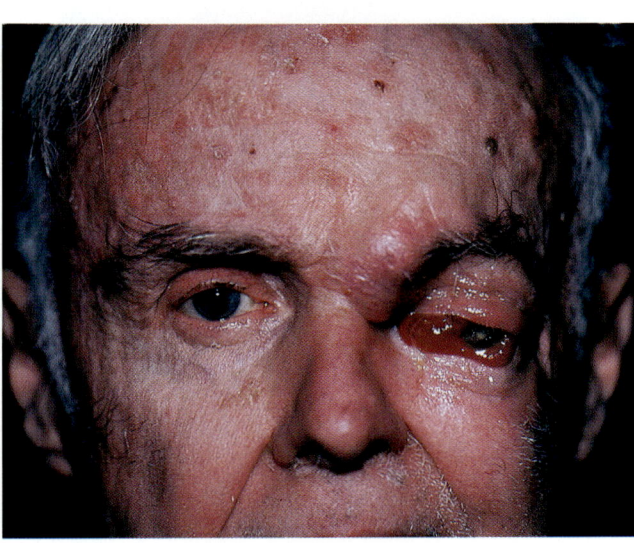

FIG. 15. Case 3. Preoperative view of a large left orbital squamous cell carcinoma involving the globe and frontal bone.

CASE 3 (Continued)

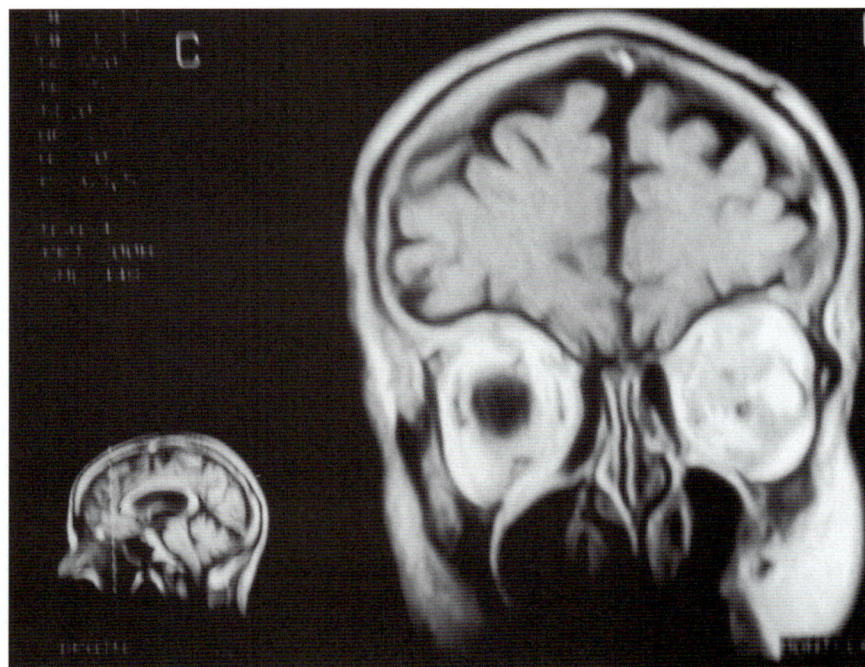

FIG. 16. Case 3. Magnetic resonance image showing gross involvement of the entire left orbital cavity with tumor.

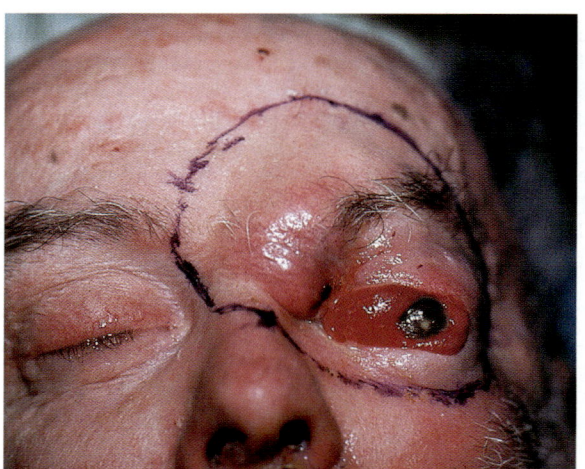

FIG. 17. Case 3. Outline of resection margin of tumor.

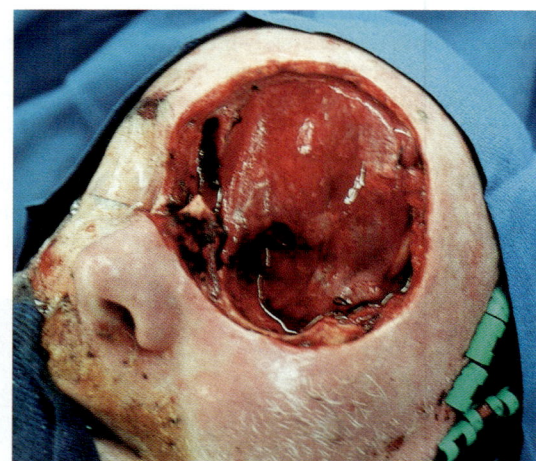

FIG. 18. Case 3. Surgical defect after *en bloc* orbital exenteration with surrounding skin, muscle, and bone.

CASE 3 (Continued)

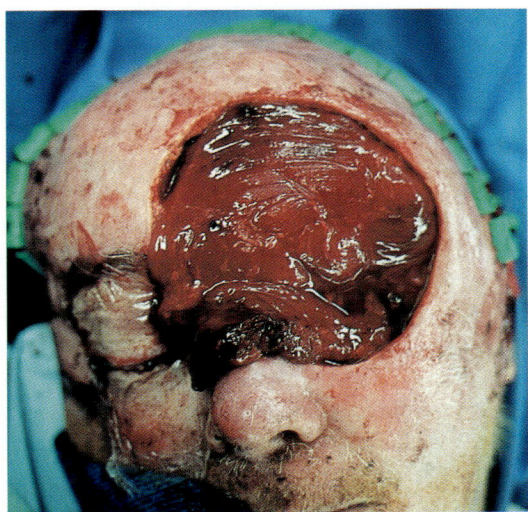

FIG. 19. Case 3. Reconstruction of defect from Fig. 18 with free rectus muscle flap.

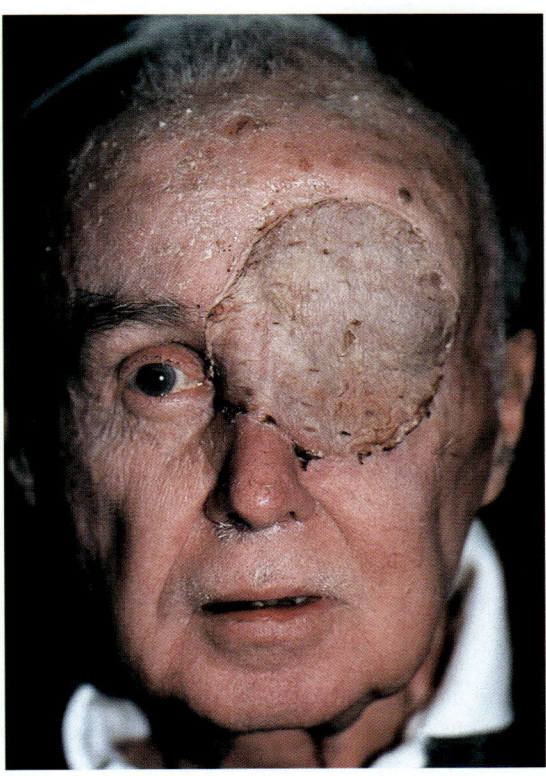

FIG. 20. Case 3. Postoperative anteroposterior view of patient 4 months after surgery.

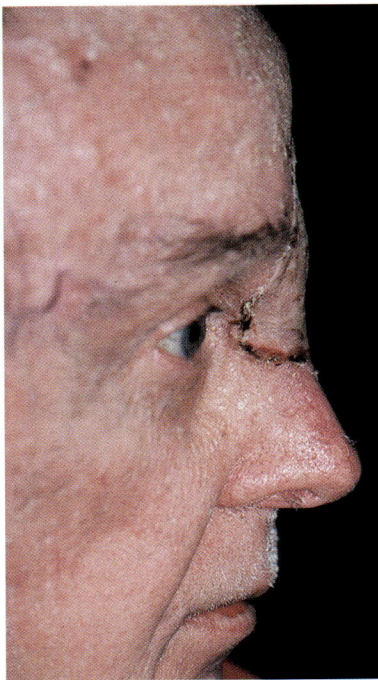

FIG. 21. Case 3. Lateral postoperative view of patient showing contralateral extent of reconstructed nasal dorsum. Note proximity of reconstructed region to remaining orbit.

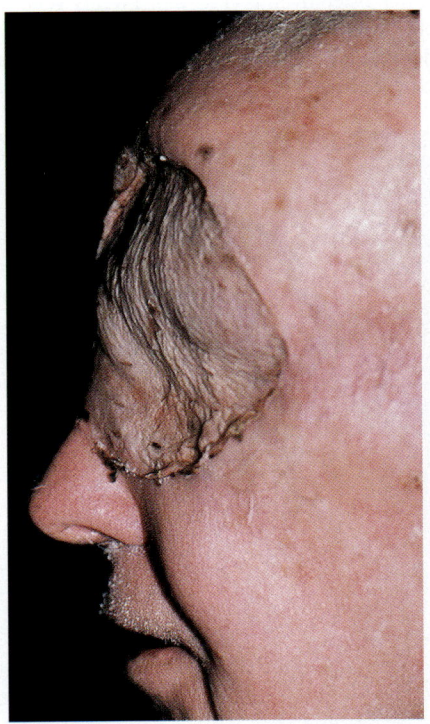

FIG. 22. Case 3. Lateral postoperative view of patient.

Advantages

The rectus abdominis free flap can be harvested with the patient in a supine or semiseated position, which is the usual position for most neurosurgical and head and neck procedures. It is located at a sufficiently remote distance from the head so that a simultaneous two-team approach can be carried out comfortably. The vascular pedicle is long and has a large diameter, and the surface area that can be harvested is extremely large, second only to the latissimus dorsi–scapula (12).

Disadvantages

The primary disadvantage of the rectus abdominis free flap is its bulk when it is used with its overlying skin because of the width of the subcutaneous tissues of the abdominal wall. This is particularly true in women or overweight patients. This may be avoided by harvesting muscle only and covering the muscle with a skin graft as needed.

LATISSIMUS DORSI AND SERRATUS ANTERIOR FREE FLAPS

Both the latissimus dorsi and serratus anterior muscles should be considered as potential donor flaps when the skull base defects are extensive. Either alone and certainly the two in combination can provide a large amount of well vascularized muscle with long vascular pedicles.

Anatomy

The latissimus dorsi muscle is a large muscle that originates from the thoracic spinous processes and posterior iliac crest and inserts into the posterior portion of the humerus. It is supplied by the thoracodorsal nerve and vessels. The vessels originate from the subscapular artery and vein. Although its function is to adduct and inwardly rotate the arm, virtually the entire muscle may be used as a flap with little impact on shoulder function (20).

The serratus anterior muscle is also a large muscle that originates from the lateral border of the upper eighth to ninth ribs and inserts on the undersurface of the scapula. The serratus anterior thus assists in stabilizing the shoulder during rotation. Because of this, the upper three or four slips of the muscle and their innervation by the long thoracic nerve should be spared whenever possible to prevent winging of the scapula. The serratus anterior is vascularized by crossing branches of the thoracodorsal vessels. The thoracodorsals are routinely included in the vascular pedicle harvest to increase its length (21).

CASE 4

A 64-year-old man presented with a frontal lobe abscess and frontal bone flap osteomyelitis (Fig. 23). Twenty years previously, he underwent resection of a frontal lobe meningioma. Five years later he underwent a second resection and radiation therapy for recurrent disease. Subsequently, he had right-sided weakness and expressive aphasia. An MRI revealed an abscess in his frontal lobe (Fig. 24). Operative debridement of all devitalized brain, the overlying bone flap, and the necrotic scalp was carried out (Fig. 25). A free latissimus muscle flap was then used to obliterate the potential space in the frontal lobe and to reconstruct the scalp (Fig. 26). The

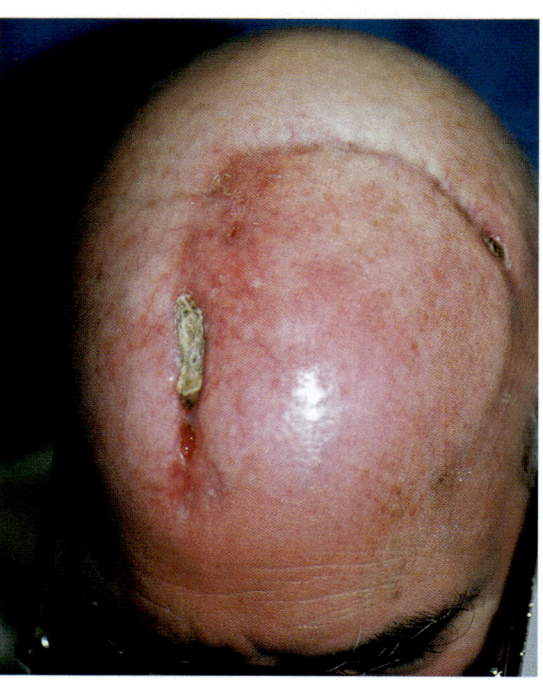

FIG. 23. Case 4. Preoperative view of scalp of patient with frontal bone osteomyelitis and frontal lobe abscess.

CASE 4 (Continued)

thoracodorsal vessels were anastomosed to the facial vessels primarily without vein grafts. The muscle was covered with split-thickness skin grafts (Figs. 27, 28). No bony reconstruction was carried out. The patient's postoperative course was uneventful.

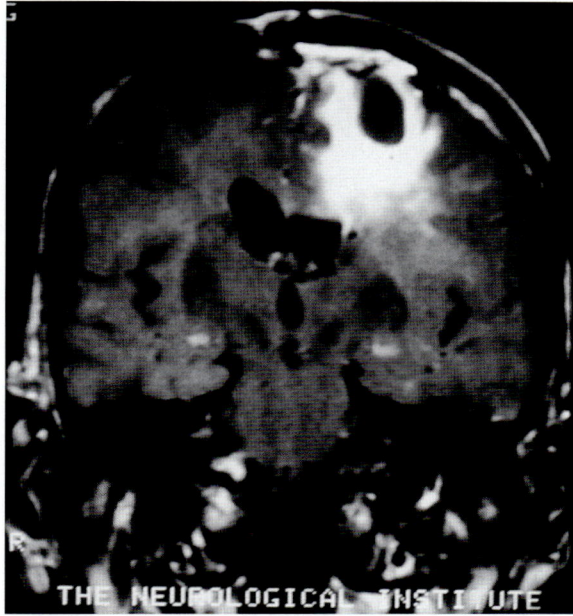

FIG. 24. Case 4. Preoperative coronal magnetic resonance image demonstrating abscess in the frontal lobe of the brain.

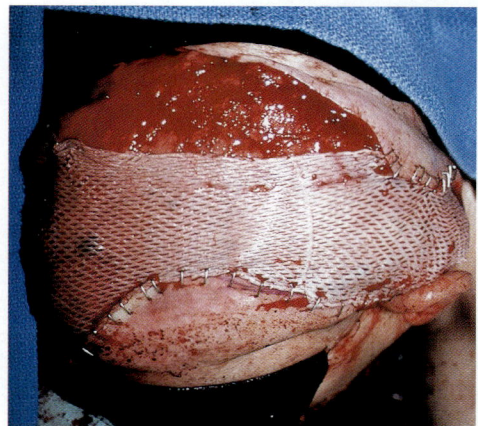

FIG. 26. Case 4. Free latissimus dorsi muscle flap inset into cranial defect with overlying split-thickness skin graft.

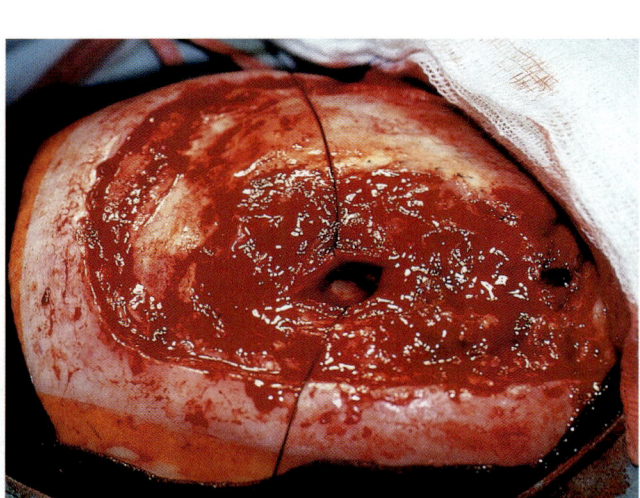

FIG. 25. Case 4. Defect after debridement of devitalized brain, overlying bone flap, and necrotic scalp.

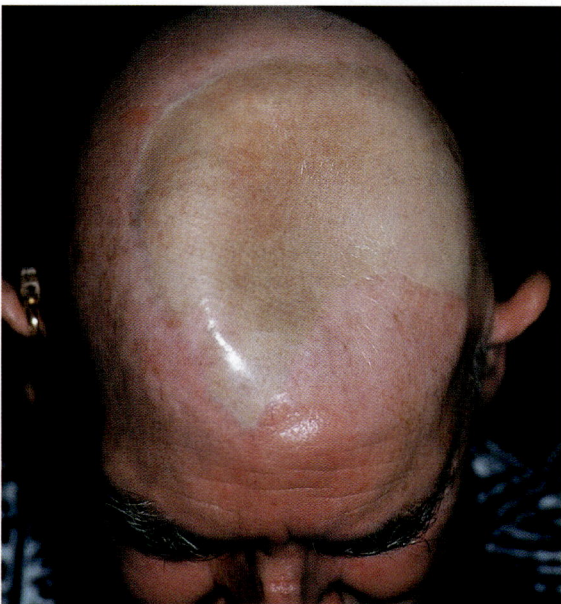

FIG. 27. Case 4. Postoperative aerial view of patient 6 months after surgery.

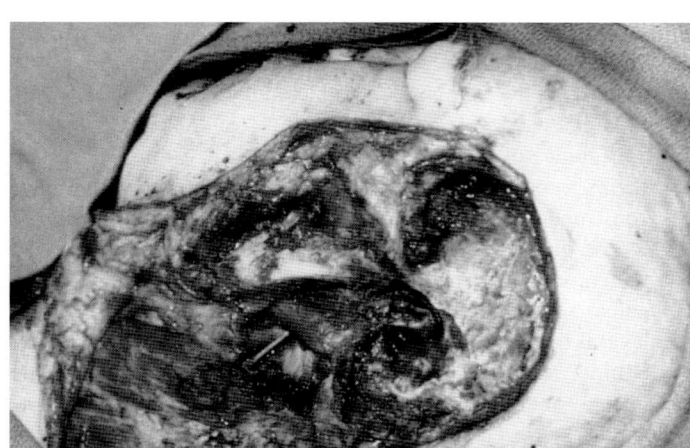
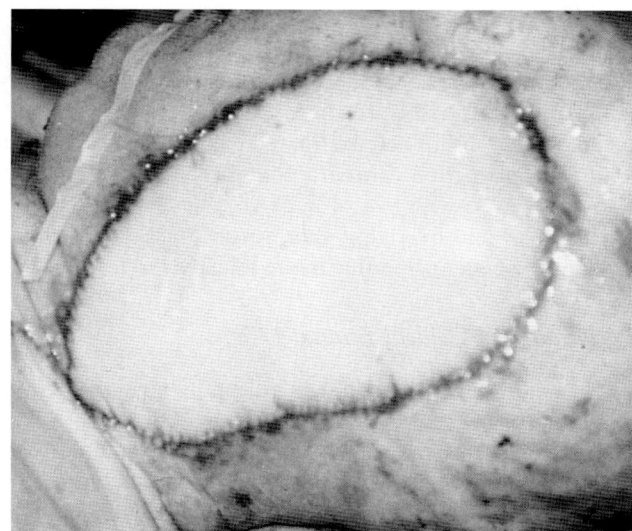
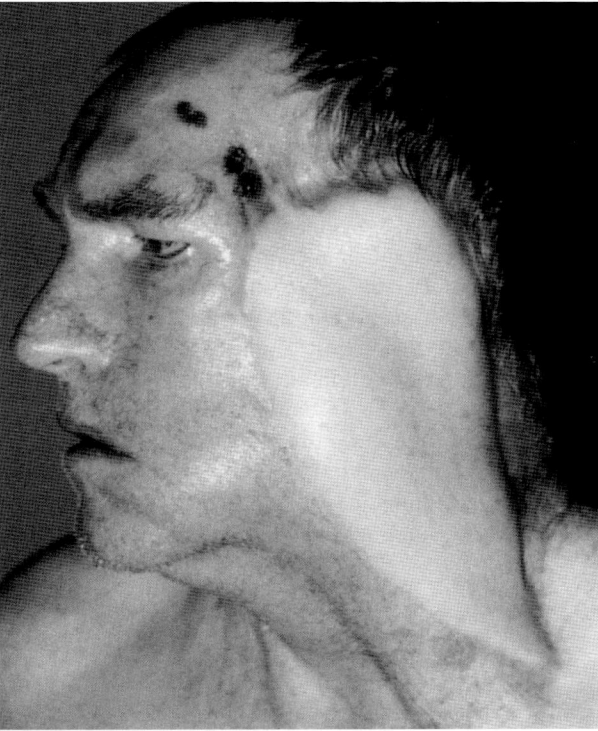

FIG. 13. **A,B:** The latissimus myocutaneous flap is large enough to cover extensive defects of the lateral skull base. **C:** Over time, revision of this flap is necessary because of the inferior pull of the pedicle, resulting in "sagging" of the skin paddle.

sion. The thoracodorsal nerve is divided only if atrophy of the muscle is desired, or if it results in venous compression during the rotation of the flap.

The flap is tailored into the defect and the back is closed primarily over several closed-suction drains. If needed, the tendinous humeral portion of the muscle is attached to the chest wall or the pectoralis minor tendon to prevent further pull on the pedicle. Rarely after harvest of an extensive flap, the defect must be resurfaced with a split-thickness skin graft. Because of the constant movement in this area of the chest wall, the results of skin graft healing are often frustrating. After surgery, the ipsilateral arm is positioned in a neutral position, resting on a pillow, for several days, to prevent venous compression.

Anterior Skull Base

With the limitation of this chapter to reconstruction of the skull base with regional and pedicled flaps, this section dedicated to the anterior skull base is very brief. This region includes defects in the frontal bone and the cribriform region. Only the latissimus flap reaches this area, but it is a poor choice for reconstruction of this region. To reach this area well, the pedicle would have to pass externally, with a second stage necessary to take down the pedicle.

Most defects encountered in anterior skull base surgery are in the region of the cribriform plate as a result of craniofacial surgery. With defects limited to the roof of the nasal vault, reconstruction can be accomplished by use of local flaps. However, with loss of large volumes of soft tissue or frontal skull and overlying skin, reconstruction can be accomplished better using free tissue transfer.

Pericranial and Galeal Frontalis Flaps

The anterior scalp provides two different layers for reconstruction of the cribriform region. The major benefit of both these flaps is that they can be easily preserved along with their inferior blood supply during the standard bicoronal approach to lesions of the anterior skull base. The length of the flaps is determined by how high up on the scalp the bicoronal incision is outlined.

The most commonly used of the two is the pericranial flap, consisting of the periosteum of the anterior skull, based on branches of the supraorbital artery. The flap can be separated from the overlying scalp at the beginning of the procedure, or it can be raised up with the bicoronal flap, elevating it off the scalp at the end of the surgical resection of the tumor (Fig. 14). The latter provides better protection of the flap during the resection. During elevation, as the supraorbital region is approached, care is taken to include several of the branches of the supraorbital artery in the flap. With care, the sensory branches of the supraorbital nerve can be preserved passing into the scalp flap. The flap is inserted through the inferior lip of the frontal craniotomy after a few millimeters of the inferior aspect of the bone flap are removed to ensure adequate room for postoperative swelling of the base of the flap. The flap can be secured in place by drilling several 1.5-mm holes in the residual planum sphenoidale, taking care not to injure the optic nerves.

The major drawback to the pericranial flap is its limited blood supply. Often during postoperative examination of the nasal roof, the flap appears to have undergone partial necrosis with eschar formation. In spite of the postoperative appearance of the flap, very few CSF leaks occur. This area seems to be a very forgiving of this poorly vascularized reconstruction.

The galeal–frontalis flap offers a better-vascularized flap with more volume to reconstruct this same region. The frontal galea is the same layer anterior as the superficial temporal layer is over the temporal region. As the temporal region is left behind, the galea divides into two leaves enveloping the frontalis muscle. The major branches of the supraorbital artery and nerve pass into this layer. The flap is raised up with the bicoronal flap and elevated away from the scalp when needed. Because of the increased thickness of this flap, a wider slit in the bone flap should be created to prevent postoperative swelling from strangulating the blood supply to the flap.

The increased bulk and vascularity of this flap make it appear to be a far superior flap than the pericranial flap for reconstruction of anterior defects. However, this loss of the galea and the frontalis muscle from the undersurface of the frontal scalp leaves a very thin, poorly vascularized flap of skin to cover the bone flap. With the transfer of this flap, sensation and animation of the frontal scalp are lost. Any defects in the frontal bone reconstruction such as bur holes and craniotomy bone cuts are readily seen through the thinned skin. Previous radiation therapy is a contraindication to the use of this flap.

The authors recommend that the pericranial flap be used as the first-line reconstruction in most anterior cranial defects, with the galeal–frontalis flap reserved for defects that warrant the extra bulk and vascularity it provides.

The superficial temporoparietal flap as outlined previously can be used in the anterior skull base as well. It is excellent for orbital lining and reconstruction after orbital exenteration. By extending the length of the flap during

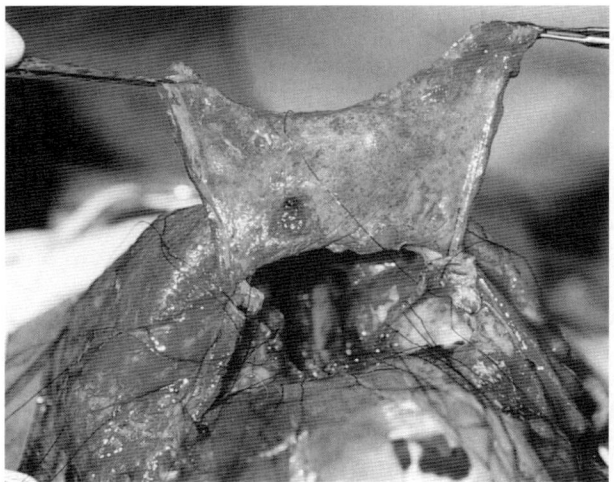
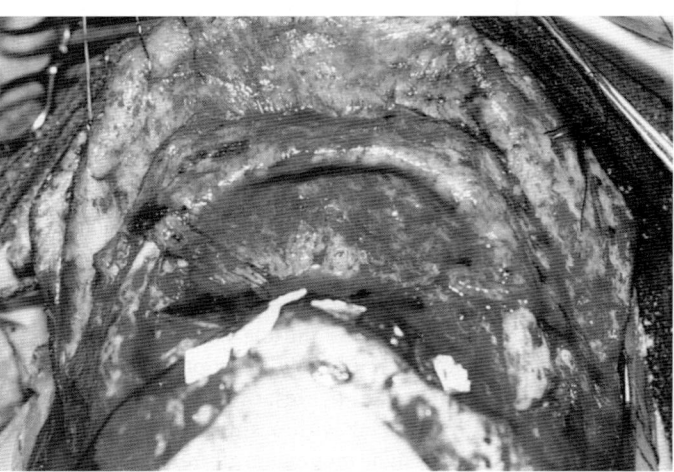

FIG. 14. A: The pericranial flap is elevated away from the scalp after the resection has been completed. **B:** It is inset over the cribriform defect and attached with sutures to small holes drilled in the remnant of the roof of the sphenoid sinus.

harvest, the flap can reach across the midline to reconstruct the cribriform region.

Nerve Grafts

Nerve grafting, a common procedure in the rehabilitation of lateral skull base surgery, is most often performed for facial nerve loss. Although cranial nerves IX, X, XI, and XII are at significant risk during the resection of glomus jugulare tumors, they are not often grafted because the proximal stumps adjacent to the brainstem are either unavailable for grafting or extremely difficult to graft to. Grafting in this situation has not been shown to be of benefit in the return of function of these nerves. However, during resection of glomus vagale tumors, if cranial nerves IX and XII are resected, their proximal stumps are often suitable for grafting. An interposition to reconstitute the vagus nerve has not been shown to effect return of laryngeal function. This was based on the observation that there was no return of vocal cord motion. No electromyographic follow-up has been performed on a group such as this to test for return of electromyographic activity. Maintenance of muscle bulk and motor tone, with the absence of motion, benefits voice and swallowing results. Thus, if the proximal stump of the vagus is available, either mobilization and proximal division of the recurrent laryngeal nerve to anastomose it directly to the vagal stump, or transfer of one of the ansa branches is recommended.

Infrequently, the facial nerve is resected in its mastoid portion secondary to malignant parotid, temporal bone, or glomus tumors, necessitating grafting. Three peripheral nerves are most often used for graft replacement in the lateral skull base: (a) the great auricular, (b) the sural, and (c) the medial antebrachial cutaneous.

Proximity to the operative site is the major advantage of the great auricular nerve. Often, it has to be divided for access to the lateral skull base, and thus no loss of function occurs with its use in these cases. The major disadvantage is the limited length of nerve available for the transfer. With proximal resection of the lower cranial nerves, its length is often insufficient for a tension-free graft. Also, if it has not been divided for tumor excision or access, the morbidity of sensory loss to the auricle is a complaint that will resurface as long as the patient is followed.

The sural nerve offers the advantage of increased length and size. It is formed by the union of the lateral sural cutaneous and the medial sural cutaneous nerves in the midcalf (9). It then descends along with the lessor saphenous vein to pass posterior and inferior to the lateral malleolus of the ankle (Fig. 15). The dissection, which is performed through a longitudinal incision to expose the nerve, is facilitated by a pressure cuff around the thigh. To gain adequate length, the branches are followed onto the dorsum of

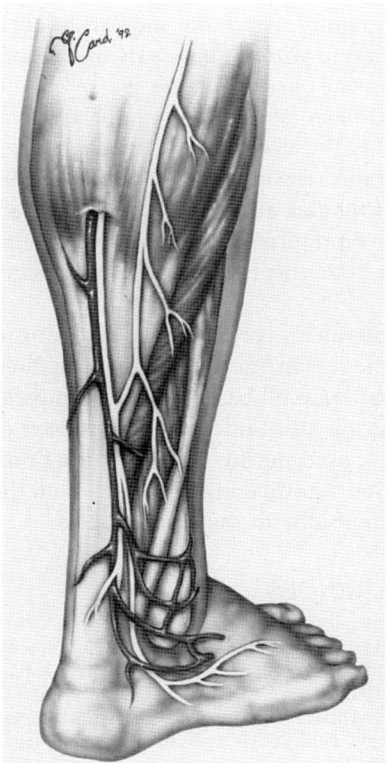
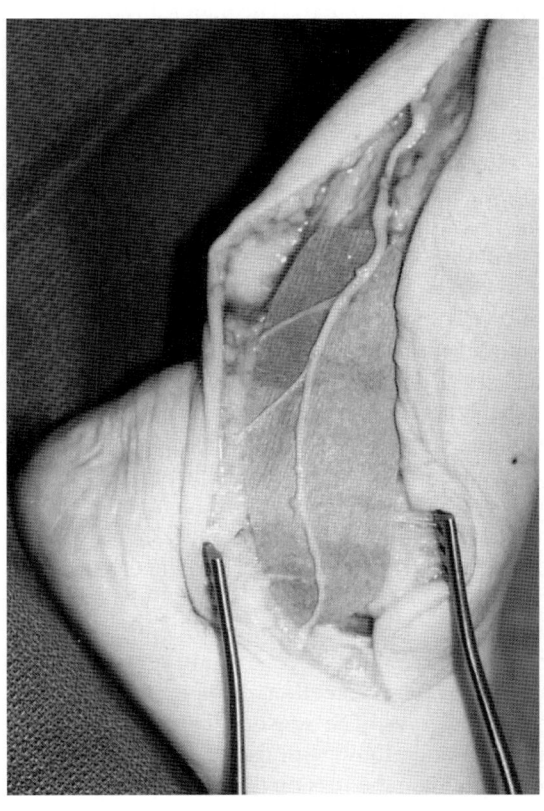

FIG. 15. A: The course of the sural nerve is demonstrated passing posteroinferior to the lateral malleolus and then ramifying onto the dorsal surface of the foot. **B:** It has excellent size, but the branching pattern is not as good a match for total facial nerve replacement as the antebrachial nerve.

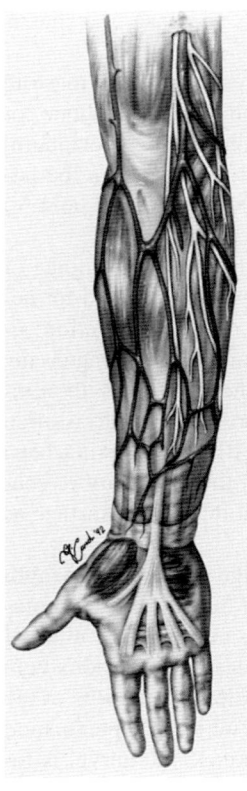 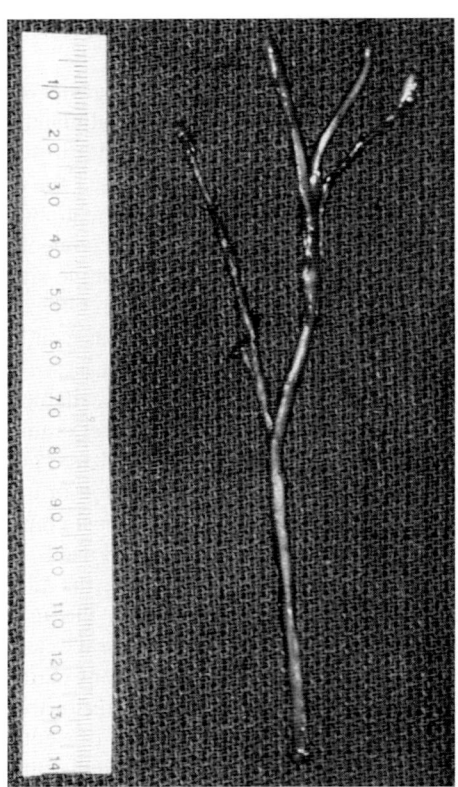

FIG. 16. A: The course of the medial antebrachial cutaneous nerve is demonstrated on the medial aspect of the arm. The use of the anterior branch is preferred over the ulnar branch. **B:** The size and branching of the nerve produce a good match for facial nerve replacement after extensive facial nerve resection.

the foot. The resultant sensory defect on the dorsal region of the foot is little noticed by the patient. The major disadvantage of this graft is the increased connective tissue-to-nerve fiber ratio seen in all nerves of the lower extremity compared with nerves of the upper extremity (10). This provides less opportunity for nerve regrowth.

Because of this, the authors' preference is the medial antebrachial cutaneous nerve, which descends through the arm, anterior and medial to the brachial artery in the medial intermuscular septum. At the junction of the middle and lower thirds of the arm, it pierces the brachial fascia along with the basilic vein and divides into an anterior and ulnar branch, providing sensation to the anterior forearm and posteromedial aspect of the forearm, respectively (Fig. 16). To dissect the nerve, a vertical incision is performed over the palpable groove between the biceps anteriorly and the triceps posteriorly on the medial aspect of the arm. The branches are identified and followed superiorly until the nerve is seen passing deep to the brachial fascia. The nerve can be followed further superior if necessary.

The distal ramification of the nerve is an excellent replacement for the facial nerve. The large size of the two major branches also makes for an excellent cable graft for any of the lower cranial nerves. The sensory loss on the medial aspect of the arm and elbow with use of the ulnar branch is more noticeable than the loss on the dorsal forearm from use of the anterior branch. For this reason, some have recommended use of the anterior division alone.

This area of sensory loss gradually decreases with time. Care must be taken not to dissect deep into the intermuscular septum where the median motor nerve lies. Nerve stimulation with no paralysis under anesthesia before resection can ensure that the sensory antebrachial nerve has indeed been isolated. Its major advantage over the sural nerve is the decrease in the connective tissue-to-nerve fiber ratio seen in upper extremity nerves. This increase in neural tubules allows for greater nerve regeneration with improved return of function. The resultant sensory defect on the forearms is better tolerated than auricular sensory loss.

In summary, preoperative planning to keep all of the possible reconstructive options available is a very important part of skull base surgery. The patient and the family are always fully informed about each of the options that may be used during the reconstruction. Adequate reconstruction significantly decreases both the short- and long-term morbidity of these procedures.

REFERENCES

1. Jackson CG, Glasscock ME, Carrasco VN, et al. Defect reconstruction and CSF management in neurotologic skull base tumors with intracranial extension. *Laryngoscope* 1992;102:1205–1214.
2. Abul-Hassan HS, Ascher GD, Acland RD. Surgical anatomy and blood supply of the fascial layers of the temporal region. *Plast Reconstr Surg* 1986;77:17–23.
3. Netterville JL, Panje WR, Maves MD. The trapezius myocutaneous flaps. *Archives of Otolaryngology* 1987;113:271–281.
4. Urken ML, Naidu RK, Lawson W, Biller HF. The lower trapezius is-

land musculocutaneous flap revisited. *Arch Otolaryngol Head Neck Surg* 1991;117:502–511.
5. Netterville JL, Wood DE. The lower trapezius flap: vascular anatomy and surgical technique. *Archives of Otolaryngology* 1991;117:73–76.
6. Maves MD, Panje WR, Shagets F. Extended latissimus dorsi myocutaneous flap reconstruction of major head and neck defects. *Otolaryngol Head Neck Surg* 1984;92:551–558.
7. Sabatier RE, Bakamjian VY. Transaxillary latissimus dorsi flap reconstruction in head and neck cancer. *Am J Surg* 1985;150:427–434.
8. Chowdhury CR, Mclean NR, Harrop-Griffiths K, Breach NM. The repair of defects in the head and neck region with the latissimus dorsi flap. *J Laryngol Otol* 1988;102:1127–1132.
9. Ortiguela ME, Wood MD, Cahill DR. Anatomy of the sural nerve complex. *J Hand Surg [Am]* 1987;12:1119–1123.
10. Slingluff CL, Terzis JK, Edgerton MT. The quantitative microanatomy of the brachial plexus in man: reconstructive relevance. In: Terzis JK, ed. *Microreconstruction of nerve injuries*. Philadelphia: WB Saunders, 1987:285–324.

Subject Index

Note: Page numbers followed by *f* indicate figures; those followed by *t* indicate tables.

A

Abducens nerve. *See* Cranial nerve VI
Abscess
  brain
    management of, 591–592
    reconstruction with free latissimus dorsi flap, 616–618, 616–618f
  with osteomyelitis, 595
  sellar/parasellar, 560t, 581
  wound complications, 603
Accessory meningeal artery, 21, 113t
Accessory nerve
  head position and, 535f
  jugular foramen, 548, 549f
  maxillotomy, extended unilateral, 230
  spinal root, 28, 28f
  vertebral artery management, 537f, 540f, 542, 542f
Acinic cell carcinoma, 209t, 331
Acoustic neuroma, 8, 9
  cerebellopontine angle lesion imaging, 98–99, 98f, 98t
  neurophysiological monitoring, 159f
Acoustic reflex testing, 445
Acoustic tumors, history, 7–9, 8–9f
ACTH-secreting adenoma, 564–565, 578
Adenocarcinoma
  anterior fossa lesion imaging, 90
  external auditory meatus/temporal bone, 383t, 384
  mid–skull base approaches, 209t
  pathophysiology, 52t
  subcranial approaches, extended anterior, 259t
  temporal bone, 380
  transfacial approach indications, 165
Adenoid cystic carcinoma, 47t
  ICA management, 367–370, 367–370f
    saphenous vein bypass graft, 361–363, 361–363f
    tumor biology and, 360
  infratemporal–middle fossa approach, 320f, 331
  mid–skull base approaches, 209t
  orbital exenteration indications, 173
  pathophysiology, 51, 52t, 56–57
  perineural extension, central skull base, 95
  presentation, 74, 78f, 79f, 84f
  radiation therapy, 406
  subcranial approaches
    extended anterior, 259t
    transbasal–Derome, 350
  temporal bone, 380, 383–384, 383t
Adenoma
  cranioorbital zygomatic approach, 274, 276–277f, 278
  external auditory meatus/temporal bone, 383–384, 383t
  pituitary, 560t, 560–562, 561t, 577–579
  subcranial approaches, extended anterior, 259t
Aditus ad antrum, 380
Adrenal paraganglioma, 473
Aesthesioneuroblastoma. *See* Esthesioneuroblastomas
Air cells
  foramen magnum region surgery, 496
  jugulotympanic paraganglioma, 474, 476, 476f, 479, 480f, 481
  lateral rhinotomy, 170
  vestibular schwannoma, 464, 464f
Air cisternography, vestibular schwannoma, 446
Air embolism, 426, 429
Airway
  infratemporal–middle fossa approach, 337
  maxillotomy complications, 234
  median labial mandibuloglossoptomy, 522
  nursing care, 121, 133
  postoperative management, 602–603
Alar ligament, 508, 509f, 510f
Alloplastic slings, 405
Al Mefty, O., 11, 11f
Alveolar artery, 229
Alveolar ridge, 85, 299, 299f, 343
Aminoglutethimide, 578
Ampulla, vestibular schwannoma, 468
Analgesia, 122
Anastomoses, 107, 107f
  therapeutic embolization considerations, 113–114, 113t, 114–115f
  vertebral artery, 534
Anatomy
  anterior skull base, 15–19
    intracranial contents, 15–16, 17–18f
    osteology, 15, 16–17f
    subcranial relationship, 16–19, 18–19f
  flap and graft construction. *See specific donor sites*
  foramen magnum region, 491–492, 507–514, 507–513f
  imaging considerations, 87
  infratemporal–middle fossa approach, subtemporal trapezoid exposure, 322, 326f
  maxillotomy, extended unilateral, 231–232t
  middle skull base, 19–27
    intracranial contents, 21–24, 22–26f
    osteology, 19–21, 20–21f
    subcranial relationships, 24–27, 24–27f
  petroclival, 424f, 425–426, 425–427f
  posterior skull base, 27–29, 28–29f
  sella/parasellar surgery, 555–560, 556–559f
    nasal cavity, 555, 557f
    parasellar structures, 558, 559f
    pituitary gland and hypothalamus, 555, 558, 558–559f
    sphenoid bone and sella, 555, 556f, 557f
  temporal bone, 377–380, 378–380f
  transcervicomastoid approach, 413
  vascular. *See also specific vessels*
    embolization, therapeutic, 113–116, 113t, 114–116f
    magnetic resonance angiography, 87
    veins of skull, skull base, and vertebral column, 67f, 68f
  vertebral artery, 533–537, 533–535f
    branches, 534, 534f
    course, 533
    dynamic changes, 534–537
    relationships, 533–534
    variations and anomalies, 534
Anemia, 108
Anesthesia. *See also* Neurologic monitoring, intraoperative; *specific procedures*
  and cerebral blood flow, 105
  cerebral blood flow requirements during, 359–360
  facial degloving approach, 197
  maxillotomy, extended unilateral, 212
  neurophysiological monitoring, 143, 145, 145f. *See also* Neurological monitoring, intraoperative
  EEG, 148
  SEPs, 149, 149f, 150
  nursing staff duties, 128, 129, 131
  petroclival surgery, 429–430
  prevention of complications, 588
  rebound hypertension, 599
  transcervicomastoid approach, 412–413

641

Aneurysms, 11
  cranioorbital approach, 278–282, 279–284f
  foramen magnum region surgery, 491, 503
  ICA, 362f, 363f
  mid–skull base approaches, 209t
  petroclival, 423, 429
  sellar/parasellar, 581
  transmandibular approach, 341
  vertebral artery, 533, 542t, 551, 552, 552t
  vertebrobasilar, 29, 230
Aneurysmal cyst, vertebral artery, 540f, 544f, 546t
Aneurysmatic bone cyst
  facial degloving approach, 205
  subcranial approaches, 357t
  transbasal approach, Derome modification, 350–351, 350–351f
Angiofibroma
  magnetic resonance angiography, 87
  mid-skull base approaches, 209t
  nasopharyngeal. *See* Nasopharyngeal angiofibromas
  pathology, 37–39, 38f
  presentation, 74, 76f, 77, 77f, 83
  subcranial approaches, extended anterior, 259t
Angiography, 87, 94f
  anastomoses, 114f
  carotid, 412f
    cerebral blood flow assessment, 105–111, 106–110f
    temporal bone tumor management, 386
  embolization, preoperative, 113–116, 113t, 114–116f, 368, 369f, 412f
  glomus jugulare/jugular foramen tumors, 410, 411, 411f
  internal carotid artery, 373
    cavernous sinus syndrome, 363, 365f, 367f
    preoperative evaluation, 360
    ICA dissection, 373
    ICA to MCA bypass, 372f
  jugular foramen tumors, 410
  jugulotympanic paraganglioma, 476
  nursing care, 121
  petroclival lesions, 428, 429f
  postoperative management, 601
  preoperative evaluation, 105–111, 106–110f
  sellar/parasellar lesions, 565–566, 573, 581
  subcranial approaches, transbasal–Derome, 357
  temporal bone tumors, 382
  vertebral artery, 534f, 541f, 550f
    aneurysm, 551
    head position/movement and, 544–545
Angiolipoma, 93, 94f, 546t
Angioma, 204f, 205f, 259t
Angiomyolipoma, 542, 542t, 543f, 550f
Annulus of Zinn, 19, 175
Anomalies, vascular, 113t
Anosmia, 77, 357, 574, 606
Antebrachial nerve, 637f, 638, 638f
Anteriolateral approach, vertebral artery, 535, 537, 538, 538f, 550
  complications, 552
  indications, 548, 548t
Anterior approaches
  complications, 586t

cranioorbital. *See* Cranioorbital approach
degloving. *See* Facial degloving
frontal crest midline ridge in, 15, 16f
history, 3–7, 4–7f
to petrous bone, 423, 425–426, 425–426f
subcranial extended, 239–260. *See also* Subcranial extended anterior approach
temporal lobe tissue removal, 62
transbasal–Derome, 347–358. *See also* Transbasal approach, Derome modification
transfacial, 165–194
transfacial subcranial, extended, 287–308. *See also* Transfacial subcranial approach, extended
subzygomatic, needle biopsy, 112f, 113
Anterior cerebral artery, 24
Anterior cerebral artery aneurysm, 281–282, 281f
Anterior choroid artery, 24
Anterior communicating artery, 279, 279f, 281–282, 281f, 369f
Anterior crest, 16f
Anterior deep temporal artery, 114, 316
Anterior ethmoid artery, 15, 230, 239
Anterior ethmoid foramen, 19f
Anterior fossa
  adenoid cystic carcinoma, 34t
  anatomy, 15–19, 22
    intracranial contents, 15–16, 17–18f
    osteology, 15, 16–17f
    subcranial relationship, 16–19, 18–19f
  cephalometrics, 521, 522f
  contraindications to transsphenoidal approach, 566, 566t
  cranioorbital zygomatic approach, trauma repair, 283
  CSF fistula, traumatic, 285, 285f
  frontal sinus tumor presentation, 81f
  history of surgical procedures, 3–7, 4–7f
  maxillotomy, extended unilateral, 231t
  pneumocephalus, 593
  reconstruction, radial forearm free flap, 608–611, 609–610f
  regions of cranial base surgery, 74f
  squamous cell carcinoma primary sites, 32t
  subcranial approaches
    extended anterior, 259f
    frontobasal, 357, 357f
    meningioma, 355–356, 355–356f
    transbasal–Derome, 347, 348, 351, 351f, 352f
  subcranial extended transfacial approach, 296f
    Type I, 292
    Type II, 299
  transmandibular approach, 341
Anterior inferior cerebellar artery (AICA), 28, 113t, 436
Anterior-infratemporal regions, transmandibular approach, 341–346, 342–345f
Anterior skull base
  anatomy, 15–19
    intracranial contents, 15–16, 17–18f
    osteology, 15, 16–17f
    subcranial relationship, 16–19, 18–19f
  imaging, 89–91, 89–92f

maxillotomy, extended unilateral, 231t
reconstruction, 624t, 635–637, 636f
Anterior spinal artery, 29, 534, 538
Anterior vertebral plexus, anatomy, 68f
Antibiotic prophylaxis
  CSF leaks, 133
  jugular foramen tumor surgery, 412
  maxillotomy, extended unilateral, 210
  petroclival surgery, 429
  transbasal–Derome approach, 348
  transoral approach to clivus and cervical spine, 513
Antibiotics
  brain abscess management, 591–592
  postoperative, 601
Anticoagulation, 107, 373
Anti-embolic stockings, 412, 601
Antrostomy, 179
Antrum, 179, 195, 426
Apex syndrome, 239
Aphasia, 134
Apical ligament of dens, 28
Apoplexy, pituitary, 564, 579
APUDoma, 383t, 385, 411
Aqueducts, 380, 450
Aquino's sign, 474
Arachnoid
  cavernous sinus, 21
  petroclival surgery, 435, 437
  petroclival tumors, 423
  vestibular schwannoma, 458, 461, 461f
Arachnoid cysts
  imaging, 98, 98t, 99
  sellar/parasellar, 560t, 563, 581
Arachnoid plane, ICA salvage/sacrifice, 360
Arcuate eminence, 21
  cranioorbital zygomatic approach, 267
  petrous bone anatomy, 425, 425f
  vestibular schwannoma, 465, 468, 468f, 469f
Arnold's nerve, 473
Arterial grafts. *See* Vascular grafts
Arteriovenous complexes. *See* Glomus/glomus jugulare tumors
Arteriovenous malformations. *See* Vascular malformations
Arthritis
  craniocervical junction, 516, 516f
  mid-skull base approaches, 209t
  odontectomy, 527–529, 528–530f, 531
  TMJ, 522
Articular eminence, 26f
Ascending pharyngeal artery
  cranial nerve blood supply, 113t
  jugulotympanic paraganglioma, 479
  maxillotomy, extended unilateral, 229
  meningeal branch, 28
  recurrent adenoid cystic carcinoma, 368, 369f
  therapeutic embolization considerations, 115, 116f
Aspiration biopsy, fine-needle, 111–113, 112f
Aspiration syndrome, 405
  glomus tumors, 411, 412
  jugulotympanic paraganglioma, 481, 486t
  nursing care, 123
  odontectomy complications, 531
  postoperative care, 602
  transoral approach complications, 522

Aspirator debulking, 352, 461, 462f, 463
Atelectasis, 602
Atherosclerosis, 107, 551t
Atlantic part of vertebral artery, 29
Atlantoaxial joint, 29, 209t
Atlantoaxial ligament, 508, 509f, 510f
Atlantooccipital joint. *See* Craniocervical junction
Atlantooccipital membranes, 28
Atlas. *See also* Foramen magnum region; Vertebral artery management
 anatomy, 23f, 29, 507–508, 509f
 condylar resection
  foramen magnum meningioma, 498f
  temporal bone resection, 387, 389
 embryology, 507
 vertebral artery management, 535, 546–548, 546t, 547f, 549, 549f
  control and mobilization, 539f
  control of segments, 538
  posterlateral approach, 536f
  posterolateral, 537f
  transposition, 540f
Atrial catheterization, 429
Atticotomy, 389, 394f, 469f
Audiography, 445
Audiovestibular complex, vestibular schwannoma, 461, 461f
Auditory brainstem response. *See* Brainstem auditory evoked potentials
Auditory canal. *See* External auditory canal; Internal auditory canal
Auditory evoked potentials (AEPs), 138, 429
 multimodal evoked potential recording, 144f, 145
 neurological monitoring, 151–152, 154, 154–155f
 vestibular schwannoma, 445–446, 458
Auditory rehabilitation, 605–606, 605f
Auricle. *See* Ear
Auricular nerve, 79, 637
Auriculotemporal nerve, 310
Axis anatomy, 508, 509–510f

B

Balloon occlusion, therapeutic, 603
Balloon occlusion test
 glomus tumors, 409
 infratemporal–middle fossa approach, 309, 311, 313
 jugular fossa surgery, 421
 jugulotympanic paraganglioma, 477–478
 limitations of, 109, 111
 nursing care, 121–122
 preoperative evaluation, 107–108, 107f, 110t, 360
 temporal bone tumor management, 386
 transbasal–Derome approach, 352
 vertebral artery, 542, 552
Barbiturate coma, 332, 360, 361, 371, 373
Barbiturates, neurophysiological monitoring, 147–148, 149
Basal cell carcinoma, 47t
 ear region, 83, 83f
 pathophysiology, 51, 52t, 57
 presentation, 73, 74, 75f, 83, 83f
 subcranial approaches, extended anterior, 259t

 temporal bone, 380, 383, 383t, 389
 transfacial approach indications, 165
Basal exposure, cranioorbital zygomatic approach, 278
Basal foramina, 24
Basilar artery. *See also* Foramen magnum region
 anatomy, 28, 29f
 aneurysm
  cranioorbital zygomatic approach, 284f
  petroclival, 423, 429
 carotid-basilar anastomosis as BTO contraindication, 107, 107f
 collateral flow in carotid artery occlusion, 359
 formation of, 533
 maxillotomy, extended unilateral, 226f, 227f
 petroclival surgery, 428f, 429, 433, 434f
 subcranial extended transfacial approach, 298
Basilar impression, 514, 514f
 acquired, 516
 clinical presentation, 521
 mid-skull base approaches, 209t
 odontectomy, 527–529, 528–530f
Basilar invagination, 29, 521
Basilar plexus
 anatomy, 22, 64, 65f, 67f, 555
 cavernous sinus resection, 334
Basilar sinus anatomy, 67f
Basilar tip aneurysm, 282, 283f, 284f
Basiocciput
 anatomy, 27
 maxillotomy, extended unilateral, 223
Basipharyngeal fascia, 335, 335, 336f
Basisphenoid
 anatomy, 27
 maxillotomy, extended unilateral, 223, 231t
Basisphenoid-basiocciput synostosis, 27
Basivertebral veins, 67f, 68f
Bicoronal craniotomy, 348, 349f
Bicoronal flap, 239
Bicoronal skin incision, 182f, 264, 264f, 278
Bifrontal cranioorbital approach, 285, 285f
Bifrontal craniotomy, 357
Bill's bar, 425, 454, 454f, 463, 463f, 468, 470f
Bill's island, 450, 452f
Biologic behavior of tumors. *See* Tumor biology
Biopsy. *See also* Frozen sections
 fine-needle aspiration, 111–113, 112f
 nursing staff duties, 127, 130
 sellar/parasellar lesions
  inflammatory, 581
  transsphenoidal approach, 571
 temporal bone tumors, 387
 vestibular schwannoma, 461
Bipolar cautery. *See* Cautery
Blair incision, 313, 314f
Bleeding. *See also* Epitaxis; Hemorrhage
 imaging, 88
 nasopharyngeal tumor presentation, 83
 prevention of complications, 588
Blindness. *See* Vision/visual deficits
Blood-borne tumor emboli, 67
Blood-brain barrier, 148
Blood degradation products, 88
Blood flow
 carotid artery assessment, 105–111, 106f–110f
 collateral. *See* Collaterals/collateral flow

 intraoperative monitoring, EEG, 145–148
 postoperative management, 599
 preoperative assessment, 105–111, 106f–110f. *See also* Carotid artery, assessment techniques
 ICA, 360
 physiology of, 359–360
 temporal bone tumor management, 386–387
 vertebral artery, 534–537
 tests of. *See* Balloon test occlusion; Doppler ultrasound; Xenon CT
Blood gases
 and cerebral blood flow, 105
 neurophysiological effects, 143, 148
 petroclival surgery, 429
 postoperative care, 600
Blood pressure
 and cerebral blood flow, 154, 405
 during ICA surgery, 373
 with jugular foramen tumors, 412
 jugulotympanic paraganglioma resection, 477
 neurophysiological effects, 143, 144f, 148, 150
 neurosecretory tumors and, 411
 postoperative management, 599, 600
Blood vessels
 anomalies and malformations. *See* Vascular malformations
 angiography. *See* Angiography
 tumor extension via, 57, 59–61, 60f
Blue lined superior semicircular canal, 468, 469f
Bogaard angle, 521, 522f
Bone cyst, 205, 357t
Bone defects. *See also* Reconstruction/defect repair
 anterior skull base lesions, 89
 prevention of complications, 588f, 589
Bone destruction, 51
 with chondrosarcomas, clival, 518f, 519
 with glomus jugulare/jugular foramen tumors, 411, 411f
 imaging
  central skull base metastasis, 95
  diffuse lesions of skull base, 102, 102t
  jugular fossa tumors, 102
 with nasal/paranasal sinus tumors, 81, 82, 167, 169
 transfacial approach, 167, 169, 304–305
 with temporal bone tumors, 381
Bone flaps and grafts. *See also* Reconstruction/defect repair
 infratemporal–middle fossa approach, 337
 reconstruction
  cosmetic rehabilitation, 604–605
  internal auditory canal, 464, 464f
  rectus abdominis free flap, 611–613, 611–613f
 subcranial extended anterior approach, 241, 244f, 245
 vestibular schwannoma, 464, 464f, 465
 zygomatic cranioorbital approach, 266–267, 266f, 271
Bone imaging, 70, 87–88, 95
Bone invasion, 61, 69
Bone window, 70, 449
Box paradigm, maxillary sinus, 78, 78f, 79
Brachial plexus SEPs, 148, 148f, 150, 151f

644 / SUBJECT INDEX

Brain
  abscess. *See* Abscess, brain
  herniation, 347
  imaging considerations, 87, 312f, 386
  tumor invasion, 62, 62t
    infratemporal–middle fossa approach, 311, 312f
    resection. *See* Brain resection; *specific structures and regions*
Brain metabolism
  cerebral blood flow, 105, 359
  EEG effects, 145
  induced coma and hypothermia, 361
Brain perfusion. *See* Blood flow; Carotid artery, assessment techniques
Brain protection
  ICA to MCA bypass, 371
  prevention of complications, 587
Brain resection, 386–387, 395f
  anterior craniotomies, 187
  infratemporal–middle fossa approach, 334–335, 334–335f
  temporal lobe, 386–387, 395f
Brain scans, 386
Brainstem, 12, 27, 28f, 29
  angioma, 204f, 205f
  basilar impression, 521
  clivus tumors and, 519
  foramen magnum region surgery
    odontectomy, 527–529, 528–530f
    tumors, 494, 501f
  infratemporal–middle fossa approach, 309
  nasopharyngeal tumor involvement, 85
  neurophysiological monitoring, 151–152, 154, 154–155f
    AEP, 138, 144f, 145
    EEG, 148, 148f
    SEP, 138, 150, 151f
  petroclival surgery, 435, 435f, 438
    anatomy, 424f
    complications, 437
    middle fossa intradural approach, 436
  temporal bone anatomy, 377
  tissue removal, 62
  transbasal–Derome approach, 354–355, 354–355f
  transoral approach, 515–516
  tumor pathophysiology, 56, 57f
  vestibular schwannoma, 444, 455, 456f, 463
Brainstem evoked potentials
  auditory, 138, 145
    multimodal evoked potential recording, 144f
    neurological monitoring, 151–152, 154, 154–155f
    petroclival surgery, 429
  somatosensory, 138, 151
Breast cancer metastases, 47, 66, 66t, 67, 67t
  imaging, 70, 71f
  infratemporal–middle fossa approach, 310
  temporal bone metastases, 386
Breathing. *See* Respiration
Breschet, frontal diploic veins of, 16
Bridging veins, 65f, 436
Bromcriptine, 577
Brown's sign, 474
Buccal branch of Cranial nerve VII, 155
Buccinator muscle, 231t
Burst suppression, 145, 147f

C

Calcification
  central skull base lesions, 92
  chordoma, 93–94, 517
  imaging, 91f, 92
  meningioma, 446
  posterior atlantooccipital membrane, 534
Caldwell-Luc approach, 195, 288
Caloric test, 445
Calvarium
  congenital anomalies, 514
  cranioorbital zygomatic approach reconstruction, 270–271
  prevention of complications, 588f, 589
  reconstruction, 588–589, 588f
  temporal bone anatomy, 378
  temporal bone resection, 395f
  tumors
    anterior approaches, 184
    infratemporal–middle fossa approach, 309
    pathophysiology, 54f, 61
    transfacial approach, 184f, 185
Cancellous bone, tumor spread, 61
Canthal ligament fixation, 244f, 245, 249f, 260
Canthal skin lesions, 73
Canthotomy, postoperative care, 602
Carbon dioxide partial pressure, 105, 148. *See also* Blood gases
Carcinoid tumors, 383t, 385, 411
Cardiac arrest, 360
Cardiorespiratory arrest, 521, 522
Cardiorespiratory monitoring, postoperative, 599
Cardiovascular function, 429
  jugular foramen surgery, 413
  jugulotympanic paraganglioma resection, 477
  neurosecretory tumors and, 411
  postoperative monitoring, 132
  prevention of complications, 588
Care plan, 119
Caroticocavernous branches of ICA, 21
Caroticoclinoid foramen, 19
Caroticojugular spine, glomus tumors, 116f
Caroticotympanic artery
  jugulotympanic paraganglioma, 479, 484, 485f
  temporal bone anatomy, 378
Caroticotympanic branch of ICA, 23
Caroticotympanic plexus, 380
Carotid artery, 25. *See also* External carotid artery; Internal carotid artery
  anomalies and malformations
    contraindications to transsphenoidal approach, 566, 566t
    persistent anastomoses, 107, 107f, 113–114, 114t, 114–115f
    sellar/parasellar region, 560t, 581
  assessment techniques, 105–111, 106–110f
    balloon test occlusion, 107–108, 107f
    ICA workup and management, 359–374. *See also* Internal carotid artery
    imaging techniques, 88
    limitations of, 109, 111
    nursing care, 121–122
    occlusion, preoperative, 107
    preoperative evaluation, 105–107, 106f
    regional blood flow, 105
  tests of cerebral blood flow reserve, 108–109, 109–110f
  cranioorbital zygomatic approach, 267–268, 268f, 270, 279
    aneurysm repair, 280, 284f
    subclinoid, 274, 278
    supraclinoid, 276f
    grafts/resection. *See also* Vascular grafts
    neurophysiological monitoring, 153f
    nursing care, 133
    postoperative management, 601
  embolization, preoperative, 113–116, 113t, 114–116f
  foramen magnum region chordoma, 501f
  infratemporal–middle fossa approach, 309, 330–333, 331–333f
    diagnosis/presentation, 311
    incisions, 315
    preoperative assessment, 309, 311, 313, 352
    tumor penetration, 331–332
  jugular fossa surgery, 421
  jugulotympanic paraganglioma, 474, 477–478
    classification, 478
    infratemporal fossa approach, 481
    spread via, 475
  maxillotomy, extended unilateral, 209
  petroclival surgery, 436, 437
  petrous bone anatomy, 426
  postoperative hemorrhage, 603
  prevention of complications, 587
  reconstruction, goals of, 623
  sellar/parasellar region approaches
    complications, 573
    pterional, 575
    subtemporal, 577
    transsphenoidal, 566, 566t, 570–571, 571f, 572, 572f
  subcranial approaches
    extended anterior, 246–248f
    extended transfacial, 301
    extended transfacial Type III, 306–307f
    transbasal–Derome, 352, 357
  temporal bone tumors and, 381
  temporal resection, 386–387
  transmandibular approach, 342, 345
  tumor spread via cavernous sinus, 66
  vertebral artery bypass graft, 551, 552
Carotid artery occlusion, 360
Carotid-basilar anastomosis, BTO contraindications, 107, 107f
Carotid body tumors, 409, 419t. *See also* Jugulotympanic paraganglioma
  paraganglioma, 473, 474
  therapeutic embolization, 115
  transcervicomastoid approach, 409–422. *See also* Transcervicomastoid approach
Carotid canal, 21f, 22, 23, 26f
  facial degloving approach, 208
  infratemporal–middle fossa approach, 332t
  jugular foramen surgery, 414, 417
  maxillotomy, extended unilateral, 207, 224, 225f
  middle ear anatomy, 380
  periosteum as barrier to tumor spread, 72
  petrous bone anatomy, 426
  subcranial extended transfacial approach Type III, 305, 305f

temporal bone tumors, 381, 382, 382t, 397
total petrosectomy, 401
tumor spread via, 58f, 59, 59f
Carotid foramen
  infratemporal–middle fossa approach, 315, 319f
  tumor spread via, 57, 58f, 59, 59f
Carotid ophthalmic artery aneurysms, cranioorbital zygomatic approach, 278
Carotid sheath, jugulotympanic paraganglioma, 476
Cartilage grafts, 245
Catecholamines, 411, 477
Catheter. See also Fogarty embolectomy catheter
  atrial catheterization, 429
  epidural, 133
  therapeutic embolization, 115
Caton, R., 3
Cautery
  foramen magnum region approaches, transoral, 524
  infratemporal–middle fossa approach
    cavernous sinus resection, 333
    craniotomy, 326, 328
    temporalis elevation, 316
  jugular foramen surgery, 414
  jugulotympanic paraganglioma, 479, 484, 486f
  maxillotomy, extended unilateral, 211t
  pituitary tumor resection, 580
  prevention of complications, 587
  transsphenoidal approach to sella, 571
  vestibular schwannoma, 454–455, 461, 463, 464
Cavernous angioma, 360, 560t
Cavernous arteries, temporal bone anatomy, 378
Cavernous fistula, sellar/parasellar, 581
Cavernous internal carotid artery. See Internal carotid artery, cavernous
Cavernous sinus, 19, 21–22, 22f, 23f, 27, 28
  anatomy, 65f, 67f
  carotid-cavernous fistula, 581
  cranioorbital zygomatic approach, 263, 269f, 274, 276–277f
  aneurysms, 278, 279f
  entry into, 269–270, 270–271f
  emissary vein from, 21
  glomus tumor, 498, 499f, 500
  hemorrhage, 595
  ICA, 24, 24f, 25, 25f
  ICA management
    adenoid cystic carcinoma recurrence, 367–370, 367–370f
    cavernous sinus syndrome, 363–367, 363–367f
  imaging, 88
    chondrosarcoma, 97f
    nasopharyngeal tumor erosion, 94–95
    inflammatory lesion, 310, 310f
  infratemporal–middle fossa approach, 309, 333–334, 333f
    carotid artery management, 331, 332
    craniotomy, 328
    diagnosis/presentation, 310–311, 311f, 312f
    preoperative assessment, 311

jugulotympanic paraganglioma spread, 475
meningioma, 106f
nasopharyngeal angiofibroma, 520, 520f
nasal/paranasal sinus tumor presentation, 82
nasopharyngeal tumor erosion, 94–95
petroclival tumors, 423, 424f, 426–427
sellar/parasellar anatomy, 555, 558, 559f
sellar/parasellar lesions
  clinical presentation, 564
  meningioma, 580
  pituitary tumor resection and, 578–579
  transcranial-intradural approaches, 574
  transsphenoidal approach, 571–572
sphenoid sinus tumor presentation, 81
subcranial approaches
  extended anterior, 239
  transbasal–Derome, 348, 350, 352, 357
  transfacial, extended, 288, 288f, 290, 291f, 296–297, 305
temporal bone anatomy, 378
total petrosectomy, 401, 402f
transfacial approaches
  extended subcranial, 288, 288f, 290, 291f, 296–297, 305
  indications, skin cancer, 167f
  maxillectomy, 173, 174f
tumor pathophysiology, 51, 53, 53f
  patterns of spread, 59, 59f, 60f, 61, 64, 66, 69f, 83
  and prognosis, 72
  nasal/paranasal sinus tumor presentation, 82
Cavernous sinus syndrome, ICA management, 363–367, 363–367f
Cavitron aspirator, 461, 462f, 463
Cavity ablation, temporal resection, 400
Cavum, 195, 197f, 199, 200, 200f
Cell of Onodi, 175
Central skull base, 74f
  imaging, 92–97, 92–97f
  reconstruction, 626–637, 626–637f
    fat-dermal and fat grafts, 626–627
    fibrin glue, 630
    latissimus dorsi myocutaneous flap, 633–635, 634–635f
    myocutaneous flaps, 630–635, 631–635f
    pectoralis myocutaneous flaps, 631
    temporal fascia, 627–630, 627–628f
    temporalis muscle, 630
    trapezius myocutaneous flap, 631–633, 631–633f
Cephalometrics, 521, 521f, 522f
Cerebellar artery
  anterior inferior, 28, 113t, 115, 436, 436f
  posterior inferior, 29, 534, 538, 551, 552
  superior. See Superior cerebellar artery
Cerebellar plate, 400, 402f
Cerebellopontine angle, 28
  anatomy
    petrous bone, 425, 426, 426f
    temporal bone, 377
  imaging, 98–99, 98–99f, 98t, 101
  petroclival surgery, 423, 426, 435–436, 435f
  vestibular schwannoma, 446, 455f, 458, 461, 461f
Cerebellopontine angle tumors. See also Petroclival lesions; Vestibular schwannoma
  history, 443

meningioma, 106f
neurophysiological monitoring, intraoperative, 159f, 446
Cerebellum, 28
  AEPs, retraction and, 154
  cerebellopontine angle lesion imaging, 98–99, 98f, 98t
  foramen magnum region surgery, 502f
  petroclival surgery, 431, 431f, 432f, 434f, 435, 435f
  petroclival tumor symptoms, 426
  petrous bone anatomy, 426f
  temporal bone anatomy, 378, 378f
  tissue removal, 62
  vestibular schwannoma, 444, 455
Cerebral arteries
  anatomy, 23f, 24
  aneurysm, 281–282, 281f, 284f
  cavernous sinus anatomy, 65f
  middle, 23f, 24
    cranioorbital zygomatic approach, 268
    embolism, 150–151, 152f
    ICA management, 361, 361f, 362
    preoperative evaluation, 360
    stroke, 359
  posterior, 28
    cranioorbital zygomatic approach, 278, 282, 283f
    petroclival surgery, middle fossa extradural approach, 436
Cerebral blood flow reserve, 108–109, 109–110f. See also Blood flow
Cerebral cortex, sellar/parasellar lesions and, 564
Cerebral edema, 599, 600. See also Intracranial pressure
Cerebral infarction, 22, 599
Cerebral perfusion. See Blood flow
Cerebral vein of Galen, 28
Cerebral veins
  anatomy, 22, 28, 65, 67f
  cavernous sinus anatomy, 65f
  infratemporal–middle fossa approach, 334, 334f, 335
Cerebromedullary cistern, 435 look cistern
Cerebromedullary syndrome, basilar impression and, 521
Cerebrovascular events. See Stroke
Ceruminous adenoma, 383, 383t, 384
Cervical blood vessels. See also Carotid artery
  anastomoses, 113t
  anatomy, 22–23, 23f
  ascending cervical artery, 534f
    therapeutic embolization considerations, 115
  vertebral artery management, 550, 550f
  ICA grafts, 360, 362f, 363f
  tumor pathophysiology, 59
Cervical hygroma, 589, 589f
Cervical incisions
  infratemporal–middle fossa approach, 313, 313f
  maxillotomy, extended unilateral, 207
Cervical lymph nodes, 380, 381
Cervical spinal cord, SEPs, 148
Cervical spine, 29. See also Foramen magnum region; Vertebral artery management

Cervical spine (contd.)
    anatomy, veins, 67f, 68f
    facial degloving, sublabial transoral, 208
    foramen magnum lesions, 102
    foramen magnum region surgery, 492
        transoral approach, 527, 527f
        vertebral artery management, 546
    ICA management, 371–373, 371–373f
    jugular foramen surgery, 415
    maxillotomy, extended unilateral, 209, 222–224, 225–227f, 231–232t
    odontectomy, 527
    petroclival surgery, 429
    prevention of complications, 587
    transbasal–Derome approach, 347–348
    transmandibular approach, 341–346, 342–345f
    vertebral artery management, 533; 546, 548, 548f, 548t
Cervical sympathetic nerves, 311
Cervicocranial junction. See Craniocervical junction
Cervicofacial skin flap, 317f
Chamberlain's line, 521, 521f
Cheesman, A. D., 6f, 7
Chemosis, 79
Chemotherapy, 357
Chiasmatic sulcus, 15, 19
Chiasmic groove, 556f
Chief cells, 473, 474
Cholesteatoma, 383t, 385, 389, 602
Cholesterol cysts, 92t, 95, 97, 97f
Chondroma
    anterior fossa
        facial degloving, 204f, 205f, 205
        nasopharyngeal tumor presentation, 83
    foramen magnum region, 518
    infratemporal–middle fossa approach, 309
    mid-skull base approaches, 209t
    pathophysiology, 52t
Chondromyxofibroma, 228t
Chondrosarcoma
    anterior approaches
        combined resection with fossa floor invasion, 168
        facial degloving, 200, 205
        maxillotomy, extended unilateral, 228t, 233
        subcranial transfacial, 287
    cavernous sinus syndrome, 363–367, 363–367f
    clival, 518f, 519
    external auditory meatus/temporal bone, 383t, 384–385
    foramen magnum region, 505
        condylectomy, 494
        pathology, 518–519
    ICA management
        surgical dissection of tumor, 361
        tumor biology and, 360
    imaging, 92t, 93, 94
        central skull base lesions, 96f, 97, 97f
        foramen magnum lesions, 102
        jugular fossa tumors, 98t, 102
    infratemporal–middle fossa approach, 309
    mid-skull base approaches, 209t
    nasopharyngeal tumor presentation, 83
    occipitoatlatoaxial region, 491

    pathology, 43, 43f
    pathophysiology, 52t
    petroclival, 423, 426, 436, 436f
    subcranial approaches, 357t
        sellar/parasellar region, 575
        transbasal–Derome, 348, 350, 351–352, 351–352f
    transcervicomastoid approach, 409–422. See also Transcervicomastoid approach
Chorda tympani, 25, 379, 479
Chorda tympani nerve, 379
Chordoma, 12
    anterior approaches
        combined resection with, 168
        cranioorbital zygomatic approach, 271, 276f
        facial degloving, extended transmaxillary, 200
        maxillectomy, subtotal, 208
        maxillotomy, extended unilateral, 208–209, 228t, 229, 233
        subcranial transfacial, 287
    clival, 519, 519f
    external auditory meatus/temporal bone, 383t, 385
    foramen magnum region
        condylectomy, 494
        imaging, 98t, 102
        lateral transcondylar approach, 500–503, 501–503f
        pathology, 516, 517, 518, 518f
        transoral approach, 527
    foramen magnum region surgery, 505
    ICA management
        surgical dissection of tumor, 361
        tumor biology and, 360
    imaging, 92t, 93–94, 98t, 102
    infratemporal–middle fossa approach, 309, 313, 314f
    mid-skull base approaches, 209t
    nasopharyngeal tumor presentation, 83
    occipitoatlatoaxial region, 491
    pathology, 43–44, 44f
    pathophysiology, 52t
    petroclival, 423, 426, 436, 436f, 441, 441f
    sellar/parasellar, 560t, 562, 575, 580–581
    subcranial approaches, 357t
        sella/parasellar region, 575
        transbasal–Derome, 348, 350, 352–354, 352–354f
    vertebral artery management, 540f, 544, 545f, 546t
Choristoma, 562, 579
Choroid artery, anterior, 24
C incision, 492, 624, 624f
Circle of Willis, 24, 28, 122
    collateral flow in carotid artery occlusion, 359
    preoperative assessment, 311, 313
    temporal bone tumor management, 386
Circular sinus, 22, 65f, 334, 571
Cisternae, 437
Cisterna magna, 455, 458
Cisternography, 446, 566
Clear cell carcinoma, 259t
Clinical nurse specialist, 120, 122, 135
Clinical presentation, 73–85

    clival and foramen magnum region tumors, 519–522, 519–521f
    ear and temporal bone, 82–83, 82–83f
    infratemporal–middle fossa approach, 309–313, 310–313f, 313t
    jugulotympanic paraganglioma, 474–476, 475f, 475t
    nasopharymx, 83–85, 84f
    nose and paranasal sinus lesions, 74–82
        central invasion, 81–82, 81–82f
        ethmoid sinus, 80, 82f
        frontal sinus, 80–81, 80–81f
        maxillary sinus, 78–80, 78–79f, 81–82f
        nose, 74, 76f, 77–78, 77f
        sphenoid sinus, 81, 81f, 82f
    oropharyngeal, upper neck, and parotid gland tumors, 84f, 85
    petroclival tumors, 426–427
    sella/parasellar lesions, 563–565
    temporal bone lesions, 381
    vestibular schwannoma, 444–445
Clinoid
    anatomy, 15, 17f, 19, 21, 24, 556f
    cephalometrics, 521, 522f
    clivus tumor erosion, 562
    cranioorbital approach, 263, 274, 276f, 278, 279
        aneurysm repair, 280–281, 280–281f, 282, 283f
        entering, 269–270, 270f
    meningioma, 580
    middle, 19
    subtemporal approach to sella, 575, 576
    total petrosectomy, 402f
    transbasal–Derome approach, 350
Clival syndrome, 69, 70
Clivus, 12. See also Petroclival lesions
    anatomy, 17f, 22, 27, 29, 424f, 425, 555
    cephalometrics, 521, 522f
    chordoma, 93, 517f, 518, 518f
    clinical presentation, 519–521
    complications, prevention of, 587
    compression of, 521
    facial degloving approach, 195, 200, 205
    foramen magnum region surgery, 498, 500, 503f, 504f
    imaging, 87–88
        chordoma, 93
        craniopharygioma, 92
        epidermoid and cholesterol cysts, 95
        foramen magnum lesions, 102
    infratemporal–middle fossa approach, 309
        dural resection, 335
        incision, 313, 314f
    maxillotomy, extended unilateral, 208, 217f, 225f, 226f, 230
        dura, 209–210, 213, 224, 226f
        exposure, 222–223, 223f
    medial subcranial structures, 27
    meningioma, ICA involvement, 106f
    nasopharyngeal carcinoma, 516–517, 517f
    odontectomy, 527
    primary lesion presentation, 85
    sellar/parasellar involvement, 560t, 562
    sellar/parasellar lesions
        chordoma, 580–581
        subtemporal approaches, 575
    sphenoid sinus tumor presentation, 81

subcranial approaches
   extended anterior, 241, 243f, 245, 246–248f
   transbasal–Derome, 347, 348, 350–353, 351f, 353f, 357
   transfacial approach, extended, 297, 298f, 299
total petrosectomy, 401
transfacial approaches
   maxillectomy, 173, 173f
   extended, 297, 298f, 299
transmandibular approach, 341
transoral approach, 507–531. See also Foramen magnum region
   operative technique, 521–531
   pathology, 514–519, 514–519f
transsphenoidal approach, 27
tumor pathophysiology, 53, 53f, 61, 64, 67t
vertebral artery management, 546–548, 546t, 547f
Cob periosteal elevator, 513, 513f
Cochlea
  ear lesion involvement, 83
  foramen magnum region surgery, 504f
  jugulotympanic paraganglioma. See Jugulotympanic paraganglioma
  petroclival surgery
    petrous bone anatomy, 425, 426f, 426
    middle fossa extradural approach, 436
  vestibular schwannoma, 450, 457f, 468
Cochlear aqueduct, 380, 450
Cochlear aqueduct vein, 413
Cochleariform process, 378
Cochlear nerve, 9
  compound action potentials, 154
  petrous bone anatomy, 425
  temporal bone anatomy, 378
  vestibular schwannoma, 463f, 463, 463f
Cochlear promontory, cautery contraindicated, 479
Cochleovestibular complications, 405
Cocke, E.W., 7, 7f
Collagenase, 61
Collaterals/collateral flow, 122
  anastomoses, 113t
  anterior communicating artery, 369f
  carotid artery occlusion, 359
  and carotid artery sacrifice, 360
  embolization, therapeutic, 114
  internal carotid artery management, 361
    preoperative evaluation, 360
    recurrent adenoid cystic carcinoma, 367–370, 367–370f
  sigmoid sinus occlusion and, 59
  temporal resection, 386, 405
  vertebral artery, 115f, 539, 544
Collateral veins, tumor pathophysiology, 59
Collet-Sicard syndrome, 386, 476
Colon cancer mets, 47
Coma
  grunting respirations, 586, 592–593
  postoperative monitoring, 586f, 600, 601t
Coma, induced, 371
  and cerebral blood flow, 105
  during ICA surgery, 373
Common carotid artery
  anastomoses, 114f
  arteriography, vertebral artery occlusion, 115f

balloon test occlusion, 107
vertebral artery bypass, 551
vertebral artery management, 540f, 541
Communicating artery, anterior
  aneurysm, cranioorbital zygomatic approach, 279, 279f, 281–282, 281f
  ICA collateralization, 369f
Complications
  balloon test occlusion, 111
  embolization, therapeutic, 114
  infratemporal–middle fossa approach, 309, 335, 596–597, 596f
  internal carotid artery resection, 387
  internal carotid artery to MCA bypass, 371
  jugulotympanic paraganglioma, 481, 486t, 487
  maxillotomy, extended unilateral, 210, 228–229, 228t, 229t
  median labial mandibuloglossoptomy, 522
  neurophysiological monitoring, 152. See also Neurologic monitoring, intraoperative
  petroclival surgery, 429, 437
  prevention and management, 585–597
    CSF leakage, 586t, 589–590, 590f, 592f
    hemorrhage, 593, 593f, 595
    infection, 586t, 590–592, 590f, 591f
    osteomyelitis, 595–597, 596f
    pericranial flap slough, 594f, 595
    pneumocephalus, 592–593
    prevention, 585–589, 586t, 586–588f
  radiation therapy, 406
  reconstruction goals, 608
  sellar/parasellar surgery, 573
  subcranial approaches
    extended anterior, 239, 260, 260t
    transbasal–Derome, 347, 357
  temporal resection, 400, 404–406, 405f
  therapeutic embolization, 113
  transbasal approach, Derome modification, 357
  transcervicomastoid approach, 419–422, 419t, 420t
  transmandibular approach, 343–346
  transoral approaches to clivus and craniocervical junction, 531–532
  vertebral artery surgery, 552
  vestibular schwannoma, 446, 448–449
  vestibular schwannoma radiotherapy, 447
Compound action potentials (CAPs), 154
Compression boots, 412
Compression syndromes, odontectomy, 527–529, 528–530f
Computed tomography. See also Imaging; SPECT; Xenon CT
  biopsy, 111
  ICA to MCA bypass, 373f
  necrosis on, 62, 63f
  squamous cell carcinoma, 69f
  techniques and general diagnostic criteria, 87
  therapeutic embolization, 116f
Conchal pneumatization of sphenoid sinus, 555, 557f
Condylar emissary veins, 28, 494
Condylar vein, 484
Congenital malformations, 6f, 7, 533
  craniocervical junction, 514
  subcranial approaches, transbasal–Derome, 347, 348

vascular. See also Anastomoses; Vascular malformations
Connective tissue, tumor extension via, 67
Connective tissue tumors
  anterior fossa, facial degloving approach, 205
  pathophysiology, 54
Consciousness, levels of, 133
Contrast enhancement, 87, 88. See also Imaging
Coronal flap, 190f, 241–242f
Coronal incision, 182f
Coronoid process
  anatomy, 24
  facial degloving, 208
  maxillotomy, extended unilateral, 213, 213f, 216f, 223f
Cortical activation, 145
Cortical bone imaging, 87–88
Cortical evoked potentials, 150
  carotid assessment, 386–387
  multimodal evoked potential recording, 144f
Cosmetic defects
  infratemporal–middle fossa approach, 313
  rehabilitation, 604–605, 604f, 605f
  subcranial approaches, 357
Costocervical trunk anastomoses, 113t
Cottle elevators, 569
Cottle speculum, 570
Cranial fossae, middle, 20
Cranial involvement. See Intracranial extension
Cranial nerve I. See Olfactory nerve
Cranial nerve II. See Optic nerve
Cranial nerve III (oculomotor)
  anatomy, 19, 21, 22, 23f, 28
    cavernous sinus, 66
    foramen magnum region, 495f
    petroclival region, 424f
  blood supply, 113, 113t
  cranioorbital zygomatic approach, 278
    aneurysm repair, 279f, 282, 283f, 284f
    exposure, 270, 271f
  EMG, 156, 158f
  imaging, 88
  infratemporal–middle fossa approach, 311, 311f
  intraoperative monitoring. See$ Neurologic monitoring, intraoperative
  nasal and paranasal sinus tumor presentation, 82
  petroclival surgery, 424f, 427, 436, 436f
  sellar/parasellar anatomy, 558, 559f
  sellar/parasellar region approaches, 575, 577
Cranial nerve IV (trochlear)
  anatomy, 19, 21–22, 22, 23f
    cavernous sinus, 66
    petroclival, 424f
    sellar/parasellar anatomy, 558, 559f
  blood supply, 113, 113t
  cavernous sinus anatomy, 66
  cavernous sinus syndrome, 363
  cranioorbital zygomatic approach, 270, 271f
  EMG, 156, 158f
  imaging, 88
  infratemporal–middle fossa approach, 311, 311f
  intraoperative monitoring. See Neurologic monitoring, intraoperative

Cranial nerve IV (contd.)
  nasopharyngeal carcinoma and, 53–54
  nasal/paranasal sinus tumor presentation, 82
  petroclival surgery, 424f, 427, 434f, 436, 436f, 437
  sellar/parasellar region approaches, 558, 559f, 577
Cranial nerve V (trigeminal)
  anatomy, 22, 25
    cavernous sinus, 66
    foramen magnum region, 495f
    petroclival, 424f, 426f
    temporal bone, 322, 379
  blood supply, 113, 113t
  cranioorbital zygomatic approach, 270
  EMG, 156
  imaging, 88, 92
  inflammatory lesion, 310, 310f
  infratemporal–middle fossa approach
    diagnosis/presentation, 311f
    otic exposure, 326f
    temporal bone anatomy, 322
  intraoperative monitoring. See Neurologic monitoring, intraoperative
  mandibular branch. See Cranial nerve V3
  maxillary branch. See Cranial nerve V2
  neuroma, 92
  oropharyngeal, parotid, and upper neck lesion involvement, 85
  petroclival surgery, 424f, 427, 433, 433f, 434f
    middle fossa extradural approach, 436
    middle fossa intradural approach, 436f, 437
    posterior fossa primary intradural approach, 435
  petrous bone anatomy, 426f
  sellar/parasellar anatomy, 559f
  subcranial approaches
    transbasal–Derome, 350
    transfacial extended Type III, 305
  temporal bone anatomy, 379
  temporal bone tumors, 386
  total petrosectomy, 401
  tumor pathophysiology, 56, 57f
  tumors of. See Trigeminal neuroma; Trigeminal schwannoma
  vestibular schwannoma and, 444–445
Cranial nerve V1 (ophthalmic)
  anatomy, 22
  cranioorbital zygomatic approach, 271f
  imaging, 88, 95
  infratemporal–middle fossa approach, 310, 311
  nasal/paranasal sinus tumor presentation, 82
  orbital syndrome, 69
  postoperative care, 602, 602f
  sellar/parasellar anatomy, 558
Cranial nerve V2 (maxillary)
  anatomy, 21, 22, 25
  clinical syndromes, 69
  extended transfacial subcranial approach, 287
  imaging, 95
  infratemporal–middle fossa approach, 310, 311
  maxillotomy, extended unilateral, 231–232t
  nasal/paranasal sinus tumor presentation, 82
  sellar/parasellar anatomy, 558
  subcranial approaches, transbasal–Derome, 350

Cranial nerve V3 (mandibular)
  anatomy, 22, 25, 27f
  clinical syndromes, 69
  cranioorbital zygomatic approach, 267, 268f, 269f
  extended transfacial subcranial approach, 287
  imaging, 88, 90f, 95
  infratemporal–middle fossa approach
    craniotomy, 328, 330
      diagnosis/presentation, 311
      temporal bone anatomy, 322
  maxillotomy, extended unilateral, 223f, 224, 225f, 231–232t
  nasal and paranasal sinus tumor spread, 82
  naspharyngeal tumor spread, 83
  oropharyngeal, parotid, and upper neck lesion involvement, 85
  subcranial approaches, transbasal–Derome, 350
  temporal bone anatomy, 378
  transmandibular approach, 342
  tumor pathophysiology, 56, 57f, 57, 57f
Cranial nerve V foramen, cavernous sinus anatomy, 65f
Cranial nerve V ganglion. See Gasserian ganglion
Cranial nerve VI (abducens)
  anatomy, 22, 23f
    cavernous sinus, 21, 66
    foramen magnum region, 495f
  clinical syndromes with metastasis, 69, 70
  clival compression and, 521
  cranioorbital zygomatic approach, 270
  EMG, 155
  imaging, 88
  infratemporal–middle fossa approach, 311, 311f
  intraoperative monitoring. See Neurologic monitoring, intraoperative
  jugular foramen tumors, 410, 410t
  jugular fossa surgery complications, 419, 419t
  maxillotomy, extended unilateral, 231–232t
  nasopharyngeal tumor presentation, 83
  petroclival surgery, 426, 427, 433f, 436, 436f
  sellar/parasellar anatomy, 559f
  temporal bone tumors, 386
  total petrosectomy, 401
  tumor pathophysiology, 61
Cranial nerve VII (facial), 8, 9. See also Facial neuropathy
  anatomy, 21, 22, 24–25, 24f, 28
    foramen magnum region, 495f, 496f
    petroclival, 425, 425f, 426, 426f, 427f
    temporal bone, 378, 378f, 379
  blood supply, 113t
  clinical syndromes with metastasis, 69, 70
  compound action potentials, 154
  cranioorbital zygomatic approach, 264
  ear tumor presentation, 82, 83
  EMG, 155, 157, 158f, 159f
  foramen magnum region surgery
    chordoma, 502f
    glomus tumor, 500f
  infratemporal–middle fossa approach, 315, 316f
  intraoperative monitoring. See Neurologic monitoring, intraoperative

jugular foramen anatomy, 413
jugular foramen surgery, 410, 410t, 414, 415–416, 416f, 417, 419f
jugular fossa surgery, 419, 419t, 421
jugular fossa tumors, 420t
jugulotympanic paraganglioma, 480, 480f, 483f, 484
  infratemporal fossa approach, 481, 484f
  mastoid-neck approach, 482f
  results, 486
meningeal branch of, 21
nerve grafts, 405, 637, 637f
neuroma, imaging, 98t, 99
petroclival anatomy, 427f
petroclival surgery, 427, 431, 433, 433f, 434f
  anatomy, 425, 425f, 426, 426f, 427f
  complications, 429
  middle fossa extradural approach, 436
  posterior fossa primary intradural, 435, 435f
resection, eye care after, 402
temporal bone anatomy, 378, 378f, 379
temporal bone resection, 391f, 393
temporal bone tumors, 381, 387
total petrosectomy, 401f
vestibular schwannoma. See Vestibular schwannoma
Cranial nerve VII paralysis
  facial reanimation for, 604f
  with infratemporal lesions, 310
  nursing care, postoperative assessments, 133–134
Cranial nerve VIII (vestibulocochlear)
  anatomy, 22, 28, 495f, 496f
  clinical syndromes with metastasis, 69, 70
  intraoperative monitoring. See Neurologic monitoring, intraoperative
  jugular foramen tumors, 410, 410t
  petroclival surgery, 427, 433, 433f, 434f, 435, 435f, 436
  petrous bone anatomy, 426f
  vestibular schwannoma, 455, 461, 463
Cranial nerve IX (glossopharyngeal), 25, 28
  anatomy, 25, 28, 379, 492, 495f, 496f
  blood supply
    ICA to MCA bypass, 371
    therapeutic embolization and, 113
  clinical syndromes with metastasis, 69, 70
  ear tumor involvement, 83
  EMG, 156
  foramen magnum region surgery, chordoma, 502f
  ICA to MCA bypass, 371
  infratemporal–middle fossa approach, 311, 315
  intraoperative monitoring. See Neurologic monitoring, intraoperative
  jugular foramen, 548
  jugular foramen syndrome, 519
  jugular foramen tumors, 410, 410t
  jugular fossa surgery complications, 419, 419t
  jugular fossa tumors, 421
  jugulotympanic paraganglioma, 474, 476, 480, 481
  maxillotomy, extended unilateral, 230
  nerve grafts, 405, 637

oropharyngeal, parotid, and upper neck lesion
        presentation, 85
    petroclival surgery, 427, 433
    temporal bone tumors, 379, 381, 386
    transmandibular approach, 343
    vertebral artery anatomy, 534
    vertebral artery control, 539
    vestibular schwannoma, 450, 461
Cranial nerve X (vagus)
    anatomy, 25, 28, 492, 495f, 496f
    blood supply
        ICA to MCA bypass, 371
        therapeutic embolization and, 113
    clinical syndromes with metastasis, 69, 70
    ear tumor involvement, 83
    EMG, 156
    foramen magnum region surgery, 496f, 502f
    glomus tumors, 409, 411
    infratemporal–middle fossa approach, 311, 315
    intraoperative monitoring. *See* Neurologic monitoring, intraoperative
    jugular foramen, 548
    jugular foramen anatomy, 413
    jugular foramen syndrome, 519
    jugular foramen tumors, 410, 410t
    jugular fossa surgery complications, 419, 419t
    jugular fossa tumors, 421
    jugulotympanic paraganglioma, 476, 480, 481
    maxillotomy, extended unilateral, 230
    nerve grafts, 637
    oropharyngeal, parotid, and upper neck lesion presentation, 85
    paraganglioma, 473
    paralysis, 519
    petroclival surgery, 427, 433
    temporal bone anatomy, 379
    temporal bone tumors, 381, 386
    transcervicomastoid approach, 409–422. *See also* Transcervicomastoid approach
    transmandibular approach, 343
    vertebral artery anatomy, 534
    vertebral artery control, 539
    vestibular schwannoma, 450, 461
Cranial nerve XI (glossopharyngeal)
    anatomy, 25, 28, 379, 492, 495f, 496f
    blood supply, therapeutic embolization and, 113
    clinical syndromes with metastasis, 69, 70
    clival compression and, 521
    ear tumor involvement, 83
    EMG, 156
    foramen magnum region surgery, 502f
    infratemporal–middle fossa approach, 311, 315
    intraoperative monitoring. *See* Neurologic monitoring, intraoperative
    jugular foramen anatomy, 413
    jugular foramen surgery, 416
    jugular foramen syndrome, 519
    jugular foramen tumors, 410, 410t
    jugular fossa surgery complications, 419, 419t
    jugular fossa tumors, 421
    jugulotympanic paraganglioma, 476, 480, 481
    neck dissection, 402–403

nerve grafts, 637
petroclival surgery, 427, 433
temporal bone tumors, 381, 386
transmandibular approach, 343
vertebral artery anatomy, 534
vertebral artery management
    complications, 552
    control, 539
    foramen magnum region lesions, 546, 547f
vestibular schwannoma, 450, 461
Cranial nerve XII (hypoglossal)
    anatomosis to facial nerve, temporal resection, 400–401
    anatomy, 25, 28, 29, 492, 495f, 496f
    blood supply, 113, 113t
    clinical presentation with tumor involvement of, 519
    clinical syndromes with metastasis, 69, 70
    EMG, 156
    foramen magnum region surgery, 502f, 504f
    infratemporal–middle fossa approach, 311, 315
    intraoperative monitoring. *See* Neurologic monitoring, intraoperative
    jugular foramen, 548
    jugular foramen anatomy, 413
    jugular foramen tumors, 410, 410t
    jugular fossa tumors, 421
    jugulotympanic paraganglioma, 476, 481
    maxillotomy, extended unilateral, 209, 223, 224, 231–232t
    nerve grafts, 405, 637
    oropharyngeal, parotid, and upper neck lesion presentation, 85
    petroclival surgery, 433
    temporal bone tumors, 386, 400–401
    transmandibular approach, 343
    vertebral artery anatomy, 534
    vertebral artery control, 539
Cranial nerves. *See also specific nerves*
    anatomy
        foramen magnum region, 492, 495f, 496f
        temporal bone, 378
    basilar impression and, 521
    blood supply, 113, 113t
    cavernous sinus, 21–22, 22f
    foramen magnum region surgery, 491, 494
        anatomy, 492, 495f, 496f
        glomus tumor, 498, 499f
        meningioma, 498f
    imaging, 70, 98t
    jugular foramen anatomy, 413
    jugular foramen surgery, 418f
    jugulotympanic paraganglioma, 475, 476, 478, 481, 484
    maxillotomy, extended unilateral, 231–232t
    monitoring, 154–159, 158–159f
        BTO, 107
        infratemporal–middle fossa approach, 313. *See also* Neurologic monitoring, intraoperative
        jugulotympanic paraganglioma, 480
        postoperative, 600
    nerve grafts, 637–638, 637–638f
    neurinoma, imaging, 98t
    petroclival surgery, 433, 433f

prevention of complications, 587
    sellar/parasellar lesions, clinical presentation, 563
    subcranial extended transfacial approach, 297
    tumor spread via, 85
    vertebral artery control, 539
    vestibular schwannoma, 448, 456f
Cranial neuropathies
    complications, 405
        jugulotympanic paraganglioma surgery, 487
        maxillotomy, 228, 228t, 229, 230
        petroclival surgery, 437
        sellar/parasellar surgery, 573, 578–579
        therapeutic embolization, 113, 114
        transmandibular approach, 345
    nursing care
        nutrition, 123
        postoperative, 133–134
    postoperative care with, 602
    rehabilitation, 606
    symptoms. *See also* Clinical presentation
        clinical presentations, 519
        foramen magnum region tumors, 500
        glomus tumor, 410, 410t
        jugulotympanic paraganglioma, 474, 474t, 480, 481
        petroclival tumors, 426
        temporal bone tumors, 381, 386
Cranial vault, tumor pathophysiology, 54
Craniocervical junction. *See also* Foramen magnum region; Vertebral artery management
    anatomy, 11, 29, 508, 511f, 514–519f
    embryology, 507, 508f
    foramen magnum region surgery, 505
    halo-type fixation, 531
    joint abnormalities
        vertebral artery effects, 536, 545, 546t
        stabilization/fusion, 496, 500, 502, 503, 503f
    maxillotomy, extended unilateral, 228t
    tumor invasion, 61
    vertebral artery and, 505
    vertebral artery lesions, 542, 542t
Craniofacial cervical incision, 313, 313f
Craniofacial resection, 5
    cranioorbital zygomatic approach, bifrontal, 274
    prosthetic rehabilitation, 605, 605f
    reconstruction, radial forearm free flap, 608–611, 609–610f
    squamous cell carcinoma, 274, 275f
    transmandibular approach, 343
Cranioorbital approach, 263–285
    for aneurysms, 278–282, 279–284f
    for trauma, 282, 284f, 285
    for tumors, 271–278
        bifrontal, 272–274, 273–275f
        supraorbital, 271–272, 272–273f
        zygomatic, 274, 276–277f, 278
    zygomatic (COZ), 263–271
        bone flap, 266–267, 266f
        carotid artery exposure, 267–268, 268f
        cavernous sinus, entering, 269–270, 270–271f
        intradural dissection, 268–269, 269f
        patient positioning, 263–264

Cranioorbital approach (contd.)
  reconstruction and closure, 270–271
    skin incision and pericranial flap, 264–265, 264–265f
    sphenoid bone, drilling, 267, 267f
Craniopharyngioma
  imaging, 92
  mid-skull base approaches, 209t
  sellar/parasellar, 560t, 562, 571, 574, 579–580
  subcranial approaches, transbasal–Derome, 348, 352, 354–356, 354–356f, 357, 357t
Craniotomy, 182f
  cranioorbital zygomatic approach, 283
  evolution of techniques, 6f, 7
  facial degloving, 195, 197, 202–205, 203–205f
  frontal and nasoorbital, 239
  frontobasal approach, 357
  infratemporal–middle fossa approach, 322, 326, 326f, 328–330. 328–330f
  with maxillotomy, extended unilateral, 229
  modified Fisch approach, 309
  petroclival surgery, 430, 430f, 435, 437
  pterional, 575, 576f
  subcranial approaches
    frontobasal, 357
    transbasal–Derome, 348, 349f
  subcranial extended transfacial approach
    Type I, 292, 297
    Type II, 296
    Type III, 305
  temporal bone resection, 395f
  transfacial approach, 183–190, 182–189f
  vestibular schwannoma, 458, 459f, 465, 467f
Craniotomy bone flaps
  infratemporal–middle fossa approach, 337
  internal auditory canal reconstruction, 464, 464f
Craniotomy flaps
  infratemporal–middle fossa approach, 335, 336f, 338f
  osteomyelitis, 595
Craniovertebral junction. See Craniocervical junction
Cribriform plate, 15, 16, 17f, 18f
  cranioorbital zygomatic approach, bifrontal, 273
  esthesioneuroblastoma, 167
  degloving, 201, 213, 213f
  imaging, 87, 88, 89, 89f
  maxillotomy, extended unilateral, 213, 213f, 214f, 223f, 232t
  subcranial extended transfacial approach, 292, 294f
  transoral approaches to foramen magnum region, 524
  tumor spread via, 51, 52f, 55, 55f
Cribroethmoid foramen, 15
Cricopharyngeal myotomy, 305
Crista galli, 15, 16, 17f, 189f
  cranioorbital zygomatic approach, bifrontal, 273, 274f
  craniotomy considerations, 186
  subcranial approaches
    extended anterior, 241–242f
    transbasal–Derome, 349
Crista transversalis, 378

Crockard, A., 11, 12f
Crockard instruments, 512f, 513f, 529
  mouth gag, 522
  odontectomy, 529
  retractor, 524f, 526, 526f
Cross facial sural nerve interposition grafts, 405
Cruciate ligament, 511f
Crumley, R., 12
Crutchfield tongs, 521
CSF
  bone dust, 454
  cochlear aqueduct, 380
  hemorrhage and, 593
  imaging, 88, 89, 89f
  petroclival surgery, 431
  pneumocephalus, 592–593
  subarachnoid space, 378
  temporal craniotomy, 397
  vestibular schwannoma, 458, 461
CSF drain
  anterior craniotomies, 186
  cranioorbital zygomatic approach, 263–264, 268, 282–283
  CSF leak detection, 590
  CSF testing for white cells or bacteria, 591
  encephalocele repair, 282–283
  foramen magnum region surgery, 496
  frontobasal subcranial approach, 357
  infratemporal–middle fossa approach, 313, 337
  jugulotympanic paraganglioma, 486
  nursing care with, 128, 129, 132
  petroclival surgery, 435
  petroclival surgery complications, 437
  postoperative monitoring, 600–601
  prevention of complications, 586, 588
  sellar/parasellar surgery, 568, 573
  subfrontal approach, 574
  temporal craniotomy, 397
  transoral approach, 522
CSF fistula, 590
  cranioorbital zygomatic approach, 285f
  foramen magnum region surgery, 496
  prevention of, 589
  sella surgery, 571, 573, 573f
  subcranial approaches, 347, 348, 356, 357, 357t
  vestibular schwannoma, 448–449, 470f
CSF leak
  anterior approach, incidence after, 586t
  infratemporal–middle fossa approach, 335
  jugular fossa tumors, 420t
  jugulotympanic paraganglioma, 486t
  management of, 586t, 589–590, 590f, 592f
  maxillotomy, 228t, 229
  nasal and paranasal sinus tumor presentation, 82
  nursing care, postoperative monitoring, 133
  odontectomy complications, 532
  petroclival surgery complications, 437
  pituitary cistern and, 555
  postoperative care, 599, 602
  postoperative monitoring, 600
  prevention of, 586
  reconstruction goals, 608, 623
  sella surgery, 555, 572
  temporal bone resection, 400, 404

dural repair, 403
  total petrosectomy reconstruction, 402
  transmandibular approach, 345
  transoral approach, 532
  vestibular schwannoma, 464
CSF rhinorrhea and otorrhea, 602
Cushing, H., 3, 5, 5f, 7–8, 443, 457
Cushing-Landau retractor, 570
Cushing's veil, 590, 591f
Cutaneous flaps, 317f, 343, See also Flaps, free; Flaps and grafts, regional
Cutaneous sensory nerves, neurotropic tumors, 165
Cyproheptadine, 578
Cystic degeneration, imaging, 87, 89f, 101, 101f
Cystic lesions, 204f, 560t, 552, 571
Cytology, 70

D
Dacryocystitis, 203, 204f
Dacryocystorhinostomy, 203, 204f
Dandy, W. E., 5, 5f, 8
DDAVP, 602
Debridement, osteomyelitis management, 597
Deep temporal arteries, 24, 115, 316
Deep temporal nerve, 231t
Defect repair. See Reconstruction/defect repair
Degloving. See Facial degloving
Denker procedure, 199
  anterior wall ostectomy as alternative to, 170, 171f
  subcranial extended transfacial approach, 293f
  transfacial approach, 168–173, 168–174f
Dens
  apical ligament, 28
  Metzger's line, 521, 521f
  odontectomy, 527–529, 528–530f
Dental ligament, 508
Dentition. See Teeth
Dermoid cysts, 560t, 562
Derome modification, anterior transbasal approach, 347–358. See also Transbasal approach, Derome modification
Dexamethasome, 456, 457
Diabetes insipidus, 573, 579, 600, 602
Diaphragma sellae, 21, 555
Diaphyseal dysplasias, imaging, 102, 102t
Diffuse lesions, imaging, 102, 102t
Digastric groove, 416
Digastric muscle, 28
  ICA course, 22
  jugular foramen surgery, 414
  jugulotympanic paraganglioma, 480, 481
  temporal bone anatomy 379
  transmandibular approach, 343
Digastric ridge, 426
Dingman mouth gag, 513, 513f, 522
Diploic bone, 61
Diplopia, 69, 80. See also Vision/visual deficits
Dissection, arterial
  BTO complications, 111
  vertebral artery, 551, 551t
Dissection, surgical. See Resection/dissection/tumor margins
Diuretics, 397
Donald, P.J., 12

SUBJECT INDEX / 651

Donor sites. *See also specific flap sites*
  infratemporal–middle fossa approach
    preparation, 313, 313f
    reconstruction, 337
  nursing care
    preoperative preparation, 128
    postoperative, 133
  ultrasound mapping, 122
  vestibular schwannoma reconstruction, 455
Dopamine, 477
Doppler ultrasound
  during ICA surgery, 373
  petroclival surgery, 429
  postoperative, 601
  preoperative evaluation, 360
  temporal bone tumor management, 386
Dorello's canal, 21, 23f, 69, 401
Dorsum sellae, 20f, 21, 559f
Doyle, B.B., 8
Drainage, nasal, 74, 78, 80
Drains
  brain abscess management, 591–592
  CSF. *See* CSF drain
  infratemporal–middle fossa approach, 337
  jugular foramen surgery, 417
  nursing care, 128, 129, 132, 134
  postoperative management, 601
  temporal bone resection, 401
Draping, 126, 129–130
Dry eye, 82
Duckbill elevator, 454
Dura
  anatomy
    cavernous sinus, 21, 22
    clivus, 29
    foramen magnum, 28
    middle fossa, 19, 21
    posterior fossa, 28
  cavernous sinus, 21, 22, 59, 173
  craniotomy, 184
  facial degloving approaches, 201
  frontal sinus tumor presentation, 81f
  imaging, 70, 87
    central skull base lesions, 92
    foramen magnum lesions, 102
    intradural compartment-paranasal sinus communication, 356
  Meckel's cave area, 20
  nasal and paranasal sinus tumor presentation, 81, 82
  pneumocephalus, 592–593
  sella, 571f
  squamous cell carcinoma spread, 383
  tumor pathophysiology, 52f, 53, 72
    imaging metastatic disease, 70, 71f
    invasion, 61
    lymphoma, 54
    nasal/paranasal sinus tumors, 167, 167f
    patterns of spread, 61–62, 62f, 62t
    squamous cell carcinoma, 383
  vertebral artery dissection, 537
Dural grafts. *See* Dural repair
Dural incisions, vestibular schwannoma, 460f, 462f
Dural invasion, 61, 167, 167f
  contraindications to transsphenoidal approach, 566, 566t

palliative radiation therapy, 407
squamous cell carcinomas, 383
Dural plate, transverse, 21
Dural repair
  complications
    pneumocephalus, 586, 593
    prevention of, 588–589, 588f
  craniorbital zygomatic approach, trauma repair, 283
  fascia lata patch, 295f
  foramen magnum region surgery, 496
  goals of, 623
  infratemporal–middle fossa approach, 335, 335f
  jugular foramen surgery, 417
  jugulotympanic paraganglioma, 484
  materials, 190, 190f
  temporal bone resection, 387, 400, 403
  tensor fascia lata graft, 619, 619f
  total petrosectomy, 402
Dural space, transbasal–Derome approach
  complications, 347, 357
Dural tail, 92, 446, 565
Dural tumors, infratemporal–middle fossa approach, 309
Dura propria, craniorbital zygomatic approach, 270
Dysphagia. *See* Swallowing/dysphagia
Dysplasias, diffuse lesions of skull base, 102, 102t

E

Ear. *See also* External auditory canal; Internal auditory canal; Middle ear
  auricle/external auditory meatus, 322, 326
    anatomy, 378
    otitis, external, 98, 381, 406
    pinna reconstruction, 405
    temporal bone anatomy, 378
    skin lesions, 73, 82, 83f
    tumor extension, 54, 67
    tumor presentation, 82–83, 82–83f, 380, 381, 389f
  craniorbital zygomatic approach, 263, 270
  CSF otorrhea, 602
  external otitis, 98, 381, 406
  infratemporal–middle fossa approach, 317f, 318f
    otologic exposure, 322, 326
    postoperative care, 337
  jugular foramen surgery, 416
  temporal bone resection, 396f
  vestibular schwannoma, 450, 451f
Edema
  and diagnosis of recurrences, 310
  imaging, 88
  with meningioma, 106f
  prevention of complications, 588
  tumor and, 64f
Elderly, dural fragility, 186, 329, 397
Electrocardiography, 429
Electroencephalography, 145
  during carotid endarterectomy, 153f
  cerebral blood flow monitoring, 107, 359
  data acquisition, 140
  ICA dissection, 373
  during ICA surgery, 373

infratemporal–middle fossa approach, 313
intraoperative monitoring, 145–158, 146–147f
Electrolytes, 600, 602. *See also* Fluids
Electromyography, 138, 145
  data acquisition, 140
  jugulotympanic paraganglioma, 480, 481
  nerve grafts, 637
  neurological monitoring, 154–159, 158–159f
  petroclival surgery, 429–430
Electronystagmography, 445, 465
Electroretinography, 154–155, 156f
Emboli, tumor, 67
Embolism
  anti-embolic stockings, 412, 601
  carotid artery sacrifice and, 111
  cerebral blood flow and, 359
  maxillotomy complications, 228, 228t
  neurophysiological monitoring
    EEG, 147
    MSPs, 150–151
  postoperative monitoring, 600
  SEP waveforms, 152f
  vertebral artery, 551
Embolization, therapeutic, 113–116, 113t, 114–116f, 116t
  adenoid cystic carcinoma, recurrent, 368, 369f
  glomus/jugular foramen tumors, 409, 420, 411, 499f
  jugulotympanic paraganglioma, 477–478, 487
  maxillotomy, extended unilateral, 222
  petroclival tumors, 428
  prevention of complications, 587
  transcervicomastoid approach, 412, 412f
  vertebral artery management, 550, 551
Embryology, craniocervical junction, 507, 508f
Embryonal rhabdomyosarcoma, 42, 42f
EMG. *See* Electromyography
Emissary veins
  cavernous sinus anatomy, 22
  condylar, 28
  hypoglossal nerve, 492
  to pterygoid plexus, 21
  tumor extension via, 61
En bloc resection, 165
  glomus tumors, 409
  petrosectomy, 401
  subcranial extended transfacial approach, 291, 304, 304f
  temporal bone resection, 397
  transbasal–Derome procedure, 348
Encephalocele
  craniorbital zygomatic approach, 282–283, 284f
  subcranial approaches, transbasal–Derome, 347, 357
Endolymphatic duct, 28, 380
  anatomy, middle ear, 380
  vestibular schwannoma, 461, 463f
Endolymphatic sac tumor, 98t
Endoscopy
  equipment, 125
  nasopharyngeal tumor presentation, 85
  nursing care, 122
  vestibular schwannoma closure, 464, 464f

Enophthalmos, 357, 604–605
Enzymes
  clinical syndromes with metastasis, 70
  tumor spread, 61
Eosinophilic granuloma, 385, 386
Ependymoma
  cerebellopontine angle lesion imaging, 98, 98t, 100
  vertebral artery involvement, 546t
Epidermoid carcinoma
  maxillotomy, extended unilateral, 228t
  mid-skull base approaches, 209t
Epidermoid cysts/tumors
  imaging, 97
    central skull base lesions, 92t, 95
    cerebellopontine angle lesions, 98, 98t, 99
  pathophysiology, 52t
  petroclival, 426, 435–436
  sellar/parasellar region, 560t, 562
  vertebral artery involvement, 546t
Epidural venous networks, tumor emboli, 67
Epinephrine, 477
Epiphora, 603
Epistaxis, 74, 77, 356, 520
  with ethmoid sinus tumors, 80
  with nasopharyngeal tumors, 83
Epithelial cysts, sellar/parasellar, 560t, 562
Epithelial tissue, anterior fossa reconstruction, 191
Erosion. *See also* Bone destruction
  imaging, 92
  presentation, 77, 82
Esthesioneuroblastoma
  anterior approaches
    cranioorbital zygomatic approach, 271
    eye region, globe-sparing procedure, 168, 168f
    facial degloving approach, 205
    transfacial approach, 165, 166f, 167
  imaging, 89f, 89t
  pathophysiology, 52t, 57
  presentation, 77f
  sellar/parasellar involvement, 574
  subcranial approaches, 357t
    combined transbasal–Derome-transfacial, 355–356, 355–356f
    extended anterior, 259t
    transbasal–Derome, 348
Ethmoid. *See also* Ethmoidectomy
  anatomy, 15, 16, 19, 19f, 557f
  coronal section, 18f
  cranioorbital zygomatic approach, 283
  ethmoid sinus tumor spread, 167, 167f
  facial degloving, 195, 199
  maxillary sinus tumor presentation, 79
  maxillectomy, 180, 180f
  maxillotomy, extended unilateral, 231–232t
  sellar/parasellar surgery, 569f, 573–574
  sphenoethmoid anterior maxillotomy-medial maxillectomy approach, 292–298, 293–298f
  subcranial approaches
    extended anterior, 239, 245, 246–248t
    extended transfacial type I, 292
    extended transfacial Type II, 299, 299f
    transbasal–Derome, 349
  tumor pathophysiology, 55, 55f
  tumor presentation, 77f

Ethmoid artery, 55f
  anastomoses, 113t
  anterior, 15, 230, 239
  cranioorbital zygomatic approach, bifrontal, 273
  posterior, 15, 17, 230
  sellar/parasellar region approaches, 574
  subcranial approaches, transbasal–Derome, 350
  therapeutic embolization considerations, 115
  tumor spread via foramina, 55–56, 55–56f
Ethmoid cells, 175, 184
Ethmoidectomy, 172
  facial degloving with, 197, 201, 201f
  lateral rhinotomy, 170, 170f
  maxillectomy, 179
  subcranial extended transfacial approach, 293f
  transmaxillary, 198
Ethmoid foramen, 19f
Ethmoid sinus, 16, 81
  facial degloving
    sublabial transoral, 208
    transmaxillary approach, 199
  imaging, 90, 91f, 92f
  maxillary sinus tumor invasion, 79–80
  maxillotomy, extended unilateral, 231t, 232t
  subcranial approaches, transbasal–Derome, 350, 354f
Ethmoid sinus tumors
  anterior cranial fossa spread, 167
  anterior craniotomies, 187f, 188f
  facial degloving-transmaxillary procedure, 201, 201f
  imaging, 88, 89, 89f, 89t
  infratemporal–middle fossa approach, 320f
  pathophysiology, 51, 52f
  presentation, 77f, 79f, 81, 82f
  routes of spread, 167
  subcranial extended transfacial approach, 288, 288f, 289f
  symptoms, 80, 82f
  transfacial approach indications, 165
Ethmosphenoidectomy, with maxillotomy, 221f, 223f
Ethmosphenoid plane, subcranial approaches, 243f, 253–254, 253–254f
Etmodiate coma, 360, 361, 373
Eustachian tube, 22, 23, 27, 589
  anatomy, 25, 380
  clinical presentation of tumors, 83, 519
  facial degloving, sublabial transoral, 208
  foramen magnum region surgery, 504f
  imaging, 96f
  infratemporal–middle fossa approach, 315, 326f, 329
  jugular foramen surgery, 416
  jugulotympanic paraganglioma spread, 474
  mandibular condylectomy/resection, 393
  mandibular displacement, 626, 626f
  maxillotomy
    extended unilateral, 209, 212, 215, 223f
    complications, 228, 228t
  postoperative care, 602
  reconstruction goals, 623
  subcranial extended transfacial approach, 301, 301f

  Type II, 302f
  Type III, 305
  temporal bone resection, 399f
  temporal bone tumors, 381, 386
  total petrosectomy, 402
  tumor pathophysiology, 53, 53f
  vestibular schwannoma, 457f
Eustachian tube line, 26f
Evoked potentials. *See also* Neurologic monitoring, intraoperative
  cerebral blood flow effects, 359
  data acquisition, 140, 142
Ewing's sarcoma, 45, 102
Excitation time, 88
Exophytic lesions, 80f, 81, 82
Extended anterior approaches
  maxillotomy, unilateral, 207–235. *See also* Maxillotomy, extended unilateral
  subcranial, 239–260. *See also* Subcranial extended anterior approach
  subcranial transfacial, 287–308. *See also* Transfacial subcranial approach, extended
  transmaxillary approach, 199–200
External auditory canal, 73
  anatomy, 379
  foramen magnum region surgery, 500, 502f
  infratemporal–middle fossa approach, 315, 318f
    craniotomy, 326, 328f
    otologic exposure, 322, 326
  jugular foramen surgery, 416
  jugular fossa surgery, 421
  jugulotympanic paraganglioma
    infratemporal fossa approach, 481
    mastoid-neck approach, 482f
  lymphatic drainage, 380
  otitis, external, 98, 381, 406
  radiation therapy complications, 406
  squamous cell carcinoma, 383, 383f
  temporal bone resection, 395f
  temporal bone tumor staging, 382, 382t
  tumor pathophysiology, 54
  vestibular schwannoma, 449, 451f, 452f, 456, 466f
External auditory meatus, 378, 380, 381
External carotid artery, 534f
  anastomoses, therapeutic embolization considerations, 113, 113t
  angiography, 116f
  embolization, therapeutic, 113, 113t, 114–116f
  glomus jugulare/jugular foramen tumors, 411, 411f, 498, 499f
  infratemporal–middle fossa approach, flap vascularization, 337
  jugulotympanic paraganglioma, 484
  maxillotomy, extended unilateral, 216f, 231t
  therapeutic embolization considerations, 115
  vertebral artery anastomoses, 534
  vertebral artery management, 550, 550f
External otitis, 98, 381, 406
Extracranial spaces, petroclival tumors, 423, 424f
Extradural approach
  petroclival region, 429–435, 430–434f, 436–437, 436f

Subject Index / 653

sella/parasellar region, 566–573, 566t, 567–574f
   chordoma, 581
   extracranial, 566–573, 566t, 567–574f
   transbasal approach, Derome modification, 349–352, 350–352f
   combined, 352–354, 352–354f
Extradural space
   petroclival anatomy, 424f, 425
   reconstruction, radial forearm free flap, 608–611, 609–610f
Extremities
   atlantoaxial compression effects, 521
   patient positioning, 126
Eye. *See also* Orbital exenteration; Orbit/periorbital structures
   blood supply, 114
   canthal skin lesions, 73
   ear lesion presentation, 82
   esthesioneuroblastoma, 167
   ethmoid sinus tumor presentation, 80
   after facial nerve resection, 402
   infratemporal–middle fossa approach, 311f
   lateral rectus palsy, 312f
   lateral rhinotomy, 170
   nasal and paranasal sinus tumor presentation, 82
   postoperative management, 601–602
   protection, 586
      nursing staff duties, 129
      temporary tarsorraphy, 587f
      with transoral approach, 522
   radiation therapy complications, 406–407
   subcranial approach
      extended anterior, 239
      transbasal–Derome, 357
   subcranial approach complications, 357
   vestibular schwannoma, 456
Eyelid
   gold implants, 405, 602
   infraorbital nerve involvement, 311, 311f
   nasal and paranasal sinus tumor presentation, 81, 82, 168f
   orbital exenteration, 175, 176f
   skin lesions, 73

F

Facial artery
   maxillotomy, extended unilateral, 229
   therapeutic embolization considerations, 115
Facial bones, free rectus muscle flap, 613–616, 614–615f
Facial canal, 380
Facial degloving, 195–205
   closure, 200
   combined surgery, 201–205, 200–205f
      craniotomy, anterior, 202–205, 203–205f
      ethmoidectomy, external, 201, 201f
      frontoethmoidectomy, external, 202, 202f
   combined transbasal–Derome-transfacial, 355–356, 355–356f
   development of, 195, 195f
   extended transmaxillary approach, 199–200
   incisions and subperiosteal elevation, 197–200, 197–199f
   maxillotomy, extended unilateral, 212–213, 213f, 222, 230

preparation, 197
sellar/parasellar region approaches, 573, 574
structures accessed by, 195–196, 196f
sublabial transoral, 208
tumor resection, 199f, 200
Facial expression, muscles of, 379
Facial hiatus, vestibular schwannoma, 465, 468
Facial muscle, 379
   maxillotomy, extended unilateral, 231t
   paralysis
      ear lesion presentation, 82
      reconstruction, 405, 604–605, 604f
      with temporal bone tumors, 381, 386
Facial nerve. *See* Cranial nerve VII
Facial neuropathy
   postoperative care, 602, 602f
   vestibular schwannoma, 445, 456, 447, 448
Facial recess, 393, 394f
   glomus tumors, 410
   jugulotympanic paraganglioma, 475, 478t, 480f, 481
   temporal bone anatomy, 379
Facial rerouting, jugulotympanic paraganglioma, 481, 482f
Facial vein, anatomy, 67f
Falciform fold, 270f
Fallopian canal
   jugular foramen anatomy, 413
   jugulotympanic paraganglioma, 473
   petroclival anatomy, 427f
   petroclival surgery, 431
   temporal bone resection, 389
   vestibular schwannoma, 456f
Falx cerebelli, 27, 67f
Falx cerebri, 15, 17f, 67f, 273, 274f
Fang, H.S.Y., 12
Fascia graft. *See also specific donor sites*
   dural dehiscence and pneumocephalus, 593
   maxillotomy, extended unilateral, 227f
   reconstruction options, 624t
   tympanic membrane reconstruction, 393
Fascia lata applicator, 241, 244f
Fascia lata grafts
   cranioorbital zygomatic approach, trauma, 283
   CSF leak management, 591, 592f
   infratemporal–middle fossa approach
      preparation, 313
      reconstruction, 335, 335f
   subcranial approaches, extended anterior, 253–254, 253–254f
Fascia lata patch, 295f
Fascia slings, 405
Fat-dermal and fat grafts, 626–627
Fatty tissue, imaging, 87–88, 93f, 94f, 95
Fetal vascular anastomoses, 113t, 534
Fibrin glue, 624t, 630
Fibrogranuloma, 527
Fibroma, mid-skull base approaches, 209t
Fibroosseous lesions, imaging, 90
Fibrosarcoma
   eye region, globe-sparing procedure, 168, 168f
   maxillotomy, extended unilateral, 228t
Fibrous dysplasia
   anterior fossa, 168, 205

clivus, 519, 519f
external auditory meatus/temporal bone, 383t, 385
facial degloving approach, 205
foramen magnum region, transoral approach, 527
imaging, 102, 102t
maxillotomy, extended unilateral, 228t
mid-skull base approaches, 209t
pathology, 37, 37f, 38f
subcranial approaches, 357t
   extended anterior, 259t
   transbasal–Derome, 348
vertebral artery involvement, 546t
Fibrous histiocytoma, mid-skull base approaches, 209t
Fibrous ring, 23f, 24f, 58f, 59, 59f
   infratemporal–middle fossa approach, 315, 319f
      barrier to invasion by tumor, 331
      carotid dissection, 330
   subcranial extended transfacial approach Type III, 305, 305f
   vestibular schwannoma, 456
Fick principle, 108
50:50 rule, 447
Fila olfactoria, 167
Filling defects, 88
Fine-needle aspiration biopsy, 111–113, 112f
Fisch, Ugo, 9–10, 10f
Fischgold's line, 521, 521f
Fisch technique, 11, 309, 315
Fissure of Santorini, 83, 381, 386
Fistula
   CSF. *See* CSF fistula
   orbital, 202, 202f
   reconstruction, radial forearm free flap, 608–611, 609–610f
   sellar/parasellar, 560t, 581
   vertebral artery, 542t, 551, 552, 552t
Flap necrosis, 601, 603
Flaps, free, 607–621
   goals of reconstruction, 608
   history, 607
   latissimus dorsi and serratus anterior, 616–618, 616–618f
   patient factors, 607–608
   radial forearm, 608–611, 609–610f
   rectus abdominis, 611–616, 611–615f
      meningioma, 611–613, 611–613f
      squamous cell carcinoma of orbit and nasal skin, 613–616, 614–615f
   subscapular system, 618–621, 619–620f
Flaps, osteplastic, 3
Flaps and grafts. *See also* Reconstruction/defect repair
   cranioorbital zygomatic approach, 264
   infratemporal–middle fossa approach
      craniotomy, 329, 330f
      elevation, 317f, 318f
      preparation, 313, 313f
   prevention of complications, 588–589, 588f
   recurrence considerations, 74
   temporal bone resection, 401
Flaps and grafts, regional, 623–638
   anterior skull base reconstruction, 635–637, 636f
   graduated sequence of options, 624t

Flaps and grafts, lateral and central skull base reconstruction (contd.)
  infratemporal–middle fossa approach, 335, 335f, 336f, 337, 337f
  lateral and central skull base reconstruction, 626–637, 626–637f
    fat-dermal and fat grafts, 626–627
    fibrin glue, 630
    latissimus dorsi myocutaneous flap, 633–635, 634–635f
    myocutaneous flaps, 630–635, 631–635f
    pectoralis myocutaneous flaps, 631
    temporal fascia, 627–630, 627–628f
    temporalis muscle, 630
    trapezius myocutaneous flap, 631–633, 631–633f
  nerve grafts, 637–638, 637–638f
  surgical exposure and incisions, 624–626, 624–626f
Fluids
  postoperative management, 573, 599, 601, 602
  prevention of complications, 588
  sellar/parasellar lesions, 573
  temporal craniotomy, 397
Fluoroscopy, sellar surgery, 570
Fogarty embolectomy catheter
  cranioorbital zygomatic approach, 269f
    aneurysm repair, 279f
    ICA exposure, 267–268
  jugular fossa tumors, 421
Foramen cecum, 17f, 26f, 186
Foramen lacerum, 22, 23f, 25, 26f, 27
  infratemporal–middle fossa approach, carotid artery dissection, 332f
  maxillotomy, extended unilateral, 217f, 223f, 224, 225f, 231t
  subcranial extended transfacial approach Type III, 305, 306–307f
  temporal bone anatomy, 378
  tumor biology
    extension via, 53, 53f, 61, 83, 517f
    nasopharyngeal tumor erosion, 94–95
Foramen magnum, 24
  anatomy, 24, 27, 28, 29, 491, 495f, 496f, 533
  Chamberlain's line, 521, 521f
  chordoma involvement, 93
  imaging, 87, 98t, 102
  vertebral artery management, 533, 550
Foramen magnum region. *See also* Vertebral artery management
  lateral transcondylar approach, extreme, 491–505
    anatomy, 491–492
    case 1. meningioma, 496–498, 497–498f
    case 2. glomus jugulare tumor, 498–500, 499–500f
    case 3. chordoma, 500–503, 501–503f
    postoperative care, 496
    principles of surgery, 492
    special problems, 503–505, 504f
    surgical approach, 492–496
  petroclival surgery. *See also* Petroclival lesions
    anatomy, 425
    posterior fossa primary intradural approach, 435
    tumors, 423, 429, 441, 441f

maxillotomy, extended unilateral, 223, 223f, 224, 225, 231t
transbasal–Derome submandibular approach, 347–348
transmandibular approach, 341
transoral approach, to clivus and upper cervical spine, 507–531
  anatomy, 507–514, 507–513f
  clinical presentation, 519–522, 519–521f
  complications, 531–532
  pathology, 514–519, 514–519f
transoral approach, operative technique, 521–531
  closure, 529–531, 531f
  ondontectomy, 529, 529f, 530f
  preparation, 522, 522f, 523f
  procedure, 522–528, 524–527f
  tumor excision, 527, 528f
vertebral artery lesions, 542, 542t, 543f
vertebral artery management, 546–548, 546t, 547f, 548t. *See also* Vertebral artery management
  indications for surgical approaches, 548t
  mobilization, 539
Foramen of Luschka, 100
Foramen of Monro obstruction, 568
Foramen of Morgagni, 27, 83
Foramen of Vesalius, 21
Foramen ovale, 20f, 21f, 25, 26f
  anatomy, 556f
  imaging, 88
  infratemporal–middle fossa approach
    craniotomy, 326, 328, 328f, 330
    diagnosis/presentation, 310
    incision, 313, 314f
    otic exposure, 326f
    temporal bone anatomy, 322
    temporalis elevation, 316
  maxillotomy, extended unilateral, 217f, 223f, 224, 225f, 231t
  subcranial extended transfacial approach, 290, 291f, 305
  temporal bone resection, 388f
  tumor pathophysiology, 53, 53f, 56, 56f, 57, 57f
  tumor spread via
    nasal and paranasal sinus tumors, 82
    nasopharyngeal lesions, 83
    oropharyngeal, parotid, and upper neck lesions, 85
Foramen rotundum, 19f, 20f, 21f, 21, 27f, 56f
  anatomy, 556f
  CSF leak, 590
  imaging, 88, 90f
  nasal and paranasal sinus tumor spread, 82
  orbital exenteration, 175, 177
  subcranial extended transfacial approach, 290, 297
    Type II, 299, 300f
    Type III, 305
  tumor pathophysiology, 56
Foramen spinosum, 20f, 21f, 25, 26f
  cranioorbital zygomatic approach, 267, 268f
  imaging, 88
  infratemporal–middle fossa approach

    craniotomy, 326, 328, 328f
    temporal bone anatomy, 322
  maxillotomy, extended unilateral, 231t
  oropharyngeal, parotid, and upper neck lesion spread, 85
  petrous bone anatomy, 425
  subcranial extended transfacial approach, 305
  temporal bone resection, 388f
  vestibular schwannoma, 465
Foramen transversum, 507, 509f
Foramina
  anatomy, 15, 19, 19f, 21, 21f, 28
  imaging, 88, 95
  tumor spread via, 54, 55–56, 55–56f, 57, 59, 67, 69, 95, 474
Forehead extension, 80–81
Foreign bodies, transmandibular approach, 341
Fossa of Rosenmüller, 83
Fourth ventricle tumors, 98, 98t, 100
Fovea ethmoidalis, 15, 52f
  ethmoid sinus tumor spread, 167, 167f
  subcranial extended transfacial approach, 294f
Fractures
  facial, 207
  mid-skull base approaches, 209t
  odontoid, 514–516, 515f, 515t, 522
  ossiculum terminale versus, 507
Frameless stereotaxy, 577
Frazier, C.H., 4f
Free flaps, 607–621. *See also* Flaps, free; Reconstruction/defect repair
Freer elevators, 569
Frontal bone, 15
  cranioorbital approach, 263, 266, 266f, 272–274, 273–275f
  facial degloving with craniotomy, 205f
  frontobasal approach, 357
  orbital process, 16, 19
  osteomyelitis, 595, 596
  reconstruction
    free latissimus dorsi flap, 616–618, 616–618f
    free rectus muscle flap, 613–616, 614–615f
    rectus abdominis free flap, 611–613, 611–613f
    subscapular graft, 619–620, 619–620f
  subcranial approaches, extended anterior, 243f, 244f, 245
Frontal craniotomy, 239, 357
Frontal crest, 15, 16f
Frontal diploic veins of Breschet, 16
Frontalis branch of facial nerve, 24f
Frontalis muscle, 315, 316f
Frontalis paralysis, 604f
Frontal lobe, 16
  craniotomy, 190
  frontal sinus tumor presentation, 81
  nasal and paranasal sinus tumor spread, 82
  orbital surface, 18f
  pericranial flap slough, 594f, 595
  resection of, 335
  sellar/parasellar lesions and, 564
  subcranial approaches
    extended anterior, 239, 253–254, 253–254f, 260
    transbasal–Derome, 357
  tissue removal, 62, 64f

Frontal nerve, 19, 81
Frontal pole retraction, and AEPs, 154
Frontal sinus, 16
  craniocorbital zygomatic approach, 266, 266f, 272, 283, 285f
  craniotomy, 185, 185f, 186, 186f, 187f, 188f, 204f
  facial degloving
    with craniotomy, 204f
    frontoethmoidectomy, 197, 202, 202f, 203f
  osteoma and fibrooseous lesion involvement, 90
  osteomyelitis, 595
  osteoplastic flap, 3
  primary squamous cell carcinoma, 167, 168f
  reconstruction, 190, 190f
  subcranial approaches
    extended anterior, 239, 243f, 244f, 245, 259f
    extradural, 353f
    transbasal–Derome, 347, 349, 357
Frontal sinus cranialization, 203, 204f
Frontal sinus fracture, 283, 285f
Frontal sinusitis, 357
Frontal sinus tumors, 5
  imaging, 88, 89, 89f, 89t, 91f
  symptoms, 80–81, 80–81f, 82
Frontobasal approach
  combined, 355–356, 355–356f
  degloving, esthesioneuroblastoma, 356, 356f
  reconstruction, 357, 357f
Frontoethmoidectomy, 197, 202, 202f, 203f
Frontolateral approaches. See Cranioorbital approach
Frontonasal orbital ostectomy, 296
Frontonasal orbital osteotomy, 239
Frontonasal segment, extended anterior subcranial approaches, 239, 241–242f, 243f, 245, 249f, 253–254, 253–254f
Frontoorbital craniotomy, transbasal–Derome, 357
Frontoorbital technique, 7
Frontotemporal approach, sellar/parasellar region, 567f
Frontotemporal bone, cranioorbital approach, 263, 266, 266f
Frontotemporal semicircular incision, 279
Frontozygomatic suture, 239
Frozen sections, 31–32, 127, 165, 347
  esthesioneuroblastoma, 355–356, 355–356f
  infratemporal–middle fossa approach, 326f
  nursing staff duties, 130
  orbital exenteration, 177
  temporal bone resection, 397
Fungal infections, 98

G
Gadolinium, 87, 88, 94
  anterior fossa imaging, 90
  cerebellopontine angle lesions, 98, 99
  diffuse lesions of skull base, 102t
  inflammation, 98
  metastases, 70
  perineural extension, central skull base, 95
Galea flap
  anterior fossa reconstruction, 191
  postoperative care, 603

Galea-frontalis flaps, 624t
Galea-periosteum flap
  anterior skull base defect repair, 357, 357f
  transbasal–Derome approach, 347, 348, 349f, 351, 351f, 352–353, 352–353f
Galen, great cerebral vein of, 28
Gangliocytoma, 562
Gasserian ganglion, 22
  anatomy, 20, 22
  craniocorbital zygomatic approach, 267, 268f
  diagnosis/presentation of lesions, 310
  eye care after resection of, 402
  imaging, 88
  nasal and paranasal sinus tumor spread, 82
  petrous bone anatomy, 425
  total petrosectomy, 401
  transbasal–Derome approach, 350
  transfacial approach indications, skin squamous cell carcinoma, 167f
  tumor pathophysiology, 56, 56f, 57f
Gastrostomy, 421
Geniculate ganglion, 21
  ear lesion presentation, 82
  foramen magnum region surgery, 504f
  imaging, 99, 99f
  jugular foramen surgery, 415–416
  jugulotympanic paraganglioma, 481
  petrous bone anatomy, 425f
  temporal bone anatomy, 378
  vestibular schwannoma, 465, 468
Geniculate ridge, 378
Germ cell tumors, 71
Germinoma, 560t
Giant adenoma, pituitary, 579
Giant aneurysm, 11
  carotid artery management, 360
  ICA, 362f, 363f
Giant cell granuloma, 89t, 90, 560t, 563, 581
Giant cell tumor, anterior
  facial degloving approach, 205
  subcranial extended anterior approach, 245, 246–248f, 259t
Gigli saw
  maxilla division, 208
  maxillotomy, extended unilateral, 215, 217–220f, 230
Giordano, 3
Glasgow Coma Scale, 600, 601t
Glassock's triangle, 267, 268f, 269f, 269
Glenoid fossa, 22, 25, 27f
  infratemporal–middle fossa approach, 322, 326, 328f
  mandibular condylectomy/resection, 393
  temporal bone resection, 394f, 399f, 400
Glenoid zygomatic complex, 626f, 626f
Glioma, 209t, 562
Globe. See Eye; Orbital exenteration
Glomus jugulare, 473
Glomus/glomus jugulare tumors, 473. See also Jugulotympanic paraganglioma
  cavernous artery supply of, 378
  embolization, therapeutic, 116f
  hemostasis, 587
  imaging, 98t, 100, 100f
  infratemporal–middle fossa approach incision, 313, 314f

  lateral transcondylar approach, 491, 498–500, 499–500f, 503, 505
  transcervicomastoid approach, 409–422. See also Transcervicomastoid approach
Glomus jugulotympanicum, 116f
Glomus tympanicum, 479f
Glomus vagale tumors, 409, 419t, 637
Glossopharyngeal nerve. See Cranial nerve IX
Glossopharyngeal paralysis, 519
Glossoptomy, median labial, 522, 523f, 526, 531, 531f
beta-Glucuronidase, 70
Gradenigo's syndrome, 386
Gradient echo imaging, 87
Grafts. See also Flaps and grafts; Reconstruction/defect repair
  nerve, 405
  osteomyelitis management, 597
  recurrence considerations, 74
  vascular. See Saphenous vein graft; Vascular grafts
Granular cell tumor, neurohypophysis, 579, 560t, 562
Granulocytes, 61
Granuloma
  imaging, 89t, 90
  sellar/parasellar, 560t, 563
Great auricular nerve, 637
Great cerebral vein anatomy, 67f
Great cerebral vein of Galen, 28
Greater auricular nerve grafts, 405
Greater palatine artery, 229, 593
Greater petrosal nerve
  petrous bone anatomy, 425
  vestibular schwannoma, 468, 468f
Great occipital nerve, 29
Greenberg retractor, 454
Growth factors, 61
Growth hormone-secreting adenoma, 564, 577–578
Grunting respiration, 586f, 586, 592–593
Gugliemi coils, 587
Gutin, P., 12
Gyrus rectus, 16, 18f, 167, 167f

H
Halo brace, 522, 531
Hamartoma, neurohypophysis, 562
Headache
  clinical syndromes with metastasis, 70
  diagnosis/presentation, 311
  nasal and paranasal sinus tumor presentation, 81
  petroclival tumors, 427
  sellar/parasellar lesions, 564, 578
  vestibular schwannoma, 445
  postoperative monitoring, 132
  vestibular schwannoma complications, 449
Head and neck surgeons, 347. See also Multidisciplinary team
  subcranial approaches, transbasal–Derome, 357
  transcervicomastoid approach, 409–422. See also Transcervicomastoid approach
Head position/movement
  clinical syndromes with metastasis, 70

Subject Index

Head position/movement (contd.)
  foramen magnum region surgery, 492
  sellar/parasellar surgery, 568
  vertebral artery effects, 535, 535f, 536, 544–545
Hearing
  AEP patterns, 152, 155f
  petroclival surgery monitoring, 429
Hearing loss
  complications
    AEP monitoring, 152
    jugular fossa surgery, 420t
    petroclival surgery, 429, 431, 437
  symptoms
    ear lesion presentation, 82, 83
    glomus tumor symptoms, 410, 410t
    jugulotympanic paraganglioma, 474, 474t
    petroclival tumors, 426, 427
    temporal bone tumors, 381, 386
    vestibular schwannoma, 443, 444, 445, 447
  rehabilitation, 406, 605–606, 605f
Hemangioblastoma, vertebral artery involvement, 546t
Hemangioma, 209t
Hemangiopericytoma, 102, 205
Hematoma, 595
  postoperative monitoring, 601
  vertebral artery, 551, 551t
Hematopoietic metastasis, 560t, 562
Hemilaminectomy, 494
Hemimandibular muscle, 305
Hemimandibulectomy, 304, 304f
Hemodynamics
  jugulotympanic paraganglioma resection, 477
  neurophysiological effects, 143
  postoperative management, 599
  prevention of complications, 588
  vertebral artery changes, 534–537
Hemorrhage
  glomus jugulare/jugular foramen tumors, 412
  ICA and jugular bulb injury, 399–400
  jugular foramen surgery, 413
  management of, 593, 593f, 595
  petrous bone surgery, 426
  postoperative care, 600, 603
  prevention of, 587, 588, 588f
  rebound hypertension and, 599
Hemostasis. See also specific procedures
  infratemporal–middle fossa approach
    cavernous sinus resection, 333
    craniotomy, 326, 328
    temporalis elevation, 316
  maxillotomy, extended unilateral, 230
  prevention of complications, 587, 588
Heparin, 107, 373
Herniation, brain, 347
Hirsch, O., 12
Histiocyosis. See also Langerhans' cell histiocytosis
  sellar/parasellar, 560t, 563
  vertebral artery involvement, 542f, 544, 544f, 546t
Histology, 31. See also$ specific tumor types
  anterior skull base lesions, 89t, 90
  and presentation, 73–74
  temporal bone tumors, 383–386
Histology slides, 585
History, cranial base surgery

anterior fossa and pituitary surgery, 3–7, 4–7f
central skull base surgery, 1–12
maxillotomy, extended unilateral, 207–209
middle fossa surgery, 9–11, 10–11f
posterior fossa and acoustic tumors, 7–9, 8–9f
History, patient, 123–124, 131, 585
  infratemporal–middle fossa lesions, 310
  with temporal bone tumor, 381
Hitselberger, W., 9, 9f
Hitselberger's sign, 445
HMPAO, 313, 278
Home care planning, 134–135
Homer's syndrome, 552
Homonomous hemianopsia, 82
Horizontal maxillotomy. See Maxillotomy, extended unilateral
Hormones, hypothalamic and pituitary, 558, 558f, 561t, 563–564, 566
Horner's syndrome, 311, 476
Horsely, Sir Victor, 3, 4f, 7
Hospice care, 122
House, H., 8
House, W.F., 8
House-Urban retractor, 465
Huschke's foramen, 386
Hydrocephalus
  clival compression and, 521
  sellar/parasellar lesions, 564, 568, 579, 580
  vestibular schwannoma, 443
Hyperbaric oxygen, 346
Hyperostosis, imaging, 92
Hypertension
  induced, 371
    collateral flow in carotid artery occlusion, 359
    ICA management, saphenous vein bypass graft, 361
    preoperative management with jugular foramen tumors, 412
  rebound, 599
Hypesthesia, 69
Hypocycloidal tomography, 381
Hypoglossal artery anastomoses, 534
Hypoglossal canal, 25, 28
  clinical presentation with tumor involvement of, 519
  facial degloving, 208
  foramen magnum region surgery, 494, 502f, 504f, 505
  jugular foramen anatomy, 413
  jugulotympanic paraganglioma, 476
  transoral approach, 208, 527
Hypoglossal foramen, maxillotomy, extended unilateral, 209
Hypoglossal nerve. See Cranial nerve XII
Hypoglossal venous plexus, 28
Hypophyseal blood supply, 281, 281f, 559f
Hypophysectomy, 578. See also Pituitary tumors; Sella/parasellar region
Hypotension
  BTO considerations, 108
  and cerebral hypoperfusion, 405
  neurosecretory tumors and, 411
  postoperative monitoring, 600
Hypothalamus, 555, 558, 558–559f, 563–564
Hypothermia
  and cerebral blood flow, 105
  induced, 360, 361

Hypotympanic triangle, 475
Hypotympanum, 394f, 479, 480f
Hypoxia
  balloon test occlusion considerations, 108
  EEG effects, 145–148

I

ICA. See Internal carotid artery
Imaging, 89t
  advances in, 3
  anatomic considerations, 87
  anterior skull base lesions, 89–91, 89–92f
  carotid artery, 105–111, 106–110f
    angiography. See Angiography
    spin-echo sequences, 88
  central skull base lesions, 92–97, 92–97f
  cerebellopontine angle tumors, 443
  clinical syndromes with metastasis, 70
  diffuse lesions, 102, 102t
  before extended transfacial subcranial approach, 287–288
  infratemporal–middle fossa approach, 310, 311, 312f
  jugular fossa tumors, 100–102, 100–101f
    jugular foramen tumors, 410–411
    jugulotympanic paraganglioma, 476–477, 476–477f, 478, 479
  metastases, 70, 70f, 71f
  nursing care, 121–122
  occipitoatlantoaxial surgery, 492
  osteolyelitis, 98
  paranasal sinus tumors, 167, 169
  petroclival, 424f, 427–428, 427–428f, 429
  posterior skull base lesions, 98–100, 99–100f
  postoperative, 600, 604
  preoperative preparation, 585
  recurrence, failure to detect, 74
  sellar/parasellar lesions, 565–566
    pituitary adenoma, 578
    vascular, 581
  sphenoid sinus tumor presentation, 81
  subcranial approaches
    extended anterior, 245, 246–248f
    extended transfacial Type III, 304
  techniques and general diagnostic criteria, 87–88
  temporal bone tumors, 377, 380–381, 381f, 387
  transcervicomastoid approach, 410–411, 410t, 411f
  tumor spread, 69f
  vestibular schwannoma, 443, 446, 461
Immunohistochemistry, 31, 32t, 70
Incisions
  coronal and bicoronal, 182f
  facial degloving, 197–200, 197–199f
  foramen magnum region surgery, 492
  infratemporal–middle fossa approach, 313–315, 313–317f
  inverted tuning fork, 3, 4f
  in maxillotomy, extended unilateral, 212, 212f, 213f
  petroclival surgery, 430, 430f
  regional flaps and grafts, 624–626, 624–626
  temporal bone resection, 390f
  Weber-Fergusson. See Weber-Fergusson incision
  zygomatic cranioorbital approach, 264–265, 264–265f

Incisura, 92, 423, 425
Incudostapedial joint
 infratemporal fossa approach, 481
 jugular foramen surgery, 416
 vestibular schwannoma, 452f, 455, 469f
Incus, 416, 452f, 455, 469f
Indium scans, 476–477
Infarction, inferior anastomotic vein of Labbé, 22
Infection
 anterior approach, incidence after, 586t
 infratemporal–middle fossa approach reconstruction considerations, 335
 jugulotympanic paraganglioma, 486t
 management of, 586t, 590–592, 590f, 591f
 mandibulotomy complications, 346
 maxillotomy complications, 228, 228t, 229, 232
 and osteomyelitis, 595–596
 otitis, external, 98, 381, 406
 postoperative monitoring, 132, 133, 601
 prevention of, 587
 reconstruction goals, 608
 sellar/parasellar, 560t, 563, 581
 sphenoid sinus tumor presentation, 81
 subcranial approaches. 347, 348, 357
 with temporal bone tumors, 381
 transmandibular approach complications, 345
 transoral approach complications, 532
 vertebral artery involvement, 542t, 546t
Inferior alveolar nerve, 85, 231t, 310
Inferior anastomotic vein of Labbé, 22, 334f, 335
Inferior-anterior approaches, subcranial extended, 239–260. *See also* Subcranial extended anterior approach
Inferior cerebellar artery, 28, 113t, 115, 436
 anterior, 28, 113t, 436
 posterior, 534
  anatomy, 29
  vertebral artery aneurysm, 551, 552
  vertebral artery management, 538
Inferior cerebral vein, 22
Inferior colliculus, 152
Inferior maxillectomy, 177
Inferior oblique muscle, 156, 492
Inferior ophthalmic vein
 anatomy, 19, 67f
 tumor extension via, 59, 59f, 60f, 61
Inferior orbital fissure, 19
 anatomy, 19, 20f, 27
 tumor pathophysiology, 55–56, 55–56f
Inferior orbital nerve, 208
Inferior petroclival space, 425
Inferior petrosal sinus
 anatomy, 22, 27, 28, 67f
  jugular foramen, 413, 418f
  sella and parasellar, 555
  temporal bone anatomy, 378, 379f
 jugulotympanic paraganglioma, 477f, 481
  infratemporal fossa approach, 484
  spread of, 475
 petroclival surgery, middle fossa extradural approach, 436
 subcranial extended transfacial approach Type III, 305, 306f
 temporal bone resection, 388f
 tumor pathophysiology, 57

Inferior petrosal sinus vein, 231t
Inferior rectus muscle, 156
Inferior saggital sinus, 15, 28, 67f
Inferior turbinates
 facial degloving approach, 198, 199f, 201, 201f
 maxillotomy, extended unilateral, 212–213
Inferior tympanic branch of ascending pharyngeal artery, 479, 479f
Inferior vestibular nerve, 425, 465
Inflammation
 craniocervical junction, 516, 516f
 imaging, 89t, 90
  foramen magnum lesions, 98t, 102
  otitis, external, 98, 381, 406
 maxillotomy complications, 228, 228t
 sellar/parasellar, 560t, 563, 581
 temporal bone tumor etiology, 381
 Tolosa-Hunt syndrome, 310
 and tumor spread, 61
Inflammatory pseudotumor, 36–37, 37f
Informed consent, 119, 120
Infraorbital artery, 114
Infraorbital canal, 56, 208
Infraorbital foramen, 198, 222, 231t
Infraorbital groove, 17
Infraorbital nerve
 facial degloving, 196f
  sublabial transoral, 208
  transmaxillary approach, 199
 infratemporal–middle fossa approach, 311, 311f
 maxillary sinus tumor presentation, 79
 maxillotomy, extended unilateral, 213, 213f, 222
 neurotropic spread, 167f
 neurotropic tumors, 165
 orbital exenteration, 177
 perineural spread of skin tumors, 75f, 76f
 subcranial extended transfacial approach Type II, 298
Infratemporal crest, maxillotomy, extended unilateral, 224
Infratemporal fossa, 9–10
 anatomy, 24, 25, 27
 complications of resecting, 603, 603f, 604f
 facial degloving approach, 195, 197f
  with craniotomy, 202, 203f
  sublabial transoral, 208
 glomus tumors, 410
 ICA to MCA bypass, 371, 371f, 372f
 maxillary sinus tumor presentation, 79f
 maxillotomy, extended unilateral, 210, 221f, 222, 223f, 225f, 230, 231t
 orbital exenteration, 175
 subcranial approaches
  combined transbasal–Derome-transfacial, 355–356, 355–356f
  extended anterior, 245
  extended transfacial, 289f, 290, 290f
  extended transfacial Type III, 304, 306–307f
  transbasal–Derome, 350
 temporal bone anatomy, 378
 temporal bone tumors, 381, 387
 transmandibular approach, 341–346, 342–345f

tumor pathology
 adenoid cystic carcinoma, 34t
 squamous cell carcinoma primary sites, 32t
 tumor spread via, 54, 85
Infratemporal fossa approach
 foramen magnum region, 504f, 505
 jugulotympanic paraganglioma, 478t, 481–486, 483–486f
 petroclival region, 423
 postoperative care, 602
 preauricular, foramen magnum region surgery, 505
 recurrent adenoid cystic carcinoma, 368
Infratemporal fossa dissection, 27f
Infratemporal fossa–middle fossa approach, 309–339
 carotid dissection, 330–333, 331–333f
 cavernous sinus, 333–334, 333f
 clinical presentation, 309–313, 310–313f, 313t
 complications, 596–597, 596f
 contraindications, 311
 craniotomy, 326, 328–330. 328–330f
 dura and brain resection, 334–335, 334–335f
 external auditory canal obliteration, 315, 318f
 incision, 313–315, 313–317f
 mandibular condylectomy, 320, 322, 325–326f
 otologic exposure, 322, 326, 327f
 preparation, 313, 313f
 reconstruction, 335–339, 336–338f
 subtemporal trapezoid exposure, 322, 326–329f
 temporalis elevation, 315–316, 316f, 319f
 zygomatic ostectomy, 319–320, 320–325f
Infratemporal space, facial degloving approach, 200, 200f
Infundibulum, 269f, 273f, 559f
Inner ear, 22, 28. *See also* Internal auditory canal
 anatomy, 380
 temporal bone tumor spread, 381
Innominate foramen, 21
Instrumentation, 527
 maxillotomy, extended unilateral, 210–211t, 222, 224
 neurological monitoring
  electrode properties, 139–140f
  monitoring system, 140–142, 141–142f
  neuroanesthetic conditions, 143, 144f, 145, 145f
  signal acquisition and processing, 142–143, 143–144f
 nursing staff, 124, 125
 nursing staff duties, 128
 subcranial approaches, extended anterior, 239, 244f, 249
 titanium plates. *See* Titanium fixtures
 transoral approach to clivus and cervical spine, 511f, 512f, 513, 525f, 526, 526f
 transsphenoidal approach to sellar region, 569, 570
 vestibular schwannoma, 458, 459f
Insurance, 119, 123
Intensive care unit management, 132–135, 135f, 599–602, 600t, 600f, 601t, 602f

Intercavernous plexuses, 22
Interhemispheric-transcallosal approach, sellar/parasellar tumors, 580
Internal acoustic meatus
  cranioorbital zygomatic approach, 263
  temporal bone anatomy, 379f
Internal auditory canal
  anatomy
    petrous bone, 425, 425f, 426, 426f
    temporal bone, 378, 378f, 379, 379f
  bypass grafts
    neurophysiological monitoring, 146–157
    saphenous vein. *See* Saphenous vein graft
  cranioorbital zygomatic approach, 270
  ear lesion involvement, 83
  glomus tumor, 500
  infratemporal–middle fossa approach, 317f
  jugulotympanic paraganglioma, 481. *See also* Jugulotympanic paraganglioma
  petroclival region
    anatomy, 427f
    middle fossa extradural approach, 436
    tumors, 423, 424f
  vestibular schwannoma. *See* Vestibular schwannoma
Internal carotid artery (ICA)
  anastomoses, 114f
    therapeutic embolization considerations, 113, 113t
    vertebral artery, 534
  anatomy, 15, 17f, 21, 22–24, 23f, 24f, 26f, 29
    cavernous sinus, 21, 22
    foramen magnum region, 495f
    middle ear, 380
    osteology, 20
    petrous bone, 426f
    tumor spread via, 58f, 59, 59f
  aneurysm, 341
  balloon test occlusion, 110f
  carotid artery salvage/sacrifice, 360
  cavernous, 64
    adenoid cystic carcinoma, recurrent, 367–368, 367–370f
    anastomoses, 113t
    anatomy, 22, 24f, 25f
    aneurysm, 362f, 363f
    cavernous sinus syndrome, 363, 364f
    infratemporal–middle fossa approach, 309
  cervical
    bypass grafts, 363f
    factors affecting salvage/sacrifice, 360
    graft anastomosis, 362f
  clinoid segment, 350
  cranioorbital zygomatic approach, 269f, 270, 279
  embolization, therapeutic, 113–116, 113t, 114–116f
  hemorrhage, 595
  infratemporal–middle fossa approach, 309, 317f, 319f
    craniotomy, 326, 329
    dissection, 330–333, 331–333f
    jugulotympanic paraganglioma, 481, 481–486, 483–486f, 485f
    preoperative assessment, 311, 313
    preparation, 313

jugular foramen/glomus tumors, 409, 410, 411, 411f, 495f, 499f
jugular fossa surgery, 421
  complications, 419
  transcervicomastoid approach, 420
jugulotympanic paraganglioma, 476, 483f
  collateral circulation assessment, 477–478
  infratemporal fossa approach, 481, 481–486, 483–486f
  management, 361–374, 361–374f
    adenoid cystic carcinoma recurrence, 367–370, 367–370f
    cavernous sinus syndrome secondary recurrent chondrosarcoma, 363–367, 363–367f
    meningioma of jugular foramen and upper cervical area, 371–373, 371–373f
  preoperative workup, 110f. *See also* Carotid artery, assessment techniques
    grafting results, 373
    operative technique, 373
    physiology of cerebral circulation, 359–360
    preoperative assessment, 360
mandibular condylectomy/resection, 393
maxillotomy, extended unilateral, 223f, 231t
medial subcranial structures, 27
middle skull base bony structures, 19
neurophysiological monitoring, EEG, 146–147, 153
ophthalmic artery, 19
orbital exenteration, 177
petrous segment
  anastomoses, 113t
  bypass grafts, 363f
  factors affecting salvage/sacrifice, 360
  foramen magnum region surgery, 500, 504f
  transmandibular approach, 343
preoperative evaluation, 106f
prevention of complications, 587
and radiation therapy, 406
sellar/parasellar lesions, 559f, 563
sigmoid curve, 19
subcranial approaches, transbasal–Derome, 348, 352, 357
subcranial approaches, transfacial extended, 291
  eustachian tube resection, 301
  Type III, 304, 305, 305f, 306f
temporal bone anatomy, 377, 378, 378f, 379f
temporal bone resection, 399–400
  assessment, 386
  complications, 387, 404
  total petrosectomy, 401, 402f
temporal bone tumors, 382
therapeutic embolization considerations, 115
transfacial subcranial approaches, extended, 288, 288f
transmandibular approach, 341, 342f
tumor involvement, and prognosis, 72
tumor pathophysiology, 53, 53f, 64, 83, 84f
vertebral artery anastomoses, 534
vestibular schwannoma, 455, 457f
Internal jugular lymph nodes, 311
Internal jugular vein
  foramen magnum region surgery, 492, 494–495, 504f
  anatomy, 28, 496f
  chordoma, 502f

infratemporal–middle fossa approach, 319f, 337
jugular foramen surgery, 414f, 416, 416f
  mobilization and ligation, 414–415
  vertebral artery management, 549, 549f
mandibular condylectomy/resection, 393
subcranial extended transfacial approach Type III, 304
temporal bone anatomy, 378, 378f
total petrosectomy, 401, 402f
transmandibular approach, 343–344
vertebral artery approaches, posterolateral, 537f
Internal labyrinthine artery, 378
Internal labyrinthine vein, 378
Internal maxillary artery, 25
  anastomoses, 113t, 114f
  hemorrhage, 593
  infratemporal–middle fossa approach, 316
  mandibular condylectomy, 392f
  maxillotomy, extended unilateral, 215, 216f, 224, 225f, 231t
  temporal bone anatomy, 378
  therapeutic embolization considerations, 115
  transfacial approaches, 173
Internal occipital protuberance, 27
Internal vertebral plexuses, 67f
Intervertebral vein anatomy, 68f
Interview, patient, 85–86, 86t
Intracranial anatomy
  anterior skull base, 15–16, 17–18f
  middle skull base, 21–24, 22–26f
Intracranial extension
  anterior fossa floor invasion, combined resection with, 168
  anterior subcranial approaches for extended, 254–255, 255f
  transfacial, 287, 290
  cranioorbital zygomatic approach, 266, 266f
  facial degloving approach, 200, 200f
  glomus tumors, 409
  jugular fossa tumors, 421
  jugulotympanic paraganglioma, 474
  nasal and paranasal sinus tumor, 81–82
  temporal bone involvement, 386
  treatment philosophy, 34
Intracranial hemorrhage. *See* Hemorrhage; Stroke
Intracranial pressure
  hemorrhage and, 593
  nasal/paranasal sinus tumor presentation, 81
  pneumocephalus prevention, 592–593
  postoperative management, 599
  postoperative monitoring, 132, 600
  prevention of CSF leaks, 586
  sella surgery, 571
Intradural approach
  petroclival region, 435–436, 435f, 436
  sella/parasellar region, 574–577, 575–576f
  transbasal approach, Derome modification, 348, 352–355, 352–355f
Intradural structures
  petroclival anatomy, 424f, 425
  zygomatic cranioorbital approach, 268–269, 269f
Intranasal flap, 212–213, 214–215f, 222

Intraoperative management
  nurse role, 124–126
  prevention of complications, 586–589
Intraoperative monitoring. *See also* Neurologic
    monitoring, intraoperative
  ICA dissection, 373
  infratemporal–middle fossa approach, 313
Intraoral approaches. *See* Foramen magnum
    region; Oral cavity
Intraorbital approach, palatine defect
    reconstruction, 254–255, 255f
Intubation
  facial degloving approach, 197
  foramen magnum region surgery, 500
  infratemporal–middle fossa approach, 337
  jugular foramen surgery, 412–413
  maxillotomy, extended unilateral, 212
  maxillotomy complications, 234
  pneumocephalus prevention, 593
  postoperative care, 602
  with transoral approach, 522
  ventilation tube, 602
Invasiveness. *See* Tumor biology; *specific tumor
    types*
Inverted tuning fork incision, 3, 4f
Inverting papilloma, 517, 517f
  facial degloving, 202–205, 203–205f
  imaging, 89t
  subcranial, extended, 259t
  transfacial, 165, 166f
    combined, 167
    subcranial extended, 292, 296f
Iodinated contrast material, 87
Irrigation, prevention of complications, 587
Ischemia
  BTO complications, 111
  EEG, 145–148

J

Jacobson's nerve, 473
Jacobson's plexus, 379
Jugular bulb, 28
  foramen magnum region surgery, 492, 494,
      500, 503
  jugulotympanic paraganglioma, 475–476, 480
    classification, 478
    infratemporal fossa approach, 481
    spread of, 475
  petrous bone anatomy, 426
  subcranial extended transfacial approach
      Type III, 306f
  temporal bone anatomy, 378f, 378, 379f
  temporal bone resection, 397, 399–400
  tumor involvement, 69f
  tumor pathophysiology, 53, 53f, 57
  vestibular schwannoma, 450, 453f, 454f, 457f
Jugular canal, 494, 505
Jugulare tumors. *See also* Glomus/glomus
    jugulare tumors; Jugulotympanic
    paraganglioma
  complications, 486t, 487
  results, 486
Jugular foramen, 22, 25, 26f, 27, 28, 84f
  clinical syndromes with metastasis, 70
  extradural subcranial approach from fronal
      sinus, 353f
  foramen magnum region surgery, 494
    anatomy, 492, 496f
  chordoma, 502f
  cranial nerves, 492
  glomus tumor, 498, 500
  ICA management, 371–373, 371–373f
  infratemporal–middle fossa approach, 315
  jugular foramen surgery, 416
  jugulotympanic paraganglioma, 476, 477f
  needle biopsy approaches, 112f, 113
  petroclival tumors, 423, 424f, 435f
  subcranial extended transfacial approach
      Type III, 305
  temporal bone anatomy, 379
  transcervicomastoid approach, 409–422. *See
      also* Transcervicomastoid approach
  tumor spread via, 57, 59, 66, 67t, 85
  vertebral artery management, 539, 548–550,
      548t, 548–550, 549f. *See also* Vertebral
      artery management
  vestibular schwannoma, 450, 456f
Jugular foramen syndrome, 69–70, 85, 409, 476,
    519
Jugular formation, vestibular schwannoma, 461
Jugular fossa
  imaging, 98t, 100–102, 100–101f
  jugular foramen anatomy, 413
  temporal bone tumors, 381, 382, 382t
  vertebral artery control, 539, 546t
Jugular fossa tumors. *See also* Glomus/glomus
    jugulare tumors; Jugulotympanic
    paraganglioma
  imaging, 100–102, 100–101f
  therapeutic embolization, 116f
Jugular lymph nodes, 311
Jugular process of occipital bone, 413, 415
Jugular spine of petrous bone, 413
Jugular tubercle, 539
Jugular vein. *See also* Internal jugular vein
  anatomy, 28
  ear tumor presentation, 83
  jugular foramen anatomy, 413
  jugulotympanic paraganglioma, 480, 483f
    infratemporal fossa approach, 481, 484,
        485f
    spread, 475
  subcranial extended transfacial approach
      Type III, 306f
  tumor spread via, 57, 59
Jugulotympanic paraganglioma, 473–487
  biology, 473–474, 474f, 474t
  classification and selection of approach, 478,
      478f
  clinical characteristics, 474–476, 475f, 475t
  complications, 486t, 487
  differential diagnosis, 478
  imaging, 476–477, 476–477f
  perioperative management, 477–478
  petroclival, 477f
  radiation therapy, 478–486, 479–486f, 487
    infratemporal fossa approach, 481–486,
        483–486f
    mastoid extended facial recess, 479, 480f
    mastoid-neck approach, 480–481, 481f
    mastoid-neck approach with limited facial
        rerouting, 481, 482f
    transcanal, 478–479
Jugum sphenoidale, 15, 556f
Juvenile nasopharyngeal angiofibroma. *See*
    Nasopharyngeal angiofibromas, juvenile
    move
Juxtacondylar approach to jugular foramen, 549,
    550

K

Kawase's approach, 436
Kawase's triangle, 263, 270, 425, 437
Kerrison rongeur, 541, 570
Ketoconazole, 578
Key hole craniotomy, 6f, 7
Kidney function, postoperative monitoring, 599
Kidney tumors, 67, 67t, 310
  craniocervical/clival metastases, 519
  temporal bone metastases, 386
Killed end response, 156, 158f
Killiani, O.G.T., 3
Klopp, C.T., 5
Kocher's incision, 207
Krause, 3, 7
Kurze, T., 9

L

Labbé, vein of, 22, 334f, 335, 397, 429, 431,
    437
Labial mandibuloglossoptomy, median, 522,
    523f, 526, 531, 531f
Labiomandibulotomy, transmandibular
    approach, 341, 342–343, 343–344f
Labyrinth
  ear lesion involvement, 83
  foramen magnum region surgery, 505
  petroclival anatomy, 426, 427f, 430f
  petroclival surgery, 431, 436, 437
  vestibular schwannoma, 447, 468
Labyrinth block, 430f, 436
Labyrinthectomy
  foramen magnum region chordoma, 500
  vestibular schwannoma, 450, 453f
Labyrinthine arteries, 28, 378
Labyrinthine nerve, 378
Lacrimal artery anastomoses, 113t
Lacrimal bone, 16
Lacrimal duct, 203, 204f, 228t
Lacrimal fossa, 574
Lacrimal nerves, 19
Lacrimal sac, 197f, 198, 199
Lamina cribrosa, 349, 357
Lamina papyracea
  facial degloving with external
      frontoethmoidectomy, 202, 202f
  imaging, 88–89
  orbital exenteration, 175
  sellar/parasellar region approaches, 574
  tumor spread via, 55, 55f
Lamina terminales, 269
Langerhans' cell histiocytosis, 383t, 385–386
  imaging, 89t, 90
  sellar/parasellar, 560t, 563, 581
Laryngeal cancer, temporal bone metastases,
    386
Laryngeal paraganglioma, 473
Laryngoplasty, 603
Laser cavitation, 224
Lateral approaches
  to foramen magnum, 28

Lateral approaches (contd.)
  maxillotomy versus, 209
  postoperative care, 602, 603
  suboccipital approach, 491
  subzygomatic approach, needle biopsy, 112f, 113
  transcondylar approach to craniocervical junction. See Foramen magnum region
Lateral compartment, 342f
  maxillotomy, extended unilateral, 210, 221f, 224, 225f
  transmandibular approach, 341–346, 342–345f
Lateral meniscus, 152
Lateral pterygoid muscle, 25, 112f, 113
Lateral pterygoid plate, 25, 26f, 27f, 215, 216f
Lateral rectus muscle, 82, 155–156
Lateral rectus palsy, 83, 311, 312f
Lateral resection, temporal bone, 387–393, 388–395f
Lateral rhinotomy, 63f
  extended transfacial subcranial approach, 287, 288f
  transfacial subcranial approaches, 288t
Lateral rhinotomy-Denker-medial maxillectomy, 168–173, 168–174f
Lateral rhinotomy incision, 168–169, 169f, 287, 293f
Lateral sinus
  temporal bone tumors, 381, 397
  vestibular schwannoma, 454
Lateral skull base
  incision, superficial temporal fascia, 624, 624f
  infratemporal fossa approach, 309
  maxillotomy, extended unilateral, 223f
  reconstruction, 626–637, 626–637f
    fat-dermal and fat grafts, 626–627
    fibrin glue, 630
    latissimus dorsi myocutaneous flap, 633–635, 634–635f
    myocutaneous flaps, 630–635, 631–635f
    pectoralis myocutaneous flaps, 631
    temporal fascia, 627–630, 627–628f
    trapezius myocutaneous flap, 631–633, 631–633f
Lateral venous sinus, temporal bone tumor involvement, 97, 397f
Latissimus dorsi flaps
  free, 616–618, 616–618f, 621
  myocutaneous, 633–635, 634–635f
  reconstruction options, 624t
  subcranial extended transfacial approach Type III, 308, 308f
  traumatic disruption, 591
Latissimus dorsi-scapular free flap, 621
Lavage, 165
Lazy-S incision, 458, 458f
  infratemporal–middle fossa approach, 313, 314f
  vestibular schwannoma, 465, 466f
LeFort classification of fractures, 207
LeFort I, 195, 199, 208, 229, 232, 245
Leiomyosarcoma, 52t
Leminiscus, AEPs, 152
Leptomeninges, imaging, 70

Lesser occipital nerve, 507
Leukocytes, 61
Levator palati muscle, 27
Levator palpebrae superioris muscle and nerve, 19
Levator scapulae, 492
Levator veli palatini, 25, 232t
Ligaments
  atlantoaxial, 508, 509f, 510f
  barriers to tumor extension, 527
Ligamentum flavum, 510f
Ligature, ICA, 481
Lingual artery, therapeutic embolization considerations, 115
Lingual nerve, maxillotomy, 231t
Lingual paralysis, 519
Lip
  degloving, 208
  labial mandibuloglossoptomy, 522, 523f, 526, 531, 531f
  oropharyngeal, parotid, and upper neck lesion involvement, 85
  subcranial extended transfacial approach Type III, 303f, 304
  sublabial incision, 196f
  transmandibular approach, labiomandibulotomy, 342–343, 343–344f
  Weber-Fergusson incision, 179, 179f, 180f
Lipoma, sellar/parasellar, 560t
Lip splitting incision, 342, 343, 343f
Longissimus capitis, 29
Longitudinal sinuses, 68f
Longus colli muscle, 507
L-shaped craniotomy, 326, 328–329, 328–329f
Lumbar drain. See CSF drain
Lumbar vein, anatomy, 68f
Lung cancer, 47, 66, 66t, 67t, 71, 386
Luschka, foramen of, 100
Lymphatic metastasis
  esthesioneuroblastoma, 166f
  infratemporal–middle fossa approach, 309, 311
  neck dissection, 402–403
  and radiation therapy, 406
  temporal bone tumors, 381
Lymph nodes
  external auditory canal and middle ear, 380
  oropharyngeal, parotid, and upper neck lesion presentation, 85
  temporal bone tumor, 380, 382, 382t
Lymphocytic hypophysitis, 581
Lymphoma
  imaging
    anterior skull base lesions, 89t
    perineural extension, central skull base, 95
  pathology, 44–45, 47t
  pathophysiology, 52t, 54, 54f
    chemo- and radiosensitivity, 71
    metastasis, 66, 66t, 67t
  sellar/parasellar region, 560t, 562
  subcranial approaches, extended anterior, 259t
  temporal bone involvement, 386
  vertebral artery involvement, 542t, 544
Lytic destruction of bone. See Bone destruction

M

MacCarty's keyhole, 272
Macrophages, 61

Magnetic resonance imaging. See also Imaging
  biopsy, 111
  carotid artery assessment, clival meningioma, 106f, 107
  infratemporal–middle fossa approach, 311
  lymphoma spread, 54f
  metastatic disease, 70, 71f
  nasopharyngeal adenoid cystic carcinoma, 84f
  nasopharyngeal carcinoma, 69f
  necrosis, 64f
  necrosis on, 62, 63f
  preoperative evaluation, 105, 107
  presentation of recurrent tumor, 76f
  skin tumor spread, 75f, 76f
  sphenoid sinus tumor presentation, 81
  subcranial approaches, extended anterior, 246–248f
  techniques and general diagnostic criteria, 87–88
  therapeutic embolization of glomus tumor, 116f
Malar bones, 221
Malar eminence, 180
Malar process, 264, 265f
Malignant external otitis, 98
Malignant fibromatosis, 205
Malignant fibrosarcoma, 52t
Malignant fibrous histiocytoma, 89t
Malignant schwannoma, 52t, 305, 306–307f
Malis cautery unit, 414
Malleus, 416, 452f, 469f
Managed care, 73
Mandible
  anatomy, 24
  alternatives to excision, 625–626, 626f
  facial degloving, 195, 208
  jugular fossa tumors, 420
  labial mandibuloglossoptomy, 522, 523f, 526, 531, 531f
  labiomandibulotomy, 342–343, 343–344f, 346
  maxillotomy, extended unilateral, 213, 213f, 216f, 219f, 221f
  needle biopsy approaches, 112f, 113
  subcranial extended transfacial approach, 290, 291f, 290–291, 291f, 291f
  Type II, 301
  Type III, 304, 304f
  temporal bone anatomy, 378f
  transfacial subcranial approaches, 288t
  transmandibular approach, 343–344, 343–344f
Mandibular artery, 115
Mandibular branch of cranial nerve V. See Cranial nerve V3
Mandibular branch of cranial nerve VII, 155
Mandibular condyle/condylectomy
  anatomy, 24
  infratemporal–middle fossa approach, 320, 322, 325–326f
  temporal bone resection, 394f, 395f, 397
  incisions for, 390f, 391–392f
  tumor involvement, 387, 389
Mandibular foramen, 219f, 221f
Mandibular nerve. See Cranial nerve V3
Mandibular swing, 341, 343. See also Transmandibular approach

Mandibulectomy, 287, 291
Mandibuloglossoptomy, median labial, 522, 523f, 526, 531, 531f
Mandibulotomyomandibular labiomandibulotomy, 342–343, 343–344f, 346
Mandibulovidian artery, 113t
Mannitol, 397
Mapping studies, 122
Margins, 165
Marrow, imaging, 87–88
Marsupialization, sellar cysts, 581
Masseter muscle
 cranioorbital zygomatic approach, 264
 EMG, 156
 maxillotomy, extended unilateral, 213, 213f, 216f, 223f, 226f
Masticator muscle myositis, 205
Mastoid, 20
 glomus tumors, 410
 imaging, 96f
 jugular foramen surgery, 414, 415f, 416, 416f, 417
 jugulotympanic paraganglioma, 475. See also Jugulotympanic paraganglioma
 petroclival surgery, 430, 430f
 petrous bone anatomy, 426
 reconstruction, 393
 stylomastoid foramen, 24–25
 temporal bone resection, 390f, 397
 temporal bone tumor, 381, 382, 382t
 tumors
  pathophysiology, 54
  radiation and, 381
 vestibular schwannoma and, 454, 455
Mastoid air cells, 380, 387
 foramen magnum region surgery, 496
 petrous bone anatomy, 426
 vestibular schwannoma, 450, 455
Mastoidectomy
 foramen magnum region surgery, 494, 500
 infratemporal–middle fossa approach, 337
 jugulotympanic paraganglioma, 479, 481
 occipital craniotomy as extension, 398f
 petroclival surgery, 431
 prevention of complications, 587
 radical, 8
 temporal bone resection, 387, 389, 393f
  complete, 393, 396f
  total petrosectomy, 401f
 vertebral artery control, 539
 vestibular schwannoma, 450, 451f
Mastoid emissary veins, 61, 378
Mastoid-extended facial recess approach, 478t, 479, 480f
Mastoid-neck approach, jugulotympanic paraganglioma, 478t, 480–481, 481–483f
Mastoid periosteal flap, 483f
Mastoid process
 pain, 519
 vertebral artery management, 538, 546, 549
Mastoid region of temporal bone, 377
Mastoid tip, 24, 26f, 28, 29
 jugular foramen surgery, 414, 414f
 Metzger's line, 521, 521f
 nasopharyngeal tumor presentation, 85

temporal bone anatomy, 378f
temporal bone resection, 388f
Mastoid vein, 28
Maxilla, 17, 19
 degloving, 195, 196, 197f. See also Facial degloving
 maxillotomy. See Maxillotomy
 subcranial extended transfacial approach, 291
  Type II, 300f
  Type III, 304
 subperiosteal dissection, 195
Maxillary antrum, imaging, 90f
Maxillary artery, 24, 25, 215, 216f. See also Internal maxillary artery
Maxillary branch of cranial nerve V. See Cranial nerve V2
Maxillary crest, 214f
Maxillary nerve, 173, 297
Maxillary ostium, facial degloving approach, 197f
Maxillary sinus
 Denker procedure, 170, 171f
 facial degloving, 199, 201–202, 201–203f
 maxillectomy, 183
 maxillotomy, extended unilateral, 214f, 215, 221f, 222, 223f, 232t
 subcranial approaches
  combined transbasal–Derome-transfacial, 355–356, 355–356f
  extended anterior, 245, 249–252, 250–252f, 254–255, 255f, 256–258, 256–258f, 260
  subcranial extended transfacial approach, 290–291, 291f
 transfacial approach indications, 165
Maxillary sinus tumors, symptoms, 77f, 78–81, 78–79f, 81–82f
Maxillary tuberosity, 27, 343
Maxillary vein, 67f
Maxillectomy, 287
 anterior maxillotomy approach, 292–298, 293–298f
 with facial degloving approach, 195, 196f
 medial
  lateral rhinotomy-Denker-medial maxillectomy, 170–172, 171–172f
  sphenoethmoid anterior maxillotomy approach, 292–298, 293–298f
 reconstruction, 192f
 sellar/parasellar region approaches, 574
 subtotal, 208. See also Maxillotomy, extended unilateral, 208
 total, 172–173, 179–180, 179–180f
 transfacial subcranial approaches, extended, 288t, 290f, 291, 293f, 295f, 297
 indications, 288, 290
 Type II, 298–299, 298–299f
 with transmandibular approach, 343
Maxillotomy
 maxillectomy, 179
 sellar/parasellar region approaches, 573, 574
 transfacial subcranial approaches, 288t
Maxillotomy, extended unilateral, 207–235
 advantages, 229–233, 231–232t
 comments, 233–234
 complications, 228–229, 228t, 229t
 facial degloving, 212–213, 213f, 222, 230

history, 207–209
indications, 209–210, 209t
landmarks, 225f
postoperative care, 224,2 28
preoperative management, 210–212, 210t, 211t
technique, 212–224, 212–221f, 225–228f
 additional technical options, 221–222, 223f
 anterior maxillary exposure, 213, 216
 closure, 224
 Gigli saw positioning, 215, 217–220f
 hard palate exposure, 212, 213f
 intranasal flap construction, 212–213, 214–215f
 lateral maxillary wall, lateral pterygoid plate, and interior maxillary artery exposure, 215, 216f
 maxillary and pterygoid plate osteotomies, 218, 221, 221f
 maxillary plating, preliminary, 218
 nasal exposure, 212, 212f
 retropharyngeal and cervical spine exposure, 222–224, 225–227f
 skull base exposure, 222, 223f
Maxillotomy-medial maxillectomy approach, 292–298, 293–298f
Mayfield head rest, 125
 infratemporal–middle fossa approach, 313
 nursing staff duties, 129
 prevention of complications, 586
 vestibular schwannoma, 449, 465
McGregor's line, 521, 521f
McRae angle, 521, 522f
Meatal branch of cranial nerve VII, 378
Meckel's cave, 20, 22, 23f
 imaging, 88, 93f
 infratemporal–middle fossa approach
  diagnosis/presentation, 310
  otic exposure, 326f
  temporal bone anatomy, 322, 326f
 meningioma, 106f
 nasal and paranasal sinus tumor spread, 82
 naspharyngeal tumor spread, 83
 petroclival surgery, 435
 subcranial extended transfacial approach, 290, 290f, 291f, 305
 temporal bone anatomy, 379
 total petrosectomy, 401
 tumor pathophysiology, 56, 57, 57f
Medial maxillectomy, 170–172, 171–172f, 292–298, 293–298f
Medial rectus muscle, 156
Median labial mandibuloglossoptomy, 12, 522, 523f, 526, 531, 531f
Median nerve, 144f, 148–151, 149–151f, 152f
Medical history, 585
Medical management
 jugulotympanic paraganglioma resection, 477
 pituitary adenoma, 577–578
Medications
 analgesic, 122
 EEG effects, 145
 home care planning, 135
 and neurophysiological monitoring, 145
Medulla oblongata, 28
 imaging, 102
 vertebral artery, 533, 534

Meibomian glands, 586
Melanoma
　chemo- and radiosensitivity, 71
　external auditory meatus/temporal bone, 383t, 385
　imaging, 89t, 90
　infratemporal–middle fossa approach, 331
　orbital exenteration indications, 173
　pathology, 45–46, 46f, 47t
　pathophysiology, 52t, 57
　presentation, 74
　sellar/parasellar, 560t
　subcranial extended anterior approach, 259t
　temporal bone, 380
　vertebral artery involvement, 546t
Membrane tectoria, 28
Meningeal artery, 28, 29
　anterior, 534, 550, 550f
　cranial nerve blood supply, 113t
　posterior, 413
Meningeal branch of ascending pharyngeal artery, 28
Meningeal branch of cranial nerve VII, 21
Meningeal carcinomatosis, 335
　esthesioneuroblastoma, 166f
　temporal bone involvement, 386
Meningeal lesions, hematopoietic metastases, 560t, 562
Meninges, imaging, 87
Meningiocele, 347, 357
Meningioma, 11
　anterior fossa
　　combined resection with floor resection, 168
　　facial degloving with craniotomy, 204f
　anterior subcranial transfacial approaches, 287
　cerebellopontine angle
　　imaging, 98, 98t, 99, 100f
　　neurophysiological monitoring, 159f
　clivus, 519. See also Meningioma, petroclival
　cranioorbital zygomatic approach, 271, 272–273, 273f, 274, 276–277f, 278, 276f, 277f, 278
　foramen magnum region, 503
　　imaging, 98t
　　lateral transcondylar approach, 496–498, 497–498f
　ICA involvement, 106f
　ICA management
　　surgical dissection of tumor, 361
　　tumor biology and, 360
　imaging, 92, 92t
　　central skull base lesions, 92
　　cerebellopontine angle lesions, 98, 98t, 99, 100f
　　foramen magnum lesions, 98t
　　jugular fossa tumors, 98t, 102
　infratemporal–middle fossa approach, 309
　internal auditory canal, 446
　jugular foramen, 549
　jugular fossa, 419t
　maxillotomy, extended unilateral, 228t, 233
　middle skull base, ICA management, 371–373, 371–373f
　occipitoatlatoaxial region, 491
　pathology, 39–40, 39f
　petroclival, 423, 424f, 426, 429, 431, 433, 438–439, 438–439f
　　complications, 437
　　middle fossa intradural approach, 436
　　posterior fossa primary intradural approach, 435–436, 435f
　rectus abdominis free flaps, 611–613, 611–613f
　sellar/parasellar, 560t, 562, 580
　　subfrontal approach, 574
　　subtemporal approaches, 575
　subcranial approaches, 355–356, 355–356f, 357t
　　extended anterior, 259t
　　transbasal–Derome, 348, 352, 357
　therapeutic embolization, preoperative, 115
　transcervicomastoid approach, 409–422. See also Transcervicomastoid approach
　vertebral artery involvement, 542t, 542, 542t, 543f, 546, 546t, 547f
　vertebral artery management, 549, 550, 550f, 550
　vestibular schwannoma versus, 446
Meningitis
　anterior approach, incidence after, 586t
　jugulotympanic paraganglioma, 486t
　maxillotomy complications, 228, 228t, 229
　postoperative monitoring, 132, 133, 601
　prevention of, 588–589, 588f, 590–591, 591f
　reconstruction goals, 608
　sellar/parasellar lesions, 581
　subcranial approaches, 356, 357
　temporal bone resection complications, 404
　transmandibular approach complications, 345
Meningocele
　imaging, 88, 89, 89f, 89t
　mid-skull base approaches, 209t
Meningoencephalocele, maxillotomy, extended unilateral, 228t
Mentalis branch of Cranial nerve VII, EMG, 158f
Mentalis muscle, EMG, 155
Mental nerve, 85, 343
Mesenchymal tumors, 36–44, 47t
Metaphyseal dysplasias, 102, 102t
Metastasis, 66–71, 66t, 67t, 67–71f. See also specific tumor types
　clivus, 517f, 519
　cranioorbital zygomatic approach, 271
　dural involvement, 61
　foramen magnum region, 527
　imaging, 70, 70f, 71f
　　central skull base lesions, 92t, 95
　　cerebellopontine angle lesions, 98, 98t, 99–100
　　diffuse lesions of skull base, 102, 102t
　　infratemporal–middle fossa approach, 313, 313t
　　jugular fossa tumors, 102
　infratemporal–middle fossa approach, 309
　　diagnosis/presentation, 311
　　imaging, 313, 313t
　jugulotympanic paraganglioma, 476–477
　oropharyngeal, parotid, and upper neck lesions, 85
　pathology, 46–47, 47f, 47t
　pituitary carcinoma, 579
　radiation therapy, 406
　sellar/parasellar region, 560t, 562
　temporal bone, 383t, 386
　temporal bone tumors, 381
　tumor biology, 66–71, 66t, 67t, 67–71f
　vertebral artery involvement, 544, 544f, 546t
Methemoglobin, 88
Methylmethacrylate, defect repair, 588f, 589
Metrapone, 578
Metzger's line, 521, 521f
Microscopes, 8
Midas Rex, 125
Midas Rex TAC attachment, 512f, 513
Midbrain, 28
　AEP, 152
　petroclival surgery, 436f
Middle compartment, 342f
　maxillotomy, extended unilateral, 210, 221f, 224, 225f
　transmandibular approach, 341–346, 342–345f
Middle concha, 18f
Middle cranial fossa. See Middle fossa
Middle ear, 20
　anatomy, 20, 379–380, 380f
　CSF leak via, 464, 464f
　foramen magnum region surgery, 496, 500, 504f, 505
　glomus tumor
　　foramen magnum region, 500
　　therapeutic embolization, 116f
　infratemporal fossa approach, 479, 481
　infratemporal–middle fossa approach, 337
　　otologic exposure, 322, 326
　　postoperative care, 337
　jugular foramen surgery, 416, 417
　jugular foramen tumors, 550
　jugulotympanic paraganglioma, 479, 481
　lymphatic drainage, 380
　postoperative care, 602
　reconstruction goals, 623
　temporal bone anatomy, 378f, 379, 379f
　temporal bone resection, 389
　temporal bone tumor etiology, 381
　temporal bone tumors, 381, 382, 382t
Middle ear tumors
　paraganglioma, 550
　pathophysiology, 54
　squamous cell carcinoma, 383, 383f
Middle ethmoid foramen, 19f
Middle fossa. See also Infratemporal fossa–middle fossa approach; Middle skull base
　anatomy, 19, 28, 380
　cranioorbital approach. See Cranioorbital approach
　facial degloving, 195, 197
　foramen magnum region surgery, chordoma, 502f
　history of surgery, 9–11, 10–11f
　imaging, 69f, 92, 95
　jugulotympanic paraganglioma, 475, 476
　maxillotomy, extended unilateral, 231t
　metastatic disease, 32t, 66, 67t, 70, 71f
　nasopharyngeal angiofibroma, 520, 520f
　orbital exenteration, 175, 177
　petroclival tumors, 423, 424f, 426, 427f, 435, 441, 441f

petrous bone anatomy, 426
posterior fossa primary intradural approach, 435
sellar/parasellar region approaches
  anatomy, 559f
  contraindications to transsphenoidal approach, 566, 566t
  subcranial approaches
    extended anterior, 259f
    combined transbasal–Derome-transfacial, 355–356, 355–356f
    transbasal–Derome, 350, 357
  subcranial extended transfacial approach, 290, 290f, 291f, 296
    Type II, 299, 301, 301, 301f
    Type III, 306f
  temporal bone tumors, 381, 382, 382t
  tumor pathophysiology, 34t, 52f, 53, 53f, 54, 56, 57f
  tumor presentation, 520, 520f
    nasal and paranasal sinus tumors, 82
    sphenoid sinus tumors, 81
Middle fossa approach
  CPA, 443
  extradural (transtentorial), petroclival region, 436–437, 436f
  intradural, 436
  petroclival region, 423, 429, 436–437, 436f
  vestibular schwannoma, 445, 447, 448, 465–470, 466–470f
Middle fossa craniotomy
  facial degloving combined with, 195
  temporal bone resection, 397, 399, 399f
  total petrosectomy after, 401f
Middle fossa floor
  infratemporal–middle fossa approach, 310, 322
    carotid dissection, 330
    craniotomy, 328
    reconstruction, 335, 336f
    temporal bone resection, 400
    temporal craniotomy, 399, 399f
Middle fossa syndrome, 69
Middle meningeal artery
  anastomoses, therapeutic embolization considerations, 113–114, 113t
  anatomy, 20, 25, 27f
  cranial nerve blood supply, 113t
  cranioorbital zygomatic approach, 267, 268f
  infratemporal–middle fossa approach, 326
  petrous bone anatomy, 425
  temporal craniotomy, 397
  tumor extension via, 61
  vestibular schwannoma, 465
Middle skull base
  anatomy, 19–27
    intracranial contents, 21–24, 22–26f
    osteology, 19–21, 20–21f
    subcranial relationships, 24–27, 24–27f
  craniospinal lesions approaches, 209t
  maxillotomy, extended unilateral, 223f, 231t
  regions of cranial base surgery, 74f
Midface degloving, 196, 573
Midface splitting, 245
Midline approaches
  foramen magnum region. *See* Foramen magnum region

maxillotomy, extended unilateral, 209
  sublabial approach, 5
Midline lesions, 7
Midline region, cranial base surgery, 74f
Midline ridge, frontal crest, 15
Midline skull base, extended maxillotomy, 224
Miniplates/microplates, 192f. *See also* Titanium fixtures
Mitotane, 578
Mohs resections, 61, 73, 389f
Monitoring
  intraoperative
    infratemporal–middle fossa approach, 313. *See also* Neurologic monitoring, intraoperative
    petroclival surgery, presigmoid approach, 429–430
    prevention of complications, 588
  nursing care. *See* Nursing care
  postoperative management, 132–133, 599
Morgagni, foramen of, 27, 83
Motor nerves, 19
Motor root of Cranial nerve V, 22
Mouth gags, 512f, 513f, 522
MSPs, 145, 150, 151
Mucoceles
  ethmoid sinus tumor presentation, 80
  imaging, 89t, 89, 90, 91f
  sellar/parasellar, 560t, 562, 581
  sinus tumor presentation, 80, 81, 81f
Mucoepidermoid carcinoma, 52t, 63f
Mucoperiosteal flap, maxillotomy, 212–213
Mucosal infection, and osteomyelitis, 595
Mullan's triangle, 270
Multidisciplinary team, 120–121, 120t, 347
  coordinator, 119, 120t
  infratemporal–middle fossa approach, 313
  sellar/parasellar surgery, 568n.
  subcranial approaches, transbasal–Derome, 357
  temporal bone resection, 377
Multifocal skin lesions, 73, 75f
Multiple myeloma, 92t, 95, 102t
Muscle
  CT imaging considerations, 87
  imaging, 88
  maxillotomy, extended unilateral, 231–232t
  tumor extension via, 67
Muscle relaxants, 145, 412, 457
Muscle transfer, 405
Musculocutaneous flaps. *See* Myocutaneous flaps; Flaps and grafts, regional; Reconstruction/defect repair
Mylohyoid muscle, 343
Myocutaneous flaps, 630–635, 631–635f
  infratemporal–middle fossa reconstruction, 335–337, 335–337f
  latissimus dorsi, 633–635, 634–635f
  pectoralis, 631
  reconstruction options, 624t
  subcranial approaches, extended anterior, 241, 244f, 245
  temporal bone reconstruction, 404
  trapezius, 631–633, 631–633f
Myositis, 205
Myotomy, palate, 208
Myringotomy, 8, 210t, 212

N

Nasal bone. *See also* Lateral rhinotomy
  maxillectomy, 179, 179f, 180, 180f, 182
  maxillotomy, extended unilateral, 232t
  subcranial approaches, extended anterior, 245
Nasal cavity
  anatomy, 555, 557f
  CSF leaks, 589–590, 602
  intranasal flap, 212–213, 214–215f, 222
  postoperative care, 603
  sellar/parasellar surgery, 569f
    closure, 572
    trassphenoidal approach, 567f, 568
  subcranial approaches, extended anterior, 239, 243
  transmandibular approach, 343
Nasal cavity lesions
  imaging, 89, 89f, 89t, 90, 92f
  symptoms, 74, 76f, 77–78, 77f
Nasal dorsum
  reconstruction, free rectus muscle flap, 613–616, 614–615f
  skin cancer. *See* Skin cancer
Nasal exposure, maxillotomy, extended unilateral, 212, 212f
Nasal-facial groove, 73
Nasal flap, 212–213, 214–215f, 222
Nasal floor
  maxillotomy, extended unilateral, 221–222
  frontobasal/degloving, 356, 356f
Nasal obstruction, 74, 519
  nasal and paranasal sinus tumor presentation, 78
  presentation, 77
Nasal packing, postoperative care, 601
Nasal paraganglioma, 473
Nasal reconstruction
  radial forearm free flap, 608–611, 609–610f
  rectus abdominis free flaps, 613–616, 614–615f
Nasal septal flaps, 590, 590f
  anterior cranial floor defect repair, 296f
  maxillotomy, extended unilateral, 210
Nasal septum
  ethmosphenoidectomy, 223f
  facial degloving, 195, 196f, 208
  foramen magnum region approaches, transoral, 523
  incisions, 3, 4f
  maxillectomy, 179, 179f, 180, 180f
  maxillotomy, extended unilateral, 214f, 217f, 222, 223f, 230, 232, 232t
  mucoperiosteal flaps, maxillotomy, 210
  subcranial approaches
    transbasal–Derome, 349
    transfacial extended type I, 292
  tumors
    degloving approach, 205
    presentation, 79f
Nasal/paranasal sinuses. *See also specific sinuses*
  anatomy, 16, 557f
  chordoma involvement, 93
  CSF leaks, 589–590
  hemorrhage, 593
  imaging, 87
  maxillotomy, extended unilateral, 232t

664 / SUBJECT INDEX

Nasal/paranasal sinuses (*contd.*)
  sinus box paradigm, 78, 78f
  subcranial approaches
    extended anterior, 239, 249–252, 250–252f
    transbasal–Derome, 347, 350, 355–356, 355–356f, 357
  transmandibular approach, 343
  tumor extension, 67
Nasal/paranasal sinus tumors, 6f, 7. *See also specific sinuses*
  adenoid cystic carcinoma, 33, 34t
  anterior subcranial transfacial approaches, 287
  direct extension, 67
  facial degloving approach, 195, 201–202, 201–203f
  facial degloving with craniotomy, 202, 203f
  imaging, 88, 89, 89f, 89t, 90, 91f, 92f
  infratemporal–middle fossa approach, 310
  pathophysiology, 51
  subcranial approaches
    extended anterior, 254–255, 255f, 256–258, 256–258f
    extended transfacial, 288, 288f
    transbasal–Derome, 347, 348, 357
  symptoms, 74–82
    central invasion, 81–82, 81–82f
    ethmoid sinus, 80, 82f
    frontal sinus, 80–82, 80–81f
    maxillary sinus, 78–80, 78–79f, 81–82f
    sphenoid sinus, 81, 81f, 82f
  transfacial approaches, 165, 288, 288f
Nasal tumors
  anterior cranial fossa spread, 167
  facial degloving, 195
    with craniotomy, 203, 204f
    transmaxillary, 199
  mid-skull base approaches, 209t
Nasal wall
  facial degloving, 208, 213, 213f
  subcranial approaches
    extended anterior, 241–243f
    extended transfacial Type II, 299, 299f
Nasofrontal duct, 80
Nasogastric tube
  infratemporal–middle fossa approach, 337
  transmandibular approach, 345
Nasolacrimal duct
  facial degloving approach, 196, 196f, 197f
  maxillotomy complications, 228, 228t
Nasoorbital osteotomy, 239
Nasopharyngeal angiofibroma
  cavernous artery supply of, 378
  facial degloving, 195, 196–200, 198–200f, 205
  juvenile, 74, 76f, 77, 77f, 115, 196, 198, 200, 198–200f, 205
    hemostasis, 587
    maxillotomy, extended unilateral, 222, 228t
  presentation, 74, 76f, 77, 77f, 520, 520f
  therapeutic embolization, preoperative, 115
Nasopharyngeal carcinoma, 27
  clivus, 517f
  cranioorbital zygomatic approach, 274, 275f
  foramen magnum region involvement
    clinical presentation, 519, 520

  pathology, 516–517, 517f
  imaging, 88, 92t, 94–95
  infratemporal–middle fossa approach, 309, 310
    carotid dissection and eustachian tube, 330
    cavernous sinus resection, 333–334, 333f
    diagnosis/presentation, 311, 312f
    incision, 313, 314f
    presentation, 310
  maxillotomy, extended unilateral, 222–223
  MRI imaging of middle fossa involvement, 69f
  pathophysiology, 53–54, 53f, 61, 69f
  presentation, 83
  subcranial extended transfacial approach, 290f, 291f, 304
  temporal bone metastases, 386
  transmandibular approach, 341–346, 342–345f
Nasopharyngeal polyps, 207
Nasopharynx, 29. *See also* Craniopharyngioma
  anatomy, 380
  chordoma involvement, 93
  facial degloving approach, 195
  imaging, 87, 92
  infratemporal–middle fossa approach, 309, 335, 336f
  maxillotomy, extended unilateral, 215, 222, 230, 232t
  subcranial approaches
    extended transfacial Type I, 292
    extended transfacial Type II, 303f
    frontobasal/degloving, 356, 356f
    transbasal–Derome, 349, 357
  symptoms with lesions of, 83–85, 84f
  total petrosectomy, 402
  transoral approaches to clivus and craniocervical junction. *See* Foramen magnum region
  transsphenoidal approach to sellar region, 570
  tumor extension, 67
Neck. *See* Transcervicomastoid approach
Neck dissection
  infratemporal–middle fossa approach
    incision, 313, 314f
  temporal bone resection, 387, 402–403
  with transfacial subcranial approach, extended, 304
Neck flexion
  and SEPs during median nerve stimulation, 150, 151f
  and vertebral artery, 535, 535f, 536, 544–545
Neck incisions, transmandibular approach, 345
Neck lesions
  maxillotomy, extended unilateral, 207
  nasopharyngeal tumor presentation, 83
  symptoms with, 84f, 85
Neck management, temporal resection, 402–403
Neck muscles
  anatomy, 507, 508
  foramen magnum region surgery, 492
  jugular foramen syndrome, 519
  vertebral artery approaches
    anterolateral, 538
    complications, 552
    posterolateral, 537f
  vestibular schwannoma, 458

Neck pain, clival lesions, 519
Necrosis
  and hemorrhage, 595
  mandibulotomy complications, 346
  maxillotomy complications, 228, 228t, 230, 234
  nasal and paranasal sinus tumor presentation, 78
  pericranial flap slough, 595
  postoperative management, 601
  radiation therapy complications, 406, 407f
  with temporal bone tumors, 381
  tumor pathophysiology, 62, 63f, 64, 64f
Needle aspiration biopsy, 111–113, 112f
Nelson's syndrome, 578
Nerve anastomosis, temporal bone resection, 400–401, 400f
Nerve grafts, 637–638, 637–638f
Nerve stimulation, SEP effects, 144f, 145f
Nervus intermedius, 28, 378, 379
Neural/perineural spread, 71–72
  CT image of, 69f
  histological tumor types, 74
  imaging, 88
    anterior fossa lesions, 90f
    nasopharyngeal tumors, 94–95
    oropharyngeal, parotid, and upper neck lesions, 85
    skin tumors, 75f, 76f
  squamous cell carcinoma, 32, 383
  temporal bone involvement, 383, 386
  total petrosectomy, 401–402
  transfacial approach indications, 165
  tumor pathophysiology, 55–56, 55f, 56, 57f
Neurilemmoma
  cranioorbital zygomatic approach, 271
  imaging, jugular fossa lesions, 101
  mid-skull base approaches, 209t
Neurinoma
  vertebral artery involvement, 542, 542f, 542t, 546t
  vertebral artery management
    control and mobilization, 539f
    jugular foramen lesions, 549, 549f
Neuroanatomy, 19
  middle fossa, 21, 21f
  posterior fossa, 28
  temporal bone anatomy, 378–379
Neuroblastoma
  mid-skull base approaches, 209t
  olfactory. *See* Esthesioneuroblastoma; Olfactory neuroblastoma
  pathology, 40, 40f
  pathophysiology, 52t, 57
Neuroendocrine tumors. *See* Jugulotympanic paraganglioma
Neurofibroma
  imaging
    central skull base lesions, 92t
    jugular fossa lesions, 101
  jugular fossa, 419t
  mid-skull base approaches, 209t
  subcranial approaches, extended anterior, 259t
  transcervicomastoid approach, 409–422. *See also* Transcervicomastoid approach
  vestibular schwannoma with, 447

Subject Index / 665

Neurogenic tumors. *See also specific tumor types*
  anterior fossa, facial degloving approach, 205
  cranial nerves. *See* Esthesioneuroblastoma; Olfactory neuroblastoma; Vestibular schwannoma
  imaging
    central skull base lesions, 92t
    foramen magnum lesions, 98t, 102
    jugular fossa tumor, 98t
    paraganglioma, 40–41, 41f
  pathophysiology, 52t, 57
Neurohypophysis
  anatomy, 558, 558f
  tumors of, 560t, 562, 579–581
Neurologic deficits/neuropathies. *See also* Cranial nerves; *specific cranial nerves*
  balloon test occlusion and, 108, 111
  brain resection, 335
  diagnosis/presentation, 311, 311f. *See also specific cranial nerves*
    nasal and paranasal sinus tumors, 82
    nasopharyngeal tumors, 83
  ICA resection complications, 387
  infratemporal–middle fossa approach, 309, 335
  jugulotympanic paraganglioma, 475
  maxillotomy complications, 228, 228t, 229, 230
  olfactory nerve, 347
  petroclival cerebellopontine angle capsule adherence and, 435–436
  recurrent cancer in infratemporal and middle fossa, 310
  subcranial approaches, transbasal–Derome, complications, 347
  vertebral artery surgery complications, 552
  vestibular schwannoma, 443
Neurologic evaluation
  balloon test occlusion, 107
  carotid artery assessment, 108, 386
  cerebral perfusion and, 359
  equipment, 124
  jugular foramen surgery, 413
  nursing care, postoperative, 132–133
  signs and symptoms with bone invasion, 69–70
Neurologic monitoring, intraoperative, 137–160
  approach, 137–139, 138f
  foramen magnum region surgery, 492
  during ICA dissection, 373
  infratemporal–middle fossa approach, 313
  jugulotympanic paraganglioma, 480, 481
  measures, 145–159
    auditory system (AEP and BAEP), 151–152, 154, 154–155f
    EEG, 145–158, 146–147f
    electromyography, cranial nerve function, 154–159, 158–159f
    somatosensory system (SEPs), 148–151, 148–153f
    visual system (VEPs), 154–155, 156–157f
  methodology/instrumentation, 139–145, 141f, 143–145f
    electrode properties, 139–140f
    monitoring system, 140–142, 141–142f
    neuroanesthetic conditions, 143, 144f, 145, 145f
  signal acquisition and processing, 142–143, 143–144f
  petroclival surgery, 429–430
  prevention of complications, 588
  vestibular schwannoma, 454, 458
Neurologic monitoring, postoperative, 600–601, 600f, 601t
Neuroma
  cranioorbital zygomatic approach, 277f, 278
  imaging, 93f
    central skull base lesions, 92, 92t
    cerebellopontine angle lesions, 99, 99f
    jugular fossa lesions, 101, 101f
  transcervicomastoid approach, 409–422. *See also* Transcervicomastoid approach
Neuronal conductivity, cerebral blood flow and, 105
NeuroNet. *See* Neurologic monitoring, intraoperative
Neuropathy. *See* Neurologic deficits/neuropathies
Neurosecretory tumors, 411, 412, 477. *See also* Glomus/glomus jugulare tumors; Jugulotympanic paraganglioma
  neurohypophysis, 560t, 562, 579–581
  preoperative management, 413
Neurosurgeon, 347. *See also* Multidisciplinary team
  infratemporal–middle fossa approach, 313
  prevention of complications, 587
  sellar/parasellar surgery, 568n.
  subcranial approaches, transbasal–Derome, 357
  temporal bone resection, 377, 387
  temporal craniotomy, 397
  transcervicomastoid approach, 409–422. *See also* Transcervicomastoid approach
Neurotropic spread. *See* Neural/perineural spread
Neurovascular structures
  petroclival tumors, 423
  tumor invasion and metastases involving, 67, 69
Nitroglycerin, 115
Nitrous oxide, 108
Node of Rouviére, 84f, 85
Non-Hodgkin's lymphoma, 44, 45, 45f, 560t, 562
Norepinephrine, 411, 412, 477
Notochord. *See* Chordomas
Nursing care, 119–135
  carotid assessment, 121–122
  clinical nurse specialist role, 120
  ICU, postoperative, 132–135, 135f
  informed consent, 120
  multidisciplinary team, 120–121, 120t
  perioperative and intraoperative, 124–132
    intraoperative procedures, 124–126
    preoperative assessment, 124
    sequence of events, 126–132
  postoperative, 601. *See also* Postoperative management
  preoperative, 121–124
  preparation and patient education, 119–120
  team coordinator, 119, 120t
Nutrition
  home care planning, 135
  nursing care, 122–123
  postoperative care, 602
Nylén, C.O., 8
Nystagmus, 445, 521

O

Obgeweser elevator, 320
Obliquuus capitis, 29
Occipital artery, 28–29
  anastomoses, 113t, 114
  cranial nerve blood supply, 113t
  jugular foramen surgery, 414
  therapeutic embolization considerations, 115
  vertebral artery aneurysm, 551
  vertebral artery occlusion, 115f
Occipital bone
  cranial surface, 27
  embryology, 507
  jugular foramen anatomy, 413, 415
  lymphoma, 54
  maxillotomy, extended unilateral, 231–232t
  MacGregor's line, 521, 521f
  petroclival lesions, 430. *See also* Petroclival lesions
  prevention of complications, 587
  squamous cell carcinoma primary sites, 32t
  synostosis with sphenoid, 27
  temporal craniotomy, 398f
  tumor involvement, CT image, 69f
  vertebral artery management, 536f
  vestibular schwannoma, 458
Occipital condyle, 24, 25, 26f, 28f, 29
  anatomy, 491, 507
  facial degloving approach, 208
  foramen magnum region surgery, 500f, 502f, 503, 503f
  glomus tumor, 500f
  ICA course, 23f
  infratemporal–middle fossa approach, 322, 326f
  joint capsule, 495f
  maxillotomy, extended unilateral, 209, 223f, 224, 225f
  tumor metastasis to, 67t
  vertebral artery management, 539, 546, 547f
Occipital condyle syndrome, 69, 70
Occipital craniotomy, with mastoidectomy, 398f
Occipital crest, 27, 538
Occipital nerve, great, 29
Occipital sinus, 27, 67f, 413
Occipitoatlantoaxial region. *See* Craniocervical junction; Foramen magnum region; Vertebral artery management
Occipitocervical fusion, 496, 500, 502f, 503, 503f
Octreotide, 577–578
Ocular ischemic syndrome, 108
Ocular motility, 69, 79
Ocular sacrifice. *See* Orbital exenteration
Oculomotor foramen, cranioorbital zygomatic approach, 270, 282, 283f
Oculomotor nerve. *See* Cranial nerve III
Odondoid anomalies, 514
Odonotoid fractures, 522
Odontectomy, 514, 521
  complications, 531
  transoral approach, 527–529, 528–530f

Odontoid ligament, 511f
Odontoid process, 29
  anatomy, 508, 509f
  clinical presentation of lesions, 519
  embryology, 507
  fracture, 514–516, 515f, 515t
  imaging, 521
  malformations, 514
  transmandibular approach, 341
  vertebral artery management, 546
Ohngren's line, 177, 178f
Olfaction, 77, 357, 574, 606
Olfactory bulbs, 16, 18f, 82
Olfactory filaments, 239
Olfactory groove tumors, 273, 274f, 348, 580
Olfactory meningioma, 574
Olfactory nerve
  anatomy, 15, 16, 17f, 18f, 29
  blood supply, 113, 113t
  anosmia, 77, 357, 574, 606
  subcranial approaches
    transbasal–Derome, 349, 352, 355f
    transbasal–Derome complications, 347
  subfrontal approach, 574
Olfactory neuroblastoma, 47t, 90. *See also*
    Esthesioneuroblastoma
  mid-skull base approaches, 209t
  pathology, 40, 40f
Oncology consultation, temporal bone tumors, 387
Ong, G.B., 12
Onodi, cell of, 175
Operculum, 461, 463f
Ophthalmic artery, 19, 24
  anastomoses, 113t, 114f
  anomalous origins, 113t
  collateral flow in carotid artery occlusion, 359
  cranioorbital zygomatic approach, 270, 278, 279f, 280
  hemorrhage, 593
  ocular ischemic syndrome, 108
  orbital exenteration, 175
Ophthalmic nerve. *See* Cranial nerve V1
Ophthalmic vein
  anatomy, 19, 22, 67f
  hemorrhage, 593
  infratemporal–middle fossa approach, cavernous sinus resection, 334
  subcranial extended transfacial approach, 297
  tumor extension via, 59–61, 60f, 64
Ophthalmologists, 347
Ophthalmoplegia, 69, 311, 311f
Optic canal, 15, 17f, 19, 20f
  cranioorbital approach, 263
  cranioorbital zygomatic approach, 269, 276f, 278, 279
    aneurysm repair, 279f
    bifrontal, 273f
  imaging, 90
  nasal and paranasal sinus tumor spread, 82
  orbital exenteration, 175, 178f
  subcranial approaches
    extended anterior, 239
    extended transfacial, 297
    extended transfacial Type II, 299, 300f
    extended transfacial Type III, 305
    transbasal–Derome, 350
  tumor biology, perineural spread, 55–56, 55–56f
Optic chiasm, 15
  cranioorbital zygomatic approach, 269, 269f
  orbital exenteration, 178f
  sellar/parasellar anatomy, 558
  sellar/parasellar lesion presentation, 563
  subcranial approaches
    extended anterior, 239
    extended transfacial, 297
    transbasal–Derome, 355f
  VEPs, 154–155, 156f
Optic foramen
  anatomy, 17, 19f
  tumor biology, perineural spread, 55–56, 55–56f
Optic nerve
  anatomy, 15, 17f, 18f, 19, 24, 558, 559f
  cranioorbital zygomatic approach, 269, 269f, 272, 272f
    aneurysm repair, 279f
    bifrontal, 273f
  facial degloving
    combined, 201
    with external frontoethmoidectomy, 202, 203f
    transmaxillary procedure, 201
  imaging, 90
  infratemporal–middle fossa approach, 311
  intraoperative monitoring. *See* Neurologic monitoring, intraoperative
  medial subcranial structures, 27
  nasal and paranasal sinus tumor presentation, 82
  orbital exenteration, 175, 178f
  petroclival tumors, 427
  sellar/parasellar region approaches, 558, 559f, 563, 574, 575
  subcranial approaches
    extended anterior, 239, 243f
    extended transfacial, 297
    extended transfacial Type II, 298, 301, 302f
    transbasal–Derome, 348, 352, 357
  VEPs, 154–155, 156f
Optic-vidian-rotundum triangle, 300f
Oral cavity. *See also* Oropharynx
  imaging, 88
  incisions, subcranial transfacial approach Type III, 303f, 304
  sella surgery, closure, 572–573
  transoral approaches, 11, 12f
    to clivus and craniocervical junction, 513. *See also* Foramen magnum region
  sellar/parasellar chordoma, 581
  sublabial facial degloving, 208
Orbicularis oculi, 155, 175, 176f
Orbicularis oris, 155
Orbital apex
  anatomy, 16, 21
  tumor imaging, 69f
  tumor pathophysiology, 52f, 55–56, 55–56f
Orbital compression, 201, 201f, 202, 203f
Orbital exenteration, 178f
  complications, 593
  deep recurrences after, 74
  with extended transfacial subcranial approach, 287–288
  maxillectomy incision with, 179
  reconstruction
    free rectus muscle flap, 613–616, 614–615f
    prosthetic rehabilitation, 605, 605f
    radial forearm free flap, 608–611, 609–610f
    subscapular graft, 619–620, 619–620f
  transfacial approach, 168, 173, 175–177, 175–178f
  transfacial approach, subcranial extended, 288t, 289f, 291, 292, 296f, 298
Orbital fissures, 20f, 55–56, 56f
Orbital paraganglioma, 473
Orbit/periorbital structures
  anatomy, 16, 18f
  cranioorbital approach. *See* Cranioorbital approach
  esthesioneuroblastoma, 167
  ethmoid sinus tumor presentation, 80
  facial degloving approach, 195, 197f, 198
    combined, 201
    with external frontoethmoidectomy, 202, 202f, 203f
    sublabial transoral, 208
  facial degloving-transmaxillary procedure, 199, 201
  frontal sinus tumor presentation, 80–81
  imaging, 88–89, 89
  infratemporal–middle fossa approach
    cavernous sinus resection, 334
    zygomatic ostectomy, 319–320, 321–324f
  intraobital approach to palatine defect reconstruction, 254–255, 255f
  maxillary sinus tumor presentation, 79
  maxillectomy, 179, 180, 183
  maxillotomy, extended unilateral, 213, 213f, 222, 231t
  reconstruction
    after orbital exenteration, Orbital exenteration, reconstruction
    rectus abdominis free flaps, 613–616, 614–615f
  sphenoid sinus tumor presentation, 81
  subcranial approaches
    extended anterior, 239, 241–243f, 244f, 245, 246–248f, 249–254, 250–254f, 259f
    extended transfacial, 288, 288f, 289f
    extended transfacial Type II, 299, 299f, 300f
    frontobasal/degloving, 356, 356f, 357
    transbasal–Derome, 348–349, 349f, 350, 351, 351f, 357
  traumatic encephalocele, 284f
  tumor pathophysiology, 55–56, 56f
    extension via, 59, 59f, 60f, 61
    metastasis to, 66, 67
    perineural spread, 55–56, 55–56f
  vascular anastomoses, 113t
Orbital process, frontal bone, 15, 19
Orbital retractor, 241, 244f
Orbital syndrome, 69
Orbital tumors, imaging, 88
Orbitocranial approach. *See* Cranioorbital approach
Orbitotomy, posterior, 266, 266f, 271, 272, 272f

SUBJECT INDEX / 667

Oritcochea flap, 597
Oropharyngeal cancers
  infratemporal–middle fossa lesions, 310
  symptoms, 84f, 85
  temporal bone metastases, 386
  transmandibular approach, 341–346, 342–345f
Oropharynx
  facial degloving approach, 198
  manfibular resection with extended transfacial subcranial approaches, 304
  maxillotomy, extended unilateral, 208–209, 215, 223, 232t
  subcranial extended transfacial approach, 291
  transoral approaches to clivus and craniocervical junction, *See* Foramen magnum region
Oscillopsia, 521
Osler-Weber-Rendue lesions, 205
Osmotic diuretics, 397
Osseointegrated implants, 404, 406
Osseointegration, 193
Osseomyocutaneous flaps, 241, 244f, 245. *See also* Bone flaps; *specific donor sites*
Osseous tumors, vertebral artery involvement, 542t, 544, 544f, 546, 546t
Ossicles, 379–380, 380f, 416
Ossiculum terminale, 507
Ossifying fibroma, 209t, 357t
Osteoblastoma, 209t, 542
Osteochondroma, 544, 546t
Osteoclastic activity, 61
Osteology
  anterior skull base, 15, 16–17f
  middle skull base, 19–21, 20–21f
  posterior skull base, 27–28
Osteoma
  anterior fossa, 168
    facial degloving, 201–202, 201–202f, 203f, 205
    imaging, 90
  mid-skull base approaches, 209t
  subcranial approaches, 348, 357t
  vertebral artery involvement, 546t, 548
Osteomyelitis
  imaging, 98
  management of, 595–597, 596f
  mandibulotomy complications, 346
  radiation therapy complications, 406
  reconstruction, free latissimus dorsi flap, 616–618, 616–618f
  sellar/parasellar involvement, 563
Osteopetrosis, 102, 102t
Osteophytes, 536
Osteoplastic flap, 3, 16f
  anterior fossa floor repair, 296
  craniotomy, 185–186, 185–187f
  transfacial, reconstruction after, 190, 190f
Osteosarcoma, 37, 383t, 385
Osteotomes, rhinotomy, 168–169, 169–170f
Osteotomies. *See also* Craniotomy; *specific bones*
  cranioorbital zygomatic approach, 264, 265f, 266f
  frontonasoorbital frame, 239
  Lefort I, 199
  subcranial approaches extended anterior, 241–243f, 246–248f
  transmandibular approach, 343f

Ostium, sphenoid, 27f
Otalgia, 410, 410t
Otic artery, 534
Otic capsule
  jugulotympanic paraganglioma, 476, 476f
  petrous bone anatomy, 426
  temporal bone tumor staging, 382, 382t
  vestibular schwannoma, 452f, 456–457, 457f, 469f
Otitis externa, 98, 381, 406
Otitis media, 8, 83, 377, 381, 597
Otolaryngologists, 347, 357, 568n.
Otologic surgery, 7–9, 7–9f
  infratemporal–middle fossa approach, 322, 326, 327f
  transcervicomastoid approach, 409–422. *See also* Transcervicomastoid approach
Otorrhea
  CSF, 602
  with temporal bone tumors, 381, 386
Oval window, 378f, 380
Oxygen, hyperbaric, 346
Oxygen tension. *See also* Blood gases
  hypoxia, 108, 145–148
  neurophysiological monitoring, EEG, 145–146

P

Paget's disease, 102, 102t
Pain management, nursing care, 121, 122
Palate
  Chamberlain's and McGregor's lines, 521, 521f
  facial degloving, 195, 208
  imaging, 88
  maxillary sinus tumor presentation, 78, 78f
  maxillectomy, 179, 180, 180f, 182, 183, 208
  maxillotomy
    complications, 234
    extended unilateral, 213, 213f, 218, 220f, 223, 223f, 224, 226f, 230, 232t
    horizontal unilateral, 208–209
  nasopharyngeal lesions, 84f, 85
  subcranial approaches
    extended anterior, 253–258, 253–258f
    extended transfacial, 291, 299, 299f, 300f, 303
  transmandibular approach, 343
  transoral approach to clivus and foramen magnum region, 523, 524, 524f, 526, 526f
  closure, 530f, 531
  complications, 532
  odontectomy, 527
  weakness of, 69
Palatine arteries, 229
Palatine branch of ascending pharyngeal artery, 229
Palatine neurovascular bundle, transoral approach to foramen magnum, 524
Palliation
  embolization techniques, 113–116, 113t, 114–116f
  glomus tumors, 409
  radiation therapy, 407
  subcranial approaches, transbasal–Derome, 348

Palsies. *See* Neurologic evaluation; Neuropathy; *specific cranial nerves*
Pannus, 529, 530f
Panse, R., 8, 9
Paraclinoid aneurysm, 280, 280f
Paraganglioma. *See also* Jugulotympanic paraganglioma
  jugular foramen, 550
  mid-skull base approaches, 209t
  pathology, 40–41, 41f
  therapeutic embolization, 115
  vertebral artery involvement, 546t
  vertebral artery management, 550, 550f
Paranasal sinuses. *See* Nasal/paranasal sinuses; Nasal/paranasal sinus tumors
Parapharyngeal lymph nodes, 311
Parapharyngeal space
  facial degloving approach, 195, 198
  imaging, 88
  jugulotympanic paraganglioma, 476
  maxillotomy, extended unilateral, 232t
  transmandibular approach, 341–346, 342–345f
Parasellar pneumatization of sphenoid sinus, 555, 557f
Parasellar structures. *See* Sella/parasellar region
Parasellar syndrome, 69
Paraspinous veins, 59
Parietal bone, pterion, 20
Parkinson, D., 11, 11f
Parkinson's triangle, 270, 271f, 278
Parotidectomy
  temporal bone resection, 387, 390f, 397
  total petrosectomy after, 401f
Parotid gland, 626
  anatomy, 24
  jugular foramen surgery, 414
  temporal bone resection planning, 387
Parotid tumors
  facial nerve paralysis with, 310
  imaging, 88
  infratemporal–middle fossa approach, 309, 313, 314f
  needle biopsy approaches, 112f, 113
  pathophysiology, 54, 56–57
  squamous cell carcinoma, 383
  symptoms, 84f, 85, 310
Pars nervosa, 413
Pars venosa, 413
Pathology, 31–47
  clival and craniocervical lesions, 514–519, 514–519f
  epithelial tumors, 32–36, 47t
    immunohistochemistry, 32t
    metastasis, 46–47, 47f, 47t
    squamous cell carcinoma, 32–33, 32t, 33f, 37t
  frozen section diagnosis, 31–32
  histological type and presentation, 73–74
  histology, 31
  imaging, 89t
  immunohistochemistry, 31, 32t
  infratemporal–middle fossa approach, 309
  lymphoma, 44–45, 47t
  melanoma, 45–46, 46f, 47t
  mesenchymal tumors, 36–44, 47t
    angiofibroma, 37–39, 38f

Pathology (contd.)
 chondrosarcoma, 43, 43f
 chordoma, 43–44, 44f
 fibrous dysplasia, 37, 37f, 38f
 inflammatory pseudotumor, 36–37, 37f
 meningioma, 39–40, 39f
 metastasis, 46–47, 47f, 47t
 olfactory neuroblastoma, 40, 40f
 paraganglioma, 40–41, 41f
 rhabdomyosarcoma, 41–42, 42f
metastasis, 46–47, 47f
nursing staff duties, 127, 130
sella/parasellar lesions, 560–563, 561–562t
 inflammation, 563
 neoplastic, 560–562, 560t, 561t
 nonneoplastic, 562–563
 vascular, 563
slide review, 585
subcranial approaches
 extended anterior, 259t
 transbasal–Derome, 348, 352
temporal bone tumors, 387
vertebral artery, 541–552, 548t, 551t, 552t
 cervical spine access, 548, 548f, 548t
 foramen magnum region access, 546–548, 547f, 548t
 jugular foramen access, 548–550, 548t
 nontumor processes, 544–545
 tumors, 541–544, 541–545f, 541t, 546t
 vascular control and revascularization, 549–550, 550g, 551t, 552t
Pathology specimens. See also Frozen sections
 nursing staff duties, 127, 130
 slide review, 585
Pathophysiology, 258. See also Tumor biology
 and carotid artery salvage/sacrifice, 360
 maxillotomy, extended unilateral, 232–233
 orbital exenteration indications, 173
Patient education, 119–120
Patient evaluation. See also Preoperative assessment
 carotid artery assessment, 105–111, 106–110f
 occipitoatlantoaxial surgery, 492
 sella/parasellar lesions, 565–566
 temporal resection, 381–382, 382f
 transcervicomastoid approach, 411–412
 transmandibular approach, 342
Patient factors, flap construction, 607–608
Patient history, 123–124
Patient position
 foramen magnum region surgery, 492, 493f
 nursing care, 125–126
 petroclival surgery, 429, 430f
 sellar/parasellar surgery, 567f
 and SEPs during median nerve stimulation, 150, 151f
 vertebral artery access, 535
 vestibular schwannoma, 457–458, 458f
 zygomatic cranioorbital approach, 263–264
Patient preparation. See also Nursing care
 facial degloving, 197
 home care planning, 134–135
 infratemporal–middle fossa approach, 313
 interview, 85–86, 86t
 jugulotympanic paraganglioma, 481
 nursing care, 119–120
 prevention of complications, 585

Patient presentation. See Clinical presentation
Patient selection, petroclival tumor, 423, 424f
Paul, F.T., 3
Pectoralis flap, 631
 infratemporal–middle fossa reconstruction, 337, 337f
 reconstruction options, 624t
 temporal bone reconstruction, 403f, 403f, 404
 with transmandibular approach, 343
Pediatric patients, temporal bone tumors, 380, 381
Pericranial flap/graft
 anterior fossa reconstruction, 191, 192f
 complications, management of, 594f, 595
 cranioorbital zygomatic approach, 283
 jugular foramen surgery, 417
 postoperative care, 603
 transfacial approaches, 190–191, 190–191f
 zygomatic cranioorbital approach, 264–265, 264–265f
Pericytoma, 209t
Perineural spread. See Neurotropic/perineural spread
Perioperative management
 jugulotympanic paraganglioma, 477–478
 nursing procedures, 124–132
Periorbital region. See Orbit/periorbital structures
Periosteal elevators, 513, 513f
Periosteal flap, 347, 348. See also Pericranial flap
Periosteum
 carotid canal, 59
 clivus, 27
 infratemporal–middle fossa approach closure, 317f, 318f
 tumor spread, 72
 vertebral artery management, 533, 541
  dissection, 537
  mobilization, 539
  posterolateral approaches, 537f
Peroneal nerve stimulation, SEP effects, 145f
Persistent trigeminal artery, 107, 107f
Persistent vascular anastomoses, 113t
PET. See Positron emission tomography
Petroclinoid folds, 21–22, 23f
Petroclival fissure, imaging, 94
Petroclival lesions, 423–441. See also Clivus; Petrous bone
 anatomy, 424f, 425–426, 425–427f
 case reports
  chordoma, 441, 441f
  meningioma, 438–439, 438–439f
  trigeminal schwannoma, 440, 440f
 clinical aspects, 426–427
 complications, 437
 jugulotympanic paraganglioma, 477f
 patient selection and surgical concept, 423, 424f
 radiology, 427–428, 427–428f
 surgical approaches, 423, 429–436
  middle fossa extradural (transtentorial), 436–437, 436f
  middle fossa intradural, 436
  posterior fossa-primary extradural-presigmoid, 429–435, 430–434f
  posterior fossa primary intradural, 435–436, 435f
  subcranial approaches, 348

Petrooccipital fissure, maxillotomy, 209, 225f
Petroocipital suture, jugulotympanic paraganglioma, 477f
Petrosal nerves, 268f, 383. See also Superficial petrosal nerve
Petrosal part of ICA, 23f
Petrosal sinuses. See also Inferior petrosal sinus
 anatomy, 22, 67f, 555
 naspharyngeal tumor spread, 83
 temporal bone anatomy, 378, 379f
 temporal bone resection, 388f
 total petrosectomy, 401–402, 401–402f
 tumor pathophysiology, 64
Petrosectomy
 petroclival surgery, middle fossa intradural approach, 436f, 437
 temporal resection, 401–402, 401–402f
Petrosphenoid fissure, maxillotomy, 223, 223f, 225f
Petrotympanic fissure, 25
Petrous apex, 27, 64
 epidermoid and cholesterol cysts, 95, 96f
 internal auditory canal reconstruction, 464
 middle fossa extradural approach, 436
 temporal bone tumors, 381
 vestibular schwannoma, 446
Petrous apex disease
 neurologic symptoms with, 379
 temporal bone resection, 404
Petrous bone. See also Petroclival lesions
 anatomy, 27, 28
 cranioorbital zygomatic approach, 239, 267
 greater superficial petrosal nerve, 22
 jugular foramen anatomy, 413
 maxillotomy, extended unilateral, 225f
 subcranial approaches, transbasal–Derome, 357
 tumor pathophysiology, 59
 vestibular schwannoma, 461, 468, 468f
Petrous bone dura
 middle fossa intradural approach, 437
 vestibular schwannoma, 462f
Petrous canal
 cranioorbital zygomatic approach, 267–268
 infratemporal–middle fossa approach, 332
 tumor pathophysiology, 59
Petrous ridge, temporal bone, 20, 21
 infratemporal–middle fossa approach, 309
 tumor involvement, 69
Petrous temporal bone, 377
 anatomy, 380
 jugular foramen anatomy, 413
 jugulotympanic paraganglioma, 476
Petrous tip
 cavernous sinus resection, 334
 cranioorbital zygomatic approach, 270
 subcranial approach, 301
 tumor pathophysiology, 53f, 54
Pharyngeal artery, ascending. See Ascending pharyngeal artery
Pharyngeal cancers. See Nasopharyngeal cancer; Oropharyngeal cancer
Pharyngeal flap, transoral approaches to clivus, 524, 526, 526f
Pharyngobasilar canal, 27
Pharyngobasilar fascia, 27

Subject Index / 669

Pharynx. *See also* Nasopharynx; Oropharynx
  maxillotomy, extended unilateral, 223, 232t
  subcranial extended transfacial approach, 291
  transmandibular approach, 341, 343
  transoral approach to clivus and foramen magnum region. *See* Foramen magnum region
Phenobarbital, 145
Pheochromocytoma, 411, 473, 477
Physaliferous cell, 517, 517f
Physical examination, 85
Pia, petroclival tumors, 423, 437
Pinna
  otitis externa, 98, 381, 406
  squamous cell carcinoma, presentation of, 83f
  tumor pathophysiology, 54
Piriform apertures, 239
Pituitary. *See also* Sella/parasellar region
  anatomy, 19, 555, 558, 558–559f
  clinical syndromes, 69
  imaging, 89f
  medial subcranial structures, 27
  sphenoid sinus tumor presentation, 81
  transsphenoidal approach, 27
  tumor spread, 64
Pituitary adenoma, 560t, 560–562, 561t, 577–579
Pituitary apoplexy, 564, 579
Pituitary carcinoma, 579
Pituitary fossa, 21
Pituitary stalk, 21, 355f, 555
Pituitary surgery, 3–7, 4–7f
Pituitary tumors
  clinical presentation, 520, 520f, 563–564
  cranioorbital zygomatic approach, 274, 276–277f, 278
  imaging, 92
  maxillotomy, extended unilateral, 228t
  mid-skull base approaches, 209t
  pathology, 560t, 560–562
  specific hormone secreting, 564–565
  subcranial approaches, 357t
    transbasal–Derome, 352
    with transfacial approach, 356, 356f
Plain films
  sellar/parasellar lesions, 565
  temporal bone tumors, 381
Planning, 585
  prevention of complications, 587
  temporal bone tumors, 387
Planum sphenoidale, 15, 17f, 18f
  cranioorbital zygomatic approach, 271, 274
  craniotomy, 184
  subcranial approaches, transbasal–Derome, 349, 350
Plasmacytoma
  imaging
    anterior skull base lesions, 89t, 90
    central skull base lesions, 92t
  mid-skull base approaches, 209t
  vertebral artery involvement, 546t
Plastic surgeons, 357, 377
Plating
  maxillotomy, extended unilateral, 218
  reconstruction. *See* Titanium fixtures
  zygomatic ostectomy, 319
Platybasia, 521, 522

Platysma, infratemporal–middle fossa approach, 315
Pneumatization
  postsellar, 52f
  sphenoid, 27
  sphenoid sinus, 555, 557f
Pneumocephalus
  management of, 592–593
  maxillotomy complications, 228, 228t
  postoperative monitoring, 600, 600f, 601
  prevention and management, 586, 586f
  reconstruction, radial forearm free flap, 608–611, 609–610f
  sellar/parasellar surgery, 573
  subcranial approach complications, 357
  transmandibular approach complications, 345
Pneumotoscopy, 474
Polyps, imaging, 89t, 92f, 89
Pons, 28, 29f
  AEP, 152
  cardiorespiratory arrest, 521
  cerebellopontine angle lesion imaging, 98–99, 98f, 98t
  cranioorbital zygomatic approach, 263
Pontine artery, 28
Pontine dura, tumor invasion, 52f, 53, 61
Pontomedullary junction, 533
Portal system, pituitary, 559f
Porus acousticus
  anatomy, 22, 28
  vestibular schwannoma, 450, 454, 456, 457
Positron emission tomography, 3, 310
  cerebral blood flow assessment, 109
  infratemporal–middle fossa approach, 313, 313t
  metastases, 70
  recurrence, failure to detect, 74
Postauricular approach, jugulotympanic paraganglioma, 483f
Postauricular artery, 115, 316
Postauricular incision, 483f
  jugular foramen surgery, 415, 415f
  vestibular schwannoma, 449, 450f
Postauricular skin, 73
Postauricular sulcus tumors, 387
Posterior approaches
  jugular bulb. *See* Jugulotympanic paraganglioma
  to petrous bone, 426, 427f
  temporal bone resection, 377–407. *See also* Temporal bone resection
  transcervicomastoid approach, 409–422. *See also* Transcervicomastoid approach
Posterior atlantooccipital membrane, 534
Posterior cervical triangle, foramen magnum region surgery, 492, 492f
Posterior communicating artery, 24
Posterior ethmoid artery, 15, 17, 230
Posterior ethmoid sinuses, 81
Posterior fossa
  cranioorbital zygomatic approach, 270
  CSF leaks, 589–590
  foramen magnum region surgery, 502f
  history of surgery, 7–9, 8–9f
  imaging, 92
  jugulotympanic paraganglioma, 476
  petroclival tumors, 424f, 426, 427

petrous bone anatomy, 426
regions of cranial base surgery, 74f
sphenoid sinus tumor presentation, 81
subcranial approaches, transbasal–Derome, 357
temporal bone tumor staging, 382, 382t
tumor involvement, involvement, contraindications to transsphenoidal approach, 566, 566t
tumor pathophysiology, 52f, 54, 54, 54f
vestibular schwannoma, 450, 454, 454f, 458. *See also* Vestibular schwannoma
Posterior fossa approach
  bony exposure, 494
  foramen magnum region surgery
    chordoma, 500
    glomus tumor, 500
  petroclival lesions, 429
    extradural-presigmoid, 429–435, 430–434f
    intradural, 435–436, 435f
Posterior fossa decompression, 458
Posterior meningeal artery, 413
Posterior pituitary. *See* Neurohypophysis
Posterior skull base
  anatomy, 27–29, 28–29f
  congenital anomalies, 514
  imaging, 98–100, 99–100f
    cerebellopontine angle lesions, 98–99, 98–99f, 98t
    foramen magnum lesions, 98t, 102
    jugular fossa tumors, 98t, 100–102, 100–101f
Posterior spinal arteries, 28
Posterior superior alveolar artery
Posterior triangle, 413
Posterolateral approach, vertebral artery, 536f, 537–538
  foramen magnum region lesions, 546, 547f
  head position/movement, 545
  indications, 548, 548t
Posterolateral (Glasscock's) triangle, 267, 268f
Postoccipital procedures, 8
Postoperative management
  infratemporal–middle fossa approach, 337
  lateral transcondylar approach to foramen magnum, 496
  maxillotomy, extended unilateral, 224, 228, 234
  maxillotomy complications, 234
  nursing care, 132–135, 135f, 601
  phases of, 599–606
    intensive care, 132–135, 135f, 599–602, 600f, 600t, 601f, 602f
    intermediate period (2 weeks-3 months postoperative), 603, 603f, 604f
    late postperative (after 3 months), 604–606, 605f
    recovery room, 599
    ward management, 602–603
  transmandibular approach, 345
  vestibular schwannoma, 455
Postradiation fibrosis, 74, 76f
Preauricular infratemporal approach
  foramen magnum region, 504f, 505
  petroclival region, 423
  recurrent adenoid cystic carcinoma, 368
Preauricular skin lesions, presentation, 82
Prechiasmal sulcus, 17f, 20f

670 / SUBJECT INDEX

Preoperative assessment, 124
　biopsies, 111–113, 112f, 113t
　carotid artery, 105–107, 106f, 105–111, 106–110f. *See also* Carotid artery, assessment techniques
　　ICA, 360
　　ICA to MCA bypass, 371
　embolization of vascular lesions, 113–116, 113t, 114–116f
　ICA to MCA bypass, 371
　imaging. *See* Imaging
　infratemporal–middle fossa approach, 309
　nursing, 124, 127
　occipitoatlantoaxial surgery, 492
　subcranial approaches, transbasal–Derome, 352, 357
　transmandibular approach, 342
　vertebral artery, 552
Preoperative management
　infratemporal–middle fossa approach, 313
　maxillotomy, extended unilateral, 210–212, 210t, 211t
　nursing care, 121–124, 126
　prevention of complications, 585
Patient preparation
　infratemporal–middle fossa approach, 313, 313f
　of operative sites, 126
　transoral approach to clivum and foramen magnum region, 522, 522f, 523f
Prepontine area, petroclival anatomy, 425
Prepontine cisterns, 437
Presentation. *See* Clinical presentation
Presigmoid approach
　intradural, 352–353, 353f
　petroclival region, 423, 429–435, 430–434f
　　combined approaches, 438–440, 438–440f
　retrosellar lesion, 354f
　vertebral artery management, 546
Prevertebral veins, tumor emboli, 67
Primary tumors
　metastases. *See specific primary sites*
　second, 61
Proatlantal artery, 534
Processus cochleariformis, 380
Processus jugularis, 28
Prolactinoma, 564
　clinical presentation, 520, 520f
　maxillotomy, extended unilateral, 228t
　treatment, 577
Proptosis, 69, 74, 76f, 520, 520f
Prostate cancer metastases, 46f, 47, 47f, 66, 66t, 67, 67t, 310
　clivus, 517f
　imaging, 70, 71, 95
　temporal bone, 386
Prosthetic rehabilitation
　anterior fossa, 193, 193f
　external ear, 405
　hearing, 605–606, 605f
　orbit, 406, 605, 605f
Proton density images, 87
Protympanum, 22, 475
Pseudoaneurysm, 111
Psychiatry, 123–124
Pterion, 20
Pterional approach, sellar/parasellar region, 567f, 575, 576f, 580

Pterional bone flap, cranioorbital zygomatic approach, 266, 266f, 278
Pterygoid base, maxillotomy, extended unilateral, 223f, 225f
Pterygoid branch of ICA, 23
Pterygoid canal, 22
Pterygoid fossa, imaging, 88
Pterygoid muscle
　infratemporal–middle fossa approach, 322
　lateral and medial, 25
　maxillary sinus tumor presentation, 79
　maxillotomy, extended unilateral, 224, 225f
　postoperative care after resection, 603
　subcranial extended transfacial approach, 290, 290f, 291, 291f
　　Type II, 301
　　Type III, 305
　temporal bone anatomy, 378
Pterygoid osteotomy, 223f
Pterygoid plate
　anatomy, 25, 26f, 27f
　erosion of, 6
　facial degloving approach, 195, 208
　infratemporal–middle fossa approach, 322, 328
　lateral, 25, 26f, 27f, 215, 216f
　maxillectomy, 180f, 183
　maxillotomy, extended unilateral, 214f, 215, 216f, 217f, 218, 219f, 221, 221f, 224, 225f
　medial
　　anatomy, 24, 25, 26f, 380
　　oropharyngeal, parotid, and upper neck lesions, 85
　　transmandibular approach, 341
　subcranial approaches, transbasal–Derome, 357
　subcranial approaches, transfacial approach, 291
　　Type II, 298–299, 299–300f
　　Type III, 304
　transfacial approaches, 173, 174f
　transmandibular approach, 341, 343
Pterygoid plexus, 22, 25
　anatomy, 67f
　emissary veins to, 21
　hemorrhage, 593
　temporal bone anatomy, 378
　temporalis elevation, 316
　tumor, patterns of spread, 64
Pterygoid process, 25
Pterygomandibular raphe, maxillotomy, extended unilateral, 223
Pterygomaxillary fissure, 25
　infratemporal–middle fossa approach, temporalis elevation, 316
　maxillotomy, extended unilateral, 215, 216f, 217f
Pterygomaxillary fossa, 27, 341
Pterygopalatine area, extended subcranial approaches, 245, 256–258, 256–258f
Pterygopalatine artery, 197f
Pterygopalatine fossa
　facial degloving, 195, 199, 199f
　imaging, 90f, 94f
　maxillotomy, extended unilateral, 215
　subcranial approaches, 355–356, 355–356f
　transmandibular approach, 343

Pterygopalatine ganglion, 379
Pulmonary embolus, 486t
Pyomucoceles, sinus tumor presentation, 80
Pyramidal bone, petroclival tumor surgery, 429
Pyramidal eminence, temporal bone anatomy, 379
Pyriform sinus
　anterior wall ostectomy, 170, 171f
　facial degloving approach, 198, 213f
　sellar/parasellar surgery, 569, 572, 572f

R

Radial artery grafting, 373
Radial forearm free flaps, 608–611, 609–610f
Radiation therapy
　and complications
　　osteomyelitis, 597
　　pericranial flap slough, 595
　and flap necrosis, 603
　ICA management, tumor biology and, 360
　jugular fossa tumors, 420, 421
　　glomus tumors, 409
　　jugulotympanic paraganglioma, 487
　maxillotomy, extended unilateral, 233
　reconstruction after, 193, 623
　recurrence, postradiation fibrosis and, 74
　sellar/parasellar lesions
　　chordoma, 581
　　pituitary tumors, 578, 579, 580
　subcranial approaches, treatment philosophy, 357
　and temporal bone resection, 377
　temporal bone tumors, 381, 387, 404, 406–407, 406–407f
　transcervicomastoid approach, 412, 412f
　vertebral artery necrosis, 551t
　vestibular schwannoma, 446
　and wound healing, 603, 603f
Radical mastoidectomy, 8
Radical neck dissection, 313, 314f
Radiculomuscular artery, 534
Radiology. *See* Imaging
Radionuclide scans
　jugulotympanic paraganglioma, 476–477
　metastases, 70
　nursing care, 122
Radiosurgery, 71, 446–447, 448
Rainey clips, 587
Rand, R.W., 9
Rathke's cleft cysts, 560t, 562, 581
Raveh, J., 7
Raveh dissectors, 513, 513f, 527
Reconstruction/defect repair, 00
　anterior approaches, craniotomy, 185–186, 186f
　anterior cranial floor defect repair, 296f
　anterior fossa after transfacial approaches, 190–193, 190–193f
　complications
　　flap dehiscence, 593
　　osteomyelitis, 595–596, 596f
　cranial/pericranial tissue, 182f, 183–184, 183–184f
　cranioorbital zygomatic approach, 270–271
　　trauma, 282–285, 284–285f
　　tumors, 277f, 278

dural dehiscence and pneumocephalus, 593
facial degloving approach, 196
free flap techniques, 607–621. *See also* Flaps, free
goals of, 608
hemorrhage, 595
infratemporal fossa approach, 484
infratemporal–middle fossa approach, 313, 335–339, 336–338f
   preparation, 313
   zygomatic ostectomy, 319, 320, 320f, 321f
jugular foramen surgery, 417
jugulotympanic paraganglioma, 484
maxillary antrum, 198
maxillectomy, 180f, 295f
maxillotomy, 210, 223, 224, 227f, 230, 234
nursing care
   donor site preparation, 128
   intraoperative, 125
   postoperative, 133
   preoperative studies, 122
   wound care, 134
orbital exenteration, 175
periocranial flap slough, 594f
postoperative monitoring, 601
prevention of complications, 588–589, 588f
recurrence considerations, 74
recurrent adenoid cystic carcinoma, 368, 370f
regional flap and graft techniques, 623–638. *See also* Flaps and grafts, regional
subcranial approaches
   extended anterior, 241, 244f, 245, 249–252, 250–252f
   extended transfacial, 297–298, 303, 305, 308
   frontobasal/degloving, 356, 356f
   transbasal–Derome, 347, 348, 351, 351f, 352–353, 352–353f, 357, 357f
temporal bone resection, 377, 387, 396f, 401
   total petrosectomy, 402
   tympanic membrane, 393
temporalis muscle limitations, 24
temporal resection, 403–404, 403–404f
transcervicomastoid approach, 416–418, 417–419f
transfacial approaches, 190–193, 190–193f
   subcranial extended, 297–298, 303, 305, 308
transmandibular approach, 343–344
transoral approach, 522, 529, 530f, 531
vestibular schwannoma, 455, 457, 464, 464f, 470
Records, medical, 585
Recovery room care, 131, 599
Rectosigmoid approach, 9
Rectus abdominis flaps, 611–616, 611–615f
   infratemporal–middle fossa approach, 338f
   preparation, 313
   reconstruction, 337, 337f
   meningioma, 611–613, 611–613f
   recurrent adenoid cystic carcinoma, 368, 370f
   squamous cell carcinoma of orbit and nasal skin, 613–616, 614–615f
   temporal bone reconstruction, 404
   total petrosectomy, 402
   transmandibular approach, 344
Rectus capitis lateralis muscle, 415

Rectus capitis posterior major, 29
Rectus gyrus, 281
Rectus muscle, tendons of, 19
Recurrence
   imaging problems, 74, 76f
   infratemporal–middle fossa approach, 310
   jugular fossa tumors, 421
   local
      en bloc technique with, 165
      indications for combined transfacial approach, 167
   perineural spread of skin tumor, 75f, 76f
   temporal bone, 382
Recurrent laryngeal nerve, 637
Referred pain, 70
Regional flaps and grafts. *See* Flaps and grafts, regional
Rehabilitation, 604
Relaxation time, 88
Renal adenocarcinoma, 47f
Renal cell carcinoma, 66, 66t, 69f
   chemo- and radiosensitivity, 71
   metastasis, 67, 67t
   pathophysiology, 52t
Renal function, postoperative monitoring, 599
Resection/dissection/tumor margins. *See also* Frozen sections
   en bloc. *See* En bloc resection
   esthesioneuroblastoma, 355–356, 355–356f
   infratemporal–middle fossa approach, brain resection, 335
   jugular foramen surgery, 418f
   Mohs, 61, 73, 389f
   petroclival tumors, 423
   and radiation therapy, 406
   subcranial approaches
      transbasal–Derome procedure, 348
      treatment philosophy, 357
   temporal bone resection, 397
   temporal bone tumors, 387
   temporal craniotomy, 397
   total petrosectomy, 401–402
   treatment philosophy, 347
   vestibular schwannoma, 455
Respiration
   grunting, 586f, 586, 592–593
   nasopharyngeal tumor presentation, 83
   postoperative management, 599
   Valsalva maneuver, 464, 571, 572
Retina, VEPs, 154–155, 156f
Retinoblastoma, 5
Retrolabyrinthine approach
   petroclival region, 423
   vertebral artery management, 546
Retromandibular approach, needle biopsy, 112f, 113
Retropharyngeal lymph nodes, 311
Retropharyngeal space
   drainage, 11
   maxillotomy, extended unilateral, 222–224, 225–227f, 230
Retrosigmoid approach
   petroclival region, 423, 435
   vestibular schwannoma, 447, 448–449, 457–465, 458–464f
Revascularization, vertebral artery management, 540f, 541, 549–550, 550f, 551t, 552t

Rhabdomyosarcoma
   imaging, 90
   mid-skull base approaches, 209t
   pathology, 41–42, 42f
   temporal bone, 380, 383t, 384
Rheumatoid arthritis. *See* Arthritis
Rhinectomy, 74
Rhinoplasty incisions, 195
Rhinorrhea, CSF, 602
Rhinotomy. *See also* Lateral rhinotomy
   complications, osteomyelitis, 595
   subcranial approaches, extended anterior versus, 245
Roll-over, vestibular schwannoma, 447
Rosenmüller, fossa of, 83
Round window, 380, 413, 450
Rouviére, node of, 84f, 85
Rubber vascular loops, 494, 587, 588f

S
Saggital sinus
   anatomy, 15, 16, 16f, 17f, 67f
   cranioorbital zygomatic approach, bifrontal, 273, 274f
   craniotomy considerations, 186
Salivary gland tumors
   adenoid cystic carcinoma, 33
   pathophysiology, 54, 56–57
   temporal bone metastases, 386
Samii, M., 11, 11f
Santorini, fissure of, 83, 381, 386
Saphenous vein graft, 332, 333f
   ICA, 361–363, 361–363f
      cavernous sinus syndrome, 363–367, 363–367f
      recurrent adenoid cystic carcinoma, 367–370, 367–370f
   infratemporal–middle fossa approach, 313, 313f
   operative technique, 373
   results, 373
   subcranial approaches
      extended transfacial Type III, 305, 305f, 306–307f
      transbasal–Derome, 352
   vertebral artery, 540f, 541, 551
Sarcoidosis, sellar/parasellar, 563, 581
Sarcomas 47t
   anterior approaches
      periorbital resection, 168
      subcranial, 259t
   external auditory meatus/temporal bone, 383t, 384–385
   imaging
      anterior skull base lesions, 89t
      foramen magnum lesions, 102
   maxillotomy, extended unilateral, 228t
   mid-skull base approaches, 209t
   pathophysiology, 52t, 54
   vertebral artery involvement, 542t, 542, 542t, 543f, 546t
Scala tympani, 380
Scalp
   skin cancer pathophysiology, 54, 61
   temporal bone resection, 387
Scapular free flaps, 619–621, 619–620f
Schramm, V., 10–11, 10f
Schramm and Sekhar modified Fisch approach, 309

Schwannoma. *See also* Vestibular schwannoma
  foramen magnum region surgery, 503
  ICA management, 360
  imaging, 92t
  infratemporal–middle fossa approach, 309
  jugulotympanic paraganglioma versus, 478
  mid-skull base approaches, 209t
  occipitoatloaxial region, 491
  pathophysiology, 52t
  petroclival, 423, 426, 429, 434f, 436
  subcranial extended transfacial approach, 305, 306f
Sclerosing basal cell carcinoma, 73
Sclerosis, imaging, 95, 102
Secondary carcinoma of temporal bone, 386
Second primary, 61
Secretions, imaging, 87, 88
Seizures, 82, 564, 580, 600
Sekhar, L.N., 10f, 11
Sella/parasellar region, 17f, 19, 20f, 20, 20f
  anatomy, 555–560, 556–559f, 558, 559f
    nasal cavity, 555, 557f
    parasellar structures, 558, 559f
    pituitary gland and hypothalamus, 555, 558, 558–559f
    sphenoid bone and sella, 555, 556f, 557f
  clinical presentation, 563–565
  craniorbital zygomatic approach, 239, 271, 276–277f, 278
  craniopharyngioma, 92
  diagnostic evaluation, 565–566
  imaging, 87, 89, 89f, 92
  management of lesions, 555–581
  metastases, 66, 67t, 70, 71f
  pathology, 560–563, 561–562t
    inflammation, 563
    neoplastic lesions, 560–562, 560t, 561t
    nonneoplastic cysts, 562–563
    vascular lesions, 563
  petroclival anatomy, 425
  pneumatization, 27, 555, 557f
  postoperative care, 602
  sphenoid sinus tumor presentation, 81
  surgical approaches, 566–577, 566t, 567–576f
    extracranial extradural, 566–573, 566t, 567–574f
    midface degloving with maxillotomy, 573
    subcranial transbasal–Derome, 347, 350, 352, 354–355, 354–355f
    transcranial-intradural, 574–577, 575–576f
    transoral, 527
    transsphenoethmoidal, 573–574
  treatment, 577–581
    apoplexy, 579
    inflammation and infection, 581
    pituitary adenoma, 577–579
    pituitary carcinoma, 579
    posterior pituitary tumors, 579–581
  tumor spread, 64, 66, 67t
  VEPs during resection, 157f
Semicircular canal, 21
  petroclival anatomy, 427f
  petroclival surgery, 431
  petrous bone anatomy, 426f, 426
  vestibular schwannoma, 450, 451f, 452f, 463f, 465, 468

Sensory evoked potentials, 138, 148, 148f
  during carotid endarterectomy, 153f
  cerebral blood flow effects, 359
  foramen magnum region surgery, 492
  nerve stimulation effects, 144f, 145f
Sensory nerves
  neurotropic tumors, 165
  temporal bone anatomy, 379
Sensory neuropathy, vestibular schwannoma, 444, 445
Sensory root of cranial nerve V, 22
Serous otitis, 345
Serratus anterior free flaps, 616–618, 616–618f
Shaw cautery knife, 414
Shoulder weakness, jugular foramen syndrome, 519
SIADH, 600, 602
Sigmoid curve, 19
Sigmoid sinus, 22, 27, 28
  anatomy, 67f
    foramen magnum region, 496f
    jugular foramen, 413
    petroclival, 427f
    temporal bone, 378, 378f
  foramen magnum region tumors, 494, 494f, 496
  jugular foramen, 549f
  jugular foramen surgery, 415, 416, 416f, 417f, 421
  jugulotympanic paraganglioma, 475, 480, 485f
  petroclival surgery, 429, 430f, 431, 435
  petrous bone anatomy, 426
  subcranial extended transfacial approach, 305
  temporal bone resection, 388f
  temporal bone tumors, 382, 397
  thrombosis, ear tumor presentation, 83
  tumor pathophysiology, 53, 53f, 57
  vertebral artery management, 539, 549, 549f
  vestibular schwannoma, 450, 451f, 452f, 454, 460f
Sinodural angle, temporal bone resection, 400
Sinonasal tract anatomy, 16
Sinus box paradigm, 78, 78f
Sinuses, paranasal. *See* Nasal/paranasal sinuses; Nasal/paranasal sinus tumors; *specific sinuses*
Sinuses, vascular. *See* Vascular sinuses; *specific structures*
Sinusitis, 78
Sinus mucosa, anterior fossa reconstruction, 191
Skin
  jugular foramen surgery, 416
  maxillary sinus tumor presentation, 78
Skin cancer, 32t. *See also* Basal cell carcinoma; Melanoma
  craniocervical/clival metastases, 519
  pathophysiology, 51, 54, 56, 57, 61, 69f
  presentation
    ear lesions, 82–83, 82–83f
    eyelid lesions, 73
  reconstruction
    rectus abdominis free flaps, 613–616, 614–615f
    subscapular graft, 619, 619f
  transfacial approach indications, 165, 167f
Skin flaps, 317f, 343. *See also* Flaps, free; Flaps and grafts, regional

Skull base conference, 124
Skull base coordinator, 130
Slings, 405
Small bowel cancer, 67
SMAS, 315, 391f
Smith, M.F.W., 9
Smith, R.R., 5
Social services, 123–124
Soft tissue compression, cephalometrics, 521, 521f, 522f
Somatosensory evoked potentials, 148–151, 148–153f
  carotid assessment, 386–387
  ICA dissection, 373
SPECT
  cerebral blood flow assessment, 108, 109, 110f, 360
  infratemporal–middle fossa approach, 309, 313
  nursing care, 121
  subcranial extended transfacial approach, 291
  temporal bone tumor management, 386
Speech problems, 82, 519
Sphenocavernous area, cavernous sinus syndrome, 363, 364f
Sphenoclival defect, maxillotomy, 213
Sphenoclival region, subcranial approaches, 239, 243f, 246–248f, 259f
Sphenoethmoid approach
  anterior maxillotomy-medial maxillectomy, 292–298, 293–298f
  sella/parasellar region, 573–574
Sphenoethmoid plane, subcranial approaches, 239, 245
Sphenoethmoid tumors, 7, 260, 287, 288f
Sphenoid
  anatomy, 15, 16–17, 17f, 19, 20f, 27f
    sellar region, 555, 556f, 557f
    temporal bone, 377
  anterior face, 27f
  craniorbital zygomatic approach, 266
  facial degloving, transmaxillary approach, 199
  maxillotomy, extended unilateral, 207, 209, 214f, 222, 223, 223f, 224, 225f, 231t
  optic canal, 19
  petroclival lesions. *See* Petroclival lesions
  pneumatization of, 27
  sellar/parasellar lesions, transsphenoidal approach, 566–575, 566t, 567–573f
  spine of, 25
  subcranial approaches
    extended anterior, 243f, 245, 246–248f, 250f, 253–254, 253–254f
    extended transfacial, 290, 291, 299, 301
  synostosis with occiput, 27
  transfacial approaches
    extended subcranial, 290, 291, 299, 301
    maxillectomy, 173
  transmandibular approach, 341
  transoral approaches to clivus, 526, 526f
  tumor invasion, 61
  zygomatic craniorbital approach, 267, 267f
Sphenoid body, 19
Sphenoidectomy, 198, 201, 201f
Sphenoidotomy, 288t
Sphenoid ridge, 6, 20, 21, 267, 267f
Sphenoid sinus
  anatomy, 15, 16, 17f, 21, 23f, 27, 59

sella and parasellar, 555, 556f, 557f, 559f
clivus tumor involvement, 562
CSF leak, 591, 592f
extended transfacial subcranial approach, 287, 288f
facial degloving, 195, 195–196, 197f
 sublabial transoral, 208
 transmaxillary approach, 199, 199f
foramen magnum region surgery, 504f, 523
hemorrhage, 593f, 595
imaging, 81, 92, 565
infratemporal–middle fossa approach, carotid artery management, 332
maxillotomy, extended unilateral, 214f, 222, 223f, 232t
middle skull base, 27
nasal and paranasal sinus tumor spread, 82
sellar/parasellar lesions, 92, 563, 565, 572
subcranial approaches
 extended transfacial, 287, 288, 288f, 292, 297
 frontobasal/degloving, 356, 356f
 transbasal–Derome, 350–351, 351f, 353f, 354f
transfacial approaches
 maxillectomy, 173, 174f
 subcranial, 287, 288, 288f, 292, 297
transmandibular approach, 343
transoral approach, 527
transsphenoidal approach to sella, 572
Sphenoid sinusitis, 563
Sphenoid sinus tumors
cranioorbital zygomatic approach, 274, 275f
facial degloving-transmaxillary procedure, 201, 201f
facial degloving with craniotomy, 202, 203f, 204f
imaging, 88, 89, 89f, 89t, 90
metastatic, 47
presentation, 82f
symptoms, 81, 81f, 82f
transfacial subcranial approaches, extended, 288, 288f
tumor pathophysiology, 54
Sphenoid spine, 26f
Sphenoid wing
anatomy, 15, 20, 27, 556f
cranioorbital approach, 263
cranioorbital zygomatic approach, 269, 277f, 279, 279f
imaging, 92
infratemporal–middle fossa approach, 309
maxillotomy, extended unilateral, 224, 225f, 231t
sellar/parasellar meningioma, 580
subcranial approaches, transbasal–Derome, 350
tumor pathophysiology, 53, 53f
Sphenoid wing, greater, 20, 27
Sphenopalatine artery, 114
Sphenopalatine foramen, 231t
Sphenopalatine ganglion, 25, 173, 231t
Sphenoparietal sinus, 15, 22
Spinal accessory nerve. See Cranial nerve XI
Spinal arteries
 anterior, 29, 534, 538
 posterior, 28

Spinal branches of accessory nerve, 28
Spinal cord
 nasopharyngeal tumor involvement, 85
 patient positioning, SEP effects, 150, 151f
 transoral approach, 515–516
Spinal cord compression, 516f
Spinal nerve, first, 507
Spinal nerve roots
 imaging, foramen magnum lesions, 102
 vertebral artery compression, 545
 vertebral artery management
  anatomy, 533–534
  anterolateral, 538
  complications, 552
  control and mobilization, 539f
  control of segments, 538
  posterolateral, 537, 537f
Spinal root of accessory nerve, 28f
Spine, cervical. See Cervical spine
Splenius capitis, 29
Squamous cell carcinoma, 47t
 cranioorbital zygomatic approach, 274, 275f
 foramen magnum region, 516–517, 517f
 frontal sinus primary, 167, 168f
 ICA management
  saphenous vein bypass graft, 361–363, 361–363f
  tumor biology and, 360
 imaging, 95
 infratemporal–middle fossa approach, 309
  carotid artery management, 331
  carotid resection, 330
  diagnosis/presentation, 311f
 nasopharyngeal carcinoma, 35, 35t
 orbital exenteration indications, 173
 pathology, 32–33, 32t, 33f, 37t
 pathophysiology, 51, 57, 69f
 perineural spread, 69f, 95
 presentation, 74, 77
  ear lesions, 82–83, 82–83f
  maxillary sinus tumors, 79f
 reconstruction, rectus abdominis free flaps, 613–616, 614–615f
 subcranial approaches, extended anterior, 259t
 temporal bone, 380, 381, 383, 383f, 383t
 transfacial approach indications, 165, 167f
Squamous temporal bone, 20
 maxillotomy landmarks, 225f
 osteomyelitis, 596–597, 596f
 vestibular schwannoma, 465, 466f, 467f
Staging, temporal bone tumors, 382–382t
Stapedial reflexes, 445
Stapedius muscle, 379
Stapes, 419
Stenosis, vertebral artery, 544
Stereotaxic radiosurgery, 448
Stereotaxy, frameless, 577
Sternocleidomastoid muscle, 28, 29
 atrophy of, 69
 jugular foramen anatomy, 413
 jugular foramen surgery, 414
 jugular foramen syndrome, 519
 jugulotympanic paraganglioma, 480
 neck dissection, 402–403
 transmandibular approach, 342
 vertebral artery management

anterolateral approach, 538
complications, 552
posterolateral approach, 537f
Sternocleidomastoid muscle flap
 incision, 625, 625f
 infratemporal–middle fossa approach, reconstruction, 337
 jugular foramen surgery, 417
Sternomastoid muscle, 413, 492, 493f
Stomach cancer metastases, 386
Straight sinus, 28, 67f
Stroke
 carotid occlusion and, 359
 embolization, therapeutic, 114
 ICA graft complications, 373
 ICA ligation and, 404
 ICA management, 361
 infratemporal–middle fossa approach
  carotid artery dissection complications, 332f
  diagnosis/presentation, 311
 jugulotympanic paraganglioma, 478, 486t
 postoperative monitoring, 133–134, 600
 therapeutic embolization complications, 113
Stryker blade, 218, 220f
Stump pressure, 107
Styloid process, 22, 24, 25f, 26f, 400
Stylomastoid artery, 113t
Stylomastoid foramen, 24
 imaging, 88
 jugular foramen anatomy, 413
 jugular foramen surgery, 415–416
 jugulotympanic paraganglioma, 481, 484f
 temporal bone anatomy, 379
Stylomastoid periosteum, 481, 484
Subarachnoid hemorrhage, 551
Subarachnoid part of vertebral artery, 29
Subarachnoid space
 ICA management, 360
 pneumocephalus, 593
 posterior atlantooccipital membrane, 29
 temporal bone anatomy, 378
 temporal bone tumor involvement, 386
 vertebral artery, 533
Subclavian artery, 29
Subcranial approaches
 anterior
  transbasal–Derome, 347–358. See also Transbasal approach, Derome modification
  transfacial extended, 287–308. See also Transfacial subcranial approach, extended
 petroclival tumors, 348
Subcranial extended anterior approach, 239–260
 complications, 258–259, 260t
 ostetomy types, 240
 preoperative evaluation, 239–240
 reconstruction, 241, 243f, 244
 results, 258–260, 259f, 260t
 technique, 240, 241–244f
 tumor location, 245–258
  anterior skull base planes with intracranial, nasal lumen, and maxillary sinus extension, 245, 249–258, 249–258f
  posterior ethmoid, sphenoid, and clivus, 245, 246–249f

Subcranial extended anterior approach (contd.)
  tumor types
    esthesioneuroblastoma, 249–252, 250–252f, 254–255, 255f
    juvenile angiofibroma, 256–258, 256–258f
    squamous cell carcinoma, 253–254, 253–254f
    survival rates, 259t
Subcranial relationships
  anterior skull base, 16–19, 18–19f
  middle skull base, 24–27, 24–27f
Subcranial tissue. See Infratemporal fossa–middle fossa approach
Subcranial trapezoid, 26f
Subfascial dissection, cranioorbital zygomatic approach, 271–272
Subfrontal approach, sellar/parasellar lesions, 567f, 574, 575f, 580
Subfrontal dissection, with cranioorbital zygomatic approach, 269
Subfrontal-lamina terminalis approach, 580
Sublabial approach, 3, 5
Sublabial incision, facial degloving approach, 196f
Sublabial transoral degloving approach, 208
Sublabial variation, transsphenoid approach, 569
Sublingual gland, 379
Submandibular ganglion, 379
Submandibular gland, 343, 379
Submastoid approach, 112f, 113
Submucous resection, septum, 3
Suboccipital approach, 9
  lateral, 491
  petroclival region, 423, 435
  vestibular schwannoma, 445, 457
Suboccipital craniectomy, 435, 494
Suboccipital muscles, 29
Suboccipital musculature, 28
Suboccipital transmeatal approach, 9
Suboccipital triangle, 29
Subperiosteal dissection
  degloving, 195
  mandibular condylectomy, 392f
  petroclival surgery, 430
Subperiosteal elevation, degloving, 197–200, 197–199f
Subscapular free flaps, 618–621, 619–620f
Subtemporal approaches
  foramen magnum region, 500, 504f, 505
  petroclival region, 423
  preauricular infratemporal, 505
  presigmoid, 440, 440f
  sellar/parasellar meningioma, 580
  transtentorial approach, 436–437, 436f
Subtemporal dissection, with cranioorbital zygomatic approach, 269
Subtemporal trapezoid, 24
Subtemporal trapezoid exposure, 322, 326–329f
Subzygomatic approaches, needle biopsy, 112f, 113
Suction drain
  infratemporal–middle fossa approach, 337
  maxillotomy, extended unilateral, 210t, 211t
  nursing care
    intraoperative, 126

wound care, 134
prevention of complications, 589
Superficial middle cerebral vein, 22
Superficial petrosal nerve
  cranioorbital zygomatic approach, 267, 268f
  greater and lesser, 21, 22
  petrous bone anatomy, 425f
  temporal bone anatomy, 379
  vestibular schwannoma, 465, 468, 468f
Superficial temporal artery, 24f, 264, 316
Superficial temporal fascia, 624, 624f, 624t
Superior anastomotic vein of Trolard, 22
Superior cerebellar artery, 28
  aneurysm, cranioorbital zygomatic approach, 278
  petroclival surgery, middle fossa intradural approach, 436f
  petrous bone anatomy, 426f
Superior cerebral vein of Trollard, 397
Superior cerebral veins, 16, 22
Superior constrictor muscle, 85, 343, 524
Superior hypophyseal artery, 559f
Superior hypophyseal artery aneurysm, 281, 281f
Superior laryngeal nerve, 230
Superior maxillectomy, 179
Superior oblique muscle, 156, 492
Superior ophthalmic vein, 19
  anatomy, 67f
  cavernous sinus, 22
  tumor extension via, 59, 59f, 60f, 61
Superior orbital fissure
  anatomy, 19, 19f, 20f, 21, 556f
  cavernous sinus anatomy, 65f
  cranioorbital zygomatic approach, 267, 267f, 269
  facial degloving approaches
    combined, 201
    transmaxillary procedure, 201
  infratemporal–middle fossa approach, 334
  nasal and paranasal sinus tumor spread, 82
  orbital exenteration, 175, 177
  subcranial approaches
    transbasal–Derome, 350
    transfacial, extended, 296–297
  tumor pathophysiology, 55–56, 55–56f
Superior petrosal sinus, 21, 22, 28
  anatomy, 67f
    petrous bone, 425
    sella and parasellar, 555
    temporal bone, 379f
  infratemporal–middle fossa approach, 334
  petroclival surgery, 431f, 431, 432f, 437
  temporal bone resection, 388f
  temporal craniotomy, 397
Superior pharyngeal constrictor muscle, 27
  maxillotomy, extended unilateral, 223, 231t, 232t
  transoral approaches to clivus, 525f
Superior rectus muscle, 19
Superior sagittal sinus
  anatomy, 15–16, 16f, 17f, 67f
  craniotomy considerations, 186
  frontal sinus tumor presentation, 81
  infratemporal–middle fossa approach, 335
Superior semicircular canal, 21
Superior thyroid artery, 115

Superior vestibular nerve, 425, 445, 454f
Superolateral cranioorbital approach, 272
Suppurative otitis media, 381
Supracavernous portion of ICA, 24f, 25f
Supraclinoid carotid, 23f
Supraorbital approach. See also Cranioorbital approach
  cranioobital, 271–272, 272–273f
  traumatic encephalocele, orbital roof, 284f
Supraorbital artery, 348, 348f
Supraorbital bone flap, 271, 272f, 278
Supraorbital foramen, 264, 265f
Supraorbital nerve
  cranioorbital zygomatic approach, 264, 265f
  craniotomy, 184
  frontal sinus tumor presentation, 81
  subcranial approaches, 348, 348f
Supraorbital–pterional bone flap, 266, 266f
Supraorbital vein, 67f
Supratentorial-presigmoid approach, petroclival tumor, 438–439, 438–439f
Supratrochlear nerve, 81, 184
Sural nerve grafts, 405, 637, 637f
Swallowing/dysphagia, 69, 519
  complications, 405. See also Aspiration
  maxillotomy, extended unilateral, 223, 230
  odontectomy, 531
  rehabilitation program, 123, 406
  transoral approach, 522
  symptoms
    ear tumor, 83
    glomus tumors, 412
    petroclival tumors, 426
  postoperative management, 602, 603
Swan-Ganz catheter, 107
Sylvian fissure, 278, 281, 575
Sylvian vein, 268
Symptoms. See Clinical presentation
Syncope, clival compression and, 521
Synostosis, basisphenoid-basiocciput, 27
Synovial cyst, 98t, 102t, 546, 546t

T
Tarsorrhaphy, temporary, 586, 587f
  maxillotomy, extended unilateral, 210t, 212
  postoperative care, 602, 602f
Team, surgical. See Multidisciplinary team
Team coordinator, 119, 120f, 122
Technetium scans. See SPECT
Tectorial membrane, 511f
Teeth
  extended anterior subcranial approaches, 254, 254f
  mandibulotomy, 343, 346
  maxillectomy, 179, 180f
  maxillotomy, extended unilateral, 220f, 230, 232t
  maxillotomy complications, 228, 228t, 234
  prosthetic rehabilitation, 605
Tegmen, 382, 382t, 451f
Tegmen mastoideum, 397, 402f
Tegmen tympani, 20, 380, 468, 469f
Temperature, body
  hypothermia, induced, 360, 361
  neurophysiological monitoring, 143
    EEG, 148
    SEPs, 149–150

Temperature, operating room, 126
Temporal arteries, deep, 24
Temporal bone
  carotid canal, 22
  cranioorbital approach, 263, 277f, 278
  foramen magnum region surgery, 494, 500, 502f, 504f, 505
  ICA, 23–24, 24f
  imaging, 69f
    central skull base lesions, 96f
    cerebellopontine angle lesions, 99f
  infratemporal–middle fossa approach, 322, 326f
  jugular foramen anatomy, 413
  jugular fossa tumors, transcervicomastoid approach, 420
  jugulotympanic paraganglioma, 474, 476
  maxillotomy, extended unilateral, 225f, 231–232t
  naspharyngeal tumor spread, 83
  petroclival lesions. See Petroclival lesions
  postoperative care, 602
  subcranial approaches, 239, 301
  subcranial relationships of posterior skull base, 28
  symptoms with lesions of, 82–83, 82–83f
  transcervicomastoid approach, 415–416, 415–416f
  tumor biology, 32t, 34t, 54, 66, 69f
    invasion,, 58f, 59, 61, 61f
    primary sites with metastases, 32t
  tympanic portion (vaginal process), 25
  vestibular schwannoma, 448–449, 465, 466f, 467f
Temporal bone, petrous ridge of, 20
Temporal bone, squamous
  anatomy, 20
  maxillotomy landmarks, 225f
  osteomyelitis, 596–597, 596f
  vestibular schwannoma, 465, 466f, 467f
Temporal bone resection
  anatomy, 377–380, 378–380f
  clinical features, 381
  complications, 404–406, 405f
  etiology, 381
  histologic types, 383–386
  incidence of malignancies, 380–381
  management, 386–404
    biopsy, 387
    carotid artery, 386–387
    cavity ablation, 400
    closure, 401
    complete resection, 393, 396–399f
    final bony cuts, 399–400, 399f
    hypoglossal-to-facial nerve anastomosis, 400–401
    lateral resection, 387–393, 388–395f
    neck management, 402–403
    reconstruction, 403–404, 403–404f
    surgical considerations, 387
    temporal craniotomy, 397, 399, 399f
    total petrosectomy, 401–402, 401–402f
  patient evaluation, 381–382, 382f
  radiation therapy, 406–407, 406–407f
  reconstruction goals, 623
  staging, 382–382t

Temporal bone tumors
  anterior extension into infratemporal fossa, 310
  imaging, 98t
  infratemporal–middle fossa approach, 309
    diagnosis/presentation, 312f
    incision, 313, 314f
  jugulotympanic paraganglioma. See Jugulotympanic paraganglioma
  pathophysiology, 61
  recurrences after resection, 74
  therapeutic embolization, 115
  transmandibular approach, 341
Temporal craniotomy, 397, 399, 399f
Temporal dura, 502f
Temporal fossa, degloving approach, 195, 198, 200, 200f
Temporalis fascia
  craniotomy, vsemicircular cuff, 183, 183f
  flaps and grafts, 627–630, 627–628f
  infratemporal–middle fossa approach
    incisions, 315, 315f, 316f
    reconstruction, 335, 335f
  subcranial approaches, transbasal–Derome approach, 348
  temporal bone resection, 389, 391f
  vestibular schwannoma, 457
Temporalis fascia graft
  internal auditory canal reconstruction, 464
  jugular foramen surgery, 417
  vestibular schwannoma, 455
Temporalis muscle, 19, 24, 25f
  cranioorbital zygomatic approach, 265f, 266, 271, 277f
  flaps and grafts, 630
    infratemporal fossa approach, 484
    infratemporal–middle fossa approach, 335, 336f, 337
    maxillotomy, extended unilateral, 210
    temporal bone reconstruction, 404
    total petrosectomy, 402
  infratemporal–middle fossa approach, 319f
    adenoid cystic carcinoma, 320f
    elevation of, 315–316, 316f, 319f
    reconstruction, 335, 336f, 337
  jugular foramen surgery, 416, 417
  maxillotomy, extended unilateral, 216f, 224, 225f, 231t
  petroclival surgery, 430, 430f
  vestibular schwannoma, 455, 465, 466f
  wasting of, 604f
Temporal lobe, 22, 27f
  anterior horn, 19
  cavernous sinus, 22
  facial degloving approach, 200, 200f
  infratemporal–middle fossa approach, 335
  nasal and paranasal sinus tumor spread, 82
  petroclival surgery, 431f, 431, 432f, 436
  resection of, 386–387, 395f
  sellar/parasellar region approaches, 575, 577f
  subcranial extended transfacial approach, 299
  temporal bone anatomy, 378, 378f
  vestibular schwannoma, 465, 470f
Temporal lobe dura
  infratemporal–middle fossa approach
    craniotomy, 328–329
    diagnosis/presentation, 311

  reconstruction, 335, 335f
  subcranial extended transfacial approach Type III, 305
  temporal craniotomy, 397
Temporal nerve, 79
Temporomandibular joint (TMJ), 377
  alternatives to excision, 625–626, 626f
  ear lesion involvement, 83
  jugulotympanic paraganglioma, 481
  mandibular condylectomy/resection, 320, 322, 325–326f, 389–393, 390–393
  maxillotomy, extended unilateral, 216f, 221f
  maxillotomy complications, 228, 228t, 233
  postoperative care, 603
  rehabilitation, 406
  squamous cell carcinoma, 383
  subcranial extended transfacial approach, Type II, 299
  temporal bone anatomy, 378f
  temporal bone tumor, 381, 387, 389, 393
  transmandibular approach complications, 345
  transoral approach to middle and posterior fossa, 522
Temporomandibular joint syndrome, 310
Temporoparietal fascia, reconstruction options, 484, 624t
Tensor palati muscle, 27
Tensor tympani, 474
Tensor veli palatini, 25, 231t
Tentorial incisura, 423, 425
Tentorium, 424f, 431, 435, 436, 500
  cranioorbital zygomatic approach, 278
  infratemporal–middle fossa approach, 309
  temporal bone resection, 397
Tentorium cerebelli, 21, 22, 27, 28, 67f
Teratogenic cysts, 209t
Teratoma, 560t
Tessier, P., 6f, 7
Testicular tumors, 67
Thalamus, 148
Third ventricle, 424f, 425, 579
Thromboembolic stockings, 412, 601
Thromboembolism/thrombosis. See also Embolism
  anti-embolic stockings, 601
  carotid artery sacrifice and, 111
  ear tumor presentation, 83
  ICA ligation and, 405
  petroclival surgery complications, 437
  postoperative monitoring, 600
Thyrocervical trunk anastomoses, 113t
Thyroid artery, 115
Thyroid cancer metastases, 47, 386
Thyroid-stimulating hormone-secreting adenoma, 565
Thyroplasty, 305
Thyrotropic adenoma, 578
Titanium fixtures, 193
  cranioorbital zygomatic approach, 278
  defect repair, 588f, 589
  subcranial approaches, 241, 242–244f, 245, 249–252, 250–252f
Tolosa-Hunt syndrome, 310, 310f, 519, 519f, 527
Tongue
  lingual paralysis, 519
  manfibular resection with extended transfacial subcranial approaches, 304

676 / SUBJECT INDEX

Tongue (contd.)
   maxillotomy, extended unilateral, 223
   median labial mandibuloglossoptomy, 522, 523f, 526
   odontectomy complications, 531–532
   subcranial approaches
      extended anterior, 253–254, 253–254f
      extended transfacial, 291, 304
Tonsils
   carcinoma, clinical presentation, 76f, 85
   degloving approach, sublabial transoral, 208
   maxillotomy, extended unilateral, 223, 223f, 226f, 232t
   subcranial extended transfacial approach, 291
Torcular Herophili, 54, 54f, 59
Trabecular structures, 64
Tracheostomy
   foramen magnum region surgery
      chordoma, 500
      transoral approach, 522, 531
   home care planning, 135
   infratemporal–middle fossa approach, 337
   nursing care, 128–129, 133
   nursing staff duties, 128–129
   pneumocephalus prevention, 593
   postoperative care, 601, 602–603
   transcervicomastoid approach, 411
Transbasal approach, 260
Transbasal approach, Derome modification, 347–358
   case reports, 350–357, 350–357f, 357t
      aneurysmatic bone cyst, 350–351, 350–351f
      chondrosarcoma, 351–352, 351–352f
      chordoma, 352–354, 352–354f
      craniopharyngioma, 354–356, 354–356f
   complications, 357
   extradural approach, 349–352, 350–352f
   extradural-intradural, combined, 352–354, 352–354f
   indications and contraindications, 347–348
   intradural approach, 352–355, 352–355f
   reconstruction, 357, 357f
   technique, 348–350, 348–350f
Transcanal approach, jugulotympanic paraganglioma, 478–479, 478t, 479f
Transcervicomastoid approach, 409–422
   anatomy, 413
   anesthesia, 412–413
   diagnosis and imaging, 410–411, 410t, 411f
   embolization and radiation therapy, 412, 412f
   evolution of procedure, 409–410
   indications and alternative treatments, 409
   preoperative evaluation, 411–412
   results and complications, 419–422, 419t, 420t
   technique, 415–418
      skull base exposure, 413–415, 414–415f
      temporal bone exposure, 415–416, 415–416f
      tumor removal and reconstruction, 416–418, 417–419f
Transcochlear approach, petroclival tumor, 441, 441f
Transcondylar approach to craniocervical junction. See Foramen magnum region
Transconjunctival approach, palatine defect reconstruction, 254–255, 255f

Transcranial approaches, 5, 6, 6f, 7, 260
   intradural, 574–577, 575–576f
   chordoma, 581
Transdural tumors, jugulotympanic paraganglioma classification, 478
Transethmoidal approach, 260, 567f
Transethnoid approach, 260
Transfacial approach, 6, 6f, 165–194
   craniotomy, 183–190, 182–189f
   indications, 165–168, 166–168f
   lateral rhinotomy-Denker-medial maxillectomy, 168–173, 168–174f
   maxillectomy, 177–183, 179–181f
   orbital exenteration, 173, 175–177, 175–177f
   reconstruction, 190–193, 190–193f
   results, 193–194
   with subcranial exposure, 355–356, 355–356f
Transfacial subcranial approach, extended, 287–308
   extended anterior versus, 260
   indications, 287–292, 287t, 288–291f
   technique
      type IA: sphenoethmoid anterior maxillotomy-medial maxillectomy approach, 292–298, 293–298f
      type IB (type IA plus orbital exenteration), 292
      type II, 298–303, 298–303f
      type III, 303–308, 304–308f
Transfrontal approach, 3
Transfusion, 131
Transition-type tumors, clival, 517, 517f
Translabyrinthine approach
   cerebellopontine angle, 443
   petroclival region, 423, 441, 441f
   vertebral artery management, 546
   vestibular schwannoma, 447, 448, 449–456, 450–456f
Translabyrinthine procedures, 8
Transmandibular approach, 341–346, 342–345f
   complications, 343–346
   indications, 341
   preoperative evaluation, 342
   technique, 342–345
      labiomandibulotomy, 342–343, 343–344f
      skull base exposure, 343–344, 345
Transmaxillary approach
   degloving, 198–200, 198–200f
   case material, 205
   with external ethmoidectomy, 201, 201f
   with external frontoethmoidectomy, 202, 202f
   inverting papilloma, 203, 204f
   sellar/parasellar region, 567f, 581
   subcranial approaches, combined transbasal–Derome-transfacial, 355–356, 355–356f
Transnasal approach, sellar/parasellar surgery, 5, 567f, 568, 568n
Transnasal flap, 214f
Transoral approaches, 11, 12f
   to clivus and craniocervical junction. See Foramen magnum region
   degloving, 208
   sellar/parasellar chordoma, 581
Transorbital approach, 5
Transoropharyngeal route, 11

Transotic approach, vestibular schwannoma, 456–457, 457f
Transpetrosal approach, petroclival region, 423, 441, 441f
Transposition of vertebral artery, 539, 540f, 552
Transseptal variation, transsphenoid approach, 569
Transsigmoid approach
   petroclival surgery, 429
   vertebral artery management, 546
Transsphenoethmoidal approach, sella/parasellar region, 573–574
Transsphenoidal approach
   nasal cavity anatomy, 555, 557f
   sellar/parasellar lesions, 566–575, 566t, 567–573f
   chordoma, 581
   meningioma, 580
   pituitary adenoma, 578, 579
Transsylvan dissection, 269
Transtentorial approach, petroclival region, 436–437, 436f
Transverse dural plate, 21
Transverse foramen, 537, 541
Transverse ligament, 529
Transverse processes, atlas, 507
Transverse sinus, 22, 28
   anatomy, 67f
   petroclival surgery, 429, 430, 431, 435
   temporal bone anatomy, 378, 378f
   vestibular schwannoma, 460f
Trapezius muscle, 25, 29
   atrophy of, 69
   flaps and grafts
      reconstruction options, 624t
      technique, 631–633, 631–633f
      temporal bone reconstruction, 404, 404f
   infratemporal–middle fossa approach, 322, 326–329f
   jugular foramen anatomy, 413
   jugular foramen syndrome, 519
   jugulotympanic paraganglioma, 480
   vertebral artery surgery complications, 552
Trauma
   craniocervical junction, 514–516, 515f, 515t
   cranioorbital approach, 282, 284f, 285
   subcranial approaches
      extended anterior, 239
      transbasal–Derome, 347, 348, 352
   vertebral artery aneurysm, 533, 551, 551t
Trautmann's triangle, 430f, 431
Treatment philosophy, 347
Trigeminal artery, 107, 107f, 534
Trigeminal ganglion. See Gasserian ganglion
Trigeminal impression, 21f
Trigeminal nerve. See Cranial nerve V
Trigeminal neuroma
   cranioorbital zygomatic approach, 277f, 278
   facial degloving approach, 205
   imaging, 93f
Trigeminal schwannoma
   infratemporal–middle fossa approach, 309
   petroclival, 426, 428f, 429, 434f, 435, 440, 440f
Trochlear nerve. See Cranial nerve IV
Trollard, superior anastomotic vein of, 22
Trollard, superior cerebral vein of, 397
Tuberculum sellae, 17f, 19, 20f, 21
   anatomy, 558

craniooorbital zygomatic approach, 272, 273f, 279f
meningioma, 580
subcranial approaches, transbasal–Derome, 348, 352, 357
subfrontal approach, 574, 575f
Tumor biology, 51–72, 258. *See also* Pathology
and carotid artery salvage/sacrifice, 331, 360, 361
foramen magnum region lesions, 516–517, 517f, 518–519
jugulotympanic paraganglioma, 473–474, 474f, 474t
maxillary sinus tumors, 79–80
maxillotomy, extended unilateral, 232–233
metastatic disease, 66–71, 66t, 67t, 67–71f
methods of nasocranial spread, 51–61, 52t, 52–61f
orbital exenteration indications, 173
patterns of spread, 61, 61f, 62–65f, 62t, 66t
petroclival tumors, 423
sellar/parasellar lesions, 560–563, 561–562t
transfacial approach indications, 165–168, 166–168f
vascularization from vertrbral artery, 550f
Tumor markers, 70
Tumor necrosis factors, 61
Tumor resection. *See* Resection/dissection/tumor margin
Tumor types
and clinical presentation. *See* Clinical presentation
infratemporal–middle fossa approach, 309
Turbinates
facial degloving approach, 196, 196f, 198, 199, 199f
maxillotomy, extended unilateral, 212–213, 221f, 222, 223f, 231t, 232, 232t, 234
maxillotomy complications, 234
sellar/parasellar region approaches, 574
sellar/parasellar surgery, 569
transnasal excision, 3
Von Eiselsberg's incision, 3, 4f
Tympanic annulus, 393
Tympanic bone
jugular foramen surgery, 416
mandibular condylectomy/resection, 393
total petrosectomy, 402f
Tympanic membrane. *See also* Middle ear
anatomy, 380
infratemporal–middle fossa approach, otologic exposure, 322, 326
jugular foramen surgery, 416
jugulotympanic paraganglioma, 479
in maxillotomy, extended unilateral, 212
reconstruction, 393
with temporal bone tumors, 381
vestibular schwannoma, 452f
Tympanic nerve. *See* Jugulotympanic paraganglioma
Tympanic region of temporal bone, 25, 377
Tympanic ring, jugulotympanic paraganglioma, 481, 483f
Tympanicum tumors. *See also* Jugulotympanic paraganglioma
classification, 478
complications, 487
results, 486

Tympanomastoid fissure, 414
Tympanomastoid tumors, 478
Tympanomeatal flap, 326f
Tympanoplasty, 479
Tympanum
infratemporal–middle fossa approach, 326f
invasion via, 397

U

Ulceration
ear lesion presentation, 82
frontal sinus tumor presentation, 80f, 81
mucosal tumors, 520
Ultrasonic aspirator
intradural tumors, 352
vestibular schwannoma debulking, 461, 462f, 463
Ultrasound
donor site mapping, 122
Doppler. *See* Doppler ultrasound
Urine output
postoperative care, 602
postoperative monitoring, 599
Uterine cancer metastasis, 386

V

Vaginal process of temporal bone, 25
Vagus nerve. *See* Cranial nerve X
Valsalva maneuver, 464, 571, 572
Vasa vasorum, 59, 360
Vascular anastomoses. *See* Anastomoses
Vascular anomalies. *See* Vascular malformations
Vascular channels
jugulotympanic paraganglioma spread, 474
tumor pathophysiology, 55–56, 55–56f
Vascular control
ICA management, 361–374, 361–374f
vertebral artery management, 549–550, 550f, 551t, 552t
Vascular grafts. *See also* Saphenous vein graft
complications, necrosis, 595
ICA, 373
nursing care, 122–123
vertebral artery, 540f, 541
Vascularity
cavernous sinus invasion by tumor, 64
imaging, 93, 94f
diffuse lesions of skull base, 102
glomus jugulare tumors, 100, 100f
jugulotympanic paraganglioma, 474
Vascular lesions
angiofibroma, 37–39, 38f
angiomas, 204f, 205f, 259t
cerebellopontine angle, 98t
embolization, preoperative, 113–116, 113t, 114–116f
mid-skull base approaches, 209t
petroclival, 429
posterior fossa, 28
sellar/parasellar, 560t, 563, 581
subcranial approaches, 347
vertebral artery, 550–552
Vascular loops, prevention of complications, 587
Vascular malformations
anterior fossa, 168

balloon test occulusion contraindications, 107, 107f
hemostasis, 587
ICA management, 360
jugulotympanic paraganglioma versus, 478
vertebral artery, 524t, 533, 534, 550–551, 552, 552t
Vascular occlusion, saphenous vein bypass graft, 361
Vascular sinuses
anatomy, 67f, 68f
cavernous sinus, 21–22, 22f
jugulotympanic paraganglioma spread, 475
sagittal, 15–16
temporal bone anatomy, 377, 378, 379f
thrombosis, petroclival surgery complications, 437
Vascular spasm, 405
Vasomotor effects
carbon dioxide partial pressure and, 105
jugular foramen tumors, 413
therapeutic embolization and vasospasm, 115
Vasopressin, 573, 602
Vein graft
results, 373. *See also* Saphenous vein graft
subcranial extended transfacial approach Type III, 305, 305f
Vein of Labbé, 22, 334f, 335, 397, 429, 431, 437
Vein of Vesalius, 334
Veins
anatomy, 67f, 68f
cavernous sinus, 22
jugular foramen anatomy, 413
pterygoid plexus, 25
tumor emboli, 67
Venous plexus
basilar, 555
vertebral artery, 29, 492, 494, 533, 535f, 541–542, 551
Ventricles
drains, nursing care, 132
fourth, 106f
third, 424f, 425
Ventriculostomy, sellar/parasellar surgery, 568, 579
Vernet's syndrome, 476
Verrucous carcinoma of middle ear, 383t, 385
Vertebrae, cervical. *See* Cervical spine
Vertebral artery. *See also* Foramen magnum region
anastomoses, 114
anatomy, 23f, 28f, 28, 29, 491, 496f
anastomoses, therapeutic embolizaiton considerations, 113, 113t
craniocervical junction, 510f
foramen magnum region access, 496f
aneurysm, 491
foramen magnum region surgery, 495f, 503, 505
anatomy, 496f
chordoma, 500, 501f, 502f
exposure of, 492–494, 492f
glomus tumor, 498, 499f, 499f
meningioma, 497f, 498f
indications for surgical approaches, 548t
lesions of, 542, 542t, 543f

Vertebral artery (contd.)
  maxillotomy, extended unilateral, 227f
  occipitoatlantoaxial approaches, 492
    therapeutic embolization
      considerations, 115
Vertebral artery management, 533–552
  anatomy, 533–537, 533–535f
    branches, 534, 534f
    course, 533
    dynamic changes, 534–537
    relationships, 533–534
    variations and anomalies, 534
  exposure, 536, 537–538
    anteriolateral approach, 537, 538, 538f
    posteriolateral approach, 536f, 537–538
  historical data, 533
  lesion locations and, 538–541, 538–541f
  mobilization, 539
  mortality and morbidity, 552
  pathology, 541–552, 548t, 551t, 552t
    cervical spine access, 548, 548f, 548t
    foramen magnum region access, 546–548, 547f, 548t
    jugular foramen access, 548–550, 548t
    nontumor processes, 544–545
    tumors, 541–544, 541–545f, 541t, 546t
    vascular control and revascularization, 549–550, 550f, 551t, 552t
Vertebral canal, 28
Vertebral plexus anatomy, 67f, 68f
Vertebral veins, 59, 67, 67f, 68f
Vertebrobasilar aneurysm, 29, 551, 552, 552t
  maxillotomy, extended unilateral, 230
  petroclival surgery, 433
Vertebrobasilar system. See also Foramen magnum region
  anatomy, 27, 29
  aneurysm, 551, 552, 552t
  petroclival tumors, 423
  therapeutic embolization considerations, 115
Vertebrobasilar veins, anatomy, 67f, 68f
Vesalius, foramen of, 21
Vesalius, vein of, 334
Vestibular aqueduct, 380
Vestibular complications, 405
Vestibular incisions, 195
Vestibular nerve, 9
  compound action potentials, 154
  petrous bone anatomy, 425
  vestibular schwannoma, 470f
Vestibular schwannoma, 443–470
  clinical presentation, 444–445
  complications, 448–449
  diagnostic testing, 445–446
  middle fossa approach, 465–470, 466f–470f
  retrosigmoid approach, 457–465, 458f–464f
  translabyrinthine approach, 449–456, 450–456f

transotic approach, 456–457, 457f
treatment options, 446–448
Vestibulocochloear nerve. See Cranial nerve VIII
Vidian artery, 113t
Vidian canal, 25, 27, 27f, 56f
  nasal and paranasal sinus tumor presentation, 82
  subcranial extended transfacial approach, 299, 300f
Vidian nerve, 25, 27
  medial subcranial structures, 27
  orbital exenteration, 177
  subcranial extended transfacial approach, 297, 298
Vision/visual deficits, 69
  aneurysmatic bone cyst, 350
  basilar impression and, 521
  chondrosarcoma, 351
  craniopharyngioma, 354
  nasal/paranasal sinus tumor presentation, 79, 80, 82
  ocular ischemic syndrome, 108
  petroclival tumors, 427
  pituitary tumor resection and, 578
  sellar/parasellar lesions, 581
    clinical presentation, 563
    evaluation, 566
    postoperative evaluation, 573
Visual evoked potentials (VEPs), 145, 154–155, 156–157f
Vocalis muscle, 480
Vomer, 555
  anatomy, 557f
  sellar/parasellar surgery, 569f
  subcranial extended transfacial approach, Type II, 303
  transsphenoidal approach to sellar region, 570
Von Eiselsberg, A.F., 3, 4f, 7
Von Langenbeck elevator, 316

W

Weber-Fergusson incision, 6, 6f, 179f, 180f
  facial degloving, 203, 204f
  maxillectomy, 179
  modifications, 195, 196f
  and scarring, 234
  subcranial approaches
    combined transbasal–Derome-transfacial, 355–356, 355–356f
    extended transfacial Type II, 298, 298f
    extended transfacial Type III, 303f, 304
  subtotal maxillectomy, 208
Weitlander retractors, 465, 466f
Whitnall's tubercle, 19
Williams, J.M., 5
Willis, circle of, 24, 28

Window craniotomy, 6f, 7
Woodson elevators, 569
Wound care, 134, 135, 337
Wound complications, 603
Wound contracture, 605

X

Xenon CT
  cerebral blood flow assessment, 108, 109, 109f, 110f, 360
  infratemporal–middle fossa approach, 311, 313
  jugulotympanic paraganglioma, 478
  subcranial extended transfacial approach, 291
  temporal bone surgery, 386

Y

Yasargil, Gazi, 10, 10f

Z

Zinn, annulus of, 19, 175
Zygoma, 17
  division of, 222
  extrusion of, 603f
  infratemporal–middle fossa approach, 309, 316
    ostectomy, 319–320, 319–325f
    reconstruction, 337, 338f
  mandibular displacement, 626, 626f
  maxillectomy, 180, 181f
  maxillotomy, extended unilateral, 216f, 218, 219f, 221f, 223f, 225f, 233
    division of, 222
    subdural clival tumor exposure, 226f
  needle biopsy approaches, 112f, 113
  osteomyelitis, 596–597, 596f
  osteotomy
    cranioorbital approach, 263
    subcranial approaches, extended anterior, 254
    subtemproal approach to sellar/parasellar region, 575, 577
  temporal bone anatomy, 378f
  temporal bone resection, 388f, 395f, 396f
Zygomatic arch, 24
Zygomatic branch of cranial nerve VII, 155
Zygomatic cranioorbital approach, 263–271, 274, 276–277f, 278
Zygomaticofrontal approach, 11
Zygomatic region of temporal bone, 377
Zygomatic root
  infratemporal–middle fossa approach, 326
  jugulotympanic paraganglioma, 484
  temporal bone resection, 394f, 397
  temporal bone tumor involvement, 387, 390f, 393, 393f
  vestibular schwannoma, 465